Clinical Tuberculosis

Clinical Tuberculosis

Fourth edition

Edited by

Peter DO Davies MA DM FRCP
Professor, Consultant Physician,
Cardiothoracic Centre and University Hospital Aintree,
Liverpool, UK

Peter F Barnes MD
Professor of Medicine, Microbiology and Immunology,
Director, Center for Pulmonary and Infectious Disease Control,
The University of Texas Health Center at Tyler, Tyler, TX, USA

Stephen B Gordon MA MD FRCP DTM&H
Senior Clinical Lecturer in Tropical Respiratory Medicine
Liverpool School of Tropical Medicine, Liverpool, UK
and
Honorary Consultant in Respiratory Medicine
Royal Liverpool University Hospital, Liverpool, UK

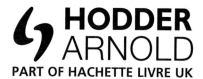
HODDER
ARNOLD
PART OF HACHETTE LIVRE UK

First published in Great Britain in 1994 by Chapman & Hall
Second edition 1998
Third edition 2003
This fourth edition published in 2008 by
Hodder Arnold, an imprint of Hodder Education, part of Hachette Livre UK,
338 Euston Road, London NW1 3BH

www.hoddereducation.com

Whilst the advice and information in this book are believed to be true
and accurate at the date of going to press, neither the author[s] nor
the publisher can accept any legal responsibility or liability for any
errors or omissions that may be made. In particular (but without
limiting the generality of the preceding disclaimer) every effort has
been made to check drug dosages; however it is still possible that
errors have been missed. Furthermore, dosage schedules are constantly
being revised and new side-effects recognized. For these reasons the
reader is strongly urged to consult the drug companies' printed
instructions before administering any of the drugs recommended in this
book.

British Library Cataloguing in Publication Data
A catalogue record for this book is available from the British Library

Library of Congress Cataloging-in-Publication Data
A catalog record for this book is available from the Library of Congress

ISBN-13   978 0 340 94840 8

1 2 3 4 5 6 7 8 9 10

Commissioning Editor: Philip Shaw
Project Editor: Amy Mulick
Production Controller: Karen Tate
Cover Designer: Andrew Campling

Typeset in 10/12 Minion by Phoenix Photosetting, Chatham, Kent
Printed and bound in Great Britain

What do you think about this book? Or any other Hodder Arnold
title? Please send your comments to **www.hoddereducation.com**

Dedication of the fourth edition

The fourth edition of *Clinical Tuberculosis* is dedicated to the brilliant workers in the fight against tuberculosis of the latter part of the twentieth century: Professor Sir John Crofton, Professor Denny Mitcheson and Professor Wallace Fox.

There were giants in the earth in those days. *Genesis 6:4*

Dedication of the third edition

The third edition of *Clinical Tuberculosis* is dedicated to the people of the United States of America in the hope that they will lead the world into greater equality of health and resources.

From those to whom much has been given will much be required. *Luke 12:48*

Dedication of the second edition

The second edition of *Clinical Tuberculosis* is dedicated to Gordon Leitch, who died while helping to rescue friends in a swimming accident in Cyprus, July 1996.

Greater love has no-one than this, that he lay down his life for his friends. *John 15:13*

Dedication of the first edition

This book is dedicated to the disadvantaged of the world, who are at greatest risk from tuberculosis, in the hope that it may help to improve their expectation of good health.

The stranger, and the fatherless and the widow, which are within the gates shall come, and shall eat and be satisfied. *Deuteronomy 14:29*

Contents

List of contributors

Paul Albert MB ChB
Specialist Registrar
University Hospital Aintree
Liverpool, UK

Jayant N Banavaliker MD DTCD MBA
Senior Consultant in Tuberculosis and Director
Rajan Babu Institute of Pulmonary Medicine
Delhi, India

John Banks MD FRCP
Princess of Wales Hospital
Bridgend, UK

Peter F Barnes
Professor of Medicine, Microbiology and Immunology,
Director, Center for Pulmonary and Infectious Disease Control,
The University of Texas Health Center at Tyler
Tyler, TX, USA

Jaime Bayona MD MPH
Department of Social Medicine
Harvard Medical School
Boston, MA, USA; and
Socios En Salud
Lima, Peru

William R Bishai MD PhD
Professor, Co-Director
Center for Tuberculosis Research, Department of Medicine
Division of Infectious Diseases
Johns Hopkins School of Medicine
Baltimore, MD, USA

Jane Buikstra
Professor of Archaeology and Director of the Center for
Bioarchaeological Research
School of Human Evolution and Social Change
Arizona State University
Tempe, AZ, USA

Ian A Campbell MD FRCP
Consultant Chest Physician
Llandough Hospital
Vale of Glamorgan, UK

Qijian Cheng MD
Fellow
Department of Medicine
Division of Infectious Diseases
Johns Hopkins School of Medicine
Baltimore, MD, USA; and
Currently Instructor in Medicine
Department of Pulmonary Disease
Ruijin Hospital
Shanghai, PR China

Victoria J Cook MD FRCPC
TB Control, BCCDC and University of British Columbia
Vancouver, BC, Canada

Charles L Daley
Head, Division of Mycobacterial and Respiratory Infections
Professor of Medicine, National Jewish Medical and Research
Center and the University of Colorado Health Sciences Center
Denver, CO, USA

Peter DO Davies MA DM FRCP
Professor, Consultant Physician
Cardiothoracic Centre and University Hospital Aintree
Liverpool, UK

Christopher Dye DPHIL
Co-ordinator
Tuberculosis Monitoring and Evaluation
HIV/AIDS, Tuberculosis and Malaria and Neglected Tropical
Diseases Cluster
World Health Organization
Geneva, Switzerland

Jerrold J Ellner MD
Department of Medicine and Ruy V Lourenco Center for the
Study of Emerging and Reemerging Pathogens
University Professor
University of Medicine and Dentistry of New Jersey
Newark, NJ, USA

Sarah England MSc DPhil(oxon) MBA
Technical Officer
Tobacco Free Initiative
World Health Organization Representative Office
Beijing, China

Marcos Espinal MD MPH DrPH
Executive Secretary
Stop TB Partnership Secretariat
World Health Organization
Geneva, Switzerland

Elizabeth L Fair PhD MPH
Francis J Curry National Tuberculosis Center
Division of Pulmonary and Critical Care Medicine
San Francisco General Hospital
University of California
San Francisco, CA, USA

Paul Farmer MD PhD
Division of Social Medicine and Health Inequalities
Brigham and Women's Hospital;
Program in Infectious Disease and Social Change
Department of Social Medicine
Harvard Medical School
Boston, MA, USA; and
Socios En Salud
Lima, Peru

J Mark FitzGerald MB FRCPI FRCPC
Centre for Clinical Epidemiology and Evaluation
Vancouver General Hospital and University of British Columbia
Vancouver, BC, Canada

Peter Goldstraw FRCS
Consultant Thoracic Surgeon
Head of Thoracic Surgery
Royal Brompton Hospital
London, UK; and
Professor of Thoracic Surgery
Imperial College
London, UK

Stephen B Gordon MA MD FRCP DTM&H
Senior Clinical Lecturer in Tropical Respiratory Medicine
Liverpool School of Tropical Medicine
Liverpool; and
Honorary Consultant in Respiratory Medicine
Royal Liverpool University Hospital
Liverpool, UK

John M Grange MSc MD
Centre for Infectious Diseases and International Health
University College London
Windeyer Institute for Medical Sciences
London, UK

Anthony D Harries OBE MA MD FRCP
Professor
HIV Unit
Ministry of Health
Lilongwe, Malawi;
Family Health International
Arlington, VA, USA; and
London School of Hygiene and Tropical Medicine
London, UK

Philip C Hopewell MD
Professor, Associate Dean
Francis J Curry National Tuberculosis Center
Division of Pulmonary and Critical Care Medicine
San Francisco General Hospital
University of California
San Francisco, CA, USA

Susan Jamieson
Team Leader
TB Specialist Nurses
Liverpool PCT
Liverpool, UK

Deborah A Lewinsohn
Associate Professor
Division of Pediatric Infectious Diseases
Oregon Health and Science University
Portland, OR, USA

David M Lewinsohn
Associate Professor
Division of Pulmonary and Critical Care Medicine
Oregon Health and Science University
and Portland VA Medical Center
Portland, OR, USA

Sebastian B Lucas FRCP FRCPATH
Professor
Department of Histopathology
King's College London School of Medicine
St Thomas' Hospital
London, UK

Dick Menzies MD FRCPC
Montreal Chest Institute
Respiratory Epidemiology Unit
McGill University
Montreal, Canada

Henry Mwandumba PhD, MRCP(UK), DTM&H
Senior Clinical Lecturer/Consultant Physician
Department of Pharmacology and Therapeutics
University of Liverpool
Liverpool, UK

Eric L Nuermberger MD
Assistant Professor of Medicine and International Health
Center for Tuberculosis Research
Johns Hopkins University
Baltimore, MD, USA

Melissa R Nyendak
Instructor
Division of Infectious Diseases
Oregon Health and Science University
Portland, OR, USA

Peter Ormerod BSc MB ChB MD DSc(Med) FRCP
Professor, Chest Clinic
Royal Blackburn Hospital
Blackburn, UK; and
Lancashire Postgraduate School of Medicine and Health
University of Central Lancashire
Preston, UK

Madhukar Pai MD, PhD
Department of Epidemiology, Biostatistics, and Occupational Health
McGill University
Montreal, Canada

Charles A Peloquin PharmD
Director, Infectious Disease Pharmacokinetics Laboratory
National Jewish Medical and Research Center
Denver, CO; and
Clinical Professor of Pharmacy and Medicine,
University of Colorado Schools of Pharmacy and Medicine
Denver, CO, USA

Dirk U Pfeiffer Tierarzt, Dr med vet, PhD, MACVSc, DipECVPH
Professor of Veterinary Epidemiology
The Royal Veterinary College
University of London
London, UK

Anton Pozniak MD FRCP
Consultant Physician
Chelsea and Westminster Hospital
London, UK

Mario Raviglione MD
Director
Stop TB Department
World Health Organization
Geneva, Switzerland

Hans L Rieder MD MPH
Department of Tuberculosis Control and Prevention of the IUATLD
Paris, France

Charlotte Roberts BA MA PhD SRN
Professor of Archaeology
Department of Archaeology
Durham University
Durham, UK

Daniel Sagebiel MD MPH
Robert Koch Institute
Department for Infectious Disease Epidemiology
Berlin, Germany

Neil W Schluger MD
Chief, Division of Pulmonary, Allergy, and Critical Care Medicine
Professor of Medicine, Epidemiology, and Environmental Health Sciences,
Columbia University College of Physicians and Surgeons
Columbia University Mailman School of Public Health
Columbia University Medical Center
New York, NY, USA

Stephan K Schwander MD PHD
Assistant Professor of Medicine
Department of Medicine and Ruy V Lourenco Center for the Study of Emerging and Reemerging Pathogens
Assistant Professor, University of Medicine and Dentistry of New Jersey
Newark, NJ, USA

Sonya Shin MD
Infectious Disease Division
Brigham and Women's Hospital
Department of Social Medicine
Harvard Medical School
Boston, MA, USA; and
Socios En Salud
Lima, Peru

Delane Shingadia MBChB DCH DTM&H MPH MRCP FRCPCH
Consultant in Paediatric Infectious Diseases
Great Ormond Street Hospital for Children
London, UK

S Bertel Squire BSc MB BChir MD FRCP
Reader in Clinical Tropical Medicine
Liverpool School of Tropical Medicine
Liverpool; and
Consultant in Infectious Diseases and Tropical Medicine
Royal Liverpool University Hospital
Liverpool, UK

Wing Wai Yew MB BS MRCP(UK) FRCP(Edin)
Chief
Tuberculosis and Chest Unit
Grantham Hospital
Aberdeen, Hong Kong, China

Rony Zachariah MBBS DTM&H DCH PhD
Médecins sans Frontières
Operational Research HIV-TB
Medical Department
Brussels Operational Center
Brussels, Belgium

Jean-Pierre Zellweger MD
Consultant Chest Physician
Department of Ambulatory Care and Community Medicine
University of Lausanne
Lausanne, Switzerland

Foreword

When I was a boy of 15, I nearly died of tuberculosis. I was in hospital for almost 2 years, often too weak to get out of bed. I was very lucky to survive.

You know for over 50 years we've had a cure for TB and many people think it's been wiped out. But this year 2 million women, men and children will die of this forgotten disease. And TB is on the increase – in Africa, it's a scourge killing those weakened by AIDS. In India, TB creates more orphans than any other infectious disease. In Britain, there are more new TB cases each year than HIV. It's shocking that people are dying of something which can so easily be cured.

Let me tell you about Judy Tembo from Zambia. Judy is one of 150 local volunteers who decided to take action against TB which was devastating their community. Judy tells people about the symptoms of TB and where to go for diagnosis. She supports them through the 8-month course of TB medicines. She even helps with chores like fetching water if patients are too weak. Judy's patients rely on her visits, as well as the food and other essentials, like soap and blankets, she brings to help make ends meet while they can't work. A small charity pays for these supplies, for Judy's training and the bicycle which she uses to travel around the villages. It's not glamorous work, but Judy will tell you with justifiable pride that it saves lives. It stops the spread of TB.

In Africa, the fight is made harder by the other deadly epidemic of HIV/AIDS, which lowers resistance to tuberculosis. Yet there is a simple cure for TB, even for someone who is HIV-positive.

You might think TB has been eradicated even in the UK. Sadly, this is not the case. In the year 2005 there were over 8000 new cases of TB in the UK. In London, numbers have doubled in 15 years and parts of the capital city have rates of TB as high as those in China. No-one can be complacent. TB cannot be controlled in one country until it is controlled worldwide.

This is the fourth edition of the reference book *Clinical Tuberculosis*, first published in 1994. It provides an essential work to those working to eliminate TB both in the developed and developing world whether they are doctors, nurses or other health workers and whether they are at the clinical, laboratory or public health interface.

I believe we *can* wipe out TB. We just need to make sure everyone who has the disease gets treated quickly, before passing it on to others.

Archbishop Desmond Tutu
South Africa, 2007

Preface

It must be a matter of concern that 20 years after it was realized that tuberculosis was out of control across much of the developing world, the tide of tuberculosis shows no sign of being controlled. As a race, human kind is still losing the fight against tuberculosis. The main reason for an apparent peaking of the incidence is a peaking of HIV incidence. There is still an annual increase in the total number of cases globally.

Though there have been some encouraging developments particularly in the area of new diagnostics for tuberculosis, the minimum of 6 months of treatment is unlikely to be modified by the introduction of new drugs in the next 5 years. New vaccine development takes time and though there are some encouraging signs of new developments, it seems unlikely that we can replace BCG for at least 10 years. In that time another 20 million people will die and 80 million be affected by what should be a preventable and treatable disease.

The setting up of such global organizations as the Global Fund to Fight AIDS, Tuberculosis and Malaria, the Global Alliance for TB Drug Development and the Green Light Committee, which oversees help with MDR-TB, are steps in the right direction.

However, despite these developments, funding for tuberculosis drug, vaccine and diagnostic development is still woefully short of requirements.

The contribution to the fight against tuberculosis by developing countries is also a matter for concern. India, for example, with the highest burden of disease from tuberculosis, has decreased the annual proportion of its GDP spending on health from 1.4 per cent in the 1950s to 0.9 per cent currently.

In the preface to the last edition, I said that the English contribution to the International Union against Tuberculosis and Lung disease was assured. I was mistaken. Unfortunately, the British Lung Foundation decided to stop its share of the funding in 2005. The British Thoracic Society membership then voted as to whether it should take over the full contribution and despite a clear bias by its officers against the contribution voted only narrowly against continuing the contribution, currently running at 25 000 Euros a year. The Department of Health is currently funding on a year by year basis.

Though disappointing for the present, I feel the up and coming generation of chest physicians may be more sym-

pathetic to the needs of the developing world than their predecessors.

The fourth edition of *Clinical Tuberculosis* is therefore published against a rather depressing background of a disease which is proving incredibly difficult to control, partly because it is not yet perceived as a national or international priority. The principal reason for this is co-infection with HIV, which renders the host uniquely susceptible to infection with tuberculosis and progression to disease. In parts of Africa where HIV infection is endemic, rates of tuberculosis have tripled over 15 years. Other factors are important to overcome if TB is to be controlled. In particular, poor medical infrastructures linked to poverty of individuals and communities render management almost impossible as it is difficult to get drugs to patients.

Even in well-resourced settings, tuberculosis does not always receive the priority it deserves and control is compromised.

As with previous editions, *Clinical Tuberculosis* is designed to provide the TB worker, whether in public health, laboratory science or clinical practice with a synoptic and definitive account of the latest methods and practice in its control.

The book is intended to be relatively short so that it is affordable to resource-poor concerns. For this reason, we have also excluded colour prints.

For the fourth edition, the main changes are in the area of laboratory-based diagnosis and management of disease. The gamma interferon-based blood tests make their appearance for the first time. The molecular techniques for diagnosing the species of mycobacterium and rifampicin resistance gene are now in first-line service provision in well-resourced settings. New developments, such as the microscopic observation for drug sensitivity (MODS), are detailed. Over the four editions of the book, the evolution of diagnostic methods has progressed so that what is being researched in one edition becomes of service use in the next. Unfortunately, the same cannot be said of drug or vaccine development.

A new chapter on the human immune response to the tubercle bacillus is included.

Increasing organization of what should be standard practice for all medical staff managing tuberculosis has resulted in clear guidelines being published on both side of the Atlantic. A new chapter on standards of care is therefore also included. However, tuberculosis cannot be controlled anywhere until it is controlled everywhere. Central co-ordination by WHO and the International Union against Tuberculosis and Chest Diseases are required. To outline this task, a new chapter on the Global Plan to Stop TB has been added.

Finally, more in hope than expectation of a change before another edition is published, a separate chapter from the standard treatment regimens is now given over to new drugs and their likely place in regimens which may become standard practice in bringing down the length of treatment in the future.

The new charity for tuberculosis in the UK, TB Alert, continues to raise the profile of tuberculosis in the UK and the founding of an interparty TB committee in the House of Commons this year is a cause for hope.

In turning to the dedication of this book I felt it was time to honour those who had given the most to the fight against tuberculosis in the UK and across the world: my former teacher and mentor Wallace Fox, his partner in the MRC TB Units sadly closed in the 1980s, Denny Mitcheson and my good friend Sir John Crofton.

Peter DO Davies

Acknowledgements

With the publication of the fourth edition I would again like to thank all the authors who have willingly contributed so much time and energy to their writing. I would especially like to thank the dozen or so who have contributed now to all four editions.

Also thanks to the new team at Hodder Arnold, Philip Shaw and Amy Mulick, whose patient toils have reaped a great reward.

PART 1

BACKGROUND

The history of tuberculosis from earliest times to the development of drugs

CHARLOTTE ROBERTS AND JANE BUIKSTRA

INTRODUCTION

Tuberculosis is now a conquered disease in the British Isles and the rest of the industrialised world.[1]

How wrong can one be? In the late 1980s, indeed, we thought that tuberculosis (TB) was an infection that had been controlled and almost eradicated in the developed world. However, both emergence and re-emergence of infectious disease plague both the developed and the developing worlds today and the medical profession struggles to cope with their persistence. It is suggested that TB today is responsible for more morbidity and mortality than any other bacterial pathogen, and that one-third of the human population is, or has been, infected by the tubercle bacillus.[2,3] Whether this was the case in the past cannot be ascertained with a great deal of accuracy as we will see. However, today, 'it appears poised to develop frequency rates with the status of the "big killer" again as we move through into the 21st century'.[4] We would argue that tuberculosis was of equal importance in our ancestors' world as it is today, but of course the difference between past and present is that we now have drugs to successfully (potentially) treat the disease, and health education programmes to prevent TB occurring. Being a 'disease of poverty', we additionally have the mechanisms and infrastructure to ensure that poverty is not a precursor to the development of the infection. Of course, having coping mechanisms does not mean that TB will be controlled, as we can see from increased rates in recent years. In some respects, they can complicate the situation, and one could argue that, because one of the major predisposing factors for TB is poverty, then if poverty could be alleviated then the disease would disappear. Of course, having drug therapy can ultimately lead to drug resistance as we know, which may occur for a variety of reasons.

Our ancestors perhaps may have been in a better position to combat TB, assuming they recognized that poverty led to the infection. They certainly did not have to deal with one of the predisposing factors today, that is HIV (human immunodeficiency virus), or so we assume. According to Raviglione et al.,[5] HIV is the most important single risk factor for the progression of dormant tuberculosis into clinical disease, the virus compromising the immune response. The combination of poverty, HIV and drug resistance makes for a challenging and terrifying situation for many people in the world today. Additionally, concepts of the causation of tuberculosis, and associated stigma, around the world in different cultures can vary considerably, which then affects what treatments are provided, opportunity for access to, and success of, available treatments, and the implementation of preventive measures (see Ref. 6, for an example). Unfortunately, as Walt indicates,[7] politics will often determine who is treated, when and how, in different countries of the world. No doubt this was the case in the past. We also have to consider that men, women and children may be treated differently, not only with TB but with any health problem. Hudelson,[8] for example, notes that women more than men in sub-Saharan Africa are at risk from contracting both HIV and TB. Of course, treating the whole patient and not just their signs and symptoms will be more likely to pro- duce a successful outcome. Unfortunately, it is the infec- tion itself, rather than the person, which is often the focus of attention in treatment. It is always easier (and quicker) to, 'look at the scientific cause of the disease rather than the related areas which actually explain why tuberculosis is more common in some parts of the world than others'.[4]

In other chapters in this book, more detailed consider- ation will be placed on the problem of TB today and the coping mechanisms in place but, for the purposes of this chapter, we will be focusing our attention on the long his- tory of tuberculosis as seen mainly in skeletal remains, and also in historical sources. First, we will consider the pri- mary evidence for tuberculosis in the past, the remains of people themselves, chart the distribution of the infection through time from a global perspective, and consider the historical data for the presence of the disease in the distant past. We will also consider recent biomolecular analysis of the tubercle bacillus in human remains that is currently shedding light on aspects of the history of tuberculosis about which, until now, we had little knowledge. Finally, we argue that studying the past history of tuberculosis can aid in understanding the problem today.

SOURCES OF EVIDENCE FOR THE PRESENCE OF TB IN THE PAST

Scholars studying TB in our ancestors draw on a number of sources of evidence. The primary evidence derives from people themselves (Figure 1.1) who were buried in ceme- teries regionally and temporally throughout the world, people who have been excavated over the years and con- tribute to our understanding of our long history. Secondary sources of evidence 'flesh out' the skeletal remains that we study. For example, we might consider historical sources that document frequencies of tuberculo- sis at particular points in time in specific parts of the world, something we cannot glean from the skeletal remains. Written accounts will also tell us something

about whether tuberculosis was treated and how. Illustrations in texts may indicate that the infection was present in the population, and the deformity and/or dis- ability that accompanied it. The following sections con- sider this evidence in more detail, highlighting the strengths and limitations of our data.

Diagnosis of TB in skeletal and mummified remains

Being able to safely identify TB in human remains from an archaeological site proves the presence of the disease in a population. This compares with a written description of the infection which may be confused with other respira- tory disease. While historical sources may provide us with more realistic estimates of the frequency of tuberculosis in the past, we have to be sure that diagnosis was precise and we would argue that this is not always possible.

The skeletal structure will be affected in around 3–5 per cent of untreated people.[9] The spine is where most people will be affected, with the hip and knee being common joints involved. Changes to the skeleton are the end result of post-primary tuberculosis spreading haematogenously or via the lymphatic system to the bones. A point to note is that, without biomolecular analysis, we cannot identify tuberculosis in the skeletons of those people who suffered primary tuberculosis. Initial introduction into a popula- tion will lead to high mortality because of lack of previous exposure. In this case, in a past skeletal population, we would expect to see no bony damage. As time goes by and generations of the population have been exposed to tuber- culosis it is at that point when we might expect to see it in their skeletons. TB in humans caused by both *Mycobacterium tuberculosis* and *Mycobacterium bovis* can cause skeletal damage, but the latter is much more likely to do this.[10] Thus, evidence in skeletal remains indicates a chronic long-term process that a person could have endured for many years, and one that their immune system was capable of dealing with. If we take a hypothet- ical skeletal population and look at people affected and not affected with TB, it is those with bone changes that could be classed as the healthy ones. Those without bone changes are those who died either from TB or one of the many other diseases that affected our ancestors, including those only affecting the soft tissues, such as the plague, cholera and smallpox. Wood *et al.*[11] is a good starting point for the reader to explore what the presence of disease indicators might mean in skeletons from archaeological sites, and the limitations of the data and its interpretation.

The first step in the diagnosis of TB in skeletal remains for a palaeopathologist is to distinguish true pathological lesions from normal variants and changes due to post- mortem damage. Post-mortem damage is an inevitable consequence of burial of human remains in the ground. If we imagine a person buried for several hundreds of years, during that time many internal and external forces may

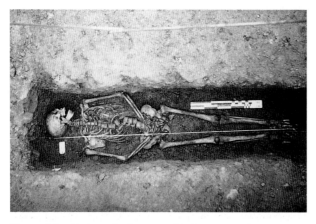

Figure 1.1   Skeleton in the ground before excavation.

compromise the survival of the remains. For example, acidic soils, water in the grave and small rodents and insects can all play their part in the eventual alteration and destruction of the body's soft tissues and skeleton.[12] As the majority of the skeletal change is the result of destruction of bone, then destruction of bone due to post-mortem damage is differentiated from destruction due to disease. However, some circumstances may preserve whole bodies very well, such as very dry, waterlogged and frozen environments.[13] In these latter cases, if soft tissues are preserved, the potential amount of data retrievable can be impressive, and diagnosis of disease can be easier. We are also careful not to ascribe disease to skeletons on the basis of 'lesions' that are actually normal. The component parts of the skeleton, i.e. individual bones, display many lumps and bumps, cavities and holes that, to the uninitiated, may appear to be pathological. However, years of experience play an enormous part in making sure that skeletons are not assigned diseases they do not have!

Funerary ritual can also have its part to play in the survival of the body for examination and analysis. For example, the cremation process, which was common in areas of the world in large parts of prehistory and history, can destroy most of the evidence for disease. For example, in Britain in the Neolithic, Bronze and Iron Ages, and the Roman and early Medieval periods, cremation was a common funerary rite which usually led to the deposition in the ground (with or without urns) of very fragmented skeletal material, often difficult to identify.[14] Evidence for TB in these types of remains is usually absent. For the most part, inhumed skeletal material provides us with the data with which palaeopathologists trace the origin, evolution and palaeoepidemiology of disease.[15] However, we must not forget that even inhumed bodies were deposited in different ways according to region of the world, time period and culture, and these factors again may compromise survival.

Disease can only affect the skeleton in two ways, bone formation and bone destruction, although both can be found together. Therefore, these changes are recorded for each bone of the skeleton, their distribution pattern noted and differential diagnoses provided. Because the skeleton can only react in these limited ways to disease then the same changes can occur in different diseases. This is why providing a detailed description of the lesions and a list of possible diagnoses, based on the presence and distribution of the lesions, is essential if diagnoses are to be verified and/or re-evaluated in the future. This is a point repeatedly emphasized (e.g. Wood et al.,[11] Roberts and Manchester,[15] Buikstra and Ublelaker,[16] Ortner[17]).

Recognition of TB, then, relies usually on the presence of, mainly, destructive lesions in the spine, termed Pott's disease (after the nineteenth century physician Percival Pott who first described the changes). The bacilli focus on the red bone marrow and there is gradual slow destruction of the bony tissue. Resnick and Niwayama[9] indicate that 25–50 per cent of people with skeletal TB will develop

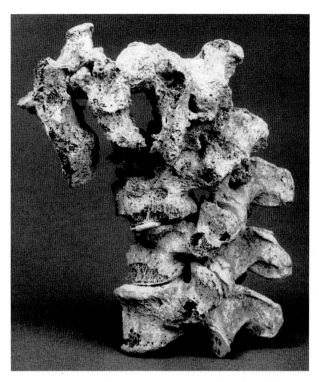

Figure 1.2 Spinal tuberculosis in an early Medieval victim from southern England.

spinal changes. Once the vertebral integrity is lost then the structure collapses and angulation (kyphosis) of the spine develops (Figure 1.2) with possible fusion of vertebrae. The lower thoracic and lumbar spine are most affected and rarely the neural arches. Central, anterior and paradiscal vertebral lesions can occur and a psoas abscess may develop as a complication of spinal tuberculosis, spreading down the fascial plane of the psoas muscle to the lesser trochanter of the femur.

In the major weight-bearing joints of the body, the hip and knee (Figure 1.3), TB similarly destroys bone tissue, but usually only affects one joint. The infection may develop in the joint itself or spread from an adjacent lesion in the long bones, especially those near the growth plate in children and the metaphysis in adults. Other joints such as the shoulder, elbow, wrist and ankle may also be affected, but not as frequently as the hip and knee. The flat bones may be involved, but rarely. The skull, for example, is affected in 0.1 per cent of people with skeletal TB,[18] and destroys both tables. Some authors suggest that meningitis caused by TB may affect the endocranial aspect of the skull by causing new bone formation,[19] although this must be seen as a possible non-specific indicator.[20] Likewise, new bone formed on the visceral surface of ribs (Figure 1.4) has been suggested by many to indicate TB of the lungs as a direct result of transmission through the pleura (e.g. Kelley and Micozzi,[21] Roberts et al.,[22] Santos and Roberts[23]). However, many chronic lung conditions could lead to this bone change, for example pneumonia, chronic bronchitis

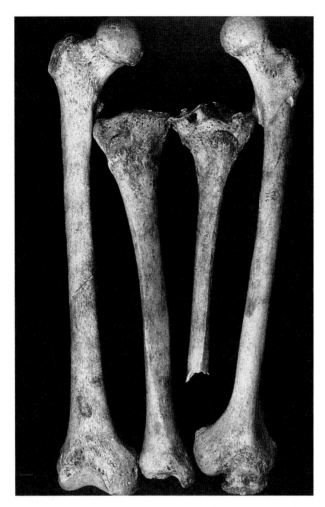

Figure 1.3 Probable tuberculosis of the left knee in a fourth century AD individual; also note the wasting of the left leg bones compared with the right.

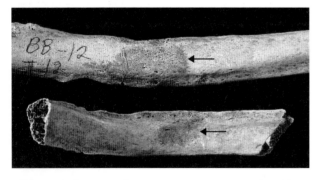

Figure 1.4 New bone formation on the visceral surface of ribs.

and even carcinoma, and thus its presence holds many possible avenues of explanation.

The short bone diaphyses may also be affected, particularly the hands and feet of infants and young children (tuberculous dactylitis). The periosteum thickens and elevates with erosion of the cortex, and osteomyelitis can

develop. Also called 'spina ventosa', this can be seen in other conditions such as congenital syphilis[24] and sickle cell anaemia.[9] In children's long bones, bone destruction is seen in the metaphyses with formation of sequestra and periosteal new bone formation on a thinned cortex.[24] In adults, secondary hypertrophic osteoarthropathy (or hypertrophic pulmonary osteoarthropathy (HOA)) may be manifest on the long bones as new bone formation. Pulmonary conditions, such as tuberculosis, can cause this change, along with many other lung diseases.[9] Interesting work by Santos[25] has recently provided a link between TB and HOA in a skeletal population with known cause of death from Portugal.

The majority of palaeopathologists will diagnose TB using spinal evidence. However, it is not possible to detect all people with TB using this approach. Over the last 10 years or so, there has been a move towards applying methods of analysis developed in biomolecular science to diagnose disease in skeletal and mummified remains. This approach, discussed in more detail below, includes focusing on human remains without any evidence of disease, as well as those with pathological changes. Tuberculosis has been the main focus of activities and its diagnosis has been achieved using the presence of ancient DNA and mycolic acids of the tubercle bacillus.[26,27] While there are inevitable problems of survival and extraction of ancient biomolecules from human remains, we are set to learn more than ever before about the history and evolution of disease from our primary evidence.

Historical and pictorial data

We are not historians or art historians, and are not trained in the analysis and interpretation of texts and illustrations related to the history of disease and medicine. However, while we recognize the limitations in the data that we are experts with, we can recognize that historical sources can generate problems in interpretation. The signs and symptoms of TB may include shortness of breath, coughing up blood, anaemia and pallor, fatigue, night sweats, evening fevers, pain in the chest and the effects of associated skeletal changes (for example, kyphosis of the back and paralysis of the limbs). Clearly, all these features, visible to an author or artist, could be associated with other health problems. For example, pallor may be seen in anaemia, shortness of breath in chronic bronchitis, and coughing up blood in cancer of the lung. Likewise, kyphotic deformities of the back (Figure 1.5) may be the result of osteoporosis of the spine or trauma. Focusing more on the historical written data for TB, and particularly cause of death rates, we have to be especially careful of the data. For example, Hardy[28] reminds us that, as TB was a sensitive disease and associated with stigma in the nineteenth century, cause of death from TB was not always recorded. People could also have had more than one cause of death and we must also not assume that those who diagnosed disease in the past

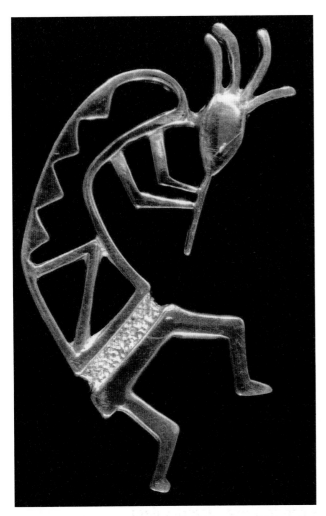

Figure 1.5 Kokopelli figure from North America with hunched back.

were competent at achieving a correct diagnosis. Even today some causes of death on death certificates may not be correct.[29] Despite the problems we will consider some of this evidence following our treatment of the skeletal data.

THE ANTIQUITY OF TB FROM A GLOBAL PERSPECTIVE

Before embarking on a temporal and global visit of TB, we should emphasize that some parts of the world have not seen the intense investigation of human remains from archaeological sites that have been applied to North America and parts of Europe. There are many areas of the world where palaeopathologists have not yet ventured and therefore evidence for TB is, to date, absent. This does not of course mean that it did not exist in that particular part of the world in the past, it is just that the evidence has not been looked for or found. It therefore becomes a little difficult at times to trace the origin, evolution and transmission of TB globally. With this caveat in mind, we would first like to consider the factors that we think were proba-

bly important in the development of TB in past human populations.

What led to TB appearing in human populations?

ANIMALS

Our assumption, until recently, has been that humans contracted TB from infected animals, probably cattle, when they were domesticated about 10 000 years ago.[30] This is when people in different parts of the world simultaneously manipulated plants and animals to their advantage. They moved from a subsistence existence as hunter-gatherers to one more reliant on growing crops and keeping animals, although it is clear that some people would have continued hunting and gathering in addition to the adoption of farming; in effect, it was not an overnight transition.

In the Near East, for example, domestication was present by 8000 years BC and sheep and goats were domesticated; this occurred by 6500 BC in Northern Europe, the Mediterranean and India.[31] In the New World, domestication is believed to have been established by 2700 BC in Central Mexico, the eastern United States in 2500 BC and the South Central Andes in South America by 2500 BC.[32] Clearly, at these times, and assuming that animals were infected by TB, the potential for transmission was present. We should not, however, forget that wild and feral animals may also be infected. Thus, hunter-gatherers could have contracted the disease through capture, butchery and consumption of their kill, if animal to human transmission is accepted. Therefore, domestication of animals may not necessarily have any part to play in the first appearance of TB in humans. Furthermore, a number of pieces of evidence have come to light recently that suggest that domestication was of less importance in the palaeoepidemiology of TB than has been previously thought. Kapur et al.[33] suggest that mycobacterial species first appeared 15 000–20 000 years ago, long before domestication, and Rothschild et al.[34] revealed M. tuberculosis complex ancient DNA from the remains of an extinct long horned bison from North America dated to 17 870 ± 230 years BP (before present) with tuberculosis-compatible pathology. The idea that M. tuberculosis developed from M. bovis following domestication of animals, and when population density was of the correct size, has also been questioned. Recent work by Brosch et al.[35] has indicated, on the basis of analysis of the genomic structure of tubercle bacilli, that M. tuberculosis did not evolve from M. bovis. Other researchers suggest that TB is the culmination of a global history extending over 3 million years in the Old World, originating in Africa, affecting our hominine ancestors.[36]

M. bovis can be transmitted from animals to humans via the gastrointestinal tract, but it can also be contracted by humans through droplet infection from animals. M.

tuberculosis is transmitted via droplet infection. Thus, in situations where infected meat and/or milk are being consumed by humans, where humans live or work in dwellings in contact with their infected animals, and where humans live or work in dwellings with other infected humans, there is an opportunity for the infection to take its hold. In hunting and gathering populations, population density is generally low[37] and therefore it is likely that the animal to human form of transmission would have been the most common. Readers may be asking whether there is evidence for TB in animal remains from archaeological sites. Unfortunately, there are only two reported cases so far in archaeozoological research and both have confirmed diagnoses using ancient DNA analysis, a dog's skeleton from North America dated to AD 1600[38] and cattle bone from a Roman site in Germany (Teegen, personal communication). The study of disease in animal bones is, however, problematic. Animal bones tend to be disarticulated and very fragmented because of butchery; they are rarely buried as individual bodies. It is therefore not possible to look at distribution patterns of pathological lesions and, furthermore, the veterinary science literature is not very helpful, probably because animals are usually slaughtered before bone changes occur.[39] Clearly, however, animals were likely very important for transmission of TB to humans in the past, as they are today in some parts of the world (see discussion in Roberts and Buikstra[4]).

HUMANS, URBANIZATION AND INDUSTRIALIZATION

The human form of TB requires close contact of people ('sneezing distance') for it to be transmitted from human to human. Before people started to live in permanent housing and practised farming, they lived in low densities and were constantly on the move, not needing the security of settled communities. Once settled and practising agriculture, population numbers and density increased rapidly as the food produced was able to support more people. Higher population densities enabled population density-dependent diseases, such as TB to flourish, although it was not until into the late Medieval period (twelfth to sixteenth centuries) when the disease really increased in Europe.[4] Add to this poverty, something many would have experienced at this time and later in the post-Medieval period and into the Industrial Revolution, and we have a potentially explosive situation for TB. The development of trade and the migration of people from rural communities to urban centres, usually for work, also enabled TB to be transmitted to previously unexposed people. Additionally, working with animals and their products may have exposed people to the infection. For example, the processing of animal skins in the tanning industry, the working of bone and horn, and processing food products from animals all predisposed people to the infection. Working in industries that produced particulate pollution, such as the textile trade, could also irritate the lungs and probably predispose people to TB. Finally,

the use of infected animal dung as a fertilizer or as a fuel may have been hazardous.

We might also ask what people ate in the past, and whether their diet was balanced and nutritious. Levels of nutrition affect people's immune systems and how strong they become at resisting infection. If a person becomes malnourished, they are more susceptible to TB. Skeletal evidence suggests that health tends to deteriorate with agricultural development.[40–42] People eat less protein which is needed to produce antibodies to fight infection, wheat lacks certain amino acids, and diets are less varied. Harvests may also fail and there is a real risk of under- and malnutrition. Along with high population density, poverty and the inevitable low levels of sanitation in urban centres, poor diet was one more load that urban populations endured, all of which potentially predisposed to TB.

As today, the appearance of TB in the past would have been determined by many factors, but most of all population density and poverty. When animals contributed to the tuberculous load is now under debate, but we suggest that it was probably late in human history rather than at the time of domestication several thousand years ago (see Chapter 30, Tuberculosis in animals).

Skeletal remains from the Old World

Human remains are the primary evidence for showing when TB first appeared. We can define the Old World as the world that was known before the European presence in the Americas, and comprising Europe, Asia and Africa.[43] Most of the evidence comes from Europe, which we believe reflects the palaeopathology activity here compared to the rest of the Old World. This may also reflect non-survival of human remains, non-excavation, and particular funerary rites that do not preserve remains well in some areas.[4] However, those Old World areas with no evidence may truly be areas with no TB. We can divide the data into three broad areas in the Old World, 'Northern Europe', the 'Mediterranean' and 'Asia and islands', which reflect similar climate and environmental features.

THE MEDITERRANEAN

In Italy, we find the earliest evidence of skeletal TB in the world. The female skeleton aged around 30 years at death, is dated to 5800 ± 90 BC, and comes from the Neolithic cave of Arma dell'Aquila in Liguria.[44]

Jordan also has two early examples of TB from Bab edh-Dhra at 3150–2200 BC,[45] although Israel does not reveal evidence until AD 600 at the monastery of John the Baptist in the Judean Desert.[46] Zias[47] suggests that Jewish populations generally have low TB frequencies and may have genetic resistance, and therefore we might not expect much evidence in Israel. This group also suffer Tay–Sachs disease, which can confer resistance to TB. Additionally, Jewish people are believed to be lactose intolerant and, therefore, if these data are accepted, then we might expect to see TB less if only the human form of transmission operated in the past.[47]

Close by, Egypt reveals evidence dated to 4500 BC,[48] although there is no evidence from sub-Saharan Africa (Santos, personal communication). Egypt and the Sudan have seen much work on all aspects of their heritage, and the analysis of human remains is no different. Data on TB in human remains have been published since early last century.[49] Probably the most famous is that of the mummy Nesperehān, excavated in Thebes, where a psoas abscess and spinal changes were recorded and established TB's presence in Egypt by between 1069 and 945 BC.[48] Derry[50] summarized the data at that time, dating from 3300 BC, while Morse *et al.*[48] record evidence from Nagada dated to as early as 4500 BC. It is in Egypt that work on soft tissue evidence for TB has been most common. For example, Nerlich *et al.*[51] and Zink *et al.*[52] isolated and sequenced DNA from tissue from the lung of a male mummy from a tomb of nobles (1550–1080 BC), providing a positive diagnosis for TB.

Spain comes next in date, with possible TB in skeletal remains dated to the Neolithic,[53] and in Greece TB appears by 900 BC.[54] Since Angel's work, there has been very few data forthcoming on TB from Greece, but, of course, by the fifth century BC Hippocratic writings are describing the infection,[55] so it is likely that TB had been around for some considerable time.

France, like Lithuania, and Austria (Northern Europe) reveals TB around the fourth century AD.[56] Data are focused in specific regions and reflect the work effort. Evidence has appeared in early, late and post-Medieval south-east France.[57–64] Northern France has probably seen the most extensive work[56,65] with nearly 2500 skeletons being examined from 17 sites dated to between the fourth and twelfth centuries AD. Twenty-nine cases of TB were identified and most came from urban sites. Other 'Mediterranean' countries, such as Serbia,[66] Turkey[67] and Portugal[68] do not have their first evidence for the infection until much later in the Medieval period (from around the twelfth century AD). In fact, it is not until that period that there appear to be significant numbers of populations with tuberculosis,[4] as described above.

NORTHERN EUROPE

In 'Northern Europe', Poland reveals the first evidence for TB from the Neolithic site of Zlota dated to 5000 BC,[69] but frequencies, as for many other countries in Europe, increased in the later Medieval period. Data from Russia suggest TB was present by 1000 BC at the Bronze Age site of Manych, southern Russia,[70] but there is much more work to be done in this huge country.

In the history of TB, Denmark became important from the Iron Age (500–1 BC) from a site at Varpelev, Sjælland,[71] and in Britain the first evidence is from an Iron Age site at Tarrant Hinton, Dorset, dated to 400–230 BC.[72,73] Austria

and Lithuania have skeletal evidence all by the fourth century AD. For Austria, this coincides with the late Roman occupation. Britain is fortunate in having had a long history of palaeopathological study and therefore the evidence for TB is much more plentiful than for other countries of the world. All the evidence recorded derives from settled agriculturally based communities of historic date (i.e. from the Iron Age). If we look at the distribution pattern for TB in Britain through time,[4] we see the earliest cases in the south and east of England, many of which may be the result of contact with the invading Roman army. This is a picture mirrored for the following early Medieval period (fifth to late eleventh century AD). By the later Medieval period (eleventh to sixteenth centuries AD), numbers of cases increase and are more evenly spread through the British Isles and reach into Scotland (Figure 1.6). Also interesting to note is that the northern sites tend to be more rural in context than the southern more urban sites. However, if we thought that TB in human populations in rural sites would be more likely to be the result of infection from animals we must think again. Recent work using ancient DNA analysis has indicated that TB at the

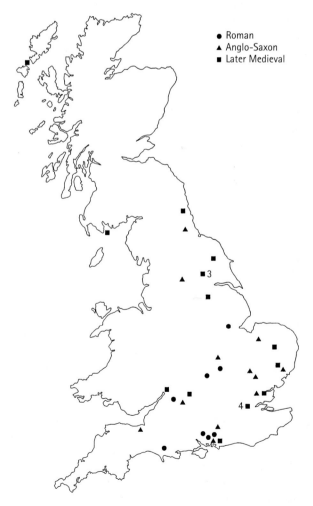

Figure 1.6 Distribution map of skeletal tuberculosis in the British Isles from the Roman to post-Medieval periods.

rural Medieval site of Wharram Percy was the result of *M. tuberculosis* and not *bovis*.[74]

Lithuania has seen extensive work documenting the frequency of TB in skeletal remains with the Marvelé site producing late Roman data;[75] this skeleton was also subject to ancient DNA analysis which produced positive results for *M. tuberculosis* complex.[76] As time goes by, frequencies increase along with population density and intensification of agriculture. Jankauskas[77] suggests that cattle probably transmitted the infection to humans but, as we have seen, this may not necessarily have been the case. Jankauskas also considered the age at death of people with and without TB in the early Medieval period and found that suffering TB did not lead to a high death rate in young people. Paradoxically, people appeared to be surviving the acute stages of the infection, which may appear surprising for that period in time, although adaptation and resistance to the organism could have developed over many years. In the fifteenth and sixteenth centuries, Jankauskas[77] notes the increase in trade, and population density again, with intensification of agriculture and the growth of towns and crafts, and a rise in TB.

Norway (Holck, personal communication) and Switzerland feature in the history of TB by the seventh century AD,[78] along with Hungary, and Sweden and the Netherlands in the eleventh and thirteenth centuries AD, respectively. In Hungary there has been extensive published work documenting the frequency of TB over time.[79] Clearly, from the data, TB was fairly common in the seventh to eighth centuries and also in the fourteenth to seventeenth centuries; an obvious gap in the evidence in the tenth century may be, it is suggested, due to the semi-nomadic way of life the population had at that time. Skeletal and mummified remains displaying TB from Hungary have also probably seen the most analysis of any country using ancient DNA. This has allowed the confirmation of possible tuberculous cases.[80,81] In Sweden, an extensive study of over 3000 skeletons from Lund dated to between AD 990 and 1536 showed TB of the spine in one individual (AD 1050–1100), although over 40 had possible TB in one or more joints.[82] The Czech Republic also provides its first evidence in the later Medieval period.[83]

ASIA AND THE ISLANDS

'Asia and the islands' reveal TB in skeletal remains much later than both the 'Mediterranean' and 'Northern European' areas. China has evidence from a mummy dated to between 206 BC and the seventh century AD,[84] but the first written description of TB treatment is dated to 2700 BC,[85] and the first accepted description of the disease to 2200 BC.[84] Japan has skeletal evidence dated to the sixth to seventh centuries AD.[86,87] Thailand is reputed to have possible evidence a little earlier and dated to 300 BC to AD 300 (Tayles, personal communication). It is much later that Papua New Guinea and Hawaii[88–90] produce data ('pre-European'), with possible TB being recorded on Tonga and the Solomon Islands (Pietruwesky, personal communication).

SUMMARY OF DATA FROM THE OLD WORLD

While the data for skeletal TB around the Old World appear quite plentiful, there are many areas where there is no evidence (Figures 1.7 and 1.8). This may be because:

● it really does not exist even though extensive skeletal analysis has been undertaken;

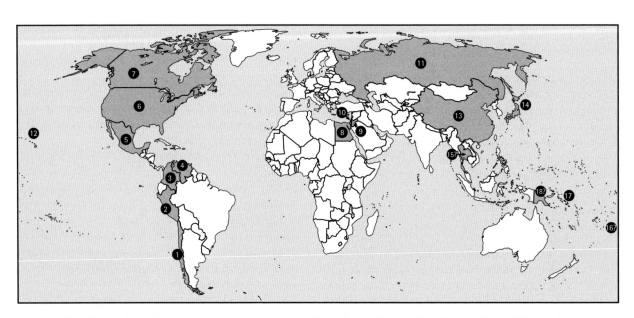

Figure 1.7   Distribution map of occurrences of skeletal tuberculosis in the world, excluding Europe. Key: 1, Chile; 2, Peru; 3, Colombia; 4, Venezuela; 5, Mexico; 6, USA; 7, Canada; 8, Egypt; 9, Jordan; 10, Israel; 11, Russia; 12, Hawaii; 13, China; 14, Japan; 15, Thailand; 16, Tonga; 17, Solomon Islands; 18, Papua New Guinea.

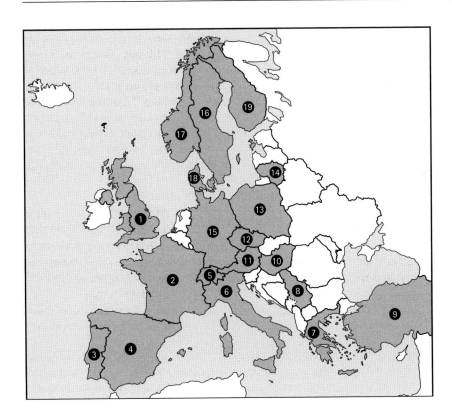

Figure 1.8 Distribution map of occurrences of skeletal tuberculosis in Europe. Key: 1, British Isles; 2, France; 3, Portugal; 4, Spain; 5, Switzerland; 6, Italy; 7, Greece; 8, Serbia; 9, Turkey; 10, Hungary; 11, Austria; 12, Czech Republic; 13, Poland; 14, Lithuania; 15, Germany; 16, Sweden; 17, Norway; 18, Denmark; 19, Finland.

- skeletal remains are not traditionally studied in a particular country;
- disposal of bodies at a particular time may not preserve them well for the evidence to be observed (e.g. cremation in Bronze Age in Britain);
- skeletal remains just do not survive burial because of the climate or environment in a specific geographic area (e.g. the freezing climate of Finland (Vuorinen, personal communication) or the acidic soils of Wales or Scotland);
- for some periods of time in some countries there just have not been any skeletal remains excavated, for whatever reason (e.g. the Roman period in Poland[69]).

There are many areas where there is very little systematic work being undertaken on identifying disease in human remains. Of course, what should also be noted is that the skeletal evidence described here is that recorded from remains that have been excavated and analysed. Thus, the picture of TB that we see will reflect these facts, and what we understand of its origin and evolution may change considerably with each new find.

However, on the basis of the evidence to date we see that TB has an early focus in the Mediterranean and Northern European areas, and specifically Italy, in the Neolithic period. There are later appearances in Asia and other parts of Northern Europe and the Mediterranean. However, it is not until urbanization and an increase in population size and density of the later Medieval period that we see a rise in the frequency of the disease in most places. Additionally, at this time, 'Touching for the King's Evil' was a practice that was developing where the monarch could apparently cure a TB victim by touching them on the head and giving them a gold piece;[91] whether all people 'touched' were tuberculous is debatable. It therefore appears to be associated with the hazards of urban living and closely packed communities, allowing the infection to be readily transmitted by droplet spread. While the early evidence has often suggested a source of TB in domesticated animals, new molecular data suggest that *M. tuberculosis* did not evolve from *M. bovis*.[35,36] However, it is argued that infection of human populations by contaminated animals would always have been a hazard and would probably have increased the absolute TB burden of human populations.[4] Interestingly, there has been no TB identified in either hunter-gatherer human populations or wild animals, and only one (as yet unpublished) report of TB in cattle bones, identified using ancient DNA analysis, from a German site dated to the Roman period (Teegen, personal communication). Currently, therefore, there is compelling evidence for TB as a 'Medieval urban disease'.

During that later Medieval period in England, for example, we understand that from the late eleventh century AD, following the Norman Conquest of 1066, there was a very rapid increase in population numbers and by the end of the thirteenth century the country was very overpopulated.[92] This would have given TB every chance to take its hold. In the urban situation, houses were built packed close together, many people lived near to their animals, and poverty and poor standards of hygiene were real issues with which to contend.[93] Compounded by harvest failures during much of the fourteenth century, urban populations were exposed to the onslaught of infectious diseases such as TB.

Skeletal remains from the New World

In the New World, particularly in North America, skeletal remains have been studied for a considerable time. For example, the first reported cases of TB were in 1886,[94] although there has been some re-evaluation of them. By the mid-twentieth century evidence had considerably increased in eastern North America,[95] the North American southwest[96] and South America.[97] There have been doubts as to its presence in terms of diagnosis,[98] and questions raised about TB's presence in pre-contact/Columbian (i.e. AD 1492) populations,[30] but TB was, without doubt, present in the prehistoric Americas. A major argument for its absence in prehistoric populations was the suggestion that large population aggregates did not exist at that time and therefore TB could not establish itself. However, this idea has been overturned with the discovery of TB in late prehistoric populations from very large communities.[4,99] For example, estimates of population size at Cahokia in the Central Mississippi Valley, around AD 1100, have ranged from 3500[100] to 35 000,[101] with a population density of 21–27 individuals per square kilometre.[100] Although there have been doubts about the need to have large populations for TB to flourish,[102] there were certainly wild and domesticated animals that could have provided a reservoir of the infection.

The evidence from the Americas can be divided into north, central and southern areas, although most of the evidence comes from the north and south.

NORTH AMERICA

There are two areas of North America where the skeletal evidence for TB derives, the Mid-continent and the southwest.[99] Both these areas had large population centres in late prehistory, i.e. before AD 1492. However, the Mid-continent (i.e. east of the Mississippi River) provides the majority of the data, with four sites in North America producing more than 10 individuals with TB: Uxbridge,[103] Norris Farms,[104] Schild[105] and Averbuch.[106] This probably reflects not only the intensity of skeletal analysis here, but also the rite of cremation in the south-west, and casual disposal, in some periods of prehistory, which would make diagnosis of TB problematic. However, the earliest cases of TB in North America do derive from the south-west region just when there were major population increases in large 'pueblos', which were permanent agricultural settlements.[107] For example, the site of Pueblo Bonito had more than 800 rooms, with some of the site having buildings up to five storeys high.[108] By the tenth century AD, when the first cases of TB are noted, a regional population in excess of 80 000 is estimated. All cases in North America thus post date AD 900 and are later than those in South America.

MESOAMERICA

Despite large numbers of people living in Mesoamerica before European contact, and considerable skeletal analy-

sis, there is a 'virtual absence' of TB.[4] This may be explained by poor preservation in some areas of Mesoamerica, but there have also been excavations and analysis of very large well-preserved cemeteries and no evidence of TB has been forthcoming.[109] One explanation for its absence is that people were dying in Mesoamerica before bone changes occurred. However, similar stresses of living are also identified in North America where evidence of TB exists.[106] One could also argue that those with TB, manifest by Pott's disease of the spine, were buried away from the main cemetery or disposed of in a different way to those without the disease. We also know that people with hunchbacks in Mesoamerica, the deformity seen in spinal TB, appear to have been awarded special status, as depicted on painted ceramics,[110] and their treatment in society may have been very different to the rest of the population, including their final disposal.[99]

SOUTH AMERICA

The earliest cases of TB in the New World are seen in South America in Peru,[111] Venezuela,[112] Chile[113] and Colombia.[114] The earliest case overall is from Caserones in the Atacama Desert in Northern Chile.[113] This individual was dated originally to around AD 290 by Allison et al.,[113] but Buikstra,[99] in considering radiocarbon dating problems, dates it to no earlier than AD 700. Within the larger South American sites, it is interesting to note that males more than females are affected (as seen generally today[115]), whereas in North American sites the sexes are equally affected.[4] An explanation suggested relates to the possibility of camelid transmission via droplet infection to males who were responsible for llama herding. Stead et al.[116] also suggest that prehistoric TB in the Americas is likely due more to the *bovis* organism from infected animal products. *M. bovis*, compared to *M. tuberculosis*, is also 10 times more likely to produce skeletal damage. Continuing from the prehistoric period in both North and South America, we see TB increasing after about AD 1000 and continuing at European contact and later into the Historic periods.[117,118]

SUMMARY OF THE DATA FROM THE NEW WORLD

It appears that the earliest evidence of skeletal TB in the New World is in South America at AD 700, with later appearances in North America, which suggests a transmission route of south to north, although Mesoamerica generally does miss the encounter. It is argued that this may be explained by transmission by sea travel.[4] Coincidentally, archaeological evidence from West Mexico documents South American trade, and the only Mesoamerican sites with multiple cases of Pott's disease are in that very area. It is also indicated that TB in the Americas may have been caused by *M. bovis* rather than *M. tuberculosis* as a result of contact with camelids, and possibly mostly the result of ingestion of infected products. However, much more work remains to be done to confirm or disprove these theories and answer the many outstanding questions about TB in the New World[119] and it will be ancient biomolecular analysis that will take us forward.

HISTORICAL AND PICTORIAL DATA

While we would argue that the evidence for TB in past communities should rely primarily on the skeletal and mummified data, there are large bodies of written and illustrative evidence that has contributed to tracing the evolution and history of this infectious disease. This type of evidence, however, is fraught with problems that differ from the skeletal data. Unfortunately, the clinical expression of pulmonary TB may mimic other lung diseases such as cancer and pneumonia, and kyphotic deformities of the spine could be caused by other spinal conditions or trauma. We also have to remember that authors and artists write about, and depict, the most common and visually disturbing diseases which may not always include TB. Thus, using historical sources as an indicator for the presence and frequency of TB remains hazardous.

Historical data

In the Old World, a Chinese text (2700 BC) provides a description of TB in the neck's lymph glands and coughing up of blood.[120] while the Ebers Papyrus (1500 BC) also describes TB of the lymph glands.[121] The Rig Veda, of the same date, in India talks of 'phthisis', and in Mesopotamia (675 BC) a disease representing TB is described.[85] Numerous references are encountered in Classical antiquity ranging from Homer (800 BC) through Hippocrates (460–377 BC) to Pliny (first century AD). Arabian writers too document the disease in the ninth to eleventh centuries AD, suggesting animals may be affected.

Later evidence appears more prolific in the Medieval period in Europe. For example, Fracastorius (1483–1553) wrote 'De Contagione' and was the first to suggest that TB was due to invisible 'germs' carrying the disease. From the beginning of the seventeenth century we get some idea, in England at least, that TB was becoming very common. The London Bills of Mortality record that 20 per cent of deaths in England by the mid-1600s were due to TB.[122] TB was also associated with romanticism and genius. By the eighteenth century, it was meant to be attractive to appear pale and thin and TB allowed this to happen;[123] for example, the heroines in some of the famous operas such as La Traviata were beautiful women with TB.[122] TB apparently also inspired genius, and during fevers it was considered that this was the best time for authors to write. In the nineteenth century, many authors and artists died of TB, thus perpetuating the myth that genius was associated with TB but, at a time when much of the population in Europe were succumbing to TB, this is hardly surprising. Whether TB can be ascribed to the reason behind the decline in the arts in the nineteenth century is debatable.

When historical data are available, it can potentially provide a window on rates of TB. However, it is suggested that the numbers actually dying from TB when historical data become available will be inaccurate. This could be due to many reasons, including non-diagnosis (some due to the stigma attached to TB and the effect on life's prospects[121]) and misdiagnosis. Until 1882, when the tubercle bacillus was identified, diagnosis was based on the analysis of signs and symptoms,[124] and then later sputum tests and radiography played their part. Of course, a post-mortem examination is the only sure way of achieving a diagnosis of cause of death.

Artistic representation

Art evidence may come in a variety of forms, including paintings, drawings, reliefs and sculpture. However, we must remember that the artistic convention of the time and region must be considered, that artists may be biased in what they portray, and that the depiction may not be accurate and will be dependent on the artists' interpretation and skills. There appear to be two types of possible depictions of TB, the kyphotic spine and pale, tired young women.[125] The former is more represented than the latter. In North Africa, Morse et al.[48] describe spinal deformities dated to before 3000 BC, and similar appearances are seen in Egyptian (3500 BC) and North American contexts. A figurine in a clay pot from Egypt (4000 BC) has, for a long time, been identified as depicting TB in the spine and emaciation, but the spinal deformity is in the cervical region (rare in TB) and we have already noted the possible differential diagnoses for these kyphotic deformities. An important point to note is that it is more likely that the angular deformities are representing TB rather than those that are more rounded.[85] In the later and post-Medieval periods in Europe, we see more illustrations of deformed spines, such as those by Hogarth in London. In Central America, of course, we have already seen similar evidence on pottery.[110] While potential evidence for TB in the past exists, both in written and in art form, we consider that their interpretation, until more recent times, is more problematic than the skeletal evidence.

BIOMOLECULAR EVIDENCE FOR TB FROM ANCIENT SKELETAL REMAINS

We would now, as a separate section, like to consider the biomolecular evidence for TB from human remains as an emerging analytical method that will shed much more light on the details of the origin, evolution and palaeoepidemiology of TB. The study of ancient biomolecules using polymerase chain reaction (PCR) analysis as a tool for diagnosing disease has had a short life, spanning the last 15 years or so (for a summary of the use of aDNA analysis in human remains, see Refs 126 and 127). While there are certainly quality control issues to consider in ancient DNA analysis,[128] and the need to have rigorous methodologies in place, it has allowed theories about the origin and evolution of infectious disease to be explored. However, it is TB that has received the most attention from biomolecular scientists. The most common problems tackled have been:

- confirmation of problematic diagnoses;[129]
- diagnosis of individuals with no pathological changes of TB;[78,130]
- the identification of the organism that caused TB in humans;[75,131] and
- attempting to confirm that bone changes are the result of TB.[132,133]

Research diagnosing TB using ancient DNA analysis started in Britain and the Americas. In 1993, Spigelman and Lemma[134] documented the amplification of *M. tuberculosis* complex DNA in Britain. Around the same time Salo *et al.*[26] successfully amplified *M. tuberculosis* DNA from the South American site of Chiribaya Alta; a calcified subpleural nodule was noticed during the autopsy of a woman who had died 1000 years ago. A 97 base pair segment of the insertion sequence (IS) 6110, which is considered specific to the *M. tuberculosis* complex, was identified and directly sequenced.[135] Three other sites have yielded the same *M. tuberculosis* complex ancient DNA, two in eastern North America (Uxbridge and Schild) and one in South America (SR1 in northern Chile). The samples came from Uxbridge (AD 1410–83): a pathological vertebra from an ossuary site;[136] Schild (AD 1000–1200): a pathological vertebra from a female;[136] and Chile (AD 800): an affected vertebra of an 11- to 13-year-old child.[137]

In the Old World, most work to date has been focused on samples from British, Lithuanian and Hungarian skeletons and mummies. For example, Gernaey *et al.*[27] confirmed a diagnosis of TB in an early Medieval skeleton from Yorkshire with Pott's disease using both ancient DNA and mycolic acid analyses. Taylor *et al.*[129,138] provided positive diagnoses for skeletons from the fourteenth century site of the Royal Mint in London. Gernaey *et al.*,[130] at the post-Medieval site at Newcastle in the north-east of England, established that 25 per cent of the population buried had suffered from TB, although the majority had no bone changes. In Hungary, Pálfi *et al.*[139] and Haas *et al.*[132] confirmed a number of TB diagnoses using ancient DNA analysis, dating from the seventh and eighth centuries AD to the seventeenth century, and the analysis of four eighteenth and nineteenth century mummies from Vac (two with TB) revealed positive results for three. Fletcher *et al.*[140] also analysed tuberculous DNA in a family group from the same site. In Lithuania, Faerman and Jankauskas[76] and Faerman *et al.*[141] have also confirmed diagnoses of TB in skeletal remains, including individuals with no skeletal changes.

The use of biomolecular analysis to identify TB in human remains is beginning to answer questions it was not possible to contemplate before. However, it is clear that there are more developments to be made utilizing ancient DNA analysis. One focuses on determining which species of the *M. tuberculosis* complex infected humans over time and in different regions of the world. The second is identifying whether the strains of the organism are the same today as in the past, i.e. compare phylogenetic relationships of organisms causing TB in the past and present and see how the organisms have evolved. Both these areas of research are currently receiving attention by the authors.

OVERVIEW OF THE SKELETAL DATA

Clearly, there is much skeletal evidence for TB from around the world, but the evidence appears to be concentrated in North America and Europe. An early focus for the infection appears in Italy in the Mediterranean area in the sixth millennium BP, in Spain and Poland in the Neolithic, and in Egypt from 4500 BC, but TB does not increase with any real frequency until the later and post-Medieval periods in the Old World. This latter observation corroborates the historical sources. There is little evidence at all in Asia and what there is remains sporadic, more likely reflecting the lack of intense skeletal analysis over the years. In the New World, TB appears for the first time in South America (AD 700) and is not seen until around AD 1000 in North America, all but missing affecting Mesoamerica. The current biomolecular evidence suggests that *M. tuberculosis* did not evolve from *M. bovis* and, thus, humans may not have contracted their TB initially from domesticated animals several thousand years ago. In the prehistoric Americas, population size and aggregation was such that TB could flourish via droplet infection. However, in both Europe and the Americas, wild and domesticated animals may also have been a reservoir of infection.

TB IN THE NINETEENTH AND TWENTIETH CENTURIES

We have considered the evidence for TB in populations from very far distant eras but, to bring us up to the introduction of antibiotics in the mid-twentieth century, we must now turn to the records of TB in the late nineteenth and early twentieth century. In the eighteenth century, John Bunyan referred to TB as the 'Captain of all these men of death'.[121,142] By the beginning of the nineteenth century, TB was the lead cause of death in most European countries, reaching up to 500–800 cases per 100 000 population.[143] In the Victorian period in Britain, it was one of the main causes of death.[144] In the late 1800s and the start of the Industrial Revolution in Britain, rapid urbanization, including rural to urban migration, favoured the spread of

TB. By the mid-nineteenth century, the concept of the sanatorium had been established.[121] Fresh air, a good healthy diet, rest and graded exercise was the regime offered to TB sufferers, with surgery, such as lung collapse and rib resection, being undertaken for some. Patients were isolated from their families in an attempt to control the infection's spread. The first was opened in Germany in 1859, with many more founded over the next 100 years.

In 1882, Robert Koch first described the tubercle bacillus, and in 1895 Conrad Roentgen discovered the x-ray, which provided a new method of diagnosing TB. By 1897, the theory of transmission of TB via droplet infection was established,[145] and by the early twentieth century it was known that animals could contract the infection. By the second half of the nineteenth century and into the twentieth, there was an obvious decline in TB.[146] This is, by most, attributed to the improvement of living conditions and diet, although Davies *et al.*[147] have shown that none of the other poverty-related diseases also showed a decline, thus making interpretations difficult. It is noted, however, that an antituberculosis campaign started once Koch had discovered the bacillus,[124] which included controls on the quality of meat and milk. In 1889, the Tuberculosis Association had been set up in the United States and in the 1890s the League Against Tuberculosis was founded in France to encourage the control of TB in Europe.[121] In 1898, the National Association for the Prevention of Tuberculosis and other forms of consumption (NAPT) was established in Britain,[121] part of an international movement. The International Union against TB was founded in 1902 to encourage a system of control; this included the notification of all cases, contact tracing and the provision of dispensaries and sanatoria.[121] Mass radiography during the wars allowed higher detection rates, while rehabilitation schemes, the BCG vaccination in the 1950s (in Britain), health education and pasteurization of milk were all seriously considered.[124] Clearly, this trend continued with the introduction of antibiotics in the middle part of the twentieth century, a situation which has recently reversed. Clearly, this infection has been with us for thousands of years and, despite once being thought of as a conquered infection, it remains a plague on a global scale.

CONCLUSION

The history of TB in earlier times has been traced through the analysis and interpretation of the evidence from human remains derived from archaeological sites around the world. While there may be limitations to using such evidence to trace the origin, epidemiology and long history of TB, this is the most reliable evidence we have at our disposal. The picture of an origin in Italy for the Old World nearly 8000 years ago, and the appearance in the Americas by AD 700 truly illustrates its antiquity. We have seen that in both worlds, TB increased with population size, which

allowed transmission of the infection through exhaled and inhaled droplets. Infection of humans by their wild and domesticated animals was also a risk, although there is much more work to be done in identifying the most frequent infecting organism for the past. TB continued to increase in frequency through time on into the Industrial Revolution of the 1800s in Europe. In the late 1900s and early twentieth century, a decline in frequency is noted which continued after the introduction of antibiotics. The reasons for this decline are hard to determine. An improvement in living conditions and diet (and its quality), better diagnosis, health education, vaccination and immunization, pasteurization of milk and isolation of people with TB away from the uninfected may all have helped to lower rates.

We have seen from the skeletal evidence that TB can provide us with a very broad temporal and geographic picture of the infection from its very earliest times. It can also point us to the areas of the world that have revealed the earliest evidence and, along with their cultural context, we can begin to explore the epidemiological factors that allowed the infection to flourish. We can see that the factors are very similar to today (poverty, high population density, urban situations, poor access to health care, infected animals and certain occupations). How much trade and contact, and travel and migration, contributed to the tuberculous load in past populations is yet to be established, but is an area of future research. Of course HIV and AIDS, and antibiotic resistance, were not issues with which our ancestors had to contend. Biomolecular studies of TB in the past will also contribute to our understanding of the palaeoepidemiology of this infection, both by identifying the causative organism and differences in strains of TB compared with today.

ACKNOWLEDGEMENTS

To the many researchers listed in Roberts and Buikstra[4] who have given freely of their time and data during the writing of our chapter. Many thanks also to Keith Manchester for allowing the use of Figure 1.1, and to the following for producing figures: Jean Brown (Bradford) for Figures 1.2 and 1.3, Trevor Woods (Durham) for the image of Figure 1.5, Yvonne Beadnell (Durham) for Figure 1.6, and the Design and Imaging Unit, University of Durham for Figures 1.7 and 1.8.

LEARNING POINTS

- Evidence of TB in history comes from two sources: the remains of the people themselves and written or other recorded evidence.
- The skeletal structure will be affected in 3–5 per cent of untreated individuals, the spine being the most common site.

- Skeletal damage implies chronic disease and therefore may be present in individuals with some resistance to TB. Those with little resistance probably died before the skeleton could be affected.
- Care must be taken to distinguish pathological lesions of the skeleton from post-mortem abnormalities.
- The most common skeletal deformity caused by TB is destruction of the vertebral bodies leading to angulation of the spine.
- The hip and knee are the next most common sites, but any bone may be affected.
- The previous belief that TB was spread from animals to humans as they were domesticated has been put in doubt by evidence of humans being infected by TB before domestication of animals took place. Genomic studies have also cast doubt on the earlier held theory.
- Study of skeletal remains of animals has not been helpful in assessing the extent of TB in ancient times and whether TB in animals presented a risk for humans.
- Evidence of skeletal TB may reflect interest in paleopathology in a given area rather than an actual high incidence of disease.
- Evidence of the earliest affected human remains is from Italy dated around 5800 BC.
- During medieval times, the incidence of TB seemed to rise with population density.
- Disease in Asia seems to have occurred much later; the earliest evidence dating to around 2700 BC.
- Evidence for TB in the New World dates to relatively recent times; around AD 1000 in North America and AD 700 in South America.
- The earliest written or pictorial evidence of TB probably refers to tuberculous lymphadenitis from Chinese manuscripts around 2700 BC.
- The most common depiction of TB from ancient times is the deformed spine.
- Biomolecular data can show evidence of TB infection where no pathological lesion is apparent; ancient DNA analysis of TB in human remains will expand our knowledge of the origin, evolution and palaeoepidemiology of TB.
- By the beginning of the nineteenth century, TB was the leading cause of death in most European countries with rates exceeding 500/100 000.
- The first sanatorium opened in Germany in 1859.
- The steady decline in the incidence of TB in European countries from the early nineteenth century cannot be completely explained by the decline in poverty and improvement of living conditions.

REFERENCES

1. Smith ER. *The retreat of tuberculosis 1850–1950*. London: Croom Helm, 1988.
2. Kochi A. *The global tuberculosis situation and the new control strategy of the World Health Organisation. Tubercle* 1991; **72**: 1–6.
3. Young DB. Blueprint for the white plague. *Nature* 1998; **393**: 515–16.
4. Roberts CA, Buikstra JE. *Bioarchaeology of tuberculosis: global perspectives on a re-emerging disease*. Gainesville, FL: University Press of Florida, 2003.
5. Raviglione MC, Snider DE, Kochi A. Global epidemiology of tuberculosis morbidity and mortality of a worldwide epidemic. *J Am Med Assoc* 1995; **273**: 220–6.
6. Vecchiato NL. Sociocultural aspects of tuberculosis control in Ethiopia. *Med Anthropol Q* 1997; **11**: 183–201.
7. Walt G. The politics of tuberculosis: the role of power and process. In: Porter JDH, Grange JM (eds). *Tuberculosis: an interdisciplinary perspective*. London: Imperial College Press, 1999, 67–98.
8. Hudelson P. Gender issues in the detection and treatment of tuberculosis. In Porter JDH, Grange JM (eds). *Tuberculosis: a interdisciplinary perspective*. London: Imperial College Press, 1999: 339–55.
9. Resnick D, Niwayama G. Osteomyelitis, septic arthritis and soft tissue infection: organisms. In: Resnick D (ed.). *Diagnosis of bone and joint disorders*. Edinburgh: WB Saunders, 1995, 2448–558.
10. Stead WW. What's in a name? Confusion of *Mycobacterium tuberculosis* and *Mycobacterium bovis* in ancient DNA analysis. *Paleopathol Assoc Newslett* 2000; **110**: 13–16.
11. Wood JW, Milner GR, Harpending HC, Weiss KM. The osteological paradox: problems of inferring prehistoric health from skeletal samples. *Curr Anthropol* 1992; **33**: 343–70.
12. Henderson J. Factors determining the state of preservation of human remains. In: Boddington A, Garland AN, Janaway RC (eds). *Death, decay and reconstruction. Approaches to archaeology and forensic science*. Manchester: Manchester University Press, 1987: 43–54.
13. Aufderheide AC. *The scientific study of mummies*. Cambridge: Cambridge University Press, 2003.
14. McKinley JI. *Spong Hill. Part VIII: The cremations*. East Anglian Archaeology Report 69. Norwich: Field Archaeology Division, Norfolk Museums Service, 1994.
15. Roberts CA, Manchester K. *The archaeology of disease*, 3rd edn. Stroud: Sutton Publishing/Ithaca, NY: Cornell University Press, 2005.
16. Buikstra JE, Ubelaker D (eds). *Standards for data collection from human skeletal remains*. Arkansas: Archeological Research Seminar Series, 1994: 44.
17. Ortner DJ. Theoretical and methodological issues in palaeopathology. In: Ortner DJ, Aufderheide AC (eds). *Human paleopathology. Current syntheses and future options*. Washington DC: Smithsonian Institution Press, 1991: 5–11.
18. Ganguli PK. Radiology of bone and joint tuberculosis. New York: Asia Publishing House, 1963.
19. Schultz M. The role of tuberculosis in infancy and childhood in prehistoric and historic populations. In: Pálfi G, Dutour O, Deák J, Hutás I (eds). *Tuberculosis. Past and present*. Szeged: Golden Book Publishers/Budapest: Tuberculosis Foundation, 1999, 503–507.
20. Lewis ME. Endocranial lesions in non-adult skeletons: understanding their aetiology. *Int J Osteoarchaeol* 2004; **14**: 82–97.
21. Kelley MA, Micozzi M. Rib lesions in chronic pulmonary tuberculosis. *Am J Phys Anthrop* 1984; **65**: 381–6.
22. Roberts CA, Lucy D, Manchester K. Inflammatory lesions of ribs: an analysis of the Terry Collection. *Am J Phys Anthropol* 1994; **85**: 169–82.
23. Santos AL, Roberts CA. Anatomy of a serial killer: differential

diagnosis of tuberculosis based on rib lesions of adult individuals from the Coimbra Identified Skeletal Collection, Portugal. *Am J Phys Anthropol* 2006; **130**: 38–49.

24. Ortner DJ. *Identification of pathological conditions in human skeletal remains*, 2nd edn. London: Academic Press, 2003.

25. Santos AL. A skeletal picture of tuberculosis. Macroscopic, radiological, biomolecular, and historical evidence from the Coimbra Identified Skeletal Collection. Portugal: Department of Anthropology, University of Coimbra, unpublished PhD thesis, 2000.

26. Salo WL, Aufderheide AC, Buikstra JE, Holcomb TA. Identification of *Mycobacterium tuberculosis* DNA in a pre-Columbia mummy. *Proc Natl Acad Sci U S A* 1994; **91**: 2091–4.

27. Gernaey A, Minnikin DE, Copley M, Dixon R, Middleton JC, Roberts CA. Mycolic acids and ancient DNA confirm an osteological diagnosis of tuberculosis. *Tuberculosis* 2001; **81**: 259–65.

28. Hardy A. Death is the cure of all diseases. Using the General Register Office cause of death statistics for 1837–1920. *Soc Hist Med* 1994; **7**: 472–92.

29. Payne D. Death keeps Irish doctors guessing. *Br Med J* 2000; **321**: 468.

30. Cockburn A. *The evolution and eradication of infectious disease*. Baltimore, MD: Johns Hopkins University Press, 1963.

31. Renfrew C, Bahn P. *Archaeology. Theories, methods and practice*. London: Thames and Hudson, 1991.

32. Smith BD. *The emergence of agriculture*. New York: Scientific American Library, 1995.

33. Kapur V, Whittam TS, Musser JM. Is *Mycobacterium tuberculosis* 15,000 years old? *J Infect Dis* 1994; **170**: 1348–9.

34. Rothschild BM, Martin LD, Lev G et al. *Mycobacterium tuberculosis* complex DNA from an extinct bison dated 17,000 years before present. *Clin Infect Dis* 2001; **33**: 305–11.

35. Brosch R, Gordon SV, Marmiesse M et al. A new evolutionary sequence for the *Mycobacterium tuberculosis* complex. *Proc Natl Acad Sci U S A* 2002; **99**: 3684–9.

36. Gutierrez MC, Brisse S, Brosch R et al. Ancient origin and gene mosaicism of the progenitor of *Mycobacterium tuberculosis*. *PLoS Pathol* 2005; **1**: e5.

37. Lee RB, De Vore I (eds). *Man the hunter*. Chicago: Aldine, 1968.

38. Bathurst R, Barta JL. Molecular evidence of tuberculosis induced hypertrophic osteopathy in a 16th century Iroquoian dog. *J Archaeological Sci* 2004; **31**: 917–25.

39. O'Connor TP. *The archaeology of animal bones*. Gloucester: Sutton Publishing, 2000.

40. Cohen MN. Health and the rise of civilisation. New York: Yale University Press, 1989.

41. Steckel R, Rose JC (eds). *The backbone of history. Health and nutrition in the western hemisphere*. Cambridge: Cambridge University Press, 2002.

42. Roberts CA, Cox M. *Health and disease in Britain. Prehistory to the present day*. Stroud: Sutton Publishing, 2003.

43. Hanks P. *Collins dictionary of the English language*. London: Collins, 1979.

44. Canci A, Minozzi S, Borgognini Tarli, S. New evidence of tuberculous spondylitis from Neolithic Liguria (Italy). *Int J Osteoarchaeol* 1996; **6**: 497–501.

45. Ortner DJ. Disease and mortality in the Early Bronze Age people of Bab edh-Dhra, Jordan. *Am J Phys Anthropol* 1979; **51**: 589–98.

46. Zias J. Leprosy and tuberculosis in the Byzantine monasteries of the Judaean Desert. In: Ortner DJ, Aufderheide AC (eds). *Human palaeopathology. Current syntheses and future options*. Washington DC: Smithsonian Institution Press, 1991, 197–9.

47. Zias J. Tuberculosis and the Jews in the ancient Near East: the biocultural interaction. In: Greenblatt CL (ed.). *Digging for pathogens*. Jerusalem: Centre for the Study of Emerging Diseases/Rehovot, PA: Balaban Publishers, 1998: 277–95.

48. Morse D, Brothwell DR, Ucko PJ. Tuberculosis in ancient Egypt. *Am Rev Respir Dis* 1964; **90**: 526–41.

49. Elliot-Smith G, Ruffer MA. Pottsche Krakheit an einer ägyptischen Mumie aus der Zeit der 21 dynastie (um 1000 v. Chr.). In: *Zur Historichen Biologie der Kranzheit Serreger*. Leipzig: 1910: 9–16.

50. Derry DE. Pott's disease in ancient Egypt. *Med Press Circ* 1938; **197**: 196–9.

51. Nerlich AG, Haas CJ, Zink A, Szeimies U, Hagdorn HG. Molecular evidence for tuberculosis in an ancient Egyptian mummy. *Lancet* 1997; **35**: 1404.

52. Zink A, Haas CJ, Hagedorn HG, Szeimies U, Nerlich AG. Morphological and molecular evidence for pulmonary and osseous tuberculosis in a male Egyptian mummy. In: Pálfi G, Dutour O, Deák J, Hutás I (eds). *Tuberculosis. Past and present*. Szeged: Golden Book Publishers/Budapest: Tuberculosis Foundation, 1999: 371–91.

53. Santoja M. Estudio antropológico. In: Excavaciones de la Cueva de la Vaquera, Torreiglesias. Segovia: Edad del Bronce, 1975, 74–87.

54. Angel JL. Health as a crucial factor in the changes from hunting to developed farming in the Eastern Mediterranean. In: Cohen MN, Armelagos GJ (eds). *Paleopathology at the origins of agriculture*. London: Academic Press, 1984: 51–74.

55. Grmek M. *Diseases in the ancient Greek world*. London: Johns Hopkins University Press, 1989.

56. Moyart V, Pavaut M. *La tuberculose dans le nord de la France du IVe à la XIIIe siecle*. Thèse pour le Diploma d'état de Docteur en Médecine. Lille 2, U du Droit et de la Santé, Faculté de Médecine Henri Warembourg, 1998.

57. Ardagna Y, Aycard P, Bérato J, Leguilloux M, Maczel M, Pálfi G. Abbaye de la Celle, Var. Sondages de diagnostic et fouille d'urgence. In: Berato J, Laurier F (eds). *Le Centre Archeologique du Var 1999*. Toulon: CAV, 1999: 159–233.

58. Bérato J, Dutour O, Pálfi G. À propos d'une spondylodiscite medievale du Xeme sièècle (La Roquebrusanne, Var). *Paleobios* 1991; **7**: 9–17.

59. Brun J-P, Bérato J, Dutour O, Panuel M, Pálfi G. Middle age tuberculosis cases from the south-east of France. Poster presented to the International Congress on the Evolution and Palaeoepidemiology of Tuberculosis, Szeged, Hungary, 1997.

60. Dutour O, Bérato JM, Williams J. Sépultures du site antique de la Porte d'Orée (Frejus). *L'Anthropologie* 1991; **95**: 651–60.

61. Dutour O, Pálfi G, Brun J-P et al. Morphological, paleoradiological and paleomicrobiological study of a French Medieval case of tuberculous spondylitis with cold abscess. In: Pálfi G, Dutour O, Deák J, Hutás I (eds). *Tuberculosis. Past and present*. Szeged: Golden Book Publishers/Budapest: Tuberculosis Foundation, 1999, 395–400.

62. Molnar E, Marcsik A, Dutour O, Berato J, Pálfi G. Skeletal tuberculosis in Hungarian and French Medieval anthropological material. In: Guerci A (ed.). *La cura della mallattie. Itinerari storici*. Genoa: Erga Edizione, 1998: 87–99.

63. Pálfi G. Rapport preliminaire sur l'anthropologie et la paleopathologie des squelettes provenant du site archaeologique de Graveson (Saint-Martin-de-Cadillan). Unpublished manuscript, 1995.

64. Pálfi G, Dutour O, Bérato J. A case of spondylodiscitis from the 10th century (La Roquebrusanne, Var). *Munibe Antropol Arkeol Suppl* 1992; **8**: 107–10.

65. Blondiaux J, Hédain P, Chastanet M, Pavaut M, Moyart V, Flipo R-M. Epidemiology of tuberculosis: a 4th to 12th cenury AD picture in a 2498-skeleton series from Northern France. In: Pálfi G, Dutour O, Deák J, Hutás I (eds). *Tuberculosis. Past and present*. Szeged: Golden Book Publishers/Budapest: Tuberculosis Foundation, 1999: 521–30.

66. Djurić-Srejić M, Roberts CA. Palaeopathological evidence of infectious disease in later medieval skeletal populations from Serbia. *Int J Osteoarchaeol* 2001; **11**: 311–20.

67. Brothwell D. The human bones. In: Harrison RM (ed.). *Excavations at Saraçhane in Istanbul. Volume 1: The excavations, structures, architetcural decoration, small finds, coins, bones and molluscs*. Princeton, NJ: Princeton University Press, 1986: 374–98.

68. Cunha E. Paleobiologia des populacoes Medievals Portuguesas-os-casos de Fão e. S. oãoda Almedina. FCT, University of Coimbra, Portugal, unpublished PhD thesis, 1994.

69. Gladykowska-Rzeczycka JJ. Tuberculosis in the past and present in Poland. In: Pálfi G, Dutour O, Deák J, Hutás I (eds). *Tuberculosis. Past and present.* Szeged: Golden Book Publishers/Budapest: Tuberculosis Foundation, 1999: 561–73.

70. Rokhlin DG. Diseases of ancient men. Bones of the men of various epochs – normal and pathologic changes. Moscow: Nauka, 1965 [in Russian].

71. Bennike P. Facts or myths? A re-evaluation of cases of diagnosed tuberculosis in Denmark. In: Pálfi G, Dutour O, Deák J, Hutás I (eds). *Tuberculosis. Past and present.* Szeged: Golden Book Publishers/Budapest: Tuberculosis Foundation, 1999: 511–18.

72. Mays S, Taylor GM. A first prehistoric case of tuberculosis from Britain. *Int J Osteoarchaeol* 2003; **13**: 189–96.

73. Taylor GM, Yound GB, Mays S. Genotypic analysis of the earliest prehistoric case of tuberculosis in Britain. *J Clin Microbiol* 2005; **43**: 2236–40.

74. Mays S, Taylor GM, Legge AJ, Young DB, Turner-Walker G. Paleopathological and biomolecular study of tuberculosis in a Medieval skeletal collection from England. American. *J Phys Anthropol* 2001; **114**: 298–311.

75. Jankauskas R. History of human tuberculosis in Lithuania: possibilities and limitations of paleoosteological evidences. *Bull Mém Soc Anthropol Paris. New Ser* 1998; **10**: 357–74.

76. Faerman M, Jankauskas R. Osteological and molecular evidence of human tuberculosis in Lithuania during the last two millenia. *Sci Israel–Technol Adv* 1999; **1**: 75–8.

77. Jankauskas R. Tuberculosis in Lithuania: palaeopathological and historical correlations. In: Pálfi G, Dutour O, Deák J, Hutás I (eds). *Tuberculosis. Past and present.* Szeged: Golden Book, 1999. Publishers/Budapest: Tuberculosis Foundation, 1999: 551–8.

78. Morel MMP, Demetz J-L, Sauetr M-R. Un mal de Pott du cimitère burgonde de Saint-Prex, canton de Vaud (Suisse) (5me, 6me, 7me siècles). *Lyon Med* 1961; **40**: 643–59.

79. Pálfi G, Marcsik A. Paleoepidemiological data of tuberculosis in Hungary. In: Pálfi G, Dutour O, Deák J, Hutás I (eds). *Tuberculosis. Past and present.* Szeged: Golden Book Publishers/Budapest: Tuberculosis Foundation, 1999, 533–9.

80. Haas CJ, Zink A, Molnár E *et al.* Molecular evidence for tuberculosis in Hungarian skeletal samples. In: Pálfi G, Dutour O, Deák J, Hutás I (eds). *Tuberculosis. Past and present.* Szeged: Golden Book Publishers/Budapest: Tuberculosis Foundation, 1999: 385–91.

81. Pap I, Józsa L, Repa I *et al.* 18th–19th century tuberculosis in naturally mummified individuals (Vác, Hungary). In Pálfi G, Dutour O, Deák J, Hutás I (eds). *Tuberculosis. Past and present.* Szeged: Golden Book Publishers/Budapest: Tuberculosis Foundation, 1999, 421–42.

82. Arcini C. *Health and disease in early Lund. Osteo-pathologic studies of 3,305 individuals buried in the first cemetery area of Lund 990–1536.* Lund: Department of Community Health Sciences, University of Lund, 1999.

83. Horácková L, Vargová L, Horváth R, Bartoš M. Morphological, roentgenological and molecular analyses in bone specimens attributed to tuberculosis, Moravia (Czech Republic). In: Pálfi G, Dutour O, Deák J, Hutás I (eds). *Tuberculosis. Past and present.* Szeged: Golden Book Publishers/Budapest: Tuberculosis Foundation, 1999: 413–17.

84. Kiple K (ed.). *The Cambridge world history of human disease.* Cambridge: Cambridge University Press, 1993.

85. Morse D. Tuberculosis. In: Brothwell D, Sandison AT (eds). *Diseases in antiquity.* Springfield, IL: Charles C Thomas, 1967: 249–71.

86. Suzuki T. A palaeopathological study of the vertebral columns of the Japanese Jomon to Edo period. *J Anthrop Soc Nipp* 1978; **86**: 321–36 [Japanese with English summary].

87. Suzuki T. Paleopathological evidence of spinal tuberculosis from the protohistoric period in Japan. *The Bone* 2000; **14**: 107–12 [Japanese].

88. Pietruwesky M, Douglas MT. An osteological assessment of health and disease in precontact and historic (1778) Hawai'i. In: Larsen CS, Milner GR (eds). *In the wake of contact. Biological responses to conquest.* New York: Wiley-Liss, 1994, 179–96.

89. Pietruwesky M, Douglas MT, Kalima PA, Ikehara R. *Human skeletal and dental remains from Honokahua burial site, Hawai'i.* Paul H Rosendahl Inc. Archaeological, Historical and Cultural Resource Management Studies and Services. Report 246-041091, 1991.

90. Trembly D. A germ's journey to isolated islands. *Int J Osteoarchaeol* 1997; **7**: 621–4.

91. Crawfurd R. *The king's evil.* Oxford: Oxford University Press, 1911.

92. Platt C. *Medieval England. A social history and archaeology from the Conquest to 1600 AD.* London: Routledge, 1997.

93. Dyer C. *Standards of living in the later Middle Ages. Social change c1200–1520,* rev edn. Cambridge: Cambridge University Press, 1989.

94. Whitney WF. Notes on the anomalies, injuries and diseases of the bones of the native races of North America. *Annu Rep Trustees Peabody Museum Am Archeol Ethnol* 1886; **3**: 433–48.

95. Lichtor J, Lichtor A. Paleopathological evidence suggesting pre-Columbian tuberculosis of the spine. *J Bone Joint Surg* 1952; **39A**: 1398–9.

96. Judd NM. *The material culture of Pueblo Bonito.* Washington DC: Smithsonian Institution Miscellaneous Collections, Volume 124, 1954.

97. Gar´cia-Frías JE. La tuberculosis en los antiguos Peruanos. *Actualidad Médica Peruana* 1940; **5**: 274–91.

98. Morse D. Prehistoric tuberculosis in America. *Am Rev Respir Dis* 1961; **85**: 489–504.

99. Buikstra JE. Paleoepidemiology of tuberculosis in the Americas. In: Pálfi G, Dutour O, Deák J Hutás I (eds). *Tuberculosis. Past and present.* Szeged: Golden Book Publishers/Budapest: Tuberculosis Foundation, 1999: 479–94.

100. Milner GR. *The Cahokia Chiefdom: the archeology of a Mississippian society.* Washington DC: Smithsonian Institution Press, 1998.

101. Gregg ML. A population estimate for Cahokia. In: *Perspectives in Cahokia archeology.* Bulletin 10. Urbana, IL: Illinois Archeological Survey, 1975, 126–36.

102. Black FL. Infectious disease in primitive societies. *Science* 1975; **187**: 515–18.

103. Pfeiffer S. Rib lesions and New World tuberculosis. *Int J Osteoarchaeol* 1991; **1**: 191–8.

104. Milner GR, Smith VG. Oneota human skeletal remains. In: Santure SK, Harn AD, Esarey D (eds). *Archeological investigations at the Morton Village and Norris Farms 36 cemetery.* Reports of Investigations 45. Springfield, IL: Illinois State Museum, 1990: 111–48.

105. Buikstra JE. Differential diagnosis. An epidemiological model. *Yearb Phys Anthropol* 1977; **20**: 316–28.

106. Eisenberg LE. Adaptation in a 'marginal' Mississippian population from Middle Tennessee. Biocultural insights from palaeopathology. New York University, unpublished PhD thesis, 1986.

107. Dean JS, Doelle WH, Orcutt JD. Adaptive stress, environment and demography. In: Gumerman GJ (ed.). *Themes in southwest prehistory.* Santa Fe, NM: School of American Research Press, 1994, 53–86.

108. Cordell LS. *Archaeology of the south-west,* 2nd edn. San Diego: Academic Press, 1997.

109. Storey R. *Life and death in the ancient city of Teotihuacan.* Tuscaloosa, AL: University of Alabama Press, 1992.

110. Kerr J. *The Maya vase book. A corpus of rollout photographs of Maya vases.* New York: Kerr Associates, 1989.

111. Buikstra JE, Williams S. Tuberculosis in the Americas: current perspectives. In: Ortner D, Aufderheide AC (eds). *Human paleopathology. Current syntheses and future options.* Washington DC: Smithsonian Institution Press, 1991: 161–72.

112. Requena A. Evidencia de tuberculosis en la América pre-Columbia. *Acta Venezolana* 1945; **1**: 1–20.

113. Allison MJ, Gerszten E, Munizaga J, Sanoro C, Mendoza D. Tuberculosis in pre-Columbian Andean populations. In: Buikstra JE (ed.). *Prehistoric tuberculosis in the Americas*. Evanston, IL: Northwestern University, 1981: 49–51.

114. Romero Arateco WM. *Estudio bioanthropologico de las momias de la Casa del Marque de San Jorge de Fondo de Promocion de la Cultura, Banco Popular, Bogota*. Carrera de Antropologia, Universidad Nacional de Colombia, 1998.

115. Murray CJL, Lopez AD. *The global burden of disease*. Cambridge, MA: Harvard University Press, 1996.

116. Stead WW, Eisenach KD, Cave MD *et al*. When did *M. tuberculosis* infection first occur in the New World? An important question for public health implications. *Am J Resp Crit Care Med* 2000; **151**: 1267–8.

117. Clabeaux MS. Health and disease in the population of an Iroquois ossuary. *Yearb Phys Anthropol* 1977; **20**: 359–70.

118. Pfeiffer S, Fairgrieve S. Evidence from ossuaries: the effect of contact on the health of Iroquians. In: Larsen CS, Milner GR (eds). *In the wake of contact. Biological responses to conquest*. New York: Wiley-Liss, 1994, 47–61.

119. Mackowiak PA, Tiesler Blos V, Aguilar M, Buikstra JE. On the origin of American tuberculosis. *Clin Infect Dis* 2005; **41**: 515–18.

120. Keers RY. Laënnec: a medical history. *Thorax* 1981; **36**: 91–4.

121. Evans CC. Historical background. In: Davies PDO (ed.). *Clinical tuberculosis*, 2nd edn. London: Chapman and Hall Medical, 1998, 1–19.

122. Lutwick LI. Introduction. In: Lutwick LI (ed.). *Tuberculosis*. London: Chapman and Hall Medical, 1995: 1–4.

123. Sontag S. *Illness as metaphor. Aids and its metaphor*. London: Penguin, 1991.

124. Bryder L. 'A health resort for consumptives'. Tuberculosis and immigration to New Zealand 1880–1914. *Medical History* 1996; **40**: 453–71.

125. Clarke HD. The impact of tuberculosis on history, literature and art. *Medical History* 1962; **6**: 301–18.

126. Brown K. Ancient DNA applications in human osteoarchaeology. In: Cox M, Mays S (eds). *Human osteology in archaeology and forensic science*. London: Greenwich Medical Media, 2000: 455–73.

127. Stone AC. Ancient DNA from skeletal remains. In: Katzenberg MA, Saunders SR (eds). *Biological anthropology of the human skeleton*. New York: Wiley-Liss, 2000, 351–71.

128. Cooper A, Poinar HN. Ancient DNA: do it right or not at all. *Science* 2000; **289**: 1139–41.

129. Taylor MM, Crossley M, Saldanha J, Waldron T. DNA from *M. tuberculosis* identified in Medieval human skeletal remains using PCR. *J Archaeol Sci* 1996; **23**: 789–98.

130. Gernaey A, Minnikin DE, Copley MS *et al*. Correlation of the occurrence of mycolic acids with tuberculosis in an archaeological population. In: Pálfi G, Dutour O, Deák J, Hutás I (eds). *Tuberculosis. Past and present*. Szeged: Golden Book Publishers/Budapest: Tuberculosis Foundation, 1999: 275–82.

131. Zink AR, Sola C, Reischel U *et al*. Molecular identification and characterisation of *Mycobacterium tuberculosis* complex DNA in Egyptian mummies. *Int J Osteoarchaeol* 2004; **14**: 404–413.

132. Haas CJ, Zink A, Molnár E *et al*. Molecular evidence for different stages of tuberculosis in ancient bone samples from Hungary. *Am J Phys Anthrop* 2000; **113**: 293–304.

133. Zink A, Grabner W, Nerlich A. Molecular identification of human tuberculosis in recent and historic bone tissue samples: the role of molecular techniques for the study of the history of tuberculosis. *Am J Phys Anthropol* 2005; **126**: 32–47.

134. Spigelman M, Lemma E. The use of polymerase chain reaction (PCR) to detect *Mycobacterium tuberculosis* in ancient skeletons. *Int J Osteoarchaeol* 1993; **3**: 137–43.

135. Eisenach KD, Cave MD, Bates JH, Crawford JT. Polymerase chain reaction amplification of a repetitive DNA sequence specific for *Mycobacterium tuberculosis*. *J Infect Dis* 1990; **161**: 977–81.

136. Braun M, Cook D, Pfeiffer S. DNA from *Mycobacterium tuberculosis* complex identified in North American pre-Columbian human skeletal remains. *J Archaeol Sci* 1998; **25**: 271–7.

137. Arriaza B, Salo W, Aufderheide AC, Holcomb TA. Pre-Columbian tuberculosis in Northern Chile: molecular and skeletal evidence. *Am J Phys Anthrop* 1995; **98**: 37–45.

138. Taylor GM, Goyal M, Legge AJ, Shaw RJ, Young D. Genotypic analysis of *Mycobacterium tuberculosis* from Medieval human remains. *Microbiology* 1999; **145**: 899–904.

139. Pálfi G, Ardagna Y, Molnár E *et al*. Coexistence of tuberculosis and ankylosing spondylitis in a 7th–8th century specimen evidenced by molecular biology. In: Pálfi G, Dutour O, Deák J, Hutás I (eds). *Tuberculosis. Past and present*. Szeged: Golden Book Publishers/Budapest: Tuberculosis Foundation, 1999, 403–409.

140. Fletcher HA, Donoghue HD, Taylor GM, Van der Zanden AG, Spigelman M. Molecular analysis of *Mycobacterium tuberculosis* DNA from a family of 18th century Hungarians. *Microbiology* 2003; **149**: 143–51.

141. Faerman M, Jankauskas R, Gorski A, Bercovier H, Greenblatt CL. Prevalence of human tuberculosis in a Medieval population of Lithuania studied by ancient DNA analysis. *Anc Biomol* 1997; **1**: 205–14.

142. Guthrie D. *A history of medicine*. London: Thomas Nelson, 1945.

143. Pesanti EL. A short history of tuberculosis. In: Lutwick LI (ed.). *Tuberculosis*. London: Chapman and Hall Medical, 1995, 5–19.

144. Howe GM. *People, environment, disease and death. A medical geography of Britain through the ages*. Cardiff, University of Wales Press, 1997.

145. Meachen NG. *A short history of tuberculosis*. London: Staples Press, 1936.

146. Bryder L. *Below the magic mountain. A social history of tuberculosis in 20th century Britain*. Oxford: Clarendon Press, 1988.

147. Davies RPO, Tocque K, Bellis MA, Rimmington T, Davies PDO. Historical declines in tuberculosis in England and Wales: improving social conditions or natural selection? *Int J Tuberc Lung Dis* 1999; **3**: 1051–4.

Epidemiology

CHRISTOPHER DYE

THE LENGTH AND BREADTH OF TB EPIDEMIOLOGY

Why did tuberculosis (TB) decline in Europe and North America for much of the nineteenth and twentieth centuries? What is the direction of the global TB epidemic at the start of the twenty-first century? Will TB become resistant to all antibiotics? This overview of TB epidemiology is structured around 10 such questions about the distribution and control of the disease in human populations (Table 2.1). The aim is not to dwell on the relatively arid methodology, but rather to focus on the chief epidemiological issues under active debate today.

Table 2.1 Ten leading questions about TB epidemiology.

1   What is the burden of TB worldwide and which countries are most affected?
2   Why does *M. tuberculosis* cause epidemics of a rare disease running over centuries?
3   Why do some people get TB and not others?
4   Why did TB decline in Europe and North America for most of the twentieth century?
5   What explains the resurgence of TB since 1990, especially in Africa and the former Soviet countries?
6   How does TB affect the distribution of other diseases?
7   Can the WHO Stop TB Strategy contain the global TB epidemic?
8   How could drugs be used more effectively?
9   Will TB become resistant to all antibiotics?
10 What is the current and potential impact of vaccination?

The chapter also has two more general themes. The first is that we cannot fully address the problems in Table 2.1 without thinking about the leading disease agent (*Mycobacterium tuberculosis*) and the principal host (humans) as dynamic, interacting populations. The conventional tools of epidemiology include cross-sectional, case–control and cohort studies and, the ultimate investigative method, experimental trials.[1] With these techniques we can assess, for example, whether drug-resistant *M. tuberculosis* is associated with certain genotypes, the relative risk of TB among cigarette smokers, and whether new drugs are effective treatments for individual patients. However, these studies tend to be static in outlook. For instance, a new TB vaccine that is found to have, in a randomized controlled trial, a protective efficacy of 70 per cent against pulmonary disease TB in adults would be a breakthrough for TB control. However, knowing only the protective efficacy, we could neither predict, nor retrospectively understand, the community-wide impact of a vaccination programme over 10 years. That understanding requires a knowledge of events that happen through population interactions and across bacterial and human generations – of processes that can be understood and measured in terms of case reproduction numbers, heterogeneity in transmission, herd immunity, feedback loops, equilibrium and evolutionary selective pressure.[2] These concepts carry traditional epidemiology into the wider, non-linear domain of population biology, including ecology (as distinct from 'ecologic' study[1]), demography and evolutionary biology.

The second theme is that successful TB control will require epidemiologists to take an imaginative and unrestricted view of the opportunities for intervention.

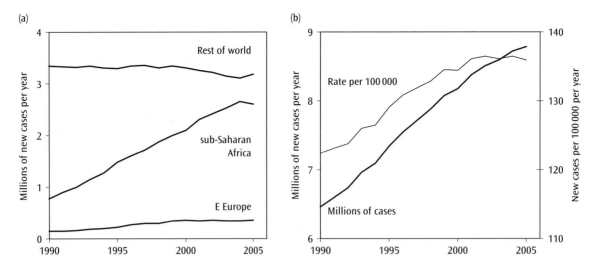

Figure 2.1 Trends in TB incidence by region of the world. The trajectories are based on annual case reports data from countries that supply reliable case notifications.[8]

Over the past decade, the chemotherapy of active TB, delivered under the rubric of the World Health Organization (WHO) DOTS strategy, has come to be accepted as the cornerstone of good TB management. As a model of delivery, standardization and evaluation, DOTS represents a major advance in the attack, not just on TB, but on the principal endemic diseases of the developing world. One example of the broader significance of DOTS is that directly observed treatment (the DOT component), though persistently controversial,[3] may be a useful model for the delivery of antiretroviral drugs for AIDS patients.[4,5] However, the world needs more than DOTS because DOTS on its own is unlikely to lead to TB eradication. For this reason, the scope of DOTS was widened as the WHO Stop TB Strategy (of which DOTS remains part) in 2006.[6] However, it is too early to tell whether the new strategy will be enough to meet the targets set within the framework of the Millennium Development Goals (MDGs). These are to ensure that the incidence rate is falling globally (MDG 6, target 8) and to halve TB prevalence and death rates by 2015 (as compared with 1990 levels).[7]

The first half of the chapter describes and attempts to explain some important patterns in the distribution of TB. The second half examines the real and potential effectiveness of TB control, given these underlying patterns. All 10 questions in Table 2.1 are ultimately about the way populations of the host and the pathogen multiply and interact in their natural and social environments.

TB BURDEN AND TRENDS AT THE START OF THE TWENTY-FIRST CENTURY

Based on notification reports, and surveys of the prevalence of infection and disease, there were an estimated 8.8 million new TB cases in 2005. Of these cases, 3.9 million were pulmonary sputum smear-positive, the most infec-

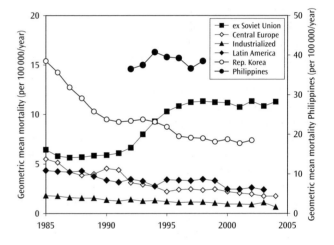

Figure 2.2 Trends in tuberculosis deaths for four regions of the world, plus the Philippines and the Republic of Korea, evaluated with vital registration data reported to the World Health Organization.

tious form of the disease.[8] Assuming lifelong infection, about one-third of humanity is infected with *M. tuberculosis*. Across regions, the WHO African region (mainly sub-Saharan Africa) had by far the highest annual incidence rate in 2005 (343/100 000 population; Figure 2.1a), but the most populous countries of Asia harboured the largest number of cases: India, China, Indonesia, Bangladesh and Pakistan together accounted for about half of the world's new TB cases in 2005. Roughly 80 per cent of new cases live in 22 high-burden countries (HBCs).

Judging from trends in case notifications, and from mathematical modelling, the global TB epidemic is on the threshold of decline. The incidence rate *per capita* was growing during the 1990s, but had stabilized or begun to fall by 2005. However, because the populations of the countries heavily affected by TB are still growing, the total

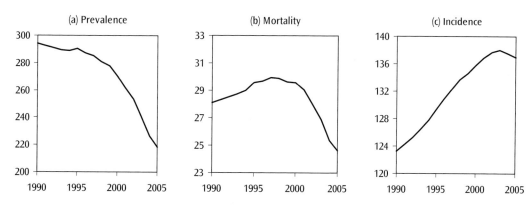

Figure 2.3 Estimated global prevalence, incidence and mortality rates, for all forms of tuberculosis per 100 000 population, 1990–2005. Mortality and incidence rates are per year. Notice the different scales on the vertical axes. From Ref. 8.

number of new TB cases arising each year was also still slowly increasing in 2005 (Figure 2.1b).[8]

This rather static picture of the global epidemic close to its peak conceals much variation in the dynamics of TB among regions (Figure 2.1). In general, while the burden of TB is carried predominantly by Asian countries (56 per cent of all new cases in 2005), it is Africa and Eastern Europe that have determined global trends. The countries of sub-Saharan Africa and the former Soviet Union showed the most striking increases in case load during the 1990s. These rises offset the fall in case numbers in other parts of the world, principally West and Central Europe, the Americas and the Eastern Mediterranean regions. Industrialized countries are typically seeing fewer cases among nationals each year, but steady or rising numbers of cases among immigrants. In 12 of 28 Western European countries providing data in 2005, the majority of TB patients were foreign-born or foreign citizens.[9]

An estimated 1.6 million people died of TB in 2005. TB is the world's second largest killer among single infectious agents, behind HIV/AIDS.[10] In terms of years of healthy life lost, TB remains among the top 10 causes of illness, death and disability. The 195 000 TB deaths in adults infected with HIV were 12 per cent of all TB deaths and 9 per cent of adult AIDS deaths in 2005, and the vast majority (159 000) were in Africa.[8] Death registrations have been increasing in former Soviet countries since the 1980s, but falling in Central Europe, Latin America and in the industrialized world (Figure 2.2). It is not possible to assess precisely the global trend in TB deaths because many countries, including most in Africa and Asia, have no system of death registration (the Republic of Korea and the Philippines are exceptions, as shown in Figure 2.2). Nevertheless, estimation methods suggest that, while TB deaths were probably increasing during the 1990s, driven mainly by the steep rise in HIV-related mortality in Africa, the global TB death rate peaked before the year 2000. This was after prevalence began to fall, but before the peak in incidence (Figure 2.3).

TB is predominantly a disease of adults. Although children of 0–14 years make up 30 per cent of the world's population, they account for only 10 per cent of TB cases.

Where transmission rates are high, such as in Peru, Haiti and Bolivia, TB incidence peaks in young adults (Figure 2.4a). As transmission falls, the average age of TB cases increases; in industrialized countries where transmission rates are now low, the majority of indigenous TB cases are found among the elderly (Figure 2.4b). Although women are less likely to seek effective TB treatment in some countries,[11–13] this is not true everywhere,[14] and it is clear that the greater part of the global TB burden is carried by men. The sex ratio of cases is exceptionally male-biased in countries of the former Soviet Union, where TB is a major cause of death among men along with alcoholism and cardiovascular disease (Figure 2.4c).[15–18]

TB incidence rates also vary on smaller spatial scales and between subpopulations classified by characteristics other than age and sex. TB notification rates vary among London boroughs by a factor of more than 10 and TB 'hotspots' changed little between 1997 and 2003.[19,20] Population surveys undertaken in China in 1979 and 1990 found that smear-positive disease was five times more prevalent among the Uygur and Zhuang peoples than among the Yi and Chaoxian.[21] The Philippines has more TB in urban areas and TB is concentrated among the urban poor.[22]

There is general agreement that TB remains among the top 10 causes of illness and disability (as measured by disability-adjusted life years, DALYs).[23] Nonetheless, the estimation of TB burden remains imprecise, especially in high-burden countries where precision is most needed.[24] Better surveys of infection and disease will increase the accuracy of these estimates, but the world as a whole cannot be surveyed. The ultimate monitoring method for all countries must be high-quality routine surveillance, building on systems already in place.[8,25]

SLOW EPIDEMICS OF A RARE DISEASE

Notwithstanding the enormous burden of disease due to TB, the interaction between *M. tuberculosis* and humans is relatively benign in at least three respects. First, as a rule of

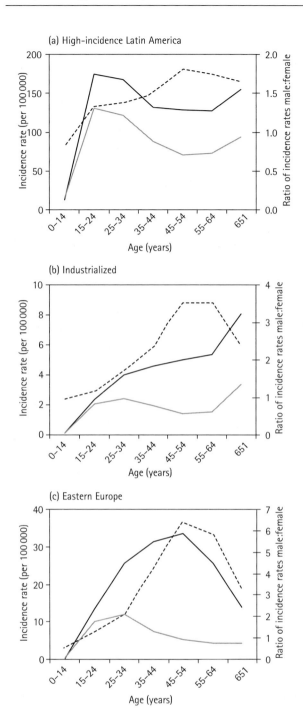

Figure 2.4 Tuberculosis case notifications by age for men (black), women (grey) and for the ratio men/women (broken) living in three regions. (a) High-incidence Latin America is Peru, Bolivia and Haiti. (b) Thirteen industrialized countries include 10 from Western Europe, with the USA, Australia and New Zealand. (c) Eastern Europe includes eight countries of the former Soviet Union, plus Hungary and Romania. Data are from the 2000 WHO report on Global Tuberculosis Control, in the same series as Ref. 8.

thumb, untreated sputum smear-positive cases infect 5–10 other individuals each year.[26,27] For a prevalence of smear-positive disease of 0.1 per cent (i.e. 100/100 000, a little less than the estimated global average of 122/100 000) an aver-

age contact rate of 10 per year would generate an annual risk of infection of 1 per cent. Second, only about 5 per cent of infected individuals (in the absence of other predisposing conditions) develop 'progressive primary' disease following infection; the proportion is lower in children and higher in adults.[28,29] Third, the progression time is slow, averaging 3–4 years.[30] After 5 years, there is a low annual risk of developing TB by 'reactivation' of infection that is then said to be 'latent'. Whether latent bacteria remain viable for the full life span of all infected people is unknown, but the risk of reactivation certainly persists into old age for many (Figure 2.4b).

Besides the strong innate resistance to developing disease, infection is associated with an acquired immune response, though this is only partially protective,[28–31] signalling the problem of developing an effective vaccine.[32,33] Consequently, infected persons living in an endemic area are at risk of TB following reinfection. The importance of reinfection remains controversial in the minds of some, but the decline of TB in Europe cannot easily be explained without it,[29,34] and molecular fingerprinting is producing a catalogue of persuasive examples.[35–38] The lifetime risk of developing TB following infection clearly depends on ambient transmission rates; it has been calculated at 12 per cent for all forms of pulmonary disease in England and Wales during the second half of the twentieth century.[39] Styblo[40] found empirically that the incidence of smear-positive disease increased by about 50/100 000/year for every 1 per cent increase in the annual risk of infection, a result that can be recreated with mathematical models.[34]

These norms and tendencies capture the essence of TB epidemiology, but rules of thumb are inevitably broken. During a TB outbreak in Leicester (UK), an unusually high proportion (23 per cent) of the children who were known to be infected developed active TB within 1 year.[41] Regarding Styblo's 1:50 rule, this is most likely to hold when TB is stably endemic, when there is no programme of drug treatment for patients with active TB, and in the absence of HIV. Thus, the rule may no longer be widely valid.[42,43]

The low incidence of infection and the low probability of breakdown to disease explain why TB is relatively rare. Its importance among infectious diseases is attributable to the high case fatality rate among untreated or improperly treated cases. About two-thirds of untreated smear-positive cases will die within 5–8 years, the majority within the first 2 years.[26] The rest will either remain chronically ill or self-cure. The case fatality rate for untreated smear-negative cases is lower, but still of the order 10–15 per cent.[44,45] Even among smear-positive patients receiving antituberculosis drugs, the case fatality rate can exceed 10 per cent if adherence is low, or if rates of HIV infection and drug resistance are high.[8]

The longer-term consequences of this host–pathogen relationship can be explored with a simple mathematical model (Figure 2.5). Individuals in a population are assigned to mutually exclusive states of infection and dis-

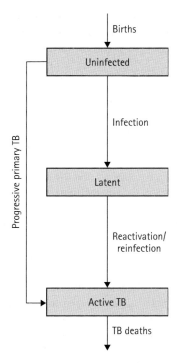

Figure 2.5 A simple compartmental model of tuberculosis (TB) epidemiology. Individuals within a population are assigned to the mutually exclusive states uninfected, latent and with active TB (boxes), and the arrows represent possible transitions between states. TB can develop soon after infection (progressive primary disease, usually taken to be within 5 years), or after a period of latency by reactivation or reinfection. Most mathematical models are more complex than the scheme represented here, distinguishing, for example, infectious from non-infectious disease, or allowing for different rates of progression among HIV-infected and uninfected individuals.

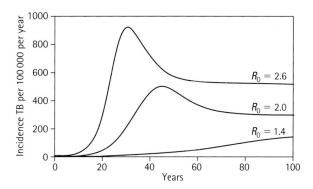

Figure 2.6 Model TB epidemics generated for three different basic case reproduction numbers (R_0). The mathematical model is described in Ref. 178.

Compared with epidemics of highly infectious childhood viral diseases, TB epidemics consume susceptibles very slowly, through low transmission rates, weak immunity and the long generation time. The rate of removal of susceptibles from a population is not much faster than the rate at which they are replaced by births, so *M. tuberculosis* does not generate persistent cycles like measles.[2] TB epidemics are characteristically more stable, showing no more than one peak at an incidence rate that is not much higher than the endemic steady state (Figure 2.6).

Although large, uninfected human populations no longer exist, and no country has yet eliminated TB altogether, the concept of R_0 remains useful because it guides thinking about a wide range of epidemiological processes, including the spread of drug resistance and the efficacy of different control methods.

VARIATIONS ON A THEME: FACTORS AFFECTING THE COURSE OF TB EPIDEMICS

While the simple model described in the previous section captures the typical behaviour of TB epidemics, there are important variations on the basic theme. Some of these variations have been discovered through investigations of epidemiological 'risk factors'. A risk factor can be represented as some link in a causal chain of processes influencing TB epidemiology. The number of possible causal chains is essentially infinite because causation can be expressed on any scale (e.g. physiological, genetic, behavioural) and focused on any part of the *M. tuberculosis* life cycle (infection, disease progression, outcome). The goal of risk factor analysis is to try to identify, out of the innumerable possibilities, the principal causal and modifiable factors in TB epidemiology.

The list of known risk factors for TB is long and growing. A small selection is given in Table 2.2, classified in terms of the *M. tuberculosis* life cycle rather than the scale on which they act. It will be clear from Table 2.2 that there are numerous identifiable risks associated with exposure

ease, and the natural history quantified above specifies the rates of flow between states. All such models of *M. tuberculosis* generate slow epidemics which peak after several decades at an incidence rate that is typically below 1 per cent (Figure 2.6).[34,46–48]

The early growth rate of the epidemic is governed by the basic case reproduction number, R_0, the average number of secondary infectious cases generated when one infectious case is introduced into an uninfected population. For an infection to spread, R_0 must exceed 1. Because active TB can arise via three different routes, and typically with a considerable time delay after infection, it is not straightforward to calculate an exact value of R_0.[49] However, rough estimates of R_0 for TB are relatively low among infectious diseases, of the order of 2 in untreated populations.[50] For $R_0 = 2$, the expected doubling time of an epidemic in its early stages is the same as the *M. tuberculosis* generation time of 4–5 years (Figure 2.6). If transmission is concentrated within certain subpopulations at higher risk, the dynamic effect is to increase R_0 locally, but to reduce the proportion of the entire population that will ever get TB.

Table 2.2 Selected risk factors for infection, progression to active tuberculosis (TB) and adverse outcomes of disease.

Risk factor	Type of study	Source
Infection		
Black Caribbeans and alcoholics are more likely to have TB as a result of recent rather than remote infection	Retrospective analysis of strain clusters	52
Increased risk of TB among health-care workers	Retrospective ecologic	53
TB among the homeless associated with recent transmission	Retrospective analysis of strain clusters	54
HIV-positive TB patients less likely to infect contacts than HIV-negatives	Cohort	55
Childhood infection linked to consumption of unpasteurized milk or cheese	Case–control	56
Progression to disease		
HIV increases the risk of recurrent TB via reinfection	Cohort	57
TB associated with smoking and low blood pressure	Case–control	58
TB associated with exposure to smoke from biomass stoves	Case–control	59
TB associated with intake of dietary iron from traditional beer	Case–control	60
Vitamin D deficiency associated with active TB, facilitated by polymorphism in the vitamin D receptor gene	Case–control	61
NRAMP1 polymorphisms associated with smear-positive pulmonary TB	Case–control	62
Adverse outcome of disease		
Malnutrition associated with early mortality in a cohort of patients with high HIV infection	Cohort	63
Women at higher risk of carrying MDR-TB	Retrospective analysis of strain clusters	64
Previously treated TB patients less likely to adhere to therapy	Cohort	65
Severity of pulmonary disease associated with death among hospitalized patients	Cross-sectional	66
Non-adherence to treatment linked to alcoholism, injection drug use and homelessness	Cohort	67

MDR-TB, multidrug-resistant TB

and the establishment of infection, with the progression from infection to active TB, and with the outcome of active disease.[45] Some risk factors are qualitatively obvious, though the magnitude of the risk may not be. For example, health-care workers who come into contact with TB patients are exposed to infection, but the risk varies from one setting to another.[51]

HIV co-infection dramatically increases the risk of disease following primary infection, and reactivates latent infection. For example, in three studies that compared HIV-infected and uninfected individuals, the average relative risk of developing TB was 28 over 25 months.[68] The risk associated with HIV infection increases as immunity is progressively impaired.[69–74] Other factors known to enhance the risk of TB include diabetes,[75] silicosis,[76] malnutrition (with or without HIV infection),[77–80] and the smoke from domestic stoves and cigarettes.[81,82]

HIV infection is massively more detrimental than all of these to the co-infected individual. However, the impact of a risk factor at population level depends on the number of people exposed, as well as the risk to each person exposed. Consequently, some adverse factors that present low risks to individuals but which are widespread in populations can be responsible for a large proportion of TB cases in a population (i.e. a high population attributable fraction). As determinants of the total number of TB cases, tobacco smoking in Asia and malnutrition in Africa could be even more important than HIV.[83]

Besides environmental factors and concomitant illness, infection and the progression to active TB are also under human genetic control. It is well known that TB runs in families, but this observation on its own confounds genes and transmission. Among the genes that have been associated with susceptibility to TB by more discerning methods (e.g. case–control studies) are those encoding the vitamin D receptor, natural resistance-associated macrophage protein (NRAMP1), HLA and mannose binding lectin (MBL).[84–88] Protection against tuberculous meningitis has been associated with certain variants of collectin molecules, and proinflammatory interleukin-1 haplotypes are over-represented in some groups of patients with tuberculous pleurisy.[89] The genetic polymorphisms associated with these conditions produce various clinical outcomes because phenotypes are typically determined by the interactions between genes and their environment.[90,91] However, the collection of epidemiological studies carried out to investigate genetic determinants has not always yielded consistent and unambiguous results, as illustrated by studies of vitamin D receptor polymorphisms.[92]

Indeed, as explanations for epidemiological patterns, and in suggesting opportunities for control, the results of risk factor studies need careful interpretation.[93] One such study in India found that exposure to smoke from biomass fuel (wood or dung) accounted for 51 per cent of active TB in persons aged 20 years or older.[94] There are three potential difficulties with results of this kind. First, even if the use of biomass fuel is a major risk, it does not preclude other major risks: in the many possible hierarchies of causal factors, risks are not additive. Second, other major risk factors will remain undiscovered unless exposure to these factors varies in the population under study: with no variation, there can be no apparent risk. The third pitfall is confounding, where the factor being investigated is correlated with, and acts as proxy for, some other causal factor. In this instance, infection rates might have been higher in households using biomass fuel. There probably is a strong causal relationship between indoor smoke and TB, but it is unlikely that the elimination of all smoke from these sources would reduce TB incidence by as much as 51 per cent.

In sum, the standard picture of *M. tuberculosis* as the agent of slow epidemics is a useful frame of reference, but certain co-factors – besides targeted control methods – can profoundly alter TB epidemiology. Though some of these factors are known, many aetiological questions remain unanswered. Above all, we still have no more than a superficial understanding of why 10 per cent of infected individuals, rather than 90 per cent, go on to develop active TB. The next two sections describe phenomena that constitute radical, but only partly explicable, departures from the simple, slow epidemic.

LONG-TERM DECLINE OF TUBERCULOSIS

The model used to generate the epidemics in Figure 2.6 shows the incidence of TB eventually reaching a steady state. Case reports suggest that TB incidence has been nearly steady for at least two decades in some South East Asian countries (Figure 2.1), but no such equilibrium was ever reached in Western Europe or North America. TB has been in decline ever since rates *per capita* peaked in industrialized countries, probably sometime during the early nineteenth century and certainly before chemotherapy began in the 1950s. Prior to the emergence of HIV/AIDS, case reports and surveys of the prevalence of infection also indicated that TB was in decline, albeit a slower decline, in Africa and the Middle East.[95] Some of this decline could be due to the natural waning of the epidemic after incidence reached a maximum (Figure 2.6),[47] but the decline in the west is almost certainly too prolonged for this to be the whole explanation. In this respect, then, the basic model appears to be wrong.

The reasons for the 150-year decline have been the subject of perennial debate (for much of that period),[96] with proposed explanations of broadly three kinds. The first is that transmission diminished as people began to live at lower density with better ventilation in improved housing, and when patients were isolated in sanatoria. Transmission could have been further reduced as the caseload shifted to older people who perhaps have fewer contacts with the rest of the population.[97] One analysis determined that the number of effective contacts per infectious case fell from 22 in England and Wales in 1900 to about 10 by 1950.[98] This is the fall in the contact rate needed to explain the observed decline in TB deaths, assuming no concomitant change in the risk of disease among infected individuals (and ignoring any changes in exposure to *M. bovis*).

Yet there may also have been a fall in susceptibility due to improved nutrition, or because concomitant illness became less common. Nutrition did improve[99] and it is linked to susceptibility,[80] so it seems reasonable to deduce that it played a part. Susceptibility is also under genetic control and, with 15–30 per cent of deaths in cities of the USA attributable to TB during the early nineteenth century,[100] most of them among young adults of reproductive age, there must have been some selective pressure. However, genetic analysis suggests that natural selection by pulmonary TB is unlikely to have played a major role in the decline of TB prior to the availability of antituberculosis drugs.[101] If nutrition and genetics did contribute, it was apparently in moderating the breakdown to disease and not in changing the outcome of a TB episode. The relationship between death and case registrations for England and Wales during the twentieth century indicates that case fatality did not fall dramatically until antituberculosis drugs were used widely from the late 1940s onwards (Figure 2.7).

The third explanation is that *M. tuberculosis* has generally become less pathogenic. Intriguingly, irreversible genetic deletions appear to have produced phenotypes of *M. tuberculosis* that are less likely to cause cavitary pulmonary disease.[102,103] It remains to be proven that these deletions accumulate more rapidly than the genome can throw up novel, virulent strains.[104] Indeed, some apparently virulent strains are associated with novel genetic deletions.[41] More generally, some emergent strains of *M. tuberculosis*, including some in the Beijing group, are relatively virulent, at least to experimental mice.[105]

It is not yet possible to disentangle the factors contributing to TB decline before the widespread introduction of chemotherapy, and it may never be possible. All of the above factors could plausibly have played some role. What is clear, however, is that these processes together caused a fall in the TB death rate in Western Europe of only 5 per cent/year in the era before chemotherapy. While environmental and nutritional improvements are highly desirable, it remains to be shown that they can be powerful instruments for TB control.

THE RESURGENCE OF TB SINCE 1990

At least two main factors and two subsidiary factors explain the resurgence of TB, or its sluggish decline, over the past two decades. Outstandingly important has been

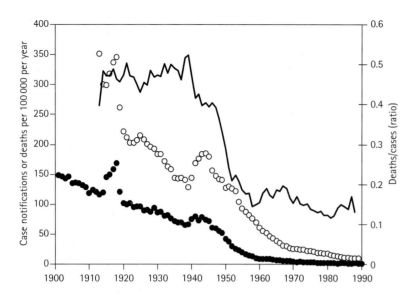

Figure 2.7 Tuberculosis (TB) case notifications (open circles) and death registrations (filled circles) for men in England and Wales, 1900–90. The ratio of cases/deaths (line) falls sharply between 1945 and 1960, probably reflecting the impact of drugs in reducing TB case fatality. Data were compiled from public records.[179]

the spread of HIV/AIDS in Africa, and social and economic deterioration in former Soviet countries. Immigration and ageing have contributed to the stagnation in middle- and high-income countries.

The spatial and temporal variation in TB incidence in Africa is strongly correlated with the prevalence of HIV infection (Figure 2.8).[8,106] HIV infection rates in TB cases are correspondingly high, estimated to be 50 per cent in countries including Mozambique, South Africa, Zambia and Zimbabwe. Around the estimated 11 per cent of all new adult TB cases infected with HIV in 2005, there were marked variations among regions: from 28 per cent in the WHO African region, through 7 per cent in industrialized countries, to 1 per cent in WHO's Western Pacific Region. HIV infection rates in adult TB patients are estimated to be less than 1 per cent in Bangladesh, China and Indonesia; they may or may not remain so. The extent to which HIV is fuelling TB transmission (in addition to provoking reactivation) remains poorly known: one analysis suggests that 1–2 per cent of all transmission events were from HIV-infected, smear-positive TB cases in 2000.[107] TB incidence has been rising especially in eastern and southern Africa since the 1980s, and is still rising. However, the rate of increase appears to be slowing, presumably because the underlying HIV epidemics are also approaching a maximum.[8]

In Russia and other ex-Soviet countries, TB incidence and deaths increased sharply between 1990 and 2000, but have since stabilized (Figures 2.1, 2.2 and 2.9a). Understanding precisely why this increase happened is as difficult as understanding the preceding decline. It is clear that there was a marked deterioration in case finding and cure rates in Russia (Figure 2.9b), but this cannot explain all of the rise.[108] Other factors that may have shaped the post-1990 epidemic in Russia include enhanced transmission due to the mixing of prison and civilian populations, an increase in susceptibility to disease following infection

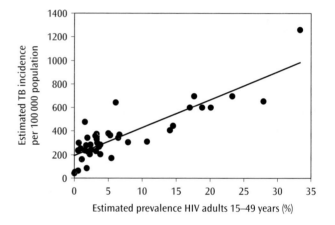

Figure 2.8 Estimated TB incidence in relation to adult HIV prevalence for 43 African countries. Updated from Ref. 180, with estimates for 2005.[8]

(possibly linked to stress and malnutrition), poor service delivery and the spread of drug resistance and, latterly, HIV infection.[18,109,110]

Immigration from high-incidence countries is part of the reason why the decline of TB in Western Europe, North America and the Gulf States has stopped or has been reversed. Many immigrants are infected in their countries of origin, and they are responsible, in varying degrees, for further transmission and outbreaks in the countries where they have come to live or work.[111–115]

TB incidence has also stopped falling in some east Asian countries, notably Hong Kong, Japan and Singapore. Part of the explanation – a part that remains to be quantified – could be that more cases are arising by reactivation from an ageing TB epidemic in an ageing human population.[116] TB deaths are not frequent enough to cause significant demographic change, but demographic changes can markedly affect TB epidemiology.

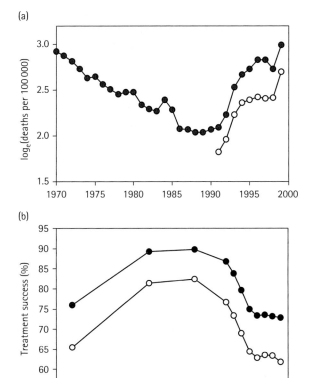

Figure 2.9 (a) Trends in tuberculosis (TB) deaths in the Russian Federation, 1970–99, as recorded by the Russian State Committee for Statistics (upper series) and the Ministry of Health TB services (lower). (b) Coincident changes in treatment success, defined by bacteriological conversion (upper) or cavity closure (lower). Trends observed in (a) are only partly due to those seen in (b). From Ref. 108.

TB AFFECTING THE DISTRIBUTION OF OTHER DISEASES

M. tuberculosis is one of a set of pathogens interacting competitively or facultatively via the human immune system. Mammalian adaptive immune responses fall into two antagonistic subclasses – T_H1 and T_H2 – each with its own set of cytokine mediators. Microbial infections have the potential to influence the balance between T_H1 and T_H2 responses by altering cytokine profiles, with positive or negative consequences for health. Bacterial infections probably have such a role in atopy, an allergic state producing mucosal inflammation characteristic of asthma, and characterized by over-reactive T_H2 responses.

Because mycobacteria elicit strong T_H1 responses, shifting the T_H1/T_H2 balance away from T_H2, *M. tuberculosis* infection could protect against asthma. One study of Japanese children found that strong tuberculin responses, probably attributable to *M. tuberculosis* exposure, were associated with less asthma, rhinoconjunctivitis and eczema in later childhood.[117] In positive tuberculin

responders the rate of current atopic symptoms was one-third the rate in negatives, and asthmatic symptoms were one-half to one-third as likely. On top of this, remission of atopy in children aged 7–12 years was six to nine times as likely in positive tuberculin responders. A study of South African children found an inverse association between *M. tuberculosis* infection and atopic rhinitis.[118] Other comparisons among countries have found that asthma tends to be more common where TB is not.[119,120] The implication of these results, taken together, is that TB has been inhibiting the spread of asthma and other atopic disorders worldwide.

As the evidence for an immunological link between TB and asthma becomes more compelling, interactions between other infections have come under investigation, leading to various propositions including the following. Vigorous T_H2 responses are seen in protective immune reactions to helminth infections, and helminths could modulate atopic disease while compromising the immune response to bacille Calmette–Guérin (BCG) and *M. tuberculosis*.[121–123] Seen from the other direction, a mycobacterial vaccine might be constructed to prevent atopy and asthma. BCG could already serve that purpose, though the evidence is ambiguous.[121] *M. tuberculosis* infection may protect against leprosy, as does BCG,[124] and natural TB transmission could have contributed to the decline of leprosy in Europe.[125]

The synergistic and antagonistic interactions between bacterial, viral and parasitic infections, mediated by immunity, are complex and unresolved. Nonetheless, the above examples at least raise the possibility that mycobacteria influence, and are influenced by, other infections to a far greater extent than hitherto appreciated.

IMPLEMENTATION AND IMPACT OF THE DOTS STRATEGY

With this epidemiological background, we can now explore the impact of various control methods. The cornerstone of TB control is the prompt treatment of symptomatic cases with short-course chemotherapy, administered as the DOTS strategy. Standard short-course regimens can cure over 90 per cent of new, drug-susceptible TB cases and high cure rates are a prerequisite for expanding case finding. DOTS is the foundation for more complex strategies for control where, for example, rates of drug resistance (DOTS-Plus) or HIV infection are high. The wider range of approaches is described by the Stop TB Strategy,[6,8] and the blueprint for implementation is the Global Plan to Stop TB (2006–15).[126]

Data submitted to WHO by the end of 2006 have been used to assess whether national tuberculosis control programmes met the 2005 targets of 70 per cent case detection and 85 per cent cure, which were set by the World Health Assembly. Many of the 187 national DOTS programmes in existence by the end of 2005 have shown that they can

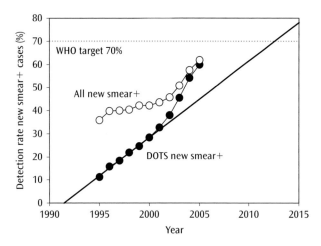

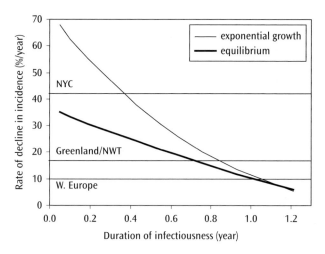

Figure 2.10 Progress towards the WHO target of 70 per cent case detection, which should have been reached by 2005. Filled circles: new smear-positive case detection rates under DOTS, 1995–2005. Open circles: new smear-positive case detection rates, with cases reported from all sources. From Ref. 8.

Figure 2.11 Theoretical relationship between the duration of infectiousness and the rate of decline in tuberculosis (TB) incidence. The two curves show the potential impact of chemotherapy applied during an exponentially growing epidemic (upper) or to stable, endemic TB (lower). The horizontal lines mark approximate rates of decline achieved for endemic TB in Western Europe, Greenland and the North Western Territories of Canada, and for epidemic TB in New York City. From Ref. 128.

achieve high cure rates: the average treatment success (i.e. patients who were cured plus those who completed treatment) in the 2004 DOTS cohort of more than 2 million patients was 84 per cent, just below the 85 per cent target. The outstanding deviations below that average were in the WHO African (74 per cent) and European regions (74 per cent). Although most TB patients probably receive some form of treatment, the estimated case detection rate of new smear-positive cases by DOTS programmes in 2005 was 60 per cent – 10 per cent below target (Figure 2.10). Both targets were met by the entire Western Pacific region, and by a total of 26 countries including China, the Philippines and Vietnam.

High case detection and cure rates are essential if incidence, prevalence and death rates are to be reduced so as to meet the TB-related Millennium Development Goals.[7] Mathematical modelling suggests that the incidence of endemic TB will decline at 5–10 per cent/year with 70 per cent passive case detection and 85 per cent cure.[127,128] In principle, TB incidence could be forced down more quickly, as much as 30 per cent/year, if new cases could be found soon enough to eliminate transmission (Figure 2.11). In general, the decline will be faster when a larger fraction of cases arises from recent infection (primary progressive or exogenous disease), i.e. in areas where transmission rates have been high. As TB transmission and incidence go down, a higher proportion of cases comes from the reactivation of latent infection, and the rate of decline in incidence slows (Figure 2.12). These facts about TB aetiology also explain why it should be easier to control epidemic rather than endemic disease: during an outbreak in an area that previously had little TB, the reservoir of latent infection will be small, and most new cases come from recent infection.

In the control of endemic TB (largely) by chemotherapy, the best results have been achieved in communities of

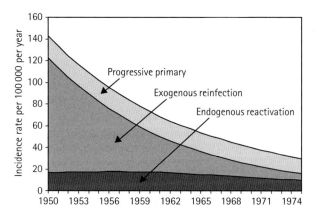

Figure 2.12 The changing aetiology of tuberculosis in decline, modelled on 45–49 year olds in the Netherlands. From Ref. 128, after Ref. 26.

Alaskan, Canadian and Greenland Eskimos, where incidence was reduced at 13–18 per cent/year from the early 1950s onwards.[26] Over a much wider area in Western Europe, TB declined at 7–10 per cent/year after drugs became available during the 1950s, though incidence was already falling at 4–5 per cent/year before chemotherapy (Figures 2.11 and 2.13).[26] For epidemic TB, as a result of aggressive intervention following an outbreak in New York City, the number of multidrug-resistant TB cases (MDR, resistant to at least isoniazid and rifampicin) fell at over 40 per cent/year.[129]

The most impressive recent examples of impact come from Morocco and Peru. In Morocco, the incidence of pulmonary TB among children aged 0–4 years fell at more

(a)

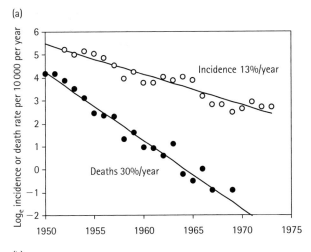

(b)

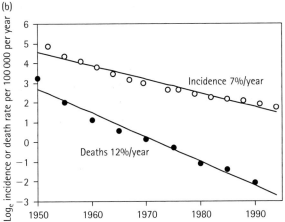

Figure 2.13 Comparative rates of decline in tuberculosis incidence (open circles) and deaths (filled circles) in (a) Alaskan Eskimos, 1950–73[181] and (b) the population of the Netherlands, 1950–95.[26,182]

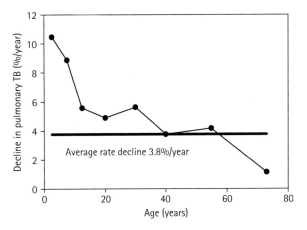

Figure 2.14 Annual rate of decline in pulmonary tuberculosis incidence by age in Morocco. The relatively rapid decline in young children may reflect a rapid fall in transmission. Data from the Moroccan National TB Control Programme.

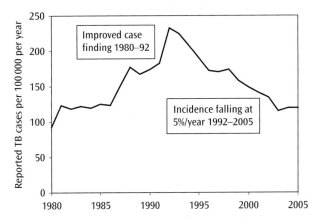

Figure 2.15 Trends in tuberculosis case reports in Peru. The incidence of disease has been falling at 5 per cent/year on average since 1992, after the introduction of DOTS. Data from Refs 8 and 130.

than 10 per cent/year between 1994 and 2000, suggesting that the risk of infection was falling at least as quickly (Figure 2.14). DOTS was launched in Peru in 1990, and high rates of case detection and cure appear to have forced down the incidence of pulmonary TB at an average of 5 per cent/year (Figure 2.15).[130] TB case notification rates are falling in many other countries, but it is not always clear that these reductions represent a real decline in incidence. Still harder to assess is the proportion of any apparent reduction in incidence that can be attributed to drug treatment programmes.

Case notification series from some countries do not show that incidence is falling in the manner anticipated by modelling studies, even though national TB control programmes have apparently achieved high rates of case detection and cure. Vietnam is a case in point. WHO targets for case detection and cure had, on the available evidence, been met by 1997, and yet the notification rate of all TB cases remained more or less stable up to 2005. Closer inspection of the data reveals that falling case rates among adults 35–64 years old (especially women) have been offset

by a rise in the age group 15–34 years old (especially men; Figure 2.16). The evident rise in incidence among young adults is partly associated with HIV infection, but this is unlikely to be the whole explanation. Data from other Asian countries indicate that this resurgence of TB among young adults may not be confined to Vietnam.[8]

Although the long-term aim of TB control is to prevent any new case of TB (incidence), the more immediate goals are to reduce prevalence (a measure of the total burden of illness) and deaths. About 90 per cent of the burden of TB, as measured in terms of years of healthy life lost (or disability-adjusted life years, DALYs) is due to premature death, and prevalence and deaths can be reduced faster than incidence in a programme of community-wide chemotherapy. Thus, the TB death rate among Alaskan Eskimos dropped at an average of 30 per cent/year in the interval 1950–70, and at 12 per cent/year throughout the Netherlands from 1950 to 1990 (faster at first, slower later;

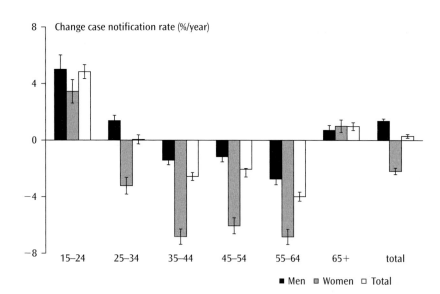

Figure 2.16 Average annual change in TB case notification rates for men (black) and women (grey) in different age classes in Vietnam, and for all age classes, 1997–2004. Error bars are 95 per cent confidence limits. The data can be found in Global Tuberculosis Control reports (e.g. Ref. 8), but this graph was drawn by KNCV Tuberculosis Foundation, The Hague.

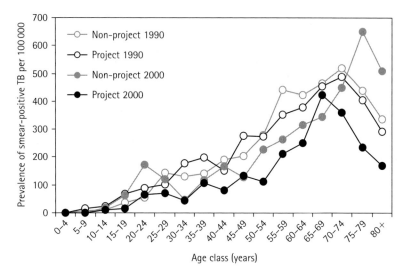

Figure 2.17 Prevalence of smear-positive TB by age in 1990 (grey) and 2000 (black) in parts of China where DOTS was (project) or was not implemented (non-project). Over the decade, DOTS reduced prevalence 37 per cent more than in non-project areas. Data from Refs 132 and 183.

Figure 2.13). Indirect assessments of DOTS impact suggest that 70 per cent of TB deaths were averted in Peru between 1991 and 2000, and more than half the expected TB deaths have been prevented each year in DOTS provinces of China.[130,131] Surveys done in China in 1990 and 2000 showed a 37 per cent reduction in the prevalence of smear-positive disease in DOTS areas, as compared with other parts of the country (Figure 2.17).[132] These observations indicate that the objective of halving the TB death rate by 2015 (as compared with 1990 levels) is technically feasible, at least in countries that are not burdened by high rates of HIV infection or drug resistance. This view is reinforced by calculations carried out for the Global Plan to Stop TB: full implementation of the plan should halve prevalence and death rates globally by 2015, and in all regions except sub-Saharan Africa and eastern Europe.

Where the prevalence of HIV infection is high, as in eastern and southern Africa, energetic programmes of chemotherapy, perhaps including active case finding, will be required to reverse the rise in TB incidence.[133,134] Mathematical modelling indicates that, even in the midst

of a major HIV epidemic, early detection and cure are the most effective ways to cut TB burden (Figure 2.18). There are at least two reasons for this. First, DOTS attacks all TB cases, not just those linked with HIV. Second, HIV is driving an epidemic in which a relatively high fraction of TB cases arises from recent rather than remote infection (compare this with an epidemic in a population not infected with HIV).[135,136] Supporting methods of TB control – the prevention of HIV infection, the treatment of latent TB infection, and antiretroviral therapy[137] – were, by the end of 2005, reaching only a small fraction of the people who could benefit from them.[8]

USING TB DRUGS MORE WIDELY AND MORE EFFECTIVELY

The DOTS strategy espouses passive case detection for three reasons: (1) the majority of smear-positive cases develop much more quickly than any reasonable interval between mass screening of symptoms or by radiography;

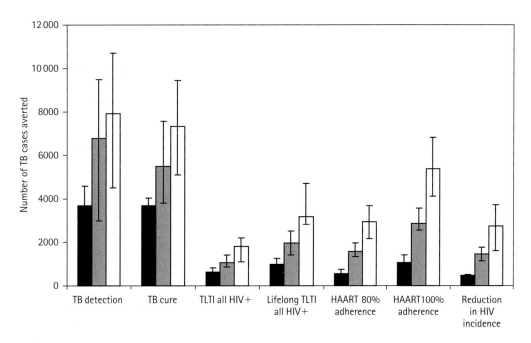

Figure 2.18 Theoretical impact of various interventions against tuberculosis (TB) in the presence of high rates of HIV infection. Each group of bars shows the number of TB cases that would be averted over 10 years in Kenya by 1 per cent increases in case detection, cure, 6 months of preventive therapy (or treatment of latent TB infection, TLTI) for all HIV-positives, lifelong TLTI for HIV-positives, lifelong highly active antiretroviral therapy (HAART) with annual dropout rates of 20 or 0 per cent, and reduced HIV incidence. The three bars within each group show results for low, medium and high HIV epidemics. Baseline detection and cure rates were 50 and 70 per cent, with zero initial coverage for all other interventions. By improving case detection and cure, DOTS compares favourably with other interventions here, and under a wider range of assumptions. From Ref. 137.

(2) the majority of patients severely ill with a life-threatening disease are likely to seek help quickly;[138] and (3) countries that have not yet implemented effective systems for passive case detection are not in a position to pursue cases more actively.

However, the drawback of passive case finding is that it is often very passive indeed. Population surveys of disease commonly find large numbers of TB patients who have not sought treatment of any kind, or have sought treatment but were not diagnosed with TB. While drug treatment after a long illness can prevent death, it may not have much impact on transmission. Going beyond passive case finding, further studies of risk can identify subpopulations in which TB tends to be relatively common, and systematic surveys of these subpopulations for active TB may be logistically feasible, affordable and cost-effective. The target populations include refugees,[139] those sleeping in shelters for the homeless,[140] contacts of active cases,[141,142] health workers,[53] drug users and prisoners,[143] in addition to people known to be HIV-positive (see above).[133]

Taking a step further, people at high risk of TB can be given a tuberculin skin test; those found to be positive are offered treatment for a latent infection (TLTI), most commonly isoniazid preventive therapy (IPT). Studies among contacts of active cases have demonstrated that 12 months of daily isoniazid gives 30–100 per cent protection against active TB,[144] and yet IPT is not widely used. The main

reason is that compliance to 6 or more months of daily treatment tends to be poor among healthy people: a relatively high risk of TB is usually still a low risk in absolute terms. In addition, active disease must be excluded (e.g. by radiography) before isoniazid is taken alone and side effects include a hepatitis risk of 1 per cent/year.

The epidemiological literature on IPT contains mixed reports of success and failure, with outcomes that are not always predictable. In the USA, for example, the practice of contact tracing and IPT has fallen short of recommendations;[145] some high-risk groups, such as the elderly,[145,146] do not receive the full benefits that IPT can provide. IPT can be hard to manage in the groups that most need it, such as illegal immigrants,[147] though supervision has helped drug users,[148,149] and financial incentives have improved completion rates among the homeless.[150]

The high risk of TB among persons co-infected with *M. tuberculosis* and HIV is a reason for encouraging wider use of preventive therapy, especially in Africa.[126] Although trials of IPT in skin test positive adults infected with HIV have averaged about 60 per cent protection, the effects have been lost soon afterwards, and there has been little or no impact on mortality.[151–157] By contrast, IPT has been shown to reduce both TB incidence and mortality among HIV-infected children.[158] However, as for HIV-negative people, there remain significant logistic hurdles to providing IPT for people who are co-infected.[159]

The challenge, in sum, is to find ways in which active case finding and preventive therapy can significantly boost the impact of DOTS programmes. Success is most likely in groups at high risk of infection or where active disease can be identified, and where treatment compliance is high.

PREVENTING AND ELIMINATING DRUG RESISTANCE

The resurgence of TB in former Soviet countries has been linked to the spread of drug resistance. More than 10 per cent of new TB cases are reported (1999–2002) or estimated (2004) to be MDR in eight former Soviet countries, including Kazakhstan, Uzbekistan and the Russian Federation.[160,161] MDR rates among previously treated cases, which typically make up the majority of the MDR caseload, were estimated to be over 25 per cent in 38 countries in 2004. Resistance is a byproduct of TB's revival in these countries, not the primary cause of it. However, such high rates of drug resistance appear, so far, to be a local phenomenon. In 2004, there were over 400 000 episodes of MDR-TB, divided more or less equally between new and previously treated cases. An average of 2–3 per cent, and a median of 1–2 per cent, of all new TB cases were MDR. Three countries – China, India and the Russian Federation – accounted for about 260 000 MDR-TB cases, or 62 per cent of the estimated global incidence in 2004.[161,162]

How far multidrug resistance spreads around the world depends crucially on the relative and absolute fitness of resistant and susceptible strains, as measured by their case reproduction numbers. At full efficacy, short-course chemotherapy can cure over 90 per cent of patients carrying bacteria classified as drug-susceptible, thereby preventing the emergence of resistant strains. The cure rate is little compromised by resistance to isoniazid alone.[163] It is significantly lowered by resistance to rifampicin, by the combination of rifampicin and isoniazid resistance (MDR), and by other forms of multiple drug resistance. Low cure rates mean that MDR strains have higher reproductive fitness when treated with first-line regimens. However, it is not obvious how much higher because mutation usually carries a cost, and because even resistant bacilli retain some ill-defined level of susceptibility.

Surveys of studies that have measured relative fitness (RF), for example by comparing the size of clusters of strains with identical genetic fingerprints, show much variability (Figure 2.19).[164,165] As yet, there are too few studies to explain how and why RF for multidrug resistance appears to vary from one setting to another, but the observed median of 1–2 per cent multidrug resistance among new cases suggests that RF is commonly less than 1. Mathematical modelling confirms that this median is consistent with a RF close to the bottom end of the observed range (Figure 2.20).[50] If this is generally correct, multidrug resistance is likely to remain a local phenomenon.

This prophecy about the spread of multidrug resistance will remain conditional until the wide variation in fitness is better understood. The case reproduction number of any strain has both genetic and environmental determinants, the latter including the choice of drug regimens and the efficiency with which they are administered. The differential response by strains to their environment is the source of differences in fitness. There is weak evidence that low RF for multidrug resistance is associated with locally high cure rates for all forms of TB, which suggests that the variation is more to do with public health practice than with biological differences among strains.[164] However, that hypothesis remains to be properly tested. Experimental studies have shown that the fitness cost of rifampicin resistance can be eliminated under prolonged treatment,[166] and some modelling studies have emphasized that strains of multidrug resistance could, given the plausible range of RF, become dominant in *M. tuberculosis* populations.[167,168]

If the goal of TB control programmes is to minimize the number of future cases and deaths on a limited budget, the solution in poorer countries might include individualized or standardized treatment for patients with drug-resistant disease.[169,170] There is no definitive, general solution to this optimization problem as yet because too little is known

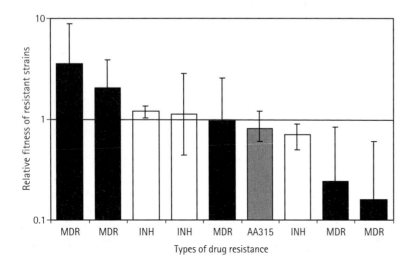

Figure 2.19 Estimated relative fitness (RF) of isoniazid (INH) and multidrug-resistant strains (MDR), and strains carrying the AA315 mutation linked to isoniazid resistance (shaded), as compared with fully sensitive strains. Error bars are 95 per cent confidence limits. There is great variability in the observed RF of MDR strains. Data are from a series of different studies described in Ref. 164.

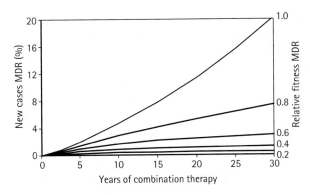

Figure 2.20 Consequences of different hypothetical levels of fitness for the spread of multidrug resistance. Both relative (RF) and absolute fitness are important, and the effect of fitness is non-linear; MDR increases much more quickly when RF grows above roughly 0.5, the point at which the basic case reproduction number of MDR exceeds 1 in this model. From Ref. 50.

about the efficacy of different drug combinations, about their effectiveness when used in real control programmes (as distinct from trials), and about the transmissibility of drug-resistant strains. To add to the uncertainty, second-line drug prices are falling rapidly.[171] Cost-effectiveness analyses have begun,[172] and will continue, to help identify the most suitable regimens of first- and second-line drugs for patients carrying resistant strains.[173,174]

CURRENT AND POTENTIAL IMPACT OF VACCINATION

If R_0 for *M. tuberculosis* is of the order of 2, then TB could be eliminated with a vaccine that can immunize more than a fraction $1 - 1/R_0 = 0.5$ children (50 per cent) at birth. In terms of generating herd immunity, this is a less demanding criterion than faced by the polio vaccination programme, which has almost succeeded in eradicating that disease.

The elimination of TB by vaccination presents problems of two kinds. The first is that the current vaccine, BCG, generally has low efficacy in preventing infectious TB in countries with a high disease burden.[175] Thus, even with the very high coverage now achieved (~100 million or 89 per cent of all infants in 2005[176]), BCG is unlikely to have any substantial impact on transmission, and hence incidence, because its main effect is to prevent serious (but non-infectious) disease in children. In parts of Europe and North America that did and did not use BCG, TB declined at rates that were not noticeably different.[26]

Second, even high coverage at birth of a vaccine that confers lifelong protection against infection would cause only a slow decline in incidence (Figure 2.21).[32] This is the expected response of a predominantly adult disease with a generation time of several years. However, the manufacture of a new, high-efficacy vaccine would certainly change immunization practice: mass vaccination campaigns

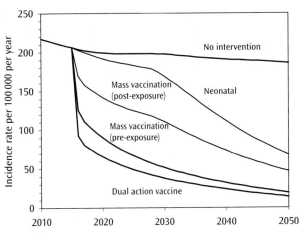

Figure 2.21 Hypothetical impact of four vaccination strategies on TB incidence rate. Calculations have been carried out with an age-structured mathematical model[31] set up to investigate the effect of vaccination on a TB epidemic like that in south Asia with an annual incidence set at about 200 per 100 000 population in 2015. Mass vaccination of uninfected populations (pre-exposure) would reduce the annual incidence to 20 per 100 000 in 2050. In a country the size of India, this would correspond to prevention of 50 million cases. A dual-action vaccine active both pre- and post-exposure would prevent a further 5 million cases, reducing the incidence to 14 per 100 000. From Ref. 32.

among adults (rather than infants) could have dramatic effects going far beyond the expectations of DOTS programmes. In general, a 'pre-exposure' vaccine that prevents infection is expected to have a greater impact than a 'post-exposure' vaccine that stops progression to disease among those already infected (Figure 2.21). However, this is theory; it will be hard to predict the impact of different kinds of vaccine until we know more about their mode of action and their efficacy from clinical trials.[33,177]

Despite the phenomenal number of BCG vaccinations given to children, there have been few assessments of BCG effectiveness at the population level. One recent analysis suggests that wide coverage of BCG should be maintained: the 100 million BCG vaccinations given to infants in 2002 are estimated to have prevented about 30 000 cases of TB meningitis and 11 000 cases of miliary TB in children during their first 5 years of life.[27] The greatest numbers of cases were prevented in South East Asia (46 per cent), sub-Saharan Africa (27 per cent) and the Western Pacific region (15 per cent).

CONCLUSIONS

The two interlocking themes of this chapter – population dynamics and interventions – were chosen in an effort to widen the discussion about how and why TB burden changes, and can be made to change, from place to place and from time to time. Our present assessment of the scale and direction of the TB epidemic, based largely on routine surveillance data supplemented by a limited number of population surveys, is a mixed report in the context of TB control.

The positive news is that the global TB epidemic appears to be on the threshold of decline. Incidence and death rates grew during the 1990s, due mainly to the spread of HIV in Africa and to social and economic decline in former Soviet countries, but had reached a maximum by or before 2005. The apparent decline in incidence rate, following earlier falls in prevalence and death rates, satisfies target 8 of the Millennium Development Goals, 10 years before the 2015 deadline.

The conclusion that the global TB epidemic is on the threshold of decline is offset by more sobering statistics. At the start of the twenty-first century, TB remains among the top 10 causes of human illness and premature death. In addition, although the burden of TB may be falling, the decline is not yet fast enough to meet other key targets, namely to halve prevalence and deaths rates by 2015.

The immediate response is to propose that the Global Plan to Stop TB (2006–15) be fully implemented in all regions of the world. Mathematical modelling suggests that, if the plan is executed as conceived, the targets will be met at the global level. However, this simple statement needs elaboration, in at least five ways. First, even if the targets are achieved globally, prevalence and death rates are unlikely to be halved in sub-Saharan Africa and eastern Europe, given the resurgence of TB during the 1990s and present resources for control in these regions – health services, funding and technology. Second, the Global Plan was not funded and implemented at the levels expected in its first year, 2006. In particular, far too little effort was made to diagnose and properly treat patients with HIV-positive and MDR-TB. Third, the aggregate success of the plan at global level depends crucially on the impact of DOTS and the Stop TB Strategy in Asia, where the majority of new TB cases arise each year. Despite meeting WHO targets for case detection and cure, TB incidence is not yet falling as fast as expected in several Asian countries. These include the world's highest-burden country – India. The reasons are not fully understood, but are likely to include the spread of HIV and chronic conditions such as diabetes, along with migration and demographic change. Fourth, the Global Plan makes no allowance for the impact of new technology before 2015 (though it does put a price on the cost of development). There is now greater investment than ever before in improving the technology for TB control, and the combination of efforts in fundamental and applied science will surely yield practical results, first perhaps in diagnostics, then to improve drug regimens, and ultimately to make a better vaccine than BCG. Fifth, while the Stop TB Strategy takes a more expansive view of TB control than DOTS, the options for control go wider still. Further study of 'risk factors' could help to quantify, for example, the impact of tobacco control and reduced air pollution (indoor and outdoor), even if TB control programmes cannot take primary responsibility for carrying out such interventions. With regard to epidemiological investigation, cross-disciplinary analyses may carry a cost in complexity, but they may also reveal new areas of vulnerability that can be exploited for better TB control.

LEARNING POINTS

- The pathogen–host relationship is central to thinking about the epidemiology of tuberculosis.
- There were an estimated 8.8 million new cases of tuberculosis in 2005. Of these, 3.9 million were sputum smear-positive.
- About a third of the human race is infected with *M. tuberculosis.*
- Eighty per cent of new cases live in 22 high-burden countries.
- About 1.6 million people died of tuberculosis in 2005, which makes TB the biggest infectious killer after HIV/AIDS.
- TB prevalence and death rates have probably been falling in recent years, at least since the turn of the millennium. In 2005, the incidence rate per capita was stable or in decline in all major regions of the world. However, the total number of cases was still rising slowly due to population growth.
- Though there is general agreement about the approximate global TB burden, estimates remain imprecise because surveillance systems are weak in many high-burden countries.
- Where transmission rates are high, the incidence rate of TB peaks in young adults. After decades of TB decline, incidence rates are highest among the elderly.
- Men carry the greater part of the global TB burden.
- Infection with TB has a low probability of breakdown into disease; about 10 per cent over a lifetime, which explains its relative rarity. The high case fatality is due to untreated or improperly treated cases.
- Two-thirds of untreated smear-positive cases will die within 5–8 years. The rest will remain chronically ill or self-cure.
- Because the number of secondary cases arising from a primary case is low (basic reproduction number, $R_0 = 2$), the doubling time of an epidemic is as much as 5 years, slower than most other infectious diseases.
- Certain risk factors increase the likelihood of infection leading to disease, therefore speeding up the development of an epidemic. For individuals, HIV co-infection is the most important risk factor yet discovered. At the level of whole populations, malnutrition, tobacco smoking and indoor air pollution could be responsible for TB cases than HIV.

- The causes of TB decline in Europe before the advent of chemotherapy are a subject of debate, but probably include factors that reduced both transmission (e.g. sanatoria, improved housing) and susceptibility to infection and disease (e.g. improved nutrition).
- The two most important factors in the resurgence of TB during the 1990s were the spread of HIV in Africa and the collapse of health and health services in countries of the former Soviet Union.
- Migration and ageing populations have contributed to the stagnation in decline in middle- and high-income countries.
- More than 26 million TB patients were treated with 'short-course' chemotherapy under the WHO DOTS strategy between 1995 and 2005.
- Although the DOTS strategy has been adopted in most countries, national TB control programmes around the world narrowly missed the 2005 targets of 70 per cent case detection (reached 60 per cent) and 85 per cent cure (reached 84 per cent).
- In theory, TB incidence could be forced down at more than 30 per cent a year, if new cases could be found soon enough to eliminate transmission. In practice, the best reduction achieved was 13–18 per cent a year among the Inuit Indians of northern America from the early 1950s.
- Active case finding and targeted prevention can add to the effectiveness of DOTS in TB elimination.
- Current data indicate that MDR-TB is less likely to emerge, and is less frequently transmitted, in TB control programmes that achieve high average cure rates. If DOTS is widely used, MDR is likely to remain a local phenomenon.
- If the basic reproduction number of (R_0) for TB is around 2, then a vaccine that can immunize more than $1 - 1/R_0 = 0.5$ (50 per cent) uninfected people would succeed in eradicating the disease. However, because of the large reservoir of latent infection, eradication will take many decades.
- Cross-disciplinary analytical models, which include economic and social factors, need to be brought to play in the study of the epidemiology of TB.

REFERENCES

1. Streiner DL, Norman GR, Blum HM. *PDQ epidemiology*. Toronto: BC Decker Inc, 1989.
2. Anderson RM, May RM. *Infectious diseases of humans: dynamics and control*. Oxford: Oxford University Press, 1991.
3. Volmink J, Garner P. Directly observed therapy for treating tuberculosis (Cochrane Review). *Cochrane Database Syst Rev* 2003: CD003343.
4. Braithwaite RS, Roberts MS, Justice AC. Incorporating quality of evidence into decision analytic modeling. *Ann Intern Med* 2007; **146**: 133–41.
5. White BL, Wohl DA, Hays RD et al. A pilot study of health beliefs and attitudes concerning measures of antiretroviral adherence among prisoners receiving directly observed antiretroviral therapy. *AIDS Patient Care STDs* 2006; **20**: 408–17.
6. Raviglione MC, Uplekar MW. WHO's new Stop TB strategy. *Lancet* 2006; **367**: 952–5.
7. Dye C, Maher D, Weil D et al. Targets for global tuberculosis control. *Int J Tuberc Lung Dis* 2006; **10**: 460–62.
8. World Health Organization. *Global tuberculosis control: surveillance, planning, financing*. Geneva: World Health Organization, 2007.
9. Euro TB and the National Coordinators for Tuberculosis Surveillance in the WHO European Region. *Surveillance of tuberculosis in Europe. Report on tuberculosis cases notified in 2005*. Paris: Institut de Veille Sanitaire, 2007.
10. Lopez AD, Mathers CD, Ezzati M, Jamison DT, Murray CJL. *Global burden of disease and risk factors*. New York: Oxford University Press/The World Bank, 2006.
11. Yamasaki-Nakagawa M, Ozasa K, Yamada N et al. Gender difference in delays to diagnosis and health cafre seeking behaviour in a rural area of Nepal. *Int J Tuberc Lung Dis* 2001; **5**: 24–31.
12. Gilks CF, Floyd K, Otieno LS, Adam AM, Bhatt SM, Warrell DA. Some effects of the rising case load of adult HIV-related disease on a hospital in Nairobi. *J Acquir Immune Defic Syndr Hum Retrovirol* 1998; **18**: 234–40.
13. Thorson A, Diwan VK. Gender inequalities in tuberculosis: aspects of infection, notification rates, and compliance. *Curr Opin Pulmon Med* 2001; **7**: 165–9.
14. Borgdorff MW, Nagelkerke NJ, Dye C, Nunn P. Gender and tuberculosis: a comparison of prevalence surveys with notification data to explore sex differences in case detection. *Int J Tuberc Lung Dis* 2000; **4**: 123–32.
15. Leon DA, Chenet L, Shkolnikov VM et al. Huge variation in Russian mortality rates 1984–94: artefact, alcohol, or what? *Lancet* 1997; **350**: 383–8.
16. Shkolnikov V, McKee M, Leon DA. Changes in life expectancy in Russia in the mid-1990s. *Lancet* 2001; **357**: 917–21.
17. Walberg P, McKee M, Shkolnikov V, Chenet L, Leon DA. Economic change, crime, and mortality crisis in Russia: regional analysis. *Br Med J* 1998; **317**: 312–8.
18. Toungoussova OS, Bjune G, Caugant DA. Epidemic of tuberculosis in the former Soviet Union: social and biological reasons. *Tuberculosis (Edinb)* 2006; **86**: 1–10.
19. McKee M, Jacobson B. Public health in Europe. *Lancet* 2000; **356**: 665–70.
20. Anderson SM, Maguire H, Carless J. Tuberculosis in London a decade and a half of no decline. *Thorax* 2006; **62**: 162–7.
21. Ministry of Public Health of the People's Republic of China. *Nationwide random survey for the epidemiology of tuberculosis in 1990*. Beijing: Ministry of Public Health of the People's Republic of China, 1990.
22. Tupasi TE, Radhakrishna S, Quelapio MID et al. Tuberculosis in the urban poor settlements in the Philippines. *Int J Tuberc Lung Dis* 2000; **4**: 4–11.
23. Lopez A, Mathers C, Ezzati M et al. *Global burden of disease and risk factors*. New York: The World Bank/Oxford University Press, 2006.
24. Dye C, Scheele S, Dolin P et al. Global burden of tuberculosis. Estimated incidence, prevalence, and mortality by country. *J Am Med Assoc* 1999; **282**: 677–86.
25. Dye C, Bassili A, Bierrenbach AL et al. Measuring tuberculosis burden, trends and the impact of control programmes. *Lancet Infect Dis* 2008; **8**: Published online 6 January.
26. Styblo K. *Epidemiology of tuberculosis*, 2nd edn. The Hague: KNCV Tuberculosis Foundation, 1991.

27. Bourdin Trunz B, Fine P, Dye C. Effect of BCG vaccination on childhood tuberculous meningitis and miliary tuberculosis worldwide: a meta-analysis and assessment of cost-effectiveness. *Lancet* 2006; **367**: 1173–80.

28. Sutherland I, Svandova E, Radhakrishna S. The development of clinical tuberculosis following infection with tubercle bacilli. 1. A theoretical model for the development of clinical tuberculosis following infection, linking from data on the risk of tuberculous infection and the incidence of clinical tuberculosis in the Netherlands. *Tubercle* 1982; **63**: 255–68.

29. Vynnycky E, Fine PEM. The natural history of tuberculosis: the implications of age-dependent risks of disease and the role of reinfection. *Epidemiol Infect* 1997; **119**: 183–201.

30. Sutherland I. The ten-year incidence of clinical tuberculosis following 'conversion' in 2,550 individuals aged 14 to 19 years. Tuberculosis Surveillance and Research Unit progress report. The Hague: KNCV, 1968.

31. Dye C, Garnett GP, Sleeman K, Williams BG. Prospects for worldwide tuberculosis control under the WHO DOTS strategy. Directly observed short-course therapy. *Lancet* 1998; **352**: 1886–91.

32. Young DB, Dye C. The development and impact of tuberculosis vaccines. *Cell* 2006; **124**: 683–7.

33. Kaufmann SH. Envisioning future strategies for vaccination against tuberculosis. *Nature Rev Immunol* 2006; **6**: 699–704.

34. Dye C, Garnett GP, Sleeman K, Williams BG. Prospects for worldwide tuberculosis control under the WHO DOTS strategy. *Lancet* 1998; **352**: 1886–91.

35. de Viedma DG, Marin M, Hernangomez S *et al.* Reinfection plays a role in a population whose clinical/epidemiological charactersitics do not favor reinfection. *Arch Intern Med* 2002; **162**: 1873–9.

36. Richardson M, Carroll NM, Engelke E *et al.* Multiple *Mycobacterium tuberculosis* strains in early cultures from patients in a high-incidence community setting. *J Clin Microbiol* 2002; **40**: 2750–54.

37. Mathema B, Kurepina NE, Bifani PJ, Kreiswirth BN. Molecular epidemiology of tuberculosis: current insights. *Clin Microbiol Rev* 2006; **19**: 658–85.

38. Chiang CY, Riley LW. Exogenous reinfection in tuberculosis. *Lancet Infect Dis* 2005; **5**: 629–36.

39. Vynnycky E, Fine PEM. Life time risks, incubation period, and serial interval of tuberculosis. *Am J Epidemiol* 2000; **152**: 247–63.

40. Styblo K. The relationship between the risk of tuberculous infection and the risk of developing infectious tuberculosis. *Bull Int Union Tuberc Lung Dis* 1985; **60**: 117–19.

41. Newton SM, Smith RJ, Wilkinson KA *et al.* A deletion defining a common Asian lineage of *Mycobacterium tuberculosis* associates with immune subversion. *Proc Natl Acad Sci U S A* 2006; **103**: 15594–8.

42. van Leth F, Van der Werf MJ, Borgdorff MW. Prevalence of tuberculous infection and incidence of tuberculosis: a re-assessment of the Styblo rule. *Bull World Health Organ* 2008; **86**: 20–6.

43. Dye C. Breaking a law: tuberculosis disobeys Styblo's rule. *Bull World Health Organ* 2008; **86**: 1.

44. Krebs W. Die Fälle von Lungentuberkulose in der aargauischen Heilstätte Barmelweid aus den Jahren 1912–1927. *Beitr Klin Tuberk Spezif Tuberkuloseforsch* 1930; **74**: 345–79.

45. Rieder HL. *Epidemiologic basis of tuberculosis control*, 1st edn. Paris: International Union Against Tuberculosis and Lung Disease, 1999.

46. Grigg ERN. The arcana of tuberculosis. With a brief epidemiologic history of the disease in the USA. *Am Rev Tubercul* 1958; **78**: 151–72.

47. Blower SM, McLean AR, Porco TC *et al.* The intrinsic transmission dynamics of tuberculosis epidemics. *Nature Med* 1995; **1**: 815–21.

48. Murray CJL, Salomon JA. Modeling the impact of global tuberculosis control strategies. *Proc Natl Acad Sci U S A* 1998; **95**: 13881–6.

49. Vynnycky E, Fine PEM. The long-term dynamics of tuberculosis and other diseases with long serial intervals: implications of and for changing reproduction numbers. *Epidemiol Infect* 1998; **121**: 309–24.

50. Dye C, Espinal MA. Will tuberculosis become resistant to all antibiotics? *Proc Roy Soc Lond Ser B, Biol Sci* 2001; **268**: 45–52.

51. Joshi R, Reingold AL, Menzies D, Pai M. Tuberculosis among health-care workers in low- and middle-income countries: a systematic review. *PLoS Med* 2006; **3**: e494.

52. Maguire H, Dale JW, McHugh TD *et al.* Molecular epidemiology of tuberculosis in London 1995–7 showing low rate of active transmission. *Thorax* 2002; **57**: 617–22.

53. Cuhadaroglu C, Erelel M, Tabak L, Kilicaslan Z. Increased risk of tuberculosis in health care workers: a retrospective survey at a teaching hospital in Istanbul, Turkey. *BioMed Central Infect Dis* 2002; **2**: 14.

54. Geng E, Kreiswirth B, Driver C *et al.* Changes in the transmission of tuberculosis in New York City from 1990 to 1999. *N Engl J Med* 2002; **346**: 1453–8.

55. Carvalho AC, DeRiemer K, Nunes ZB *et al.* Transmission of *Mycobacterium tuberculosis* to contacts of HIV-infected tuberculosis patients. *Am J Respir Crit Care Med* 2001; **164**: 2166–71.

56. Besser RE, Pakiz B, Schulte JM *et al.* Risk factors for positive mantoux tuberculin skin tests in children in San Diego, California: evidence for boosting and possible foodborne transmission. *Pediatrics* 2001; **108**: 305–10.

57. Sonnenberg P, Murray J, Glynn JR, Shearer S, Kambashi B, Godfrey-Faussett P. HIV-1 and recurrence, relapse, and reinfection of tuberculosis after cure: a cohort study in South African mineworkers. *Lancet* 2001; **358**: 1687–93.

58. Tocque K, Bellis MA, Beeching NJ, Syed Q, Remmington T, Davies PD. A case-control study of lifestyle risk factors associated with tuberculosis in Liverpool, North-West England. *Eur Respir J* 2001; **18**: 959–64.

59. Perez-Padilla R, Perez-Guzman C, Baez-Saldana R, Torres-Cruz A. Cooking with biomass stoves and tuberculosis: a case control study. *Int J Tuberc Lung Dis* 2001; **5**: 441–7.

60. Gangaidzo IT, Moyo VM, Mvundura E *et al.* Association of pulmonary tuberculosis with increased dietary iron. *J Infect Dis* 2001; **184**: 936–9.

61. Wilkinson RJ, Llewelyn M, Toossi Z *et al.* Influence of vitamin D deficiency and vitamin D receptor polymorphisms on tuberculosis among Gujarati Asians in west London: a case–control study. *Lancet* 2000; **355**: 618–21.

62. Bellamy R, Ruwende C, Corrah T, McAdam KP, Whittle HC, Hill AV. Variations in the NRAMP1 gene and susceptibility to tuberculosis in West Africans. *N Engl J Med* 1998; **338**: 640–4.

63. Zachariah R, Spielmann MP, Harries AD, Salaniponi FM. Moderate to severe malnutrition in patients with tuberculosis is a risk factor associated with early death. *Trans R Soc Trop Med Hyg* 2002; **96**: 291–4.

64. Toungoussova OS, Caugant DA, Sandven P, Mariandyshev AO, Bjune G. Drug resistance of *Mycobacterium tuberculosis* strains isolated from patients with pulmonary tuberculosis in Archangels, Russia. *Int J Tuberc Lung Dis* 2002; **6**: 406–14.

65. Sevim T, Aksoy E, Atac G *et al.* Treatment adherence of 717 patients with tuberculosis in a social security system hospital in Istanbul, Turkey. *Int J Tuberc Lung Dis* 2002; **6**: 25–31.

66. Abos-Hernandez R, Olle-Goig JE. Patients hospitalised in Bolivia with pulmonary tuberculosis: risk factors for dying. *Int J Tuberc Lung Dis* 2002; **6**: 470–4.

67. Pablos-Méndez A, Knirsch CA, Barr RG, Lerner BH, Frieden TR. Nonadherence in tuberculosis treatment: predictors and consequences in New York City. *Am J Med* 1997; **102**:164–70.

68. Shafer RW, Edlin BR. Tuberculosis in patients infected with human immunodeficiency virus: perspective on the past decade. *Clin Infect Dis* 1996; **22**: 683–704.

69. Freedberg KA, Losina E, Weinstein MC et al. The cost effectiveness of combination antiretroviral therapy for HIV disease. New England Journal of Medicine 2001; 344: 824–31.

70. Badri M, Wilson D, Wood R. Effect of highly active antiretroviral therapy on incidence of tuberculosis in South Africa: a cohort study. Lancet 2002; 359: 2059–64.

71. Antonucci G, Girardi E, Raviglione MC, Ippolito G. Risk factors for tuberculosis in HIV-infected persons. A prospective cohort study. The Gruppo Italiano di Studio Tubercolosi e AIDS (GISTA). J Am Med Assoc 1995; 274: 143–8.

72. Selwyn PA, Hartel D, Lewis VA et al. A prospective study of the risk of tuberculosis among intravenous drug users with human immunodeficiency virus infection. N Engl J Med 1989; 320: 545–50.

73. Williams BG, Dye C. Antiretroviral drugs for tuberculosis control in the era of HIV/AIDS. Science 2003; 301: 1535–7.

74. Yazdanpanah Y, Chene G, Losina E et al. Incidence of primary opportunistic infections in two human immunodeficiency virus-infected French clinical cohorts. Int J Epidemiol 2001; 30: 864–71.

75. Stevenson CR, Forouhi NG, Roglic G et al. Diabetes and tuberculosis: the impact of the diabetes epidemic on tuberculosis incidence. BMC Public Health 2007; 7: 234.

76. Corbett EL, Churchyard GJ, Clayton T et al. Risk factors for pulmonary mycobacterial disease in South African gold miners. A case–control study. Am J Respir Crit Care Med 1999; 159: 94–9.

77. van Lettow M, Fawzi WW, Semba RD. Triple trouble: the role of malnutrition in tuberculosis and human immunodeficiency virus co-infection. Nutr Rev 2003; 61: 81–90.

78. Cegielski JP, McMurray DN. The relationship between malnutrition and tuberculosis: evidence from studies in humans and experimental animals. Int J Tuberc Lung Dis 2004; 8: 286–98.

79. Comstock GW, Palmer CE. Long-term results of BCG vaccination in the southern United States. Am Rev Respir Dis 1966; 93: 171–83.

80. Edwards LB, Livesay VT, Acquaviva FA, Palmer CE. Height, weight, tuberculous infection, and tuberculous disease. Arch Environ Health 1971; 22: 106–12.

81. Lin HH, Ezzati M, Murray M. Tobacco smoke, indoor air pollution and tuberculosis: a systematic review and meta-analysis. PLoS Med 2007; 4: e20.

82. International Union Against Tuberculosis And Lung Disease and World Health Organization. Association between exposure to tobacco smoke and tuberculosis: a qualitative systematic review. 2007 (unpublished report).

83. World Health Organization, Stop TB Department. Expanding the global tuberculosis control paradigm – the role of TB risk factors and social determinants. Unpublished Report for the Priority Public Health Condition Knowledge Network, Commission on Social Determinants of Health. Geneva: World Health Organization 2008.

84. Grange JM, Gandy M, Farmer P, Zumla A. Historical declines in tuberculosis: nature, nurture and the biosocial model. Int J Tuberc Lung Dis 2001; 5: 208–12.

85. Goldfeld AE, Delgado JC, Thim S et al. Association of an HLA-DQ allele with clinical tuberculosis. J Am Med Assoc 1998; 279: 226–8.

86. Hill AV. Aspects of genetic susceptibility to human infectious diseases. Ann Rev Genet 2006; 40: 469–86.

87. Fernando SL, Britton WJ. Genetic susceptibility to mycobacterial disease in humans. Immunol Cell Biol 2006; 84: 125–37.

88. Liu PT, Stenger S, Li H et al. Toll-like receptor triggering of a vitamin D-mediated human antimicrobial response. Science 2006; 311: 1770–3.

89. Hoal EG. Human genetic susceptibility to tuberculosis and other mycobacterial diseases. IUBMB Life 2002; 53: 225–9.

90. Alm JS, Sanjeevi CB, Miller EN et al. Atopy in children in relation to BCG vaccination and genetic polymorphisms at SLC11A1 (formerly NRAMP1) and D2S1471. Gene Immun 2002; 3: 71–7.

91. Schurr E. Is susceptibility to tuberculosis acquired or inherited? J Intern Med 2007; 261: 106–11.

92. Lewis SJ, Baker I, Davey Smith G. Meta-analysis of vitamin D receptor polymorphisms and pulmonary tuberculosis risk. Int J Tuberc Lung Dis 2005; 9: 1174–7.

93. World Health Organization. The world health report: reducing risks, promoting healthy life. Geneva: World Health Organization, 2002.

94. Mishra VK, Retherford RD, Smith KR. Biomass cooking fuels and prevalence of tuberculosis in India. Int J Infect Dis 1999; 3: 119–29.

95. Cauthen GM, Pio A, ten Dam HG. Annual risk of infection. World Health Organization Document 1988; WHO/TB/88.154: 1–34.

96. Davies RPO, Tocque K, Bellis MA, Rimmington T, Davies PDO. Historical declines in tuberculosis in England and Wales: improving social conditions or natural selection? Int J Tuberc Lung Dis 1999; 3: 1051–4.

97. McFarlane N. Hospitals, housing and tuberculosis in Glasgow. Soc Hist Med 1989; 2: 259–85.

98. Vynnycky E, Fine PEM. Interpreting the decline in tuberculosis: the role of secular trends in effective contact. Int J Epidemiol 1999; 28: 327–34.

99. McKeown T, Record RG. Reasons for the decline in mortality in England and Wales in the nineteenth century. Popul Stud 1962; 16: 94–122.

100. Lowell AM, Edwards LB, Palmer CE. Tuberculosis. Vital and health statistics monographs. American Public Health Association. Cambridge: Harvard University Press, 1969.

101. Lipsitch M, Sousa AO. Historical intensity of natural selection for resistance to tuberculosis. Genetics 2002; 161: 1599–607.

102. Kato-Maeda M, Rhee JT, Gingeras TR et al. Comparing genomes within the species Mycobacterium tuberculosis. Genome Res 2001; 11: 547–54.

103. Mostowy S, Cousins D, Brinkman J, Aranaz A, Behr MA. Genomic deletions suggest a phylogeny for the Mycobacterium tuberculosis complex. J Infect Dis 2002; 186: 74–80.

104. Valway SE, Sanchez MP, Shinnick TF et al. An outbreak involving extensive transmission of a virulent strain of Mycobacterium tuberculosis. N Engl J Med 1998; 338: 633–9.

105. Lopez B, Aguilar D, Orozco H et al. A marked difference in pathogenesis and immune response induced by different Mycobacterium tuberculosis genotypes. Clin Exp Immunol 2003; 133: 30–37.

106. Corbett EL, Steketee RW, ter Kuile FO, Latif AS, Kamali A, Hayes RJ. HIV-1/AIDS and the control of other infectious diseases in Africa. Lancet 2002; 359: 2177–87.

107. Corbett EL, Watt CJ, Walker N et al. The growing burden of tuberculosis: global trends and interactions with the HIV epidemic. Arch Intern Med 2003; 163: 1009–21.

108. Shilova MV, Dye C. The resurgence of tuberculosis in Russia. Philos Trans R Soc Lond B Biol Sci 2001; 356: 1069–75.

109. Atun RA, Samyshkin YA, Drobniewski F et al. Barriers to sustainable tuberculosis control in the Russian Federation health system. Bull World Health Organ 2005; 83: 217–23.

110. Stone R. Social science. Stress: the invisible hand in Eastern Europe's death rates. Science 2000; 288: 1732–3.

111. Borgdorff MW, Nagelkerke N, van Soolingen D, de Haas PE, Veen J, van Embden JD. Analysis of tuberculosis transmission between nationalities in the Netherlands in the period 1993–1995 using DNA fingerprinting. Am J Epidemiol 1998; 147: 187–95.

112. Murray MB. Molecular epidemiology and the dynamics of tuberculosis transmission among foreign-born people. CMAJ 2002; 167: 355–6.

113. Lillebaek T, Andersen AB, Dirksen A, Smith E, Skovgaard LT, Kok-Jensen A. Persistent high incidence of tuberculosis in immigrants in a low-incidence country. Emerg Infect Dis 2002; 8: 679–84.

114. Verver S, van Loenhout-Rooyackers JH, Bwire R et al. Tuberculosis infection in children who are contacts of immigrant tuberculosis patients. Eur Respir J 2005; 26: 126–32.

115. Borgdorff MW, Nagelkerke NJ, de Haas PE, van Soolingen D. Transmission of Mycobacterium tuberculosis depending on the age and sex of source cases. Am J Epidemiol 2001; 154: 934–43.

116. Borgdorff M, Yamada N. *WHO/WPRO country/area profiles on possible stagnation of tuberculosis decline.* Manila: World Health Organization, 2002: 21.

117. Shirakawa T, Enomoto T, Shimazu S, Hopkin JM. The inverse association between tuberculin responses and atopic disorder. *Science* 1997; **275**: 77–9.

118. Obihara CC, Beyers N, Gie RP *et al.* Inverse association between *Mycobacterium tuberculosis* infection and atopic rhinitis in children. *Allergy* 2005; **60**: 1121–5.

119. von Mutius E, Pearce N, Beasley R *et al.* International patterns of tuberculosis and the prevalence of symptoms of asthma, rhinitis, and eczema. *Thorax* 2000; **55**: 449–53.

120. Shirtcliffe P, Weatherall M, Beasley R. An inverse correlation between estimated tuberculosis notification rates and asthma symptoms. *Respirology* 2002; **7**: 153–5.

121. Hopkin JM. Atopy, asthma, and the mycobacteria (editorial). *Thorax* 2000; **55**: 443–5.

122. Obihara CC, Beyers N, Gie RP *et al.* Respiratory atopic disease, Ascaris-immunoglobulin E and tuberculin testing in urban South African children. *Clin Exp Allergy* 2006; **36**: 640–8.

123. Ferreira AP, Aguiar AS, Fava MW, Correa JO, Teixeira FM, Teixeira HC. Can the efficacy of bacille Calmette-Guérin tuberculosis vaccine be affected by intestinal parasitic infections? *J Infect Dis* 2002; **186**: 441–2.

124. Group KPT. Randomised controlled trial of single BCG, repeated BCG, or combined BCG and killed *Mycobacterium leprae* vaccine for prevention of leprosy and tuberculosis in Malawi. *Lancet* 1996; **348**: 17–24.

125. Lietman T, Porco T, Blower S. Leprosy and tuberculosis: the epidemiological consequences of cross-immunity. *Am J Public Health* 1997; **87**: 1923–7.

126. Stop TB Partnership and World Health Organization. *The global plan to stop TB, 2006–2015.* Geneva: Stop TB Partnership, 2006.

127. Dye C, Garnett GP, Sleeman K, Williams BG. Prospects for worldwide tuberculosis control under the WHO DOTS strategy. Directly observed short-course therapy. *Lancet* 1998; **352**: 1886–91.

128. Dye C. Tuberculosis 2000–2010: control, but not elimination. *Int J Tuberc Lung Dis* 2000; **4**: S146–52.

129. Frieden TR, Fujiwara PI, Washko RM, Hamburg MA. Tuberculosis in New York City – turning the tide. *N Engl J Med* 1995; **333**: 229–33.

130. Suarez PG, Watt CJ, Alarcon E *et al.* The dynamics of tuberculosis in response to 10 years of intensive control effort in Peru. *J Infect Dis* 2001; **184**: 473–8.

131. Dye C, Zhao F, Scheele S, Williams BG. Evaluating the impact of tuberculosis control: number of deaths prevented by short-course chemotherapy in China. *Int J Epidemiol* 2000; **29**: 558–64.

132. China Tuberculosis Control Collaboration. The effect of tuberculosis control in China. *Lancet* 2004; **364**: 417–22.

133. Golub JE, Mohan CI, Comstock GW, Chaisson RE. Active case finding of tuberculosis: historical perspective and future prospects. *Int J Tuberc Lung Dis* 2005; **9**: 1183–203.

134. Nunn P, Williams BG, Floyd K, Dye C, Elzinga G, Raviglione MC. Tuberculosis control in the era of HIV. *Nat Rev Immunol* 2005; **5**: 819–26.

135. Sonnenberg P, Murray J, Glynn JR, Shearer S, Kambashi B, Godfrey-Faussett P. HIV-1 and recurrence, relapse, and reinfection of tuberculosis after cure: a cohort study in South African mineworkers. *Lancet* 2001; **358**: 1687–93.

136. Casado JL, Moreno S, Fortun J *et al.* Risk factors for development of tuberculosis after isoniazid chemoprophylaxis in human immuno-deficiency virus-infected patients. *Clin Infect Dis* 2002; **34**: 386–9.

137. Currie CS, Williams BG, Cheng RC, Dye C. Tuberculosis epidemics driven by HIV: is prevention better than cure? *AIDS* 2003; **17**: 2501–8.

138. Toman K. *Tuberculosis case-finding and chemotherapy. Questions and answers*, 1st edn. Geneva: World Health Organization, 1979.

139. Marks GB, Bai J, Stewart GJ, Simpson SE, Sullivan EA. Effectiveness of postmigration screening in controlling tuberculosis among refugees: a historical cohort study, 1984–1998. *Am J Public Health* 2001; **91**: 1797–9.

140. Solsona J, Cayla JA, Nadal J *et al.* Screening for tuberculosis upon admission to shelters and free-meal services. *Eur J Epidemiol* 2001; **17**: 123–8.

141. Noertjojo K, Tam CM, Chan SL, Tan J, Chan-Yeung M. Contact examination for tuberculosis in Hong Kong is useful. *Int J Tuberc Lung Dis* 2002; **6**: 19–24.

142. Claessens NJM, Gausi FF, Meijnen S, Weismuller MM, Salaniponi FM, Harries AD. High frequency of tuberculosis in households of index TB patients. *Int J Tuberc Lung Dis* 2002; **6**: 266–9.

143. Nyangulu DS, Harries AD, Kang'ombe C *et al.* Tuberculosis in a prison population in Malawi. *Lancet* 1997; **350**: 1284–7.

144. Cohn DL, El-Sadr WM. Treatment of latent tuberculosis infection. In: Reichman LB, Herschfield ES (eds). *Tuberculosis: a comprehensive international approach.* New York: Marcel Dekker, 2000.

145. Reichler MR, Reves R, Bur S *et al.* Evaluation of investigations conducted to detect and prevent transmission of tuberculosis. *J Am Med Assoc* 2002; **287**: 991–5.

146. Sorresso DJ, Mehta JB, Harvill LM, Bentley S. Underutilization of isoniazid chemoprophylaxis in tuberculosis contacts 50 years of age and older. A prospective analysis. *Chest* 1995; **108**: 706–11.

147. Matteelli A, Casalini C, Raviglione MC *et al.* Supervised preventive therapy for latent tuberculosis infection in illegal immigrants in Italy. *Am J Respir Crit Care Med* 2000; **162**: 1653–5.

148. Gourevitch MN, Alcabes P, Wasserman WC, Arno PS. Cost-effectiveness of directly observed chemoprophylaxis of tuberculosis among drug users at high risk for tuberculosis. *Int J Tuberc Lung Dis* 1998; **2**: 531–40.

149. Chaisson RE, Barnes GL, Hackman J *et al.* A randomized, controlled trial of interventions to improve adherence to isoniazid therapy to prevent tuberculosis in injection drug users. *Am J Med* 2001; **110**: 610–15.

150. Tulsky JP, Pilote L, Hahn JA *et al.* Adherence to isoniazid prophylaxis in the homeless: a randomized controlled trial. *Arch Intern Med* 2000; **160**: 697–702.

151. Wilkinson D, Squire SB, Garner P. Effect of preventive treatment for tuberculosis in adults infected with HIV: systematic review of randomised placebo controlled trials. *Br Med J* 1998; **317**: 625–9.

152. Bucher HC, Griffith LE, Guyatt GH *et al.* Isoniazid prophylaxis for tuberculosis in HIV infection: a meta-analysis of randomized controlled trials. *AIDS* 1999; **13**: 501–7.

153. Johnson JL, Okwera A, Hom DL *et al.* Duration of efficacy of treatment of latent tuberculosis infection in HIV-infected adults. *AIDS* 2001; **15**: 2137–47.

154. Quigley MA, Mwinga A, Hosp M *et al.* Long-term effect of preventive therapy for tuberculosis in a cohort of HIV-infected Zambian adults. *AIDS* 2001; **15**: 215–22.

155. Whalen CC, Johnson JL, Okwera A *et al.* A trial of three regimens to prevent tuberculosis in Ugandan adults infected with the human immunodeficiency virus. Uganda-Case Western Reserve University Research Collaboration. *N Engl J Med* 1997; **337**: 801–8.

156. Mwinga A, Hosp M, Godfrey-Faussett P *et al.* Twice weekly tuberculosis preventive therapy in HIV infection in Zambia. *AIDS* 1998; **12**: 2447–57.

157. Woldehanna S, Volmink J. Treatment of latent tuberculosis infection in HIV infected persons. *Cochrane Database Syst Rev* 2004: CD000171.

158. Zar HJ, Cotton MF, Strauss S *et al.* Effect of isoniazid prophylaxis on mortality and incidence of tuberculosis in children with HIV: randomised controlled trial. *Br Med J* 2007; **334**: 136.

159. Ayles H, Muyoyeta M. Isoniazid to prevent first and recurrent episodes of TB. *Trop Doct* 2006; **36**: 83–6.

160. Aziz MA, Wright A, Laszlo A *et al.* Epidemiology of antituberculosis drug resistance (the Global Project on Anti-

tuberculosis Drug Resistance Surveillance): an updated analysis. *Lancet* 2006; **368**: 2142–54.

161. Zignol M, Hosseini MS, Wright A *et al.* Global incidence of multidrug-resistant tuberculosis. *J Infect Dis* 2006; **194**: 479–85.

162. Dye C, Espinal MA, Watt CJ, Mbiaga C, Williams BG. Worldwide incidence of multidrug-resistant tuberculosis. *J Infect Dis* 2002; **185**: 1197–202.

163. Espinal MA, Kim SJ, Suarez PG *et al.* Standard short-course chemotherapy for drug-resistant tuberculosis. Treatment outcomes in 6 countries. *J Am Med Assoc* 2000; **283**: 2537–45.

164. Dye C, Williams BG, Espinal MA, Raviglione MC. Erasing the world's slow stain: strategies to beat multidrug-resistant tuberculosis. *Science* 2002; **295**: 2042–6.

165. Cohen T, Sommers B, Murray M. The effect of drug resistance on the fitness of *Mycobacterium tuberculosis*. *Lancet Infect Dis* 2003; **3**: 13–21.

166. Gagneux S, Long CD, Small PM, Van T, Schoolnik GK, Bohannan BJ. The competitive cost of antibiotic resistance in *Mycobacterium tuberculosis*. *Science* 2006; **312**: 1944–6.

167. Cohen T, Murray M. Modeling epidemics of multidrug-resistant *M. tuberculosis* of heterogeneous fitness. *Nature Med* 2004; **10**: 1117–21.

168. Blower SM, Chou T. Modeling the emergence of the 'hot zones': tuberculosis and the amplification dynamics of drug resistance. *Nature Med* 2004; **10**: 1111–16.

169. Espinal MA, Dye C, Raviglione M, Kochi A. Rational 'DOTS plus' for the control of MDR-TB. *Int J Tuberc Lung Dis* 1999; **3**: 561–3.

170. Farmer P, Bayona J, Becerra M *et al.* The dilemma of MDR-TB in the global era. *Int J Tuberc Lung Dis* 1998; **2**: 869–76.

171. Gupta R, Kim JY, Espinal MA *et al.* Responding to market failures in tuberculosis control. *Science* 2001; **293**: 1049–51.

172. Dye C, Floyd K. Tuberculosis. In: Jamieson DT, Alleyne GAO, Breman JG *et al.* (eds). Disease control priorities in developing countries, 2nd edn. Washington DC: Oxford University Press 2006; pp. 289–309.

173. Suarez PG, Floyd K, Portocarrero J *et al.* Feasibility and cost-effectiveness of standardised second-line drug treatment for chronic tuberculosis patients: a national cohort study in Peru. *Lancet* 2002; **359**: 1980–89.

174. Resch SC, Salomon JA, Murray M, Weinstein MC. Cost-effectiveness of treating multidrug-resistant tuberculosis. *PLoS Med* 2006; **3**: 1048–57.

175. Fine PEM. BCG vaccines and vaccination. In: Reichman LB, Hershfield ES (eds). *Tuberculosis: a comprehensive international approach*. New York: Marcel Dekker, 2001.

176. World Health Organization. *WHO vaccine preventable diseases: monitoring system. 2006 global summary*. Geneva: World Health Organization, Immunization, Vaccines and Biologicals, 2006.

177. Kaufmann SHE, Baumann S, Nasser Eddine A. Exploiting immunology and molecular genetics for rational vaccine design against tuberculosis. *Int J Tuberc Lung Dis* 2006; **10**: 1068–79.

178. Dye C, Williams BG. Criteria for the control of drug-resistant tuberculosis. *Proc Natl Acad Sci U S A* 2000; **97**: 8180–85.

179. Vynnycky E. *An investigation of the transmission dynamics of M. tuberculosis*. Department of Epidemiology and Population Sciences, London School of Hygiene and Tropical Medicine. London: London University, 1996.

180. Corbett EL, Watt CJ, Walker N *et al.* The growing burden of tuberculosis: global trends and interactions with the HIV epidemic. *Arch Intern Med* 2003; **163**: 1009–21.

181. Grzybowski S, Styblo K, Dorken E. Tuberculosis in Eskimos. *Tubercle* 1976; **57** (Suppl.): S1–S58.

182. Styblo K, Broekmans JF, Borgdorff MW. Expected decrease in tuberculosis incidence during the elimination phase. How to determine its trend? *Tuberc Surveil Res Unit Prog Rep* 1997; **1**: 17–78.

183. China MoHotPsRo. *Report on nationwide random survey for the epidemiology of tuberculosis in 2000*. Beijing: Ministry of Health of the People's Republic of China, 2000.

PART 2

PATHOLOGY AND IMMUNOLOGY

3

Genotyping and its implications for transmission dynamics and tuberculosis control

CHARLES L DALEY

INTRODUCTION

One of the primary goals of tuberculosis control programmes is to interrupt the transmission of *Mycobacterium tuberculosis*. The most effective way to accomplish this goal is to identify and treat individuals with active tuberculosis. Unfortunately, most transmission of *M. tuberculosis* occurs prior to diagnosis and initiation of therapy and thus, even in effective tuberculosis control programmes, transmission continues to occur. The ability to track specific strains of *M. tuberculosis* as they spread through a community would allow us to identify chains of transmission and provide a powerful tool for outbreak investigations and for furthering our understanding of the transmission and pathogenesis of tuberculosis. Several genotyping methods now provide us with such a tool. Molecular epidemiology studies that couple routine epidemiologic investigations with genotyping have identified episodes of laboratory cross-contamination, described the rates of tuberculosis due to recent versus remote infection, identified people at risk for rapid progression to disease, differentiated recurrent tuberculosis as relapse versus reinfection, described the dynamics of tuberculosis transmission and uncovered outbreaks and unrecognized transmission.

The field of molecular epidemiology has evolved rapidly over the past decade and is likely to continue to do so. Genotyping methods that were initially laborious and required viable bacilli have evolved to the point of rapid amplification based methods that can be done on non-viable organisms. Although a detailed discussion of genotyping is beyond the scope of this chapter, a brief review of the most commonly used methods is necessary in order to understand the strengths and weaknesses of the various techniques. The primary focus of this chapter will be to review what we have learned from using these methods and the implications for understanding the transmission dynamics of tuberculosis and the impact on tuberculosis control activities.

GENOTYPING METHODS

Several genotyping methods have been developed that allow us to distinguish between different strains of *M. tuberculosis*. In general, most methods identify repetitive units in the mycobacterial genome, either interspersed repeats (direct repeats or insertion sequence-like repeats) or tandem repeats.[1] The most commonly used methods are compared and contrasted in Table 3.1. Each method has its strengths and weaknesses and the choice of which method to use should be based on the epidemiologic question(s) being asked. For example, if one wishes to conduct an outbreak investigation, the genotyping method should be stable enough to detect changes in the genotype pattern over a period of a few years, whereas if one wishes to evaluate the global epidemiology of *M. tuberculosis*, a method that is stable over decades or centuries would be more useful.

IS *6110*-based restriction fragment length polymorphisms

One of the most widely used methods of genotyping, referred to as restriction fragment length polymorphism

Table 3.1 Advantages and limitations of the three most commonly used genotyping methods.

Method	Advantages	Limitations	Technical issues
IS6110-based RFLP analysis	Gold standard	Requires subculturing and DNA isolation	Target DNA – IS6110
	Most discriminatory method	Slow turnaround time	Amount of DNA – >2 mg
	Patterns can be computerized for analysis	Laborious process	Technique for detection – Southern blot
	Rate of mutation appropriate for transmission studies	Poor discrimination for isolates with <6 copies	
Spoligotyping	Simplest method	Less discriminatory than IS6110-based RFLP and MIRU-VNTR analysis, particularly in areas with predominant or endemic strains	Target DNA – Spacers between repeated DNA sequences in the DR locus
	Data in binary format, so data can be easily exchanged		Amount of DNA – nanograms
	Can be performed on cell lysate and non-viable bacteria		Technique for detection – PCR
MIRU-VNTR	Rapid, high throughput method	Less discriminatory than IS6110-based RFLP analysis when using 12 loci	Target DNA – Scattered repeat loci in the genome in variable numbers
	More discriminatory than spoligotyping		Amount of DNA – nanograms
	Digitized results make sharing of data easy		Technique for detection – PCR
	Can be performed on cell lysate		
	Automated analysis possible		

MIRU-VNTR, mycobacterial interspersed repetitive units-variable number tandem repeats; PCR, polymerase chain reaction; RFLP, restriction fragment length polymorphism.

(RFLP) analysis, uses restriction endonucleases to cleave the mycobacterial DNA at the sites of specific repetitive sequences, producing DNA restriction fragments of different lengths that can be separated by gel electrophoresis (Figure 3.1).[2] The genomic DNA restriction fragments that are complementary to and hybridize with specific probes are visible, resulting in a specific band pattern on the gel. A standardized protocol for RFLP genotyping of the *M. tuberculosis* complex takes advantage of a specific, well-characterized, repetitive element, insertion sequence 6110 (IS6110).[2] This insertion sequence, first described by Thierry *et al.*,[3] is unique to the *M. tuberculosis* complex and randomly dispersed throughout the genome although 'hot spots', where insertion is more common, have been reported. Most strains of *M. tuberculosis* have between 1 and 26 copies of the IS6110 insertion sequence that are located in different sites within the genome. IS6110-based genotyping is characterized by significant diversity to the patterns that are generated, making it one of the most discriminatory of the genotyping methods.

The patterns generated by IS6110-based RFLP analysis are relatively stable over the time-frames typically used for epidemiological studies. The half-life of the RFLP pattern has been estimated to be between 3 and 8 years,[4–6] although the rate of change may be more rapid early in disease when the mycobacterial load and replication rate is highest.[6]

Despite its widespread use, there are several disadvantages with IS6110-based RFLP genotyping. First, it can only be done on cultures of *M. tuberculosis* and thus can take 6–8 weeks from the time of specimen collection to generation of an RFLP pattern. Second, it is a slow, labour-intensive and technically demanding technique. Finally, it has relatively poor discriminatory power for isolates with fewer than six copies of IS6110 and should be supplemented with other genotyping methods.[7]

Spacer oligonucleotide typing (spoligotyping)

Spoligotyping is a polymerase chain reaction (PCR)-based method that interrogates a small direct repeat (DR) sequence with 36 base pair (bp) repeats interspersed with unique, non-repetitive sequences ranging in size from 35 to 41 bp (Figure 3.2).[8] All of the unique, non-repetitive sequences, or 'spacers,' between the direct repeats can be amplified simultaneously using one set of primers. These spacer sequences can be detected by hybridizing labelled-PCR-amplified DR loci with membranes spotted with 43 synthetic oligonucleotides resulting in a pattern that can be detected by chemiluminescence.[9] Strains are differentiated by the number and position of the spacers that are missing from the complete spacer set. Unlike IS6110-based

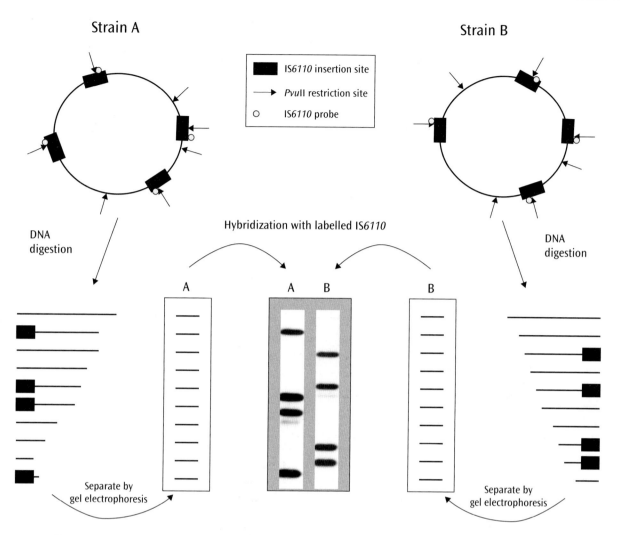

Figure 3.1 IS*6110*-based restriction fragment length polymorphism analysis. The DNA from two strains of *Mycobacterium tuberculosis* are depicted schematically. After the DNA has been extracted from the mycobacteria (this step is not illustrated), the DNA is cleaved using *Pvu*II, a specific restriction endonuclease (*Pvu*II) (arrows). In reality, thousands of fragments of DNA are created and then separated according to molecular weight by gel electrophoresis. At this stage, the thousands of bands produce a nearly confluent image which is difficult to interpret. By hybridization with an IS*6110* probe (circle), only those fragments containing IS*6110* will be visible on the gel. In this example, the two strains each have four copies of IS*6110*, but they differ in location on the gel.

RFLP analysis, smaller amounts of DNA are needed with spoligotyping so the procedure can be performed on clinical samples or on strains of *M. tuberculosis* shortly after inoculation into liquid culture, and the results can be expressed in a digital format.[10] However, spoligotyping is less discriminatory than IS*6110*-based genotyping. Spoligotyping can be used as either a secondary genotyping method, or as a primary genotyping method followed by another genotyping method with greater discriminatory power.[11,12]

VNTR/MIRU analysis

A promising PCR-based method is a high-resolution genotyping technique that characterizes the number and size of the variable number tandem repeats (VNTR) in

each of 12 independent mycobacterial interspersed repetitive units (MIRU) (Figure 3.3).[13,14] As with IS*6110*-based RFLP analysis, a standardized nomenclature has been proposed based on the four digits of the locus position on the H37Rv genome. The discriminatory power of MIRU-VNTR using 12 loci is less than that of IS*6110*-based RFLP typing, but more discriminatory for those strains with few copies of the IS*6110* sequence. The stability of MIRU-VNTR depends on which locus is used since the rate of change appears to vary between loci.[14]

MIRU-VNTR profiling is appropriate for strains regardless of their IS*6110* RFLP copy number, can be automated for large-scale genotyping, and permits rapid comparison of results from independent laboratories using a digital classification system.[15,16] The Centers for Disease Control and Prevention use this methodology, along with spoligotyping, for all initial isolates of *M. tuberculosis* in

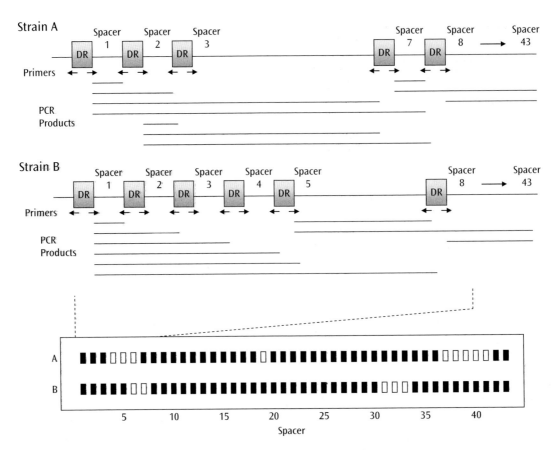

Figure 3.2 Spoligotyping. In the upper part of the figure, the DR region is illustrated for two strains of *Mycobacterium tuberculosis*. In this example, only spacers 1–8 are illustrated in detail. Strain A is missing spacers 4–6 and strain B is missing 6–7 (additional spacers are missing but not highlighted in the figure). Polymerase chain reaction (PCR) amplification of the conserved DR locus is performed using two sets of primers depicted with the arrows. The resulting PCR products are hybridized to a membrane containing covalently bound oligonucleotides corresponding to each of the 43 spacers. Each strain of *M. tuberculosis* produces a positive (black) or negative (white) signal at each spacer location. In this example, strain A is missing eight spacers and strain B is missing five. The resulting genotype pattern can be converted into a binary code for easy data sharing.

the United States as part of a national genotyping programme. Despite the many technical advantages, more studies are needed to understand better the role of MIRU typing in the molecular epidemiology of tuberculosis.

OTHER GENOTYPING METHODS

Polymorphic GC-rich repetitive sequence (PGRS) analysis can distinguish strains of *M. tuberculosis* using a PGRS-specific probe cloned in the plasmid pTBN12.[17] The pattern that is generated by PGRS typing is complex and more difficult to read than other methods. Moreover, the pattern is less discriminatory than IS*6110*-based typing and the method is labour intensive. The primary role of PGRS typing has been as a secondary typing method in low copy number strains typed by IS*6110*.[18,19]

Single nucleotide polymorphism (SNP) analysis has been used to genotype isolates and create phylogenetic trees of *M. tuberculosis*.[1] Synonymous and non-synony-

mous polymorphisms have been used to differentiate strains of *M. tuberculosis*. Synonymous polymorphisms do not alter the amino acid sequence and thus, are functionally neutral. These polymorphisms can be used to develop phylogenetic trees and examine evolutionary relationships of *M. tuberculosis*.[1,20] In contrast, non-synonymous polymorphisms alter the amino acid sequence and can be associated with phenotypic changes, such as drug resistance.

The sequencing of multiple strains of *M. tuberculosis* has provided opportunities for comparative genomic analysis and large sequence polymorphisms (LSPs) have been identified in *M. tuberculosis*.[21] LSPs are thought to occur through genomic deletion and once this occurs, the subsequent strains can be identified by the presence/absence of these deletions. Analysis of chromosomal deletions has been useful in investigating the global evolution and phylogeny of *M. tuberculosis*, but its use as an epidemiologic tool is not well studied. A rapid throughput system, analogous to spoligotyping and termed 'deligotyping' has been developed.[22]

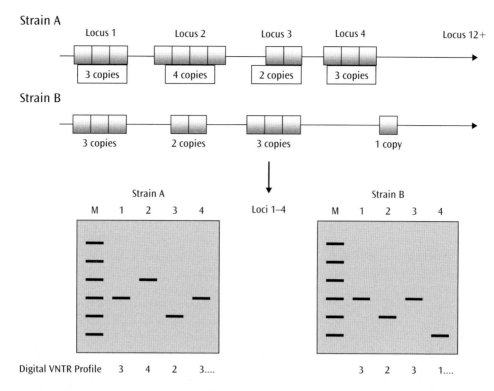

Figure 3.3 Mycobacterial interspersed repetitive units (MIRU)-variable tandem number repeats (VNTR). Portions of the DNA from two hypothetical strains of *Mycobacterium tuberculosis* are depicted. Only four of the standard 12 loci are illustrated. In this example, strains A and B have three copies of the repeat at locus 1, whereas strain A has four copies at locus 2 and strain B has only two copies. In the lower half of the figure, the loci are depicted along the top of the gels. There is a molecular weight standard (M) on the left side of each gel. The loci move down the gel, based on molecular weight, so those at the top of the gels are larger pieces of DNA that contain more copies of the repeat than those at the bottom of the gel. This information can be digitized to provide an easy way to share information between laboratories. For example, strain A would be given the identifier 3423 and strain B would be 3231.

COMPARISON OF GENOTYPING METHODS

Isolates from different patients who have the same genotype, based on one or more methods, are said to be 'clustered', indicating that the same strain has infected more than one patient. The selection of a specific genotyping method will depend on a number of factors, such as the epidemiologic questions to be answered, the discriminatory capability of the method, whether viable bacilli are needed, and the speed with which a result is needed. Therefore, it is very important to understand how the different methods compare to each other. In a study from Quebec, 302 clinical isolates were evaluated with three different genotyping methods: IS6110-based genotyping categorized 27 per cent of the isolates as clustered, MIRU 61 per cent, and spoligotyping 77 per cent.[23] When all three methods were used, only 14 per cent were clustered which was closer to what would have been expected in the study population. In a subsequent report,[24] the investigators compared IS6110-based RFLP analysis, MIRU typing, spoligotyping and the combination of MIRU and spoligotyping. With each method, the isolates were assigned into clusters, the percentage of isolates with matched genotypes and the percentage of cases due to recent transmission was

determined. IS6110-based typing grouped 347 isolates into 12 clusters and transmission was felt to have occurred in 4 per cent of cases. In contrast, MIRU typing identified 40 clusters and transmission occurred in 33 per cent, spoligotyping identified 34 clusters with transmission in 53 per cent and the combination of MIRU and spoligotyping identified 29 clusters and 23 per cent transmission. Considering IS6110-based typing as the gold standard, the investigators estimated the sensitivity of MIRU-VNTR for identifying clustered isolates to be 52 per cent and that of spoligotyping, 83 per cent. The estimated specificity of MIRU-VNTR for identifying isolates with unique IS6110-based genotypes was 56 per cent and that of spoligotyping, 40 per cent. In a similar study,[15] isolates were genotyped with IS6110-based typing, MIRU, spoligotyping and various combinations of these methods. Of the three methods, RFLP divided the isolates into the fewest number of clusters and had the lowest percentage of clustering. The combination of spoligotyping and MIRU approached that of IS6110-based typing in terms of clustering, but divided the isolates into more clusters. Using all three methods, the isolates were categorized into the fewest number of clusters and the lowest percentage of clustering. It is clear from these studies and others that IS6110-based RFLP typing is the most specific followed by the combination of spoligotyping and MIRU profiling (12 loci).

More recent studies have evaluated the discriminatory power of MIRU-VNTR using additional loci. Supply et al.[25] evaluated 29 loci and excluded five because of lack of robustness and/or stability. The use of the 24 remaining loci provided additional discriminatory power and reduced the clustering rate four-fold compared with the standard 12-loci approach. They then identified the 15 loci with the highest evolutionary rates and reported that their predictive value for identifying transmission of M. tuberculosis was similar to that of IS6110-based RFLP analysis. Based on these observations, they proposed that these 15 loci be used instead of the standard 12 loci. In a subsequent population-based study in Hamburg, Germany, the investigators evaluated the 24- and 15-loci approach among 154 isolates.[26] They reported that both the 24- and the 15-loci approach showed a comparable to slightly better predictive value than IS6110-based RFLP analysis, particularly when combined with spoligotyping.

Methodologic considerations

Regardless of which genotyping method is used to interpret the results, we assume that epidemiologically related strains will have the same genotype pattern and epidemiologically unrelated strains will have different patterns. Clustering has often been equated with recent or ongoing transmission, and the factors associated with clustering have been sought as a means to identify and target subpopulations with substantial ongoing transmission.[27] In contrast, patients whose isolates of M. tuberculosis have genotype patterns that do not match any other isolates in the community are considered to be unique and likely represent disease caused by reactivation of latent tuberculosis infection (LTBI). Thus, genotyping enables us to distinguish tuberculosis due to recent or ongoing infection versus reactivation of LTBI and to estimate the proportion of ongoing tuberculosis transmission in a community.

It is important to note that in some instances there is not always an epidemiological link between patients whose isolates have identical genotype patterns. Some studies have demonstrated that clustered cases often have no discernible contact or other epidemiological links among themselves, even in relatively stable populations,[28,29] while others have shown that most patients do have epidemiological links.[30]

The amount of transmission represented by genotypic clustering will depend on the sampling strategy and duration of the study.[31,32] Undersampling can bias the estimates of the proportion of tuberculosis cases that were likely caused by recent or ongoing transmission and it can bias the estimates of the risk factors associated with clustering. Modelling studies suggest that clustering of cases based on identical matching of genotype patterns will lead to underestimates of clustering in the young and an overestimate in the elderly.[33] Biases may also be introduced if a molecular epidemiologic study does not cover an adequate time period. For example, two population-based cohort studies in San Francisco[34] and the Netherlands[35] reported that the percentage of clustered strains was high during the first 2 years and declined thereafter. Thus, clustering based on less than 2 years of sampling will likely underestimate the amount of ongoing transmission. Despite the limitations noted above, genotyping has provided investigators and tuberculosis control programmes with new tools to understand transmission of M. tuberculosis in our communities.

TRANSMISSION DYNAMICS

Genotyping has revolutionized our ability to track strains of M. tuberculosis as they spread through a community, and allows us to describe chains of transmission. When combined with standard epidemiologic investigations, genotyping provides insights into the transmission and pathogenesis of M. tuberculosis and, in the process, teaches important lessons for tuberculosis control. Studies evaluating the community epidemiology of tuberculosis have identified high rates of transmission in some areas, as well as risk factors for recent infection with rapid progression to disease. The frequency of mixed infections and exogenous reinfection have been elucidated, as has the impact of underlying drug resistance on the transmission and pathogenesis of tuberculosis. These and other lessons from molecular epidemiology will be reviewed below.

Community epidemiology and risk factors for clustering

Tuberculosis develops by rapid progression from a recently acquired infection, reactivation of LTBI or from exogenous reinfection. Prior to the availability of genotyping tools, epidemiologic studies estimated that approximately 90 per cent of pulmonary tuberculosis in adults resulted from reactivation of latent infection, 10 per cent from recent infection and very little from exogenous reinfection.[36] However, genotyping studies have demonstrated that these suppositions were often incorrect.

Most molecular epidemiology studies have assumed that the proportion of clustered isolates in a population estimates the amount of recent or ongoing transmission of M. tuberculosis. In many studies, this estimate is refined by subtracting one case from each group of clustered cases $(n - 1)$ assuming that at least one of these patients developed tuberculosis as a result of reactivation from remotely acquired infection. For example, if there are 10 patients whose isolates have the same genotype pattern, then one is considered the index case and the subsequent cases as secondary cases. If you subtract the index case from the total number of clustered cases, then nine cases are considered to have resulted from recent infection with rapid progression to disease.

Using the approach described above, community-based studies have attempted to describe the burden of tuberculosis due to recent or ongoing transmission and identify risk factors for transmission (Table 3.2).[35,37–56] The frequency of clustering has ranged from 17 per cent in low incidence areas, such as Vancouver, BC,[41] to 34–46 per cent in urban areas in the United States[37,38] and Western Europe.[35,43] In high-incidence settings and populations, such as gold miners in South Africa, 50 per cent of tuberculosis patients were in clusters[50] and in Botswana 42 per cent of the cases were clustered.[51]

Whether or not clustered cases represent tuberculosis due to recent transmission has remained a controversial point. In one of the first population-based studies using IS6110-based genotyping, investigators in San Francisco performed an intensive investigation of the largest cluster in the city. Of the 30 patients whose isolate had an identical genotype pattern, only three lacked epidemiological links.[38] Additional evidence supporting the belief that clustering results from recent or ongoing transmission comes from the Netherlands, where 29 per cent (20 per cent using the $n – 1$ approach) of 481 patients were clustered, suggesting recent transmission. The authors reported that 86 per cent of the cases had epidemiologic links consistent with recent transmission.[30]

Clearly, in some areas, clustering may not always represent recent infection with rapid progression to disease. In these settings, there may be endemic ancestral strains that are prevalent and shared in the region. Thus, just because two individuals have isolates with identical strains, it does not mean that transmission occurred between them in the absence of epidemiologic connections. For example, Braden et al.[28] reported that most cases with matching RFLP patterns in Arkansas were not epidemiologically linked and that clustering in a low-incidence state such as Arkansas did not necessarily represent recent transmission.

Conventional epidemiological methods can be used in combination with molecular genotyping techniques to identify the risk factors associated with recent infection and rapid progression to disease (Table 3.3). In studies in low-incidence areas, young age, being in an ethnic minority group, homelessness and substance abuse have been associated with recent infection with rapid progression to disease.[37–39,57] In New York City, birth outside the United States, age ≥60 years and diagnosis after 1993 were factors independently associated with having a unique strain, while homelessness was associated with clustering or recent transmission.[58] Tuberculosis among foreign-born people was more likely to result from recent transmission among those who were HIV-infected and more likely to result from the reactivation of LTBI among those who were not infected with HIV. These data suggest that tuberculosis prevention and control strategies need to be targeted to the large number of foreign-born people in New York City who have LTBI. Among foreign-born people with tuberculosis in Hamburg, Germany, risk factors for

recent infection included a history of contact tracing, intravenous drug use, alcohol dependence, asylum and unemployment.[59] Thus, the risk factors associated with recent infection and rapid progression to disease have varied from study to study partly because of differences in populations, methodologies and definitions.

There are relatively few population-based studies from high-incidence areas. In a study of South African gold miners, tuberculosis patients who had failed treatment at entry to the study were more likely to be in clusters (adjusted OR = 3.41), and patients with MDR-TB were more likely to have failed tuberculosis treatment but less likely to be clustered than those with a drug-susceptible strain (OR = 0.27).[50] HIV infection, although common (53.6 per cent), was not associated with clustering. Apparently, persistently infectious individuals who had previously failed treatment were responsible for one-third of the tuberculosis cases in this population. In a study from Cape Town, South Africa, 72 per cent of cases were clustered, suggesting high rates of transmission in the community.[53] In general, the rates of clustering are higher in high-incidence areas than in low-incidence areas and the risk factors for clustering often differ.

Exogenous reinfection and mixed infection

For many years, it was argued that patients developed tuberculosis through either progression of primary disease or reactivation of latent infection.[60] However, Romeyn[61] argued that in high incidence areas, exogenous reinfection with a new strain of M. tuberculosis was another way that someone could develop tuberculosis. Evidence to support exogenous reinfection comes from epidemiologic studies[62] and outbreaks in which patient isolates were demonstrated to have different phage types.[63]

Molecular genotyping, because of its increased discriminatory power compared with phage typing, has made the identification of exogenous reinfection easier. Studies have reported evidence of reinfection in both immunocompromised and immunocompetent persons.[64–81] Exogenous reinfection in areas with a low incidence of tuberculosis is less common than in high-to-moderate incidence regions. Jasmer et al.[72] evaluated 1244 patients with culture-confirmed pulmonary tuberculosis who participated in clinical trials sponsored by the Centers for Disease Control and Prevention. Seventy-nine patients with tuberculosis had recurrent disease, of whom 75 had paired isolates available for analysis. In only three cases was reinfection felt to be the cause of the recurrence. The rate of reinfection in all patients was 0.15 per 100 patient-years compared with 3.63 for relapse. The rates did not vary significantly by HIV status (one case was HIV+ and two were HIV−). In contrast, in Houston, Texas, among 100 patients with recurrent tuberculosis who completed therapy for a first episode of tuberculosis, exogenous reinfection was reported to cause a surprisingly high 24–31 per cent of the second

Table 3.2 Frequency of clustering and risk factors for clustering in selected studies by tuberculosis incidence rate.

Study location, dates (Ref.)	Study population	N (ever clustered)	Risk factors for clustering
Low to moderate incidence areas (<50/100 000 population)			
New York, NY, 1989–92[37]	Hospital based	104 (38%)	HIV seropositive
			Hispanic ethnicity
			Younger age
			Drug-resistant disease
			Low income
San Francisco, CA, 1991–92[38]	Community based	473 (40%)	Acquired immunodeficiency syndrome
			Born in the United States
Baltimore, MD, 1994–96[39]	Community based	182 (46%)	Intravenous drug use
The Netherlands, 1993–97[35]	Country based	4266 (46%)	Male gender
			Urban residence
			Dutch and Surinamese nationality
			Long-term residence in the Netherlands
Norway, 1994–98[40]	Country based	698 (18%)	Analysis not performed
Vancouver, BC, 1995–99[41]	Community based	793 (17%)	Canadian-born aboriginals
			Canadian-born non-aboriginals
			Injection drug users
Montreal, Quebec, 1997–98[42]	Community based	243 (25%)	Haitian birth
Hamburg, Germany, 1997–99[43]	Community based	423 (34%)	Alcohol abuse
			History of contact tracing
			Unemployment
London, UK, 1995–97[44]	Community based	2042 (23%)	Young age
			Birth in UK
			Black Caribbean ethnic group
			Alcohol dependence
			Streptomycin resistance
Western Canada, 1995–97[45]	Regionally based	944 (32%)	Younger age
			Male gender
			Pulmonary disease
			Living in shelter
			Drug susceptible disease
			Predisposing factors for tuberculosis
			Prior contact
			Prior skin test
Manitoba, Canada, 1992–99[46]	Province based	629 (7%)	Male gender
			Younger age
			Treaty aboriginals
			Living on reserve land
Belgrade, Central Serbia, 1998–99[47]	Random sample	176 (31%)	Multidrug-resistant disease
Slovenia, 2001[48]	Country based	306 (38%)	Younger age
			Alcohol abuse
			Homelessness
Madrid, Spain, 1992–2001[49]	Community based	448 (50.7%)	Younger age
			Pleural effusion
High incidence areas (≥50/100 000 population)			
South Africa, 2000[50]	Gold miners	419 (50%)	Treatment failure
			Time spent working in mines
Botswana, 1997–98[51]	Community based	301 (42%)	Imprisonment
Tiruvallur District, India, 1999–2000[52]	Community based	378 (38%)	Identified by house-to-house survey
Cape Town, South Africa, 1993–98[53]	Community based	797 (72%)	Smear-positive
			Defaulted retreatment cases
			Specific community
Hong Kong, 1999–2002[54]	Community based	1553 (29%)	Younger age
			Permanent residents
			Previous treatment default
Karonga, Malawi, 1995–2003[55]	Community based	1044 (74%)	Not reported
Quagadougou, Burkina Faso, 2001[56]	Community based	120 (79%)	No factors associated with clustering

Table 3.3 The frequency of exogenous reinfection in selected studies by tuberculosis (TB) incidence rates.

Study location	Study population	Patients with two episodes of TB or two isolates	Patients with genotyping	Patients with reinfection
Low to moderate incidence areas (<50/100 000 population)				
Kings County Hospital, New York City[64]	AIDS patients with positive culture for >1 year *or* increasing drug resistance	17 31	6 11	0 4 (36%)
Switzerland[65]	HIV cohort with two isolates	20	20	2 (10%)
Madrid, Spain[66]	HIV-infected Spanish inmates who remained culture positive for >4 months	11	9	2 (22%)
Lombardy, Italy[67]	TB recurrences separated >6 months	NA	32	5 (16%)
Gran Canaria Island, Spain[68]	Two positive cultures >12 months apart	23	18	8 (44%)
Tartu, Estonia[69]	Treatment failures	35	11	11 (100%)
Madrid, Spain[70]	HIV+ and HIV– cases with two isolates >100 days apart	172	43	14 (33%)
Houston, Texas[71]	TB recurrences	100	100	24–31%
United States[72]	TB recurrences in two large randomized clinical trials	85	75	3 (4%)
San Francisco, CA[73]	TB recurrences in HIV+ cases	13	8	0
High incidence areas (≥50/100 000 population)				
Nairobi, Kenya[74]	TB recurrences	NA	4	1 (20%)
Madras, India[75]	Recurrence *or* isolated positive culture in randomized clinical trial	30 32	30 32	11 (37%) 29 (91%)
Cape Town, South Africa[76]	Recurrent TB	48	16	12 (75%)
Gauteng Province, South Africa[77]	HIV+ and HIV– gold miners	57	48	2 (4%)
Rio de Janeiro, Brazil[78]	HIV+ patients with multiple isolates	12	12	3 (25%)
Kampala, Uganda[79]	HIV+ and HIV– TB recurrences	NA	40	9 (23%)
Western Cape, South Africa[80]	Recurrent TB in HIV+ children	9	4	1 (25%)
Shanghai, China[81]	Recurrent TB	202	52	32 (61%)

NA, not available; HIV+, seropositive for the human immunodeficiency virus (HIV); HIV–, seronegative for HIV; TB, tuberculosis.

episodes of tuberculosis.[71] The higher rate of exogenous reinfection in the latter study may be related to the proximity of Houston to Mexico, where the incidence of tuberculosis is higher than that in the United States.

In high-incidence areas, exogenous reinfection is likely to be more common than in low-incidence areas, although a recent review was unable to confirm this.[82] In Cape Town, South Africa, where there is a high incidence of tuberculosis and ongoing transmission, 16 of 698 patients had more than one episode of tuberculosis, of whom 75 per cent (12/16) had pairs of isolates of *M. tuberculosis* with different genotyping patterns.[76] All but one of these cases was HIV seronegative. Sonnenberg *et al.*[77] reported the incidence of reinfection in a cohort of 65 gold miners with recurrent disease. Of these, 39 had isolates available for genotyping and 14 were thought to have been reinfected. The miners with HIV infection were 2.4 times more likely to suffer a recurrence due to reinfection than the HIV seronegative miners. Another study[83] reported that

the rate of reinfection was four times higher in patients who have been previously treated, compared with the rate in new TB cases in Cape Town, South Africa. Among patients who were cured, 90 per cent of the recurrences with genotyping data were felt to be due to reinfection compared with 50 per cent of those who completed therapy and 11 per cent in defaulters. The authors concluded that previous TB strongly predicted an increased risk of developing TB when reinfected.

Recent studies have reported the presence of mixed infection with different strains of *M. tuberculosis*. Multiple infections were demonstrated in a patient in San Francisco, California,[84] in two patients who worked in a medical-waste processing plant in Washington State,[85] and among prisoners in Spain.[86] In South Africa, a country with a high frequency of exogenous reinfection, mixed infections appear to be common. Warren *et al.*,[87] using a PCR-based strain classification method, reported that 19 per cent of all patients were simultaneously infected with

Beijing and non-Beijing strains, and that 57 per cent of patients infected with Beijing strains were also infected with a non-Beijing strain. These observations indicate that simultaneous infections with multiple strains of *M. tuberculosis* occur and may be responsible for conflicting drug-susceptibility results[88] or episodes of recurrence thought to be caused by exogenous reinfection. As with exogenous reinfection, the frequency of mixed infection is likely to vary between low- and high-incidence areas.

Impact of drug resistance on transmission and pathogenesis

Before the availability of genotyping, studies suggested that isoniazid-resistant strains of *M. tuberculosis* were less likely to result in disease in animals.[89–91] More recently, mutations or deletions within the *katG* gene of isoniazid-resistant strains of *M. tuberculosis* have been associated with decreased pathogenicity in animal models.[92] In contrast, studies evaluating skin test reactivity among contacts of drug-susceptible or drug-resistant source cases have failed to demonstrate significant differences in tuberculin reactivity or development of disease.[93,94]

With the global increase in drug-resistant tuberculosis including MDR and extensively drug-resistant (XDR) strains, it is critical that we understand how drug resistance may impact the transmission and pathogenesis of tuberculosis.[95] Several molecular epidemiologic studies have reported that patients with drug-resistant strains were less likely to be in clusters, implying that drug-resistant strains could be less likely to being transmitted and/or to cause active tuberculosis.[35,50,96] Because genotyping studies require the development of active tuberculosis, they cannot determine if drug resistance affects the transmission of the bacteria, establishment of infection and/or progression to disease. Burgos *et al.*[97] reported that the number of secondary cases generated by isoniazid-resistant cases of tuberculosis was significantly less than that generated by drug-susceptible cases, regardless of HIV serostatus and place of birth. In a subsequent study from San Francisco, investigators evaluated clustering based on specific mutations that cause isoniazid resistance.[98] The investigators divided the patients into four groups, based on whether or not their isolates had (1) a specific *katG* mutation (S315T), (2) a *katG* mutation other than S315T, (3) an *inhA* mutation or (4) no mutations or other mutations. None of the isolates with non-S315T *katG* mutation were clustered, compared with 44 per cent of those with S315T mutations, 44 per cent of those with *inhA* mutations and 13 per cent of those with no mutation or another mutation. This study demonstrated that while drug resistance may produce an underlying fitness cost, this reduction in fitness may be related to specific mutations.

Similar findings have been reported from the Netherlands where the 315 mutation in *katG* has been associated with transmission of isoniazid-resistant tuberculosis.[99] Among 8332 patients diagnosed from 1992 to 2002, isoniazid resistance was found in 592 (7 per cent) isolates, of which 323 (55 per cent) carried a S315T mutation. The degree of clustering by RFLP analysis was the same in the S315T isolates and drug susceptible isolates. In contrast, other isoniazid-resistant strains clustered significantly less than drug-susceptible strains.

In Spain, 118 mycobacteriology laboratories participated in a study of 189 MDR *M. tuberculosis* isolates from January 1998 to December 2000. IS*6110*-based RFLP analysis, spoligotyping, rifotyping (typing based on the sequence of the *rpoB* gene) and PCR amplification of a 620-bp portion of the *katG* gene were performed on all isolates.[100] One hundred and five (58 per cent) were unique by RFLP and 75 (42 per cent) were in 20 different clusters. The authors reported that there was less transmission associated with MDR strains than with drug-susceptible strains (33 versus 47 per cent). In Singapore, investigators reported that 22 of 230 drug-resistant strains were likely the result of recent transmission. The estimated transmission rate for drug-resistant tuberculosis was only 10 per cent and that for MDR tuberculosis was 8 per cent.[101]

Although these findings support the hypothesis that drug-resistant strains are less likely than drug-susceptible strains to result in disease, there are populations in which drug resistance is neither detected nor treated effectively, and where the longer duration of infectiousness for patients with drug-resistant organisms treated with standard regimens might offset the bacterium's diminished capacity to cause secondary cases.[97] In areas with high-prevalence rates of HIV, the increased host susceptibility, even to strains with diminished virulence, may offset bacterial differences. Several nosocomial outbreaks in New York City in the early 1990s[102] with the MDR strain of *M. tuberculosis*, strain W, as well as recent outbreaks of XDR tuberculosis,[95] provide examples of how these strains can disseminate. It is possible that some organisms could experience a subsequent mutation that increases their virulence back to the pre-drug-resistant state.[103]

Geographical distribution and global dissemination of *M. tuberculosis*

Genotyping has permitted the tracking of strains of *M. tuberculosis* as they spread both locally within communities and globally. Some strains of *M. tuberculosis* are infrequently encountered while others are widely dispersed both geographically and temporally, suggesting the strains are either older, more transmissible, or they are more likely than other strains to cause disease. In general, most strains are not widely disseminated. For example, most clusters (66 per cent) from the National Tuberculosis Genotyping and Surveillance Network in the USA were restricted to a single site with 25 per cent of the clusters in two sites, 5 per cent in three, 2 per cent in four and 1 per cent each in five and six sites.[104]

The Beijing family of strains have been detected in high proportions among strains collected throughout the world,[105] including China,[106,107] other parts of Asia,[108] the former Russian Federation,[109,110] Estonia,[111] Europe[112–114] and South Africa.[115] Among 408 randomly selected isolates throughout China, 65 per cent were of the Beijing genotype, as assessed by spoligotyping.[107] The 'W strain', a MDR strain of *M. tuberculosis* that caused many cases of TB among patients and healthcare workers in nosocomial outbreaks and other institutional settings in New York City[101,116–119] is a member of the Beijing family. The reason for the Beijing strains's global success is not known, but it is possible that the Beijing genotype has a selective advantage and is more readily aerosolized, can establish infection more effectively or can progress more rapidly from infection to disease.[10,120] It is also possible that the Beijing genotype was introduced into multiple locations before other strains and had more time to spread.

Other non-Beijing strains have also been demonstrated to predominate in some areas. For example, a drug resistant non-Beijing strain was demonstrated to account for 10 per cent of cases of tuberculosis over 2 years in the Western Province of South Africa.[121] Interestingly, the isolates shared a rare mutation in *katG*315. In Zambia and Zimbabwe, a specific strain with a unique spoligotype signature was the cause of approximately half of the cases of tuberculosis studied.[122]

Gagneux *et al.*[123] recently reported findings on the global population structure and geographic distribution of *M. tuberculosis,* based on LSPs. They were able to divide isolates collected from across the globe into six phylogeographic lineages. They then looked at the correlation between the lineages and the birth place of patients with tuberculosis diagnosed in San Francisco. In this remarkable study, they noted a close correlation between the lineage of *M. tuberculosis* and the place of birth. More remarkable, they showed that the *M. tuberculosis* was more likely to be spread in sympatric versus allopatric populations. When transmission did occur in allopatric hosts, it was more likely to involve high-risk subjects with impaired host defences. The authors concluded that *M. tuberculosis* lineages have adapted to human populations. If true, these findings will have significant impact on future vaccine development.

TUBERCULOSIS CONTROL AND PUBLIC HEALTH

The impact of genotyping on tuberculosis control activities has been difficult to measure directly. Most studies have utilized genotyping information retrospectively, with often weeks to months of delay from diagnosis of tuberculosis to availability of genotyping results. With such delays, some information is inevitably lost and some connections within chains of transmission missed. Despite these problems, studies have been able to identify instances of laboratory cross-contamination, identify sites or settings in which transmission has been occurring, and more recently, to evaluate the performance of a tuberculosis control programme.

Identifying laboratory cross-contamination

Before the availability of genotyping tools, false-positive cultures of *M. tuberculosis* were thought to be rare. An early study by Small *et al.*[124] reported incidents of false-positive cultures due to laboratory cross-contamination and suggested that contamination should be considered when two patients with identical genotype patterns are diagnosed within 7 days of each other in the same laboratory. Subsequently, false-positive culture results were reported in 13 of 14 molecular epidemiologic studies that evaluated more than 100 patients.[125] The median false-positive rate in these studies was 3.1 per cent. In New York City, from 2001 to 2003, 2.4 per cent of 2437 patient isolates were considered falsely positive.[126]

Laboratory cross-contamination occurs when *M. tuberculosis* is introduced into a specimen that does not contain the bacillus. This can occur at several points in the mycobacteriology laboratory, including through aerosolization during specimen processing, through contaminated equipment or reagents, and when specimens are reprocessed because of bacterial or fungal contamination. In addition to laboratory errors leading to false-positive cultures, mishandling/mislabelling of specimens can also lead to false-positive cultures.

The possibility of a false-positive culture should be considered when there is a single positive culture, particularly if the specimen is AFB smear-negative, few colonies and growth in liquid media only. In these settings, the clinician should request that the laboratory determine if the cultures in question have identical genotype patterns. Since laboratory cross-contamination has become accepted, laboratories have taken measures to minimize this phenomenon and allow for more rapid detection.

Infectiousness of patients

Studies that have assessed tuberculin skin test reactivity among contacts to cases of pulmonary tuberculosis have documented the variation in infectivity among source cases, based on the bacteriologic status of the source, the extent of disease and the frequency of cough.[36] Not unexpectedly, patients with more extensive pulmonary tuberculosis, as evidenced by cavitary changes on the chest radiograph and/or the identification of acid-fast bacilli on sputum smear examination, are more likely to transmit *M. tuberculosis* to contacts. Molecular epidemiology studies have confirmed the variation in infectivity that exists between patients with tuberculosis and highlighted the infectivity of patients with smear-positive pulmonary tuberculosis. For example, a single patient with smear-positive pulmonary tuberculosis was directly or indirectly responsible for 6 per cent of the tuberculosis cases in San Francisco during a 2-year period.[38] In another report, investigators showed that a single homeless tuberculosis patient with highly infectious pulmonary tuberculosis who was a regular patron of a neighbourhood bar likely infected 42 per cent (41/97) of the contacts who were regular customers and employees of the bar and caused disease in 14 (34 per cent) of them. Among 12 patients whose isolates of *M. tuberculosis* were available, all had identical IS*6110* RFLP band patterns.[127]

Although most infection control policies and recommendations prioritize smear-positive pulmonary tuberculosis over smear-negative cases, it is important to realize that patients with sputum smears that are negative for acid-fast bacilli, but culture-positive for *M. tuberculosis*, can transmit infection to others. Molecular epidemiology studies[128,129] have reported that patients with smear-negative, culture-positive pulmonary tuberculosis are responsible for approximately 20 per cent of cases. Investigators in San Francisco reported that patients with pleural tuberculosis who had negative sputum cultures were very unlikely to generate secondary cases of tuberculosis.[130]

The potential for transmitting tuberculosis should be considered in all pulmonary tuberculosis patients/suspects, particularly in settings and environments that facilitate transmission, such as shelters, hospices, healthcare facilities, prisons and other institutional or crowded settings.[27] It would be prudent to treat smear-negative pulmonary tuberculosis suspects for some period before removing them from isolation or sending them into high-risk settings, like jails and prisons. In addition, pulmonary tuberculosis should be carefully ruled out in patients with extrapulmonary disease. Although international guidelines for the diagnosis and treatment of tuberculosis prioritize the detection and treatment of infectious sputum smear-positive patients,[131] timely diagnosis and treatment of sputum smear-negative cases should be considered when resources permit.

Contact investigations

Conventional tuberculosis contact investigations use the 'stone-in-the-pond' or concentric circle approach to collect information and to screen household contacts, coworkers and increasingly distant contacts for tuberculosis infection and disease.[132] Studies in low-incidence areas such as San Francisco[38] and Amsterdam[57] demonstrated that a relatively small proportion (5–10 per cent) of tuberculosis cases with identical IS*6110*-based genotyping patterns were named as a contact by the source case. One explanation for these findings is that unsuspected transmission of *M. tuberculosis* occurred and was not easily detected by conventional contact-tracing investigations. In a 5-year, population-based study in the Netherlands, contact investigations of persons in five of the largest clusters identified epidemiological links between them based on time, place and risk factors.[35] However, tuberculosis transmission also occurred through only short-term, casual contact that was not easily identified in routine contact investigations. That casual contact can result in transmission has also been demonstrated by others.[133]

In a more recent study from the Netherlands,[30] patients were divided into one of five 'transmission groups' based on the results of contact investigations, genotyping and in some cases, a second interview: (1) clear epidemiologic links, confirmed by genotyping and contact tracing (24 per cent), (2) clear epidemiologic links, confirmed by genotyping and second interview, but not contact tracing (6 per cent), (3) initially unclear epidemiologic links that became likely after genotyping and second interview (55 per cent), (4) no epidemiologic links but genotyping indicated clustering and (5) patients who were part of a different cluster than expected (1 per cent). Combining groups 1 and 2 would suggest that the best contact investigations could have done was to identify about 30 per cent of the clustered cases. However, 55 per cent of the clustered cases had an epidemiologic link identified after the genotyping results became available and a second interview was performed. These data suggest that as newer, more rapid amplification-based genotyping methods become available we might be able to improve contact investigations using this approach.[134]

Genotyping has also demonstrated that, even when another case is identified through a contact investigation, the contact-case may be unrelated to the index case.[135–137] For example, Behr *et al.*[135] in San Francisco reported that 30 per cent of case–contact pairs had different strains of *M. tuberculosis*. Unrelated strains were more common among foreign-born, particularly Asian, contacts. Of 538 similar case pairs in a study[138] involving seven sites in the USA, 29 per cent did not have matching genotype patterns, similar to the finding in San Francisco. Importantly, case-pairs from the same household were no more likely to have confirmed transmission than those linked elsewhere. Among patients <5 years of age, 15 per cent of culture-confirmed cases and their suspected source patient had different genotype patterns.[136] In a recent study from South Africa, investigators evaluated 129 households in which genotyping data were available for more than one patient.[137] They identified 313 patients of whom 145 (46 per cent) had a genotype pattern matching that of another member of the household. These studies would suggest that contact investigations should not focus solely on the household but on all settings frequented by the index case.

Contact tracing in the community can be ineffective in tuberculosis outbreaks if patients do not live in stable settings and either do not know or are unwilling to reveal the names and locations of contacts. Fortunately, studies which incorporate genotyping are able to provide information about the chains of transmission in these groups.[139,140] A prospective study of tuberculosis transmission in Los Angeles, California, identified 162 patients who had culture-positive tuberculosis, and interviewed the patients to identify their contacts and whereabouts.[141] Traditional contact investigations did not reliably identify patients infected with the same strain of *M. tuberculosis*: only 2 of the 96 clustered cases named others in the cluster as contacts. However, the degree of homelessness and having used daytime services at three shelters were independently associated with clustering. This study and others[142] demonstrated that locations where the homeless congregate are important sites of tuberculosis transmission.

Several studies support the idea that specific locations can be associated with recent or ongoing transmission of *M. tuberculosis*. In a 30-month prospective study of all tuberculosis cases in Baltimore, Maryland, using traditional contact investigations and IS*6110*-based genotyping, 46 per cent (84/182) of initial isolates were clustered and 32 per cent (58/182) of the cases were considered to have tuberculosis that was recently transmitted.[39] Only 24 per cent (20/84) of clustered cases had an identifiable epidemiologic link of recent contact with an infectious tuberculosis patient. Using geographic information system data, the 20 clustered cases with epidemiologic links in geographic areas of the city with low socioeconomic status and high drug use were spatially aggregated. Such studies suggest that location-based control efforts may be more effective in some populations than traditional concentric circle-based contact tracing for early identification of cases.

Studies in both low-incidence and high-incidence areas have demonstrated that a significant amount of transmission occurs outside the household. Bennett *et al.*[138] evaluated transmission between epidemiologically linked pairs identified during contact investigations. Among 538 case pairs in which the source case and secondary case were identified, 29 per cent did not have matching genotypes. Of the 260 pairs that shared the same household, 30 per cent did not have matching genotypes. In South Africa, approximately 50 per cent of households with more than one tuberculosis case had different genotypes.[143]

DETECTION OF UNSUSPECTED TRANSMISSION

Genotyping has been particularly useful to identify otherwise unsuspected and undetected transmission in the community. Molecular epidemiologic studies have confirmed suspected and unsuspected transmission of tuberculosis in places such as residential care facilities,[144] bars,[127,145–147] crack houses,[148] sites of illegal floating card games,[149] schools,[150,151] hospitals[152,153] and jails and prisons.[66,109,154,155] Tuberculosis transmission has also been demonstrated among groups such as church choirs,[156] interstate transgender social networks,[157] renal transplant patients,[158] from patient to health-care providers,[130,159]

and from health-care provider to patients.[160,161] Processing contaminated medical waste resulted in transmission of *M. tuberculosis* to at least one medical waste treatment facility worker.[162] Genotyping was also used to document unsuspected bronchoscopy-related transmission and the cross-contamination of patients.[163,164] Without the availability of genotyping, it would have been very difficult to confirm that transmission had occurred in such settings.

Integration of genotyping into the state's tuberculosis control programme allowed Alabama, a low-incidence state in the USA, to detect unsuspected sites of transmission.[165] The system identified a cluster of 25 cases, 12 of whom were in the same county and the others were spread across nine counties. Once the genotyping information became available, a second contact investigation was initiated. The primary sites of transmission were found to be a correctional facility and two homeless shelters.

COMMUNITY EPIDEMIOLOGY

Community-based studies have demonstrated different epidemiological patterns of disease among different ethnic and racial groups. Studies in New York and San Francisco have reported high rates of transmission with recent infection among US-born populations with low rates of clustering among foreign-born populations.[58,166] Whether or not there is transmission occurring between these groups has varied from study to study. In San Francisco[166] and Maryland,[167] no significant transmission could be identified between foreign-born and US-born patients. Similarly, in Denmark, only 0.9 per cent of Danish-born cases were infected by Somali-born patients and 1.8 per cent of Somali cases were infected by Danish-born cases.[168] In contrast, 17 per cent of 623 Dutch-born patients were infected by foreign-born cases between 1993 and 1995.[169] These studies highlight the fact that transmission patterns vary among and between ethnic and racial groups and that these patterns can also vary by location.

Even when the essential elements of tuberculosis control are in place, ongoing transmission of *M. tuberculosis* will continue to occur until tuberculosis is diagnosed and the patient is started on therapy. In a population-based molecular epidemiological study in an urban community in the San Francisco Bay area, 75 (33 per cent) of 221 cases had the same strain of *M. tuberculosis*.[170] Thirty-nine (53 per cent) of the 73 patients developed tuberculosis because they were not identified as contacts of source case-patients; 20 case-patients (27 per cent) developed tuberculosis because of delayed diagnosis of their sources; 13 case-patients (18 per cent) developed tuberculosis because of problems associated with the evaluation or treatment of contacts; and one case-patient (1 per cent) developed tuberculosis because of delays identifying the person as a contact.

Measuring the performance of a tuberculosis control programme

As noted previously, tuberculosis can develop through three mechanisms: recent transmission with rapid progression to disease, reactivation of latent infection or exogenous reinfection. Because clustering is considered a measure of recent or ongoing transmission, the decline in the rate of clustering could be used to evaluate interventions aimed at reducing recent transmission.[171] In an evaluation of tuberculosis transmission over a 7-year period in San Francisco, the number and proportion of clustered tuberculosis cases declined, particularly among the US-born population.[34] This decline was attributed to the implementation of targeted tuberculosis prevention and control programmes such as screening high-risk populations and implementation of directly observed therapy (DOT) to ensure high cure rates. A follow-up study from San Francisco demonstrated significant declines in tuberculosis case rates in San Francisco in both clustered and non-clustered cases.[172] The rate of clustered and non-clustered tuberculosis cases declined from 1992 to 1999, although the decline in clustered cases was significantly greater than in the non-clustered cases (95 versus 51 per cent, $p < 0.0001$). There were no further declines in the case rates after 1999 in the population as a whole or any subgroup analysed. The authors concluded that the case rates had reached a plateau despite continuing application of control measures begun in 1993 and that to see further reduction, more aggressive diagnosis and treatment of latent TB infection would be necessary. A similar study in New York City showed that, as tuberculosis case rates fell from recent high levels, the proportion of tuberculosis cases caused by recent transmission dropped from 63 per cent in 1993 to 31 per cent in 1999.[58] Tuberculosis was unlikely to result from recent transmission in people born outside the United States. Investigators in Denver[173] used clustering to measure the impact of a skin-testing programme among homeless people and showed that clustering decreased from 49 per cent during the implementation of the programme to 14 per cent in the 4-year period after the programme.

By contrast, an 8-year study in Greenland showed that the annual incidence of tuberculosis doubled from 1990 to 1997 and the percentage of culture-positive tuberculosis cases in RFLP-defined clusters increased to 85 per cent, reflecting micro-epidemics among adults and young children in small, isolated settlements.[174] Thus, genotyping was a useful indicator of changes in the proportion of cases that resulted from recent transmission with rapid progression to disease.

THE FUTURE OF MOLECULAR EPIDEMIOLOGY

Molecular genotyping, in combination with conventional epidemiologic investigations, has contributed greatly to our understanding of the transmission and pathogenesis of tuberculosis. The development of real-time amplification-based genotyping techniques should improve our ability to rapidly define a genotype and undertake effective, timely contact and outbreak investigations. Future genotyping studies will likely include evaluation of specific mutations that are associated with phenotypic difference, such as underlying drug resistance and virulence. In addition, new approaches to genotyping should improve our understanding of the phylogenetic history of the organism and provide insight into the global dissemination of certain strains. From a public health perspective, genotyping should be integrated into new surveillance systems that will allow more rapid responses to potential outbreaks of tuberculosis. Only with the widespread availability of rapid real-time genotyping will the promise of molecular epidemiology be realized in tuberculosis control activities.

LEARNING POINTS

- Molecular epidemiology can be defined as 'using the analysis of nucleic acids and proteins in the study of health and disease determinants in human populations'.
- Genotyping methods, such as IS6110-based RFLP analysis, spoligotyping and MIRU-VNTR typing have revolutionized our ability to track strains of M. tuberculosis as they spread through our communities and globally.
- IS6110-based RFLP analysis is the most discriminatory of the currently available genotyping methods.
- Spoligotyping and MIRU-VNTR typing use PCR to amplify sequences of DNA. Unlike RFLP analysis, they do not require DNA extraction or viable bacilli.
- Genotyping methods, in combination with routine epidemiologic investigations, have helped to describe outbreaks, uncover unsuspected transmission and identify sites of transmission outside the home.
- Genotyping has helped us to understand better the transmission and pathogenesis of tuberculosis, particularly in the setting of HIV infection.
- Studies have identified risk factors for recent infection with rapid progression to disease. These risk factors have varied in different communities and settings.
- The finding that 'clustered' isolates make up more than one-third of all isolates in many countries indicates that considerable amounts of tuberculosis are due to recent and ongoing transmission, and that a significant proportion of transmission of M. tuberculosis occurs outside the household.

- Recurrent tuberculosis can be due to exogenous reinfection, which is probably more common in high incidence areas.
- Mixed infections are more common than previously recognized.
- Certain mutations that confer drug resistance may result in a less fit organism. Nevertheless, drug-resistant organisms can be widely transmitted and cause disease, particularly in immunocompromised hosts.
- Certain strains of *M. tuberculosis*, such as the Beijing family, appear to be very successful and have disseminated globally. The reason for this success is not known.
- Approximately 3 per cent of tuberculosis cases are false positive and result from laboratory cross-contamination.
- Genotyping has allowed tuberculosis control programmes to evaluate how they are performing in reducing transmission within their community.

REFERENCES

1. Mathema B, Kurepina NE, Bifani PJ, Kreiswirth BN. Molecular epidemiology of tuberculosis:current insights. *Clin Micro Rev* 2006; **19**: 658–85.
2. van Embden JD, Cave MD, Crawford JT *et al.* Strain identification of *Mycobacterium tuberculosis* by DNA fingerprinting: recommendations for a standardized methodology. *J Clin Microbiol* 1993; **31**: 406–409.
3. Thierry D, Cave MD, Eisenach KD *et al.* IS6110, an IS-like element of *Mycobacterium tuberculosis* complex. *Nucleic Acids Res* 1990; **18**: 188.
4. de Boer AS, Borgdorff MW, de Haas PE *et al.* Analysis of the rate of change of IS6110 RFLP patterns in *Mycobacterium tuberculosis* based on serial patient isolates. *J Infect Dis* 1999; **180**: 1238–44.
5. Yeh RW, Ponce de Leon A, Agasion CB. Stability of *Mycobacterium tuberculosis* DNA genotypes. *J Infect Dis* 1998; **177**: 1107–11.
6. Warren RM, van der Spuy GD, Richardson M *et al.* Calculation of the stability of the IS6110 banding pattern in patients with persistent *Mycobacterium tuberculosis* disease. *J Clin Microbiol* 2002; **40**: 1705–708.
7. Yang ZH, Ijaz K, Bates JH *et al.* Spoligotyping and polymorphic GC-rich repetitive sequence fingerprinting of *Mycobacterium tuberculosis* strains having few copies of IS6110. *J Clin Microbiol* 2000; **38**: 3572–6.
8. Groenen PM, Bunschoten AE, van Soolingen D, van Embden JD. Nature of DNA polymorphism in the direct repeat cluster of *Mycobacterium tuberculosis*: application for strain differentiation by a novel typing method. *Mol Microbiol* 1993; **10**: 1057–65.
9. Kamerbeek J, Schouls L, Kolk A. Simultaneous detection and strain differentiation of *Mycobacteriuim tuberculosis* for diagnosis and epidemiology. *J Clin Microbiol* 1997; **35**: 907–14.
10. Barnes PF, Cave MD. Molecular epidemiology of tuberculosis. *N Engl J Med* 2003; **349**: 1149–56.
11. Soini H, Pan X, Amin A *et al.* Characterization of *Mycobacterium tuberculosis* isolates from patients in Houston, Texas, by spoligotyping. *J Clin Microbiol* 2000; **38**: 669–76.
12. Wilson SM, Goss S, Drobniewski F. Evaluation of strategies for molecular fingerprinting for use in the routine work of a *Mycobacterium tuberculosis* reference unit. *J Clin Microbiol* 1998; **36**: 3385–8.
13. Mazars E, Lesjean S, Banuls AL *et al.* High-resolution minisatellite-based typing as a portable approach to global analysis of *Mycobacterium tuberculosis* molecular epidemiology. *Proc Natl Acad Sci U S A* 2001; **98**: 1901–906.
14. Supply P, Lesjean S, Savine E *et al.* Automated high throughput genotyping for study of global epidemiology of *Mycobacterium tuberculosis* based on mycobacterial interspersed repetitive units. *J Clin Microbiol* 2001; **39**: 3563–71.
15. Cowan LS, Mosher L, Diem L *et al.* Variable-number tandem repeat typing of *Mycobacterium tuberculosis* isolates with low copy numbers of IS6110 by using mycobacterial interspersed repetitive units. *J Clin Microbiol* 2002; **40**: 1592–602.
16. Kwara A, Schiro R, Cowan LS *et al.* Evaluation of the epidemiologic utility of secondary typing methods for differentiation of *Mycobacterium tuberculosis* isolates. *J Clin Microbiol* 2003; **41**: 2683–5.
17. Ross BC, Raoios K, Jackson K, Dwyer B. Molecular cloning of a highly repeated DNA element from *Mycobacterium tuberculosis* and its use as an epidemiological tool. *J Clin Microbiol* 1992; **30**: 942–6.
18. Rhee JT, Tanaka MM, Behr MA *et al.* Use of multiple markers in population-based molecular epidemiologic studies of tuberculosis. *Int J Tuberc Lung Dis* 2000; **4**: 1111–19.
19. Yang ZH, Bates JH, Eisenach KD, Cave MD. Secondary typing of *Mycobacterium tuberculosis* isolates with matching IS6110 fingerprints from different regions of the United States. *J Clin Microbiol* 2001; **39**: 1691–5.
20. Sreevatsan S, Pan X, Stockbauer KE. Restricted structural gene polymorphism in the *Mycobacterium tuberculosis* complex indicates evolutionary recent global dissemination. *Proc Natl Acad Sci U S A* 1997; **94**: 9869–74.
21. Fleischmann R, Alland DD, Eisen JA. Whole genome comparison of *Mycobacterium tuberculosis* clinical and laboratory strains. *J Bacteriol* 2002; **184**: 5479–90.
22. Goguet de la Salmoniere YO, Kim CC, Tsolaki AG *et al.* High-throughput method for detecting genomic-deletion polymorphisms. *J Clin Microbiol* 2004; **42**: 2913–18.
23. Nguyen D, Brassard P, Menzies D *et al.* Genomic characterization of an endemic *Mycobacterium tuberculosis* strain:evolutionary and epidemiologic implications. *J Clin Microbiol* 2004; **42**: 2573–80.
24. Scott AN, Menzies D, Tannenbaum TN. Sensitivities and specificities of spoligotyping and mycobacterial repetitive unit-variable-number tandem repeat typing methods for studying molecular epidemiology of tuberculosis. *J Clin Microbiol* 2005; **43**: 89–94.
25. Supply P, Allix C, Lesjean S. Proposal for standardization of optimized mycobacterial interspersed repetitive unit-variable-number tandem repeat typing of *Mycobacterium tuberculosis*. *J Clin Microbiol* 2006; **44**: 4498–510.
26. Oelemann MC, Diel R, Vatin V. Assessment of an optimized mycobacterial interspersed repetitive-unit-variable-number tandem repeat typing system combined with spoligotyping for population-based molecular epidemiology studies of tuberculosis. *J Clin Microbiol* 2007; **45**: 691–7.
27. DeRiemer K, Daley CL. Tuberculosis transmission based on molecular epidemiologic research. *Semin Respir Crit Care Med* 2004; **25**: 297–306.
28. Braden CR, Templeton GL, Cave MD *et al.* Interpretation of restriction fragment length polymorphism analysis of *Mycobacterium tuberculosis* isolates from a state with a large rural population. *J Infect Dis* 1997; **175**: 1446–52.
29. Godfrey-Faussett P, Stoker NG. Aspects of tuberculosis in Africa. 3. Genetic 'fingerprinting' for clues to the pathogenesis of tuberculosis. *Trans R Soc Trop Med Hyg* 1992; **86**: 472–5.
30. van Deutekom H, Hoijng SP, de Haas PEW *et al.* Clustered

tuberculosis cases: do they represent recent transmission and can they be detected earlier? *Am J Respir Crit Care Med* 2004; **169**: 806–10.

31. Murray M, Alland D. Methodological problems in the molecular epidemiology of tuberculosis. *Am J Epidemiol* 2002; **155**: 565–71.

32. Glynn JR, Vynnycky E, Pine PE. Influence of sampling on estimates of clustering and recent transmission of *Mycobacterium tuberculosis* derived from DNA fingerprinting techniques. *Am J Epidemiol* 1999; **149**: 366–71.

33. Vynnycky EN, Nagelkerke NJ, Borgdorff MW *et al*. The effect of age and study duration on the relationship between 'clustering' of DNA fingerprint patterns and the proportion of tuberculosis disease attributable to recent transmission. *Epidemiol Infect* 2001; **126**: 43–62.

34. Jasmer RM, Hahn JA, Small PM *et al*. A molecular epidemiologic analysis of tuberculosis trends in San Francisco, 1991–1997. *Ann Intern Med* 1999; **130**: 971–8.

35. van Soolingen D, Borgdorff MW, de Haas PE *et al*. Molecular epidemiology of tuberculosis in the Netherlands: a nationwide study from 1993 through 1997. *J Infect Dis* 1999; **180**: 726–36.

36. Hopewell PC. Factors influencing transmission and infectivity of *Mycobacterium tuberculosis*: Implications for clinical and public health management. In: Sande MA, Hudson LD, Root RK (eds). *Respiratory infections*. New York: Churchill Livingstone, 1986: 191–216.

37. Alland D, Kalkut GE, Moss AR *et al*. Transmission of tuberculosis in New York City. An analysis by DNA fingerprinting and conventional epidemiologic methods. *N Engl J Med* 1994; **330**: 1710–16.

38. Small PM, Hopewell PC, Singh SP *et al*. The epidemiology of tuberculosis in San Francisco. A population-based study using conventional and molecular methods. *N Engl J Med* 1994; **330**: 1703–709.

39. Bishai WR, Fraham NM, Harrington S *et al*. Molecular and geographic patterns of tuberculosis transmission after 15 years of directly observed therapy. *J Am Med Assoc* 1998; **280**: 1679–84.

40. Dahle UR, Sandven P, Heldal E, Cavgant DA. Molecular epidemiology of *Mycobacterium tuberculosis* in Norway. *J Clin Microbiol* 2001; **39**: 1802–807.

41. Hernandez-Garduno E, Kunimoto D, Wang L *et al*. Predictors of clustering of tuberculosis in Greater Vancouver: a molecular epidemiologic study. *CMAJ* 2002; **167**: 349–52.

42. Kulaga S, Behr M, Musana K *et al*. Molecular epidemiology of tuberculosis in Montreal. *CMAJ* 2002; **167**: 353–4.

43. Diel R, Schneider S, Meywald-Walter K *et al*. Epidemiology of tuberculosis in Hamburg, Germany: long-term population-based analysis applying classical and molecular epidemiologic techniques. *J Clin Microbiol* 2002; **40**: 532–9.

44. Maguire H, Dale JW, McHugh TD. Molecular epidemiology of tuberculosis in London 1995–7 showing low rate of active transmission. *Thorax* 2002; **57**: 617–22.

45. FitzGerald JM, Fanning A, Hoepnner V *et al*. Canadian Molecular Epidemiology of TB Study Group. The molecular epidemiology of tuberculosis in western Canada. *Int J Tuberc Lung Dis* 2003; **7**: 132–8.

46. Blackwood KS, Al-Azem A, Elliott LJ *et al*. Conventional and molecular epidemiology of tuberculosis in Manitoba. *BMC Infect Dis* 2003; **3**: 18.

47. Vukovic D, Rusch-Gerdes S, Savic B, Niemann S. Molecular epidemiology of pulmonary tuberculosis in Belgrade, Central Serbia. *J Clin Microbiol* 2003; **41**: 4372–7.

48. Zolnir-Dovc M, Poljak M, Erzen D, Sorli J. Molecular epidemiology of tuberculosis in Slovenia: results of a one-year (2001) nation-wide study. *Scand J Infect Dis* 2003; **35**: 863–8.

49. Calvo JC, Mochales JA, Meixeira AP. Ten-year population-based molecular epidemiologic study of tuberculosis transmission in the metropolitan area of Madrid, Spain. *Int J Tuberc Lung Dis* 2005; **9**: 1236–41.

50. Godfrey-Faussett P, Sonnenberg P, Shearer SC *et al*. Tuberculosis control and molecular epidemiology in a South African goldmining community. *Lancet* 2000; **356**: 1066–71.

51. Lockman S, Sheppard JD, Braden CR *et al*. Molecular and conventional epidemiology of *Mycobacterium tuberculosis* in Botswana: a population-based prospective study of 301 pulmonary tuberculosis patients. *J Clin Microbiol* 2001; **39**: 1042–7.

52. Narayanan S, Das S, Garg R *et al*. Molecular epidemiology of tuberculosis in a rural area of high prevalence in south India:Implications for disease control and prevention. *J Clin Microbiol* 2002; **40**: 4785–8.

53. Verver S, Warren RM, Munch Z *et al*. Transmission of tuberculosis in a high incidence urban community in South Africa. *Int J Epidemiol* 2004; **33**: 351–7.

54. Chan-Yeung M, Tam C-M, Wong H *et al*. Molecular and conventional epidemiology of tuberculosis in Hong Kong: a population-based prospective study. *J Clin Microbiol* 2003; **41**: 2706–708.

55. Crampin AC, Glynn JR, Traore H. Tuberculosis transmission attributable to close contacts and HIV status, Malawi. *Emerg Infect Dis* 2006; **12**: 729–35.

56. Godreuil S, Torrea G, Terru D. First molecular epidemiology study of *Mycobacterium tuberculosis* in Burkina, Faso. *J Clin Microbiol* 2007; **45**: 921–7.

57. van Deutekom H, Gerritsen JJ, van Soolingen D *et al*. A molecular epidemiological approach to studying the transmission of tuberculosis in Amsterdam. *Clin Infect Dis* 1997; **25**: 1071–7.

58. Geng E, Kreiswirth B, Driver C *et al*. Changes in the transmission of tuberculosis in New York City from 1990 to 1999. *N Engl J Med* 2002; **346**: 1453–8.

59. Diel R, Rusch-Gerdes S, Niemann S. Molecular epidemiology of tuberculosis among immigrants in Hamburg, Germany. *J Clin Microbiol* 2004; **42**: 2952–60.

60. Stead WW. Pathogenesis of a first episode of chronic pulmonary tuberculosis in man: recrudescence of residuals of the primary infection or exogenous reinfection? *Am Rev Respir Dis* 1967; **95**: 729–45.

61. Romeyn JA. Exogenous reinfection in tuberculosis. *Am Rev Respir Dis* 1970; **101**: 923–7.

62. Cannetti G, Sutherland I, Sandova E. Endogenous reactivation and exogenous reinfection:their relative importance with regard to the development of non-primary tuberculosis. *Bull Int Union Tuberc* 1972; **47**: 116–34.

63. Nardell E, McInnis B, Thomas B, Weidhaas S. Exogenous reinfection with tuberculosis in a shelter for the homeless. *N Engl J Med* 1986; **18**: 1570–5.

64. Small PM, Shafer RW, Hopewell PC *et al*. Exogenous reinfection with multidrug-resistant *Mycobacterium tuberculosis* in patients with advanced HIV infection. *N Engl J Med* 1993; **328**: 1137–44.

65. Sudre P, Pfyffer GE, Bodmer T *et al*. Molecular epidemiology of tuberculosis among HIV-infected persons in Switzerland:a country-wide 9-year cohort study. Swiss HIV Cohort Study. *Infection* 1999; **27**: 323–30.

66. Chaves F, Dronda F, Alonso-Sanz M, Noriega AR. Evidence of exogenous reinfection and mixed infection with more than one strain of *Mycobacterium tuberculosis* among Spanish HIV-infected inmates. *AIDS* 1999; **13**: 615–20.

67. Bandera A, Gori A, Catozzi L *et al*. Molecular epidemiology study of exogenous reinfection in an area with a low incidence of tuberculosis. *J Clin Microbiol* 2001; **39**: 2213–18.

68. Caminero JA, Pena MJ, Campos-Herrero MI *et al*. Exogenous reinfection with tuberculosis on a European island with a moderate incidence of disease. *Am J Respir Crit Care Med* 2001; **163**: 717–20.

69. Kruuner A, Pehme L, Ghebremichael S *et al*. Use of molecular techniques to distinguish between treatment failure and exogenous reinfection with *Mycobacterium tuberculosis*. *Clin Infect Dis* 2002; **35**: 146–55.

70. Garcia de Viedma DG, Marin M, Hernangomez S et al. Tuberculosis recurrences: reinfection plays a role in a population whose clinical/epidemiological characteristics do not favor reinfection. Arch Intern Med 2002; 162: 1873–9.

71. El Sahly HM, Wright JA, Soini H et al. Recurrent tuberculosis in Houston, Texas: a population-based study. Int J Tuberc Lung Dis 2004; 8: 333–40.

72. Jasmer RM, Bozeman L, Schwartzman K et al. Recurrent tuberculosis in the United States and Canada: relapse or reinfection? Am J Respir Crit Care Med 2004; 170: 1360–6.

73. Nahid P, Gonzalez LC, Rudoy I. Treatment outcomes of patients with HIV and tuberculosis. Am J Respir Crit Care Med 2007; 175: 1199–206.

74. Godfrey-Faussett P, Githui W, Batchelor B et al. Recurrence of HIV-related tuberculosis in an endemic area may be due to relapse or reinfection. Tuber Lung Dis 1994; 75: 199–202.

75. Das S, Paramasivan CN, Lowrie DB, Prabhakar R, Narayanan PR. IS6110 restriction fragment length polymorphism typing of clinical isolates of Mycobacterium tuberculosis from patients with pulmonary tuberculosis in Madras, south India. Tuber Lung Dis 1995; 76: 550–4.

76. van Rie A, Warren R, Richardson M et al. Exogenous reinfection as a cause of recurrent tuberculosis after curative treatment. N Engl J Med 1999; 341: 1174–9.

77. Sonnenberg P, Murray J, Glynn JR, Shearer S, Kambashi B, Godfrey-Faussett P. HIV-1 and recurrence, relapse, and reinfection of tuberculosis after cure:a cohort study in South African mineworkers. Lancet 2001; 358: 1687–93.

78. Lourenco MC, Grinsztejn B, Fadinho-Montes FC, da Silva MG, Saad MH, Fonseca LS. Genotypic patterns of multiple isolates of M. tuberculosis from tuberculous HIV patients. Trop Med Int Health 2000; 5: 488–94.

79. Fitzpatrick LK, Okwera A, Mugerwa R, Ridzon R, Ehiner J, Onorato I. An investigation of suspected exogenous reinfection in tuberculosis patients in Kampala, Uganda. Int J Tuberc Lung Dis 2002; 6: 550–2.

80. Schaaf HS, Krook S, Hollemans DW. Recurrent culture-confirmed tuberculosis in human immunodeficiency virus-infected children. Pediatr Infect Dis J 2005; 24: 685–91.

81. Shen G, Xue Z, Shen X. Recurrent tuberculosis and exogenous reinfection, Shanghai, China. Emerg Infect Dis 2006; 12: 1776–8.

82. Lambert ML, Hasker E, van Deun A et al. Recurrence in tuberculosis: relapse or reinfection? Lancet Infect Dis 2003; 3: 282–7.

83. Verver S, Warren RM, Beyers N et al. Rate of reinfection tuberculosis after successful treatment is higher than rate of new tuberculosis. Am J Respir Crit Care Med 2005; 171: 1430–35.

84. Yeh RW, Hopewell PC, Daley CL. Simultaneous infection with two strains of Mycobacterium tuberculosis identified by restriction fragment length polymorphism analysis. Int J Tuberc Lung Dis 1999; 3: 537–9.

85. Braden CR, Morlock GP, Woodley CL et al. Simultaneous infection with multiple strains of Mycobacterium tuberculosis. Clin Infect Dis 2001; 33: 42–7.

86. Chaves F, Dronda F, Cave MD et al. A longitudinal study of transmission of tuberculosis in a large prison population. Am J Respir Crit Care Med 1997; 155: 719–25.

87. Warren RM, Victor TC, Streicher EM et al. Patients with active tuberculosis often have different strains in the same sputum specimen. Am J Respir Crit Care Med 2004; 169: 610–14.

88. Niemann S, Richter E, Rusch-Gerdes S et al. Double infection with a resistant and a multidrug-resistant strain of Mycobacterium tuberculosis. Emerg Infect Dis 2000; 6: 548–51.

89. Middlebrook G. Isoniazid resistance and catalase activity of the tubercle bacilli. Am Rev Tuberc 1954; 69: 471–2.

90. Cohn M, Kovitz C, Oda U. Studies on isoniazid and tubercle bacilli: the growth requirements, catalase activities, and pathogenic properties of isoniazid resistant mutants. Am Rev Tuberc 1954; 70: 641–64.

91. Riley RL, Mills CC, O'Grady F et al. Infectiousness of air from a tuberculosis ward: comparative infectiousness of different patients. Am Rev Respir Dis 1962; 85: 511–25.

92. Pym AS, Domenech P, Honore N et al. Regulation of catalase-peroxidase (KatG) expression, isoniazid sensitivity and virulence by furA of Mycobacterium tuberculosis. Mol Microbiol 2001; 40: 879–89.

93. Snider DE Jr, Kelly GD, Cauthen GM et al. Infection and disease among contacts of tuberculosis cases with drug-resistant and drug-susceptible bacilli. Am Rev Respir Dis 1985; 132: 125–32.

94. Texeira L, Perkins MD, Johnson JL. Infection and disease among household contacts of patients with multidrug-resistant tuberculosis. Int J Tuberc Lung Dis 2001; 5: 321–8.

95. Centers for Disease Control and Prevention. Emergence of Mycobacterium tuberculosis with extensive resistance to second-line drugs – worldwide, 2000–2004. MMWR Morb Mortal Wkly Rep 2006; 55: 301–305.

96. Garcia-Garcia ML, Ponce-de-Leon A, Jimenez-Corona ME et al. Clinical consequences and transmissibility of drug-resistant tuberculosis in southern Mexico. Arch Intern Med 2000; 160: 630–6.

97. Burgos M, DeRiemer K, Small PM et al. Effect of drug-resistance on the generation of secondary cases of tuberculosis. J Infect Dis 2003; 188: 1878–84.

98. Gagneux S, Burgos MV, DeRiemer K et al. Impact of bacterial genetics on the transmission of isoniazid-resistant Mycobacterium tuberculosis. PLoS Pathog 2006; 2: 603–10.

99. van Doorn HR, de Haas PEW, Kremer K. Public health impact of isoniazid resistant Mycobacterium tuberculosis strains with a mutation at amino-acid positive 315 of katG: a decade of experience in the Netherlands. Clin Microbiol Infect 2006; 12: 769–75.

100. Samper S, Iglesias MJ, Rabanaque MJ et al. Systematic molecular characterization of multidrug-resistant Mycobacterium tuberculosis complex isolates from Spain. J Clin Microbiol 2005; 43: 1220–7.

101. Sun YJ, Lee AS, Wong SY et al. Genotype and phenotype relationships and transmission analysis of drug-resistant tuberculosis in Singapore. Int J Tuberc Lung Dis 2007; 11: 436–42.

102. Munsiff SS, Nivin B, Sacajiu G et al. Persistence of a highly resistant strain of tuberculosis in New York City during 1990–1999. J Infect Dis 2003; 188: 356–63.

103. Cohen T, Sommers B, Murray M. The effect of drug resistance on the fitness of Mycobacterium tuberculosis. Lancet Infect Dis 2003; 3: 13–21.

104. Ellis BA, Crawford JT, Braden CR et al. Molecular epidemiology of tuberculosis in a sentinel surveillance population. Emerg Infect Dis 2002; 8: 1197–209.

105. Bifani PJ, Mathema B, Kurepina NE, Kreiswirth BN. Global dissemination of the Mycobacterium tuberculosis W-Beijing family strains. Trends Microbiol 2002; 10: 45–52.

106. van Soolingen D, Qian L, de Haas PE et al. Predominance of a single genotype of Mycobacterium tuberculosis in countries of east Asia. J Clin Microbiol 1995; 33: 3234–8.

107. Li WM, Wang SM, Liu YH et al. Molecular epidemiology of Mycobacterium tuberculosis in China: a nationwide random survey in 2000. Int J Tuberc Lung Dis 2005; 9: 1314–19.

108. Anh DD, Borgdorff MW, Van LN et al. Mycobacterium tuberculosis Beijing genotype emerging in Vietnam. Emerg Infect Dis 2000; 6: 302–305.

109. Toungoussova OS, Mariandyshev A, Bjune G et al. Molecular epidemiology and drug resistance of Mycobacterium tuberculosis isolates in the Archangel prison in Russia: predominance of the W-Beijing clone family. Clin Infect Dis 2003; 37: 665–72.

110. Drobniewski F, Balabanova Y, Nikolayevsky V et al. Drug-resistant tuberculosis, clinical virulence, and the dominance of the Beijing strain family in Russia. J Am Med Assoc 2005; 293: 2726–31.

111. Kruuner A, Hoffner SE, Sillastu H et al. Spread of drug-resistant

pulmonary tuberculosis in Estonia. *J Clin Microbiol* 2001; **39**: 3339–45.

112. Niemann S, Rusch-Gerdes S, Richter E. IS*6110* fingerprinting of drug-resistant *Mycobacterium tuberculosis* strains isolated in Germany during 1995. *J Clin Microbiol* 1997; **35**: 3015–20.

113. Caminero JA, Pena MJ, Campos-Herrero MI *et al.* Epidemiological evidence of the spread of a *Mycobacterium tuberculosis* strain of the Beijing genotype on Gran Canaria Island. *Am J Respir Crit Care Med* 2002; **164**: 1165–70.

114. Borgdorff MW, de Haas P, Kremer K, van Soolingen D. *Mycobacterium tuberculosis* Beijing genotype, the Netherlands. *Emerg Infect Dis* 2003; **9**: 1310–13.

115. Richardson M, van Lill SW, van der Spuy GD *et al.* Historic and recent events contribute to the disease dynamics of Beijing-like *Mycobacterium tuberculosis* isolates in a high incidence region. *Int J Tuberc Lung Dis* 2002; **6**: 1001–11.

116. Bifani PJ, Plikaytis BB, Kapur V *et al.* Origin and interstate spread of a New York City multidrug-resistant *Mycobacterium tuberculosis* clone family. *J Am Med Assoc* 1996; **275**: 452–57.

117. Bifani PJ, Mathema B, Liu Z *et al.* Identification of a W variant outbreak of *Mycobacterium tuberculosis* via population-based molecular epidemiology. *J Am Med Assoc* 1999; **282**: 2321–7.

118. Agerton TB, Valway SE, Blinkhorn RJ *et al.* Spread of strain W, a highly drug-resistant strain of *Mycobacterium tuberculosis,* across the United States. *Clin Infect Dis* 1999; **29**: 85–92.

119. Glynn JR, Whiteley J, Bifani PJ *et al.* Worldwide occurrence of Beijing/W strains of *Mycobacterium tuberculosis*: a systematic review. *Emerg Infect Dis* 2002; **8**: 843–9.

120. Lopez B, Aguilar D, Orozco H *et al.* A marked difference in pathogenesis and immune response induced by different *Mycobacterium tuberculosis* genotypes. *Clin Exp Immunol* 2003; **133**: 30–7.

121. Victor TC, Streicher EM, Kewley C *et al.* Spread of an emerging *Mycobacterium tuberculosis* drug-resistant strain in the western Cape of South Africa. *Int J Tuberc Lung Dis* 2007; **11**: 195–201.

122. Chihota V, Apers L, Mungofa S *et al.* Predominance of a single genotype of *Mycobacterium tuberculosis* in regions of Southern Africa. *Int J Tuberc Lung Dis* 2007; **11**: 311–18.

123. Gagneux S, DeRiemer K, Van T *et al.* Variable host–pathogen compatibility in *Mycobacterium tuberculosis. Proc Natl Acad Sci U S A* 2006; **103**: 2869–73.

124. Small PM, McClenny NB, Singh SP *et al.* Molecular strain typing of *Mycobacterium tuberculosis* to confirm cross-contamination in the mycobacteriology laboratory and modification of procedures to minimize occurrence of false-positive cultures. *J Clin Microbiol* 1994; **31**: 1677–82.

125. Burman WJ, Reves RR. Review of false-positive cultures for *Mycobacterium tuberculosis* and recommendations for avoiding unnecessary treatment. *Clin Infect Dis* 2000; **31**: 1390–5.

126. Clark CM, Driver CR, Munsiff SS *et al.* Universal genotyping in tuberculosis control program, New York City, 2001–2003. *Emerg Infect Dis* 2006; **12**: 719–24.

127. Kline SE, Hedemark LL, Davies SF. Outbreak of tuberculosis among regular patrons of a neighborhood bar. *N Engl J Med* 1995; **333**: 222–7.

128. Behr MA, Warren SA, Salamon H *et al.* Transmission of *Mycobacterium tuberculosis* from patients smear-negative for acid-fast bacilli. *Lancet* 1999; **353**: 444–9.

129. Hernandez-Garduno E, Cook V, Kunimoto D *et al.* Transmission of tuberculosis from smear negative patients: a molecular epidemiology study. *Thorax* 2004; **59**: 286–90.

130. Ong A, Creasman J, Hopewell PC *et al.* A molecular epidemiological assessment of extrapulmonary tuberculosis in San Francisco. *Clin Infect Dis* 2004; **38**: 25–31.

131. World Health Organization Global Tuberculosis Programme. *Global strategic plan.* Geneva: World Health Organization, 2006.

132. Veen J. Microepidemics of tuberculosis: the stone-in-the-pond principle. *Tuberc Lung Dis* 1992; **73**: 73–6.

133. Golub JE, Cronin WA, Obasanjo OO *et al.* Transmission of *Mycobacterium tuberculosis* through casual contact with an infectious case. *Arch Intern Med* 2001; **161**: 2254–8.

134. Daley CL. Tuberculosis contact investigations. Please don't fail me now. *Am J Respir Crit Care Med* 2004; **169**: 779–81.

135. Behr MA, Hopewell PC, Paz EA *et al.* Predictive value of contact investigation for identifying recent transmission of *Mycobacterium tuberculosis. Am J Respir Crit Care Med* 1998; **158**: 465–9.

136. Sun SJ, Bennett DE, Flood J *et al.* Identifying the sources of tuberculosis in young children: a multistate investigation. *Emerg Infect Dis* 2002; **8**: 1216–23.

137. Wootton SH, Gonzalez BE, Pawlak R *et al.* Epidemiology of pediatric tuberculosis using traditional and molecular techniques: Houston, Texas. *Pediatrics* 2005; **116**: 1141–7.

138. Bennett DE, Onorato IM, Ellis BA *et al.* DNA fingerprinting of *Mycobacterium tuberculosis* isolates from epidemiologically linked case pairs. *Emerg Infect Dis* 2002; **8**: 1224–9.

139. Kimerling ME, Benjamin WH, Lok KH *et al.* Restriction fragment length polymorphism screening of *Mycobacterium tuberculosis* isolates: population surveillance for targeting disease transmission in a community. *Int J Tuberc Lung Dis* 1998; **2**: 655–62.

140. Lemaitre N, Sougakoff W, Truffot-Pernot C *et al.* Use of DNA fingerprinting for primary surveillance of nosocomial tuberculosis in a large urban hospital: detection of outbreaks in homeless people and migrant workers. *Int J Tuberc Lung Dis* 1998; **2**: 390–96.

141. Barnes PF, Yang Z, Preston-Martin S *et al.* Patterns of tuberculosis transmission in central Los Angeles. *J Am Med Assoc* 1997; **278**: 1159–63.

142. Barnes PF, Yang Z, Pogoda JM *et al.* Foci of tuberculosis transmission in central Los Angeles. *Am J Respir Crit Care Med* 1999; **159**: 1081–6.

143. Verver S, Warren RM, Munch Z *et al.* Proportion of tuberculosis transmission that takes place in households in a high incidence area. *Lancet* 2004; **363**: 212–14.

144. Daley CL, Small PM, Schecter GF *et al.* An outbreak of tuberculosis with accelerated progression among persons infected with the human immunodeficiency virus. An analysis using restriction-fragment-length polymorphisms. *N Engl J Med* 1992; **326**: 231–5.

145. Yaganehdoost A, Graviss EA, Ross MW *et al.* Complex transmission dynamics of clonally related virulent *Mycobacterium tuberculosis* associated with barhopping by predominantly human immuno-deficiency virus-positive gay men. *J Infect Dis* 1999; **180**: 1245–51.

146. Garcia-Garcia M, Palacios-Martinez M, Ponce-de-Leon A *et al.* The role of core groups in transmitting *Mycobacterium tuberculosis* in a high prevalence community in Southern Mexico. *Int J Tuberc Lung Dis* 2000; **4**: 12–17.

147. Diel R, Meywald-Walter K, Gottschalk R *et al.* Ongoing outbreak of tuberculosis in a low incidence community: a molecular-epidemiologic evaluation. *Int J Tuberc Lung Dis* 2004; **8**: 855–61.

148. Leonhardt KK, Gentile F, Gilbert BP, Aiken M. A cluster of tuberculosis among crack house contacts in San Mateo County, California. *Am J Public Health* 1994; **84**: 1834–6.

149. Bock NN, Mallory JP, Mobley N *et al.* Outbreak of tuberculosis associated with a floating card game in the rural south: lessons for tuberculosis contact investigations. *Clin Infect Dis* 1998; **27**: 1221–6.

150. Bauer J, Kok-Jensen A, Faurschou P *et al.* A prospective evaluation of the clinical value of nation-wide DNA fingerprinting of tuberculosis isolates in Denmark. *Int J Tuberc Lung Dis* 2000; **4**: 295–9.

151. Kim SJ, Bai GH, Lee H *et al.* Transmission of *Mycobacterium tuberculosis* among high school students in Korea. *Int J Tuberc Lung Dis* 2001; **5**: 824–30.

152. Edlin BR, Tokars JI, Grieco MH *et al.* An outbreak of multidrug-resistant tuberculosis among hospitalized patients with the acquired immunodeficiency syndrome. *N Engl J Med* 1992; **326**: 1514–21.

153. Haas DW, Milton S, Kreiswirth BN et al. Nosocomial transmission of a drug-sensitive W-variant Mycobacterium tuberculosis strain among patients with acquired immunodeficiency syndrome in Tennessee. Infect Control Hosp Epidemiol 1998; 19: 635–9.

154. Hanau-Bercot B, Gremy I, Raskine L et al. A one-year prospective study (1994–1995) for a first evaluation of tuberculosis transmission in French prisons. Int J Tuberc Lung Dis 2000; 4: 853–9.

155. Mohle-Boetani JC, Miguelino V, Dewsnup D et al. Tuberculosis outbreak in a housing unit for human immunodeficiency virus-infected patients in a correctional facility: transmission risk factors and effective outbreak control. Clin Infect Dis 2002; 34: 668–76.

156. Mangura BT, Napolitano EC, Passannante MR, McDonald RJ, Reichman LB. Mycobacterium tuberculosis miniepidemic in a church gospel choir. Chest 1998; 113: 234–7.

157. Centers for Disease Control and Prevention. HIV-related tuberculosis in a transgender network – Baltimore, Maryland and New York City area, 1998–2000. MMWR Morb Mortal Wkly Rep 2000; 49: 317–20.

158. Jereb JA, Burwen DR, Dooley SW et al. Nosocomial outbreak of tuberculosis in a renal transplant unit: application of a new technique for restriction fragment length polymorphism analysis of Mycobacterium tuberculosis isolates. J Infect Dis 1993; 168: 1219–24.

159. Wilkinson D, Crump J, Pillay M, Sturm AW. Nosocomial transmission of tuberculosis in Africa documented by restriction fragment length polymorphism. Trans R Soc Trop Med Hyg 1997; 91: 318.

160. Frieden TR, Woodley CL, Crawford JT et al. The molecular epidemiology of tuberculosis in New York City: the importance of nosocomial transmission and laboratory error. Tuberc Lung Dis 1996; 77: 407–13.

161. Ikeda RM, Birkhead GS, DiFerdinando GT Jr et al. Nosocomial tuberculosis: an outbreak of a strain resistant to seven drugs. Infect Control Hosp Epidemiol 1995; 16: 152–9.

162. Johnson KR, Braden CR, Cairns KL et al. Transmission of Mycobacterium tuberculosis from medical waste. J Am Med Assoc 2000; 284: 1683–8.

163. Agerton T, Valway S, Gore B et al. Transmission of a highly drug-resistant straing (strain W1) of Mycobacterium tuberculosis. Community outbreak and nosocomial transmission via a contaminated bronchoscope. J Am Med Assoc 1997; 278: 1073–7.

164. Michele TM, Cronin WA, Graham NM et al. Transmission of Mycobacterium tuberculosis by a fiberoptic bronchoscope. Identification by DNA fingerprinting. J Am Med Assoc 1997; 278: 1093–5.

165. Dobbs KG, Lok KH, Bruce F et al. Value of Mycobacterium tuberculosis fingerprinting as a tool in a rural state surveillance program. Chest 2001; 120: 1877–82.

166. Chin DP, DeRiemer K, Small PM et al. Differences in contributing factors to tuberculosis incidence in US-born and foreign-born persons. Am J Respir Crit Care Med 1998; 158: 1797–803.

167. Cronin WA, Golub JE, Lathan MJ et al. Molecular epidemiology of tuberculosis in a low-to moderate-incidence state: Are contact investigations enough? Emerg Infect Dis 2002; 8: 1271–9.

168. Lillebaek T, Andersen AB, Dirksen A et al. Mycobacterium tuberculosis Beijing genotype. Emerg Infect Dis 2003; 9: 1553–7.

169. Borgdorff MW, Nagelkerke NJ, van Soolingen D et al. Analysis of tuberculosis transmission between nationalities in the Netherlands in the period 1993–1995 using DNA fingerprinting. Am J Epidemiol 1998; 15: 187–95.

170. Chin DP, Crane CM, Diul MY et al. Spread of Mycobacterium tuberculosis in a community implementing recommended elements of tuberculosis control. J Am Med Assoc 2000; 283: 2968–74.

171. McNabb SJN, Braden CR, Navin TR. DNA fingerprinting of Mycobacterium tuberculosis: lessons learned and implications for the future. Emerg Infect Dis 2002; 8: 1314–19.

172. Cattamanchi A, Hopewell PC, Gonzalez LC et al. A 13-year molecular epidemiological analysis of tuberculosis in San Francisco. Int J Tuberc Lung Dis 2006; 10: 297–304.

173. Kong PM, Tapy J, Calixto P et al. Skin-test screening and tuberculosis transmission among the homeless. Emerg Infect Dis 2002; 8: 1280–4.

174. Soborg C, Soborg B, Pouelsen S et al. Doubling of the tuberculosis incidence in Greenland over an 8-year period (1990–1997). Int J Tuberc Lung Dis 2001; 5: 257–65.

4

Mycobacterium tuberculosis: the organism

JOHN M GRANGE

INTRODUCTION

The question of whether tuberculosis was due to a transmissible agent or to an inherited disposition was a subject of controversy in the nineteenth century. The establishment of the germ theory of disease by Louis Pasteur and the demonstration by Pasteur's pupil Jean Antoine Villemin in 1868 that inoculation of tuberculous material from humans and cattle into rabbits elicited characteristic granulomatous lesions swung the argument strongly in favour of an infectious cause. The matter was finally and irrefutably settled on 24 March 1882, when Robert Koch described the series of meticulous studies in which he had not only isolated the causative bacillus but, by means of his well-known postulates, clearly confirmed its aetiological role in tuberculosis.

Koch simply termed his isolate *Tuberkelbazillus* (tubercle bacillus) but in 1891 this, and the leprosy bacillus, was included in the genus *Mycobacterium*. This name, meaning 'fungus-bacterium', refers to the fungus-like pellicles formed by tubercle bacilli on liquid media. The leprosy bacillus, *Mycobacterium leprae*, has resisted attempts to this day to cultivate it on laboratory media, but was included in this genus as it shares a characteristic staining property with the tubercle bacillus, namely acid-fastness.

It originally appeared that all strains of *Mycobacterium tuberculosis*, whether isolated from humans or cattle, were identical but in 1898 Theobald Smith reported small but constant differences between isolates from these two sources.[1] He therefore termed them human and bovine tubercle bacilli but it was only many years later, in 1970, that the species name *Mycobacterium bovis* was formally introduced.

During the late nineteenth and early twentieth centuries, acid-fast bacilli were isolated from mammals, birds, reptiles and amphibians and also from environmental sources such as grass, water and compost. Initially these were regarded as 'atypical tubercle bacilli', but were later recognized as distinct species. The classification of these other mycobacteria was chaotic and many species names were introduced, but some degree of order emerged in the 1950s when Ernest Runyon assigned them to four groups according to their pigmentation and growth rate *in vitro*, as shown in Table 4.1.[2] Runyon's pioneering work led to the establishment of the International Working Group on Mycobacterial Taxonomy (IWGMT), which clearly characterized and defined the then-known species.[3]

Despite this work, many anomalies and confusions lingered in the nomenclature of the mycobacteria, as well as in other areas of bacterial taxonomy, so in 1980 the

Table 4.1 Runyon's four groups of mycobacteria.

Group	Pigmentation	Growth rate	Examples
I	Photochromogens	Slow	*M. kansasii, M. marinum*
II	Scotochromogens	Slow	*M. scrofulaceum, M. gordonae*
III	Nonchromogens	Slow	*M. avium, M. malmoense*
IV	Rapid growers	Rapid[a]	*M. fortuitum, M. chelonae*

[a]Defined as visible growth on solid culture media within 1 week on subculture.

Approved Lists of Bacterial Names were published to serve as the reference point for all further nomenclature.[4] This list contained 41 species of mycobacteria, but many more have since been described and by 2007 well over 100 species had been formally published. For many years mycobacterial species were defined by a wide range of cultural and metabolic characteristics until this approach was supplemented and largely superseded by nucleic acid-based technology. Currently, the method of choice for defining mycobacterial species is 'ribotyping', based on differences in highly conserved regions of the genome, the DNA coding for 16S and 23S ribosomal RNA.[5]

The genus *Mycobacterium* contains the obligate pathogens responsible for human and mammalian tuberculosis and leprosy, but most of the many named species live freely in the environment, particularly in watery situations such as marshes, rivers and piped water systems.[6,7] As described in Chapter 29, Environmental mycobacteria, some of these species cause opportunist human disease, particularly in those whose immune systems are compromised. There is also evidence that exposure of the human population to these other species may affect immune responses manifesting as low degrees of tuberculin reactivity,[8] and they may also, in various ways, interfere with protective immunity conferred by bacille Calmette–Guérin (BCG) vaccination.[9,10] This may well explain the wide regional variation in the protective efficacy of BCG.

THE 'TUBERCLE BACILLUS'

The nomenclature of the causative organisms of human and mammalian tuberculosis is a source of some confusion and is not entirely logical. As described below, analysis of their genomes has shown that these bacilli, grouped in the *M. tuberculosis* complex, are very closely related, with less than 0.1 per cent genomic difference between them, and thus they clearly belong to what should be regarded as a single species. Nevertheless, they are currently allocated to seven named species (listed in Table 4.2), partly for historical reasons and partly on account of their considerable differences in host ranges and epidemiological behaviour.

The great majority of strains of *M. tuberculosis* produce rough colonies resembling bread crumbs or small cauliflowers on solid media, but one very uncommon variant, termed the Canetti type and also but unofficially '*Mycobacterium canettii*',[11] produces smooth colonies. As described below, this variant is closely related to an ancestral form of *M. tuberculosis*.

Strains of *M. bovis* differ from *M. tuberculosis* in several respects, including resistance to the antituberculosis agent pyrazinamide, but isolates susceptible to this agent though in most other respects similar to *M. bovis* have been isolated from animals, principally goats, in Spain and Germany. As there are genomic differences between these strains and *M. bovis* they have been allocated to the separate species *Mycobacterium caprae*.[12] Very rare strains of otherwise typical *M. bovis* are also susceptible to pyrazinamide.

Table 4.2 Members of the *Mycobacterium tuberculosis* complex with specific names.

Species	Principal hosts	Humans as secondary hosts
M. tuberculosis	Humans	–
M. bovis	Cattle, deer, elk, bison, badger, opossum	Yes
M. caprae	Goats	Yes
M. africanum	Humans	–
M. microti	Vole, hyrax, llama	Very rare
'*M. canettii*'	Humans	–
M. pinnipedii	Seal	Very rare

Tuberculosis caused by *M. caprae* has also been reported in humans, notably in Germany where one-third of 166 strains of human origin initially identified as *M. bovis*, isolated between 1999 and 2001 from patients principally living in south Germany, were found to be *M. caprae*.[13] The patients were in the same elderly age range as those infected with classical *M. bovis*, suggesting that disease due to both types represent reactivation of old infections.

An important 'man-made' variant of *M. bovis* is the BCG vaccine which was derived by 230 subcultivations on a potato-bile medium between the years 1908 and 1921, from a strain ('Lait Nocard') isolated from a case of bovine mastitis. The Institut Pasteur initially maintained three lines of this vaccine on different media, but from 1932 only one line, grown on an antigen-free medium, has been maintained. Some currently available daughter strains of BCG, including the Brazilian, Japanese, Romanian, Russian and Swedish strains, were issued before 1932. These differ from those daughter strains issued after this date in their cell wall structure, their active secretion of an antigenic protein MPB70 and in having two copies, rather than one, of the insertion sequence IS*6110* (see below).[14] As the efficacy of BCG varies so much from region to region, it is not known whether these two groups of daughter strains differ in their ability to induce protective immunity to tuberculosis.

A group of tubercle bacilli principally isolated from humans in equatorial Africa and in migrants from that region have properties intermediate between *M. tuberculosis* and *M. bovis* and have been given the separate species name *Mycobacterium africanum*. There are geographical differences in this species with Type I strains, principally from West Africa, resembling *M. bovis* and Type II, common in East Africa, resembling *M. tuberculosis* (Table 4.3).[15] Human disease due to *M. africanum* appears to be identical to that caused by classical *M. tuberculosis*.

In addition to *M. bovis*, strains clearly belonging to the *M. tuberculosis* complex but with unique distinguishing

Table 4.3 Differentiation of *Mycobacterium africanum* Types I and II from *Mycobacterium tuberculosis* and *Mycobacterium bovis* on the basis of simple cultural properties.[17]

Species	Nitratase activity	Oxygen preference	Susceptibility to pyrazinamide	Pyrazinamidase activity	Susceptibility to TCH[a]
M. tuberculosis	Positive	Aerobic	Susceptible	Positive	Resistant
M. africanum I	Negative	Micro-aerophilic	Susceptible	Positive	Susceptible
M. africanum II	Positive	Micro-aerophilic	Susceptible	Positive	Susceptible
M. bovis	Negative	Micro-aerophilic	Resistant	Negative	Susceptible
BCG	Negative	Aerobic	Resistant	Negative	Susceptible

[a]Thiophen-2-carboxylic acid hydrazide. The Asian or South Indian variants of *M. tuberculosis* are susceptible.
BCG, bacille Calmette–Guérin.

properties cause disease in various animals, with humans as very rare secondary hosts. The first to be described was *Mycobacteria microti*, so named because it was first isolated from the vole, *Microtus agrestis*, and originally termed the vole tubercle bacillus. It is attenuated in humans, having the same order of virulence as BCG vaccine, and for this reason it was evaluated as a vaccine for human use in comparison with BCG in clinical trials conducted by the British Medical Research Council.[16] The two vaccines were equally protective against tuberculosis but *M. microti* was associated with a slightly higher incidence of local complications. A very similar organism has been isolated from the dassie or rock hyrax and the llama.[17]

A very few cases of human tuberculosis due to *M. microti* have been described in immunocompromised patients but also, surprisingly in view of their low virulence, in those who were apparently immunocompetent.[18]

Another cluster of strains with sufficient genomic differences to justify the separate species name *Mycobacterium pinnipedii* were isolated from tuberculous lesions in free and captive seals and sea lions in Australia, New Zealand and South America, and in an Australian seal trainer.[19] Strains with distinct features have been isolated from tuberculous lesions in other animals including oryx, water buffalo and cats, but have not been given separate species names.

In the past, certain mycobacteria causing tuberculosis-like disease in birds, amphibia, reptiles and fish were termed tubercle bacilli, but they are now recognized as distinct species of environmental mycobacteria. The bird or avian tubercle bacillus is a member of the *Mycobacterium avium* complex which, as described in Chapter 29, is the most important group of environmental mycobacteria causing opportunist human disease.

THE GENOME OF *M. TUBERCULOSIS*

Among the greatest achievements in the study of *M. tuberculosis* was the huge collaborative effort to sequence its entire genome. This cooperative study, published in 1998,[20] was based on a widely used reference strain, H37Rv, of *M. tuberculosis* and revealed that the genome of this strain contains 4 411 529 base pairs and around 4000 genes. This genome is not as large as that of *Escherichia coli*, but is larger than that of many bacteria.

The genome of *M. bovis* has been sequenced and shows over 99.95 per cent similarity with that of *M. tuberculosis* although it is very slightly smaller, with 4 345 492 base pairs.[21] Other species whose genomes have been sequenced include the leprosy bacillus, *M. leprae*. With 3.27 million base pairs, the genome of this species is considerably smaller than that of *M. tuberculosis* and it differs from the latter in that many of its genes, around half, are defective and non-functional,[22] explaining why this organism has never been cultivated *in vitro* and is an obligate intracellular pathogen.[23]

The chemical structure of the genome of *M. tuberculosis* is remarkably uniform with a high guanine + cytosine content (65.6 per cent) throughout, indicating that it has evolved with minimal incorporation of DNA from extraneous sources. Other notable differences between this genome and those of other bacteria have been determined. In particular, *M. tuberculosis* has a very large number of genes coding for enzymes involved in lipid metabolism, around 250 compared with only 50 in *E. coli*. All known lipid biosynthetic pathways encountered elsewhere in nature, and in addition several unique ones, are detectable in the mycobacteria. Most of these enzymes are involved in the synthesis of the extremely complex lipid-rich mycobacterial cell walls.

The mycobacterial genome is also unique in containing a large number of genes, up to 10 per cent of the total coding potential, containing polymorphic GC-repetitive sequences (PGRS). These genes code for two unrelated families (PE and PPE) of acidic, glycine-rich proteins. The function of most of these genes and their products is unknown,[20,24] but there is evidence that these genes are responsible for diversity in antigenic structure and virulence and, as they undergo frequent genetic remodelling by gene duplication, recombination and other mechanisms, they may have contributed substantially to the evolution of the *M. tuberculosis* complex and adaptation of its various members to different hosts.[25,26]

Four main types of genomic differences between strains within the *M. tuberculosis* complex have been described: those involving just a single nucleotide variation, the so-called single nucleotide polymorphisms (SNPs),[27] those involving several sequential nucleotides and termed large sequence polymorphisms (LSPs), minisatellites and microsatellites. Although there are 1075 SNP differences between *M. tuberculosis* H37Rv and a recent clinical isolate, CDC1551, and 2437 between H37Rv and the sequenced strain of *M. bovis*, these differences are small in relation to the 4 million or more nucleotide pairs in the genomes of these strains.

The LSPs are much fewer in number than the SNPs in the *M. tuberculosis* complex and include 20 well-defined regions of difference (RD) which are described below.

Minisatellites and microsattelites are unstable regions found in the genomes of all forms of life and consist of small, often repetitive, chains of nucleotides, which are respectively of 40–100 base pairs and up to 6 base pairs in length. The function of bacterial minisatellites is unknown, but their analogues in eukaryotic genomes appear to contribute to genetic diversity by mediating chromosome recombination during mitosis.[28] In the mycobacteria they often occur as tandem repeats in the regions between functional genes and some are designated 'mycobacterial interspersed repetitive units' (MIRU). Minisatellites are utilized in a typing system known as variable number tandem repeat (VNTR) analysis, as described in Chapter 3, Genotyping and its implications for transmission dynamics and tuberculosis control. Microsatellites, by insertion or deletion, cause reversible frame shift mutations at a relatively high rate. It is thought that satellite activity imparts a genetic 'plasticity' to the genomes of pathogens, enabling them to adapt readily to different hosts.[29]

In addition to its relatively stable structure, the genome of *M. tuberculosis* contains a number of mobile units of DNA, also known as 'jumping genes', which contribute to genetic variation and evolution. These mobile elements include a class termed insertion sequences (IS) of which 56 different types, belonging to various families, are present in the genome of strain H37Rv. Most, but not all, strains of *M. tuberculosis* contain copies, usually numbering from 4 to 14, of the insertion sequence IS*6110*.[30] With some exceptions, strains of *M. bovis* contain fewer copies of IS*6110* than *M. tuberculosis*, with daughter strains of BCG containing either one or two copies. The considerable variation in the numbers and position of copies of IS*6110* between strains forms the basis of the restriction fragment length polymorphism (RFLP) typing system used for epidemiological purposes as described in Chapter 3.

An additional typing scheme which is gaining increasing popularity is spacer oligonucleotide typing or 'spoligotyping',[31] which has the advantage that it can be performed on PCR products, thereby avoiding the need for isolating the strains in culture. This typing scheme is based on the characterization of repeated sequences in structurally unique regions of the genome of members of the *M. tuberculosis* complex termed the direct repeat (DR) locus. This locus consists of repetitive 36 base-pair units of DNA separated by non-repetitive 34–41 base-pair spacer oligonucleotides which can be amplified by just one pair of PCR primers. There are numerous possible combinations of spacer oligonucleotides and these are very stable, providing a highly discriminative typing scheme as described in Chapter 3. There is evidence that variation in the DR locus is due to mutational events in the spacer oligonucleotides, including their disruption by translocations of the insertion sequence IS*6110*.[32] These mutational events occur at a very slow rate and serve as an evolutionary 'clock'.

The DR region of *M. tuberculosis* is an example of a region present in all bacterial genomes and termed 'clustered regularly interspaced short palindromic repeats' (CRISPA). The function of this region is unknown, but it may be the bacterial analogue of the centromere found in euykaryocyte chromosomes.

THE 'DEVOLUTION' OF THE *M. TUBERCULOSIS* COMPLEX

Two widely held assumptions concerning the origin of the various species within the *M. tuberculosis* complex have been seriously challenged. The first assumption was that the ancestral form of the complex was *M. bovis* and that *M. tuberculosis* developed by mutations, resulting in the more restricted host range, following an animal-to-human jump of the ancestral type at that period in human history when animals were domesticated. The second assumption was that, in common with all forms of life, the variants within this complex, as well as those within other mycobacterial species, developed principally by a process of evolution and natural selection.

In 1973 it was postulated that, on the basis of simple cultural and biochemical differences, variation within a mycobacterial species is not so much due to the evolutionary acquisition of new properties as to deletional loss of properties from an ancestral 'common progenitor type'.[33] Developments in nucleic acid technology made it possible to confirm that this is indeed the principal way that the present-day variants within the *M. tuberculosis* complex arose. It thus appears highly likely that the ancestral member of the complex, '*Mycobacterium prototuberculosis*', appeared around 3 million years ago and may have caused disease in the ancestors of modern humans.[34] It also appears that this ancestral form more closely resembled *M. tuberculosis* than *M. bovis* as the latter differs from that of the former only by genetic deletion, having no unique genes of its own. Most of the differences between the two species are in genes determining synthesis of cell wall lipids, secreted antigenic proteins and cell wall PE proteins (see above) which may play a role in determining the different host ranges.[26] In general, the differences between the two species appear more due to variations in gene expression and regulation than in the genes themselves.

The various species in the *M. tuberculosis* complex principally differ from each other by presence or absence of the regions of difference, described above.[35] Fourteen such regions, designated RD1 to RD14, varying in size from 2 to 12.7 kilobases, are present in *M. tuberculosis* H37Rv, the strain selected for sequencing of the entire genome, and a further six regions, designated RvD1 to RvD5 and TbD1, are absent from strain H37Rv, but present to a varying extent in other, more recently isolated, strains of *M. tuberculosis*.

Strains of *M. microti* and *M. bovis* possess the six regions that are absent in H37Rv, but they lack several of the other RDs, principally RD7 to RD10, and *M. microti* has a specific deletion, RD[mic]. Strains of *M. africanum* mostly possess the six regions absent in H37Rv, but lack some other RDs, principally RD9. The Institut Pasteur strain of BCG shows a particularly large number of deletions lacking RD1 to RD14 present in H37Rv. The loss of RD1, which is present in *M. bovis*, but not in any of the daughter strains of BCG may explain the loss of virulence of the latter, especially as it is also absent from *M. microti*, which is of the same order of virulence for humans as BCG.[36] In this context, genes coding for the early secreted antigenic target, 6 kDa (ESAT-6), an important determinant of virulence in humans, are located in RD1.

The various species within the *M. tuberculosis* complex may be differentiated one from another and distinguished from other mycobacterial species on the basis of their RD profiles by use of a PCR-based technique.[37,38]

Most of the strains of '*M. canettii*' possess the full complement of the RD and RvD regions and TbD1 and it has thus been postulated that they are the closest genetically to the common progenitor form of the *M. tuberculosis* complex. Strains of *M. tuberculosis* are divisible into 'ancestral' and 'modern' strains according, respectively, to the presence or absence of the RD TbD1.[34,35]

It appears likely that '*M. canetti*' and the ancestral form of *M. tuberculosis* diverged from the common progenitor at an early stage, followed later by the divergence of *M. africanum*, *M. bovis* and *M. microti* (Figure 4.1). Subsequently, the 'modern' genotypes of *M. tuberculosis* arose from the 'ancestral' strains by deletional events, notably the loss of the TbD1 region of difference. Although 'ancestral' strains are still encountered in some parts of the world, the global spread of tuberculosis has been mostly due to 'modern' strains.

LINEAGES WITHIN THE *M. TUBERCULOSIS* COMPLEX

Once thought to be homogeneous, the human tubercle bacillus, *M. tuberculosis*, has been shown to contain several types that appear to have differing implications for human health. One of the first major variants in this species to be

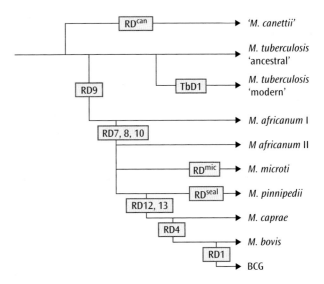

Figure 4.1 The devolutionary pathway of diversification within the *Mycobacterium tuberculosis* complex by loss of the indicated RDs.

described was the so-called Asian or south Indian type which differs from the predominant strains in Europe in several characteristics, including low virulence in the guinea pig, unique cell wall lipids and a distinct bacteriophage type.[39] This type is much more common among immigrants of Indian subcontinent ethnic origin than among the indigenous population in the United Kingdom and, although the former have a higher incidence of nonpulmonary manifestations of tuberculosis, the type of disease is not determined by the causative organism.[40]

The subsequent development of techniques for genomic analysis has revealed that *M. tuberculosis* and related species within the complex are divisible into various groups, termed lineages, families, superfamilies or clades.

There is, at the time of writing, no agreed definition of, or nomenclature for, the described lineages. Thus, they have been variously defined on the basis of spoligotyping,[41] single nucleotide polymorphisms[42] or large sequence polymorphisms,[28] but grouping by these several methods does not completely coincide. Recognized lineages include Beijing (or W/Beijing), Central Asian, East Asian (which includes the Beijing lineage), East African-Indian, West African 1 and 2 (including some strains of *M. africanum*) Indo-Oceanic, Haarlem, Euro-American, Latin American Mediterranean, Manu, S, T and X. By application of spoligotyping, a total of 62 lineages and sublineages within the *M. tuberculosis* complex have been defined and include three sublineages of *M. bovis* and two of *M. pinnipedii*.[41] Several simplified schemes for the division of *M. tuberculosis* into lineages have been proposed, including one that delineates six lineages of practical relevance to epidemiology, pathogenesis and the development of new tools for tuberculosis control.[43] There is also evidence that strains with high and low copy numbers of IS*6110* demonstrated by RFLP typing reflect different evolutionary pathways.[41]

Division of *M. tuberculosis* into lineages is of considerable epidemiological interest as there is evidence that strains within the various lineages differ in their virulence and their ability to progress from infection to overt and infectious disease.[43] The ability of lineages to spread worldwide is expressed mathematically as their spreading index (SI).[42] Those with a high SI are defined as 'epidemic' and include the Beijing lineage which is now found in many parts of the world.[44] Maps of the distribution of six common lineages throughout the world are available.[41] There is also evidence that even within the Beijing lineage there are distinct evolutionary groups that differ in their pathogenic characteristics.[45]

In addition, there is evidence that lineages vary in the extent to which they lose virulence on acquisition of drug or multidrug resistance.[46] Multidrug resistant strains of the Beijing lineage appear to retain high virulence and have thus been implicated in the epidemic spread of multidrug-resistant tuberculosis in certain regions.[47]

GROWTH CHARACTERISTICS AND METABOLISM OF MYCOBACTERIA

The mycobacteria are non-sporing and non-flagellate. In clinical specimens, members of the *M. tuberculosis* usually appear microscopically as slightly curved rods, singly or in small clumps. Members of some other mycobacterial species may be spherical (coccoid) or, particularly in the case of *Mycobacterium xenopi*, *Mycobacterium marinum* and *Mycobacterium kansasi*, may be long and filamentous. The presence of lipid storage granules may give mycobacterial cells a distinct banded or beaded appearance. In practice, though, the cellular morphology of mycobacteria in clinical specimens is so variable, particularly in patients who have received any form of antimicrobial therapy, that laboratory reports should merely state whether or not acid-fast bacilli were seen. Within the living host, tubercle bacilli produce tubular protein structures resembling the pili or fimbriae of other pathogenic bacteria and which facilitate adherence to host cells.[48]

Although mycobacteria are Gram positive, they stain poorly by this method. They do, however, have a staining property that is almost unique to them; namely, acid-fastness, which is based on their ability to retain the red colour imparted by staining with carbol fuchsin or a related arylmethane dye when treated with a dilute mineral acid. Mycobacteria are therefore commonly called acid-fast bacilli (AFB). Some workers use a mixture of acid and alcohol in the staining procedure as this reduces the number of stained artefacts, but does not, as is sometimes erroneously claimed, differentiate between members of the *M. tuberculosis* complex and species of environmental mycobacteria. Bacterial spores and members of the genus *Nocardia* are weakly acid-fast.

The original acid-fast staining technique was described by Paul Ehrlich who used it to visualize tubercle bacilli in sputum, including his own! The widely used method today is named after Ziehl and Neelsen, who introduced certain modifications to Ehrlich's technique, and is therefore termed the Ziehl–Neelsen (ZN) method. In this procedure, slides are stained with hot carbol fuchsin, decolourized with a dilute mineral acid in water or alcohol and counterstained with a dye, such as malachite green or methyl blue, so that mycobacteria appear as red organisms against a background of contrasting colour. Fluorescent staining techniques are likewise based on the acid-fast property and are more user-friendly than the standard method as specimens may be screened under low magnification, with more careful examination of fluorescing spots under higher power. Technical details for tuberculosis microscopy as well as the organization of laboratory services are given elsewhere.[49]

With few exceptions mycobacteria have simple nutritional requirements. The most widely used medium for tuberculosis bacteriology is Löwenstein–Jensen (LJ) medium, which contains glycerol, mineral salts and chicken eggs. The latter supply various nutrients and enable the medium to be solidified by heating at 80–85°C. This medium also contains malachite green, which aids the visualization of colonies of *M. tuberculosis* which are 'buff', creamy or off-white in colour and thus of a similar colour to the medium without the dye. Colonies of *M. tuberculosis* on LJ medium are usually visible after 2–6 weeks' incubation and have been described as heaped-up or 'eugonic', resembling small cauliflowers or breadcrumbs. By contrast, *M. bovis* grows poorly, or not at all, on standard LJ medium with, at best, small and flat 'dysgonic' colonies. This is due to defects in several genes of *M. bovis* involved in the phosphorylation of glucose and the formation of pyruvate,[20] and growth may be enhanced by using medium in which glycerol is replaced by sodium pyruvate. Other species within the *M. tuberculosis* complex vary in their preference for glycerol and pyruvate so ideally both types of media should be used for diagnostic purposes.

Egg is not essential for mycobacterial growth, and various simple synthetic media, either liquid or solidified with agar, are used for various purposes.[49] In particular, liquid media are used in automated mycobacterial culture systems (see Chapter 5, The diagnosis of tuberculosis).

Most species within the *M. tuberculosis* complex are strict aerobes. A notable exception is *M. bovis*, which is microaerophilic, growing preferably in conditions of low oxygen tension. A simple test for distinguishing between *M. tuberculosis* and *M. bovis* is based on this property as, when inoculated into a soft agar-based medium, the former grows on the surface and the latter a few millimetres below the surface.

THE CELL ENVELOPE OF *M. TUBERCULOSIS*

The most characteristic and distinguishing feature of the genus *Mycobacterium*, the one responsible for its acid-fastness and several other unique properties, is its extremely

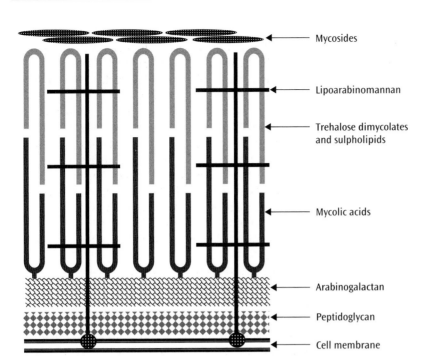

— Mycosides

— Lipoarabinomannan

— Trehalose dimycolates and sulpholipids

— Mycolic acids

— Arabinogalactan

— Peptidoglycan

— Cell membrane

Figure 4.2 A diagrammatic representation of the mycobacterial cell wall.

complex and lipid-rich cell wall. Indeed, the mycobacterial cell wall is the most complex in all of nature and, as discussed above, an unusually large number of biosynthetic pathways are involved in its synthesis.

The cell membrane which lies deep to the cell wall has much in common with that of other bacteria, essentially consisting of two phospholipid layers and incorporating various enzymes involved in energy production.

The structure of the complex cell wall is shown diagrammatically in Figure 4.2.[50] The innermost layer is composed of peptidoglycan or murein consisting of long polysaccharide chains cross-linked by short peptides consisting of four amino acids. This net-like macromolecule is very similar to that of other bacteria and contributes to the shape and rigidity of the bacterial cells.

External to the peptidoglycan is another net-like macromolecule, a branched polysaccharide consisting of arabinose and galactose, and termed arabinogalactan.[51] External to this structure is one of the principal components of the mycobacterial cell wall – a dense palisade of mycolic acids, long-chain fatty acids that give the cell wall its thickness and acid-fast staining properties. In their basic structure, the mycolic acids are aliphatic fatty acids with two chains, a short one containing 22–26 carbon atoms and a long one containing 50–56 carbon atoms. The cell walls of related genera such as *Nocardia* and *Corynebacterium* contain similar structures, but with shorter chains. The basic aliphatic chains of the mycolic acids may contain methyl side chains, oxygen-containing (methoxy) groups, unsaturated bonds and cyclopropane rings. The latter contribute to the structural integrity of the cell wall and play a role in virulence by protecting the mycobacteria against toxic oxygen derivatives.[52] The genes and enzymes involved in the synthesis of mycolic acids

have been well characterized,[53] but the processes involved in their transportation to, and assembly in, the cell wall is less well understood. In the *M. tuberculosis* complex, a group of three structurally related antigenically dominant secreted proteins forming the antigen 85 (Ag85) group are involved in the final stages of cell wall synthesis.[54] As outlined below, cell wall synthesis and assembly are important actual and potential targets for antituberculosis drugs.

External to the mycolic acid palisade is a layer formed by related long-chain fatty acids, the trehalose dimycolates and sulpholipids. The former are termed 'cord factors' as they were thought to be responsible for the characteristic 'serpentine cord' arrangement of cells of *M. tuberculosis* in

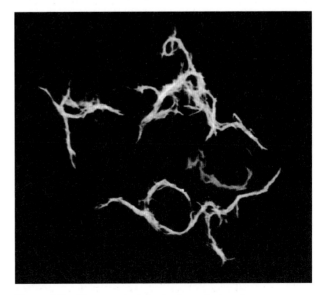

Figure 4.3 Fluorescent-stained microcolonies of *Mycobacterium tuberculosis* showing cord formation.

microcolonies (Figure 4.3). These lipids were once thought to be major determinants of virulence of *M. tuberculosis*, but this is now controversial, although, by inducing various cytokines, they have a number of effects on the host–pathogen relationship.[55] In addition, trehalose dimycolates appear to play a role in virulence by adversely influencing early interactions of the infecting organism with the innate immune system.[55]

Lipoarabinomannan (LAM), composed of arabinose and mannan, is another branched polysaccharide in the mycobacterial cell wall. It is anchored by a phospholipid to the cell membrane and reaches up to the surface of the cell wall, possibly acting as an anchor for other cell wall molecular structures. As both an adjuvant and an antigen, LAM has a crucial role in determining the nature of the host immune response.[56,57] As an adjuvant it determines the pattern and regulation of the immune response by interacting with effector molecules of the innate immune system, the Toll-like receptors, on antigen-presenting cells.[58] Two types of LAM have been described – AraLAM and ManLAM – with their branches being capped with, respectively, arabinose and mannan. The ManLAM variant, found in the *M. tuberculosis* complex, has been shown to enhance entry of the bacilli into macrophages and their survival within these cells.[59]

Complex molecules termed 'mycosides' are located on the surface of the mycobacterial cell wall.[50] Most mycosides are peptidoglycolipids, consisting of peptides, lipids (mycoserosic acids) and carbohydrates. A related class, the phenolic glycolipids or phenol-phthiocerol dimycoserosates, lack the peptide component. They appear as ribbon-like structures under the electron microscope and they may be abundant enough in some species, but not the *M. tuberculosis* complex, to form pseudo-capsules.

Being situated on the surface, the mycosides serve as receptors for bacteriophages and form the cell-surface antigens that determine agglutination serotypes in some species (see below). Their role in virulence is uncertain, but a phenolic glycolipid isolated from a particularly virulent strain of *M. tuberculosis* has been shown to inhibit innate immune responses.[60]

The mycobacterial cell wall is 100 to 1000 times less permeable to hydrophilic molecules than most other bacteria. Permeability is facilitated by channel-forming protein structures termed 'porins', of which there are at least two types in *M. tuberculosis*.[61] Some forms of pyrazinamide resistance are due to mutational changes in porin structure.[62]

Mycobacteria are dependent on iron for growth and a group of cell wall lipids termed 'mycobactins', which show considerable structural variation between species, are involved in the chelation, transport and storage of this element.[63]

ANTIGENIC STRUCTURE OF MYCOBACTERIA

The mycobacteria express a large range of antigens, some of which are in the cytoplasm, some in the cell wall and some are actively secreted. They play a key role in eliciting the various immune responses to mycobacteria and have been utilized in a number of diagnostic tests. In some cases, antigens are well defined chemically, such as the cell wall polysaccharides and the mycosides, while antigenic proteins, of which around 200 are demonstrable by two-dimensional immunoelectrophoresis in gel, are characterized and defined by their size in kilodaltons, their amino acid sequences and their mass spectroscopic patterns.[64]

Antigenic analysis has been used to classify the genus *Mycobacterium*. Antigens demonstrable by double immunodiffusion in gel are divisible into those shared by all mycobacteria and to some extent by related genera (group I), those restricted to slowly growing species (group II), those found in rapidly growing species and shared with nocardiae (group III) and those unique to each species (group IV).[65] Group I antigens contain the so-called chaperone proteins, or chaperonins, including a class known as heat-shock proteins (HSPs). These have a high amino acid sequence homology with HSPs in mammalian cells and thus, by cross-reactivity, may induce various autoimmune phenomena seen in mycobacterial disease.[66]

Old tuberculin is a crude preparation of antigens prepared by heat concentration of old and autolysed broth cultures of *M. tuberculosis* and contains the groups of antigens described above. Purified protein derivative (PPD) used in tuberculin testing is similar to old tuberculin, except that protein antigens are separated from carbohydrate antigens and components of the medium, thereby reducing the incidence of non-specific tuberculin reactions, but not cross-reactions due to prior BCG vaccination or contact with environmental mycobacteria. More recent immunodiagnostic tests for tuberculosis are based on T-cell recognition of purified antigens that are specific, or almost specific, for *M. tuberculosis* such as the secreted antigen ESAT-6 which is not produced by BCG. These tests are described in Chapter 6, Immunodiagnostic tests.

Strains of mycobacteria from which smooth suspensions can be prepared are divisible into serotypes by agglutination serology which detects antigenic differences in the mycosides on the cell surfaces. Now superseded by nucleic acid-based technology, agglutination typing was principally used to subdivide the *M. avium* complex for epidemiological purposes.[67] The technique could not be applied to the strains within the *M. tuberculosis* complex as suspensions of these readily auto-agglutinate.

A few protein antigens are actively secreted and are thus encountered by the immune system soon after infection. These include the 6 kDa early secreted antigenic target (ESAT-6) described below.

MECHANISMS OF RESISTANCE TO ANTITUBERCULOSIS AGENTS

Members of the *M. tuberculosis* complex are naturally resistant to many of the antibiotics and other agents used

Table 4.4 Targets of antituberculosis agents and the genes encoding them.

Agent	Target molecule or function	Genes encoding targets or the site of resistance–determining mutations
Isoniazid	Mycolic acid synthesis	katG, inhA and its promoter region, oxyR-ahpC intergenic region
Rifampicin	DNA-dependent RNA polymerase	rpoB
Pyrazinamide	Cell membrane energy function	pncA
Ethambutol	Arabinogalactan synthesis	embA, embB, embC
Streptomycin	Ribosomal protein S12	rpsL
Ethionamide and prothionamide	Mycolic acid synthesis	ethA, inhA and its promoter region
Capreomycin and viomycin	50S and 30S ribosomal subunit	vicA (50S), vicB (30S)
Cycloserine	Peptidoglycan synthesis	alrA
Clofazimine	? RNA polymerase	Unknown
p-aminosalicylic acid	Folic acid synthesis	Unknown

to treat bacterial disease. There are, on the other hand, several synthetic agents used specifically for the treatment of tuberculosis, notably three of the four first-line drugs – isoniazid, ethambutol and pyrazinamide – and also ethionamide and the closely related prothionamide.

The modes of action and the target structures of most of the antituberculosis agents have been characterized and are listed in Table 4.4. The characterization of the mutations responsible for drug resistance has led to the development of rapid molecular methods for detecting such resistance,[68] and kits for determining resistance to rifampicin and isoniazid are commercially available.[69]

Rifampicin

The mechanism of action of this antibiotic against mycobacteria is the same as in other bacterial genera; namely, blocking the activity of bacterial DNA-dependent RNA polymerase, thereby inhibiting synthesis of mRNA and new protein chains. Resistance is determined by one of several single amino acid mutations tightly clustered in a short region of the rpoB gene, which encodes for the b subunit of the polymerase enzyme.[70]

Isoniazid

This is a pro-drug requiring oxidative activation by the mycobacterial catalase peroxidase enzyme KatG. The most frequent mutations determining isoniazid resistance occur in the katG gene, but resistance is also due to mutations in the inhA locus or its promoter region and in the intergenic region of the oxyR-ahpC locus. The inhA locus codes for the enzyme enoyl-acyl carrier protein reductase which is involved in mycolic acid synthesis and is a target for isoniazid. The oxyR-ahpC locus is, like the katG locus, involved in protection against oxidative stress, but it is not clear why

mutations in this locus cause resistance to isoniazid. The relative frequency of the various mutations conferring resistance to isoniazid vary according to the lineages, described above, of M. tuberculosis and therefore show geographical differences in their distribution.[71]

Isoniazid is inactivated in vivo by acetylation and humans are divisible into rapid and slow inactivators.[72] In addition, mycobacteria possess a polymorphic arylamine N-acetyltransferase enzyme involved in mycolic acid synthesis which, by local acetylation of INH, may contribute to resistance to this agent.[73]

Pyrazinamide

The mode of action of this unusual drug is not fully understood, but there is evidence that it disrupts energy-generating processes in the bacterial membrane.[74] It has a powerful sterilizing activity against slowly replicating tubercle bacilli in acidic and anoxic or hypoxic inflammatory lesions,[75] and is therefore most effective during the early stage of therapy before inflammation has subsided. Pyrazinamide is a pro-drug which passively diffuses into the bacterial cell where it is converted to the active metabolite pyrazinoic acid by mycobacterial pyrazinamidase enzymes encoded by the pncA gene.

No pyrazinamidase activity is detectable in most pyrazinamide-resistant mutants of M. tuberculosis or in strains of M. bovis and BCG, which are naturally resistant to this agent. A wide range of point mutations in the 600 base-pair pncA gene confer resistance to pyrazinamide and, despite technical difficulties, straightforward techniques for the detection of these mutations have been developed.[76,77]

A few pyrazinamide-resistant strains lack mutations in the pncA gene, indicating alternative mechanisms for resistance to this agent, including defects in transportation of the agent into the bacterial cell due to mutational changes in the porins.[63]

Ethambutol

This agent inhibits the enzyme arabinosyl transferase involved in the synthesis of the major cell wall polysaccharide arabinogalactan. Acquisition of resistance is a multi-step mutational process involving several genes in the *embA*, *embB* and *embC* gene cluster (principally *embB*), which code for this enzyme. A rather bizarre finding is that mutations in codon 306 of the *embB* gene not only cause resistance to ethambutol, but appear to predispose the bacterial cell to develop resistance to a range of antituberculosis agents, thereby generating multidrug-resistant strains which have been shown by clustering studies to be readily transmissible.[78] There is only a weak association between resistance to isoniazid and ethambutol, although isoniazid-resistant strains with one particular mutation in the *katG* gene are more likely to acquire high-level resistance to ethambutol.[79]

Ethionamide

This and the closely related agent prothionamide are structurally similar to isoniazid and have the same target molecule – the enoyl-acyl carrier protein reductase enzyme coded by the *inhA* locus.[80] Also, in common with isoniazid, they are pro-drugs requiring enzymic activation, but complete sequencing of the *ethA* gene coding for the enzyme in ethionamide-resistant isolates revealed mutations in only about half of them, indicating that other mechanisms of resistance occur.[81] Thus, mutations in the *inhA* locus or its promoter region are also associated with resistance to these agents and explain the partial cross-resistance with isoniazid seen in some strains though, in contrast to isoniazid, mutants in the *katG* locus do not induce resistance to ethionamide.

MYCOBACTERIOPHAGES, LYSOGENY AND PHAGE TYPING

Several bacteriophages able to replicate in and lyse mycobacteria have been isolated from environmental sources, including soil and water, and a few have been isolated from naturally lysogenic environmental mycobacteria. No whole phages have been isolated from *M. tuberculosis*, but genomic sequencing studies have confirmed that the H37Rv strain contains two defective prophages, phiRv1 and phiRv2.[20] This was predicted in 1968 by the finding that a phage producing a single plaque type on *Mycobacterium smegmatis* regularly produced three plaque types on *M. tuberculosis* H37Rv, indicating genetic recombination between the infecting phage and phage DNA within the latter host.[82] Whether phage-mediated recombination has contributed to the evolutionary diversity seen within the *M. tuberculosis* complex is an intriguing question requiring further investigation.[83]

Most mycobacteriophages have broad host ranges and several that are propagated on certain rapidly growing mycobacteria lyse strains of the *M. tuberculosis* complex and, before the advent of more discriminating systems such as spoligotyping, were used to type members of this complex for epidemiological purposes. Three major phage types of *M. tuberculosis* have been delineated – A, B and I – and these correlate with other major biological differences between the strains, with those of type I corresponding to the variant of *M. tuberculosis* which is of low virulence in the guinea pig and is known as the Asian or south Indian type.[39] It has been postulated, but not confirmed, that this type corresponds to the 'ancestral' type of *M. tuberculosis* characterized by the possession of the TbD1 region of difference as described above.[84]

As described in Chapter 5, the diagnosis of tuberculosis, a mycobacteriophage genetically engineered to contain the gene coding for firefly luciferase has been utilized in an ingenious technique for the rapid detection of viable *M. tuberculosis* in clinical specimens and for determination of drug resistance.

PLASMIDS OR EPISOMES

In common with many other bacteria, some environmental mycobacteria contain small extra-chromosomal circles of DNA, termed plasmids or episomes. Some bacterial plasmids carry genes that determine drug resistance, but this has not been demonstrated in the genus *Mycobacterium* and no plasmids have been detected in the *M. tuberculosis* complex.

DETERMINANTS OF VIRULENCE AND PATHOGENICITY

Ever since the discovery of the tubercle bacillus in 1882, there have been numerous attempts to unravel the mechanisms of virulence of members of the *M. tuberculosis* complex. Numerous putative determinants of virulence, including almost every class of compound within these bacilli, have been described and reviewed in detail.[85] It has indeed been postulated that most of the genes of *M. tuberculosis* are, in some way or another and however minor, required for the establishment of the pathogen in the human host and the subsequent development of overt transmissible disease.[86] The development of disease passes through several distinct stages – initial infection, entry of the pathogen into tissues and cells, survival and replication within macrophages, subversion of immune defence mechanisms, establishment of dormancy or latency and induction of the gross tissue necrosis that is responsible for pulmonary cavity formation, entry of bacilli into the sputum and transmissibility of infection. Not unsurprisingly, these various stages of the disease process require quite different virulence-determining factors (Table 4.5).

Table 4.5 Major putative determinants of virulence in the *Mycobacterium tuberculosis* complex.

Stage of disease	Process	Determinants
Initial infection	Binding to tissues Entry into macrophages	PE proteins binding to fibronectin Lipoarabinomannan Complement-fixing molecules
	Local toxicity and inhibition of innate immune responses	Early secreted antigens including ESAT-6, sulpholipids, trehalose dimycolate, phenolic glycolipids
Survival within macrophages	Prevention of phagosome–lysosome fusion Neutralization of toxic oxygen derivatives	Lipoarabinomannan Catalase, peroxidase and superoxide dismutase enzymes
Latency	Adaptation to hypoxic environments	Transcription regulators including the DosR regulon Nitrate reductase enzyme
Post-primary disease	Gross tissue necrosis resulting in pulmonary cavity formation	Adjuvants inducing T_H2-determined hypersensitivity reactions

There is also evidence of strain-to-strain variation in the mechanisms of virulence of *M. tuberculosis*, in particular between the lineages and even the sublineages described above. It has indeed been postulated that the evolutionary drive for the diversification of *M. tuberculosis* into various lineages was the need to adapt to a range of human populations with differing genetic constitutions. In support of this postulate, there is evidence that infection by a strain of *M. tuberculosis* of a given lineage is more likely to proceed to overt tuberculosis in a person from a population to which it has adapted (sympatric host) than from a different population (allopatric host).[25,46] This may explain reports of limited transmission of disease between ethnic groups in the same urban region.[25]

An important practical consequence of diversity in mechanisms of virulence between the lineages of *M. tuberculosis* is the varying impact of mutation to drug or multidrug resistance. Mathematical models describing the spread of multidrug resistance have assumed that mutations determining resistance deprive the strains of 'fitness' to cause disease, but there is evidence that multidrug-resistant strains in some lineages, notably in the Beijing lineage, retain full, or almost full, virulence. The appearance and spread of the Beijing lineage in many parts of the world is therefore a source of concern.[44]

Although *M. tuberculosis* contains some toxic molecules, such as the trehalose dimycolates,[30] these do not appear to be major determinants of virulence. A possible exception is a secreted antigen (ESAT-6) of *M. tuberculosis* which has a toxic effect on host cell membranes, resulting in lysis of infected cells, spread of infection from cell to cell and possibly escape of intracellular pathogens from the phagosomes. In general, though, virulence of members of the *M. tuberculosis* complex appears to be the result of a multifactorial subversion of the various immune defence mechanisms that they encounter.

Being intracellular pathogens, members of the *M. tuberculosis* complex have mechanisms facilitating their phagocytosis by macrophages and, in common with other bacteria, this may involve complement activation and mannose binding. A key mechanism of survival within macrophages is the ability of the bacilli to inhibit phagosome maturation and to block phagosome–lysosome fusion.[87] These processes inhibit the acidification of phagosomes and the generation of various reactive oxygen and nitrogen molecules.[88] Mannose-capped lipoarabinomannan (ManLAM) of *M. tuberculosis* facilitates entry into macrophages by binding to mannose receptors and also inhibits phagosomal activity.[59]

Early secreted antigens have attracted attention as determinants of virulence and inducers of protective immunity. Particular attention has been focused on a group of early secreted antigenic proteins coded for by the *esx* locus in the RD1 region of the genome which is missing from BCG, *M. microti* and other strains that are attenuated for humans.[89] These include ESAT-6 which, as mentioned above, disrupts host cell membranes.

Initial infection leads to the development of the primary tuberculosis complex which, in most people, is clinically 'silent' and resolves, but the infection may enter a latent or dormant state that lasts for years or decades. The physiological nature of the tubercle bacilli in latent tuberculosis remains a mystery,[90] and various rather artificial animal models have shed very little light on the subject. It has been postulated that bacilli during the latent phase are sequestered in dense, anoxic, scar tissue and are in a state of dormancy,[91] determined by a regulatory system, termed DosR, that activates genes involved in dormancy and subsequent 'awakening'.[92] There is evidence that upregulation of DosR regulon in members of the W-Beijing lineage confers an advantage by enabling them to replicate under hypoxic conditions within host tissues.[93]

On the other hand, there is evidence that persisting bacilli are not strictly dormant, but are in a balanced state of replication and destruction by immune mechanisms. This would explain why lowered immune responses lead to reactivation of disease and why there is a continued production of gamma-interferon in those with latent tuberculosis.[90] The morphological nature of the persisting bacilli and their location in the host tissues also remain a mystery. While they may well be 'normal' acid-fast bacilli, a range of alternative morphological forms have been postulated, but none have been isolated and characterized.[94] Although assumed to reside in the dense and anoxic healed tuberculous lesions, there is evidence from *in situ* PCR studies that they may be scattered throughout normal lung tissue.[95]

The final stage of the evolution of tuberculosis is the post-primary form characterized by gross tissue necrosis. This stage is essential for transmission of the disease as it generates pulmonary cavities that communicate with the bronchial tree so that bacilli enter the sputum resulting in 'open' tuberculosis. The progression of the disease process to resolution and healing or to progression with extensive necrosis is determined by the nature of the host immune system which, in turn, is determined by the balance between various regulatory and effecter T lymphocytes as described in Chapter 8, Human immune response to *M. tuberculosis*. Many factors affect the immune responsiveness, including the various adjuvants in the complex mycobacterial cell wall that, by activating the innate immune system, determine subsequent immune reactivity.

It is thus evident that the pathogenicity, virulence and host range of a member of the *M. tuberculosis* complex is affected by many different components of the bacilli, and varies considerably between species, lineages and sublineages. In addition, the expression of disease in a host depends critically on numerous environmental factors affecting overall immune responsiveness. Such a huge variation in the causative factors of tuberculosis poses an enormous challenge to those seeking novel therapeutic approaches and vaccination strategies.

LEARNING POINTS

- The announcement of the discovery of the 'tubercle bacillus' was made by Robert Koch on 24 March 1882.
- The causative agents of human and mammalian tuberculosis, grouped in the *M. tuberculosis* complex, are very closely related genetically, but for historical reasons they are divided into a number of named species.
- The genome of *M. tuberculosis* has been completely sequenced and this has revealed several characteristic features, especially a high number of genes involved in lipid biosynthesis.
- Species within the *M. tuberculosis* complex are very closely related genetically and differ in single base-pair variations (single nucleotide polymorphisms), the less frequent variations in several sequential nucleotides (large sequence polymorphisms), minisatellites and microsatellites.
- Species within this complex contain many insertion sequences of DNA ('jumping genes') of which one, IS6110, has been widely studied for typing or 'fingerprinting' purposes.
- Variation within the *M. tuberculosis* complex is not so much due to evolution as to devolution from a common progenitor type by loss of units of genetic material termed 'regions of difference' (RD). Thus *M. bovis* appears to have devolved from *M. tuberculosis* by a process of genetic depletion.
- *M. tuberculosis* is divisible into a number of lineages and sublineages which differ in their virulence, their ability to cause epidemic spread and their ability to retain virulence on mutation to multidrug resistance.
- Members of the *M. tuberculosis* complex are susceptible to some antibiotics and also synthetic agents specifically used for treating mycobacterial disease. The genetic basis of susceptibility and resistance to these agents and their target molecules are mostly known.
- Virulence of tubercle bacilli is multifactorial, involving many genes and their products, and varies across the species and lineages. Different virulence-determining factors are involved in the various clinical forms of tuberculosis.

REFERENCES

1. Smith T. A comparative study of bovine tubercle bacilli and of human bacilli from sputum. *J Exp Med* 1898; **3**: 451–511.
2. Runyon EH. Anonymous mycobacteria in pulmonary disease. *Med Clin North Am* 1959; **43**: 273–90.
3. Wayne LG, Good RC, Krichevsky MI *et al.* Fourth report of the cooperative, open-ended study of slowly growing mycobacteria by the International Working Group on Mycobacterial Taxonomy. *Int J Syst Bacteriol* 1991; **41**: 463–72.
4. Skerman VDB, McGowan V, Sneath PHA. Approved lists of bacterial names. *Int J Syst Bacteriol* 1980; **30**: 225–420.
5. Tortoli E. Impact of genotypic studies on mycobacterial taxonomy: the new mycobacteria of the 1990s. *Clin Microbiol Rev* 2003; **16**: 319–54.
6. Schulze-Robbicke R, Janning B, Fischeder R. Occurrence of mycobacteria in biofilm samples. *Tuberc Lung Dis* 1992; **73**: 141–4.
7. Falkinham JO, Norton CD, Lechavallier MW. Factors influencing numbers of *Mycobacterium avium, Mycobacterium intracellulare*, and other mycobacteria in drinking water systems. *Appl Environ Microbiol* 2001; **67**: 1225–31.
8. Palmer CE, Long MW. Effects of infection with atypical mycobacteria on BCG vaccination and tuberculosis. *Am Rev Respir Dis* 1969; **94**: 553–68.
9. Stanford JL, Shield MJ, Rook GAW. How environmental mycobacteria may predetermine the protective efficacy of BCG. *Tubercle* 1981; **62**: 5–62.
10. Fine PEM. Variation in protection by BCG: implications of and for heterologous immunity. *Lancet* 1995; **346**: 1339–45.
11. Pfyffer GE, Auckenthaler R, van Embden JD, van Soolingen D. *Mycobacterium canettii*, the smooth variant of *M. tuberculosis*, isolated from a Swiss patient exposed in Africa. *Emerg Infect Dis* 1998; **4**: 631–4.

12. Aranaz A, Cousins D, Mateos A, Domínguez L. Elevation of *Mycobacterium tuberculosis* subsp. *caprae* Aranaz et al. 1999 to species rank as *Mycobacterium caprae* comb. nov., sp. nov. *Int J Syst Evol Microbiol* 2003; **53**: 1785–9.

13. Kubica T, Rüsch-Gerdes S, Niemann S. *Mycobacterium bovis* subsp. *caprae* caused one-third of human *M. bovis*-associated tuberculosis cases reported in Germany between 1999 and 2001. *J Clin Microbiol* 2003; **41**: 3070–7.

14. Fomukong NG, Dale JW, Osborn TW, Grange JM. Use of gene probes based on the insertion sequence IS986 to differentiate between BCG vaccine strains. *J App Bacteriol* 1992; **72**: 126–33.

15. Grange JM, Yates MD, de Kantor IN. *Guidelines for speciation within the Mycobacterium tuberculosis complex*, 2nd edn. Geneva: World Health Organization, WHO/EMC/ZOO/96.4, 1996.

16. Hart PD, Sutherland I. BCG and vole bacillus vaccines in the prevention of tuberculosis in adolescence and early adult life. *Br Med J* 1977; **2**: 293–5.

17. Lutze-Wallace C, Turcotte C, Glover G et al. Isolation of a *Mycobacterium microti*-like organism from a rock hyrax (*Procavia capensis*) in a Canadian zoo. *Can Vet J* 2006; **47**: 1011–13.

18. Niemann S, Richter E, Dalugge-Tamm H et al. Two cases of *Mycobacterium microti* derived tuberculosis in HIV-negative immunocompetent patients. *Emerg Infect Dis* 2000; **6**: 539–42.

19. Cousins DV, Bastida R, Cataldi A et al. Tuberculosis in seals caused by a novel member of the *Mycobacterium tuberculosis* complex: *Mycobacterium pinnipedii* sp. nov. *Int J Syst Evol Microbiol* 2003; **53**: 1305–14.

20. Cole ST, Brosch R, Parkhill J et al. Deciphering the biology of *Mycobacterium tuberculosis* from the complete genome sequence. *Nature* 1998; **393**: 537–44.

21. Garnier T, Eiglmeier K, Camus J-C et al. The complete genome sequence of *Mycobacterium bovis*. *Proc Natl Acad Sci U S A* 2003; **100**: 7877–82.

22. Cole ST, Eiglmeier K, Parkhill J et al. Massive gene decay in the leprosy bacillus. *Nature* 2001; **409**: 1007–11.

23. Sassetti CM, Boyd DH, Rubin EJ. Genes required for mycobacterial growth defined by high density mutagenesis. *Mol Microbiol* 2003; **48**: 77–84.

24. Talarico S, Cave MD, Marrs CF et al. Variation of the *Mycobacterium tuberculosis* PE_PGRS33 gene among clinical isolates. *J Clin Microbiol* 2005; **43**: 4954–60.

25. Brennan MJ, Delogu G. The PE multigene family: a 'molecular mantra' for mycobacteria. *Trends Microbiol* 2002; **10**: 246–9.

26. Karboul A, Gey van Pittius NC, Namouchi A et al. Insights into the evolutionary history of tubercle bacilli as disclosed by genetic rearrangements within a PE_PGRS duplicated gene pair. *BMC Evol Biol* 2006; **6**: 107.

27. Filliol I, Motiwala AS, Cavatore M et al. Global phylogeny of *Mycobacterium tuberculosis* based on single nucleotide polymorphism (SNP) analysis: insights into tuberculosis evolution, phylogenetic accuracy of other DNA fingerprinting systems, and recommendations for a minimal standard SNP set. *J Bacteriol* 2006; **188**: 759–72.

28. Supply P, Mazars E, Lesjean S et al. Variable human minisatellite-like regions in the *Mycobacterium tuberculosis* genome. *Mol Microbiol* 2000; **36**: 762–71.

29. Sreenu VB, Kumar P, Nagaraju J, Nagarajaram HA. Microsatellite polymorphism across the *M. tuberculosis* and *M. bovis* genomes: implications on genome evolution and plasticity. *BMC Genomics* 2006; **7**: 78 (Epub).

30. Cave MD, Eisenach KD, Templeton G et al. Stability of DNA fingerprint pattern produced with IS6110 in strains of *Mycobacterium tuberculosis*. *J Clin Microbiol* 1994; **32**: 262–6.

31. Groenen PM, Bunchoten D, van Soolingen D et al. Nature of DNA polymorphism in the direct repeat cluster of *Mycobacterium tuberculosis* and its use as an epidemiological tool. *Mol Microbiol* 1993; **10**: 1057–65.

32. Legrand E, Filliol I, Sola C, Rastogi N. Use of spoligotyping to study the evolution of the direct repeat locus by IS6110 transposition in *Mycobacterium tuberculosis*. *J Clin Microbiol* 2001; **39**: 1595–9.

33. Grange JM. Intra-specific variation in the mycobacteria – a taxonomic aid. *Ann Soc Belge Med Trop* 1973; **53**: 339–46.

34. Gutierrez MC, Brise S, Brosch R et al. Ancient origin and gene mosaicism of the progenitor of *Mycobacterium tuberculosis*. *PLoS* 2005; **1**: e5.

35. Brosch R, Gordon SV, Marmiesse M et al. A new evolutionary scenario for the *Mycobacterium tuberculosis* complex. *Proc Natl Acad Sci U S A* 2002; **99**: 3684–9.

36. Mahairas GG, Sabo PJ, Hickey MJ et al. Molecular analysis of genetic differences between *Mycobacterium bovis* BCG and virulent *M. bovis*. *J Bacteriol* 1996; **178**: 1274–82.

37. Huard RC, Lazzarini C de O, Butler WR et al. PCR-based method to differentiate the subspecies of the *Mycobacterium tuberculosis* complex on the basis of genomic deletions. *J Clin Microbiol* 2003; **41**: 1637–50.

38. Huard RC, Fabre M, de Haas P et al. Novel genetic polymorphisms that further delineate the phylogeny of the *Mycobacterium tuberculosis* complex. *J Bacteriol* 2006; **188**: 4271–87.

39. Goren MB, Grange JM, Aber VR et al. Role of lipid content and hydrogen peroxide susceptibility in determining the guinea-pig virulence of *Mycobacterium tuberculosis*. *Br J Exp Pathol* 1982; **63**: 693–700.

40. Yates MD, Collins CH, Grange JM. 'Classical' and 'Asian' variants of *Mycobacterium tuberculosis* isolated in South-East England, 1977–1980. *Tubercle* 1982; **63**: 55–61.

41. Brudey K, Driscoll JR, Rigouts L et al. *Mycobacterium tuberculosis* complex genetic diversity: mining the fourth international spoligotyping database (SpolDB4) for classification, population genetics and epidemiology. *BMC Microbiol* 2006; **12**: 719–24.

42. Filliol I, Driscoll JR, van Soolingen D et al. Snapshot of moving and expanding clones of *Mycobacterium tuberculosis* and their global distribution assessed by spoligotyping in an international study. *J Clin Microbiol* 2003; **41**: 1963–70.

43. Gagneux S, Small PM. Global phylogeography of *Mycobacterium tuberculosis* and implications for tuberculosis product development. *Lancet Infect Dis* 2007; **7**: 328–37.

44. Drobniewski F, Balabanova Y, Nikolayevsky V et al. Drug-resistant tuberculosis, clinical virulence, and the dominance of the Beijing strain family in Russia. *J Am Med Assoc* 2005; **293**: 2726–31.

45. Hanekom M, van der Spuy GD, Streicher E et al. A recently evolved sublineage of the *Mycobacterium tuberculosis* Beijing strain family was associated with an increased ability to spread and cause disease. *J Clin Microbiol* 2007; **45**: 1483–90.

46. Gagneux S, DeRiemer K, Van T et al. Variable host–pathogen compatibility in *Mycobacterium tuberculosis*. *Proc Natl Acad Sci U S A* 2006; **103**: 2869–73.

47. Toungoussova OS, Caugant DA, Sandven P et al. Impact of drug resistance on fitness of *Mycobacterium tuberculosis* strains of the W-Beijing genotype. *FEMS Immunol Med Microbiol* 2004; **42**: 281–90.

48. Alteri CJ, Xicohtencatl-Cortes J, Hess S et al. *Mycobacterium tuberculosis* produces pili during human infection. *Proc Natl Acad Sci U S A* 2007; **104**: 5145–50.

49. Collins CH, Grange JM, Yates MD. *Tuberculosis bacteriology. Organization and practice*, 2nd edn. Oxford: Butterworth Heinemann, 1997.

50. Brennan PJ, Nikaido H. The envelope of mycobacteria. *Annu Rev Biochem* 1995; **64**: 29–63.

51. Dean C, Crick DC, Mahapatra S, Brennan PJ. Biosynthesis of the arabinogalactan-peptidoglycan complex of *Mycobacterium tuberculosis*. *Glycobiology* 2001; **11**: 107R–118R.

52. Glickman MS, Cox JS, Jacobs WR. A novel mycolic acid cyclopropane synthetase is required for coding persistence, and virulence of *Mycobacterium tuberculosis*. *Mol Cell* 2000; **5**: 717–27.

53. Takayama K, Wang C, Besra GS et al. Pathway to synthesis and processing of mycolic acids in *Mycobacterium tuberculosis. Clin Microbiol Rev* 2005; **18**: 81–101.

54. Armitige LY, Jagannath C, Wanger AR, Norris SJ. Disruption of the genes encoding antigen 85A and antigen 85B of *Mycobacterium tuberculosis* H37Rv: effect on growth in culture and in macrophages. *Infect Immun* 2000; **68**: 767–78.

55. Geisel RE, Sakamoto K, Russell DG, Rhoades ER. *In vivo* activity of released cell wall lipids of *Mycobacterium bovis* bacillus Calmette–Guérin is due principally to trehalose mycolates. *J Immunol* 2005; **174**: 5007–5015.

56. Rook GAW, Zumla A. Advances in the immunopathogenesis of pulmonary tuberculosis. *Curr Opin Pulmon Med* 2001; **7**: 116–23.

57. Means TK, Jones BW, Schromm AB et al. Differential effects of a Toll-like receptor antagonist on *Mycobacterium tuberculosis*-induced macrophage responses. *J Immunol* 2001; **166**: 4074–82.

58. Jo EK, Yang CS, Choi CH, Harding CV. Intracellular signalling cascades regulating innate immune responses to *Mycobacteria*: branching out from Toll-like receptors. *Cell Microbiol* 2007; **9**: 1087–98.

59. Kang PB, Azad AK, Torrelles JB et al. The human macrophage mannose receptor directs *Mycobacterium tuberculosis* lipoarabinomannan-mediated phagosome biogenesis. *J Exp Med* 2005; **202**: 987–99.

60. Reed MB, Domenech P, Manca C et al. A glycolipid of hypervirulent tuberculosis strains that inhibits the innate immune response. *Nature* 2004; **431**: 84–7.

61. Kartmann B, Stengler S, Niederweis M et al. Porins in the cell wall of *Mycobacterium tuberculosis. J Bacteriol* 1999; **181**: 6543–6.

62. Raynaud C, Laneelle MA, Senaratne RH et al. Mechanisms of pyrazinamide resistance in mycobacteria: importance of lack of uptake in addition to lack of pyrazinamidase activity. *Microbiology* 1999; **145**: 1359–67.

63. Ratledge C. Iron, mycobacteria and tuberculosis. *Tuberculosis (Edinb)* 2004; **84**: 110–30.

64. Sonnenberg MG, Belisle JT. Definition of *Mycobacterium tuberculosis* culture filtrate proteins by two-dimensionsl polyacrylamide gel electrophotesis, N-terminal amino acid sequencing, and electrospray mass spectroscopy. *Infect Immun* 1997; **65**: 4515–24.

65. Stanford JL, Grange JM. The meaning and structure of species as applied to mycobacteria. *Tubercle* 1974; **55**: 143–52.

66. Karopoulos C, Rowley MJ, Handley CJ, Strugnell RA. Antibody reactivity to mycobacterial 65 kDa heat shock protein: relevance to autoimmunity. *J Autoimmun* 1995; **8**: 235–48.

67. Schaefer WB. Serologic identification and classification of the atypical mycobacteria by their agglutination. *Am Rev Respir Dis* 1965; **92** (Suppl.): 85–93.

68. Pai M, Kalantri S, Dheda K. New tools and emerging technologies for the diagnosis of tuberculosis: Part II. Active tuberculosis and drug resistance. *Exp Rev Mol Diagn* 2006; **6**: 423–32.

69. Aragon LM, Navarro F, Heiser V et al. Rapid detection of specific gene mutations associated with isoniazid or rifampicin resistance in *Mycobacterium tuberculosis* clinical isolates using non-fluorescent low-density DNA microarrays. *J Antimicrob Chemother* 2006; **57**: 825–31.

70. Williams DL, Waguespack C, Eisenach K et al. Characterization of rifampin resistance in pathogenic mycobacteria. *Antimicrob Agents Chemother* 1994; **38**: 2380–6.

71. Gagneux S, Burgos MV, Kathryn DeRiemer K et al. Impact of bacterial genetics on the transmission of isoniazid-resistant *Mycobacterium tuberculosis. PLoS Pathog* 2006; **2**: e61.

72. Price-Evans DA, Manley KA, McKusick VA. Genetic control of isoniazid metabolism in man. *Br Med J* 1960; **2**: 485–91.

73. Bhakta S, Besra GS, Anna M et al. Arylamine N-Acetyltransferase is required for synthesis of mycolic acids and complex lipids in *Mycobacterium bovis* BCG and represents a novel drug target. *J Exp Med* 2004; **199**: 1191–9.

74. Wade MM, Zhang Y. Effects of weak acids, UV and proton motive force inhibitors on pyrazinamide activity against *Myocbacterium tuberculosis* in vitro. *J Antimicrob Chemother* 2006; **58**: 936–41.

75. Zhang Y, Mitchison D. The curious characteristics of pyrazinamide: a review. *Int J Tuberc Lung Dis* 2003; **7**: 6–21.

76. McCammon MT, Gillette JS, Derek P et al. Detection by denaturing gradient gel electrophoresis of pncA mutations associated with pyrazinamide resistance in *Mycobacterium tuberculosis* isolates from the United States–Mexico border region. *Antimicrob Agents Chemother* 2005; **49**: 2210–17.

77. Denkin S, Volokhov D, Chizhikov V, Zhang Y. Microarray-based PncA genotyping of pyrazinamide-resistant strains of *Mycobacterium tuberculosis. J Med Microbiol* 2005; **54**: 1127–31.

78. Hazbón MH, del Valle MB, Guerrero MI et al. Role of embB codon 306 mutations in *Mycobacterium tuberculosis* revisited: a novel association with broad drug resistance and IS6110 clustering rather than ethambutol resistance. *Antimicrob Agents Chemother* 2005; **49**: 3794–802.

79. Parsons LM, Salfinger M, Clobridge A et al. Phenotypic and molecular characterization of *Mycobacterium tuberculosis* isolates resistant to both isoniazid and ethambutol. *Antimicrob Agents Chemother* 2005; **49**: 2218–25.

80. Larsen MH, Vilcheze C, Kremer L et al. Overexpression of inhA, but not kasA, confers resistance to isoniazid and ethionamide in *Mycobacterium smegmatis, M. bovis* BCG and *M. tuberculosis. Mol Microbiol* 2002; **46**: 453–66.

81. Morlock GP, Metchock B, Sikes D et al. ethA, inhA, and katG loci of ethionamide-resistant clinical *Mycobacterium tuberculosis* isolates. *Antimicrob Agents Chemother* 2003; **47**: 3799–805.

82. Mankiewicz E, Redmond WB. Lytic phenomena of phage LEO isolated from a sarcoid lesion. *Am Rev Respir Dis* 1968; **98**: 41–6.

83. Liu X, Gutacker MM, Musser JM et al. Evidence for recombination in *Mycobacterium tuberculosis. J Bacteriol* 2006; **188**: 8169–77.

84. Ahmed N, Leblebicioglu H. India's 'gold mine' of ancestral bacilli and the looming TB-HIV pandemic. *Ann Clin Microbiol Antimicrob* 2006; **5**: 31.

85. Smith I. *Mycobacterium tuberculosis* pathogenesis and molecular determinants of virulence. *Clin Microbiol Rev* 2003; **16**: 463–96.

86. Yesilkaya H, Dale JW, Strachan NJC, Forbes KJ. Natural transposon mutagenesis of clinical isolates of *Mycobacterium tuberculosis*: how many genes does a pathogen need? *J Bacteriol* 2005; **187**: 6726–32.

87. Deretic V, Singh S, Master S et al. *Mycobacterium tuberculosis* inhibition of phagolysosome biogenesis and autophagy as a host defence mechanism. *Cell Microbiol* 2006; **8**: 719–27.

88. Wei J, Dahl JL, Moulder JW et al. Identification of a *Mycobacterium tuberculosis* gene that enhances mycobacterial survival in macrophages. *J Bacteriol* 2000; **182**: 377–84.

89. Fortune SM, Jaeger A, Sarracino DA et al. Mutually dependent secretion of proteins required for mycobacterial virulence. *Proc Natl Acad Sci U S A* 2005; **102**: 10676–81.

90. Orme IM. The latent tubercle bacillus (I'll let you know if I ever meet one). *Int J Tuberc Lung Dis* 2001; **5**: 589–93.

91. He H, Zahrt TC. Identification and characterization of a regulatory sequence recognized by *Mycobacterium tuberculosis* persistence regulator MprA. *J Bacteriol* 2005; **187**: 202–12.

92. Wisedchaisri G, Wu M, Rice AE et al. Structures of *Mycobacterium tuberculosis* DosR and DosR–DNA complex involved in gene activation during adaptation to hypoxic latency. *J Mol Biol* 2005; **354**: 630–41.

93. Reed MB, Gagneux S, Deriemer K et al. The W-Beijing lineage of *Mycobacterium tuberculosis* overproduces triglycerides and has the DosR dormancy regulon constitutively upregulated. *J Bacteriol* 2007; **189**: 2583–9.

94. Grange JM. Would you know one if you met one? *Int J Tuberc Lung Dis* 2001; **5**: 1162–3.

95. Hernandez-Pando R, Jeyanathan M, Mengistu G et al. Persistence of DNA from *Mycobacterium tuberculosis* in superficially normal lung tissue during latent infection. *Lancet* 2000; **356**: 2133–8.

5

The diagnosis of tuberculosis

NEIL W SCHLUGER

INTRODUCTION

Diagnosis of tuberculosis is a crucial but often overlooked aspect of efforts to control the global tuberculosis epidemic. In most parts of the world, diagnostic methods rely on techniques developed over a century ago, with small modifications, such as the acid-fast smear of an expectorated sputum specimen. Unfortunately, only about half of all cases of tuberculosis are sputum smear-positive. As a result, a substantial percentage of the world's tuberculosis cases are probably undiagnosed, or are diagnosed only when the index patient has an advanced stage of disease and significant transmission has occurred in the community.

Recently, a decision analysis estimated that a rapid, widely available diagnostic test for tuberculosis with a sensitivity of >85 per cent and a specificity of 97 per cent could save about 400 000 lives annually by reducing the global burden of tuberculosis disease.[1] This analysis also stated that the ideal new diagnostic would require no electricity, refrigeration or access to clean water, and should be easy to use with little or no training, and that results should be available within 1 hour. While such an ideal test is not within reach in the very near term, several available tests are markedly more sensitive than sputum smear examination, with good specificity. This chapter will review current approaches to tuberculosis diagnostics and discuss several newer approaches in various stages of development. I will focus on the diagnosis of active pulmonary tuberculosis (PTB), although comments about diagnosis of extrapulmonary tuberculosis are also included.

DIAGNOSIS OF PULMONARY TUBERCULOSIS

Clinical suspicion and chest radiography

As with any clinical syndrome or condition, the diagnosis of tuberculosis begins with clinical suspicion. The classic symptoms of tuberculosis are fever, cough and weight loss, but they are non-specific, and can be mimicked by other conditions, including malignancy and other pulmonary infections. Still, in the right setting, any patient with these classic symptoms should be considered at risk for tuberculosis, particularly if they have the following demographic characteristics: current or recent residence in a high-prevalence country, recent contact with an active case of tuberculosis, residence in a congregate setting, such as a nursing home, homeless shelter, prison or jail in which occult exposure to tuberculosis might have occurred, or underlying immunosuppression due to HIV infection, other illness, or the administration of drugs which reduce immune defences, particularly antagonists of tumour necrosis factor (TNF).[2–4]

Studies have shown that failure to consider tuberculosis in the differential diagnosis of patients at risk leads to long delays in the institution of proper therapy.[5] This points out the need for continued education about tuberculosis, both in regions where the disease is uncommon and in high-burden countries.

When a physician develops a clinical suspicion, based on patient history, that tuberculosis is a possible diagnosis, chest radiography is usually the next step in the diagnostic algorithm, although this modality is not universally available. Radiographic findings in tuberculosis have been well described.[6] However, given the increasing prevalence of HIV co-infection in tuberculosis patients around the world, it is critical to recognize radiographic presentations of tuberculosis that are more common in immunocompromised hosts, such as mediastinal or hilar adenopathy without lung parenchymal abnormalities.[7]

Sputum-based diagnosis

Sputum examination is still the mainstay of the diagnostic evaluation for tuberculosis, although as described below, the optimal means to examine sputum is in considerable flux. Importantly, the technique used to obtain the respiratory sample strongly influences the ability to detect PTB. Expectorated sputum is generally the starting point. Three samples are collected on 3 separate days and stained for acid-fast bacilli (AFB).[8,9] Although the utility of collecting three samples has been questioned,[10] the overall yield for smear and culture is superior to collecting fewer specimens.[11,12] Samples are generally sent simultaneously for smear and culture, as culture is essential to confirm the diagnosis. However, in resource-poor countries, the cost of culture is often too great, resulting in reliance solely on AFB smears.

The sensitivity of sputum AFB smears for detecting PTB is limited by the threshold of detection, which is 5000 to 10 000 bacilli per millitre of specimen.[13] The sensitivity of expectorated sputum ranges from 34 to 80 per cent,[10,13-25] and is highest in patients with cavitary disease, and lowest in those with weak cough or less advanced disease. In no way does a negative sputum smear eliminate the diagnosis of active tuberculosis, particularly if the clinical suspicion is high. Instituting therapy in such cases is often warranted while awaiting culture results. If a patient with suspected PTB is smear-negative on expectorated sputum or is unable to produce sputum (30 per cent of patients in one series[26]), further diagnostic evaluation may be considered, including sputum induction (SI), fibreoptic bronchoscopy (FOB) and perhaps gastric washings. The following discussion refers specifically to patients who are expectorated sputum smear-negative or who cannot produce an expectorated sputum sample.

Sputum induction

SI for diagnosis of PTB was first described in 1961 by Hensler and colleagues,[26] who adapted an earlier technique used to obtain sputum for cytology to diagnose lung cancer. Early studies compared SI with the well-established method of gastric aspiration.[26-28] In patients unable to expectorate or with smear-negative sputum samples, SI was superior to gastric washings in obtaining a suitable sample for culture, although the two techniques were complementary[28] and gastric washings likely add to overall diagnostic yield.[29] Nevertheless, the role of gastric washings in adults is probably limited. SI, on the other hand, is very effective in patients clinically suspected of having PTB who are either unable to produce sputum or are sputum smear-negative.

SI has performed well in resource-poor countries with little added cost.[30-32] In South Africa, SI performed on 51 patients yielded a suitable sample in 36.[32] Fifteen of the 36 patients (42 per cent) were smear-positive and 12 were also culture-positive. In Malawi, Parry and colleagues[31] obtained induced sputum in 73 of 82 patients. Of these 73, 18 (25 per cent) were smear-positive and 30 (42 per cent) were culture-positive. Similarly, of 1648 patients in China

who provided induced sputum samples, 558 (34 per cent) were smear-positive, with a direct cost per SI of $0.37 (£0.18).[30] SI in these studies provided appropriate samples for diagnosis, increased the early diagnostic yield significantly, and appears to be cost-effective in resource-poor settings.

Some studies have found SI to be less helpful. In a retrospective review of 114 patients with culture-positive PTB at an urban New York hospital, 1566 SIs in 1 year yielded only 16 positive smears in 10 patients. The annual cost of $45,000 (£22,441) ($29 (£14.46) per SI) was extremely high and difficult to justify.[33] A UK study confirmed a low yield, but suggested that there might be a role for SI.[34] It is likely that indiscriminate use of SI unfavourably affected the cost–benefit equation, but most evidence indicates that the test is valuable when judiciously used, primarily in smear-negative patients with a moderate to high likelihood of tuberculosis. In addition, retrospective studies are necessarily limited in their power. Prospective studies, as discussed below, more consistently demonstrate benefit of SI.

What then is the role for SI in resource-rich countries? A large prospective study from Montreal performed repeated SI in 500 patients who were either smear-negative (5 per cent) or could not produce sputum (95 per cent).[35] An adequate sample was obtained in 99 per cent of patients and a positive culture was obtained in 43 patients (9 per cent). Among those with a smear-positive induced sputum sample, the cumulative yield with successive attempts was 64, 81, 91 and, after four inductions, 98 per cent. Among those with positive cultures of induced sputum samples, the cumulative yield also increased with each attempt from 70 to 91, 99 and 100 per cent. This study suggests that repeated SI is superior to obtaining a single sample and has a very high yield in this setting. Repeated SI should be considered in smear-negative patients for whom an experienced clinician judges the likelihood of tuberculosis to be high.[35]

The role of fibreoptic bronchoscopy

FOB encompasses bronchoalveolar lavage (BAL), bronchial washings, bronchial brushings, transbronchial biopsy and post-bronchoscopy sputum collection. FOB has been studied in PTB suspects who are smear-negative or unable to produce a sputum sample. The utility of FOB (or SI) in this setting is two-fold. First, in patients without spontaneous sputum, a sample is generated which provides the potential for making a diagnosis. Second, in either subset of patients, by providing a means of rapid diagnosis (positive smear or histopathology) while awaiting culture results, there is the potential for earlier intervention and treatment.

Chawla et al.[36] prospectively studied 50 PTB suspects in India who were smear-negative or unable to produce sputum. Cultures of Mycobacterium tuberculosis from FOB were positive in 90 per cent. More significantly, a rapid diagnosis was made in 72 per cent of cases. Smear-positive samples were obtained in 28 per cent of post-bronchoscopy sputum specimens, 24 per cent of bronchial washings and 56 per cent of bronchial brushing specimens. Ten patients (20 per cent of those studied) were rapidly diagnosed exclusively by bronchial brushing specimens. Post-bronchoscopy sputum and bronchial washings each provided the exclusive diagnosis for 6 per cent of patients. Transbronchial biopsy was performed in 30 patients and histopathology was positive in nine, with three diagnosed exclusively on biopsy. The authors comment that the high yield of bronchial brushing smears resulted from brushing caseous material in the bronchi when visible.[36]

In three prospective studies of a total of 370 PTB suspects in Hong Kong, India and South Africa, samples from FOB provided a rapid diagnosis in 65–76 per cent of cases.[37–39] Transbronchial biopsy yielded a rapid diagnosis in 43–58 per cent of patients in whom it was performed,[37,38] and was the exclusive means of rapid diagnosis in 12 per cent.[37] In two retrospective studies of a total of 71 patients with culture-proven PTB who underwent FOB, a rapid diagnosis was obtained in 34–60 per cent of patients.[21,40]

Kennedy et al.[41] retrospectively reviewed 67 HIV-positive and 45 HIV-negative patients with culture-proven PTB. Of those with smear-negative sputum, BAL provided a rapid diagnosis in 24 per cent of HIV-positive and 8 per cent of HIV-negative patients. Transbronchial biopsy yielded a rapid diagnosis in 16 per cent of HIV-positive and 42 per cent of HIV-negative patients, and provided the exclusive early diagnosis in 10 per cent of patients.[41]

While some studies report lower yields from FOB than those cited above,[42–47] the potential of FOB to make a rapid diagnosis, a crucial step in the management of PTB, generally ranges from 30 to 70 per cent, and the overall yield of culture from FOB specimens is much higher.[21,22,36,37,39–41,48–52] While the yield of the different techniques varied between studies, each technique clearly contributed to the overall yield of FOB.

The most productive use of FOB is in PTB suspects who produce no sputum or who are smear-negative, or in patients in whom there is considerable diagnostic uncertainty, where lung biopsy may produce an alternative diagnosis. These benefits must be weighed against the costs of the procedure, infection control concerns and the risk of transbronchial biopsy.

Sputum induction versus fibreoptic bronchoscopy

How does SI compare with FOB in the diagnosis of PTB in patients with smear-negative expectorated sputum or in patients unable to produce sputum? A study by McWilliams et al.[53] from New Zealand prospectively compared repeated SI with FOB in 129 patients who had negative sputum smears or produced no sputum, 27 of whom had culture-positive tuberculosis. Ninety-six per cent of patients tolerated SI without difficulty. Each successive SI increased the yield for culture-positive samples significantly, with an overall yield of 96 per cent after three tests. By contrast, the culture yield of FOB was only 52 per cent and the cost was three times that of doing three SIs. In this study, FOB alone was too insensitive and SI alone was very sensitive, missing only one case, and very cost-effective. The combination of SI and FOB would have captured all culture-confirmed cases of PTB, but at four times the cost of SI alone. The authors' preferred strategy was to employ SI, followed by FOB only in those patients who were negative on SI but had features of PTB on chest radiograph. This approach missed no cases, was only two and a half times the cost of SI alone[53] and may be worthwhile in resource-rich settings. It may be less applicable to resource-poor settings where repeated SI alone would diagnose most cases at substantially reduced cost.

Anderson et al.[54] prospectively compared SI and FOB with BAL in 101 patients with suspected PTB in Montreal, 26 of whom had culture-positive tuberculosis. SI and FOB yielded a positive smear in 19 and 12 per cent of cases, respectively, and positive cultures in 87 and 73 per cent, respectively. Overall, SI performed better than FOB and direct costs of FOB were more than eight times those of SI.[54] In a Brazilian study of 24 HIV-infected and 119 HIV-negative patients with PTB, SI and FOB showed equivalent sensitivity in both populations, yielding positive smears in 34–40 per cent of HIV-infected and HIV-negative patients.[55]

Most recently, Schoch et al.[56] evaluated the role of expectorated sputum, SI and FOB in a cohort of asylum seekers in Switzerland. They concluded that both SI and FOB offered an incremental yield over expectorated sputum, although in this study, FOB performed better than SI.

SI performs well in resource-poor and resource-rich countries, is useful in HIV-infected and HIV-negative patients, and compares favourably with FOB in diagnostic yield and cost. Some authors argue that neither SI nor FOB should be performed 'unless absolutely necessary', given the risk of exposure of health-care workers and other patients to the aerosol-generating procedures.[57] However, this warning applies mostly to places where respiratory protective equipment, exhaust ventilation devices or appropriate isolation rooms are in short supply.[57]

Cultures

Because cultures of mycobacteria require only 10–100 organisms in order to detect M. tuberculosis, the sensitivity of culture is excellent, ranging from 80 to 93 per cent.[13,16] Moreover, the specificity is 98 per cent.[13] Cultures increase the sensitivity for diagnosis of tuberculosis, allow speciation, drug susceptibility testing and, if needed, genotyping for epidemiologic purposes.[13] All specimens should therefore be cultured.

There are three types of culture media: solid media, including egg-based (Löwenstein–Jensen), agar-based (Middlebrook 7H10 and 7H11) and liquid media (Middlebrook 7H12 and other broths). Solid media – long the standard for culturing mycobacteria – yield *M. tuberculosis* more slowly than liquid media, which are now widely employed alongside solid media to increase sensitivity and decrease recovery time.[58,59] Löwenstein–Jensen, 7H10 and 7H11 media may detect mycobacteria in less than 4 weeks,[58,60,61] but they require incubation for 6–8 weeks before they can be classified as negative. In contrast, broth media combined with DNA probes for rapid species identification typically provide results in under 2 weeks with smear-positive samples and somewhat longer with smear-negative samples.[58,61,62] Broth media formulations include both manual and automated systems, using radiometric or colorimetric methods for detection of mycobacteria. Examples of broth media include the BACTEC 460TB and BACTEC MB9000 radiometric methods, the Mycobacterial Growth Indicator Tube non-radiometric method, the manual Septi-Chek AFB system (all from Becton Dickinson Microbiology Systems, Franklin Lakes, NJ, USA), and the Extra Sensing Power and Myco-ESPculture System II (Trek Diagnostic Systems, Cleveland, OH, USA).

Broth media may allow more rapid determination of drug susceptibilities as well, particularly if direct susceptibility testing is used. Direct susceptibility testing may be done with smear-positive samples which are simultaneously inoculated into bottles lacking or containing antibiotics, allowing drug susceptibilities to be known at the same time as culture results.

Newer culture technologies are in development, such as TK Medium (Salubris, Cambridge, MA), which uses multiple colour dye indicators to rapidly identify *M. tuberculosis*. It can also be used for drug susceptibility testing and can identify a contaminated specimen (www.salubrisinc.com).

Nucleic acid amplification assays

Nucleic acid amplification (NAA) assays amplify *M. tuberculosis*-specific nucleic acid sequences with a nucleic acid probe, enabling direct detection of *M. tuberculosis* in clinical specimens. Such assays complement the conventional laboratory approach to the diagnosis of active disease. Whereas AFB smears are rapid but lack sensitivity and specificity, and culture is both sensitive and very specific but may take from 2 to 8 weeks to produce results, NAA assays allow for rapid detection of *M. tuberculosis* that is both sensitive and specific. The sensitivity of commercially available NAA assays is at least 80 per cent in most studies, and as few as 10 bacilli in a sample yield a positive result under research conditions.[13] Although the sensitivity of

these assays is lower in AFB smear-negative samples than in smear-positive ones, newer assays are considerably more sensitive than earlier versions in smear-negative specimens, increasing overall sensitivity.[14,17] NAA assays are also highly specific (98–99 per cent) for *M. tuberculosis*.

Two NAA assays are approved by the United States Food and Drug Administration and are widely available for commercial use: the AMPLICOR MTB (Roche Diagnostic Systems, Branchburg, NJ, USA), and the Amplified Mycobaterium Tuberculosis Direct (MTD) test (Gen-Probe, San Diego, CA, USA). The AMPLICOR assay uses DNA polymerase chain reaction (PCR) to amplify nucleic acid targets. The COBAS AMPLICOR is an automated version of the AMPLICOR test. The MTD assay uses an isothermal strategy to amplify and detect *M. tuberculosis* ribosomal RNA. The AMPLICOR and MTD tests are approved by the Food and Drug Administration for use with smear-positive respiratory specimens. A reformulated MTD test (AMTDII or E-MTD, for enhanced MTD) was subsequently approved for detection of *M. tuberculosis* in both smear-positive and smear-negative respiratory specimens.

In clinical and laboratory studies, the sensitivity of the original MTD assay was 83–98 per cent for smear-positive respiratory samples[16,63–70] and 70–81 per cent for smear-negative respiratory samples. In one of the few studies undertaken in a resource-poor country, Zambia, the sensitivity of the MTD test in 78 culture-positive sputum specimens, half of which were smear-positive, was only 64 per cent.[25] The specificity in these studies was 98–99 per cent. The AMPLICOR assay performed similarly, with sensitivity ranging from 74–92 per cent for smear-positive,[15,16,18,67,71–76] and 40–73 per cent for smear-negative respiratory samples.[15,16,71,74–76] Specificity was 93–99 per cent in these studies. Laifer *et al.*[77] in Switzerland found that the AMPLICOR assay had only 64 per cent sensitivity for PTB in 3119 war refugees from Kosovo. However, the negative predictive value of three consecutive PCR tests (in two sputum and one brochoalveolar lavage sample) was 100 per cent. In studies comparing MTD and AMPLICOR, MTD has consistently had a small advantage.[16,67,69]

The E-MTD test has improved sensitivity,[14,17,63,78] especially in smear-negative specimens.[14,17] In a study of 1004 respiratory specimens from 489 inmates, 22 of whom were diagnosed with PTB (10 smear-positive, 12 smear-negative), Bergmann *et al.*[14] found that the E-MTD test had a sensitivity of 95 per cent and a specificity of 99 per cent. In smear-positive patients, the sensitivity and specificity were both 100 per cent. In smear-negative patients, the sensitivity was 90 per cent and the specificity 99 per cent.[14] A study from Ontario evaluated 823 specimens (616 respiratory) from unique patients, 255 of whom were diagnosed with tuberculosis, based on a positive culture or clinical criteria. The authors found that the specificity and sensitivity of the E-MTD was 100 per cent in both smear-positive and smear-negative respiratory samples, an exceptionally high value, especially for smear-negative specimens.[17] Of note, smear-negative specimens were preselected for testing with the E-MTD based on a clinical determination that the patients were at high risk for tuberculosis. Pre-selection no doubt contributed to the high sensitivity and specificity in this study, suggesting the utility of selecting appropriate patients for testing.[17]

Catanzaro et al.[79] performed a multicentre, prospective trial of particular clinical relevance, in which the E-MTD was evaluated in the context of a patient's clinical risk for PTB, which was stratified into low, intermediate or high, as determined by physicians with expertise in evaluating patients for PTB. For 338 patients, the E-MTD test had very high specificity in all groups and the sensitivities were 83, 75 and 87 per cent, respectively. However, the positive predictive value was only 59 per cent in the low-risk group, compared with 100 per cent in the other two groups. In contrast, the negative predictive value was 99 per cent in the low-risk group, and remained high at 91 per cent in the intermediate- and high-risk groups. These results compared favourably with the AFB smear, which had positive predictive values of 36, 30 and 94 per cent, and negative predictive values of 96, 71 and 37 per cent. This study demonstrates the utility of the E-MTD test and suggests that it is particularly helpful for confirming disease in intermediate- and high-risk patients and for excluding disease in low-risk patients.[79]

Other NAA assays are the LCx test, based on the ligase chain reaction (Abbott Diagnostics Division, Abbott Park, IL), and the BDProbeTec ET Mycobacterium tuberculosis Complex Direct Detection Assay (DTB) (Becton Dickinson Biosciences, Sparks, MD), a 1-hour assay that couples strand displacement amplification to a fluorescent energy transfer detection system, and performs similarly to the E-MTD test.[80,81] Several less standardized PCR assays have been developed and tested.[82–85] Real-time PCR assays have compared favourably with AMPLICOR[84,85] and E-MTD.[83] None of these tests has been approved for use in the United States.

In 2000, the Centers for Disease Control and Prevention published recommendations that an AFB smear and NAA assay should be performed on the first sputum sample collected from all tuberculosis suspects.[86] If the smear and NAA assay are both positive, PTB is diagnosed with near certainty. If the smear is positive and the NAA assay is negative, the sputum should be tested for inhibitors by spiking the sample with lysed M. tuberculosis and repeating the assay. If inhibitors are present, the NAA assay is not useful for diagnosis. If inhibitors are not detected, additional specimens are tested, and if still smear-positive, NAA-negative and without inhibitors, the patient can be presumed to have non-tuberculous mycobacterial disease. If a sputum sample is smear-negative but E-MTD-positive (only the E-MTD is approved for smear-negative specimens), the Centers for Disease Control and Prevention recommends sending additional samples. If they are E-MTD-positive, the patient can be presumed to have PTB. If both the smear and E-MTD of the initial specimen are negative, an additional specimen should be tested by E-MTD. If negative, the patient can be presumed not to be infectious, but could still have tuberculosis. The recommendations note that clinical judgement is critical and that definitive diagnosis rests on response to therapy and culture results.[86] Although these recommendations are logical, they are expensive and based on few published data.

Overall, a reasonable use of NAA assays for rapid diagnosis of PTB is as follows. For AFB smear-positive samples, the strategy outlined above by the Centers for Disease Control and Prevention is reasonable.[87] If smears are negative, but experienced observers assess the clinical suspicion of PTB to be intermediate or high,[79,88,89] NAA should be performed on a sputum sample, and a presumptive diagnosis of PTB made if the test is positive. NAA should not be performed on sputum samples from cases in which the AFB smear is negative and the clinical index of suspicion is low.[79,89,90] Testing should also be limited to those who have not been recently treated for active disease because nucleic acids from dead organisms can be shed for variable periods after successful therapy and a positive test is not diagnostic of active disease.[87]

Cost is the main consideration limiting the use of the NAA assays, particularly in the developing world. A study in Nairobi found that the AFB smear was 1.8 times as cost-effective as the AMPLICOR test.[91] However, the authors concluded that AMPLICOR could be cost-effective if the costs of the PCR kit could be reduced substantially. A cost-effectiveness analysis in Finland showed that addition of the COBAS AMPLICOR test to smear and culture was more cost-effective if limited to smear-positive specimens.[92] However, extending this to smear-negative specimens may be possible with the E-MTD, given its superior sensitivity in smear-negative patients with PTB. Furthermore, centralized laboratories can invest in technology, use batch testing, develop expertise and benefit from economies of scale. In such settings,[17,93] regular NAA testing may be economically feasible.

A major limitation of NAA tests is the lack of drug susceptibility information. In addition, they detect nucleic acids from both living and dead organisms and may be falsely positive in patients who have recently been adequately treated for tuberculosis.[66,94–96] In contrast to NAAs that detect DNA or ribosomal RNA, assays that detect M. tuberculosis mRNA, with a half-life of only minutes, remain positive only when viable mycobacteria persist and could be sensitive indicators of adequate treatment and provide means to rapidly determine drug susceptibility.[97] This technology is under study.

EXTRAPULMONARY TB

Diagnosing extrapulmonary tuberculosis presents many challenges. In most cases, the samples are paucibacillary, decreasing the sensitivity of diagnostic tests. Testing for extrapulmonary tuberculosis follows the same principles as for PTB. However, as accuracy of diagnosis is reduced in extrapulmonary disease, clinicians rely more heavily on clinical judgement and response to treatment. Meanwhile, the increased incidence of extrapulmonary tuberculosis in HIV-infected patients makes it urgent to improve diagnostic strategies for this entity.

AFB smear and culture are used but are generally less sensitive in non-respiratory samples, and respiratory samples are sometimes of benefit in extrapulmonary tuberculosis. In pleural tuberculosis, isolation of *M. tuberculosis* from sputum is diagnostic of tuberculosis in patients with an effusion. However, such patients may not provide expectorated sputum samples. Induced sputum in this setting is 52 per cent sensitive for tuberculosis,[98] compared with 60–80 per cent sensitivity of the more invasive pleural biopsy.[99]

In miliary tuberculosis, sputum smears are warranted, but if negative, FOB may play a significant role. In 41 patients with miliary disease and smear-negative sputum, FOB provided the diagnosis in 83 per cent.[100] Bronchial brushings captured 57 per cent of cases, transbronchial biopsy was diagnostic in 73 per cent, and a rapid diagnosis was made in 79 per cent of cases.[100] In another study of 22 patients with smear-negative miliary tuberculosis, FOB with brushings, aspirate and transbronchial biopsy diagnosed tuberculosis in 73 per cent. A rapid diagnosis was made in 64 per cent, transbronchial biopsy alone making 32 per cent of these.[101] Sampling multiple sites may also be of benefit in miliary disease.

NAA assays can clearly contribute in the diagnosis of extrapulmonary tuberculosis, but this role needs to be better defined. The overall sensitivity in non-respiratory specimens for the MTD or E-MTD tests ranges from 67 to 100 per cent.[17,63–65,70,78,80,102] In smear-negative samples, the sensitivity was 52 per cent in one study[70] and 100 per cent in another.[17] The AMPLICOR test had a similar sensitivity[72,103] and the specificity of both tests remains very high in non-respiratory samples. The assays do not perform equally well in all sample types, being much more sensitive in cerebrospinal fluid[102,104] than in pleural fluid.[64] However, the sensitivities vary significantly between studies, as shown in recent meta-analyses of the use of NAA tests in tuberculous meningitis[105] and pleuritis.[106] In one study of cerebrospinal fluid, the combination of AFB smear and MTD test had a sensitivity of 64 per cent, increasing to 83 per cent by the third sample tested.[107] The strand displacement amplification assay (BDProbeTec ET system) delivers similar sensitivity to the E-MTD test in non-respiratory samples.[80,108,109]

Adenosine deaminase (ADA) levels show great promise for the diagnosis of extrapulmonary tuberculosis, especially in pleural fluid samples. Two recent meta-analyses of a total of 71 studies investigating ADA for the diagnosis of tuberculous pleuritis concluded that, by using optimal cut-off values, sensitivity and specificity of ADA measurements were 92–93 per cent.[110,111] However, the performance of ADA is inconsistent across studies. In one report, the sensitivity and specificity were both 55 per cent,[112] and in another, 88 and 86 per cent, respectively.[113] There is also controversy over whether the combination of ADA determinations and PCR analysis yields superior results.[114,115] ADA may also be of limited value in diagnosing tuberculous meningitis[116] and was very sensitive for detection of tuberculous pericarditis in one study.[117]

Interferon-γ levels have been used to diagnose pleural and pericardial tuberculosis, with sensitivity and specificity similar to or better than ADA in some studies.[111,113,117] Finally, the IFN-γ release assays, discussed in Chapter 6, can also contribute to the diagnosis of extrapulmonary tuberculosis.

RAPID DETECTION OF DRUG RESISTANCE

Multidrug-resistant tuberculosis poses a major public health problem in many parts of the world. Traditional methods of drug susceptibility testing rely on cultures of *M. tuberculosis* in antibiotic-containing media and can take weeks for results to be known. Rapid detection of drug resistance is vital to tuberculosis control efforts, enabling expeditious administration of appropriate therapy and a decrease in transmission of drug-resistant strains. Rifampin resistance may be used as a surrogate for multidrug resistance since most rifampicin-resistant isolates are also isoniazid-resistant.[118,119] Rifampicin resistance therefore generally signals the need for treatment with second-line drugs. It is currently feasible to rapidly detect rifampicin resistance. One approach identifies mutations, primarily in the *rpoB* gene, that are associated with the vast majority of rifampicin-resistant *M. tuberculosis* strains. Coupling a variety of assays that identify genetic mutations (such as line probe assays and molecular beacons, described below) to PCR or related technologies allows rapid detection of the drug-resistant mutations from smear-positive respiratory specimens or from pure cultures.[118,120–124] Another approach, such as the luciferase reporter phage assay, detects phenotypic resistance, seen as persistence of the organism in a rifamycin-containing medium.

Cost and requirements for advanced technology and laboratory skills limit the applicability of many of these technologies. However, efforts to reduce costs and simplify the technology may make these tests practical for widespread use in the near future in resource-rich and perhaps in resource-poor countries.

Line probe assays

Line probe assays use PCR and reverse hybridization with specific oligonucleotide probes fixed to nitrocellulose strips in parallel lines. These assays may be used for the detection and identification of mycobacterial species or for rapid identification of mutations in the *rpoB* gene. The Inno-LiPA Mycobacteria v2 (Innogenetics, Ghent, Belgium) and GenoType Mycobacterium (Hain Diagnostika, Nehren, Germany) are very sensitive line probe assays for the simultaneous detection and identification of mycobacteria.[125] The Inno-LiPA Rif.TB assay is very sensitive for detecting rifampicin resistance.[122–124,126,127]

Molecular beacons

Molecular beacons are nucleic acid hybridization probes, designed to bind to target DNA sequences in regions, such as the *rpoB* gene, where resistance mutations are known to occur. Molecular beacons fluoresce only when bound to their targets, so that a mutation – even a single nucleotide substitution – will prevent fluorescence. A PCR assay utilizing molecular beacons can identify drug resistance in sputum samples in less than 3 hours and is both sensitive and specific.[128] Lin *et al.*[120] designed molecular beacons to detect isoniazid- and rifampicin-resistant mutations in *M. tuberculosis* from both culture- and smear-positive respiratory specimens. The sensitivity and specificity for detection of isoniazid resistance were 83 and 100 per cent, respectively, and those for rifampicin resistance were 98 and 100 per cent, respectively. Similar findings were reported by Piatek *et al.*[129]

Phage amplification

Phage amplification uses a bacteriophage to detect *M. tuberculosis* in a sample within 48 hours. FASTPlaqueTB (Biotec, Ipswich, UK) uses phage amplification to detect viable *M. tuberculosis* in sputum samples and has excellent specificity (96–99 per cent), but less sensitivity (70–87 per cent),[25,130–132] with 49 per cent of smear-negative cases detected in one study.[132] Albert *et al.*[119,133] found that the FASTPlaqueTB-RIF assay, which uses phage amplification to determine rifampicin resistance, had 100 per cent sensitivity and 94–99 per cent specificity for identifying rifampicin-resistant strains in solid or liquid culture media. More recently, they showed that this assay has 100 per cent sensitivity and specificity for determining rifampicin resistance directly from 145 smear-positive sputum samples, 11 of which contained rifampicin-resistant organisms.[134] No complex dedicated equipment or expensive supplies are needed, making it particularly suitable for use in resource-poor countries, and the results are available within 48 hours.

Luciferase reporter phages

Firefly luciferase catalyses the reaction of luciferin with ATP to generate photons and emit light. When mycobac-teriophages expressing the firefly luciferase gene are introduced into mycobacteria,[135] cellular ATP in viable mycobacteria causes light to be emitted when exogenous luciferin is added. The light is measured by a luminometer or film.[136,137] In the presence of antituberculosis drugs, drug-susceptible mycobacteria are rendered non-viable and the light is extinguished, whereas drug-resistant strains continue to produce light. This method is both sensitive and specific, and determines drug susceptibility in 1–4 days. It is also a sensitive means to identify *M. tuberculosis*.[137–141]

LEARNING POINTS

- The diagnosis of tuberculosis in most of the world still relies on the acid-fast smear, which is only about 50 per cent sensitive.
- For patients with negative sputum smears or who cannot produce sputum, SI and FOB can permit a rapid diagnosis and provide organisms for culture. SI has a comparable or higher diagnostic yield than FOB, is less costly and is preferred in resource-poor countries. FOB is indicated in selected patients in resource-rich countries.
- NAA tests are much more sensitive than the acid-fast smear. In the USA, the AMPLICOR and MTD tests are approved for use in smear-positive respiratory specimens. The E-MTD test has increased sensitivity and is approved for use in smear-negative samples.
- A reasonable diagnostic strategy in resource-rich countries is to perform a NAA assay and AFB smear on the first sputum sample. If both are positive, the patient has tuberculosis. If the smear is positive and the NAA test is negative, the sputum should be tested for inhibitors. If inhibitors are present, the NAA assay is not useful. If inhibitors are absent, more specimens are tested. If they are smear-positive, NAA-negative and without inhibitors, non-tuberculous mycobacterial disease is diagnosed. If smears are negative but the clinical suspicion for PTB is intermediate or high, NAA tests should be done, and if positive, PTB is diagnosed. If smears are negative but the clinical suspicion for tuberculosis is low, NAA assays should not be performed.
- NAA assays should not be undertaken in patients who have been recently treated for tuberculosis because nucleic acids from dead organisms can yield false-positive results.
- Extrapulmonary tuberculosis is usually paucibacillary and AFB smears are less sensitive than for PTB. SI and FOB are useful for diagnosis of pleural and miliary tuberculosis, respectively. NAA assays can contribute to the diagnosis, but their role is not clearly defined.

- Elevated adenosine deaminase levels are a promising means to diagnose pleural tuberculosis, but test performance is inconsistent across studies.
- Rifampicin resistance, a surrogate marker for multidrug resistance, can be identified by detecting mutations in the *rpoB* gene, using the line probe assay and molecular beacons. Alternatively, phage amplification and luciferase reporter phages can detect viable *M. tuberculosis* in rifampicin-containing media, providing phenotypic evidence of resistance. The roles of these new tests are being defined.

REFERENCES

1. Keeler E, Perkins MD, Small P *et al.* Reducing the global burden of tuberculosis: the contribution of improved diagnostics. *Nature,* 2006; **444** (Suppl. 1): 49–57.
2. Mohan AK, Cote TR, Block JA *et al.* Tuberculosis following the use of etanercept, a tumor necrosis factor inhibitor. *Clin Infect Dis* 2004; **39**: 295–9.
3. Centers for Disease Control and Prevention. Tuberculosis associated with blocking agents against tumor necrosis factor-alpha – California, 2002–2003. *MMWR Morb Mortal Wkly Rep* 2004; **53**: 683–6.
4. Keane J, Gershon S, Wise RP *et al.* Tuberculosis associated with infliximab, a tumor necrosis factor alpha-neutralizing agent. *N Engl J Med* 2001; **345**: 1098–104.
5. Okur E, Yilmaz A, Saygi A *et al.* Patterns of delays in diagnosis amongst patients with smear-positive pulmonary tuberculosis at a teaching hospital in Turkey. *Clin Microbiol Infect* 2006; **12**: 90–2.
6. Ellis SM. The spectrum of tuberculosis and non-tuberculous mycobacterial infection. *Eur Radiol* 2004; **14** (Suppl. 3): E34–42.
7. Geng E, Kreiswirth B, Burzynski J *et al.* (2005). Clinical and radiographic correlates of primary and reactivation tuberculosis: a molecular epidemiology study. *J Am Med Assoc* 2005; **293**: 2740–5.
8. Centers for Disease Control and Prevention. Guidelines for preventing the transmission of *Mycobacterium tuberculosis* in health-care facilities, 1994. *MMWR Rec Rep* 1994; **43** (RR-13), 1–132.
9. Jacubowiak W. *TB manual national tuberculosis programme guidelines.* Geneva: World Health Organization, 2001.
10. Mathew P, Kuo YH, Vazirani B *et al.* Are three sputum acid-fast bacillus smears necessary for discontinuing tuberculosis isolation? *J Clin Microbiol* 2002; **40**: 3482–4.
11. Craft DW, Jones MC, Blanchet CN *et al.* Value of examining three acid-fast bacillus sputum smears for removal of patients suspected of having tuberculosis from the 'airborne precautions' category. *J Clin Microbiol* 2000; **38**: 4285–7.
12. Wu ZL, Wang AQ. Diagnostic yield of repeated smear microscopy examinations among patients suspected of pulmonary tuberculosis in Shandong province of China. *Int J Tuberc Lung Dis* 2000; **4**: 1086–7.
13. Diagnostic standards and classification of tuberculosis in adults and children, 1999. *Am J Respir Crit Care Med* 2000; **161**: 1376–95.
14. Bergmann JS, Yuoh G, Fish G *et al.* Clinical evaluation of the enhanced Gen-Probe Amplified Mycobacterium Tuberculosis Direct Test for rapid diagnosis of tuberculosis in prison inmates. *J Clin Microbiol* 1999; **37**: 1419–25.
15. Cohen RA, Muzaffar S, Schwartz D *et al.* Diagnosis of pulmonary tuberculosis using PCR assays on sputum collected within 24 hours of hospital admission. *Am J Respir Crit Care Med* 1998; **157**: 156–61.
16. Dalovisio JR, Montenegro-James S, Kemmerly SA *et al.* Comparison of the amplified *Mycobacterium tuberculosis* (MTB) direct test, Amplicor MTB PCR, and IS*6110*-PCR for detection of MTB in respiratory specimens. *Clin Infect Dis*, 1996; **23**: 1099–106; discussion 1107–108.
17. Chedore P, Jamieson FB. Routine use of the Gen-Probe MTD2 amplification test for detection of *Mycobacterium tuberculosis* in clinical specimens in a large public health mycobacteriology laboratory. *Diagn Microbiol Infect Dis* 1999; **35**: 185–91.
18. Rajalahti I, Vuorinen P, Nieminen MM *et al.* Detection of *Mycobacterium tuberculosis* complex in sputum specimens by the automated Roche Cobas Amplicor Mycobacterium Tuberculosis Test. *J Clin Microbiol* 1998; **36**: 975–8.
19. Murray PR, Elmore C, Krogstad DJ. The acid-fast stain: a specific and predictive test for mycobacterial disease. *Ann Intern Med* 1980; **92**: 512–13.
20. Strumpf IJ, Tsang AY, Sayre JW. Re-evaluation of sputum staining for the diagnosis of pulmonary tuberculosis. *Am Rev Respir Dis* 1979; **119**: 599–602.
21. Mehta J, Krish G, Berro E *et al.* Fiberoptic bronchoscopy in the diagnosis of pulmonary tuberculosis. *South Med J* 1990; **83**: 753–5.
22. Baughman RP, Dohn MN, Loudon RG *et al.* Bronchoscopy with bronchoalveolar lavage in tuberculosis and fungal infections. *Chest* 1991; **99**: 92–7.
23. Kim TC, Blackman RS, Heatwole KM *et al.* Acid-fast bacilli in sputum smears of patients with pulmonary tuberculosis. Prevalence and significance of negative smears pretreatment and positive smears post-treatment. *Am Rev Respir Dis* 1984; **129**: 264–8.
24. Sputum-smear-negative pulmonary tuberculosis: controlled trial of 3-month and 2-month regimens of chemotherapy. *Lancet* 1979; **1**: 1361–3.
25. Mbulo GM, Kambashi BS, Kinkese J *et al.* (2004). Comparison of two bacteriophage tests and nucleic acid amplification for the diagnosis of pulmonary tuberculosis in sub-Saharan Africa. *Int J Tuberc Lung Dis* 2004; **8**: 1342–7.
26. Hensler NM, Spivey CG Jr, Dees TM. The use of hypertonic aerosol in production of sputum for diagnosis of tuberculosis. Comparison with gastric specimens. *Dis Chest* 1961; **40**: 639–42.
27. Jones FL Jr. The relative efficacy of spontaneous sputa, aerosol-induced sputa, and gastric aspirates in the bacteriologic diagnosis of pulmonary tuberculosis. *Dis Chest* 1966; **50**: 403–408.
28. Carr DT, Karlson AG, Stilwell GG. A comparison of cultures of induced sputum and gastric washings in the diagnosis of tuberculosis. *Mayo Clin Proc* 1967; **42**: 23–5.
29. Dickson SJ, Brent A, Davidson RN *et al.* Comparison of bronchoscopy and gastric washings in the investigation of smear-negative pulmonary tuberculosis. *Clin Infect Dis* 2003; **37**: 1649–53.
30. Li LM, Bai LQ, Yang HL *et al.* Sputum induction to improve the diagnostic yield in patients with suspected pulmonary tuberculosis. *Int J Tuberc Lung Dis* 1999; **3**: 1137–9.
31. Parry CM, Kamoto O, Harries AD *et al.* The use of sputum induction for establishing a diagnosis in patients with suspected pulmonary tuberculosis in Malawi. *Tuber Lung Dis* 1995; **76**: 72–6.
32. Hartung TK, Maulu A, Nash J *et al.* Suspected pulmonary tuberculosis in rural South Africa – sputum induction as a simple diagnostic tool? *S Afr Med J*, 2002; **92**: 455–8.
33. Merrick ST, Sepkowitz KA, Walsh J *et al.* Comparison of induced versus expectorated sputum for diagnosis of pulmonary tuberculosis by acid-fast smear. *Am J Infect Control* 1997; **25**: 463–6.
34. Bell D, Leckie V, McKendrick M. The role of induced sputum in the diagnosis of pulmonary tuberculosis. *J Infect* 2003; **47**: 317–21.
35. Al Zahrani K, Al Jahdali H, Poirier L *et al.* Yield of smear, culture and amplification tests from repeated sputum induction for the

diagnosis of pulmonary tuberculosis. *Int J Tuberc Lung Dis* 2001; **5**: 855–60.

36. Chawla R, Pant K, Jaggi OP *et al.* Fibreoptic bronchoscopy in smear-negative pulmonary tuberculosis. *Eur Respir J* 1988; **1**: 804–806.

37. So SY, Lam WK, Yu DY. Rapid diagnosis of suspected pulmonary tuberculosis by fiberoptic bronchoscopy. *Tubercle* 1982; **63**: 195–200.

38. Willcox PA, Benatar SR, Potgieter PD. Use of the flexible fibreoptic bronchoscope in diagnosis of sputum-negative pulmonary tuberculosis. *Thorax* 1982; **37**: 598–601.

39. Sarkar SK, Sharma GS, Gupta PR *et al.* Fiberoptic bronchoscopy in the diagnosis of pulmonary tuberculosis. *Tubercle* 1980; **61**: 97–9.

40. Danek SJ, Bower JS. Diagnosis of pulmonary tuberculosis by flexible fiberoptic bronchoscopy. *Am Rev Respir Dis* 1979; **119**: 677–9.

41. Kennedy DJ, Lewis WP, Barnes PF. Yield of bronchoscopy for the diagnosis of tuberculosis in patients with human immuno-deficiency virus infection. *Chest* 1982; **102**: 1040–4.

42. Russell MD, Torrington KG, Tenholder MF. A ten-year experience with fiberoptic bronchoscopy for mycobacterial isolation. Impact of the Bactec system. *Am Rev Respir Dis* 1986; **133**: 1069–71.

43. Palva T, Elo R, Saloheimo M. Bronchoscopy in pulmonary tuberculosis. *Acta Tuberc Scand* 1957; **33**: 241–64.

44. Ip M, Chau PY, So SY *et al.* The value of routine bronchial aspirate culture at fibreoptic bronchoscopy for the diagnosis of tuberculosis. *Tubercle* 1989; **70**: 281–5.

45. Chan HS, Sun AJ, Hoheisel GB. Bronchoscopic aspiration and bronchoalveolar lavage in the diagnosis of sputum smear-negative pulmonary tuberculosis. *Lung* 1990; **168**: 215–20.

46. al-Kassimi FA, Azhar M, al-Majed S *et al.* Diagnostic role of fibreoptic bronchoscopy in tuberculosis in the presence of typical X-ray pictures and adequate sputum. *Tubercle* 1991; **72**: 145–8.

47. Palenque E, Amor E, Bernaldo de Quiros JC. Comparison of bronchial washing, brushing and biopsy for diagnosis of pulmonary tuberculosis. *Eur J Clin Microbiol* 1987; **6**: 191–2.

48. Uddenfeldt M, Lundgren R. Flexible fiberoptic bronchoscopy in the diagnosis of pulmonary tuberculosis. *Tubercle* 1981; **62**: 197–9.

49. Wallace JM, Deutsch AL, Harrell JH *et al.* Bronchoscopy and transbronchial biopsy in evaluation of patients with suspected active tuberculosis. *Am J Med* 1981; **70**: 1189–94.

50. Fujii H, Ishihara J, Fukaura A *et al.* Early diagnosis of tuberculosis by fibreoptic bronchoscopy. *Tuber Lung Dis* 1992; **73**: 167–9.

51. Wongthim S, Udompanich V, Limthongkul S *et al.* Fiberoptic bronchoscopy in diagnosis of patients with suspected active pulmonary tuberculosis. *J Med Assoc Thai* 1989; **72**: 154–9.

52. de Gracia J, Curull V, Vidal R *et al.* Diagnostic value of bronchoalveolar lavage in suspected pulmonary tuberculosis. *Chest* 1988; **93**: 329–32.

53. McWilliams T, Wells AU, Harrison AC *et al.* Induced sputum and bronchoscopy in the diagnosis of pulmonary tuberculosis. *Thorax* 2002; **57**: 1010–14.

54. Anderson C, Inhaber N, Menzies D. Comparison of sputum induction with fiber-optic bronchoscopy in the diagnosis of tuberculosis. *Am J Respir Crit Care Med* 1995; **152**: 1570–4.

55. Conde MB, Soares SL, Mello FC *et al.* Comparison of sputum induction with fiberoptic bronchoscopy in the diagnosis of tuberculosis: experience at an acquired immune deficiency syndrome reference center in Rio de Janeiro, Brazil. *Am J Respir Crit Care Med* 2000; **162**: 2238–40.

56. Schoch OD, Rieder P, Tueller C *et al.* Diagnostic yield of sputum, induced sputum, and bronchoscopy after radiologic tuberculosis screening. *Am J Respir Crit Care Med* 2007; **175**: 80–6.

57. Larson JL, Ridzon R, Hannan MM. Sputum induction versus fiberoptic bronchoscopy in the diagnosis of tuberculosis. *Am J Respir Crit Care Med* 2001; **163**: 1279–80.

58. Morgan MA, Horstmeier CD, DeYoung DR *et al.* Comparison of a radiometric method (BACTEC) and conventional culture media for

recovery of mycobacteria from smear-negative specimens. *J Clin Microbiol* 1983; **18**: 384–8.

59. Sharp SE, Lemes M, Sierra SG *et al.* Lowenstein–Jensen media. No longer necessary for mycobacterial isolation. *Am J Clin Pathol* 2000; **113**: 770–3.

60. Ichiyama S, Shimokata K, Takeuchi J. Comparative study of a biphasic culture system (Roche MB Check system) with a conventional egg medium for recovery of mycobacteria. Aichi Mycobacteriosis Research Group. *Tuber Lung Dis* 1993; **74**: 338–41.

61. Kanchana MV, Cheke D, Natyshak I *et al.* Evaluation of the BACTEC MGIT 960 system for the recovery of mycobacteria. *Diagn Microbiol Infect Dis* 2000; **37**: 31–6.

62. Sharp SE, Lemes M, Erlich SS *et al.* A comparison of the Bactec 9000MB system and the Septi-Chek AFB system for the detection of mycobacteria. *Diagn Microbiol Infect Dis* 1997; **28**: 69–74.

63. Gamboa F, Fernandez G, Padilla E *et al.* Comparative evaluation of initial and new versions of the Gen-Probe Amplified Mycobacterium Tuberculosis Direct Test for direct detection of *Mycobacterium tuberculosis* in respiratory and nonrespiratory specimens. *J Clin Microbiol* 1998; **36**: 684–9.

64. Vlaspolder F, Singer P, Roggeveen C. Diagnostic value of an amplification method (Gen-Probe) compared with that of culture for diagnosis of tuberculosis. *J Clin Microbiol* 1995; **33**: 2699–703.

65. Pfyffer GE, Kissling P, Jahn EM *et al.* Diagnostic performance of amplified *Mycobacterium tuberculosis* direct test with cerebrospinal fluid, other nonrespiratory, and respiratory specimens. *J Clin Microbiol* 1996; **34**: 834–41.

66. Bradley SP, Reed SL, Catanzaro A. Clinical efficacy of the amplified *Mycobacterium tuberculosis* direct test for the diagnosis of pulmonary tuberculosis. *Am J Respir Crit Care Med* 1996; **153**: 1606–10.

67. Della-Latta P, Whittier S. Comprehensive evaluation of performance, laboratory application, and clinical usefulness of two direct amplification technologies for the detection of *Mycobacterium tuberculosis* complex. *Am J Clin Pathol* 1998; **110**: 301–10.

68. Pfyffer GE, Kissling P, Wirth R *et al.* Direct detection of *Mycobacterium tuberculosis* complex in respiratory specimens by a target-amplified test system. *J Clin Microbiol* 1994; **32**: 918–23.

69. Wang SX, Tay L. Evaluation of three nucleic acid amplification methods for direct detection of *Mycobacterium tuberculosis* complex in respiratory specimens. *J Clin Microbiol* 1999; **37**: 1932–4.

70. Coll P, Garrigo M, Moreno C *et al.* Routine use of Gen-Probe Amplified Mycobacterium Tuberculosis Direct (MTD) test for detection of *Mycobacterium tuberculosis* with smear-positive and smear-negative specimens. *Int J Tuberc Lung Dis* 2003; **7**: 886–91.

71. Wobeser WL, Krajden M, Conly J *et al.* Evaluation of Roche Amplicor PCR assay for *Mycobacterium tuberculosis*. *J Clin Microbiol* 1998; **34**: 134–9.

72. Carpentier E, Drouillard B, Dailloux M *et al.* Diagnosis of tuberculosis by Amplicor *Mycobacterium tuberculosis* test: a multicenter study. *J Clin Microbiol* 1995; **33**: 3106–10.

73. Dilworth JP, Goyal M, Young DB *et al.* Comparison of polymerase chain reaction for IS6110 and Amplicor in the diagnosis of tuberculosis. *Thorax* 1996; **51**: 320–2.

74. Tevere VJ, Hewitt PL, Dare A *et al.* Detection of *Mycobacterium tuberculosis* by PCR amplification with pan-Mycobacterium primers and hybridization to an *M. tuberculosis*-specific probe. *J Clin Microbiol* 1996; **34**: 918–23.

75. Lim T. Relationship between estimated pretest probability and accuracy of automated *Mycobacterium tuberculosis* assay in smear-negative pulmonary tuberculosis. *Chest* 2000; **118**: 641–7.

76. Bergmann JS, Woods GL. Clinical evaluation of the Roche AMPLICOR PCR *Mycobacterium tuberculosis* test for detection of *M. tuberculosis* in respiratory specimens. *J Clin Microbiol* 1996; **34**: 1083–5.

77. Laifer G, Widmer AF, Frei R et al. Polymerase chain reaction for *Mycobacterium tuberculosis*: impact on clinical management of refugees with pulmonary infiltrates. *Chest* 2004; **125**: 981–6.

78. Piersimoni C, Callegaro A, Scarparo C et al. Comparative evaluation of the new Gen-probe *Mycobacterium tuberculosis* amplified direct test and the semiautomated abbott LCx *Mycobacterium tuberculosis* assay for direct detection of *Mycobacterium tuberculosis* complex in respiratory and extrapulmonary specimens. *J Clin Microbiol* 1998; **36**: 3601–604.

79. Catanzaro A, Perry S, Clarridge JE et al. The role of clinical suspicion in evaluating a new diagnostic test for active tuberculosis: results of a multicenter prospective trial. *J Am Med Assoc* 2000; **283**: 639–45.

80. Piersimoni C, Scarparo C, Piccoli P et al. Performance assessment of two commercial amplification assays for direct detection of *Mycobacterium tuberculosis* complex from respiratory and extrapulmonary specimens. *J Clin Microbiol* 2002; **40**: 4138–42.

81. Visca P, De Mori P, Festa A et al. Evaluation of the BDProbeTec strand displacement amplification assay in comparison with the AMTD II direct test for rapid diagnosis of tuberculosis. *Clin Microbiol Infect* 2004; **10**: 332–4.

82. Sperhacke RD, Mello FC, Zaha A et al. Detection of *Mycobacterium tuberculosis* by a polymerase chain reaction colorimetric dot-blot assay. *Int J Tuberc Lung Dis* 2004; **8**: 312–17.

83. Lemaitre N, Armand S, Vachee A et al. Comparison of the real-time PCR method and the Gen-Probe amplified *Mycobacterium tuberculosis* direct test for detection of *Mycobacterium tuberculosis* in pulmonary and nonpulmonary specimens. *J Clin Microbiol* 2004; **42**: 4307–309.

84. Miller N, Cleary T, Kraus G et al. Rapid and specific detection of *Mycobacterium tuberculosis* from acid-fast bacillus smear-positive respiratory specimens and BacT/ALERT MP culture bottles by using fluorogenic probes and real-time PCR. *J Clin Microbiol* 2002; **40**: 4143–7.

85. Cleary TJ, Roudel G, Casillas O et al. Rapid and specific detection of *Mycobacterium tuberculosis* by using the Smart Cycler instrument and a specific fluorogenic probe. *J Clin Microbiol* 2003; **41**: 4783–6.

86. Update: Nucleic acid amplification tests for tuberculosis. *MMWR Morb Mortal Wkly Rep* 2000; **49**: 593–4.

87. Sloutsky A, Han LL, Werner BG. Practical strategies for performance optimization of the enhanced Gen-probe amplified *Mycobacterium tuberculosis* direct test. *J Clin Microbiol* 2004; **42**: 1547–51.

88. Divinagracia RM, Harkin TJ, Bonk S et al. Screening by specialists to reduce unnecessary test ordering in patients evaluated for tuberculosis. *Chest* 1998; **114**: 681–4.

89. Lim TK, Mukhopadhyay A, Gough A et al. Role of clinical judgment in the application of a nucleic acid amplification test for the rapid diagnosis of pulmonary tuberculosis. *Chest* 2003; **124**: 902–908.

90. Van den Wijngaert S, Dediste A, VanLaethem Y et al. Critical use of nucleic acid amplification techniques to test for *Mycobacterium tuberculosis* in respiratory tract samples. *J Clin Microbiol* 2004; **42**: 837–8.

91. Roos BR, van Cleeff MR, Githui WA et al. Cost-effectiveness of the polymerase chain reaction versus smear examination for the diagnosis of tuberculosis in Kenya: a theoretical model. *Int J Tuberc Lung Dis* 1998; **2**: 235–41.

92. Rajalahti I, Ruokonen EL, Kotomaki T et al. Economic evaluation of the use of PCR assay in diagnosing pulmonary TB in a low-incidence area. *Eur Respir J* 2004; **23**: 446–51.

93. Dowdy DW, Maters A, Parrish N et al. Cost-effectiveness analysis of the Gen-probe amplified *Mycobacterium tuberculosis* direct test as used routinely on smear-positive respiratory specimens. *J Clin Microbiol* 2003; **41**: 948–53.

94. Yuen KY, Chan KS, Chan CM et al. Use of PCR in routine diagnosis of treated and untreated pulmonary tuberculosis. *J Clin Pathol* 1993; **46**: 318–22.

95. Walker DA, Taylor IK, Mitchell DM et al. Comparison of polymerase chain reaction amplification of two mycobacterial DNA sequences, IS6110 and the 65 kDa antigen gene, in the diagnosis of tuberculosis. *Thorax* 1992; **47**: 690–94.

96. Schluger NW, Kinney D, Harkin TJ et al. Clinical utility of the polymerase chain reaction in the diagnosis of infections due to *Mycobacterium tuberculosis*. *Chest* 1994; **105**: 1116–21.

97. Hellyer TJ, DesJardin LE, Teixeira L et al. Detection of viable *Mycobacterium tuberculosis* by reverse transcriptase-strand displacement amplification of mRNA. *J Clin Microbiol* 1999; **37**: 518–23.

98. Conde MB, Loivos AC, Rezende VM et al. Yield of sputum induction in the diagnosis of pleural tuberculosis. *Am J Respir Crit Care Med* 2003; **167**: 723–5.

99. Menzies D. Sputum induction: simpler, cheaper, and safer – but is it better? *Am J Respir Crit Care Med* 2003; **167**: 676–7.

100. Willcox PA, Potgieter PD, Bateman ED et al. Rapid diagnosis of sputum negative miliary tuberculosis using the flexible fibreoptic bronchoscope. *Thorax* 1986; **41**: 681–4.

101. Pant K, Chawla R, Mann PS et al. Fiberbronchoscopy in smear-negative miliary tuberculosis. *Chest* 1989; **95**: 1151–2.

102. Lang AM, Feris-Iglesias J, Pena C et al. Clinical evaluation of the Gen-Probe Amplified Direct Test for detection of *Mycobacterium tuberculosis* complex organisms in cerebrospinal fluid. *J Clin Microbiol* 1998; **36**: 2191–4.

103. Shah S, Miller A, Mastellone A et al. Rapid diagnosis of tuberculosis in various biopsy and body fluid specimens by the AMPLICOR Mycobacterium tuberculosis polymerase chain reaction test. *Chest* 1998; **113**: 1190–4.

104. Cloud JL, Shutt C, Aldous W et al. Evaluation of a modified Gen-probe amplified direct test for detection of *Mycobacterium tuberculosis* complex organisms in cerebrospinal fluid. *J Clin Microbiol* 2004; **42**: 5341–4.

105. Pai M, Flores LL, Pai N et al. Diagnostic accuracy of nucleic acid amplification tests for tuberculous meningitis: a systematic review and meta-analysis. *Lancet Infect Dis* 2003; **3**: 633–43.

106. Pai M, Flores LL, Hubbard A et al. Nucleic acid amplification tests in the diagnosis of tuberculous pleuritis: a systematic review and meta-analysis. *BMC Infect Dis* 2004; **4**: 6.

107. Thwaites GE, Caws M, Chau TT et al. Comparison of conventional bacteriology with nucleic acid amplification (amplified mycobacterium direct test) for diagnosis of tuberculous meningitis before and after inception of antituberculosis chemotherapy. *J Clin Microbiol* 2004; **42**: 996–1002.

108. Mazzarelli G, Rindi L, Piccoli P et al. Evaluation of the BDProbeTec ET system for direct detection of *Mycobacterium tuberculosis* in pulmonary and extrapulmonary samples: a multicenter study. *J Clin Microbiol* 2003; **41**: 1779–82.

109. Johansen IS, Lundgren B, Tabak F et al. Improved sensitivity of nucleic acid amplification for rapid diagnosis of tuberculous meningitis. *J Clin Microbiol* 2004; **42**: 3036–40.

110. Goto M, Noguchi Y, Koyama H et al. Diagnostic value of adenosine deaminase in tuberculous pleural effusion: a meta-analysis. *Ann Clin Biochem* 2003; **40**: 374–81.

111. Greco S, Girardi E, Masciangelo R et al. Adenosine deaminase and interferon gamma measurements for the diagnosis of tuberculous pleurisy: a meta-analysis. *Int J Tuberc Lung Dis* 2003; **7**: 777–86.

112. Nagesh BS, Sehgal S, Jindal SK et al. Evaluation of polymerase chain reaction for detection of *Mycobacterium tuberculosis* in pleural fluid. *Chest* 2001; **119**: 1737–41.

113. Villegas MV, Labrada LA, Saravia NG. Evaluation of polymerase chain reaction, adenosine deaminase, and interferon-gamma in pleural fluid for the differential diagnosis of pleural tuberculosis. *Chest* 2000; **118**: 1355–64.

114. Lima DM, Colares JK, da Fonseca BA. Combined use of the polymerase chain reaction and detection of adenosine deaminase activity on pleural fluid improves the rate of diagnosis of pleural tuberculosis. *Chest* 2003; **124**: 909–14.

115. Trajman A, Kaisermann MC, Kritski AL *et al*. Diagnosing pleural tuberculosis. *Chest* 2004; **125**: 2366; author reply 2366-7.

116. Corral I, Quereda C, Navas E *et al*. Adenosine deaminase activity in cerebrospinal fluid of HIV-infected patients: limited value for diagnosis of tuberculous meningitis. *Eur J Clin Microbiol Infect Dis* 2004; **23**: 471-6.

117. Burgess LJ, Reuter H, Carstens ME *et al*. The use of adenosine deaminase and interferon-gamma as diagnostic tools for tuberculous pericarditis. *Chest* 2002; **122**: 900-905.

118. Fan XY, Hu ZY, Xu FH *et al*. Rapid detection of *rpoB* gene mutations in rifampin-resistant *Mycobacterium tuberculosis* isolates in Shanghai by using the amplification refractory mutation system. *J Clin Microbiol* 2003; **41**: 993-7.

119. Albert H, Trollip AP, Mole RJ *et al*. Rapid indication of multidrug-resistant tuberculosis from liquid cultures using FASTPlaqueTB-RIF, a manual phage-based test. *Int J Tuberc Lung Dis* 2002; **6**: 523-8.

120. Lin SY, Probert W, Lo M *et al*. Rapid detection of isoniazid and rifampin resistance mutations in *Mycobacterium tuberculosis* complex from cultures or smear-positive sputa by use of molecular beacons. *J Clin Microbiol* 2004; **42**: 4204-208.

121. Mokrousov I, Otten T, Vyshnevskiy B *et al*. Allele-specific *rpoB* PCR assays for detection of rifampin-resistant *Mycobacterium tuberculosis* in sputum smears. *Antimicrob Agents Chemother* 2003; **47**: 2231-5.

122. Cooksey RC, Morlock GP, Glickman S *et al*. Evaluation of a line probe assay kit for characterization of *rpoB* mutations in rifampin-resistant *Mycobacterium tuberculosis* isolates from New York City. *J Clin Microbiol* 1997; **35**: 1281-3.

123. Hirano K, Abe C, Takahashi M. Mutations in the *rpoB* gene of rifampin-resistant *Mycobacterium tuberculosis* strains isolated mostly in Asian countries and their rapid detection by line probe assay. *J Clin Microbiol* 1999; **37**: 2663-6.

124. Marttila HJ, Soini H, Vyshnevskaya E *et al*. Line probe assay in the rapid detection of rifampin-resistant *Mycobacterium tuberculosis* directly from clinical specimens. *Scand J Infect Dis* 1999; **31**: 269-73.

125. Padilla E, Gonzalez V, Manterola JM *et al*. Comparative evaluation of the new version of the INNO-LiPA Mycobacteria and genotype *Mycobacterium* assays for identification of *Mycobacterium* species from MB/BacT liquid cultures artificially inoculated with mycobacterial strains. *J Clin Microbiol* 2004; **42**: 3083-8.

126. Johansen IS, Lundgren B, Sosnovskaja A *et al*. Direct detection of multidrug-resistant *Mycobacterium tuberculosis* in clinical specimens in low- and high-incidence countries by line probe assay. *J Clin Microbiol* 2003; **41**: 4454-6.

127. Watterson SA, Wilson SM, Yates MD *et al*. Comparison of three molecular assays for rapid detection of rifampin resistance in *Mycobacterium tuberculosis*. *J Clin Microbiol* 1998; **36**: 1969-73.

128. El-Hajj HH, Marras SA, Tyagi S *et al*. Detection of rifampin resistance in *Mycobacterium tuberculosis* in a single tube with molecular beacons. *J Clin Microbiol* 2001; **39**: 4131-7.

129. Piatek AS, Telenti A, Murray MR *et al*. Genotypic analysis of *Mycobacterium tuberculosis* in two distinct populations using molecular beacons: implications for rapid susceptibility testing. *Antimicrob Agents Chemother* 2000; **44**: 103-10.

130. Butt T, Ahmad RN, Kazmi SY *et al*. Rapid diagnosis of pulmonary tuberculosis by mycobacteriophage assay. *Int J Tuberc Lung Dis* 2004; **8**: 899-902.

131. Albay A, Kisa O, Baylan O *et al*. The evaluation of FASTPlaqueTB test for the rapid diagnosis of tuberculosis. *Diagn Microbiol Infect Dis* 2003; **46**: 211-15.

132. Albert H, Heydenrych A, Brookes R *et al*. Performance of a rapid phage-based test, FASTPlaqueTB, to diagnose pulmonary tuberculosis from sputum specimens in South Africa. *Int J Tuberc Lung Dis* 2002; **6**: 529-37.

133. Albert H, Heydenrych A, Mole R *et al*. Evaluation of FASTPlaqueTB-RIF, a rapid, manual test for the determination of rifampicin resistance from *Mycobacterium tuberculosis* cultures. *Int J Tuberc Lung Dis* 2001; **5**: 906-11.

134. Albert H, Trollip A, Seaman T *et al*. Simple, phage-based (FASTPplaque) technology to determine rifampicin resistance of *Mycobacterium tuberculosis* directly from sputum. *Int J Tuberc Lung Dis* 2004; **8**: 1114-19.

135. Jacobs WR Jr, Barletta RG, Udani R *et al*. Rapid assessment of drug susceptibilities of *Mycobacterium tuberculosis* by means of luciferase reporter phages. *Science* 1993; **260**: 819-22.

136. Riska PF, Su Y, Bardarov S *et al*. Rapid film-based determination of antibiotic susceptibilities of *Mycobacterium tuberculosis* strains by using a luciferase reporter phage and the Bronx Box. *J Clin Microbiol* 1999; **37**: 1144-9.

137. Hazbon MH, Guarin N, Ferro BE *et al*. Photographic and luminometric detection of luciferase reporter phages for drug susceptibility testing of clinical *Mycobacterium tuberculosis* isolates. *J Clin Microbiol* 2003; **41**: 4865-9.

138. Carriere C, Riska PF, Zimhony O *et al*. Conditionally replicating luciferase reporter phages: improved sensitivity for rapid detection and assessment of drug susceptibility of *Mycobacterium tuberculosis*. *J Clin Microbiol* 1997; **35**: 3232-9.

139. Riska PF, Jacobs WR Jr, Bloom BR *et al*. Specific identification of *Mycobacterium tuberculosis* with the luciferase reporter mycobacteriophage: use of p-nitro-alpha-acetylamino-beta-hydroxy propiophenone. *J Clin Microbiol* 1997; **35**: 3225-31.

140. Banaiee N, Bobadilla-Del-Valle M, Bardarov S Jr *et al*. Luciferase reporter mycobacteriophages for detection, identification, and antibiotic susceptibility testing of *Mycobacterium tuberculosis* in Mexico. *J Clin Microbiol* 2001; **39**: 3883-8.

141. Banaiee N, Bobadilla-del-Valle M, Riska PF *et al*. Rapid identification and susceptibility testing of *Mycobacterium tuberculosis* from MGIT cultures with luciferase reporter mycobacteriophages. *J Med Microbiol* 2003; **52**: 557-61.

6

Immunodiagnostic tests

MELISSA R NYENDAK, DEBORAH A LEWINSOHN AND DAVID M LEWINSOHN

BACKGROUND

Until recently, the tuberculin skin test (TST) was the only method to assess infection with *Mycobacterium tuberculosis* (MTB). Because tuberculin contains >200 antigens, cross-reactivity with environmental mycobacteria and bacillus Calmette–Guérin (BCG) vaccination limits test specificity. Improper subcutaneous administration of tuberculin and digit preference also confound accurate interpretation.[1,2] The interferon-γ release assays (IGRAs) are T cell-based assays that measure interferon (IFN)-γ release by sensitized T cells in response to highly MTB-specific antigens. This chapter will review the literature and current indications for the commercially available IGRAs.

IGRAs utilize the potent MTB-specific antigens, early secretory antigen (ESAT)-6 and culture filtrate protein (CFP)-10, which elicit responses from people with active tuberculosis[3–5] and latent tuberculosis infection (LTBI),[6–8] and are absent from BCG and most non-tuberculous mycobacteria, except *Mycobacterium kansasii*, *Mycobacterium szulgai* and *Mycobacterium marinum*.[9–11] IGRAs primarily test CD4+ T-cell immunity. After exposure to mycobacterial antigen, some naive CD4+ T cells develop into effector memory T cells, which can respond rapidly to subsequent antigenic exposure by rapid release of IFN-γ, which is detected by IGRAs. In contrast, ongoing antigenic exposure, due to active tuberculosis or LTBI, may maintain IGRA responses.

The acquisition of CD4+ T-cell memory is strongly influenced by the original antigenic encounter, a phenomenon termed 'immunodominance'. For a given individual, the immune response is often tightly focused on a limited number of antigens and/or epitopes. Following the acquisition of cellular memory, the initial dominance hierarchy can have a profound impact on the response to subsequent antigenic exposures, and has three implications. First, in the absence of ongoing antigenic stimulation, the population of effector memory T cells (those capable of responding in a short-term IGRA) would be expected to decrease. Therefore, the TST (a 2- to 5-day assay) may better reflect remote exposures. Second, the original context of mycobacterial exposure may influence the acquisition of subsequent MTB-specific responses. For example, initial exposure to BCG or environmental mycobacteria may skew the response towards antigens found within BCG (such as antigen 85) and away from those unique to MTB, resulting in negative IGRA results. Third, ongoing antigenic exposure (either due to active tuberculosis or persistent latent infection) might drive and maintain high frequency T-cell responses and positive IGRA results.

METHODS

There are two commercially available IGRAs. The QuantiFERON®-TB Gold assay (Cellestis, Carnegie, Australia) (QFT-Gold) measures IFN-γ concentrations by enzyme-linked immunosorbent assay (ELISA), while the T-SPOT®.TB assay (Oxford Immunotec, Oxford, UK) (T-SPOT) assay enumerates T cells releasing IFN-γ by an enzyme-linked immunoblot (ELISPOT) assay. The more recent QuantiFERON®-TB Gold in-tube assay (QFT-Gold-IT) is similar to the QFT-Gold, but blood is collected directly into tubes containing the MTB-specific antigens, ESAT-6, CFP-10 and TB7.7(p4). Detailed test methodology is provided in the package inserts.[12,13]

QFT-Gold assays

For the QFT-Gold, aliquots of blood are placed in two wells, each containing peptides from ESAT- 6 or CFP-10; a negative control well containing media alone and a positive control well containing a mitogen, which stimulates T-cell division and determines whether viable, functional cells are present. After incubation overnight, IFN-γ release is assayed by ELISA. Specimen processing must be completed within 12 hours of collection. The QFT-Gold-IT test is used outside the USA and has recently been approved by the United States Food and Drug Administration. Here, blood is drawn directly into three heparinized tubes, one containing peptides from ESAT-6, CFP-10 and TB7.7, the other two containing the mitogen control and negative control. After incubation overnight, plasma is collected and the IFN-γ concentration is determined by ELISA. Perhaps because of the nearly immediate exposure of T cells to antigen, as well as the addition of the TB7.7 peptide, the QFT-Gold IT may be more sensitive than the QFT-Gold test (Richeldi, personal communication, 2006).

The QFT-Gold assays are considered positive if the IFN-γ concentration in response to the MTB antigens is ≥0.35 international units (IU)/mL above and 50 per cent more than the negative control value. The result is indeterminate if the mitogen well yields ≤0.5 IU/mL over the negative control of IFN-γ or the negative control well has a high background (>7) and both MTB antigens are <50% of the negative control value.

ELISPOT and T-SPOT assays

The T-SPOT assay is available in Europe and Canada. Blood is drawn into a CPT (cell preparation tube) Ficoll tube®, and must be processed within 12 hours. Peripheral blood mononuclear cells (PBMCs) are separated, enumerated and added to wells coated with monoclonal antibodies to IFN-γ. Peptides from ESAT-6 and CFP-10 are added to some wells, mitogen to positive control wells and media alone to negative control wells. After overnight incubation, cells are washed away and 'captured' IFN-γ is detected by secondary antibodies to IFN-γ, revealing spots, each of which represents an effector T cell.[14] Results are expressed as the number of spots per 250 000 cells initially placed in the well.[13,15]

The T-SPOT assay is considered positive if (1) the negative control well contains fewer than five spot-forming units (SFU) and either antigen well has greater than six SFU more than the negative control well; (2) the negative control well has greater than six SFU and either antigen well has at least twice the number of SFU in the negative control well. An indeterminate response is defined as high background in the negative control well (≥10 SFU) or unresponsiveness to mitogen (<20 SFU).

Indeterminate IGRA responses

Unlike the binary results of a tuberculin skin test, IGRAs can yield positive, negative or indeterminate results. If the indeterminate result is due to a poor response to mitogen,

there are two explanations. The first is a problem with performing the test, such as delayed specimen processing or technical errors. A repeat assay should correct this problem. A persistently diminished response to mitogen strongly suggests anergy from immunosuppresion,[16–18] although it may occur in healthy individuals. An indeterminate response due to a high background often persists on retesting and limits the utility of IGRAs in these patients. Thus, the reason for an indeterminate result and its reproducibility may provide clinically useful information.

In 318 unselected hospitalized patients, patients receiving immunosuppressive therapy were 3.5 times more likely to have an indeterminate QFT-Gold result than patients not receiving such therapy.[16] Two recent studies suggested that the T-SPOT has fewer indeterminate results than the QFT-Gold test.[17,18] Among 383 patients with suspected tuberculosis or LTBI, including many immunocompromised by cancer, ongoing chemotherapy, immunosuppressive drugs or the extremes of age, 12 (3 per cent) T-SPOT results versus 43 (11 per cent) QFT-Gold results were indeterminate.[17] In HIV+ patients, indeterminate QFT-Gold-IT results due to low IFN-γ responses to mitogen stimulation were significantly associated with CD4 counts <100.[19] In contrast, indeterminate T-SPOT assays were independent of CD4 count in 29 HIV+ patients.[20]

There are two possible explanations for these findings. First, by placing a defined number of PBMCs in each well, the T-SPOT test can compensate for a reduced CD4 count. Second, the T-SPOT test may use less stringent criteria than the QFT assays for an indeterminate result. We require 100 spots in the mitogen well to ensure that T cells are functional and the assay is valid (DM Lewinsohn, unpublished data), and others defined 150 SFU as a minimum threshold.[21] Therefore, the T-SPOT cut-off of 20 SFU may require additional validation.

Reproducibility

Results of two QFT-Gold tests, 1 month apart, in 562 military recruits agreed in 99.3 per cent.[12] However, almost all tests were negative. The manufacturers of the T-SPOT assay report a reproducibility of 97.9 per cent.[13]

Boosting

'Boosting' refers to stimulating a senescent immune response to antigen. Because tuberculin contains many antigens, TST placement could theoretically boost an IFN-γ response, confounding interpretation of IGRA results. TSTs and T-SPOT assays were performed in 44 contacts of a tuberculosis case at 0, 9, 15 and 24 months after exposure. All people remained T-SPOT–, but three became TST+, presumably from boosting.[22] Other studies suggest that the TST does not affect subsequent QFT-Gold-IT results.[23] In summary, repeat skin testing does not boost an IGRA response.

STUDIES SUPPORTING IGRA USE

IGRAs are more specific than the TST, but both tests reflect cellular immunity. Therefore, factors that affect cellular immunity, such as age and immunosuppression, can yield false-negative IGRAs. In addition, the TST is often negative in patients with advanced tuberculosis, and T-cell production of IFN-γ is inversely related to disease severity.[24–27] Therefore, a negative IGRA does not exclude tuberculosis. This section reviews published studies using IGRAs for the diagnosis of tuberculosis and LTBI in different populations, as well as their cost-effectiveness. We focus primarily on studies of the commercially available IGRAs. The findings of selected studies are presented in Table 6.1 and Table 6.2 (page 96).

Adults

SPECIFICITY

Numerous studies demonstrate exceptional specificity for the QFT-Gold and QFT-Gold-IT assays.[18,28–30] The QFT assays had 98 per cent specificity in heavily BCG-vaccinated nursing students in Japan, where the tuberculosis burden is low,[29] and 92 per cent specificity in BCG-vaccinated healthy controls in South Korea, where the tuberculosis burden is intermediate.[18] Although lower specificities have been reported with the QFT-Gold, 68% in one study,[31] the control group consisted of hospitalized patients with other conditions, slightly less than one half of which were TST positive.

Studies using an 'in-house' ELISPOT assay, similar to that of the T-SPOT test, report specificity of 92–100 per cent in cohorts with ≥75 per cent BCG vaccination rates.[15,32,33] However, limited data using the commercial T-SPOT assay suggest a slightly lower specificity of 92 per cent in 12 patients with pulmonary disease,[34] and 85 per cent in BCG-vaccinated high school students thought not to be at risk for LTBI.[18] Similarly, in a large contact investigation, 19 (5 per cent) of 414 subjects were T-SPOT+, but were at low risk of exposure to the active case and negative for either TST or QFT.[35] Additional data are needed to define the specificity of the T-SPOT assay in various clinical settings.

SENSITIVITY FOR DIAGNOSIS OF TUBERCULOSIS

The QFT-Gold and QFT-Gold-IT assays are 64–89 per cent sensitive in adults with culture-confirmed pulmonary tuberculosis, depending on practice setting, geographic region and rates of HIV infection.[18,28–31,36–38] The sensitivity for extrapulmonary tuberculosis was lower than that for pulmonary disease in one study,[36] but the QFT-Gold test was 92 per cent sensitive for extrapulmonary disease in another small series.[30]

Using an 'in-house' ESAT-6-based ELISPOT assay, two studies reported 92–96 per cent sensitivity in patients with pulmonary tuberculosis, some with extrapulmonary disease.[15,33] The commercial T-SPOT assay was positive in 95–97 per cent of a total of 152 pulmonary tuberculosis cases in Germany and South Korea.[18,34] All five patients with extrapulmonary tuberculosis were T-SPOT+ and TST+.[34] These data suggest that the T-SPOT test has excellent sensitivity for detecting tuberculosis, but highlights the need for larger studies.

LTBI

Because TST converters are at high risk for progression to active tuberculosis, treatment is strongly recommended.[39] However, treatment completion rates in converters are as low as 30 per cent, partly because the low specificity of the TST reduces confidence in the diagnosis of LTBI and diminishes provider and patient enthusiasm for treatment. The excellent specificity of the IGRAs could augment compliance with LTBI treatment recommendations.

Several investigations support the use of IGRAs for diagnosis of LTBI in contacts of tuberculosis cases. In a Danish school contact investigation, using an assay similar to the QFT-Gold, with recombinant ESAT-6 and CFP10, rather than their peptides, a positive assay correlated with exposure to the active case and with TST results (93 per cent concordant positive in the high-exposure group, 90 per cent concordant negative in the low-exposure group).[40] Because exposure to BCG and atypical mycobacteria was uncommon in Denmark, the authors argued that TST conversion likely reflected LTBI. In Japan, where BCG vaccination is uniform, QFT-Gold results correlated well with increasing exposure to tuberculosis in contact investigations at a high school,[41] universities[42,43] and a maternity ward.[44] The QFT-Gold test and TST were positive in 10 and 93 per cent, respectively, of Japanese health-care workers, 95 per cent of whom were BCG vaccinated. QFT-Gold results were significantly associated with age and a history of working with tuberculosis patients, while the TST was not.[45]

Exposure to tuberculosis also correlates with QFT-Gold results in regions with high rates of LTBI. Among health-care workers in India, the TST and the QFT-Gold-IT assay were associated with years in the health profession and age, with 81 per cent agreement between the tests.[46] In South Korea, where BCG vaccination rates were high, both the TST and the QFT were also associated with increasing risk of exposure to tuberculosis, but agreement between the tests was poor.[37]

'In house' ELISPOT assays have been useful to detect people with LTBI in low-incidence countries.[14,15,47–51] Using an ESAT-6-based ELISPOT assay in an office tuberculosis outbreak, contacts with greatest exposure to the case had higher odds of being ELISPOT+, not confounded by BCG vaccination, whereas TST results were confounded by receipt of BCG.[14] Similarly, in a school tuberculosis outbreak in which 87 per cent of students were BCG-vaccinated, the ESAT-6-based ELISPOT correlated better with exposure than the Heaf skin test.[47] However, because a higher cut-off for a positive Heaf test was used in BCG-vaccinated people, the sensitivity of the Heaf test

Table 6.1   Sensitivity and specificity of interferon-γ release assays (IGRAs)

Author	Ref./Year	Assay	Design	Sensitivity	Specificity	Key findings
Chapman[a]	32/2002	Modified T-SPOT	50 Zambian tuberculosis patients (39 HIV+); controls: 75 Zambian and 40 British adults	90% (HIV+)	See text	LTBI highly prevalent by ELISPOT; 69% of HIV-healthy Zambian patients, 80% TST+; ELISPOT 100% specific for British adults
Dewan	36/2007	QFT-Gold	Retrospective; 37 persons with culture+ tuberculosis	64%	Not done	Patients with false-negative QFT-Gold more likely to have extrapulmonary disease
Dheda[a]	20/2005	T-SPOT	29 HIV+, 19 HIV- patients	Not done	Not done	97% of HIV+ patients had evaluable results, independent of CD4 count; HIV + persons with CD4 <200 had lower response to mitogen
Dogra[b]	67/2006	QFT-Gold-IT	Cross-sectional study of 105 children admitted with suspected TB or LTBI in India	See text		TST and QFT-Gold with high agreement; 5 of 8 culture+ cases detected by QFT-Gold-IT and TST
Ferrara	17/2006	T-SPOT/ QFT-Gold	Prospective study of patients with suspected tuberculosis or LTBI	See text	Not done	High agreement between the two tests ($K = 0.69$). More indeterminate QFT-Gold than T-SPOT tests. T-SPOT identified all 11 cases of extrapulmonary tuberculosis
Goletti	31/2005	QFT-Gold	27 culture+ tuberculosis cases; controls: hospitalized patients with other conditions,[a] half of whom were TST+	89%	68%	High sensitivity for QFT-Gold in culture+ tuberculosis cases; specificity 90% for TST- subgroup
Kang	37/2005	QFT-Gold	Prospective comparison	81%	Not done	TST: 70% sensitive in comparison
Kobashi	28/2006	QFT-Gold	50 cases of tuberculosis and 100 of disease due to non-tuberculous myco-bacteria, 50 healthy volunteers	86%	94%	Specificity for non-tuberculous mycobacterial disease 85% Rate of false-negative QFT-Gold (4%). Of the six people with indeterminate (4) and negative QFT, all six diagnosed clinically with tuberculosis
Lalvani	15/2001	Modified T-SPOT	Prospective recruitment of 47 culture+ tuberculosis cases; 47 matched controls (77% BCG-vaccinated with variety of infections and rheumatologic illnesses	96%	92%	Early sensitivity and specificity paper prior to T-SPOT; included 22 cases of extrapulmonary tuberculosis
Lee[a]	18/2006	QFT-Gold	Prospective study of 87 patients with tuberculosis (63% culture+, 33.3% immunocompromised); low-risk group: 131 BCG-vaccinated male high school students	70%	92%	The IGRAs appeared superior in detecting MTB compared with the TST (sensitivity at 10 mm 67%); immunocompromised subgroup ($n = 29$), T-SPOT sensitivity 100%, QFT-Gold 62%
Liebeschuetz[a,b]	59/2004	ELISPOT	Prospective blinded study of 293 South African children with suspected tuberculosis	83%	Not done	ELISPOT sensitivity maintained in those with HIV infection, age <3 years, or malnutrition, but TST sensitivity was significantly reduced

Table 6.1 *Continued*

Author	Ref./Year	Assay	Design	Sensitivity	Specificity	Key findings
Meier	34/2005	T-SPOT	Prospective recruitment at German referral hsopital; 65 pulmonary, 58 of which were culture+; 7 extra-pulmonary	97%	92% (n = 12)	70/72 confirmed tuberculosis cases were T-SPOT+, including 7/7 cases of extrapulmonary disease; specificity based on only 12 patients
Mori	29/2004	QFT-Gold	Prospective recruitment of 216 BCG-vaccinated nursing students (just starting training) and 118 culture confirmed tuberculosis patients	89%	98%	Major paper documenting sensitivity and specificity for QFT-Gold
Nicol[b]	60/2006	ELISPOT	Hospitalized South African children with suspected tuberculosis (12 definite, 47 probable)	83% (culture positive)	Not done	Detectable ESAT-6 or CFP-10 responses in 49/70 children with clinical tuberculosis
Pathan	33/2001	Modified T-SPOT	Different clinical subgroups; 25 culture+ tuberculosis, 32 unexposed controls	92%	100%	ESAT-6 responses in 10/11 with tuberculous lymphadenitis and 7/8 with culture negative pulmonary tuberculosis
Ravn	30/2005	QFT-ESAT-6/CFP-10	Blinded prospective study; 48 tuberculosis cases (27 culture+); 39 BCG-vaccinated healthy donors	85%	97%	QFT-ESAT-6/CFP-10 detected 12/13 cases of extrapulmonary tuberculosis
Tsiouris[a]	38/2006	QFT-Gold-IT	154 culture+ adults in South Africa (70 HIV+); 131 with interpretable results	82% (when limited to new pulmonary cases 62/76); 81% (HIV+ 17/21)	Not done	Combined sensitivity for TST and IGRA 96% in culture+ cases; TST sensitivity in this cohort 90%

[a]Immunosuppressed.
[b]Children.
CFP, culture filtrate protein; ESAT, early secretory antigen.

may have been underestimated in this subgroup. Among 416 contacts of tuberculosis patients, both the TST and a modified T-SPOT assay, with different cut-offs for a positive test, were significantly associated with extent of exposure to the case.[49] In the Gambia, where the prevalence of LTBI is high, a multivariate analysis of 735 household contacts of 130 tuberculosis cases showed that those with the greatest exposure had significantly increased odds of having a positive ESAT-6/CFP-10-based ELISPOT result.[21]

The IGRAs do not detect all cases of LTBI, as the QFT-Gold-IT and T-SPOT tests were only 42 and 51 per cent sensitive, respectively, in identifying Danish individuals with TST >15 mm.[35] It is possible that remote infection is more readily detected by the TST than the IGRAs.

COST-EFFECTIVENESS

The use of IGRAs where the prevalence of tuberculosis is low, such as screening health-care workers, is attractive, as evaluation of false-positive TST results is costly. In a Markov modelling analysis, screening contacts with either the TST or QFT-Gold assay was cost-effective. Due to false-positive TST results from BCG vaccine, QFT-Gold testing in populations with high rates of BCG vaccination was less costly. Using QFT-Gold testing only in TST+ people yielded savings if the prevalence of LTBI was low.[52] A cost analysis in Switzerland also found stepwise testing with the TST, followed by T-SPOT for TST+ results, to be more cost-effective than the TST alone.[53] Stepwise testing (TST followed by IGRA if TST+) misses people who are IGRA+/TST−. The clinical significance of patients with such results is currently unclear.

COMPARISON OF IGRA SENSITIVITY AND SPECIFICITY

In the few published studies comparing the commercial IGRAs, the T-SPOT test appears to be more sensitive, but less specific, than the QFT-Gold assays for detecting LTBI

Table 6.2 Use of interferon-γ release assays (IGRAs) in latent tuberculosis infection (LTBI)

Author	Ref./Year	Assay	Design	Key findings
Arend	35/2006	T-SPOT/ QFT-Gold-IT	Supermarket contact investigation ($n = 785$)	QFTGold-IT and T-SPOT associated with exposure, whereas TST associated with increasing age; both IGRAs lacked sensitivity in those with TST >15 mm
Brock[a]	19/2006	QFT-Gold-IT	Cross-sectional study of HIV+ adults in Denmark	4.6% were QFT+ (78% had risk factors for LTBI); lower CD4 count associated with indeterminate results and low mitogen response
Brock	40/2004	QFT-ESAT-6/ CFP10	125 contacts at Danish school; (85 BCG unvaccinated)	High agreement between TST and QFT in high-exposure and low-exposure BCG-unvaccinated groups
Diel	50/2006	ELISPOT - ESAT-6	56 TST+ contacts and 27 controls	ELISPOT and TST were associated with close case exposure
Dogra[b]	67/2006	QFT-Gold-IT	Chiliden with suspected tuberculosis or LTBI from rural hospital in India	TST and QFT highly comparable, neither was confounded by BCG vaccination; age was correlated with positive TST and QFT
Ewer[a]	47/2003	ELISPOT - ESAT-6	Secondary school contact investigation	TST and ELISPOT had 89% agreement; ELISPOT correlated better with measures of exposure; TST correlated with BCG vaccination
Ferrara	17/2006	T-SPOT/ QFT-Gold	114 contacts of tuberculosis cases	TST, QFT and T-SPOT were positive in 54, 22, 34%, respectively; the number of T-SPOT+ in close contacts was significantly higher than that of QFT-Gold
Harada	42/2004	QFT-Gold	Contact investigation in Japan; most BCG-vaccinated	45% of high exposure group QFT-Gold+ versus 7% in low-exposure group; QFT-Gold reduced the number of people who needed treatment for LTBI from 28%, based on the TST, to 7%
Harada	45/2006	QFT-Gold	332 health-care workers in a hospital tuberculosis ward	10% QFT-Gold+, significantly associated with age and with history of working in a tuberculosis ward. 93% TST+, but not associated with risk factors for exposure
Higuchi	41/2006	QFT-Gold	Contacts in Japanese high school	TST positivity same in high and low exposure groups; Only 4 of 88 TST+ students were QFT+. No cases of tuberculosis in 3.5 years of follow up of TST+QFT- students
Hill	21/2004	ELISPOT	735 contacts of 130 sputum smear-positive TB cases	In multivariate analysis, positive ELISPOT and TST were associated with sleeping proximity. Positive TST was associated with proximity and sputum smear. People with TST+/ELISPOT- results, however, were associated with increasing exposure
Kang	37/2005	QFT-Gold	Prospective comparison of three groups with increasing TB exposure	As exposure category increased, odds of a positive QFT-Gold increased by 5.3 and odds of a positive TST also increased, with smaller odds ratios
Lalvani	14/2001	ELISPOT - ESAT-6	50 contacts	T-SPOT results correlated better than TST results with degree of exposure
Lalvani	15/2001	ELISPOT - ESAT-6	Household contracts of index cases	22 of 26 TST+ household contacts were ELISPOT+; none of 26 healthy BCG-vaccinated controls were ELISPOT+
Lalvani	54/2001	ELISPOT - ESAT-6, CFP-10	100 healthy adults in Mumbai	80% of healthy adults in Mumbai had a positive ELISPOT, suggesting an 80% prevalence of LTBI in urban India; by comparison, none of 40 healthy, largely BCG vaccinated, adults in the UK were ELISPOT+
Luetkemeyer[a]	71/2007	QFT-Gold-IT	Comparison of TST, QFT-GOLD-IT in 294 HIV+ adults in San Franscisco	5% had indeterminate tests, 4.2 times more likely if CD4 <100; QFT and TST had 89% agreement
Miyashita	44/2005	QFT-Gold	Contact investigation of health-care workers in maternity hospital	TST likely overestimated the prevalence of LTBI (highly BCG-vaccinated group)
Nakaoka[b]	66/2006	QFT-Gold-IT	Child contacts in Nigeria	More QFT+ than TST+ in the high-exposure group and among children of smear+ adults. Discordance noted in the high-exposure group with two children TST+/QFT- and six children TST-/QFT+

Table 6.2 *Continued*

Author	Ref./Year	Assay	Design	Key findings
Pai	46/2006	QFT-Gold-IT	Prospectively followed 216 medical and nursing students for 18 months	TST conversions in 9.5%; QFT conversions in 11.6% with good agreement with the TST. Reversions also reported
Pai	89/2005	QFT-Gold-IT	Cross-sectional comparison study of 726 health-care workers in India	81% agreement between QFT and TST; increasing age, years in health profession associated with positive TST and QFT; BCG vaccination did not confound TST results
Piana[a]	73/2006	T-SPOT	Contact evaluation of 138 haematology/oncology patients in Italy	44% of contacts were T-SPOT+ compared with 17% TST+. Although not significant the TST+ proportion fell with increasing immunosuppression whereas the T-SPOT did not. Only 6 had indeterminate results, 4 of whom were not leucopenic
Porsa	57/2006	QFT-Gold	Cross-sectional study of 409 inmates in USA	90% concordance between TST and QFT; African American ethnicity associated with TST+/QFT– discordance
Rangaka[a]	72/2006	T-SPOT/ QFT-Gold-IT	Cross-sectional study of 160 adults in South Africa (half HIV+)	The proportion of INGRA+ was not significantly different in HIV+/– persons. T-SPOT was less affected at lower CD4 counts, although the test for trend was not significant
Richeldi	48/2004	ELISPOT-ESAT-6, CFP-10	Contacts (41 neonates; 47 adults)	ELISPOT, but not TST correlated with exposure; 15 adults and 2 neonates ELISPOT+
Shams	49/2005	ELISPOT-ESAT-6, CFP-10	413 recent contacts, aged 12 years and older; prospectively defined contact score	Likelihood of a positive ELISPOT increased significantly with contact scores. The TST was less strongly associated with contact score
Soysal[b]	64/2005	ELISPOT-ESAT-6, CFP-10	979 household contacts of adult tuberculosis cases in Turkey	Positive TST and ELISPOT associated with increasing age and degree of exposure to tuberculosis cases
Zellweger	90/2005	T-SPOT	92 contacts in group home	44% TST+, 15% T-SPOT+; Odds ratio for positive T-SPOT, but not TST significantly associated with case exposure

[a]Immunosuppressed.
[b]Children.

and tuberculosis.[17,18,35] However, it is unclear if a negative QFT assay, defined as an IFN-γ concentration <0.35 IU/mL is equivalent to a negative T-SPOT assay, defined as <6 SFU. Cut-offs of 0.2 IU/mL for QFT and 13 spots for T-SPOT may offer the best agreement.[35]

Among inpatients and outpatients with suspected LTBI and tuberculosis at an Italian hospital, agreement between the T-SPOT and QFT-Gold assays was high ($K = 0.69$).[17] Both IGRAs were positive in 9 of 13 patients with pulmonary tuberculosis. Of 11 extrapulmonary cases, all were T-SPOT+ and 8 were QFT-Gold+. Fewer indeterminate responses were reported for the T-SPOT test. However, for both assays, indeterminate tests were associated with patients on chemotherapy.

The T-SPOT assay may be less specific than the QFT-Gold-IT test. In 785 non-BCG-vaccinated contacts of a tuberculosis case in Denmark, there was 90 per cent agreement between these IGRAs,[35] but the QFT-Gold-IT and T-SPOT tests were negative in 42 and 51 per cent of contacts with a TST ≥15 mm, who presumably had LTBI. However, in a multivariate analy-

sis, only the blood tests were associated with increasing levels of exposure. Overall, positive QFT-Gold-IT and T-SPOT tests were found in 10 and 19 per cent of subjects, respectively. People who were T-SPOT+/QFT-Gold-IT– were significantly more likely to have a TST ≥5 mm and to be immunosuppressed. However, in people with low risk of exposure, 5 per cent were T-SPOT+/TST–/QFT-Gold-IT–.

In summary, the studies comparing the T-SPOT and QFT assays offer some preliminary messages. First, inter-assay agreement is high and both IGRAs were sensitive in detecting tuberculosis and were associated with degree of exposure to an active case. Second, the T-SPOT assay may have greater sensitivity for tuberculosis and LTBI, particularly in immunosuppressed people, but the QFT assays may be more specific.

EFFECTS OF GEOGRAPHIC REGION AND ETHNICITY

The clinical utility of IGRAs in intermediate- or high-burden countries is less clear than in low-burden countries. Eighty per cent of Mumbai residents were ELISPOT+, using an earlier version of the T-SPOT test.[54] Because IGRAs cannot distinguish recent from remote infection, they are unlikely to diagnose recent infection in populations where most individuals have a baseline positive test. Second, because of significant regional variation in the immune response to ESAT-6 and CFP-10,[21,55] IGRA cut-offs have varied in different locations.[18,56] Third, limited evidence suggests that endemic mycobacteria may attenuate immune responses to MTB-specific antigens. For example, infection with *M. africanum* is associated with a reduced response to ESAT-6.[55] In the Gambia, discordant TST+/ELISPOT– results were more common in contacts with extensive exposure to tuberculosis patients,[21] suggesting that the TST may be more sensitive than ELISPOT in detecting new infection where tuberculosis is endemic. Finally, ethnicity may influence IGRA results, as one study of incarcerated, and thus high risk, adults in the United States found that African Americans were significantly more likely to have TST+/QFT– results.[57]

Children

Young children have immature immune responses and are at increased risk for developing tuberculosis after infection.[58] The need for improved diagnostics for tuberculosis is greater in children than adults since cultures are negative in most children with tuberculosis, and the youngest children have greatest risk of developing disseminated disease.

TUBERCULOSIS

Using an ELISPOT assay similar to the T-SPOT test, more South African children with confirmed or probable tuberculosis had positive ELISPOT assays than TSTs (83 versus 63 per cent overall, 81 versus 35 per cent for culture-confirmed cases).[59] These differences were most striking in very young (<2 years old), HIV+ and malnourished children, who have suppressed immune responses. However, the ELISPOT missed 11 TST+ children, 10 with pulmonary tuberculosis.[59] Another study of HIV-negative South African children found positive ELISPOT responses in 83 per cent of those with culture-confirmed tuberculosis and only 46 per cent of those with possible tuberculosis.[60] Thus, limited evidence suggests that IGRAs may be equivalent or better than the TST in diagnosing tuberculosis in children.

As in adults, a positive IGRA cannot distinguish tuberculosis disease from LTBI. Therefore, IGRAs have limited specificity for diagnosing tuberculosis, particularly where LTBI is common. For example, the ELISPOT assay was positive in 31 per cent of children without tuberculosis, all of whom had negative TSTs.[59]

Two reports suggest that IGRAs may facilitate diagnosis of tuberculosis in infants. Positive QFT-Gold results allowed early detection of tuberculosis in two TST–

infants,[61] and the ELISPOT detected infection with multidrug-resistant tuberculosis after neonatal exposure, months before development of a positive TST.[62]

LTBI

Accurate diagnosis of LTBI in children is critical because LTBI progresses to tuberculosis in 50 per cent of infants and 15 per cent of older children.[63] Furthermore, because BCG vaccination administered at birth is more likely to cause a false-positive TST within 2 years of vaccination, the increased specificity of the IGRAs may enhance accurate diagnosis of LTBI in young children.

In a contact investigation on a maternity unit, 2 of 41 neonates were T-SPOT+ and TST–,[48] suggesting increased sensitivity of the ELISPOT for LTBI in this vulnerable population. In contact investigations in older school children in England and in 979 child household contacts of tuberculosis patients in Turkey, a positive ELISPOT assay strongly correlated with increased exposure to the source case.[47,64] In the Gambia, similar findings were reported with an 'in house' ELISPOT assay.[65] However, increasing exposure was associated with a higher frequency of TST+/ELISPOT– results, particularly in the youngest children. Thus, the ELISPOT may be useful in identifying LTBI in children during contact investigations. However, the Gambian study raises concerns that the ELISPOT may be less sensitive than the TST in high-incidence countries.

The QFT-Gold assays have also been used for diagnosis of LTBI in children. In child household contacts of Nigerian adult tuberculosis cases, positive QFT-Gold-IT results were more common than positive TSTs in those with more extensive exposure. However, two children in the high-exposure group were TST+QFT–.[66] Among 105 child contacts and tuberculosis suspects in India,[67] there was 95 per cent agreement between the TST 10-mm cut-off and the QFT-Gold-IT result. However, two children with pulmonary tuberculosis were TST+QFT-Gold–. In a South African study of 184 school children, the TST was more often positive than the QFT-Gold-IT test in students with high exposure to tuberculosis, but this was not statistically significant.[68] Finally, an evaluation of LTBI in children found poor correlation between the TST and the QFT-Gold assay, confounded by a high rate of indeterminate assays.[69]

ROLE OF IGRAS IN CHILDREN

As detailed above, both IGRAs may facilitate the diagnosis of tuberculosis and LTBI in children. However, a positive IGRA cannot distinguish tuberculosis from LTBI. In the only published study comparing two IGRAs in children,[17] there were fewer indeterminate T-SPOT results than QFT-Gold assays in those <5 years old. However, these data are not conclusive, because the QFT-Gold-IT test may be superior to the QFT-Gold test. In summary, limited studies indicate that IGRAs will complement, but not replace, the TST in evaluating tuberculosis and LTBI in children.

Immunosuppressed populations

It is critical to identify and treat LTBI in immunocompromised patients because they are at increased risk for progression of LTBI to tuberculosis.[70] Unfortunately, the TST has low sensitivity in these patients. Several studies suggest that advanced immunosuppression is associated with indeterminate QFT results.[16,19,30,38,71] Among HIV+ patients in Denmark and San Francisco, indeterminate QFT-Gold-IT test results were associated with a CD4 count <100 cells/mm^3.[19,71] In 318 hospitalized patients, QFT-Gold assays were 3.5 times more likely to be indeterminate in immunosuppressed patients than in those without immunosuppresion.[16]

The T-SPOT test has fewer indeterminate results than the QFT in immunocompromised patients.[17,18] In adults immunosuppressed by different illnesses, 3 per cent of T-SPOT tests were indeterminate, compared with 11 per cent of QFT-Gold tests.[17] In addition, in HIV+ people, low CD4 counts were associated with indeterminate QFT-Gold tests,[19] but not with indeterminate T-SPOT tests.[20] A South African study found that positive QFT-Gold and T-SPOT tests were equally common in HIV+ and HIV– people, but the rate of positive TSTs was significantly lower in HIV+ people,[72] suggesting that both IGRAs are more sensitive than the TST in HIV+ people. The T-SPOT assay was less affected than the QFT-Gold test by low CD4 counts. Sixty-one (44 per cent) haematology/oncology patients exposed to a tuberculosis case had positive T-SPOT tests, compared with 24 (17 per cent) patients with a positive TST. Furthermore, only the T-SPOT results correlated with degree of exposure to the index case.[73] Other case reports have documented early detection of tuberculosis in immunosuppressed patients, using the T-SPOT assay.[74,75] The T-SPOT assay was also more sensitive than the TST in identifying dialysis patients with previous tuberculosis, based on history and radiographic findings.[76]

In summary, IGRAs, like the TST, depend on cellular immunity, and are affected by immunosuppression. The T-SPOT assay shows a lower rate of indeterminate results and a higher rate of positive results than the QFT-Gold test in immunosuppressed patients.

Occupational health

In countries with a low incidence of tuberculosis, healthcare workers often have TSTs yearly to identify converters for treatment of LTBI. Compared with the TST, the IGRA requires only one visit, test results are more easily documented, and improved specificity allows more accurate diagnosis, may increase treatment completion rates, and may enhance cost-effectiveness in low-risk populations. While IGRAs are more expensive than the TST, they reduce the cost of chest radiographs and staff time needed to evaluate false-positive TST results.

CURRENT NATIONAL GUIDELINES

The Centers for Disease Control and Prevention recommends that the QFT-Gold test, the only IGRA approved for use in the United States, may be generally substituted for a TST for the diagnosis of tuberculosis and LTBI.[77] These guidelines do not recommend using both tests, but note the relative absence of data in young children and those with immunosuppression and refrain from rendering an opinion on the use of QFT-Gold in these groups. Therefore, both the TST and QFT-Gold tests can be used in individuals at high risk of disease progression.

In the United Kingdom, The National Institute for Health and Clinical Excellence recommends the TST for diagnosis of LTBI. For TST+ patients and for those in whom the TST is less reliable, testing should be considered with the QFT-Gold or T-SPOT test.[78]

FUTURE DIRECTIONS

Quantitative aspects of IGRAs

The current IGRAs are interpreted as either positive, negative or indeterminate using a threshold. However, each test provides quantitative information that may have clinical utility. For example, some studies suggest that quantitative IGRA results may be used to monitor therapy, as effective treatment reduces the bacillary burden and antigen load driving the T-cell response, decreasing IFN-γ production. Eighty-six per cent of tuberculosis patients were initially QFT-Gold+, compared with 48 and 33 per cent after 6 and 12 months of treatment, respectively.[28] In 10 South African children with tuberculosis, ESAT-6 and CFP-10 responses declined after 3 and 6 months of therapy.[60] An ESAT-6-based ELISPOT result reverted from positive to negative in 13 of 18 tuberculosis patients after 3 months of therapy. Three HIV+ patients had persistently positive ELISPOT assays at 3 months, and all had positive cultures for MTB,[79] suggesting that IGRAs may predict response to therapy. Finally, in 89 tuberculosis cases, responses to ESAT-6 and CFP-10 were significantly diminished after 1 year, and tests reverted from positive to negative in 55 per cent.[80] These data strongly suggest that successful therapy is associated with decreased IFN-γ responses.

Depressed IGRA responses may be associated with severe tuberculosis and high bacillary burdens. Treatment reduces the bacterial burden and improves immune function, so therapy of severe disease may reduce or increase IFN-γ production. Several studies found augmented IFN-γ responses after treatment of tuberculosis,[81,82] and two studies described an initial rise and subsequent fall in effector cell frequencies.[83,84]

Little is known about the change in IGRA results with treatment of LTBI. In one small study, persistently positive QFT-Gold-IT responses were noted in health-care workers after 10 months of therapy for LTBI.[46] However, a large study found that 38 per cent of contacts with LTBI reverted from positive to negative T-SPOT tests after completing therapy.[85]

Redefining the natural history of LTBI

Information derived from IGRAs may provide a more nuanced understanding of LTBI and perhaps additional insight into those at risk of progression to disease. Three questions are of special interest: (1) Does transient infection with MTB occur? This is suggested by a report that 32 (35 per cent) of 92 household contacts of tuberculosis patients in the Gambia reverted their ELISPOT tests from positive to negative after 3 months.[86] (2) Is bacterial burden related to quantitative IGRA responses? We predict that quantitative MTB-specific responses will parallel bacterial burden. For example, household contacts of tuberculosis patients who initially had ESAT-6-specific IFN-γ-producing T-cell responses were more likely to have active tuberculosis after two years.[87] Conversely, treatment of LTBI can eliminate IGRA responses.[85] (3) How are IGRA responses related to the time of infection? It has been suggested that the short-term IGRAs reflect memory-effector T-cell responses. Without further antigen exposure, this population should decay and IGRA results will be negative. Longer-term assays, such as the TST, may better reflect remote infection. Conversely, ongoing antigenic exposure may maintain high frequencies of effector T cells.[88] A better understanding of the relationship between bacterial burden and IGRA responses will help to define the risk of disease progression.

RECOMMENDATIONS

Based on current published evidence, we have developed guidelines for using IGRAs in different clinical circumstances in low-incidence countries. Because LTBI is common in high-prevalence regions and is generally not treated, and because IGRAs cannot distinguish tuberculosis from LTBI, we do not recommend the use of IGRAs in high-prevalence regions, except in the case of children under 5 years of age (see recommendation 5 below).

1 *LTBI and contact investigations.* IGRAs perform as well or better than the TST in identifying those with recent infection after exposure to a tuberculosis case. Therefore, we favour use of IGRAs instead of the TST in most contacts. If the risk of disease progression is high (young children, immunocompromised hosts), the risk of a false-negative IGRA is greater than that of a false-positive TST, and both the TST and IGRA should be used. If either test is positive, treatment of LTBI is indicated. We do not endorse the UK guidelines of a stepwise approach with a TST, followed by an IGRA if TST+, as this would not detect IGRA+TST− people who may have recent infection.

2 *Targeted LTBI screening: low risk.* In countries where tuberculosis is not endemic, screening is often employed for low-risk people who may be exposed to tuberculosis, such as health-care workers. In these cases, most positive TSTs represent false-positives, and we favour using an IGRA in place of the TST.

3 *Targeted LTBI screening: moderate to high risk.* This includes new immigrants from countries where tuberculosis is common, prison inmates and the homeless. The IGRAs have operational advantages over the TST and their sensitivity is probably equal to or better than that of the TST. On the other hand, logistical considerations in some facilities may not permit performance of IGRAs. We believe that either test is reasonable in this setting.

4 *Tuberculosis in immunocompetent hosts.* Negative IGRA results do not rule out tuberculosis. However, due to their excellent specificity, a positive IGRA in a tuberculosis suspect increases the likelihood of tuberculosis in low-incidence countries. The IGRAs are at least as sensitive as the TST and the T-SPOT test is more sensitive than the QFT assays in this setting. The IGRAs are an adjunctive test for active tuberculosis, supplementing nucleic acid amplification assays, acid-fast smears and mycobacterial cultures. This recommendation is based on a higher quality of published evidence than that supporting our other recommendations.

5 *Children.* Young children are at high risk for progression of infection to disseminated tuberculosis, and the risk of a false-negative IGRA or TST can be devastating. Therefore, both tests should be used to aid in diagnosis of LTBI or tuberculosis in children <5 years of age. For older children, IGRAs and the TST should be used as in adults.

6 *Immuncompromised hosts.* The role of IGRAs in immunocompromised hosts depends on the level of immunosuppression and on the likelihood that the person has LTBI. In severely immunocompromised people, particularly in those at significant risk for LTBI, we recommend using both an IGRA and a TST to reduce the likelihood of failure to diagnose LTBI. In less severely immunocompromised people, we favour use of the IGRA over the TST because indeterminate IGRA results may provide useful information, as outlined above.

   • *Immunocompromised hosts without HIV infection.* This group has a higher rate of negative TSTs and negative or indeterminate IGRA results than immunocompetent people. Current evidence indicates that the T-SPOT test is more sensitive than the QFT-Gold assay in diagnosing LTBI in this population. Furthermore, indeterminate IGRA results may provide useful information. We recommend use of the IGRA in these patients. In patients who are severely immunocompromised or who are at high risk for LTBI, such as the contacts of a tuberculosis patient, clinicians can consider using both an IGRA and a TST.

- *HIV+ patients.* HIV-infected people with CD4 cell counts $<200/mm^3$ have higher rates of negative TSTs and negative or indeterminate IGRA results than immunocompetent individuals. Studies suggest that the T-SPOT test is more sensitive than the QFT-Gold assay for diagnosing LTBI in this population and may be less affected by a decreasing CD4 count. We therefore recommend that clinicians either use the T-SPOT test alone, or the QFT-Gold/IT assay together with a TST. HIV+ patients with CD4 cell counts $>200/mm^3$ can be tested in the same manner as immunocompetent individuals.

7 *Pre-immunosuppression.* In these patients, the risk that a false-positive TST will delay immunosuppressive treatment of a life-threatening disease, while LTBI is treated, must be weighed against the risk of missing the diagnosis of LTBI, because of TST anergy or an indeterminate IGRA result. If a patient is to be immunosuppressed and is at risk for reactivation of tuberculosis, we recommend performing an IGRA. If the IGRA is positive and tuberculosis is excluded, patients should be treated for LTBI. If the IGRA is negative and the clinical suspicion for LTBI is high (e.g. if the patient is a close contact of an active case), TST testing should also be considered.

LEARNING POINTS

- IGRAs are blood tests to diagnose LTBI and active tuberculosis, based on detecting IFN-γ production by effector memory T cells that recognize MTB-specific antigens that are absent from BCG and most environmental mycobacteria.
- The commercially available IGRAs are the QFT-Gold tests, which are based on measurement of IFN-γ by ELISA and the T-SPOT test, which is based on measurement of IFN-γ-producing cells by ELISPOT.
- IGRAs have substantial logistical advantages over the TST. They require a single visit and the criteria for a positive test are more objective.
- Because IGRA results are more specific than the TST and are particularly advantageous in diagnosing LTBI in BCG-vaccinated people.
- IGRAs are either positive, negative or indeterminate. Indeterminate results are more common in immunosuppressed patients. A persistently indeterminate IGRA due to a poor response to mitogen strongly suggests that the patient is anergic.
- For diagnosing tuberculosis, IGRAs are generally as sensitive as the TST and are useful adjunctive tests in low-incidence countries. Their utility in high-incidence countries is uncertain because they do not distinguish tuberculosis from LTBI.
- For diagnosing LTBI in low-incidence countries, IGRAs perform as well or better than the TST in people with recent tuberculosis infection, chil-

dren and hosts with mild to moderate immunosuppression. The T-SPOT test may be more sensitive but less specific than the QFT-Gold test. However, both the IGRAs and the TST depend on cellular immunity and are more frequently false-negative in young children and immunosuppressed patients.

REFERENCES

1. Huebner RE, Schein MF, Bass JB Jr. The tuberculin skin test. *Clin Infect Dis* 1993; **17**: 968–75.
2. Kendig EL Jr, Kirkpatrick BV, Carter WH *et al.* Underreading of the tuberculin skin test reaction. *Chest* 1998; **113**: 1175–7.
3. Arend SM, Andersen P, van Meijgaarden KE *et al.* Detection of active tuberculosis infection by T cell responses to early-secreted antigenic target 6-kDa protein and culture filtrate protein 10. *J Infect Dis* 2000; **181**: 1850–4.
4. Johnson PD, Stuart RL, Grayson ML *et al.* Tuberculin-purified protein derivative-, MPT-64-, and ESAT-6-stimulated gamma interferon responses in medical students before and after *Mycobacterium bovis* BCG vaccination and in patients with tuberculosis. *Clin Diagn Lab Immunol* 1999; **6**: 934–7.
5. Ulrichs T, Munk ME, Mollenkopf H *et al.* Differential T cell responses to *Mycobacterium tuberculosis* ESAT6 in tuberculosis patients and healthy donors. *Eur J Immunol* 1998; **28**: 3949–58.
6. Ravn P, Demissie A, Eguale T *et al.* Human T cell responses to the ESAT-6 antigen from *Mycobacterium tuberculosis*. *J Infect Dis* 1999; **179**: 637–45.
7. Demissie A, Ravn P, Olobo J *et al.* T-cell recognition of *Mycobacterium tuberculosis* culture filtrate fractions in tuberculosis patients and their household contacts. *Infect Immun* 1999; **67**: 5967–71.
8. Arend SM, Engelhard AC, Groot G *et al.* Tuberculin skin testing compared with T-cell responses to *Mycobacterium tuberculosis*-specific and nonspecific antigens for detection of latent infection in persons with recent tuberculosis contact. *Clin Diagn Lab Immunol* 2001; **8**: 1089–96.
9. Harboe M, Oettinger T, Wiker HG *et al.* Evidence for occurrence of the ESAT-6 protein in *Mycobacterium tuberculosis* and virulent *Mycobacterium bovis* and for its absence in *Mycobacterium bovis* BCG. *Infect Immun* 1996; **64**: 16–22.
10. Mahairas GG, Sabo PJ, Hickey MJ *et al.* Molecular analysis of genetic differences between *Mycobacterium bovis* BCG and virulent *M. bovis*. *J Bacteriol* 1996; **178**: 1274–82.
11. Arend SM, de Haas P, Leyten E *et al.* ESAT-6 and CFP-10 in clinical versus environmental isolates of *Mycobacterium kansasii*. *J Infect Dis*, 2005; **191**: 1301–10.
12. QuantiFERON-TB Gold. *The whole blood IFN-gamma test measuring responses to ESAT-6 and CFP-1 peptide antigens*. Cellestis Package Insert: Cellestis Ltd (Australia) and Cellestis Inc. (USA).
13. T-Spot.TB. An aid in the diagnosis of tuberculosis infection. Package insert for *in vitro* diagnostic use. Oxford: Oxford Immunotech, 2006.
14. Lalvani A, Pathan AA, Durkan H *et al.* Enhanced contact tracing and spatial tracking of *Mycobacterium tuberculosis* infection by enumeration of antigen-specific T cells. *Lancet* 2001; **357**: 2017–21.
15. Lalvani A, Pathan AA, McShane H *et al.* Rapid detection of *Mycobacterium tuberculosis* infection by enumeration of antigen-specific T cells. *Am J Respir Crit Care Med* 2001; **163**: 824–8.
16. Ferrara G, Losi M, Meacci M *et al.* Routine hospital use of a new commercial whole blood interferon-gamma assay for the diagnosis of tuberculosis infection. *Am J Respir Crit Care Med* 2005; **172**: 631–5.

17. Ferrara G, Losi M, D'Amico R et al. Use in routine clinical practice of two commercial blood tests for diagnosis of infection with *Mycobacterium tuberculosis*: a prospective study. *Lancet* 2006; 367: 1328–34.

18. Lee JY, Choi HJ, Park IN et al. Comparison of two commercial interferon-gamma assays for diagnosing *Mycobacterium tuberculosis* infection. *Eur Respir J* 2006; 28: 24–30.

19. Brock I, Ruhwald M, Lundgren B et al. Latent tuberculosis in HIV positive, diagnosed by the *M. tuberculosis* specific interferon-gamma test. *Respir Res* 2006; 7: 56.

20. Dheda K, Lalvani A, Miller RF et al. Performance of a T-cell-based diagnostic test for tuberculosis infection in HIV-infected individuals is independent of CD4 cell count. *AIDS* 2005; 19: 2038–41.

21. Hill PC, Brookes RH, Fox A et al. Large-scale evaluation of enzyme-linked immunospot assay and skin test for diagnosis of *Mycobacterium tuberculosis* infection against a gradient of exposure in The Gambia. *Clin Infect Dis* 2004; 38: 966–73.

22. Richeldi L, Ewer K, Losi M et al. Repeated tuberculin testing does not induce false positive ELISPOT results. *Thorax* 2006; 61: 180.

23. Leyten EM, Prins C, Bossink AW et al. Effect of tuberculin skin testing on a *Mycobacterium tuberculosis*-specific IFN-γ assay. *Eur Respir J* 2007; 29: 1282–3.

24. Sodhi A, Gong J, Silva C, Qian D, Barnes PF. Clinical correlates of interferon gamma production in patients with tuberculosis. *Clin Infect Dis* 1997; 25: 167–20.

25. Subronto YW, van Meijgaarden KE, Geluk A et al. Interferon-gamma production in response to *M. tuberculosis* antigens in TB patients in Indonesia. In: Marzuki S, Verhoef J, Snippe H (eds). *Tropical diseases: from molecule to bedside*. New York: Kluwer Academic, 2003: 249–60.

26. Vekemans J, Lienhardt C, Sillah JS et al. Tuberculosis contacts but not patients have higher gamma interferon responses to ESAT-6 than do community controls in The Gambia. *Infect Immun* 2001; 69: 6554–7.

27. Ulrichs T, Anding P, Porcelli S et al. Increased numbers of ESAT-6- and purified protein derivative-specific gamma interferon-producing cells in subclinical and active tuberculosis infection. *Infect Immun* 2000; 68: 6073–6.

28. Kobashi Y, Obase Y, Fukuda M et al. Clinical reevaluation of the QuantiFERON TB-2G test as a diagnostic method for differentiating active tuberculosis from nontuberculous mycobacteriosis. *Clin Infect Dis* 2006; 43: 1540–6.

29. Mori T, Sakatani M, Yamagishi F et al. Specific detection of tuberculosis infection: an interferon-gamma-based assay using new antigens. *Am J Respir Crit Care Med* 2004; 170: 59–64.

30. Ravn P, Munk ME, Andersen AB et al. Prospective evaluation of a whole-blood test using *Mycobacterium tuberculosis*-specific antigens ESAT-6 and CFP-10 for diagnosis of active tuberculosis. *Clin Diagn Lab Immunol* 2005; 12: 491–6.

31. Goletti D, Vincenti D, Carrara S et al. Selected RD1 peptides for active tuberculosis diagnosis: comparison of a gamma interferon whole-blood enzyme-linked immunosorbent assay and an enzyme-linked immunospot assay. *Clin Diagn Lab Immunol* 2005; 12: 1311–16.

32. Chapman AL, Munkanta M, Wilkinson KA et al. Rapid detection of active and latent tuberculosis infection in HIV-positive individuals by enumeration of *Mycobacterium tuberculosis*-specific T cells. *AIDS* 2002; 16: 2285–93.

33. Pathan AA, Wilkinson KA, Klenerman P et al. Direct *ex vivo* analysis of antigen-specific IFN-gamma-secreting CD4 T cells in *Mycobacterium tuberculosis*-infected individuals: associations with clinical disease state and effect of treatment. *J Immunol* 2001; 167: 5217–25.

34. Meier T, Eulenbruch HP, Wrighton-Smith P et al. Sensitivity of a new commercial enzyme-linked immunospot assay (T SPOT-TB) for diagnosis of tuberculosis in clinical practice. *Eur J Clin Microbiol Infect Dis* 2005; 24: 529–36.

35. Arend SM, Thijsen SF, Leyten EM et al. Comparison of two interferon-gamma assays and tuberculin skin test for tracing TB contacts. *Am J Respir Crit Care Med* 2007; 175: 529–31.

36. Dewan PK, Grinsdale J, Kawamura LM. Low sensitivity of a whole-blood interferon-gamma release assay for detection of active tuberculosis. *Clin Infect Dis* 2007; 44: 69–73.

37. Kang YA, Lee HW, Yoon HI et al. Discrepancy between the tuberculin skin test and the whole-blood interferon gamma assay for the diagnosis of latent tuberculosis infection in an intermediate tuberculosis-burden country. *J Am Med Assoc* 2005; 293: 2756–61.

38. Tsiouris SJ, Coetzee D, Toro PL et al. Sensitivity analysis and potential uses of a novel gamma interferon release assay for diagnosis of tuberculosis. *J Clin Microbiol* 2006; 44: 2844–50.

39. Anonymous. Targeted tuberculin testing and treatment of latent tuberculosis infection. American Thoracic Society. *MMWR Morb Mortal Wkly Rep* 2000; 49: 1–51.

40. Brock I, Weldingh K, Lillebaek T et al. Comparison of tuberculin skin test and new specific blood test in tuberculosis contacts. *Am J Respir Crit Care Med* 2004; 170: 65–9.

41. Higuchi K, Harada N, Mori T, Sekiya Y. Use of QuantiFERON((R))-TB Gold to investigate tuberculosis contacts in a high school. *Respirology* 2007; 12: 88–92.

42. Harada N, Mori T, Shishido S et al. [Usefulness of a novel diagnostic method of tuberculosis infection, QuantiFERON TB-2G, in an outbreak of tuberculosis]. *Kekkaku* 2004; 79: 637–43.

43. Funayama K, Tsujimoto A, Mori M et al. [Usefulness of QuantiFERON TB-2G in contact investigation of a tuberculosis outbreak in a university]. *Kekkaku* 2005; 80: 527–34.

44. Miyashita H, Higuchi K, Higashiyama N et al. [Detection of tuberculosis infection using a whole blood interferon gamma assay in a contact investigation–evaluation using quantiFERon TB-2G]. *Kekkaku* 2005; 80: 557–64.

45. Harada N, Nakajima Y, Higuchi K et al. Screening for tuberculosis infection using whole-blood interferon-gamma and Mantoux testing among Japanese healthcare workers. *Infect Control Hosp Epidemiol* 2006; 27: 442–8.

46. Pai M, Joshi R, Dogra S et al. Serial testing of health care workers for tuberculosis using interferon-gamma assay. *Am J Respir Crit Care Med* 2006; 174: 349–55.

47. Ewer K, Deeks J, Alvarez L et al. Comparison of T-cell-based assay with tuberculin skin test for diagnosis of *Mycobacterium tuberculosis* infection in a school tuberculosis outbreak. *Lancet* 2003; 361: 1168–73.

48. Richeldi L, Ewer K, Losi M et al. T cell-based tracking of multidrug resistant tuberculosis infection after brief exposure. *Am J Respir Crit Care Med* 2004; 170: 288–95.

49. Shams H, Weis SE, Klucar P et al. Enzyme-linked immunospot and tuberculin skin testing to detect latent tuberculosis infection. *Am J Respir Crit Care Med* 2005; 172: 1161–8.

50. Diel R, Ernst M, Doscher G et al. Avoiding the effect of BCG-vaccination in detecting MTB infection with a blood test. *Eur Respir J* 2006; 28: 16–23.

51. Leyten EM, Mulder B, Prins C et al. Use of enzyme-linked immunospot assay with *Mycobacterium tuberculosis*-specific peptides for diagnosis of recent infection with *M. tuberculosis* after accidental laboratory exposure. *J Clin Microbiol* 2006; 44: 1197–201.

52. Oxlade O, Schwartzman K, Menzies D. Interferon-gamma release assays and TB screening in high-income countries: a cost-effectiveness analysis. *Int J Tuberc Lung Dis* 2007; 11: 16–26.

53. Wrighton-Smith P, Zellweger JP. Direct costs of three models for the screening of latent tuberculosis infection. *Eur Respir J* 2006; 28: 45–50.

54. Lalvani A, Nagvenkar P, Udwadia Z et al. Enumeration of T cells specific for RD1-encoded antigens suggests a high prevalence of latent *Mycobacterium tuberculosis* infection in healthy urban Indians. *J Infect Dis* 2001; 183: 469–77.

55. de Jong BC, Hill PC, Brookes RH *et al*. *Mycobacterium africanum* elicits an attenuated T cell response to early secreted antigenic target, 6 kDa, in patients with tuberculosis and their household contacts. *J Infect Dis* 2006; **193**: 1279–86.

56. Jeffries DJ, Hill PC, Fox A *et al*. Identifying ELISPOT and skin test cut-offs for diagnosis of *Mycobacterium tuberculosis* infection in The Gambia. *Int J Tuberc Lung Dis* 2006; **10**: 192–8.

57. Porsa E, Cheng L, Seale MM *et al*. Comparison of a new ESAT-6/CFP-10 peptide-based gamma interferon assay and a tuberculin skin test for tuberculosis screening in a moderate-risk population. *Clin Vaccine Immunol* 2006; **13**: 53–8.

58. Lewinsohn DA, Gennaro ML, Scholvinck L, Lewinsohn DM. Tuberculosis immunology in children: diagnostic and therapeutic challenges and opportunities. *Int J Tuberc Lung Dis* 2004; **8**: 658–74.

59. Liebeschuetz S, Bamber S, Ewer K *et al*. Diagnosis of tuberculosis in South African children with a T-cell-based assay: a prospective cohort study. *Lancet* 2004; **364**: 2196–203.

60. Nicol MP, Pienaar D, Wood K *et al*. Enzyme-linked immunospot assay responses to early secretory antigenic target 6, culture filtrate protein 10, and purified protein derivative among children with tuberculosis: implications for diagnosis and monitoring of therapy. *Clin Infect Dis* 2005; **40**: 1301–308.

61. Connell T, Bar-Zeev N, Curtis N. Early detection of perinatal tuberculosis using a whole blood interferon-gamma release assay. *Clin Infect Dis* 2006; **42**: e82–5.

62. Richeldi L, Ewer K, Losi M *et al*. T-cell-based diagnosis of neonatal multidrug-resistant latent tuberculosis infection. *Pediatrics* 2007; **119**: e1–5.

63. Shingadia D, Novelli V. Diagnosis and treatment of tuberculosis in children. *Lancet Infect Dis* 2003; **3**: 624–32 (erratum appears in *Lancet Infect Dis* 2004; **4**: 251, correction refers to dosage error).

64. Soysal A, Millington KA, Bakir M *et al*. Effect of BCG vaccination on risk of *Mycobacterium tuberculosis* infection in children with household tuberculosis contact: a prospective community-based study. *Lancet* 2005; **366**: 1443–51.

65. Hill PC, Brookes RH, Adetifa IMO *et al*. Comparison of enzyme-linked immunospot assay and tuberculin skin test in healthy children exposed to *Mycobacterium tuberculosis*. *Pediatrics* 2006; **117**: 1542–8.

66. Nakaoka H, Lawson L, Squire SB *et al*. Risk for tuberculosis among children. *Emerg Infect Dis* 2006; **12**: 1383–8.

67. Dogra S, Narang P, Mendiratta DK *et al*. Comparison of a whole blood interferon-gamma assay with tuberculin skin testing for the detection of tuberculosis infection in hospitalized children in rural India. *J Infect* 2007; **54**: 267–76.

68. Tsiouris SJ, Austin J, Coetzee D *et al*. Diagnosis of latent tuberculosis infection with a whole blood interferon-γ release assay using ESAT-6 and CFP-10 and tuberculin skin test in children from Gugulethu, South Africa. *Int J Tuberc Lung Dis* 2005; **10**: 939–41.

69. Connell TG, Curtis N, Ranganathan SC, Buttery JP. Performance of a whole blood interferon gamma assay for detecting latent infection with *Mycobacterium tuberculosis* in children. *Thorax* 2006; **61**: 616–20.

70. Woldehanna S, Volmink J. Treatment of latent tuberculosis infection in HIV infected persons. *Cochrane Database Syst Rev* 2004; CD000171 (update of *Cochrane Database Syst Rev*. 2000; (4): CD000171).

71. Luetkemeyer AF, Charlebois ED, Flores LL *et al*. Comparison of an interferon-γ release assay to tuberculin skin testing in HIV-infected individuals. *Am J Respir Crit Care Med* 2007; **175**: 737–42.

72. Rangaka MX, Wilkinson KA, Seldon R *et al*. The effect of HIV-1 infection on T cell based and skin test detection of tuberculosis infection. *Am J Respir Crit Care Med* 2007; **175**: 514–20.

73. Piana F, Codecasa LR, Cavallerio P *et al*. Use of a T-cell-based test for detection of tuberculosis infection among immunocompromised patients. *Eur Respir J* 2006; **28**: 31–4.

74. Richeldi L, Ewer K, Losi M *et al*. Early diagnosis of subclinical multidrug-resistant tuberculosis. *Ann Intern Med* 2004; **140**: 709–13.

75. Richeldi L, Luppi M, Losi M *et al*. Diagnosis of occult tuberculosis in hematological malignancy by enumeration of antigen-specific T cells. *Leukemia* 20: 379–81.

76. Passalent L, Khan K, Richardson R *et al*. Detecting latent tuberculosis infection in hemodialysis patients: a head-to-head comparison of the T-SPOT.TB test, tuberculin skin test, and an expert physician panel. *Clin J Am Soc Nephrol* 2007; **2** 68–73.

77. Mazurek GH, Jereb J, Lobue P *et al*. Guidelines for using the QuantiFERON-TB Gold test for detecting *Mycobacterium tuberculosis* infection, United States. *MMWR Morb Mort Rec Rep* 2005; **54**: 49–55.

78. National Institute of Health and Clinical Excellence. *Tuberculosis: Clinical diagnosis and management of tuberculosis, and measures for its prevention and control*. London: Royal College of Physicians, 2006: 215 (www.nice.org.uk/page.aspx?o=CG033).

79. Carrara S, Vincenti D, Petrosillo N *et al*. Use of a T cell-based assay for monitoring efficacy of antituberculosis therapy. *Clin Infect Dis* 2004; **38**: 754–56.

80. Aiken AM, Hill PC, Fox A *et al*. Reversion of the ELISPOT test after treatment in Gambian tuberculosis cases. *BMC Infect Dis* 2006; **6**: 66.

81. Al-Attiyah R, Mustafa AS, Abal AT *et al*. Restoration of mycobacterial antigen-induced proliferation and interferon-gamma responses in peripheral blood mononuclear cells of tuberculosis patients upon effective chemotherapy. *FEMS Immunol Med Microbiol* 2003; **38**: 249–56.

82. Ferrand RA, Bothamley GH, Whelan A, Dockrell HM. Interferon-gamma responses to ESAT-6 in tuberculosis patients early into and after anti-tuberculosis treatment. *Int J Tuberc Lung Dis* 2005; **9**: 1034–9.

83. Ewer K, Millington KA, Deeks JJ *et al*. Dynamic antigen-specific T-cell responses after point-source exposure to *Mycobacterium tuberculosis*. *Am J Respir Crit Care Med* 2006; **174**: 831–9.

84. Wilkinson KA, Kon OM, Newton SM *et al*. Effect of treatment of latent tuberculosis infection on the T cell response to *Mycobacterium tuberculosis* antigens. *J Infect Dis* 2006; **193**: 354–9.

85. Chee CB, Khinmar KW, Gan SH *et al*. Latent tuberculosis infection treatment and T-cell responses to *Mycobacterium tuberculosis*-specific antigens. *Am J Respir Crit Care Med* 2007; **175**: 282–7.

86. Hill PCL, Fox A, Jackson-Sillah D *et al*. ELISPOT conversion and reversion after 3 months in TB case contacts in the Gambia. Keystone Symposium on Tuberculosis: Integrating Host and Pathogen Biology, Whistler, BC, 2005.

87. Doherty TM, Demissie A, Olobo J *et al*. Immune responses to the *Mycobacterium tuberculosis*-specific antigen ESAT-6 signal subclinical infection among contacts of tuberculosis patients. *J Clin Microbiol* 2002; **40**: 704–706.

88. Wu-Hsieh BA, Chen CK, Chang JH *et al*. Long-lived immune response to early secretory antigenic target 6 in individuals who had recovered from tuberculosis. *Clin Infect Dis* 2001; **33**: 1336–40.

89. Pai M, Gokhale K, Joshi R *et al*. *Mycobacterium tuberculosis* infection in health care workers in rural India: comparison of a whole-blood, interferon-γ assay with tuberculin skin testing. *J Am Med Assoc* 2005; **293**: 2746–55.

90. Zellweger JP, Zellweger A, Ansermet S *et al*. Contact tracing using a new T-cell-based test: better correlation with tuberculosis exposure than the tuberculin skin test. *Int J Tuberc Lung Dis* 2005; **9**: 1242–7.

Histopathology

SEBASTIAN B LUCAS

BACKGROUND

Tuberculosis is the prototypical granulomatous inflammatory disease caused by an intracellular infection. Its morbid anatomy has been examined for over a century and was ably summarized in 1951 by Arnold Rich.[1] Yet for variety in the patterns of its interaction with human tissues and complicated chronology, tuberculosis has few equals (Table 7.1, Figure 7.1). With the recent pandemic of co-infection of *Mycobacterium tuberculosis* with the human immunodeficiency viruses (HIV-1 and HIV-2), further impetus has been given to studying the detailed pathology of this infection and the underlying mechanisms of resistance, latent infection, tissue damage, healing, reactivation and mortality.[2–5]

This chapter describes the macroscopic and microscopic patterns of *M. tuberculosis* infection, with reference to the inflammatory and immune reactions that cause them. In addition to the 'normal' tuberculosis histopathology, 'atypical' host reactions to *M. tuberculosis* infection, often in immunosuppressed patients, are also considered. The impact of HIV on tuberculosis pathology is highly significant, and the effects of anti-HIV chemotherapy on

Table 7.1 Schema of various patterns of histopathology caused by interactions between *Mycobacterium tuberculosis* and the human host, with suggestions as to their pathogenesis.

Type of lesion	Pathogenetic mechanisms			
	CMI	DTH	Liquefaction	Bacterial toxicity
EC granuloma, no necrosis	++	–	–	–
EC granuloma + caseation necrosis	++	++	+?	?
Necrotizing granulomatous vasculitis	+	++	–	–
Liquefaction	?	+?	++	?
Non-reactive multibacillary	–	+?	?	++?
Histoid-like (rare)	–	–	–	–
Malakoplakia (rare)	?	?	–	–
Serous effusion	+	++	–	–
Leuco-encephalopathy	+?	++	–	–
Post-therapy expansion	++?	++?	–	–

The range of lesions indicated here is broader than the Ridley immunopathological spectrum of tuberculosis (see Table 7.4).
EC, epithelioid cell; CMI, cell-mediated immunity; DTH, delayed-type hypersensitivity. ++, strong; +, moderate; –, absent; +?, uncertainly present.

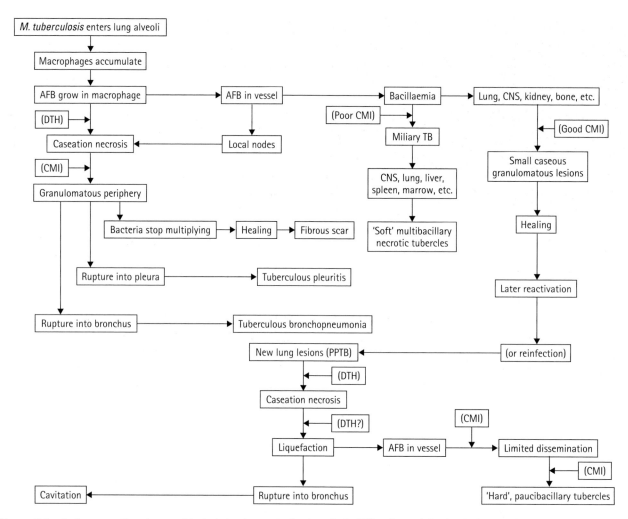

Figure 7.1 A diagrammatic scheme of typical development of tuberculosis (TB): primary infection in lung and subsequent post-primary pulmonary tuberculosis (PPTB), including some of the possible sequelae in primary disease. The immunopathological inputs – cell-mediated immunity (CMI) and delayed-type hypersensitivity (DTH) – are indicated. CNS, central nervous system; AFB, acid-fast bacilli of *M. tuberculosis*.

the clinical pathology of tuberculosis, such as the immune reconstitution inflammatory syndrome,[6] have revived interest in the treatment-related effects of tuberculosis chemotherapy. The immunopathogenesis of *M. tuberculosis* infection is considered in more detail in Chapter 8, Human immune response to *M. tuberculosis*.

The pathogenesis of tuberculosis is not well understood even now. The most coherent accounts derive from the experimental and human observation work of Lurie[7] and Dannenberg.[8–11] More recently, with a resurgence of surgical resection of lung tuberculosis taking place in Russia (because of multidrug-resistant infection), there have been further observations on the morphological and immunopathological dynamics of the host reaction by Ulrichs and colleagues.[12]

THE CLASSICAL TUBERCULOID GRANULOMA

The basic inflammatory response to infection by *M. tuberculosis* is the formation of a granuloma. A granuloma is a

focal aggregate of activated macrophages. The latter cells arise in the bone marrow, circulate in the blood as monocytes and populate the tissues as macrophages. As such they are the most effective phagocytic cells in the body. The term 'activation' describes the phenotypic, morphological and metabolic changes of macrophages into epithelioid cells, usually under the stimulus of cytokines. The most important cytokine here is interferon-γ.

Epithelioid cells are large with abundant eosinophilic mitochondria- and lysosome-rich cytoplasm, a large pale-staining round or elongated nucleus with a prominent eosinophilic nucleolus, and they have indistinct, ruffled interdigitating cell membranes seen best by electron microscopy. There are morphological schemes for differentiating immature and mature epithelioid cells.[13] In epithelioid cells, the rate of production and secretion of enzymes,[10] cytokines and free radicals is increased, and epithelioid cells are thus capable of inhibiting, killing and digesting agents such as *M. tuberculosis* more readily than unactivated macrophages.

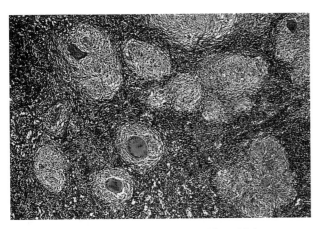

Figure 7.2 Tuberculous lymphadenitis with multiple epithelioid cell and Langhans giant cell granulomas. There is no necrosis at this stage. H&E, medium power.

In addition to epithelioid cells, many granulomas contain multinucleated giant cells (Figure 7.2). If the nuclei are randomly distributed through the cytoplasm they are often termed 'foreign body giant cells' (FBGCs); if the nuclei form a peripheral rim within the cell, the term 'Langhans giant cell' (LGC) is used, and this is the typical form seen in tuberculosis. FBGCs and LGCs form by fusion of macrophages (several cells attempting to phagocytose the same bacillus or fragment of necrotic tissue at the same time[8]), but probably by different mechanisms.[14] Their functions are unclear. Like epithelioid cells they have an enhanced oxidative and enzymatic capacity compared with macrophages.[15] They can destroy bacilli phagocytosed by prefusion macrophages and also function as antigen presenting cells.[16] When tuberculous lesions resolve, spontaneously or through treatment, the LGCs become smaller and the nuclei shrink.

Interestingly, when *M. tuberculosis* bacilli are scanty in active tissue lesions, they are more likely to be detected within LGCs than in other cells. Other inflammatory cells in and around granulomas include lymphocytes and, in

many infections, such as mycoses and parasitic worms, there are polymorphs, plasma cells and eosinophils.

Granulomas in tuberculosis characteristically fuse to form larger, visible masses, and characteristically undergo necrosis within single or fused lesions. The macroscopic appearance of such a necrotic lesion is firm, pale and yellowish (Figure 7.3), from which derives the description 'caseous' (cheese-like). Histologically, the ghosts of dead macrophages are visible within the eosinophilic mass, along with variable numbers of apoptotic nuclear fragments. The pathogenesis of this form of cell death is discussed below.

The focal activation of macrophages to form granulomas may also be accompanied by a systemic macrophage activation and clinically deleterious sequelae, such as pancytopenia from the haemophagocytic syndrome,[17,18] diagnosed on bone marrow biopsy.

HISTOLOGICAL DEMONSTRATION OF *M. TUBERCULOSIS* ACID-FAST BACILLI

Mycobacteria are bacilli that are weakly Gram positive and are classically identified in histological sections by stains that exploit their resistance to decoloration by acid, i.e. acid-fast bacilli (AFB).[19] All mycobacteria, apart from the leprosy bacillus, are well stained by the standard Ziehl–Neelsen (ZN) technique. It is worth noting that the histological detection of AFB is relatively insensitive. From the geometry of bacillus distribution in tissues and the thickness of histological sections, it can be calculated that the minimum density of bacilli for detection by the ZN method is 1000 per mL of tissue. Because of this generic insensitivity and because 'tuberculous' tissue is often not submitted for culture but put straight into mycobactericidal fixative, histopathology laboratories increasingly utilize polymerase chain reaction (PCR) technology to confirm mycobacterial infection in tissues and to identify the species.[20] However, the sensitivity of in-house or commercially available methods using formalin-fixed and paraffin-embedded tissue is not perfect: published sensitivity rates range from 43 to 63 per cent.[21,22] The sensitivity appears to decline over time of storage in paraffinized tissues.[23]

THE IMMUNOHISTOLOGY OF TUBERCULOUS GRANULOMAS

The immunological response to *M. tuberculosis* infection is cell-mediated hypersensitivity, with allergized T cells secreting cytokines that activate tissue macrophages into granulomas. Studies of the lymphocyte distribution patterns in and around early non-necrotic tuberculous granulomas shed light on how this takes place. As with granulomas in paucibacillary tuberculoid leprosy and sarcoidosis,[24,25] CD4$^+$ T cells are found throughout and around the granuloma, and CD8$^+$ T cells are mainly

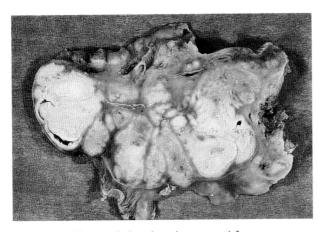

Figure 7.3 Mesenteric lymph nodes removed from a tuberculous HIV-infected cadaver showing massive caseous necrosis.

restricted to a marginal rim around the epithelioid cells.[26,27] The overall distribution and proportions of CD8[+] and CD4[+] T cells may also be differentiated according to the immune type of tuberculosis: in HIV-infected (but not HIV-negative) patients who can still form granulomas, CD8[+] cells are found throughout lymph node granulomas;[27,28] in skin lesions, the ratio of CD4[+]/CD8[+] T cells is higher in lupus vulgaris than in scrofuloderma.[29] A major function of the CD4[+] T cells is the secretion of interferon-γ (IFN-γ),[30] which activates macrophages and induces granuloma formation, so contributing to cell-mediated immunity (CMI).

However, this is probably a simplistic explanation of granuloma formation; in murine experimental *M. tuberculosis* infection, several phenotypically (and possibly functionally) distinct subsets of CD4[+] T cells emerge during the course of disease[31] and correlate with macrophage activation and mycobacterial load. Other involved murine cells include the CD11 series.[32] In man, the situation is presumably comparable. Tissue analysis of mRNA expression in human tuberculosis shows that granulocyte–macrophage colony-stimulating factor (GM-CSF) expression is correlated with florid granulomatous response, tumour necrosis factor (TNF)-γ expression with necrosis in granulomas, and IL-8 expression with occurrence of neutrophils within tuberculous granulomas.[33]

In HIV-infected people whose CD4[+] T cells are progressively destroyed, the ability to form granulomas is occasionally retained with no apparent CD4[+] T cells available. In such patients, there may be production of IFN-γ by natural killer (NK) cells to provide the activating stimulus to macrophages.[30,34]

The role of the CD8[+] T cells is unclear in the usual tuberculous granuloma.[35] The formation of multinucleate giant cells is also under the control of various cytokines including TNF-α, IFN-γ and interleukin (IL)-4 and IL-6.[15,36]

PRIMARY TUBERCULOSIS

Infection with *M. tuberculosis* occurs most commonly via the lungs, and less frequently the oropharynx, intestine and skin (through inoculation). In lung, the bacilli arrive in alveoli, inducing the local lesion usually in subpleural locations. With human infection, the initial local reactions are unclear, and it presumed that, as with experimental animals, an early neutrophil reaction is unable to contain the bacilli, and monocyte-derived macrophages phagocytose them. Within hours, bacilli are carried in cells to the local lymph nodes. In both sites, the macrophages aggregate to form enlarging but poorly defined lesions, whilst the mycobacteria continue multiplying (the primary complex).

The infected macrophage lesion enlarges through recruitment from the blood monocytes. After a few weeks, the T cell-mediated immune responses start and caseation necrosis develops in the centre of the lesion.[10,11]

This is synchronous with the acquisition of delayed-type hypersensitivity (DTH) and Dannenberg invokes DTH as the process to explain caseation; a cellular reaction to tuberculous antigen. Some of this necrosis is actually apoptosis of macrophages and T cells.[37] Some is infarction, through local microvascular thrombosis following endothelial cell activation and triggering of clotting factors.[9] It is possible that toxic products of *M. tuberculosis* bacilli are also tissue damaging, but experimentally it has never been demonstrated that the bacilli are directly cytopathic to macrophages – unlike the well-proven tissue-damaging mycolactone toxins secreted by *Mycobacterium ulcerans*.[38] The complex cytokine-mediated mechanisms of DTH are also considered in Chapter 8, Human immune response to *M. tuberculosis*. This necrotizing response is a means of stopping bacillary multiplication (they cannot replicate in the anoxic environment of the solid necrotic mass) but at the expense of destroying host tissues. The bacilli do not necessarily die, but may remain latent for a long period.

Histologically, caseation is eosinophilic smooth tissue where the ghosts of the previously existing macrophages are barely visible, there are no nuclei and nuclear karyorrhectic debris is sparse or absent. At the periphery of the necrosis, macrophages become activated into epithelioid cells – granulomas (Figure 7.4). This represents T CMI and is a distinct process from the DTH response with its tissue destruction.[8,9,11,39] Epithelioid cells are more able to kill bacilli and inhibit the expansion of the infected lesion. Nevertheless, in primary tuberculosis, a bacillaemia is characteristic at this stage through erosion into a vessel, with seeding of *M. tuberculosis* into distant organs such as kidney, adrenal and bone marrow, and locally into other parts of the lungs.

At this stage, the usual sequence in immunocompetent people is healing of the lung lesion, the hilar nodes and the small peripheral foci that have ensued from the bacillaemia. The CMI stops further bacterial replication; many

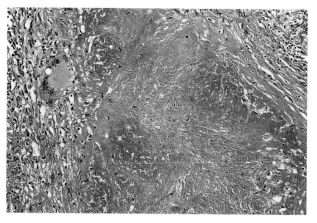

Figure 7.4 Tuberculous lymphadenitis showed caseous necrosis with minimal karyorrhectic debris and a Langhans giant cell. H&E, high power.

or even all the bacilli within the necrotic material may die; the caseous material is gradually removed by a chronic granulation tissue and phagocytic process; the granulomas are replaced by fibrosis – and the whole lesion becomes a scar with or without a residual necrotic centre. Dystrophic calcification, or even ossification, can follow within the scar; in many people the scars are reabsorbed entirely. Exaggerated and persistent fibrosis in pulmonary tuberculosis occurs in patients with co-existent pulmonary silicosis, where the fibrosing tendencies of both disease become additive (and also lead to higher mortality).[40,41]

The bloodstream dissemination of bacilli evokes different reactions according to the level of infection and the degree of CMI to *M. tuberculosis* in the patient. If the bacillaemia is low grade and CMI relatively high, the lesions are histologically epithelioid cell granulomas with LGCs but few or no bacilli and little caseation (the 'hard' tubercles described by Rich[1]). This is one form of miliary tuberculosis, where small numbers of granulomas are seen in lung, liver, spleen and nodes ('miliary' refers to the macroscopic appearance of seeing small pale seed-like nodules – the granulomas). They heal as described above, but surviving bacilli may reactivate later to cause end-organ tuberculous lesions. Clinical miliary tuberculosis is a more aggressive disease that is fatal if untreated, affecting those with lower CMI and/or a higher level of bacillaemia. In addition to the organs mentioned above, the meninges are infected. Compared with hard tubercles, these miliary lesions are more necrotic, with fewer or no activated macrophages, and bacilli are more obvious – these are the 'soft' tubercles of Rich,[1] and represent a form of non-reactive tuberculosis (see below).

The bacillaemia of primary tuberculosis is also probably the cause of tuberculosis that arises at sites of trauma when there is no evidence for direct inoculation of *M. tuberculosis*. Examples of infection in bone, joint and soft tissues, 2–4 months after injury, are described in patients with clinically inapparent primary or post-primary internal disease.[42,43]

DTH versus CMI responses

It is important to emphasize the difference between DTH and CMI responses.[9] Both are mediated via T cells, with (at least) CD8[+] T cells probably required for DTH and (at least) CD4[+] T cells needed for CMI response.[10] DTH is a means of killing an infected macrophage mass and rendering the bacilli – temporarily at least – non-multiplying. CMI is the means of controlling bacterial multiplication by intracellular inactivation or killing, the phenomenon taking place around caseous necrotic masses in primary infection, in the distant sites where the bacillaemia has seeded the infection, and around the cavitating lesions of post-primary pulmonary tuberculosis. CMI, as in granulomatous disease of any cause, is a potent inducer of fibrosis via cytokines such as IL-1.[44]

POST-PRIMARY PULMONARY TUBERCULOSIS

Tuberculous disease later in life follows primary lung infection more often than infection via the bowel or oropharynx (congruent with Marfan's 'law' which noted the infrequency with which individuals who had cervical tuberculous lymphadenitis subsequently develop pulmonary tuberculosis[1]). Some 5–10 per cent of non-immunosuppressed people who have inapparent tuberculosis in childhood develop active pulmonary disease later. Host factors that predispose to recrudescence of disease include age, malnutrition, cirrhosis and diabetes;[45] HIV infection is almost a special case in its vastly increased risk of active tuberculosis (see Chapters 17, Directly observed therapy and other aspects of management of tuberculosis care, and Chapter 18, DOTS and DOTS-Plus). The origin of the infection is still debated: whether it represents a new infection or a reactivation of old latent infection.[46] In the days of mycobacterial culture as the only means of identifying specific strains of *M. tuberculosis*, instances of proven endogenous reactivation and exogenous reinfection were documented.[45,46] With the recent technique of restriction fragment length polymorphism (RFLP) analysis of *M. tuberculosis*, it is now evident that a significant number of recrudescent episodes of pulmonary tuberculosis result from reinfection.[47,48]

The pathological basis of reactivation is the phase of haematogenous dissemination of bacilli during a first infection. They locate in the apices of the lung where oxygen tension is high, as it is in other favoured sites of dissemination, such as cerebral cortex, renal cortex and metaphysis of bones. In the lung, it can be argued that the greater vascular supply and oxygen turnover in the lower zones enable macrophages to be more metabolically effective, thus reducing the likelihood of bacilli there remaining, compared with the apices.[8] These pulmonary metastatic foci follow the usual granulomatous sequence and heal as fibrocaseous scars (the radiologically visible 'Simon foci'), but the bacilli remain viable within the macrophages, unlike the bacilli in the primary foci which more usually die off. Microbiological studies into the pathogenesis of reactivation, using guinea pig inoculation of post-mortem tissues, produced interesting results. Old healed tuberculous lesions in lung and hilar nodes contained viable bacilli in only 1/68 cases, whilst macroscopically normal tissue nearby old lesions harboured bacilli in 3/51 cases.[49] Conversely, pulmonary caseous and calcified nodules, apical fibrous scars, and nearly normal-looking lung and hilar node tissue were all found to contain viable bacilli in between one-quarter and one-third of cases, with more isolations proportionally in the non-pathological tissues.[50] This supports the contention that the apical Simon foci are the location of viable bacilli that later reactivate to cause post-primary lung disease. Recent studies suggest that the viable bacilli in these dormant lesions are more likely to be found in the peripheral cell rim rather than in the necrotic centre.[12]

Pathologically, post-primary pulmonary tuberculosis (PPTB) presents as a pneumonia, usually in the upper zones. Hilar lymphadenopathy is not a prominent feature, and histology of such nodes reveals small or no lesions. The large lung lesions show marked caseous necrosis (i.e. mass of dead inflammatory cells and host lung tissue) with peripheral granulomas and B-cell follicles.[51] AFB are not usually numerous in stained sections. Around the lesion is a fibrous capsule, hence the term 'fibrocaseous lesion'.

The lesions characteristically liquefy and then cavitate when the necrotizing process involves a bronchus and the soft material is coughed up (Figure 7.5). In liquefied material and particularly in cavitated lesions, the bacilli multiply and are readily seen on ZN stains. The lining of the cavity is ragged granulomatous necrosis, with bacilli proliferating at the tissue/air interface. Peripheral is a rim of granulation tissue and fibrous tissue. If the liquefying lesions erode and disseminate peripherally in a bronchus, there may be a

tuberculous bronchopneumonia, with diffuse granulomatous and caseating lesions affecting lung lobules and lobes. Tuberculous empyema results if the pleura is involved. The mechanisms of liquefaction are unclear, but a DTH response to *M. tuberculosis* antigens is involved, with increased hydrolytic enzymatic activity that breaks down the caseous material into osmotically active, water-absorbing medium that permits bacillary multiplication again.[8,11,52]

Recent morphological studies on PPTB lung cavities have shown a low rate of mononuclear cell multiplication in the areas around cavities, in contrast to the high rate around non-progressive tuberculomas.[53]

The florid pulmonary lesion has more destruction and cavitation than is usually seen in primary TB, along with the less marked involvement of draining lymph nodes – these features parallel the Koch phenomenon following *M. tuberculosis* infection in guinea pigs.[52] To account for the increased tissue destruction and local containment of

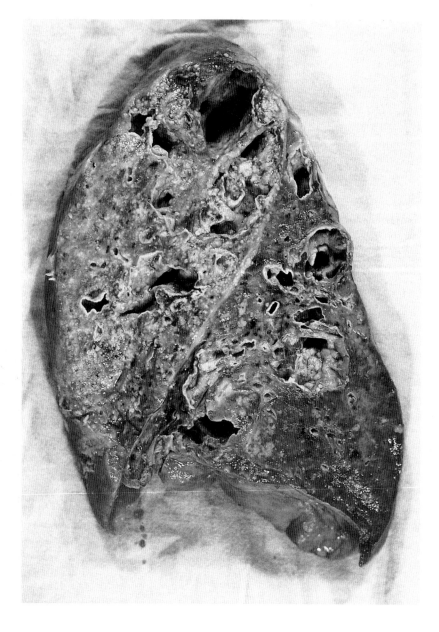

Figure 7.5 Pulmonary tuberculosis with apical cavitation and tuberculous bronchopneumonia.

infection, both the DTH-associated liquefactive reaction and CMI responses are presumed to be elevated in comparison with a primary infection.

Despite the better containment of infection to the lungs in most PPTB patients, due to heightened CMI, bacillaemia does frequently occur, as evidenced by low-grade chronic miliary lesions in many organs. These include liver and bone marrow, and often show Rich's 'hard' tubercles[1] on histology: non-necrotic epithelioid and giant cell granulomas with few or no visible bacilli.[54] Depending on host factors and levels of bacillaemia, other end-organ tuberculous lesions may occur in later tuberculous disease, with large caseous lesions in spleen, kidneys and adrenals, and tuberculomas in the brain.

The longer-term consequences of pulmonary tuberculosis include scar-related carcinoma within the lung. If there is chronic pyothorax, a non-Hodgkin B-cell lymphoma may develop.[55] These oncogenic processes are not directly due to *M. tuberculosis*, but presumably represent cellular transformation as a byproduct of chronic inflammation and scarring.

OTHER ORGANS IN TUBERCULOSIS

Figure 7.1 provides a diagrammatic schema of the sequence, pathology and outline immunopathogenesis of tuberculosis. A complete description of tuberculous lesions in other organs is not possible here, but there are features of *M. tuberculosis* infection in the central nervous system and in the skin that demonstrate interesting and varied histopathological features.

Central nervous system tuberculosis

Two main lesions are seen in the brain and spinal cord – tuberculous meningitis (TBM) and tuberculoma.[1] A small focus of tuberculosis seeds in the meninges, ependyma or superficial cerebral cortex from haematogenous spread. In the meninges, an extensive exudative (cellular) reaction follows and the base of the brain is particularly affected.[56] The reaction may be granulomatous and/or polymorphonuclear, and necrosis is frequent. In a study of 19 HIV-infected patients with tuberculous meningitis, an acute inflammatory reaction was noted in 13, fibrinoid necrosis in 18 and giant cell granulomas in only 2 cases. AFB were seen in all cases and interestingly were 10- to 100-fold more densely numerous in the meninges than in the extracerebral lesions in lung and nodes[57] (and personal observations). The finding of purely polymorphonuclear inflammation in the cerebrospinal fluid (CSF) of patients with TBM is not novel,[1] but may be misleading diagnostically.[58] Further, some TBM patients may have bacilli but no cellular exudate in CSF at all,[59] a form of neurotuberculosis previously termed 'serous tuberculosis'.[60] HIV-infected patients have a significantly high prevalence of TBM.[61]

TBM induces a granulomatous vasculitis and also the non-specific endarteritis obliterans (intimal hyperplasia) in arteries passing through the meninges. These vascular lesions obstruct blood flow and frequently cause small foci of cortical necrosis and larger cerebral infarctions.[62] The inflammation and necrosis of TBM can obstruct CSF flow, with consequent hydrocephalus. HIV-infected patients with TBM, with their less granulomatous histopathology, tend to demonstrate less communicating hydrocephalus compared with HIV-negative patients.[63] Treated TBM may fibrose and result in entrapment of the cranial nerves.[56]

A tuberculoma is a macroscopically visible caseous necrotic mass, often up to 5–6 cm in diameter, with peripheral granulomatous rim and moderate gliosis. It develops in the cerebrum, cerebellum or brain stem, and behaves as a space-occupying lesion.[62]

Some patients with CNS tuberculosis manifest an acute encephalopathy with vascular necrosis, perivascular demyelination and petechial haemorrhages.[60] This is analogous to acute haemorrhagic leukoencephalopathy, and since it usually follows recent chemotherapy, is considered to represent a hypersensitivity reaction to *M. tuberculosis* antigens. Encephalopathy with extensive cerebral demyelination is also reported in association with extracranial tuberculosis;[64] again, this is usually a manifestation after commencement of antituberculous chemotherapy and may occur in HIV-infected patients.[65]

Skin tuberculosis and tuberculids

Cutaneous tuberculosis, due to active *M. tuberculosis* infection, is a series of clinicohistopathological entities which in reality are often difficult to distinguish.[66,67] Infection occurs by three routes: (1) direct inoculation into the skin (causing a primary chancre, or tuberculosis verrucosa cutis, or tuberculosis cutis orificialis lesions); (2) haematogenous spread from an internal lesion (causing lupus vulgaris, miliary tuberculosis, and tuberculous gumma lesions); and (3) from an underlying tuberculous lymph node by direct extension (causing scrofuloderma). For descriptive purposes, the tuberculous dermatitides are delineated by a modified 'Beyt classification'.[68] Tuberculids are another group of skin lesions which result indirectly from *M. tuberculosis* infection.

Histopathologically, skin tuberculosis demonstrates many patterns. At the high-immune end of the spectrum is lupus vulgaris, with giant cells. Caseation necrosis within the tubercles is slight or absent.[69] The inflammation is most pronounced in the upper dermis, but in some areas it may extend into the subcutaneous layer, and there is destruction of the cutaneous appendages. In areas of healing, extensive fibrosis may be present. Tubercle bacilli are present in such small numbers that they can only rarely be demonstrated by staining methods. PCR detection of mycobacterial DNA is often positive.[70] Conversely, in miliary tuberculosis of the skin in infants and immuno-suppressed adults, the centre of the papule shows a micro-abscess containing neutrophils, cellular debris, numerous tubercle bacilli and there may vascular thrombi.[67]

Tuberculids are skin lesions in patients with tuberculosis, often occult, elsewhere in the body. The most common sites of active infection are lymph nodes.[71] By definition, stains for AFB and culture for mycobacteria are negative; delayed hypersensitivity skin tests for tuberculosis are positive, and the lesions heal on antituberculous therapy. The four clinicopathological patterns of tuberculids are papulonecrotic (histology: foci of infarction due to dermal necrotizing granulomatous vasculitis[72]), lichen scrofulosorum (non-necrotic granulomas adjacent to hair shafts[73]), erythema induratum (panniculitis with granulomatous vasculitis[74]) and nodular granulomatous phlebitis (granulomas in vein wall[75]). Recently, using the PCR technique, mycobacterial DNA has been identified in a proportion of lesions.[74,75] This supports the concept of tuberculids as immunological reactions to degenerate bacilli or antigenic fragments thereof that have been deposited haematogenously in the skin and subcutis.

Skin lesions associated with tuberculosis may, furthermore, contain no mycobacterial antigens or DNA at all. Erythema nodosum (a septal panniculitis with minor secondary endothelial changes) is a well-known example. Less common is cutaneous leucocytoclastic vasculitis – a common purpuric lesion associated with diverse infections and drug reactions – which may occur in patients with intrathoracic tuberculosis.[76] These indirect pathologies presumably represent systemic immune reactions where the most susceptible vessels are in the skin.

TUBERCULOSIS IN HIV-INFECTED PATIENTS

Tuberculosis differs clinically, radiologically and pathologically in those with defective cellular immunity compared with immunocompetent patients.[77] HIV infection is the most significant contemporary cause of immunosuppression. Overall, there is more frequent extrapulmonary disease, less cavitation in the lungs and a higher mortality most notable in those with the most severe immunosuppression.[78] Bizarre and previously rare clinicopathological lesions are increasingly noted, such as diffuse tuberculous myocarditis[79] and pulmonary artery thrombosis due to intramedial tuberculous vasculitis.

When infection presents early in the course of HIV infection (near normal CD4[+] T-cell counts in the blood), the clinicopathological features are similar to those of TB in HIV-negative patients; in terminal HIV disease, they are quite different.[78] Studies of HIV-associated tuberculosis show a consistent pattern of organ disease correlating with CD4[+] T-cell counts (Figure 7.6).

Autopsy studies of HIV-associated tuberculosis in Zaire, Ivory Coast and India showed that tuberculosis was the most common prime cause of death[57,80,81] in those

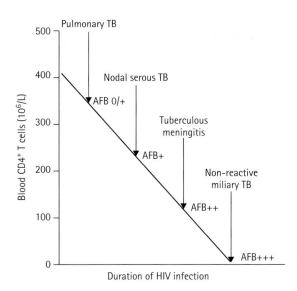

Figure 7.6 Clinical and immunopathological course of HIV-associated tuberculosis (TB). The figure does not represent one patient, but is a composite of cross-sectional data correlated with blood CD4[+] T-cell counts (10[6]/L). The CD4 data are drawn from Refs 2 and 3. AFB, semi-quantitative density of *M. tuberculosis* bacilli in lesions.

populations. In 87 per cent of the cadavers in Ivory Coast with tuberculosis, the disease was disseminated to more than one organ, nearly always involving the lungs, liver, spleen, internal lymph nodes and bone marrow. The most common gross pulmonary patterns were miliary nodules (55 per cent), miliary plus bronchopneumonia (22 per cent) and cavitating lesions seen in only 15 per cent of those with lung tuberculosis. The meninges were involved in 18 per cent of tuberculosis cases.[57]

Follow-up studies of treated tuberculosis patients in Africa and Brazil show that patients with miliary non-reactive tuberculosis (see below) who succumb early in therapy die of the disease, whereas those who survive therapy die of other HIV-related diseases.[4,82]

Histopathology of HIV-associated tuberculosis

Before profound immunodeficiency occurs in HIV-positive co-infected patients, the histopathology of tuberculosis is indistinguishable from that in HIV-negative patients[27,83,84] – typical caseating granulomatous lesions with scanty or no bacilli found on routine ZN stains. From autopsy studies of disseminated tuberculosis, as immune function fails (measured by blood CD4[+] T-cell counts), the numbers of giant cells and the degree of activation of the macrophages decline, and the number of detectable bacilli increases (Tables 7.2 and 7.3). Single organ studies, such as with pleural biopsy, produce less consistent monotonic relationships between histopathology and CD4 count, although the trend of high bacillary density with lower CD4 count is maintained.[84] The necrosis within lesions contin-

Table 7.2 Density of Langhans giant cells in tuberculosis lesions of HIV-positive cadavers correlated with pre-mortem blood CD4+ T-cell counts.[3]

Langhans giant cells	CD4+ T-cell count (10⁶/L)		
	No. of patients	Median	Range
Absent	15	34	4–221
Scanty	12	72	14–359
More than one per granuloma	11	167	26–537

Table 7.3 Density of acid-fast bacilli (AFB) in untreated tuberculosis lesions in HIV-positive cadavers, correlated with blood CD4+ T-cell counts.

No. AFB/HPF	No. of patients	CD4+ T-cell count (10⁶/L)	
		Median	Range
>100	16	28	4–130
≤100	22	151	26–537

HPF, high power microscope field at ×400 magnification.

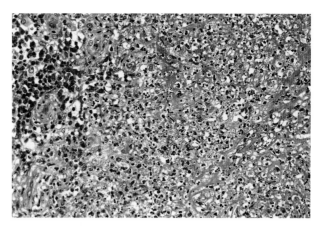

Figure 7.7 Non-reactive tuberculosis in a lymph node, showing much necrosis and karyorrhectic debris, no epithelioid or giant cells. H&E, high power.

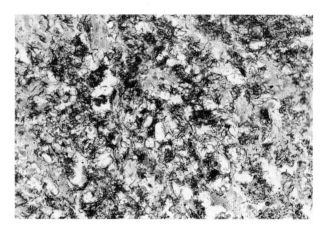

Figure 7.8 Ziehl–Neelsen stain of the node in Figure 7.7. There are large numbers of acid-fast bacilli in the necrosis; high-power view.

ues to look caseous, but histologically it becomes less homogeneously eosinophilic: polymorphs are commonly seen and the quantity of apoptotic nuclear debris increases. These represent dead macrophage nuclei. Eventually, the pattern of 'non-reactive tuberculosis' is reached, where there is no macrophage activation, and the surviving cells around the necrotic lesions have pale watery cytoplasm due to hydropic change (sublethal or early lethal damage). The necrosis is basophilic and granular, and vast numbers of bacilli are present (Figures 7.7 and 7.8). In many lesions, the cellular infiltrate includes abundant neutrophil polymorphs forming abscesses.[58] Descriptions of this pattern of tuberculosis pathology predate the HIV pandemic, being seen in the elderly and those immunosuppressed by malignancy, steroid and cytotoxic chemotherapy.[1,85] Sometimes the necrotic lesions are notably haemorrhagic as seen in the liver in HIV-infected patients.[86]

HISTOPATHOLOGICAL CLASSIFICATION OF TUBERCULOSIS

The histopathology of HIV-associated tuberculosis – particularly at the late stages of AIDS – is thus very different from that seen in immunocompetent patients. This has been a stimulus to better categorize tuberculosis pathology by organizing a comprehensive histopathological schema.[13,83,87] Since the 1960s, leprosy has been recognized as a disease that has an immunopathological spectrum, with clinical, microbiological, immunological and histopathological data correlating well within and between patients.[88] The determinants in *Mycobacterium leprae*

infection revolve around the host's CD4+ T-cell CMI, resulting in descriptions of paucibacillary granulomatous lesions at the tuberculoid pole and multibacillary non-granulomatous macrophage accumulations at the lepromatous pole. Leprosy is easier to organize than tuberculosis in this respect, since (1) *M. leprae* is definitely non-toxic and replicates more slowly than *M. tuberculosis* and (2) necrosis and the process of liquefaction of granulomatous masses are relatively uncommon. Similarly, the host reaction in children to disseminated bacillus Calmette–Guérin (BCG) infection can be divided into granulomatous paucibacillary lesions (with good survival) and non-activated multibacillary parasitism of macrophages (non-necrotic, but still with poor survival) – determined by the host's genetic constitution for CMI, such as absent receptor for IFN-γ on macrophages.[89]

Earlier attempts to rationalize tuberculosis histopathology along an immunopathological spectrum were inconclusive. One scheme arranged a spectrum by analysing the character and spread of infiltration on chest x-rays in adult patients. Although the resulting four groups showed monotonic relationships with skin hypersensitivity tests, circulating antibody, immune complexes and leucocyte migration inhibition tests, the histopathological data were not so tractable.[90] At the highest immune position, the histology of pulmonary lesions showed classical tuberculous granulomas, whilst at the least reactive pole there were many mycobacteria with polymorphs, but no epithelioid cell response. The problem lies with the intermediate groups, where the authors felt that the histology did not correlate well with the other variables. Part of the variability lies in the variation of tuberculosis histology within a patient at the same time: granulomas arise and heal over time, with therefore differing appearances of maturity and bacillary density, some are necrotic and some are not; and in some locations there will be varying bacillary counts and constraints upon cell proliferation because of physical differences in tissue structure (e.g. solid lymph nodes versus aerated lung versus liquid cerebrospinal spinal fluid and serous cavities).

More recently, Ridley[13] proposed a histopathology classification of tuberculosis that correlated with evidence of resistance to mycobacterial multiplication, and focused on the maturity of the macrophages/epithelioid cells in a lesion, the presence and character of necrosis, and the presence of polymorphs, (but omitting LGCs as criteria) (see Table 7.4).

Under this scheme, the most resistant pole is histopathologically represented by lupus vulgaris and non-caseating tuberculous lymphadenitis; the least resistant pole is non-reactive tuberculosis. In practice, most lesions encountered in daily practice fall into the intermediate groups. From observations of HIV-related tuberculous histology, two other rather similar schemes have been proposed, focusing on the density of bacilli, the numbers of surrounding epithelioid and giant cells, the amount of nuclear debris within necrosis and vacuolation (hydropic damage) of macrophages.[83,87]

Finally, there is a single case report of an immunosuppressed HIV-negative transplant patient who died with multiple pulmonary nodular lesions due to *M. tuberculosis* infection. Histologically, the response was neither a necrotic lesion with abundant bacilli, nor a granulomatous response with fewer bacilli, but a non-necrotic spindle-cell macrophage lesion teeming with bacilli.[91] This resembles the similar lesions in immunosuppressed patients with *M. avium* complex infection and leprosy patients with histoid lesions.[45,92]

Other rare atypical patterns of tuberculosis histopathology continue to be observed, such as malakoplakia in a neck abscess.[93] This pattern is normally found with Gram-negative bacteria and is characterized by Michaelis–Gutmann bodies within macrophages, indicating a phagocytosis-disposal defect within phagosomes.

TREATMENT OF TUBERCULOSIS AND ASSOCIATED REACTIONS

Repeat biopsies from tuberculous patients are infrequent, but observations of lymph nodes after the start of therapy and of lung resection and autopsy specimens enable descriptions of the normal healing changes in treated tuberculosis. Within caseous lesions, the necrosis hardens and often seems to separate from the surrounding inflammatory mantle which become more fibrotic and may develop an elastic tissue inner rim. The necrosis is slowly reabsorbed by granulation tissue. The granulomas slowly disappear, being replaced by scar tissue.[44] In many treated lymph nodes, one sees – transiently – very large LGCs around the necrosis, reminiscent of reversal reactions in leprosy. Eventually, all granulomas and giant cells have gone, leaving bland fibrosis and residual non-specific lymphocytic inflammation.

In leprosy, one of the challenges in management is controlling the tendency of patients to increase their CMI response to *M. leprae* antigens once anti-mycobacterial treatment has commenced. The result is a 'reversal reaction', where skin lesions swell, spread and become painful, new lesions develop at the sites of antigen deposition, and peripheral nerves become more inflamed, swollen and often necrotic.[94] The underlying histopathology is a notable oedema within and around the inflammatory cells, activation of macrophages to more mature epithelioid cells, larger granulomas, larger multi-nucleate giant cells and foci of fibrinoid or destructive caseation-type necrosis.[45,95,96] Immunohistological studies indicate an augmentation of CMI responses with increased production of IFN-γ in such reactions.[97]

Table 7.4 Ridley's classification of the immune spectrum of tuberculosis histology.[13]

Group	Main cell type	Necrosis	Bacilli
1a	EC organized	None	0
1b	EC + IEC unorganized	Fibrinoid	Rare
2a	IEC	Homogenous eosinophilic; no nuclear debris	Scanty
2b	Undifferentiated histiocytes	Basophilic; polymorphs present	1–2+
3a	Macrophages	Coarse nuclear debris, basophilic extensive	2–3+
3b	Scanty macrophages	Coarse eosinophilic, very extensive	>3+

EC, mature epithelioid cell; IEC, immature epithelioid cell.

A similar phenomenon occurs in *M. tuberculosis* infection. Before specific anti-mycobacterial therapy was introduced, the deleterious effects (including death) of injecting tuberculin into patients with tuberculosis (the 'Koch treatment') were widely known.[98] Skin lesions of lupus vulgaris became further inflamed and ulcerated; autopsy data showed that bowel ulcers enlarged and perforated; and tuberculin injection induced widespread inflammation, disintegration and destruction of tissue in the brain and lungs – not, as Koch hoped, the envelopment and imprisonment of bacilli in caseous cocoons to prevent further damage.[99] Patients with tuberculous lymphadenitis may experience lymph node swelling on chemotherapy;[100] similarly, neurotuberculosis patients on treatment may show expansion of intracranial tuberculomas and even development of new lesions.[101–103] Unlike the situation in leprosy where repeat biopsies establish the qualitative and quantitative changes in inflammation in such a reaction, comparative data in *M. tuberculosis* infection is sparse, but it is probable that similar processes occur: intragranuloma and perigranuloma oedema, increased cell numbers within granulomas, and perhaps more necrosis.

Patients with advanced disseminated tuberculosis have a high mortality on treatment,[78,104,105] and clinicopathological data often indicate the syndrome of acute respiratory distress (shock lung, ARDS).[106–108] In addition to the hyaline membranes, histologically some cases show necrotic epithelioid cells granulomas;[109] others show non-reactive tuberculosis.[110] It is reasonable to predict that these post-therapy reactions reflect, in part, the overproduction of tissue-damaging cytokines. The contribution of the proposed adrenal deficit in some tuberculosis patients[52] to these shock syndromes is unclear.

IMMUNE RECONSTITUTION INFLAMMATORY SYNDROME

The advent, since the mid-1990s, of highly active antiretroviral therapy (HAART) for HIV disease has provided more convincing demonstration of 'reversal reaction'-type clinical pathology. The therapy for advanced HIV disease reduces the blood HIV viral load to undetectable or very low levels (although the virus is never completely eliminated from tissues), and concomitantly the antigen-specific cell-mediated immune responses are partially restored, as monitored by rising CD4+ T-lymphocyte counts in the blood.[111] Patients being treated for tuberculosis who are also commenced on HAART, may suffer a paradoxical worsening of clinical disease locally and systemically.[5,6]

Increasing lymph node size and sinus formation, respiratory failure (with occasional mortality – personal observation) and perforation of the bowel are examples.[112–114] Histopathologically, a variable picture ensues: granuloma formation, local oedema, tissue necrosis and sometimes acute inflammation are more pronounced than in the pre-

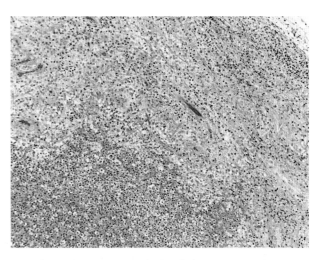

Figure 7.9 Immune reconstitution inflammatory syndrome. Lymph node biopsy. The central purulent necrosis has a moderate granulomatous macrophage surrounding reaction. No acid-fast bacilli were seen. H&E (medium power).

reaction state, and the bacillary density is less (Figure 7.9). In lung, there is much oedema, ARDS and sometimes more prominent macrophage aggregations.

The phenomenon is termed the immune reconstitution inflammatory syndrome (IRIS). Despite the florid clinical manifestation, the peripheral blood markers of cellular immune function – peripheral blood monocyte proliferation in response to tuberculosis antigen, IFN-γ secretion, increased secretion of IL-2, IL-10 and IL-12 – do not reach the levels found in normal HIV-uninfected controls.[115] However, blood levels of TNF-α are raised in IRIS.[6] Augmentation of DTH responses has been found to correlate with a decrease in plasma HIV viraemia.[111] The pathogenesis of IRIS is controversial. In all cases, the HIV viral load has declined, but the blood CD4 count is not significantly raised in all cases. The relative contribution of enhanced CD4+ T-cell activity (following redistribution of CD45Ro T cells with HAART) versus the recovery and increased activation of macrophages (whose function is also directly damaged by HIV) is debated.[6,116]

OVERVIEW OF *M. TUBERCULOSIS* HISTOPATHOLOGY

It is not yet possible to comprehend the overall histopathology and pathogenesis of *M. tuberculosis* infection. From the wide range of lesions (Table 7.1), there appear to be several mechanisms operating: CMI, DTH, necrosis, apoptosis and liquefaction. Several questions stand out:

1 In people with defective CD4+ T-cell CMI, such as those with HIV infection, there is poor or no activation of macrophages and consequent poor control of bacillary multiplication. This explains the large organ lesions, the

dissemination and the high bacillary densities. However, if T cells are also involved in the necrotizing responses, how does this necrosis occur when there is T-cell lymphopenia? Are CD8$^+$ cells (which are retained in HIV disease) involved? Are the *M. tuberculosis* bacilli themselves cytotoxic? There is evidence that they sensitize macrophages to the necrotizing effects of TNF-α (which may even be produced by the actual infected macrophages).[11,117] Such a process may underlie in part the extensive hypocellular necrotic reactions seen in non-reactive tuberculosis. On the other hand, in the rare non-necrotizing multibacillary spindle cell lesions caused by *M. tuberculosis*,[91] there is obviously no evidence of cytotoxicity; or was there no circulating TNF-α to induce necrosis?

2 In some patients with late AIDS, epithelioid cell granulomas are still formed, in response to both *M. tuberculosis* and *M. avium* infections.[118] If there are no CD4$^+$ T cells to secrete IFN-γ and activate macrophages, how do granulomas form? Do NK cells provide the cytokines?[30,34]

3 How does liquefaction of caseous lesions occur?[11,52] This is a key event in tuberculosis pathology from the public health viewpoint since it underlies the high infectivity of those with cavitating lung lesions.

LEARNING POINTS

- Tuberculosis is the prototypical granulomatous inflammatory disease, and the activated macrophage is the key cellular response.
- Granulomas are a manifestation of T-cell-mediated immunity (CMI) and function to kill or control intracellular organisms such as *M. tuberculosis*.
- The caseous necrosis seen in tuberculous lesions is another manifestation of T-cell-mediated immune response, but a necrotizing one termed 'delayed-type hypersensitivity' (DTH).
- Caseation is a compromise response: it stops bacilli multiplying, but damages host tissue in the process.
- In primary tuberculosis, there is a bacillaemia which seeds the organisms in many organs – lung, kidney, bone, etc., which can develop contemporaneously, or reactivate later to cause disease.
- In primary infection, the lesions heal asymptomatically in most people; but if the host resistance is poor, miliary bacillaemic spread and multi-organ damage occur.
- In post-primary pulmonary tuberculosis, whether due to reactivation or reinfection, there is cavitation. This is caused by liquefaction of the caseous necrotic mass, but the mechanism of this is not known.

- Liquefaction and erosion of airways permit the bacilli (now replicating readily) to be coughed up and so spread the infection to others. In contrast, non-cavitating tuberculous patients (i.e. most with primary tuberculosis) are essentially non-infective.
- In all chronic inflammatory destructive lesions of tuberculosis, there is residual scarring of the affected organs.
- In immunocompromised states such as HIV infection, the granulomatous (and CMI) reaction is abrogated and a necrotizing response with vast bacillary loads is seen in visceral lesions.
- In HIV/tuberculosis co-infected patients on anti-HIV therapy, there is frequently an immune reconstitution inflammatory syndrome (IRIS) of increased lymph node size and/or respiratory failure. Pathologically there is oedema, enhanced granulomatous response and necrosis as a consequence of recovery of the DTH and CMI responses.

REFERENCES

1. Rich AR. *The pathogenesis of tuberculosis.* Springfield: CC Thomas, 1951.
2. De Cock KM, Soro B, Coulibaly I-M, Lucas SB. Tuberculosis and HIV infection in sub-Saharan Africa. *J Am Med Assoc* 1992; **268**: 1581–7.
3. Lucas SB, Nelson AM. Pathogenesis of tuberculosis in HIV-infected people. In: Bloom BR (ed.). *Tuberculosis: pathogenesis, protection, and control.* Washington, DC: American Society for Microbiology, 1994: 503–13.
4. Greenberg AE, Lucas SB, Tossou O *et al.* Autopsy-proven causes of death in HIV-infected patients treated for tuberculosis in Abidjan, Côte d'Ivoire. *AIDS* 1995; **9**: 1251–4.
5. Meya DB, McAdam KPWJ. The TB pandemic: an old problem seeking new solutions. *J Int Med* 2006; **261**: 309–29.
6. Lawn SD, Bekker L-G, Miller RF. Immune reconstitution disease associated with mycobacterial infections in HIV-infected individuals receiving antiretrovirals. *Lancet Infect Dis* 2005; **5**: 361–73.
7. Lurie MB. *Resistance to tuberculosis: Experimental studies in native and acquired defensive mechanisms.* Cambridge, MA: Harvard University Press, 1964.
8. Dannenberg AM. *Pathogenesis of human pulmonary tuberculosis. Insights from the rabbit model.* Washington: ASM Press, 2006.
9. Manabe YC, Dannenberg AM. Pathophysiology: basic aspects. In Schlossberg D (ed.). *Tuberculosis and non-tuberculous mycobacterial infections.* New York: McGraw-Hill, 2006: 18–51.
10. Dannenberg AM. Delayed-type hypersensitivity and cell-mediated immunity in the pathogenesis of tuberculosis. *Immunol Today* 1991; **12**: 228–33.
11. Dannenberg AM, Rook GAW. Pathogenesis of pulmonary tuberculosis: interplay of tissue-damaging and macrophage-activating immune responses – dual mechanisms that control bacillary multiplication. In: Bloom BR (ed.). *Tuberculosis: pathogenesis, protection and control.* Washington: American Society for Microbiology, 1994: 459–83.
12. Ulrichs T, Kaufman SHE. New insights into the function of granulomas in human tuberculosis. *J Pathol* 2006; **208**: 261–9.
13. Ridley DS, Ridley MJ. Rationale for the histological spectrum of tuberculosis. A basis for classification. *Pathology* 1987; **19**: 186–92.

14. McNally AK, Anderson JM. Interleukin 4 induces foreign body giant cells from human monocytes/macropahges. Differential lymphokine regulation of monophage fusion leads to morophological variants of mulltinucleated giant cells. *Am J Pathol* 1995; **147**: 1487–99.

15. Seitzer U, Scheel-Toellner D, Toellner K-M *et al*. Properties of multinucleated giant cells in a new *in vitro* model for human granuloma formation. *J Pathol* 1997; **182**: 99–105.

16. Lay G, Poquet Y, Salek-Peyron P *et al*. Langhans giant cells from *Mycobacterium tuberculosis*-induced human granulomas cannot mediate mycobacterial uptake. *J Pathol* 2007; **211**: 76–85.

17. Basu S, Mohan H, Malhotra H. Pancytopaenia due to hemophagocytic syndrome as the presenting manifestation of tuberculosis. *J Assoc Phys India* 2000; **48**: 845–6.

18. Fisman DN. Hemophagocytic syndromes and infection. *Emerg Infect Dis* 2000; **6**: 601–8.

19. Draper P. The anatomy of mycobacteria. In: Ratledge C, Stanford J (eds). *The biology of the mycobacteria*. London: Academic Press, 1982: 9–52.

20. Richter E, Schlütter C, Duchrow M *et al*. An improved method for the species-specific assessment of mycobacteria in routinely formalin-fixed and paraffin-embedded tissues. *J Pathol* 1995; **175**: 85–92.

21. Li JY, Lo ST, Ng CS. Molecular detection of *Mycobacterium tuberculosis* in tissues showing granulomatous inflammation without demonstrable acid-fast bacilli. *Diag Molec Pathol* 2000; **9**: 67–74.

22. Ruiz-Manzano J, Manterola JM, Gamboa F *et al*. Detection of *Mycobacterium tuberculosis* in paraffin-embedded pleural biopsy specimens by commercial robosomal RNA and DNA amplification kits. *Chest* 2000; **118**: 648–55.

23. Hirunwiwatkul P, Tumwasorn S, Chanttanauwat C, Sirichai U. A comparative study of diagnostic tests for tuberculous lymphadenitis: PCR vs histopathology and clinical diagnosis. *J Med Assoc Thai* 2002; **85**: 320–6.

24. Modlin RL, Hofman FM, Meyer PR *et al*. *In situ* demonstration of T lymphocyte subsets in granulomatous inflammation: leprosy, rhinoscleroma and sarcoidosis. *Clin Exp Immunol* 1983; **51**: 430–8.

25. Modlin RL, Melancon-Kaplan J, Young SMM *et al*. Learning from lesions: patterns of tissue inflammation in leprosy. *Proc Natl Acad Sci U S A* 1988; **85**: 1213–7.

26. van den Oord JJ, De Wolf-Peeters C, Facchetti F, Desmet VJ. Cellular composition of hypersensitivity-type granulomas: immunocytochemical analysis of tuberculous and sarcoidal lymphadenitis. *Hum Pathol* 1984; **15**: 559–65.

27. Shen J-Y, Barnes PF, Rea TH, Meyer PR. Immunohistology of tuberculous adenitis in symptomatic HIV infection. *Clin Exp Immunol* 1988; **72**: 186–9.

28. Muller H, Kruger S. Immunohistochemical analysis of cell composition and *in situ* cytokine expression in HIV- and non-HIV-associated tuberculous lymphadenitis. *Immunobiology* 1994; **191**: 354–68.

29. Sehgal VN, Gupta R, Bose M, Saha K. Immunohistopathological spectrum in cutaneous tuberculosis. *Clin Exp Immunol* 1991; **18**: 309–13.

30. Zhang M, Gong J-H, Iyer DV, Jones BE, Modlin RL, Barnes PF. T-cell cytokine responses in persons with tuberculosis and HIV infection. *J Clin Invest* 1994; **94**: 2435–42.

31. Griffin JP, Orme IM. Evolution of CD4+ T-cell subsets following infection of naive and memory immune mice with Mycobacterium tuberculosis. *Infect Immun* 1994; **62**: 1683–90.

32. Ordway D, Harton M, Henao-Tamayo M, Montoya R, Orme IM, Gonzalez-Juarrero M. Enhanced macrophage activity in granulomatous lesions of immune mice challenged with *Mycobacterium tuberculosis*. *J Immunol* 2006; **176**: 4931–9.

33. Bergeron A, Bonay M, Kambouchner M *et al*. Cytokine patterns in tuberculous and sarcoid granulomas: correlations with histopathologic features of the granulomatous response. *J Immunol* 1997; **159**: 3034–43.

34. Hansch HC, Smith DA, Mielke ME *et al*. Mechanisms of granuloma formation in murine *Mycobacterium avium* infection: the contribution of CD4+ T-cells. *Int Immunol* 1996; **8**: 1299–310.

35. Cooper AM, D'Souza C, Frank AA, Orme IM. The course of *Mycobacterium tuberculosis* infection in the lungs of mice lacking expression of either perforin- or granzyme-mediated cytolytic mechanisms. *Infect Immun* 1997; **65**: 1317–20.

36. Lemaire I, Yang H, Lafont V *et al*. Differential effects of macrophage- and granulocyte–macrophage colony-stimulating factors on cytokine gene expression during rat alveolar macropahge differentiation into multinucleate giant cells (MGC): a role for IL-6 in type 2 MGC formation. *J Immunol* 1996; **157**: 118–25.

37. Fayyazi A, Eichmeyer B, Soruri A *et al*. Apoptosis of macrophages and T-cell in tuberculosis associated caseous necrosis. *J Pathol* 2000; **191**: 417–25.

38. Rondini S, Horsfield C, Mensah-Quainoo E *et al*. Contiguous spread of *Mycobacterium ulcerans* in Buruli ulcer lesions analysed by histopathology and real-time-PCR quantification of mycobacterial DNA. *J Pathol* 2006; **208**: 119–28.

39. Cooper AM, Dalton DK, Stewart TA *et al*. Disseminated tuberculosis in interferon gamma gene-disrupted mice. *J Exp Med* 1993; **178**: 2243–7.

40. Churchyard GJ, Kleinschmidt I, Corbett EL *et al*. Factors associated with an increased case-fatality rate in HIV-infected and non-infected South African gold miners with pulmonary tuberculosis. *Int J Tuberc Lung Dis* 2000; **4**: 705–12.

41. Charalambous S, Churchyard GJ, Murray J *et al*. Persistent radiological changes following miliary tuberculosis in miners exposed to silica dust. *Int J Tuberc Lung Dis* 2001; **5**: 1044–50.

42. Weir WRC, Muraleedharan MV. Tuberculosis arising at the site of physical injury: 8 case histories. *J Infect* 1983; **7**: 63–6.

43. Stead WW, Bates JH. Evidence of a 'silent' bacillaemia in primary tuberculosis. *Ann Intern Med* 1971; **74**: 559–61.

44. Mornex JF, Leroux C, Greenland T, Ecochard D. From granuloma to fibrosis in interstitial lung disease: molecular and cellular interactions. *Eur Resp J* 1994; **7**: 779–85.

45. Lucas SB. Mycobacteria and the tissues of man. In: Ratledge C, Stanford J (eds). *The biology of the mycobacteria*, vol. 3. London: Academic Press, 1988: 107–76.

46. Stead WW. Pathogenesis of a first episode of chronic pulmonary tuberculosis in man: recrudescence of residuals of the primary infection or exogenous reinfection? *Am Rev Respir Dis* 1967; **95**: 729–45.

47. Small PM, Shafer RW, Hopewell PC *et al*. Exogenous reinfection with multidrug-resistant *Mycobacterium tuberculosis* in patients with advanced HIV infection. *N Engl J Med* 1993; **328**: 1137–44.

48. Hawken M, Nunn PP, Gathua SN *et al*. Increased recurrence of tuberculosis in HIV-1-infected patients in Kenya. *Lancet* 1993; **342**: 332–7.

49. Feldman WH, Baggenstoss AH. The occurrence of virulent tubercle bacilli in presumably non-tuberculous lung tissue. *Am J Pathol* 1939; **15**: 501–15.

50. Opie EL, Aaronson JD. Tubercule bacilli in latent tuberculous lesions and in lung tissue withour tuberculous lesions *Arch Pathol* 1996; **4**: 1–21.

51. Ulrichs T, Kosmiadi GA, Trusov V *et al*. Human tuberculous granulomas induce peripheral lymphoid follicle-like structures to orchestrate defence in the lung. *J Pathol* 2004; **204**: 217–28.

52. Rook GAW, Bloom BR. Mechanisms of pathogenesis of tuberculosis. In: Bloom BR, (ed.). *Tuberculosis. Pathogenesis, protection and control*. Washington DC: American Society for Microbiology Press, 1994: 485–501.

53. Ulrichs T, Kosmiadi GA, Jorg S *et al*. Differential organisation of the local immune response in patients with active cavitary tuberculosis or with non-progressive tuberculoma. *J Infect Dis* 2005; **192**: 89–97.

54. Guckian JC, Perry JE. Granulomatous hepatitis. *Ann Intern Med* 1966; **65**: 1081–110.

55. Nakatsuka S, Yao M, Hoshida Y *et al.* Pyothorax-associated lymphoma: a review of 106 cases. *J Clin Oncol* 2002; **20**: 4255–60.

56. Auerbach O. Tuberculous meningitis: correlation of therapeutic results with the pathogenesis and pathologic changes. II Pathologic changes in treated and untreated cases. *Am Rev Tuberc* 1951; **64**: 419–29.

57. Lucas SB, Hounnou A, Peacock CS *et al.* The mortality and pathology of HIV disease in a West African city. *AIDS* 1993; **7**: 1569–79.

58. Smith MB, Boyars MC, Veasey S, Woods GL. Generalised tuberculosis in AIDS. *Arch Pathol Lab Med* 2000; **124**: 1267–74.

59. Laguna F, Adrados M, Ortega A, González-Lahoz JM. Tuberculous meningitis with acellular cerebrospinal fluid in AIDS patients. *AIDS* 1992; **6**: 1165–7.

60. Udani PM, Dastur DK. Tuberculous encephalopathy with and without meningitis. Clinical features and pathologic consdierations. *J Neurol Sci* 1970; **10**: 541–61.

61. Berenguer J, Moreno S, Laguna F *et al.* Tuberculous meningitis in patients infected with the human immunodeficiency virus. *N Engl J Med* 1992; **326**: 668–72.

62. Dastur DK, Manghani DK, Udani PM. Pathology and pathogenetic mechanisms in neurotuberculosis. *Radiol Clin N Am* 1995; **33**: 733–52.

63. Katrak SM, Shembalkar PK, Bijwe SR, Bhandarkar LD. The clinical, radiological and pathological profile of tuberculous meningitis in patient with and without HIV infection. *J Neurol Sci* 2000; **181**: 118–26.

64. Char G, Morgan OS. Tuberculous encephalopathy. A rare complication of pulmonary tuberculosis. *West Indian Med J* 2000; **49**: 70–2.

65. Chetty KG, Kim RC, Mahutte CK. Acute haemorrhagic leukoencephalitis dring treatment for disseminated tuberculosis in a patient with AIDS. *Int J Tuberc Lung Dis* 1997; **1**: 579–81.

66. Santa Cruz DJ, Strayer DS. The histopathologic spectrum of the cutaneous mycobacteriosis. *Hum Pathol* 1982; **13**: 485–95.

67. Saxe N. Mycobacterial skin infections. *J Cutan Pathol* 1985; **12**: 300–12.

68. Beyt BE, Ortbals DW, Santa Cruz DJ *et al.* Cutaneous mycobacteriosis: analysis of 34 cases with a new classification of disease. *Medicine* 1980; **60**: 95–109.

69. Marcoral J, Servitje O, Moreno A *et al.* Lupus vulgaris. Clinical, histologic, and bacteriologic study of 10 cases. *J Am Acad Dermatol* 1992; **26**: 404–7.

70. Serfling U, Penneys NS, Loenardi CL. Identification of *Mycobacterium tuberculosis* DNA in a case of lupus vulgaris. *J Am Acad Dermatol* 1993; **28**: 318–22.

71. Breathnach SM, Black MM. Atypical tuberculide (acne scrofulosorum) secondary to tuberculous lymphadenitis. *Clin Exp Dermatol* 1981; **6**: 339–44.

72. Wilson-Jones E, Winkelmann RK. Papulonecrotic tuberculid: a neglected disease in Western countries. *J Am Acad Dermatol* 1986; **14**: 815–26.

73. Smith NP, Ryan TJ, Sanderson RV *et al.* Lichen scrofulosorum. A report of four cases. *Br J Dermatol* 1976; **94**: 319–25.

74. Schneider JW, Jordaan HF, Geiger DH *et al.* Erythema induratum of Bazin. A clinicopathological study of 20 cases and detection of *M. tuberculosis* DNA in skin lesions by PCR. *Am J Dermatopathol* 1995; **17**: 350–6.

75. Hara K, Tsuzuki T, Takagi N, Shimokata K. Nodular granulomatous phlebitis of the skin: a fourth type of tuberculid. *Histopathology* 1997; **30**: 129–34.

76. Minguez P, Pintor E, Buron R *et al.* Pulmonary tuberculosis presenting with cutaneous leukocytoclastic vasculitis. *Infection* 2000; **28**: 55–7.

77. Barnes PF, Bloch AB, Davidson PT, Snider DE. Tuberculosis in patients with human immunodeficiency virus infection. *N Engl J Med* 1991; **324**: 1644–50.

78. Ackah AN, Coulibaly D, Digbeu H *et al.* Response to treatment, mortality, and CD4 lymphocyte counts in HIV-infected persons with tuberculosis in Abidjan, Côte d'Ivoire. *Lancet* 1995; **345**: 607–10.

79. Diaz-Peromingo JA, Marino-Callejo AI, Gonzalez-Gonzalez C *et al.* Tuberculous myocarditis presenting as a long QT syndrome. *Eur J Intern Med* 2000; **11**: 340–2.

80. Nelson AM, Perriëns JH, Kapita B *et al.* A clinical and pathological comparison of the WHO and CDC case definitions for AIDS in Kinshasa, Zaire: is passive surveillance valid? *AIDS* 1993; **7**: 1241–5.

81. Lanjewar DN, Duggal R. Pulmonary pathology in patients with AIDS: an autopsy study from Mumbai. *HIV Med* 2001; **2**: 266–71.

82. Gutierrez EB, Zanetta DM, Salvida PH, Capelozzi VL. Autopsy-proven determinants of death in HIV-infected patients treated for pulmonary tuberculosis in Sao Paolo, Brazil. *Path Res Pract* 2002; **198**: 339–46.

83. Nambuya A, Sewankambo NK, Mugerwa J *et al.* Tuberculous lymphadenitis associated with human immunodeficiency virus (HIV) in Uganda. *J Clin Pathol* 1988; **41**: 93–6.

84. Heyderman RS, Makunike R, Muza T *et al.* Pleural tuberculosis in Harare, Zimbabwe: the relationship between HIV, CD4 lymphocyte count, granuloma formation and disseminated disease. *Trop Med Int Health* 1998; **3**: 14–20.

85. O'Brien JR. Non-reactive tuberculosis. *J Clin Pathol* 1954; **7**: 216–25.

86. Brmbolic BJ, Boricic I, Salemovic DR *et al.* Focal tuberculosis of the liver with local haemorrhage in a patient with AIDS. *Liver* 1996; **16**: 218–20.

87. Yang GCH, Schinella RA. The histopathology of tuberculosis in the acquired immunodeficiency syndrome: a study of nine cases. In: Rotterdam H, Racz P, Greco MA, Cockerell CJ (eds). *Progress in AIDS pathology*, vol. II. New York: Field & Wood, 1990: 103–10.

88. Ridley DS. Histological classification and the immunological spectrum of leprosy. *Bull WHO* 1974; **51**: 451–65.

89. Emile J-F, Patey N, Altare F *et al.* Correlation of granuloma structure with clinical outcomes defines two types of idiopathic disseminated BCG infections. *J Pathol* 1997; **181**: 25–30.

90. Lenzini L, Rottoli P, Rottoli L. The spectrum of human tuberculosis. *Clin Exp Immunol* 1977; **27**: 230–7.

91. Sekosan M, Cleto M, Sensang C *et al.* Spindle cell pseudotumors in the lungs due to *Mycobacterium tuberculosis* in a transplant patient. *Am J Surg Pathol* 1994; **18**: 1065–8.

92. Wade HW. The histoid variety of lepromatous leprosy. *Int J Lepr* 1963; **31**: 129–42.

93. Govender D, Essa AS. Malakoplakia and tuberculosis. *Pathology* 1999; **31**: 280–3.

94. Pfaltzgraff RE, Ramu G. Clinical leprosy. In: Hastings RC (ed.). *Leprosy*. Edinburgh: Churchill Livingstone, 1994: 237–87.

95. Ridley DS, Radia KB. The histological course of reactions in borderline leprosy and their outcome. *Int J Lepr* 1981; **49**: 383–92.

96. Job CK. Pathology of leprosy. In: Hastings RC (ed.). *Leprosy*. Edinburgh: Churchill Livingstone, 1994: 193–224.

97. Modlin RL, Rea TH. Immunopathology of leprosy. In: Hastings RC (ed). *Leprosy*. Edinburgh: Churchill Livingstone, 1994: 225–34.

98. Stanford JL. Immunotherapy for mycobacterial disease. In: Ratledge C, Stanford J, Grange JM (eds). *Biology of the mycobacteria*, vol 3. London: Academic Press Ltd, 1989: 567–96.

99. Bristowe JS. The Koch method for treatment of tuberculosis. *Br Med J* 1891; **i**: 893–6.

100. Editorial. Immune reactions in tuberculosis. *Lancet* 1984; **ii**: 204.

101. Chambers ST, Hendrickse WA, Record C *et al.* Paradoxical expansion of intracranial tuberculomas during chemotherapy. *Lancet* 1984; **ii**: 181–4.

102. Teoh R, Humphries MJ, O'Mahony G. Symptomatic intracranial tuberculoma developing during treatment of tuberculosis: a report

of 10 patients and review of the literature. *Q J Med* 1987; **241**: 449–60.

103. Lees AJ, MacLeod AF, Marshall J. Cerebral tuberculomas developing during treatment of tuberculous meningitis. *Lancet* 1980; **ii**: 1208–11.

104. Barss P. Unexpected deaths in pulmonary tuberculosis. *Lancet* 1983; **1**: 1437.

105. Ellis ME, Webb AK. Cause of death in patients admitted to hospital for pulmonary tuberculosis. *Lancet* 1983; **1**: 665–7.

106. Onwubalili JK, Scott GM, Smith H. Acute respiratory distress syndrome related to chemotherapy of advanced pulmonary tuberculosis: a study of 2 cases and review of the literature. *Q.J Med* 1986; **230**: 599–610.

107. Dyer RA, Potgieter PD. The adult respiratory distress syndrome and bronchogenic pulmonary tuberculosis. *Thorax* 1984; **39**: 383–7.

108. Huseby JS, Hudson LD. Miliary tuberculosis and respiratory distress syndrome. *Ann Intern Med* 1976; **85**: 609–11.

109. Hsu JT, Padula JP, Ryan SF. Miliary tuberculosis and respiratory distress syndrome. *Ann Intern Med* 1978; **89**: 140–1.

110. Corbett EL, Davidson RN, Lucas SB, Miller RF. Occult miliary tuberculosis in advanced HIV disease. *Genitourin Med* 1996; **72**: 187–93.

111. Wendland T, Furrer T, Vernazza PL *et al.* HAART in HIV-infected patients: restoration of antigen specific CD4 T-cell responses *in vitro* is correlated with CD4 memory T-cell reconstitution, whereas improvement in delayed type hypersensitivity is related to a decrease in viraemia. *AIDS* 1999; **13**: 1857–62.

112. Chien JW, Johnson JL. Paradoxical reactions in HIV and pulmonary tuberculosis. *Chest* 1998; **114**: 933–6.

113. Kunimoto DY, Chui L, Nobert E, Houston S. Immune mediated 'HAART' attack during treatment for tuberculosis. *Int J Tuberc Lung Dis* 1999; **3**: 947.

114. Guex AC, Bucher HC, Demartines N *et al.* Inflammatory bowel perforation during immune reconstitution after one year of antiretroviral and antituberculous therapy in an HIV-1 infected patient: report of a case. *Dis Colon Rectum* 2002; **45**: 977–8.

115. Schluger NW, Perez D, Liu YM. Reconstitution of immune responses to tuberculosis in patients with HIV infection who receive antiretroviral therapy. *Chest* 2002; **122**: 602.

116. Van den Berg R, Vanham G, Raes G *et al. Mycobacterium*-associated immune reconstitution disease: macrophages running wild? *Lancet Infect Dis* 2006; **6**: 2–5.

117. Placido R, Mancino G, Amendola A *et al.* Apoptosis of human macrophages in *Mycobacterium tuberculosis* infection. *J Pathol* 1997; **181**: 31–8.

118. Jagadha V, Andavolu RH, Huang CT. Granulomatous infection in the acquired immune deficiency syndrome. *Am J Clin Pathol* 1985; **84**: 598–602.

8

Human immune response to *M. tuberculosis*

STEPHAN K SCHWANDER AND JERROLD J ELLNER

INTRODUCTION

Over 70 per cent of tuberculosis (TB) cases worldwide are pulmonary TB cases, which constitute a tremendous public health problem. *Mycobacterium bovis* bacille Calmette–Guérin (BCG) vaccination provides variable protection against pulmonary TB, and widespread use of this vaccine has not markedly reduced the public health problem posed by TB.

Infection with *Mycobacterium tuberculosis* (MTB) results in a dynamic interaction of host, environmental and bacterial factors that lead to heterogeneous clinical manifestations and several distinct stages of infection and disease. Elucidating the pathogenesis of an evolving, stage-dependent process that often produces equilibrium between host and pathogen requires measuring a variety of bacteriologic and host immunologic variables over time from carefully defined populations. Substantial progress in understanding innate and adaptive immunity to MTB has been made in murine models;[1] however, much less is known about human responses. Deciphering the protective immune response has taken on additional importance in an era in which new antituberculous vaccines are undergoing early trials in humans. Characterization of correlates of protective immunity in humans would provide a rational basis for vaccine development and testing.

Epidemiological evidence suggests that protective immunity against MTB infection and against progression from infection to disease exists in most exposed humans. The proportion of non-immunocompromised individuals that undergo primary infection or if infected develop reactivation disease is low. For example, only 5–10 per cent of MTB-infected individuals develop TB disease during their life time.[2] It is likely that innate immunity protects some heavily exposed contacts of infectious TB patients from developing MTB infection, but the mechanisms of this protection are unknown. It also is likely that

innate/adaptive immunity maintains latent foci of MTB infection clinically silent and prevents progression to disease by unknown mechanisms. Immunosuppressive comorbidities, such as HIV-1 infection, upset the balance between host protective immunity and bacterial replication, leading to reactivation of TB. This implies that active immunologic surveillance in health is compromised in HIV-1 infection, but here too, the protective mechanisms are undefined.

The study of human immunity to MTB infection is critical to understanding the mechanisms that contain the initial tuberculous focus and maintain clinical latency. It further potentially validates certain basic concepts established in animal models, as differences are apparent between experimental models in cell function, effector molecules and disease expression. Further and perhaps most importantly, immunological markers of protection in humans provide target end points and read-outs for the evaluation of new antituberculous vaccines, vaccine delivery strategies and adjuvant immunotherapeutic interventions. Progress in understanding the components of protective immunity has been slow, as protection is complex and may involve multiple cell types, receptors, cytokines and chemokines, including those not yet characterized, as well as antibody, complement, inflammatory factors and other host proteins not traditionally studied. A critical limitation of clinical study designs used to investigate protective immunity is lack of access to specimens before the occurrence of MTB exposure, infection and disease, as disease, infection and even exposure, may confound efforts to define the pre-existing immune status. Further, studies in the past two decades have provided evidence that local and systemic immune responses vary considerably.

It is possible that broad rather than targeted studies, employing modern screening approaches such as DNA micro-array and proteomic analysis will provide insights into the complex host–pathogen interactions and permit identification of protective profiles rather than individual protective biomarkers. Several broad screening studies in limited numbers of subjects have been performed to identify biomarkers associated with TB disease, and MTB infection.[3–5] Gene expression profiles were studied using DNA microarray technology to identify recurrent TB,[3] and to distinguish active TB from MTB infection.[5] Similarly, using proteomic fingerprinting and pattern recognition, potential biomarkers were identified in TB patient sera that may contribute to the development of new TB diagnostic tests.[4] Careful selection of subject populations and experimental conditions will be crucial to identify new diagnostic, vaccine or therapeutic targets from reliable, and generalizable gene and/or protein expression profiles.

NATURAL HISTORY OF MTB INFECTION IN HUMANS

Primary infection

Initial infection with MTB usually occurs by inhalation of droplet nuclei (1–5 μm) that contain MTB and are aerosolized from the lung of TB patients.[6,7] Infectious droplet nuclei are then deposited in the terminal airspaces of the exposed patient contacts. The frequency with which aerogenic exposure induces latent MTB infection or results in clearance of the infection is unknown. Typically, 30–50 per cent of exposed household contacts of patients with infectious sputum smear-positive pulmonary TB acquire MTB infection as evidenced by a positive tuberculin skin test (TST) to purified protein derivative (PPD), or MTB antigen-specific lymphocyte proliferation or interferon gamma (IFN-γ) release *in vitro*. The latter is the basis for modern immunodiagnostic approaches to detect MTB infection with IFN-γ release assays. The risk of developing active TB is greatest in the first 2 years following initial infection and decreases thereafter; the initial risk is higher following contact with sputum smear-positive TB cases[8] and with more intense exposure to MTB.[8,9] Particularly intense exposure, as in submarines or sharing a bed in households, is associated with greater risk of early development of TB.[10] Among untreated TST-positive household contacts of patients with TB, active pulmonary TB occurs at a rate of 0.74 per cent per year in the first 2 years after new MTB infection, 0.31 per cent per year in the next 3 years and 0.16 per cent per year in years 6 and 7 post exposure.[9] People who become infected in infancy, adolescence or old age are more likely to progress to active TB. Overall, 5–10 per cent of immunocompetent infected people develop active TB during their life time.

In a recent study of household contacts of infectious TB cases in Uganda, MTB culture filtrate-specific IFN-γ levels produced by whole blood *in vitro* at baseline were greater among individuals who converted their TST than among those who did not convert. Interestingly, in contacts with BCG vaccination, when baseline IFN-γ concentrations increased 10-fold, the risk of TST conversion increased four-fold.[11]

Primary tuberculosis

Most immunocompetent people develop an effective immune response that contains the primary MTB infection and results in a small fibrotic parenchymal scar (Ghon complex). Following primary infection, immunocompetent people develop adaptive immunity, which prevents reinfection with MTB. This immunity is long-lasting, maintained by memory T cells and possibly restimulated by low-level endogenous bacterial replication or exogenous exposure. For example, the majority of individuals studied 19 years after they were documented to be TST-positive maintained skin test reactivity and strong *in vitro* responses to PPD despite a lack of ongoing exogenous exposure to MTB.[12] In high-prevalence areas, repeated exogenous exposure to MTB may maintain and boost adaptive protective immunity.

Progressive primary tuberculosis

People who fail to develop specific adaptive immune responses following primary MTB infection may develop progressive primary TB. This form of disease is most common in young children, immunocompromised individuals and the elderly. Miliary or meningeal disease may result after widespread haematogenous dissemination of MTB. In young adults, progressive primary disease is manifest by typical symptoms of TB and upper lobe cavitary lesions. This can be reliably distinguished from reactivation TB only when recent TST conversion has been documented.[13]

Reactivation tuberculosis

The lungs are the most common sites of reactivation TB. In areas of high TB prevalence, exogenous reinfection may occur and progress to active disease. The risk of developing post-primary or reactivation TB following infection with MTB is increased in immunocompromised people. The risk varies with the underlying disease and the degree with which it impairs host defences.

Exogenous reinfection

Recent molecular epidemiologic studies confirm earlier suggestions that exogenous reinfection with MTB is important in the pathogenesis of TB in high-prevalence areas.[14] This finding raises the issue as to whether natural infection with MTB is immunizing – a relevant question for development of new vaccines. Following treatment of pulmonary TB, individuals show heightened susceptibility to reinfection disease,[14] indicating that an important component of host susceptibility may be genetic or acquired. The finding of TB disease caused by more than one strain[14] raises the possibility that apparent reinfection following treatment may represent eradication of one but not all MTB strains.

HUMAN IMMUNITY TO MTB

The classical belief that progression of MTB infection to primary or reactivation TB is solely a function of the extent and efficiency of protective human immunity is no longer tenable. There is increasing appreciation for a complex interplay between the host and pathogen and for a major role that differences in MTB isolates play in triggering different host responses (Figure 8.1).

Most of the current concepts of human immunity to MTB are based on studies of blood cells in patients with pulmonary TB, as blood cells are most accessible. Blood cells are recruited to and compartmentalized at the inflammatory focus and form the building blocks of the granulomatous tissue reaction. Protective immunity appears to be operative in household contacts who remain disease free or even show no sign of MTB infection (TST conversion) despite exposure to TB patients. Pulmonary TB in the adult, on the other hand, represents a good model to delineate pathogenesis, immunopathology and concomitants of reactivation disease and to test concepts concerning immunotherapy that may be particularly relevant in the setting of extreme drug resistance.

In exposed household contacts and individuals with latent MTB infection, both innate and adaptive immune mechanisms prevent the establishment, respectively, of infection and progression to disease. Stimulation of Toll-

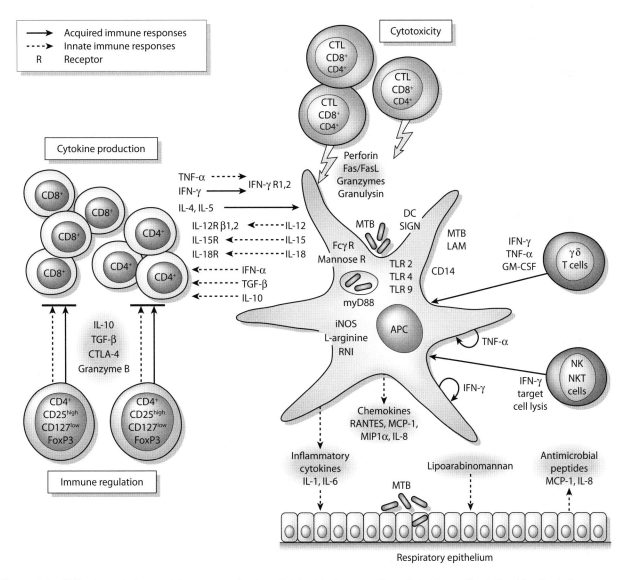

Figure 8.1 Cell subpopulations and immune mechanisms involved in human cell-mediated immunity during *Mycobacterium tubrculosis* infection.

like receptors (TLRs) on monocytes, alveolar macrophages and dendritic cells by MTB and its constituents is a key component of innate immunity. Subsequent specific adaptive immunity is characterized by a predominant T helper (T_H)1 response (interleukin (IL)-2, IFN-γ, tumour necrosis factor (TNF)-α) and suppression of T_H2 responses (IL-4, IL-5, IL-13). The initial interaction of MTB with antigen-presenting cells (APCs) determines the balance between T_H1 and T_H2 immunity, which may be modified by genetic and acquired factors. Clinically latent foci of MTB infection may break down and result in reactivation disease due to immunosuppression, ageing, comorbidities (such as diabetes mellitus) or unknown factors.

The systemic immune response during TB is dominated by immunosuppression that may avert deleterious effects of systemic immune activation, such as septic shock. However, immunosuppression may also increase susceptibility to progression of exogenous reinfection to active disease, as in TB patients from high-prevalence areas who show inordinately increased risk of exogenous reinfection.

The local immune response in active TB shows enhanced immune activation with inflammatory mediators that are present in the blood, bronchoalveolar lavage fluid, pleural fluid and sputum. Some of these mediators are immunosuppressive or pro-apoptotic. They disappear early during TB chemotherapy. Immune activation is a dominant finding in studies of bronchoalveolar lavage cells from radiographically involved lungs of TB patients. The occurrence of high local levels of potentially protective cytokines such as IFN-γ during active disease suggests that the response to these cytokines may be blocked.

Innate immunity

MTB infection usually begins with inhalation of MTB-containing aerosol droplets into the alveoli. Here, MTB enters resident alveolar macrophages, dendritic cells, recently recruited monocytes and respiratory epithelial cells. Multiple receptors, such as complement receptors, the mannose receptor, CD14, surfactant protein A receptors and scavenger receptors, all have the potential to recognize and bind MTB *in vitro*.[15] MTB can also activate the alternative pathway of complement and become opsonized by complement products that facilitate uptake by complement receptors 1, 3 and 4;[16–18] MTB also expresses surface polysaccharides that can directly interact with complement receptors.[18] Complement and/or mannose receptors on macrophages[19,20] and a C-type lectin dendritic cell-specific intercellular adhesion molecule-3 grabbing nonintegrin (DC-SIGN)[21,22] on dendritic cells are the primary receptors for MTB uptake. The role of antibody-mediated uptake of MTB has not been studied sufficiently. Following uptake of MTB into macrophages and dendritic cells, mycobacterial antigens are processed and presented in the context of major histocompatibility complex (MHC) class I or II molecules to CD8$^+$ T cells and

CD4$^+$T cells, respectively. Presentation of mycobacterial antigens occurs also through the unconventional CD1 molecule[23,24] or through undefined receptors to double negative (Vα24CD4$^-$CD8$^-$) T cells, natural killer T cells (NKTs) or γδ T cells. Macrophages and dendritic cells also express TLRs that recognize conserved antigenic patterns expressed on pathogens,[25] triggering the first line of defence against infection[25] and initiating a signal transduction pathway in the host cell that culminates in NFκb activation and induction of cytokines and chemokines.[26] These cytokines and chemokines are crucial to eliciting the adaptive immune response against MTB. Activation of TLRs and TLR signalling initiates inflammatory responses that recruit other innate cells to sites of infection and therefore represent an important link between innate cellular responses and subsequent adaptive immune defences against MTB. Besides these indirect TLR-mediated mechanisms, activation of TLRs with synthetic agonists directly enhances host resistance against intracellular infections in murine models.[27,28] Recently, TLR-2/1 activation of primary human macrophages has been found to trigger antibacterial activity by upregulating expression of the vitamin D receptor and the vitamin D-1-hydroxylase genes. Addition of 1,25(OH)$_2$D$_3$ to MTB-infected macrophages leads to induction of the antimicrobial peptide cathelicidin, and cathelicidin-induced killing of intracellular MTB.[29] Increasing appreciation of the importance of innate immunity suggests that the ability of certain individuals to resist MTB infection following exposure may be due to differences in TLR signalling.

MONOCYTES AND MACROPHAGES

The macrophage functions as a critical effector cell. Monocytes and macrophages express inducible nitric oxide synthase, which produces nitric oxide, low concentrations of which can kill MTB. Nitric oxide is released from MTB-infected blood monocytes,[30] alveolar macrophages,[31–33] and respiratory epithelial cells,[34] and is increased in exhaled air of TB patients.[35] Inducible nitric oxide synthase is present at high levels in lung granulomas from TB patients and is expressed in macrophages and multi-nucleated cells.[36] Nitric oxide production, as measured by expression of mRNA for inducible nitric oxide synthase, can be triggered in human alveolar macrophages by BCG[37] and confers antimycobacterial activity against MTB[33] and BCG.[37] Levels of nitric oxide production from alveolar macrophages vary greatly between individuals and correlate with the degree of growth inhibition of MTB within the alveolar macrophages.[33] Increased generation of nitric oxide by alveolar macrophages[31,32] or monocytes[30] from TB patients amplifies the synthesis of pro-inflammatory cytokines, such as TNF-α[30,31] and IL-1[31] in an autoregulatory manner. Conversely, the release of reactive nitrogen intermediates in human cells is triggered by IFN-γ, TNF-α and IL-1 receptor[38] and mycobacterial components, such as lipoarabinomannan and the 19 kDa lipoprotein.[39] Studies in mice also suggest that production of reactive nitrogen intermediates may be mediated by the interaction of pathogens with TLRs.[40]

Following intracellular infection with MTB[41,42] or exposure to mycobacterial products such as the secreted protein ESAT-6,[43] monocytes and alveolar macrophages undergo apoptosis,[42] a programmed cell death. Apoptosis likely represents a protective immune response to decrease viability and the spread of mycobacteria by sequestering the pathogens within apoptotic bodies.[44] This notion is supported by the fact that virulent strains of MTB suppress macrophage apoptosis *in vitro*.

High-density DNA micro-arrays allow the simultaneous assessment of the expression patterns of thousands of mRNAs (the transcriptome). The macrophage transcriptome reacts to MTB infection with non-specific and pathogen-specific expression signatures, some of which depend on TLR-induced signalling pathways.[45] Initial studies of the monocyte transcriptome during *in vitro* MTB infection indicate that MTB interferes with the human macrophage activation programme.[45–48] For example, MTB upregulates interleukins and receptors for chemokines and downregulates molecules that are necessary to respond to IL-12 and the immunosuppressive cytokine transforming growth factor (TGF)-β.[47] These responses may enhance the survival of MTB.

DENDRITIC CELLS

The differentiation of naive T cells to effector T_H1 and T_H2 subtypes is greatly influenced by dendritic cells, which phagocytose MTB and are the most potent APCs for activation of $CD4^+$ T cells and $CD8^+$ T cells in both primary and recall immune responses.[49] Dendritic cell maturation is induced by microbial lipopeptides that engage TLR-2.[50] Dendritic cells are present in the respiratory tract,[51] constitute 1 per cent of airway epithelial cells, and are found peripherally in the human lung as far distally as the alveolar septa.[52] *In vitro* infection of human monocyte-derived dendritic cells with live MTB induces co-stimulatory signals (CD54, CD40 and B7.1), MHC class I surface molecule expression[53] and secretion of TNF-α, IL-1, IL-12,[53] IL-6 and IL-10.[54] The capacity of dendritic cells to control growth of MTB appears, however, to be inferior to that of macrophages.[55]

UNCONVENTIONAL CELLS

Unconventional cells are of increasing interest in human MTB immunity because of their roles in local innate immunity and in inducing adaptive immune responses. Besides macrophages and dendritic cells, natural killer (NK) cells and CD1d-restricted NKT cells also function as effector cells in the early innate immune response to pathogens. Injection of the CD1d ligand α-galactosylceramide into mice enhances their resistance against MTB infection.[56] Upon stimulation, the $CD4^+$NKT subset produces a mixture of T_H1 and T_H2 cytokines, whereas $CD4^-CD8^-$NKT cells predominantly produce T_H1

cytokines.[57] Human NKT cells are non-MHC-restricted and recognize the non-classical APC molecule CD1d that is expressed on human monocyte-derived cells.[58] NKT cells secrete IFN-γ and IL-13 and have bactericidal effects that appear to be mediated by granulysin.[24,58]

NK cells co-regulate human $CD8^+$ T cell effector function (lysis) against MTB-infected target cells that depend on the release of IFN-γ by NK cells and of IL-15 and IL-18 from monocytes.[59] NK cells express TLRs and respond to a large number of TLR ligands.[60] Direct NK-mediated killing of MTB *in vitro* occurs within 24 hours and requires direct cell-to-cell contact.[61] NK cells can be activated *in vitro* by monocyte-derived immature dendritic cells in the presence of MTB or IFN-α and reciprocally enhance dendritic cell maturation and IL-12 production.[62] The NK cell-activating receptors, NKp46 and NKG2D, and their ligands on monocytes are involved in the lysis of mononuclear phagocytes infected with MTB.[63,64]

Human T cells with a γδ rather than the usual αβ T-cell receptor account for <10 per cent of T cells in blood and in the lungs and respond to stimulation with unusual, non-peptide phosphoantigens from MTB.[65,66] γδ T cells proliferate in response to whole MTB, are unrestricted by MHC class I or II molecules,[67] are competent cytotoxic effector cells, and recognize antigen that is presented by both alveolar macrophages[68] and monocyte-derived macrophages.[65] γδ T cells contribute to immunity by producing IFN-γ, GM-CSF, IL-3 and TNF-α, which activate macrophages to eliminate MTB.[66,69] A subgroup of human γδ T cells that recognize mycobacterial non-peptide phosphoantigens express Vγ9Vδ2 T-cell receptors on their surface.[65,66] In blood and lung cells from TB patients, these Vγ9Vδ2+ cells are decreased in numbers,[70] perhaps because of MTB-triggered apoptosis.[71] BCG vaccination, on the other hand, expands and activates this cell population to provide helper functions for MTB-specific $CD4^+$ T cells and $CD8^+$ T cells.[72] These findings suggest a potential role for γδ T cells in the protective immune response to MTB infection that may be particularly expressed in the respiratory epithelium.

Differentiation of T cells to T_H1 or T_H2 cells is controlled by the balance of expression of costimulatory receptors, receptor signalling and cytokine production by macrophages and dendritic cells, and perhaps by MTB strain differences. The resulting predominance of T_H1 or T_H2 cytokine profiles impacts on the efficiency of control of MTB infection.

Adaptive immunity

T cells play a central role in adaptive antimycobacterial host defence and mucosal immunity in adults[73] and children.[74] MHC class II-restricted $CD4^+$ T cells are the predominant source of IFN-γ and IL-2 and are critical for the induction of delayed-type hypersensitivity responses during MTB infection and the development and maintenance of $CD8^+$ cytotoxic T-lymphocyte (CTL) responses.[75]

CD4[+] T cells are directly involved in inhibiting MTB growth in human monocytes.[76] The dominant importance of CD4[+] T cells in MTB immunity is apparent during HIV-1 infection as reduced CD4[+] T-cell number and function confers the greatest known risk for reactivation of latent and progression of primary MTB infection to active TB disease. Activated CD4[+] T cells can differentiate into T_H1 or T_H2 cells. T_H1 cells secrete specific subsets of cytokines (IFN-γ, IL-2, TNF-α). The T_H1 cell product of greatest relevance to MTB immunity is IFN-γ, the predominant activator of macrophages and monocytes.[77] T_H2 cells principally produce IL-4, IL-5 and IL-13.

CD8[+] T cells have important roles in human MTB immunity[78–84] both by producing IFN-γ and acting as CTLs. We have recently shown that CD8[+] T cells from contacts of patients with TB contribute to the control of MTB growth in autologous alveolar macrophages.[84] CD8[+] T cells recognize several MTB antigens, including ESAT-6, antigens 85A and 85B, the 38 kDa protein and 19 kDa lipoprotein.[85–88] Human peripheral blood CD8[+] effector T cells also contribute to production of IFN-γ and TNF-α upon stimulation with MTB.[84]

CTLs, most of which are CD8[+], are essential for lysis of MTB-infected cells,[78] via a Fas-independent granule exocytosis pathway[80,89,90] and a Fas–FasL interaction[91] that results in apoptotic death of MTB-infected cells. Cytotoxic effector molecules, such as granulysin, perforin and granzyme, are released by CD8[+] and CD4[+] CTLs upon interaction with infected cells.[24,80] CD4[+] T cells and CD8[+] T cells from bronchoalveolar lavage[92] lyse MTB-infected macrophages from healthy individuals,[79] suggesting that either or both of these cell types in the alveoli can act as CTLs in the lung during active TB. The overlap in function of T-cell populations suggests that events which affect their localization and differentiation at sites of bacterial replication may determine their specific roles in acquired resistance.

Following MTB infection, effector T cells such as CTLs are stimulated and mediate effector mechanisms in peripheral organs such as the lungs. Subsequently, MTB antigen-specific memory T cells are generated, which can be separated into effector memory and central memory T cells. Effector memory T cells are predominantly present in peripheral tissue and at sites of inflammation, where they exhibit rapid effector function. Central memory T cells reside primarily in lymphoid organs and cannot be immediately activated. Upon re-exposure to MTB, reinfection or vaccination, central memory T cells are thought to rapidly expand and differentiate to resupply the effector T cell pool at peripheral sites.

Regulatory mechanisms and concomitants of disease

In the vast majority of individuals, the interaction of MTB with TLRs and other receptors activates a protective T_H1 dominant immune response, characterized by production of IFN-γ. Several lines of evidence support an essential role for IFN-γ in control of MTB infection. IFN-γ knockout mice fail to produce reactive nitrogen intermediates and succumb rapidly after experimental MTB infection.[93] Children with hereditary IFN-γR deficiencies are predisposed to dissemination of mostly avirulent,[94,95] but also virulent mycobacteria.[96,97] IFN-γ induces macrophages to kill intracellular pathogens[77] by regulating host genes that are involved in antimycobacterial effector mechanisms (antigen processing and presentation, generation of reactive nitrogen intermediates). Multiple factors, however, appear to interfere with the protective T_H1 response. Although T_H1 responses can contain initial MTB infections, they do not achieve sterilizing immunity and leave the host vulnerable to disease reactivation. Our work[92,98] and that of others has provided clear evidence that T_H1 immunity with antigen-specific IFN-γ and IL-12 production is enhanced in the lungs of TB patients despite unabated lung pathology and MTB growth. IFN-γ thus is not sufficient to protect from disease and T_H1 immunity invokes immunopathology, such as lung cavitation, which in turn increases infectivity and transmission of MTB to new hosts. T_H1 immunity also does not prevent individuals in high MTB transmission areas from becoming reinfected with MTB. These observations raise important questions as to what interferes with protective T_H1 immunity.

T_H2 CYTOKINES

Interference with T_H1 immunity and alteration of the extent of TB disease can result from a dominant T_H2 cytokine immune profile, or from chronic infection and immune stimulation.[99,100] Long-term control of MTB infection is associated with elevated T_H1 responses, but also with inhibition of T_H2 responses.[101,102] In a recent study of MTB-exposed health-care workers, increased median percentages of IL-4-producing CD8[+] and γδ T cells were associated with progression to active TB, whereas individuals who remained healthy had more IFN-γ-producing and fewer IL-4-producing T cells.[102] As IL-4 also modulates expression of TLRs,[103] TLR-dependent immune mechanisms may be affected.

Chronic infections with parasites, such as helminths, cause widespread immune activation and dysregulation, and a dominant T_H2 cytokine immune profile. Immunologic alterations associated with helminth co-infection appear to be responsible for increased susceptibility to MTB infection, development of TB disease and reduced BCG vaccine efficacy.[104] This is of great relevance in tropical countries, which often are endemic for TB. Antihelminthic treatment increases *in vitro* PPD-specific cell proliferation and IFN-γ production, TST reactivity and post-BCG vaccination PPD-specific immune responses.[105] Intestinal helminth infection affects anti-MTB immunity by decreasing absolute numbers of CD3[+], CD4[+], CD8[+], NKT and CD4[+]CD25[high] T cell subsets, compared to either TB patients without helminth co-infection or healthy controls. In addition, TB patients with helminth co-infection have lower IFN-γ and elevated and sustained interleukin IL-10 levels in whole blood cultures, compared with those from TB patients.[106] The immune response of co-infected patients is skewed toward a T_H2 profile, with increased IL-4 production, which favours persistent MTB infection and may explain the more severe radiologic manifestations of disease in co-infected patients.[106]

REGULATORY T CELLS

Regulatory T cells (Tregs) represent an important component of regulatory mechanisms that prevent and minimize tissue damage from autoreactive and over-exuberant immune responses to pathogens.[107,108] Tregs are a distinct T-cell subset that suppress T-cell proliferation, and T_H1 and T_H2 responses. Tregs express specific molecular and functional markers, such as high membrane expression of CD25 (IL-2Rα chain) and cytoplasmic expression of the DNA binding fork-head family transcription factor (FoxP3) protein, and some secrete IL-10 and TGF-β. Two major Treg subpopulations are naturally occurring CD4$^+$ Tregs and peripheral inducible (adaptive) antigen-specific CD4$^+$ Tregs. Additional T cells with regulatory function are the IL-10-producing Tr1, and the TGF-β1-producing T_H3 cells, as well as TGF-β1- and T_H2 cytokine-producing CD8$^+$ Tregs. It remains unclear whether naturally occurring and inducible CD4$^+$ Treg cells represent distinct lineages or phenotypic variants induced at different anatomical sites.

Naturally occurring CD4$^+$ Tregs express high levels of CD25 (CD4$^+$CD25^{high}).[109,110] The mechanisms of suppression of T-effector cells by Tregs are not fully understood, but are typically correlated in *in vitro* studies with reduced proliferation or antigen-specific IFN-γ responses. The suppressive function of CD4$^+$CD25^{high} Tregs depends critically on proximity and cell–cell interaction,[111] and can involve the action of IL-10, TGF-β1 and the costimulatory molecule, cytotoxic T lymphocyte-associated protein 4.[107,108,112] Because some Tregs express FoxP3 and are CD25^{low}, IL-7Rα chain (CD127) surface expression has recently been suggested as a marker of human Tregs.[113] FoxP3 directly downregulates CD127 expression,[113,114] so that the majority of FoxP3-positive cells are CD127$^{low/negative}$ and CD4$^+$CD25$^{intermediate/high}$.

The role for Tregs in controlling immune responses during infectious diseases[115] and particularly during human antimycobacterial immunity is not clearly defined.[116–119] Patients with advanced TB disease who lack TST reactivity have increased numbers of IL-10-secreting CD8$^+$ Tr1 cells[117,120] that inhibit MTB antigen-specific T cell responses.[117,118] Neutralizing antibodies to IL-10 increase IFN-γ production in these conditions by enhancing IL-12 production from monocytes of TB patients.[121]

An underexplored research area is how, during MTB infection, Tregs arrive and mediate suppression at sites of disease such as the lungs, where inflammation is most prominent. Evidence is accumulating that Tregs play a key role in regulating inflammation in several respiratory diseases. Both natural and inducible Tregs effectively limit the immune response in the airway mucosa during asthma.[122,123] Site-specific accumulation of FoxP3-expressing Treg cells has recently been described in a murine model of chronic *Leishmania* infection,[124] in which the chemokine CCR5 contributed to homing of CD4$^+$CD25$^+$ Tregs to the dermal sites of infection.[125] In TB patients, FoxP3-expressing CD4$^+$CD25^{high} cells may be increased and play a role in local immunity at sites of MTB-induced inflammation (pleural, pericardial effusions).[119] Interestingly, depletion of Tregs from peripheral blood mononuclear cells (PBMCs) of TB patients increased numbers of MTB antigen-induced IFN-γ-producing cells.[119] Similarly increased levels of CD4$^+$CD25^{hi} Tregs have been reported in bronchoalveolar lavage cells of untreated TB patients.[116] It is not yet known if the activity of Tregs during human TB may contribute to persistence and proliferation of MTB and if their accumulation at sites of inflammation may interfere with local protective immunity. Recent evidence from a murine model indicates that adoptive cell transfer of Tregs prevents eradication of MTB by suppressing an otherwise efficient CD4$^+$ T-cell response.[126]

Humoral immunity

Humoral immunity has been broadly considered to have little or no impact on the course of MTB infection and development of disease. However, there is recent evidence in the murine model that arabinomannan-specific antibodies alter the course of MTB infection and increase survival.[127] Antibodies to MTB lipoarabinomannan are also associated with resistance to dissemination of disease in children.[128] Antibodies may play a pathogenic role during adult TB by enhancing pro-inflammatory and by blocking downregulatory cytokines. PPD-specific IgG1 antibodies augmented secretion of TNF-α,[129] IL-6 and IL-10[129] by PPD-stimulated monocytes from patients with TB. Absorption of IgG1 removes the augmenting activity for TNF-α and IL-6, but paradoxically increases IL-10 secretion. The role of antibodies during the initial encounter between MTB and host cells in the alveolar spaces, as well as induction of anti-MTB antibodies following vaccination are important areas of active research.[130]

Antibody responses may vary during the course of MTB infection and disease. Titres of specific antibodies become detectable at stages of infection associated with increased antigen burden. Recent infection (TST conversion) appears to be associated with a measurable antibody response.[131] In contrast, latent MTB infection is usually seronegative,[132,133] presumably due to insufficient antigenic stimulus. Antibodies to MTB antigens become detectable as latent infection progresses to active TB, well before bacteriological and clinical signs of disease are seen.[134] A second aspect of the antibody response is that antibody profiles presumably vary with the stage of MTB infection. For example, the antibody response to the secreted 38-kDa antigen of MTB correlates with advanced pulmonary TB,[132] and antibodies reactive with the 16 kDa α-crystallin antigen are present in asymptomatic contacts of active TB cases.[135] Thus, specific antibody markers may be predictive of incipient disease.

Systemic immunity

Studies of blood cells from patients with smear-positive pulmonary TB provide information concerning systemic concomitants of active pulmonary TB. Blood monocytes of TB patients are increased in number and activated to selectively depress PPD-stimulated lymphocyte transformation[136,137] and production of the $T_H 1$ cytokines IL-2 and IFN-γ.[138,139] Monocytes from patients with active TB are activated, releasing cytokines[137] and expressing markers of activation such as Fcγ receptor type I and III and HLA-DR on their cell surface.[140] Constitutive expression of functional IL-2 receptors in monocytes from TB patients may be a factor in their immunoregulatory function.[141] MTB cell wall lipoglycans and culture filtrate proteins directly stimulate monocytes to produce cytokines including TNF-α[142] and TGF-β.[143] This, in part, accounts for the decreased responsiveness of blood T cells during TB and for the antigen specificity of this suppression.[144] TGF-β and IL-10 are important monocyte- and macrophage-, as well as T cell-derived mediators of cytokine-mediated suppression.[139,145] *In vitro* depletion of adherent cells[146] and neutralization of TGF-β[139] normalize lymphocyte proliferation in response to PPD, and significantly increase PPD-stimulated production of IFN-γ in TB patients. IL-10 inhibition has a similar effect on IFN-γ production. Kinetic studies performed during treatment of patients showed that overproduction of TGF-β and IL-10 was a transient phenomenon, most active during the first 3 months of treatment.[145] However, it was superimposed on a more protracted primary T-cell defect in MTB-stimulated production of IFN-γ which was still seen in some patients 18 months after the diagnosis of TB, and could contribute to the previously noted susceptibility of TB patients to reinfection disease.[145] This primary T-cell defect could be due to increased apoptosis of T cells in TB patients. The predisposition of CD4+ T cells to apoptosis may involve both low expression of the anti-apoptotic protein, Bcl-2, and excessive expression of TGF-β, TNF-α and FasL.[147] The uncontrolled immune activation during active TB is associated with high levels of cytokines in plasma, sputum, bronchoalveolar lavage fluid and pleural fluid. These inflammatory markers disappear rapidly during treatment,[148] but may contribute to programmed cell death and the protracted primary defect in T-cell function in pulmonary TB.

Early studies indicated that two populations of T cells suppressed antigen specific T-cell responses in TB patients.

T cells with surface expression of the Fcγ fragment of IgG were increased in number and functioned as suppressor cells.[149] Their activity paralleled that of suppression by monocytes. In patients with low responses, one-third demonstrated suppression by monocytes and the remainder suppression by Fcγ receptor+ T cells. In contrast, a population of CD16+ cells, which are large granular lymphocytes with NK cell activity, are increased in number in pulmonary TB and function in monocyte suppressive pathways.[150] There is now renewed focus on Tregs, as described above. A recent study of whole blood of patients with TB suggests that immunosuppression after BCG stimulation *in vitro* is associated with increased expression of TGF-β, IL-4 and FoxP3 RNA.[151] Other studies showed that the percentages of CD4+CD25+ T cells are increased in TB patients.[116,119]

Local immunity

TUBERCULOUS PLEURITIS

Tuberculous pleuritis is most common in primary TB and usually resolves spontaneously.[152] Immune responses occurring here thus likely represent protective immunity that controls multiplication of MTB. Compartmentalization of PPD-specific immune cells in TB was first described with pleural effusion cells on the basis of increased antigen-specific DNA synthesis,[146,153,154] compared to that by autologous blood cells. $T_H 1$ cytokine responses are increased and CD4+ T cells with a CD45RO memory phenotype accumulate locally,[147,155,156] and contain increased numbers of cells responding to PPD.[146,154] These cells express multiple homing receptors, such as CD11a, CCR5 and CXCR3.[156] IFN-γ[41,157,158] and TNF-α production by pleural fluid cells is increased constitutively,[147,157,158] and in response to lipoarabinomannan[155] and MTB.[157] The increases in IFN-γ production are paralleled by increases in IL-6,[159] free IL-12p40 and heterodimeric IL-12 by pleural fluid cells both constitutively and when stimulated with heat-killed MTB.[160] Pleural effusion cells from TB patients also show increased production of IL-10[157] and TGF-β.[161] IL-10 and TGF-β might limit the inflammation in this compartment. As levels of IFN-γ and of the pro-apoptotic molecules TNF-α, FasL and Fas are increased in pleural fluid, relative to plasma, spontaneous apoptosis of CD4+ T cells and non-CD4+ T cells is augmented in pleural fluid from TB patients. This suggests that immune activation and loss of antigen-responsive T cells may occur concomitantly, favouring persistence of MTB infection.[147] It is not clear how these mechanisms evolve over time, and if initially elevated pleural antigen-specific immune reactivity may be decreased by suppressive local cytokine release or apoptosis of antigen-reactive cells. These factors in combination may lead to the transient 'self-cure' of this type of pleuritis that is known to occur. In HIV-1 seronegative patients with pleural TB, vigorous immune responses usually are associated with negative MTB cultures. In HIV-1 seropositive patients with pleural TB, MTB cultures are usually positive. Therefore, the finding that levels of IFN-γ pro-apoptotic molecules and apoptosis are increased further in HIV-1 seropositive patients with pleural TB suggests a block in the protective response to IFN-γ.[162]

BRONCHOALVEOLAR SPACES

Studies of local lung immunity at the entry site of aerosolized MTB provide a window into the fundamental biologic interactions of MTB with the human host. The interplay of activating and suppressive immune mechanisms determines whether infection remains confined in latency or whether TB disease will develop. Bronchoalveolar cells obtained by bronchoalveolar lavage permit the study of localized immunoregulatory functions during TB disease and in MTB-exposed healthy household contacts. The procedure generally samples approximately 1 million alveoli, the walls of which contain the granulomas. Bronchoalveolar cells provide insight into immunologic compartmentalization and are thought to reflect processes in granulomatous tissue that is adjacent to the bronchoalveolar spaces. In health, bronchoalveolar cells are composed of 90–95 per cent alveolar macrophages and 5–10 per cent alveolar lymphocytes, with occasional neutrophils and eosinophils.

The most prominent finding of bronchoalveolar lavage studies in TB patients is a compartmentalized pulmonary immune response. Unstimulated total bronchoalveolar cells in TB contain increased numbers of cells expressing IFN-γ[163,164] and IL-12 mRNA,[164] but not IL-4 or IL-5 mRNA,[163,164] and release increased amounts of IL-1β, IL-6 and TNF-α.[165] Spontaneous TNF-α secretion by alveolar macrophages is associated with reduced MTB growth in normal alveolar macrophages in vitro.[166] Bronchoalveolar cells in pulmonary TB are also characterized by an alveolitis of αβ T-cell receptor bearing alveolar lymphocytes that are activated as manifest by membrane expression of HLA-DR and CD69.[92] Upon stimulation with PPD, these bronchoalveolar cells produce T_H1 type cytokines.[98]

Compartmentalization of mycobacterial antigen-specific responses to the lung in TB is due in part to recruitment of T cells from the blood to the lungs, as well as mycobacterial antigen-specific expansion in situ. Recruitment of MTB-specific cells to the lung is mediated by chemokines with lymphocyte chemotactic activity, such as RANTES (regulated on activation, normal T cell expressed and secreted), IL-8 and monocyte chemoattractant protein-1 (MCP-1), for which levels are increased in the bronchoalveolar lavage fluid of patients with pulmonary TB.[167,168] We have also shown that alveolar macrophages produce and release significantly higher levels than monocytes of RANTES, MCP-1 and macrophage inflammatory protein-1α[167] in response to stimulation with MTB in vitro.

There is evidence for a role for CTL in cell-mediated immunity against MTB in the human lung. Alveolar and blood CD4+ T cells and CD8+ T cells express MTB antigen-specific CTL activity when stimulated by MTB-infected alveolar macrophages from healthy TST-positive donors.[79] Mycobacterial antigen-pulsed alveolar macrophages are significantly more resistant to cytotoxicity than antigen-pulsed autologous blood monocytes.[79] Because both CD4+ T cells and CD8+ T cells are increased in number and activated in alveoli during active pulmonary TB,[92] these cell types may be antigen-specific CTLs in the lung during disease.

In healthy household contacts of patients with TB, MTB antigen 85-specific alveolar lymphocyte cell numbers were significantly increased, compared with healthy MTB-unexposed community controls,[168] suggesting induction of protective local antigen-specific immunity upon MTB exposure.

As mediators of innate and adaptive immune responses, alveolar macrophages contribute to the production of cytokines, and of chemokines that facilitate recruitment of lymphocytes and monocytes. Alveolar macrophages also provide accessory function for MTB-specific T-cell activation.[68] About 20 per cent of alveolar macrophages during active TB are immature by cytochemical criteria and may represent recently recruited monocytes.[92] MTB-infected alveolar macrophages release TNF-α, IL-1, IL-6, IL-12, IL-15, IL-18,[169–171] granulocyte–macrophage colony-stimulating factor (GM-CSF) and the deactivating cytokines IL-10 and TGF-β.[171,172] Alveolar macrophages of TB patients express IFN-γ mRNA ex vivo[163] and alveolar macrophages from normal donors produce IFN-γ upon infection with MTB in vitro.[173] Upon infection with MTB in vitro, alveolar macrophages release different amounts of RANTES, MCP-1, macrophage inflammatory protein-1α and IL-8[167,174] depending on the virulence of the infecting MTB strain.[174]

Alveolar macrophages, dendritic cells and monocytes express TLRs. Qualitative and quantitative differences in the protein expression of these TLRs have profound implications on the modulation of both innate and adaptive immunity, e.g. by mediating production of TNF-α, IL-1 and IL-6, killing of MTB[175] and probably production of reactive nitrogen intermediates.[40] Innate resistance against MTB is thought to critically depend on the engagement of TLR-2, TLR-4 and TLR-9. TLR-2 agonists include a variety of bacterial cell wall components, such as peptidoglycan and lipoarabinomannan, which is a major cell wall-associated glycolipid of MTB. Arabinose-capped lipoarabinomannan, purified from rapidly growing mycobacteria, induces TNF-α production by macrophages, in a TLR-2-dependent manner.[176,177] The major TLR-4 and TLR-9 agonists are Gram-negative bacterial LPS and unmethylated CpG-containing DNA,[176] respectively. TLRs 1–5 are expressed in almost all granulomas from TB patients. All TLRs can utilize myD88 to propagate signals to target genes and generate rapid protective responses.

THE ALVEOLAR–EPITHELIAL BARRIER

Epithelial cells play an important role in antibacterial mucosal innate immunity and MTB presumably interacts with epithelial cells after entry of infectious droplet nuclei into the alveolar spaces. However, the mechanisms by which MTB crosses the alveolar wall to establish infection in the lung parenchyma or gain access to the lymphatic and circulatory system are not well defined. The MTB laboratory strains, avirulent H37Ra and virulent H37Rv, can invade human A549 type II alveolar epithelial cell line in a microfilament- and microtubule-dependent manner, using the antivitronectin receptor, CD51, and β_1 integrin (CD29) as receptors.[178] Within these cells, MTB can replicate and survive.[178,179] Infection of A549 cells with H37Ra induces production of human beta defensin 2,[180] a peptide with antimicrobial and chemokine activities. MTB can cross epithelial–endothelial barriers and trigger the release of IL-8 and MCP-1[181] from both epithelial and endothelial cells. Following exposure to MTB, respiratory epithelium thus may create a gradient for infected mononuclear cells to migrate across the alveolar barrier. Alveolar and other respiratory epithelial cells thus are involved in the initiation and linkage of innate and adaptive antimycobacterial immune responses.

THE GRANULOMATOUS TISSUE RESPONSE

Granuloma formation is the pathologic hallmark of TB. Immunohistochemically, TB granulomas comprise monocytes, macrophages and T cells (mainly CD4[+] and CD8[+]). During human pulmonary TB, the cell distribution and their activation status differs in early granulomas, central caseating cavities or tuberculomas.[182] Developing granulomas are characterized by an inner cell layer with few CD8[+] T cells that surround the necrotic centre and an outer area infiltrated with CD4[+], CD8[+] and B lymphocytes, as well as MTB-containing APC.[183] Studies are currently under way to assess the presence and role of Tregs in human TB granulomas.

Granuloma formation in human TB is associated with the expression of characteristic cytokine profiles. mRNA expression of IFN-γ, IL-12p40, IL-1β, TNF-α, GM-CSF and lymphotoxin-β are increased between two-fold (IL-1β) and 19-fold (IFN-γ) in granulomatous TB lymph nodes, compared with lymph nodes of patients with carcinomas or chronic organizing pneumonias.[184] One half of TB granulomata express mRNA of the T_H2 cytokines, IL-4 and IL-5.[103] Levels of GM-CSF expression are tightly linked to the intensity of the granulomatous response and GM-CSF is present in epitheloid cells and lymphocytes surrounding granulomatous lesions.[184] In contrast, levels of TNF-α and lymphotoxin-β mRNA correlate negatively with the extent of caseous necrosis.[184] In surgically removed lung granulomas from five TB patients, *in situ* hybridization revealed IFN-γ and TNF-α mRNA in all and IL-4 mRNA in three of five subjects. Granulomas from two patients who exhibited IFN-γ, no IL-4, but low levels of TNF-α had more necrotic lesions than the granulomas of three TB patients which were positive for both IFN-γ and IL-4. Lung granuloma macrophages express TGF-β, which may interfere with antimycobacterial mechanisms and the efficiency of granuloma formation.[185] Interestingly, granulomas in different stages of maturity are present simultaneously in TB. These stages correlate with patterns of cytokine mRNA expression. Newer, less mature granulomas exhibit IFN-γ and TNF-α but no IL-4; intermediate granulomas exhibit IFN-γ, TNF-α and IL-4; and mature granulomas show greater expression of TNF-α, intermediate amounts of IL-4 and little IFN-γ. TNF-α appears to correlate positively with IL-4 gene expression and negatively with caseous necrosis. Granuloma cells stained with the myeloid marker CD68, probably macrophages, show mRNA production for IFN-γ and IL-4.[186] The latter observation coincides with the finding that alveolar macrophages from patients with TB[163] and alveolar macrophages infected with MTB *in vitro* express IFN-γ mRNA.[173]

The formation and plasticity of granulomatous tissue reactions depends on the regulation of apoptosis via death-inducing signals, such as lack of survival factors, metabolic supplies and binding to death signal transmitting receptors,[187] which are in turn controlled by members of the TNF-α superfamilies of TNF-α receptor and TNF-α-ligands. TNF-α induces apoptosis of MTB-infected alveolar macrophages.[41,188] Whether TNF-α induces or prevents the development of necrosis within MTB-induced granulomas is controversial[41,184] and may depend on specific local factors that regulate the apoptosis of granuloma-forming cells.

MTB virulence and protective human immunity

Human immune responses can control, but not fully eliminate, MTB in the majority of infected subjects, strongly indicating that MTB avoids detection or modulates immunity in order to evade human immune responses. MTB varies or maintains its degree of virulence in the human host and exploits and circumvents host immunoregulatory mechanisms to promote chronic infection, persistence and transmission to other hosts.[189,190] More specifically, MTB lipids arrest phagosome maturation and target host cell membrane-trafficking processes and organelle biogenesis.[191] These alterations allow escape from lysosomal bactericidal mechanisms and prevent efficient antigen presentation in phagocytic host cells. Early studies indicated a suppressive activity of the MTB polysaccharides D-arabinomannan and D-arabinogalactan. D-Arabinogalactan suppressed antigen-induced blastogenesis by a monocyte- and cyclooxygenase-dependent process. Plasma from TB patients had a similar effect, apparently through its content of D-arabinogalactan.[192]

As discussed above, enhanced T_H1 immunity and IFN-γ production, despite ongoing disease and infection at local sites of TB, represents a conundrum that urgently awaits resolution. A mechanism by which MTB avoids macrophage killing might be through inhibition of IFN-γ-mediated signalling and gene expression. In the THP-1 human monocytic cell line, induction of CD64 (Fcγ receptor 1, an IFN-γ-induced gene) surface expression and transcription are impaired following MTB infection, despite normal activation of STAT1.[193] Similarly in human monocyte-derived macrophages, MTB interferes with IFN-γ-induced genes. IL-6 release from MTB-infected macrophages decreases the transcription of class II transactivator (CIITA) and the expression of IFN-γ-induced MHC class II molecules in both infected and uninfected macrophages by a bystander effect.[194] This finding showed that inflammatory cytokines induced at the site of infection by MTB may interfere with important protective effects of IFN-γ.

An example of a MTB product with immunomodulatory capacity is the secreted 19-kDa lipoprotein, a cell wall peptidoglycan that interacts with macrophage receptors and modulates signalling systems used by infected macrophages and dendritic cells to activate innate immune responses. In mice, the 19-kDa lipoprotein exhibits immunosuppressive effects and modifies antimycobacterial immune responses via TLR-2- and myD88-dependent mechanisms that inhibit macrophage responses to IFN-γ at a transcriptional level and IFN-γ activation of murine macrophages to kill MTB.[195] In addition, the 19-kDa lipoprotein inhibits human macrophage expression of MHC class II molecules, antigen processing and antigen presentation. The 19-kDa lipoprotein binds to TLR-2, and represses IL-12 and the MHC class II presentation pathways.[196] It also inhibits the expression of several IFN-γ-regulated genes,[99,197] including HLA-DR[198] and Fcγ receptor I, thus altering processing and presentation of soluble-protein antigens to MHC-class II-restricted CD4$^+$ T cells.[199] An additional MTB cell wall lipoprotein (LprG, 24-kDa) was recently described that inhibits MHC class II antigen processing in a TLR-2-dependent manner.[200]

Other immunosuppressive mechanisms of MTB may be its inhibition of the phenotypic and functional maturation of human monocyte-derived dendritic cells.[201] For example, MTB targets DC-SIGN[21,22,202] that is an important receptor for interaction of dendritic cells with T cells. DC-SIGN is a coreceptor for HIV-1 and for mycobacterial uptake. Binding and internalization of mycobacteria through the cell wall component mannosylated lipoarabinomannan also prevents mycobacteria-induced dendritic cell maturation.[202,203]

These examples of a broad array of MTB-induced alterations of host cell function and immune responses provide important clues to the failure of protective immunity in MTB-infected subjects that progress to active TB. Lack of control of MTB growth with subsequent progression of MTB-induced pathology at sites of infection may occur despite the activation of potentially protective immune mechanisms, such as high local pulmonary IFN-γ levels.

MTB strain variation and host response

MTB strains differ in their virulence and induction of host immunity. Consequently, bacterial factors can modify epidemiological and clinical features. For example, the laboratory strain H37Rv and the clinical strain CDC1551 have different effects on TST reactivity in humans[204] and elicit production of different amounts of TNF-α, IL-6, IL-10 and IL-12 by human monocytes and of TNF-α by human alveolar macrophages during infection in vitro.[205] There is also substantial variability in the capacity of clinical MTB isolates to replicate within human cells.[206] In the murine model, an isolate of the W-Beijing family of MTB (HN878) was associated with hyperlethality, and the production of a polyketide synthase-derived phenolic glycolipid.[207] Interference with the synthesis of the phenolic glycolipid of HN878 increased TNF-α, IL-6 and IL-12 release from murine bone marrow macrophages following infection in vitro. Furthermore, studies with the avirulent H37Ra and the virulent H37Rv laboratory strains of MTB indicate that they induce release of different levels of chemokines such as RANTES, MCP-1, macrophage inflammatory protein1α and IL-8.[174] Taken together, it is clear that individual MTB components exert effects on host immune cells that affect function and recruitment of inflammatory cells, thus ultimately impacting MTB growth control mechanisms. MTB manipulates its environment by interfering with the host immune response on multiple levels. The redundancy of multiple MTB products and strain-dependent effects suggests their importance for the survival of MTB during its coevolution with humans.

Host immunogenetics and susceptibility to MTB

Genetic variation influences immune responses and may contribute to differential development of TB.[208,209] Resistance to TB disease and MTB infection is polygenic in nature. Associations with the development of mycobacterial infections and TB disease in population-based studies have been described for polymorphisms in multiple genes: human leucocyte antigen,[210–212] IFN-γ,[213,214] NRAMP,[215–217] TGF-β and IL-10,[218,219] mannose binding protein,[220,221] IFN-γ receptor,[222] TLR-2,[223,224] vitamin D receptor[225–227] and IL-1.[228,229] The identification of patients with mutations in single receptor genes that are involved in IL-12 and IFN-γ binding and signalling provided evidence for the importance of T_H1 cytokines in human resistance to mycobacteria. Defects in the IL-12 receptor,[230–232] IL-12 receptor β1,[96,233] and complete or partial defects in the IFN-γ receptor[194,233–237] have been found worldwide in individuals with disseminated infections caused primarily by

BCG, following vaccination, or nontuberculous mycobacteria of low virulence. Studies with blood cells from such individuals often show reduced or absent production of IFN-γ[238] or TNF-α[236] upon stimulation *in vitro*. Interestingly, infections with MTB or TB disease in association with the IL-12 or IFN-γ receptor defects have rarely been reported.[96,97] It is not clear if the reported preponderance of disseminated BCG and non-tuberculous mycobacterial infection in these hereditary cases is due to a specific biologic defect or to a lack of preceding exposure to MTB in the subjects studied.

Conditions favouring progression of MTB infection

HIV-1 INFECTION

In patients with concurrent HIV-1 infection, the risk that MTB infection will progress to progressive primary or reactivation TB is strikingly increased to 5–10 per cent per year,[239] indicating that CD4$^+$ T cells are required to maintain infectious foci in clinical latency. It further indicates that 'latency' is a misnomer because there is a dynamic balance between bacterial replication and host immune response at the infectious site(s). The risk of reactivation TB is 79-fold greater in HIV-1-infected people than in uninfected people[239] and may be up to 170-fold higher in patients with AIDS.[240] HIV-1 infection also strongly increases the risk of exogenous MTB reinfection, which is inversely related to the degree of immunosuppression.[241] TB is the most frequent opportunistic infection in patients with HIV-1 infection globally.

Development of TB during HIV-1 infection is associated with skin test anergy and CD4$^+$ T cell depletion,[242] and the frequency of extrapulmonary tuberculosis is increased, compared to patients without HIV-1 infection. Development of extrapulmonary TB is associated with compromised granulomatous tissue reactions[243,244] from HIV-1-induced alterations of cellular-mediated immunity. MTB-induced granuloma formation correlates with the degree of immunocompetence and peripheral CD4$^+$ T-cell depletion. In early stages of HIV-1 infection, TB granulomas are characterized by abundant epitheloid macrophages, Langhans giant cells, and a peripheral rim of CD4$^+$ T cells. MTB numbers are low. With moderate immunodeficiency, Langhans giant cells, epitheloid differentiation and activation of macrophages are absent. CD4$^+$ T cells are depleted and MTB numbers are increased. In advanced HIV-1 disease and AIDS, granuloma formation, cavitary tissue damage and number and size of cavitary lesions in the lungs are reduced, and there is little cellular recruitment and few CD4$^+$ T cells. MTB numbers are high.[245]

In vivo, the HIV-1 viral load is increased in MTB-co-infected people, compared with people infected with HIV-1 alone, if the CD4$^+$ count is >500/μL. This suggests that TB, as an early HIV-1 opportunistic infection, increases viral repli-

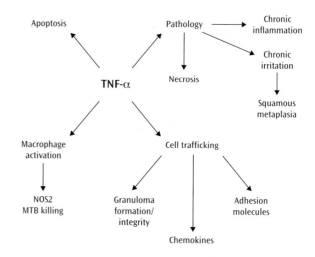

Figure 8.2 The central role of TNF-α in antimycobacterial immunity. MTB, *Mycobacterium tuberculosis*; NOS2, nitric oxide synthase.

cation and dissemination, and thus progression of HIV-1 disease.[246] IFN-γ production is preserved in HIV-1-infected TB patients with CD4$^+$ T-cell counts of 200–500/μL. TNF-α levels are similar in HIV-1 co-infected TB patients, regardless of the CD4$^+$ T-cell numbers.[247] Interestingly, among TST-positive, HIV-1-infected subjects, the incidence of TB is high and development of TB associated with an IL-10 response to PPD or with IL-5 responses when a BCG scar is present[248] In MTB-stimulated PBMCs from TST-negative donors, IL-10 significantly decreases replication of T cell-tropic HIV-1 isolates in MTB antigen-stimulated cells.[120] This may result from inhibition of TNF-α, a key enhancer of HIV-1 replication. Increased numbers of IL-10-producing CD4$^+$ T cells in TST-negative TB patients[117] suggest that HIV-1 replication in MTB-co-infected individuals is co-regulated by Tregs. Inducible Tregs may enhance host susceptibility to infection as they suppress appropriate CD4$^+$ and CD8$^+$ T-cell responses against foreign antigens. HIV-1 can infect Tregs and may impact control of inflammatory processes, such as those during HIV-1-associated TB. Interestingly, removal of Tregs from PBMCs of HIV-1-infected individuals enhances cytokine production from HIV-1 antigen-specific CD4$^+$ and CD8$^+$ T cells.[249] Upon stimulation of PBMCs from HIV-1-infected TB patients with MTB, *in vitro* proliferative and T$_H$1 responses are reduced, due to CD4$^+$ T-cell depletion and increased IL-10 production.[250] We also found that expression of TGF-β and IL-10 was higher in HIV-1-associated TB than in TB alone. However, neutralization of these cytokines *in vitro* improved, but did not completely reverse the profoundly impaired PPD-specific IFN-γ response.[145] On the other hand, TNF-α production is increased, compared with healthy individuals, suggesting that HIV-1-associated TB is accompanied by immune activation that triggers increased HIV-1 expression and accelerated progression to AIDS.[140,251]

Blood monocytes from TB patients are highly permissive to productive infection with HIV-1 *in vitro*.[252] Both

MTB and PPD increase HIV-1 replication in monocytes *in vitro* via transcriptional activation[253] and activation of NF-κB.[254] Conversely, growth of MTB is increased in HIV-1-infected human monocyte-derived macrophages.[255] As the decreased antimycobacterial immunity is HIV-1-associated, it is not surprising that *in vitro* killing of mycobacteria by blood cells and overall immune responses to mycobacteria significantly improve once highly active antiretroviral therapy (HAART) is initiated.[256] These findings coincide with the reduced susceptibility to TB in adults receiving HAART.

INHIBITORS OF TNF-α

The importance and complexity of the role of TNF-α as a regulator of local antimycobacterial host defence (Figure 8.2) has been clearly demonstrated in TNF-α antibody-treated or TNF-α receptor gene-disrupted or transgenic mice. Such mice show decreased numbers of granulomas, delayed granuloma formation and reduced containment and elimination of infecting mycobacteria,[257] an accelerated lethal course of MTB infection, delay in iNOS production,[258] widespread pulmonary inflammation,[259] necrosis and dysregulation of cytokine and chemokine production.[260] TNF-α is essential for granuloma formation[261] and maintenance, and prevents reactivation of latent MTB infection.[262] Exogenous TNF-α induces apoptosis in alveolar macrophages,[41] a mechanism that may be triggered by MTB and affect the macrophage–pathogen interaction *in vivo*. With the increased use of TNF-α inhibitors to treat inflammatory conditions, such as rheumatoid arthritis and Crohn's disease, reports of simultaneous occurrence of granulomatous infectious diseases have increased in the past 5 years.[263] Patients receiving TNF-α inhibitors are at increased risk for TB reactivation disease,[263–268] and disseminated non-reactive TB is much more common than would be expected in an adult population.[266] Currently under investigation are the relative risk of therapy with monoclonal anti-TNF-α antibodies and TNF-α receptor antagonists, and *in vitro* mechanisms of their interference with protective host immune mechanisms. We have recently shown that the anti-TNF-α antibodies, infliximab and adalimumab, reduce the proportion of MTB-responsive CD4+ cells, and suppress antigen-induced IFN-γ production, whereas the TNF-α receptor antagonist, etanercept, did not. IL-10 production was equally suppressed by all drugs. The reported risk of TB development posed by infliximab may reflect its combined effects on TNF-α and IFN-γ production.[269]

Immune restoration syndrome

A subgroup of people treated with HAART exhibits paradoxical deterioration in their clinical status, despite satisfactory control of HIV-1 replication and usually despite improvements in their CD4+ T-cell counts. This phenomenon, known as the immune restoration syndrome (IRS), immune reconstitution disease (IRD) or immune reconstitution inflammatory syndrome, results from an exuberant inflammatory response, directed towards previously diagnosed or latent opportunistic pathogens, as well as undefined antigens. In the context of MTB, IRS represents a paradoxical exacerbation with clinical or radiological deterioration of pre-existing tuberculous lesions or the development of new lesions in patients initially responding to effective treatment. This can present as fever and minor lymph node enlargement, new pulmonary infiltrates, respiratory failure or neurological deterioration. IRS is observed among 2–23 per cent of HIV-seronegative patients receiving treatment for TB,[270] the majority of cases occurring during the first 2–3 months of treatment.[270–273] Paradoxical worsening or reappearance of previous manifestations of TB or appearance of new manifestations (such as fever, lymph node enlargement, cough, pulmonary infiltrates) despite administration of effective antituberculous therapy have been reported in HIV-1-infected patients after the initiation of antiretroviral therapy.[87,88,273,274]

Patients who develop IRS are more likely to present with disseminated TB, CD4+ counts <100 cells/mm³ and with a prompt rise in CD4+ T-cell counts, TST conversion and a rapid fall of the HIV-1 viral load in the initial 3 months of HAART.[272] However, rises in CD4+ cell counts are neither diagnostic nor essential for the diagnosis of IRD.[270] CD4+ T cell increases largely represent a redistribution of activated CD45RO+ memory cells previously sequestered in lymphoid tissue and a reduction in apoptotic cell death.[275,276] Individuals starting treatment for disseminated TB and HIV-1 co-infection quickly increase frequencies of IFN-γ-producing peripheral MTB-specific blood CD4+ T cells.[277]

The incidence of IRS will rise in TB-endemic regions with high rates of HIV-1 infection, such as sub-Saharan Africa, as HAART becomes increasingly available. There is ongoing research to define the clinical and/or immunological predictors of IRS development, which would be of considerable help in the diagnosis of IRS and the identification of candidates for preventive strategies.

Approaches to vaccination against tuberculosis

The targeted design of modern antituberculous vaccines, as well as the evaluation of their protective efficacy, is based on the current understanding of antimycobacterial immunity and the correlates of immunological protection. Following comparative trials with BCG both in murine and guinea pig MTB challenge models, several new anti-TB vaccine candidates are currently undergoing phase I and II trials in humans. The vaccines target neonates for primary prevention or will be used to boost waning immunity following initial BCG vaccination in adolescents. Two of the four most advanced candidate vaccines represent genetically modified BCG strains, listeriolysin-secreting recombinant live BCG (rBCGDelta UreC:Hly)[278,279] and recombinant BCG secreting the 30-kDa protein (rBCG30).[280,281] One is a subunit vaccine (MTB-secreted Ag85B-TB10.4 fusion)[282] and one is a MTB Ag85-expressing modified vaccinia virus Ankara construct (MVA85).[283,284] The last vaccine is already in phase II testing. Because field trials are complex, costly and risky, vaccine efficacy is currently assessed by measuring components of the cell-mediated immune response, such as MTB antigen-specific cytokine production, using ELISA or ELISPOT assays.

LEARNING POINTS

- MTB infection results in a dynamic interaction of host and bacterial factors that result in heterogeneous clinical manifestations and distinct stages of infection and disease. The molecular make up of the MTB strains contributes to the subsequent host response and clinical outcome.
- HIV-1 is the strongest known single factor increasing susceptibility to infection with MTB and the development of reactivation disease from latent infection.
- Innate immunity against MTB involves the interplay of the bacterium and/or its products with host cell receptors, such as TLRs, on dendritic cells, monocytes/macrophages, epithelial cells and natural killer cells. Subsequent intracellular signalling induces processes that lead to intracellular killing of MTB and attraction of additional immune cells to sites of infection.
- Macrophages can function as effector cells against MTB, employing molecules such as nitric oxide, reactive nitrogen intermediates and cathelicidins.
- Imbalances between the effector cell subsets that mediate protective immunity and regulatory pathways may contribute to susceptibility to disease. A switch from T_H1 to T_H2 profiles is associated with the development of reactivation disease.
- Adaptive immunity primarily involves $CD4^+$ and $CD8^+$ T cells. During MTB infection, T cells that recognize a multitude of MTB antigens are expanded. When restimulated by antigen, these cells release cytokines such as IFN-γ. This mechanism is the basis of modern diagnostic approaches to detect MTB infection.
- $CD8^+$ cytotoxic T lymphocytes, NK cells and γδ T cells are involved in the killing of MTB by lysing MTB-infected target cells, such as macrophages or epithelial cells, utilizing effector molecules, such as granulysin, perforin and granzymes.
- Tregs suppress T effector cell function in a cell-contact-dependent manner that can involve IL-10, TGF-β and other molecules. Tregs are likely to be involved in suppressing MTB-induced inflammation and may adversely affect killing of MTB.
- Immune responses in TB are compartmentalized to sites of MTB infection, which most often are in the lungs. Lung immunity during TB is characterized by enhanced MTB antigen-specific T_H1 immune responses, while systemic MTB antigen-specific immune responses are suppressed.
- TB is a chronic granulomatous disease. The granulomatous tissue reaction, composed of epithelioid cells, dendritic cells and T cells, is determined by the host immune response and the molecular make up of the infecting MTB strain.
- TNF-α together with other apoptotic regulatory processes, modulate the dynamic structure of TB granulomas. TNF-α is also a major component of antimycobacterial immunity.
- The increasing clinical use of TNF-α inhibitors for treatment of chronic inflammatory diseases requires that clinically silent MTB infection be identified and treated appropriately.
- Immune restoration syndromes need to be considered in patients receiving HAART for HIV-1 co-infection. These syndromes are characterized by paradoxical clinical or radiological deterioration of pre-existing tuberculous lesions or the development of new lesions in patients initially responding to effective treatment.
- Correlates of human immunological protection are required for the evaluation of new antituberculous vaccines, as well as for the identification of new diagnostic targets.
- The current major antituberculous vaccine candidates are genetically modified MTB antigen-expressing BCG strains, vaccinia virus constructs expressing MTB antigens or subunit vaccines of composite MTB antigens. These vaccines are currently entering human phase I and II trials.

ACKNOWLEDGEMENTS

Support: NHLBI 2R01HL51630.

REFERENCES

1. North RJ, Jung YJ. Immunity to tuberculosis. *Annu Rev Immunol* 2004; **22**: 599–623.
2. Bates JH. Transmission and pathogenesis of tuberculosis. *Clin Chest Med* 1980; **1**: 167–74.
3. Mistry R, Cliff JM, Clayton CL *et al.* Gene-expression patterns in whole blood identify subjects at risk for recurrent tuberculosis. *J Infect Dis* 2007; **195**: 357–65.

4. Agranoff D, Fernandez-Reyes D, Papadopoulos MC *et al.* Identification of diagnostic markers for tuberculosis by proteomic fingerprinting of serum. *Lancet* 2006; **368**: 1012–21.

5. Jacobsen M, Repsilber D, Gutschmidt A *et al.* Candidate biomarkers for discrimination between infection and disease caused by *Mycobacterium tuberculosis*. *J Mol Med* 2007; **85**: 613–21.

6. Houk VN, Baker JH, Sorensen K, Kent DC. The epidemiology of tuberculosis infection in a closed environment. *Arch Environ Health* 1968; **16**: 26–35.

7. Riley RL, Mills CC, O'Grady F *et al.* Infectiousness of air from a tuberculosis ward. Ultraviolet irradiation of infected air: comparative infectiousness of different patients. *Am Rev Respir Dis* 1962; **85**: 511–25.

8. Grzybowski S, Barnett GD, Styblo K. Contacts of cases of active pulmonary tuberculosis. *Bull Int Union Tuberc* 1975; **50**: 90–106.

9. Ferebee SH, Mount FW. Tuberculosis morbidity in a controlled trial of the prophylactic use of isoniazid among household contacts. *Am Rev Respir Dis* 1962; **85**: 490–510.

10. Guwatudde D, Nakakeeto M, Jones-Lopez EC *et al.* Tuberculosis in household contacts of infectious cases in Kampala, Uganda. *Am J Epidemiol* 2003; **158**: 887–98.

11. Whalen CC, Chiunda A, Zalwango S *et al.* Immune correlates of acute *Mycobacterium tuberculosis* infection in household contacts in Kampala, Uganda. *Am J Trop Med Hyg* 2006; **75**: 55–61.

12. Havlir DV, van der Kuyp F, Duffy E *et al.* A 19-year follow-up of tuberculin reactors. Assessment of skin test reactivity and *in vitro* lymphocyte responses. *Chest* 1991; **99**: 1172–6.

13. Tead WW, Kerby GR, Schlueter DP, Jordahl CW. The clinical spectrum of primary tuberculosis in adults. Confusion with reinfection in the pathogenesis of chronic tuberculosis. *Ann Intern Med* 1968; **68**: 731–45.

14. Verver S, Warren RM, Beyers N *et al.* Rate of reinfection tuberculosis after successful treatment is higher than rate of new tuberculosis . *Am J Respir Crit Care Med* 2005; **171**: 1430–5.

15. Ernst JD. Macrophage receptors for *Mycobacterium tuberculosis*. *Infect Immun* 1998; **66**: 1277–81.

16. Schlesinger LS, Bellinger-Kawahara CG, Payne NR, Horwitz MA. Phagocytosis of *Mycobacterium tuberculosis* is mediated by human monocyte complement receptors and complement component C3. *J Immunol* 1990; **144**: 2771–80.

17. Schorey JS, Carroll MC, Brown EJ. A macrophage invasion mechanism of pathogenic mycobacteria. *Science* 1997; **277**: 1091–3.

18. Cywes C, Hoppe HC, Daffe M, Ehlers MR. Nonopsonic binding of *Mycobacterium tuberculosis* to complement receptor type 3 is mediated by capsular polysaccharides and is strain dependent. *Infect Immun* 1997; **65**: 4258–66.

19. Schlesinger LS. Entry of *Mycobacterium tuberculosis* into mononuclear phagocytes. *Curr Top Microbiol Immunol* 1996; **215**: 71–96.

20. Hirsch CS, Ellner JJ, Russell DG, Rich EA. Complement receptor-mediated uptake and tumor necrosis factor-alpha-mediated growth inhibition of *Mycobacterium tuberculosis* by human alveolar macrophages. *J Immunol* 1994; **152**: 743–53.

21. Tailleux L, Schwartz O, Herrmann JL *et al.* DC-SIGN is the major *Mycobacterium tuberculosis* receptor on human dendritic cells. *J Exp Med* 2003; **197**: 121–7.

22. Kaufmann SH, Schaible UE. A dangerous liaison between two major killers: *Mycobacterium tuberculosis* and HIV target dendritic cells through DC-SIGN. *J Exp Med* 2003; **197**: 1–5.

23. Sieling PA, Chatterjee D, Porcelli SA *et al.* CD1-restricted T cell recognition of microbial lipoglycan antigens. *Science* 1995; **269**: 227–30.

24. Stenger S, Hanson DA, Teitelbaum R *et al.* An antimicrobial activity of cytolytic T cells mediated by granulysin. *Science* 1998; **282**: 121–5.

25. Takeda K, Kaisho T, Akira S. Toll-like receptors. *Annu Rev Immunol* 2003; **21**: 335–76.

26. Krutzik SR, Sieling PA, Modlin RL. The role of Toll-like receptors in host defense against microbial infection. *Curr Opin Immunol* 2001; **13**: 104–8.

27. Cluff CW, Baldridge JR, Stover AG *et al.* Synthetic toll-like receptor 4 agonists stimulate innate resistance to infectious challenge. *Infect Immun* 2005; **73**: 3044–52.

28. Baldridge JR, Cluff CW, Evans JT *et al.* Immunostimulatory activity of aminoalkyl glucosaminide 4-phosphates (AGPs): induction of protective innate immune responses by RC-524 and RC-529. *J Endotoxin Res* 2002; **8**: 453–8.

29. Liu PT, Stenger S, Li H *et al.* Toll-like receptor triggering of a vitamin D-mediated human antimicrobial response. *Science* 2006; **311**: 1770–3.

30. Sharma S, Sharma M, Roy S *et al.* Mycobacterium tuberculosis induces high production of nitric oxide in coordination with production of tumour necrosis factor-alpha in patients with fresh active tuberculosis but not in MDR tuberculosis. *Immunol Cell Biol* 2004; **82**: 377–82.

31. Kuo HP, Wang CH, Huang KS *et al.* Nitric oxide modulates interleukin-1beta and tumor necrosis factor-alpha synthesis by alveolar macrophages in pulmonary tuberculosis. *Am J Respir Crit Care Med* 2000; **161**: 192–9.

32. Nicholson S, Bonecini-Almeida M, Lapa e Silva JR *et al.* Inducible nitric oxide synthase in pulmonary alveolar macrophages from patients with tuberculosis. *J Exp Med* 1996; **183**: 2293–302.

33. Rich EA, Torres M, Sada E *et al.* Mycobacterium tuberculosis (MTB)-stimulated production of nitric oxide by human alveolar macrophages and relationship of nitric oxide production to growth inhibition of MTB. *Tuber Lung Dis* 1997; **78**: 247–55.

34. Roy S, Sharma S, Sharma M *et al.* Induction of nitric oxide release from the human alveolar epithelial cell line A549: an in vitro correlate of innate immune response to *Mycobacterium tuberculosis* *Immunology* 2004; **112**: 471–80.

35. Wang CH, Liu CY, Lin HC *et al.* Increased exhaled nitric oxide in active pulmonary tuberculosis due to inducible NO synthase upregulation in alveolar macrophages. *Eur Respir J* 1998; **11**: 809–15.

36. Choi HS, Rai PR, Chu HW *et al.* Analysis of nitric oxide synthase and nitrotyrosine expression in human pulmonary tuberculosis. *Am J Respir Crit Care Med* 2002; **166**: 178–86.

37. Nozaki Y, Hasegawa Y, Ichiyama S *et al.* Mechanism of nitric oxide-dependent killing of *Mycobacterium bovis* BCG in human alveolar macrophages. *Infect Immun* 1997; **65**: 3644–7.

38. Bose M, Farnia P, Sharma S *et al.* Nitric oxide dependent killing of *Mycobacterium tuberculosis* by human mononuclear phagocytes from patients with active tuberculosis. *Int J Immunopathol Pharmacol* 1999; **12**: 69–79.

39. Brightbill HD, Libraty DH, Krutzik SR *et al.* Host defense mechanisms triggered by microbial lipoproteins through toll-like receptors. *Science* 1999; **285**: 732–6.

40. Campos MA, Closel M, Valente EP *et al.* Impaired production of proinflammatory cytokines and host resistance to acute infection with *Trypanosoma cruzi* in mice lacking functional myeloid differentiation factor 88. *J Immunol* 2004; **172**: 1711–18.

41. Keane J, Balcewicz-Sablinska MK, Remold HG *et al.* Infection by *Mycobacterium tuberculosis* promotes human alveolar macrophage apoptosis. *Infection and Immunity* 1997; **65**: 298–304.

42. Lee J, Remold HG, Ieong MH, Kornfeld H. Macrophage apoptosis in response to high intracellular burden of *Mycobacterium tuberculosis* is mediated by a novel caspase-independent pathway. *J Immunol* 2006; **176**: 4267–74.

43. Derrick SC, Morris SL. The ESAT6 protein of *Mycobacterium tuberculosis* induces apoptosis of macrophages by activating caspase expression. *Cell Microbiol* 2007; **9**: 1547–55.

44. Kornfeld H, Mancino G, Colizzi V. The role of macrophage cell death in tuberculosis. *Cell Death Diff* 1999; **6**: 71–8.

45. Schnappinger D, Schoolnik GK, Ehrt S. Expression profiling of host pathogen interactions: how *Mycobacterium tuberculosis* and the

macrophage adapt to one another. *Microbes Infect* 2006; **8**: 1132–40.

46. Volpe E, Cappelli G, Grassi M *et al.* Gene expression profiling of human macrophages at late time of infection with *Mycobacterium tuberculosis. Immunology* 2006; **118**: 449–60.

47. Nau GJ, Richmond JF, Schlesinger A *et al.* Human macrophage activation programs induced by bacterial pathogens. *Proc Natl Acad Sci U S A* 2002; **99**: 1503–8.

48. Schnappinger D, Ehrt S, Voskuil MI *et al.* Transcriptional adaptation of *Mycobacterium tuberculosis* within macrophages: insights into the phagosomal environment. *J Exp Med* 2003; **198**: 693–704.

49. Ni K, O'Neill HC. The role of dendritic cells in T cell activation. *Immunol Cell Biol* 1997; **75**: 223–30.

50. Hertz C, Kiertscher S, Godowski P *et al.* Microbial lipopeptides stimulate dendritic cell maturation via Toll-like receptor 2. *J Immunol* 2001; **166**: 2444–50.

51. Holt PG. Antigen presentation in the lung. *Am J Respir Crit Care Med* 2000; **162**: S151–6.

52. Sertl K, Takemura T, Tschachler E *et al.* Dendritic cells with antigen-presenting capability reside in airway epithelium, lung parenchyma, and visceral pleura. *J Exp Med* 1986; **163**: 436–51.

53. Henderson RA, Watkins SC, Flynn JL. Activation of human dendritic cells following infection with *Mycobacterium tuberculosis. J Immunol* 1997; **159**: 635–43.

54. Giacomini E, Iona E, Ferroni L *et al.* Infection of human macrophages and dendritic cells with *Mycobacterium tuberculosis* induces a differential cytokine gene expression that modulates T cell response. *J Immunol* 2001; **166**: 7033–41.

55. Fortsch D, Rollinghoff M, Stenger S. IL-10 converts human dendritic cells into macrophage-like cells with increased antibacterial activity against virulent *Mycobacterium tuberculosis. J Immunol* 2000; **165**: 978–87.

56. Chackerian A, Alt J, Perera V, Behar SM. Activation of NKT cells protects mice from tuberculosis. *Infect Immun* 2002; **70**: 6302–9.

57. Yu KO, Porcelli SA. The diverse functions of CD1d-restricted NKT cells and their potential for immunotherapy. *Immunol Lett* 2005; **100**: 42–55.

58. Gansert JL, Kiessler V, Engele M *et al.* Human NKT cells express granulysin and exhibit antimycobacterial activity. *J Immunol* 2003; **170**: 3154–61.

59. Vankayalapati R, Klucar P, Wizel B *et al.* NK cells regulate CD8+ T cell effector function in response to an intracellular pathogen. *J Immunol* 2004; **172**: 130–7.

60. O'Connor GM, Hart OM, Gardiner CM. Putting the natural killer cell in its place. *Immunology* 2006; **117**: 1–10.

61. Brill KJ, Li Q, Larkin R *et al.* Human natural killer cells mediate killing of intracellular *Mycobacterium tuberculosis* H37Rv via granule-independent mechanisms. *Infect Immun* 2001; **69**: 1755–65.

62. Gerosa F, Baldani-Guerra B, Nisii C *et al.* Reciprocal activating interaction between natural killer cells and dendritic cells. *J Exp Med* 2002; **195**: 327–33.

63. Vankayalapati R, Wizel B, Weis SE *et al.* The NKp46 receptor contributes to NK cell lysis of mononuclear phagocytes infected with an intracellular bacterium. *J Immunol* 2002; **168**: 3451–7.

64. Vankayalapati R, Garg A, Porgador A *et al.* Role of NK cell-activating receptors and their ligands in the lysis of mononuclear phagocytes infected with an intracellular bacterium. *J Immunol* 2005; **175**: 4611–17.

65. Rojas RE, Torres M, Fournie JJ *et al.* Phosphoantigen presentation by macrophages to *Mycobacterium tuberculosis* – reactive Vgamma9Vdelta2+ T cells: modulation by chloroquine. *Infect Immun* 2002; **70**: 4019–27.

66. Rojas RE, Chervenak KA, Thomas J *et al.* V delta 2+ gamma delta T cell function in *Mycobacterium tuberculosis*- and HIV-1-positive patients in the United States and Uganda: application of a whole-blood assay. *J Infect Dis* 2005; **192**: 1806–14.

67. Boom WH, Chervenak KA, Mincek MA, Ellner JJ. Role of the mononuclear phagocyte as an antigen-presenting cell for human gamma delta T cells activated by live *Mycobacterium tuberculosis. Infect Immun* 1992; **60**: 3480–8.

68. Balaji KN, Schwander SK, Rich EA, Boom WH. Alveolar macrophages as accessory cells for human gamma delta T cells activated by *Mycobacterium tuberculosis. J Immunol* 1995; **154**: 5959–68.

69. Barnes PF, Grisso CL, Abrams JS *et al.* Gamma delta T lymphocytes in human tuberculosis. *J Infect Dis* 1992; **165**: 506–12.

70. Li B, Rossman MD, Imir T *et al.* Disease-specific changes in gammadelta T cell repertoire and function in patients with pulmonary tuberculosis. *J Immunol* 1996; **157**: 4222–9.

71. Li B, Bassiri H, Rossman MD *et al.* Involvement of the Fas/Fas ligand pathway in activation-induced cell death of mycobacteria-reactive human gamma delta T cells: a mechanism for the loss of gamma delta T cells in patients with pulmonary tuberculosis. *J Immunol* 1998; **161**: 1558–67.

72. Hoft DF, Brown RM, Roodman ST. Bacille Calmette-Guérin vaccination enhances human gamma delta T cell responsiveness to mycobacteria suggestive of a memory-like phenotype. *J Immunol* 1998; **161**: 1045–54.

73. Boom WH, Canaday DH, Fulton SA *et al.* Human immunity to *M. tuberculosis*: T cell subsets and antigen processing. *Tuberculosis (Edinb)* 2003; **83**: 98–106.

74. Tena GN, Young DB, Eley B *et al.* Failure to control growth of mycobacteria in blood from children infected with human immunodeficiency virus and its relationship to T cell function. *J Infect Dis* 2003; **187**: 1544–51.

75. Serbina NV, Lazarevic V, Flynn JL. CD4(+) T cells are required for the development of cytotoxic CD8(+) T cells during *Mycobacterium tuberculosis* infection. *J Immunol* 2001; **167**: 6991–7000.

76. Silver RF, Li Q, Boom WH, Ellner JJ. Lymphocyte-dependent inhibition of growth of virulent *Mycobacterium tuberculosis* H37Rv within human monocytes: requirement for CD4+ T cells in purified protein derivative-positive, but not in purified protein derivative-negative subjects. *J Immunol* 1998; **160**: 2408–17.

77. Nathan CF, Murray HW, Wiebe ME, Rubin BY. Identification of interferon-gamma as the lymphokine that activates human macrophage oxidative metabolism and antimicrobial activity. *J Exp Med* 1983; **158**: 670–89.

78. Cho S, Mehra V, Thoma-Uszynski S *et al.* Antimicrobial activity of MHC class I-restricted CD8+ T cells in human tuberculosis. *Proc Natl Acad Sci U S A* 2000; **97**: 12210–15.

79. Tan JS, Canaday DH, Boom WH *et al.* Human alveolar T lymphocyte responses to *Mycobacterium tuberculosis* antigens: role for CD4+ and CD8+ cytotoxic T cells and relative resistance of alveolar macrophages to lysis. *J Immunol* 1997; **159**: 290–7.

80. Canaday DH, Wilkinson RJ, Li Q *et al.* CD4(+) and CD8(+) T cells kill intracellular *Mycobacterium tuberculosis* by a perforin and Fas/Fas ligand-independent mechanism. *J Immunol* 2001; **167**: 2734–42.

81. Canaday DH, Ziebold C, Noss EH *et al.* Activation of human CD8+ alpha beta TCR+ cells by *Mycobacterium tuberculosis* via an alternate class I MHC antigen-processing pathway. *J Immunol* 1999; **162**: 372–9.

82. Heinzel AS, Grotzke JE, Lines RA *et al.* HLA-E-dependent presentation of *M. tuberculosis*-derived antigen to human CD8+ T cells. *J Exp Med* 2002; **196**: 1473–81.

83. Lewinsohn DA, Heinzel AS, Gardner JM *et al. Mycobacterium tuberculosis*-specific CD8+ T cells preferentially recognize heavily infected cells. *Am J Respir Crit Care Med* 2003; **168**: 1346–52.

84. Carranza C, Juarez E, Torres M *et al. Myobacterium tuberculosis* growth control by lung macrophages and CD8 cells from patient contacts. *Am J Respir Crit Care Med* 2005; **173**: 238–45.

85. Lalvani A, Brookes R, Wilkinson RJ *et al.* Human cytolytic and interferon gamma-secreting CD8+ T lymphocytes specific for

Mycobacterium tuberculosis. Proc Natl Acad Sci U S A 1998; **95**: 270–5.

86. Smith SM, Klein MR, Malin AS *et al.* Human CD8(+) T cells specific for *Mycobacterium tuberculosis* secreted antigens in tuberculosis patients and healthy BCG-vaccinated controls in The Gambia. *Infect Immun* 2000; **68**: 7144–8.

87. Mohagheghpour N, Gammon D, Kawamura LM *et al.* CTL response to *Mycobacterium tuberculosis*: identification of an immunogenic epitope in the 19-kDa lipoprotein. *J Immunol* 1998; **161**: 2400–406.

88. Geluk A, van Meijgaarden KE, Franken KL *et al.* Identification of major epitopes of *Mycobacterium tuberculosis* AG85B that are recognized by HLA-A*0201-restricted CD8+ T cells in HLA-transgenic mice and humans. *J Immunol* 2000; **165**: 6463–71.

89. Stenger S, Modlin RL. Cytotoxic T cell responses to intracellular pathogens. *Curr Opin Immunol* 1998; **10**: 471–7.

90. Ernst WA, Thoma-Uszynski S, Teitelbaum R *et al.* Granulysin, a T cell product, kills bacteria by altering membrane permeability. *J Immunol* 2000; **165**: 7102–108.

91. Brookes RH, Pathan AA, McShane H *et al.* CD8+ T cell-mediated suppression of intracellular *Mycobacterium tuberculosis* growth in activated human macrophages. *Eur J Immunol* 2003; **33**: 3293–302.

92. Schwander SK, Sada E, Torres M *et al.* T lymphocytic and immature macrophage alveolitis in active pulmonary tuberculosis. *J Infect Dis* 1996; **173**: 1267–72.

93. Flynn JL, Chan J, Triebold KJ *et al.* An essential role for interferon gamma in resistance to *Mycobacterium tuberculosis* infection. *J Exp Med* 1993; **178**: 2249–54.

94. Jouanguy E, Lamhamedi-Cherradi S, Altare F *et al* Partial interferon-gamma receptor 1 deficiency in a child with tuberculoid bacillus Calmette–Guérin infection and a sibling with clinical tuberculosis *J Clin Invest* 1997; **100**: 2658–64.

95. Jouanguy E, Altare F, Lamhamedi-Cherradi S, Casanova JL. Infections in IFNGR-1-deficient children. *J Interferon Cytokine Res* 1997; **17**: 583–7.

96. Caragol I, Raspall M, Fieschi C *et al.* Clinical tuberculosis in 2 of 3 siblings with interleukin-12 receptor beta1 deficiency. *Clin Infect Dis* 2003; **37**: 302–306.

97. Picard C, Fieschi C, Altare F *et al.* Inherited interleukin-12 deficiency: IL12B genotype and clinical phenotype of 13 patients from six kindreds. *Am J Hum Genet* 2002; **70**: 336–48.

98. Schwander SK, Torres M, Sada E *et al.* Enhanced responses to *Mycobacterium tuberculosis* antigens by human alveolar lymphocytes during active pulmonary tuberculosis. *J Infect Dis* 1998; **178**: 1434–45.

99. Pai RK, Pennini ME, Tobian AA *et al.* Prolonged toll-like receptor signaling by *Mycobacterium tuberculosis* and its 19-kilodalton lipoprotein inhibits gamma interferon-induced regulation of selected genes in macrophages. *Infect Immun* 2004; **72**: 6603–14.

100. Seah GT, Rook GA. IL-4 influences apoptosis of mycobacterium-reactive lymphocytes in the presence of TNF-alpha. *J Immunol* 2001; **167**: 1230–7.

101. Demissie A, Abebe M, Aseffa A *et al.* Healthy individuals that control a latent infection with *Mycobacterium tuberculosis* express high levels of Th1 cytokines and the IL-4 antagonist IL-4delta2. *J Immunol* 2004; **172**: 6938–43.

102. Ordway DJ, Costa L, Martins M *et al.* Increased interleukin-4 production by CD8 and gammadelta T cells in health-care workers is associated with the subsequent development of active tuberculosis. *J Infect Dis* 2004; **190**: 756–66.

103. Fenhalls G, Squires GR, Stevens-Muller L *et al.* Associations between toll-like receptors and interleukin-4 in the lungs of patients with tuberculosis. *Am J Respir Cell Mol Biol* 2003; **29**: 28–38.

104. Borkow G, Weisman Z, Leng Q *et al.* Helminths, human immunodeficiency virus and tuberculosis. *Scand J Infect Dis* 2001; **33**: 568–71.

105. Elias D, Wolday D, Akuffo H *et al.* Effect of deworming on human T cell responses to mycobacterial antigens in helminth-exposed individuals before and after bacille Calmette–Guérin (BCG) vaccination. *Clin Exp Immunol* 2001; **123**: 219–25.

106. Resende CT, Hirsch CS, Toossi Z *et al.* Intestinal helminth co-infection has a negative impact on both anti-*Mycobacterium tuberculosis* immunity and clinical response to tuberculosis therapy. *Clin Exp Immunol* 2007; **147**: 45–52.

107. O'Garra A, Vieira PL, Vieira P, Goldfeld AE. IL-10-producing and naturally occurring CD4+ Tregs: limiting collateral damage. *J Clin Invest* 2004; **114**: 1372–8.

108. Bluestone JA, Abbas AK. Natural versus adaptive regulatory T cells. *Nat Rev Immunol* 2003; **3**: 253–7.

109. Stassen M, Fondel S, Bopp T *et al.* Human CD25+ regulatory T cells: two subsets defined by the integrins alpha 4 beta 7 or alpha 4 beta 1 confer distinct suppressive properties upon CD4+ T helper cells. *Eur J Immunol* 2004; **34**: 1303–11.

110. Cederbom L, Hall H, Ivars F. CD4+CD25+ regulatory T cells down-regulate co-stimulatory molecules on antigen-presenting cells. *Eur J Immunol* 2000; **30**: 1538–43.

111. Fehervari Z, Sakaguchi S. CD4+ Tregs and immune control. *J Clin Invest* 2004; **114**: 1209–17.

112. Bluestone JA, St Clair EW, Turka LA. CTLA4Ig: bridging the basic immunology with clinical application. *Immunity* 2006; **24**: 233–8.

113. Liu W, Putnam AL, Xu-Yu Z *et al.* CD127 expression inversely correlates with FoxP3 and suppressive function of human CD4+ T reg cells. *J Exp Med* 2006; **203**: 1701–11.

114. Seddiki N, Santner-Nanan B, Martinson J *et al.* Expression of interleukin (IL)-2 and IL-7 receptors discriminates between human regulatory and activated T cells. *J Exp Med* 2006; **203**: 1693–700.

115. Belkaid Y, Rouse BT. Natural regulatory T cells in infectious disease. *Nat Immunol* 2005; **6**: 353–60.

116. Ribeiro-Rodrigues R, Resende CT, Rojas R *et al.* A role for CD4+CD25+ T cells in regulation of the immune response during human tuberculosis. *Clin Exp Immunol* 2006; **144**: 25–34.

117. Boussiotis VA, Tsai EY, Yunis EJ *et al.* IL-10-producing T cells suppress immune responses in anergic tuberculosis patients. *J Clin Invest* 2000; **105**: 1317–25.

118. Delgado JC, Tsai EY, Thim S *et al.* Antigen-specific and persistent tuberculin anergy in a cohort of pulmonary tuberculosis patients from rural Cambodia. *Proc Natl Acad Sci U S A* 2002; **99**: 7576–81.

119. Gong JH, Zhang M, Modlin RL *et al.* Interleukin-10 downregulates *Mycobacterium tuberculosis*-induced Th1 responses and CTLA-4 expression. *Infect Immun* 1996; **64**: 913–18.

120. Guyot-Revol V, Innes JA, Hackforth S *et al.* Regulatory T cells are expanded in blood and disease sites in patients with tuberculosis. *Am J Respir Crit Care Med* 2006; **173**: 803–10.

121. Ranjbar S, Ly N, Thim S *et al.* *Mycobacterium tuberculosis* recall antigens suppress HIV-1 replication in anergic donor cells via CD8+ T cell expansion and increased IL-10 levels. *J Immunol* 2004; **172**: 1953–9.

122. Umetsu DT, Dekruyff RH. The regulation of allergy and asthma. *Immunol Rev* 2006; **212**: 238–55.

123. Hawrylowicz CM, O'Garra A. Potential role of interleukin-10-secreting regulatory T cells in allergy and asthma. *Nat Rev Immunol* 2005; **5**: 271–83.

124. Suffia IJ, Reckling SK, Piccirillo CA *et al.* Infected site-restricted Foxp3+ natural regulatory T cells are specific for microbial antigens. *J Exp Med* 2006; **203**: 777–88.

125. Yurchenko E, Tritt M, Hay V *et al.* CCR5-dependent homing of naturally occurring CD4+ regulatory T cells to sites of *Leishmania major* infection favors pathogen persistence. *J Exp Med* 2006; **203**: 2451–60.

126. Kursar M, Koch M, Mittrucker HW *et al.* Cutting edge: regulatory T cells prevent efficient clearance of *Mycobacterium tuberculosis*. *J Immunol* 2007; **178**: 2661–5.

127. Teitelbaum R, Glatman-Freedman A, Chen B *et al.* A mAb

recognizing a surface antigen of *Mycobacterium tuberculosis* enhances host survival. *Proc Natl Acad Sci U S A* 1998; **95**: 15688–93.

128. Costello AM, Kumar A, Narayan V *et al.* Does antibody to mycobacterial antigens, including lipoarabinomannan, limit dissemination in childhood tuberculosis? *Trans R Soc Trop Med Hyg* 1992; **86**: 686–92.

129. Hussain R, Shiratsuchi H, Phillips M *et al.* Opsonizing antibodies (IgG1) up-regulate monocyte proinflammatory cytokines tumour necrosis factor-alpha (TNF-alpha) and IL-6 but not anti-inflammatory cytokine IL-10 in mycobacterial antigen-stimulated monocytes-implications for pathogenesis. *Clin Exp Immunol* 2001; **123**: 210–18.

130. Glatman-Freedman A. Advances in antibody-mediated immunity against *Mycobacterium tuberculosis*: implications for a novel vaccine strategy. *FEMS Immunol Med Microbiol* 2003; **39**: 9–16.

131. Bothamley GH, Rudd R, Festenstein F, Ivanyi J. Clinical value of the measurement of *Mycobacterium tuberculosis* specific antibody in pulmonary tuberculosis. *Thorax* 1992; **47**: 270–5.

132. Bothamley GH. Serological diagnosis of tuberculosis. *Eur Respir J* 1995; **20** (Suppl.): 676s–88s.

133. Davidow A, Kanaujia GV, Shi L *et al.* Antibody profiles characteristic of *Mycobacterium tuberculosis* infection state. *Infect Immun* 2005; **73**: 6846–51.

134. Laal S, Samanich KM, Sonnenberg MG *et al.* Surrogate marker of preclinical tuberculosis in human immunodeficiency virus infection: antibodies to an 88-kDa secreted antigen of *Mycobacterium tuberculosis*. *J Infect Dis* 1997; **176**: 133–43.

135. Daniel TM, McDonough JA, Huebner RE. Absence of IgG or IgM antibody response to *Mycobacterium tuberculosis* 30,000-Da antigen after primary tuberculous infection. *J Infect Dis* 1991; **164**: 821.

136. Ellner JJ. Regulation of the human immune response during tuberculosis. *J Lab Clin Med* 1997; **130**: 469–75.

137. Fujiwara H, Kleinhenz ME, Wallis RS, Ellner JJ. Increased interleukin-1 production and monocyte suppressor cell activity associated with human tuberculosis. *Am Rev Respir Dis* 1986; **133**: 73–7.

138. Toossi Z, Kleinhenz ME, Ellner JJ. Defective interleukin 2 production and responsiveness in human pulmonary tuberculosis. *J Exp Med* 1986; **163**: 1162–72.

139. Hirsch CS, Hussain R, Toossi Z *et al.* Cross-modulation by transforming growth factor beta in human tuberculosis: suppression of antigen-driven blastogenesis and interferon gamma production. *Proc Natl Acad Sci U S A* 1996; **93**: 3193–8.

140. Vanham G, Edmonds K, Qing L *et al.* Generalized immune activation in pulmonary tuberculosis: co-activation with HIV infection. *Clin Exp Immunol* 1996; **103**: 30–4.

141. Toossi Z, Sedor JR, Lapurga JP *et al.* Expression of functional interleukin 2 receptors by peripheral blood monocytes from patients with active pulmonary tuberculosis. *J Clin Invest* 1990; **85**: 1777–84.

142. Wallis RS, Amir-Tahmasseb M, Ellner JJ. Induction of interleukin 1 and tumor necrosis factor by mycobacterial proteins: the monocyte western blot. *Proc Natl Acad Sci U S A* 1990; **87**: 3348–52.

143. Toossi Z, Young TG, Averill LE *et al.* Induction of transforming growth factor beta 1 by purified protein derivative of *Mycobacterium tuberculosis*. *Infect Immun* 1995; **63**: 224–8.

144. Ellner JJ. Suppressor adherent cells in human tuberculosis. *J Immunol* 1978; **121**: 2573–9.

145. Hirsch CS, Toossi Z, Othieno C *et al.* Depressed T-cell interferon-gamma responses in pulmonary tuberculosis: analysis of underlying mechanisms and modulation with therapy. *J Infect Dis* 1999; **180**: 2069–73.

146. Fujiwara H, Okuda Y, Fukukawa T, Tsuyuguchi I. *In vitro* tuberculin reactivity of lymphocytes from patients with tuberculous pleurisy. *Infect Immun* 1982; **35**: 402–409.

147. Hirsch CS, Toossi Z, Johnson JL *et al.* Augmentation of apoptosis and interferon-gamma production at sites of active *Mycobacterium tuberculosis* infection in human tuberculosis. *J Infect Dis* 2001; **183**: 779–88.

148. Hirsch CS, Toossi Z, Vanham G *et al.* Apoptosis and T cell hyporesponsiveness in pulmonary tuberculosis. *J Infect Dis* 1999; **179**: 945–53.

149. Kleinhenz ME, Ellner JJ. Antigen responsiveness during tuberculosis: regulatory interactions of T cell subpopulations and adherent cells. *J Lab Clin Med* 1987; **110**: 31–40.

150. Toossi Z, Edmonds KL, Tomford JW, Ellner JJ. Suppression of purified protein derivative-induced interleukin-2 production by interaction of CD16 (Leu 11 reactive) lymphocytes and adherent mononuclear cells in tuberculosis. *J Infect Dis* 1989; **159**: 352–6.

151. Roberts T, Beyers N, Aguirre A, Walzl G. Immunosuppression during active tuberculosis is characterized by decreased interferon-gamma production and CD25 expression with elevated forkhead box P3, transforming growth factor-beta, and interleukin-4 mRNA levels. *J Infect Dis* 2007; **195**: 870–8.

152. Roper WH, Waring JJ. Primary serofibrinous pleural effusion in military personnel. *Am Rev Tuberc* 1955; **71**: 616–34.

153. Ellner JJ. Pleural fluid and peripheral blood lymphocyte function in tuberculosis. *Ann Intern Med* 1978; **89**: 932–3.

154. Fujiwara H, Tsuyuguchi I. Frequency of tuberculin-reactive T-lymphocytes in pleural fluid and blood from patients with tuberculous pleurisy. *Chest* 1986; **89**: 530–2.

155. Barnes PF, Mistry SD, Cooper CL *et al.* Compartmentalization of a CD4+ T lymphocyte subpopulation in tuberculous pleuritis. *J Immunol* 1989; **142**: 1114–19.

156. Mitra DK, Sharma SK, Dinda AK *et al.* Polarized helper T cells in tubercular pleural effusion: phenotypic identity and selective recruitment. *Eur J Immunol* 2005; **35**: 2367–75.

157. Barnes PF, Lu S, Abrams JS *et al.* Cytokine production at the site of disease in human tuberculosis. *Infect Immun* 1993; **61**: 3482–9.

158. Barnes PF, Fong SJ, Brennan PJ *et al.* Local production of tumor necrosis factor and IFN-gamma in tuberculous pleuritis. *J Immunol* 1990; **145**: 149–54.

159. Yokoyama A, Maruyama M, Ito M *et al.* Interleukin 6 activity in pleural effusion. Its diagnostic value and thrombopoietic activity. *Chest* 1992; **102**: 1055–9.

160. Zhang M, Gately MK, Wang E *et al.* Interleukin 12 at the site of disease in tuberculosis. *J Clin Invest* 1994; **93**: 1733–9.

161. Maeda J, Ueki N, Ohkawa T *et al.* Local production and localization of transforming growth factor-beta in tuberculous pleurisy. *Clin Exp Immunol* 1993; **92**: 32–8.

162. Hodsdon WS, Luzze H, Hurst TJ *et al.* HIV-1-related pleural tuberculosis: elevated production of IFN-gamma, but failure of immunity to *Mycobacterium tuberculosis*. *AIDS* 2001; **15**: 467–75.

163. Robinson DS, Ying S, Taylor IK *et al.* Evidence for a Th1-like bronchoalveolar T-cell subset and predominance of interferon-gamma gene activation in pulmonary tuberculosis. *Am J Respir Crit Care Med* 1994; **149**: 989–93.

164. Taha RA, Kotsimbos TC, Song YL *et al.* IFN-gamma and IL-12 are increased in active compared with inactive tuberculosis. *Am J Respir Crit Care Med* 1997; **155**: 1135–9.

165. Law K, Weiden M, Harkin T *et al.* Increased release of interleukin-1 beta, interleukin-6, and tumor necrosis factor-alpha by bronchoalveolar cells lavaged from involved sites in pulmonary tuberculosis. *Am J Respir Crit Care Med* 1996; **153**: 799–804.

166. Day RB, Wang Y, Knox KS *et al.* Alveolar macrophages from HIV-infected subjects are resistant to *Mycobacterium tuberculosis in vitro*. *Am J Respir Cell Mol Biol* 2004; **30**: 403–10.

167. Sadek MI, Sada E, Toossi Z *et al.* Chemokines induced by infection of mononuclear phagocytes with mycobacteria and present in lung alveoli during active pulmonary tuberculosis. *Am J Respir Cell Mol Biol* 1998; **19**: 513–21.

168. Schwander SK, Torres M, Carranza CC *et al.* Pulmonary

mononuclear cell responses to antigens of *Mycobacterium tuberculosis* in healthy household contacts of patients with active tuberculosis and healthy controls from the community. *J Immunol* 2000; 165: 1479–85.

169. Law K, Weiden M, Harkin T *et al.* Increased release of interleukin-1 beta, interleukin-6, and tumor necrosis factor-alpha by bronchoalveolar cells lavaged from involved sites in pulmonary tuberculosis. *Am J Respir Crit Care Med* 1996; 153: 799–804.

170. Vankayalapati R, Wizel B, Lakey DL *et al.* T cells enhance production of IL-18 by monocytes in response to an intracellular pathogen. *J Immunol* 2001; 166: 6749–53.

171. Zissel G, Baumer I, Schlaak M, Muller-Quernheim J. *In vitro* release of interleukin-15 by broncho-alveolar lavage cells and peripheral blood mononuclear cells from patients with different lung diseases. *Eur Cytokine Netw* 2000; 11: 105–12.

172. Bonecini-Almeida MG, Ho JL, Boechat N *et al.* Down-modulation of lung immune responses by interleukin-10 and transforming growth factor beta (TGF-beta) and analysis of TGF-beta receptors I and II in active tuberculosis. *Infect Immun* 2004; 72: 2628–34.

173. Fenton MJ, Vermeulen MW, Kim S *et al.* Induction of gamma interferon production in human alveolar macrophages by *Mycobacterium tuberculosis*. *Infect Immun* 1997; 65: 5149–56.

174. Saukkonen JJ, Bazydlo B, Thomas M *et al.* Beta-chemokines are induced by *Mycobacterium tuberculosis* and inhibit its growth. *Infect Immun* 2002; 70: 1684–93.

175. Thoma-Uszynski S, Stenger S, Takeuchi O *et al.* Induction of direct antimicrobial activity through mammalian toll-like receptors. *Science* 2001; 291: 1544–7.

176. Means TK, Wang S, Lien E *et al.* Human toll-like receptors mediate cellular activation by *Mycobacterium tuberculosis*. *J Immunol* 1999; 163: 3920–7.

177. Means TK, Jones BW, Schromm AB *et al.* Differential effects of a Toll-like receptor antagonist on *Mycobacterium tuberculosis*-induced macrophage responses. *J Immunol* 2001; 166: 4074–82.

178. Bermudez LE, Goodman J. *Mycobacterium tuberculosis* invades and replicates within type II alveolar cells. *Infect Immun* 1996; 64: 1400–6.

179. Mehta PK, King CH, White EH *et al.* Comparison of *in vitro* models for the study of *Mycobacterium tuberculosis* invasion and intracellular replication. *Infect Immun* 1996; 64: 2673–9.

180. Rivas-Santiago B, Schwander SK, Sarabia C *et al.* Human beta-defensin 2 is expressed and associated with *Mycobacterium tuberculosis* during infection of human alveolar epithelial cells. *Infect Immun* 2005; 73: 4505–11.

181. Bermudez LE, Sangari FJ, Kolonoski P *et al.* The efficiency of the translocation of *Mycobacterium tuberculosis* across a bilayer of epithelial and endothelial cells as a model of the alveolar wall is a consequence of transport within mononuclear phagocytes and invasion of alveolar epithelial cells. *Infect Immun* 2002; 70: 140–6.

182. Ulrichs T, Kosmiadi GA, Jorg S *et al.* Differential organization of the local immune response in patients with active cavitary tuberculosis or with nonprogressive tuberculoma. *J Infect Dis* 2005; 192: 89–97.

183. Ulrichs T, Kosmiadi GA, Trusov V *et al.* Human tuberculous granulomas induce peripheral lymphoid follicle-like structures to orchestrate local host defence in the lung. *J Pathol* 2004; 204: 217.

184. Bergeron A, Bonay M, Kambouchner M *et al.* Cytokine patterns in tuberculous and sarcoid granulomas: correlations with histopathologic features of the granulomatous response. *J Immunol* 1997; 159: 3034–43.

185. Toossi Z, Gogate P, Shiratsuchi H *et al.* Enhanced production of TGF-beta by blood monocytes from patients with active tuberculosis and presence of TGF-beta in tuberculous granulomatous lung lesions. *J Immunol* 1995; 154: 465–73.

186. Fenhalls G, Wong A, Bezuidenhout J *et al. In situ* production of gamma interferon, interleukin-4, and tumor necrosis factor alpha mRNA in human lung tuberculous granulomas. *Infection Immun* 2000; 68: 2827–36.

187. Agostini C, Perin A, Semenzato G. Cell apoptosis and granulomatous lung diseases. *Curr Opin Pulm Med* 1998; 4: 261–6.

188. Oddo M, Renno T, Attinger A *et al.* Fas ligand-induced apoptosis of infected human macrophages reduces the viability of intracellular *Mycobacterium tuberculosis*. *J Immunol* 1998; 160: 5448–54.

189. Pieters J, Gatfield J. Hijacking the host: survival of pathogenic mycobacteria inside macrophages. *Trends Microbiol* 2002; 10: 142–6.

190. Young D, Hussell T, Dougan G. Chronic bacterial infections: living with unwanted guests. *Nat Immunol* 2002; 3: 1026–32.

191. Chua J, Vergne I, Master S, Deretic V. A tale of two lipids: *Mycobacterium tuberculosis* phagosome maturation arrest. *Curr Opin Microbiol* 2004; 7: 71–7.

192. Kleinhenz ME, Ellner JJ, Spagnuolo PJ, Daniel TM. Suppression of lymphocyte responses by tuberculous plasma and mycobacterial arabinogalactan. Monocyte dependence and indomethacin reversibility. *J Clin Invest* 1981; 68: 153–62.

193. Kincaid EZ, Ernst JD. *Mycobacterium tuberculosis* exerts gene-selective inhibition of transcriptional responses to IFN-gamma without inhibiting STAT1 function. *J Immunol* 2003; 171: 2042–9.

194. Nagabhushanam V, Solache A, Ting LM *et al.* Innate inhibition of adaptive immunity: *Mycobacterium tuberculosis*-induced IL-6 inhibits macrophage responses to IFN-gamma. *J Immunol* 2003; 171: 4750–7.

195. Fortune SM, Solache A, Jaeger A *et al. Mycobacterium tuberculosis* inhibits macrophage responses to IFN-gamma through myeloid differentiation factor 88-dependent and -independent mechanisms. *J Immunol* 2004; 172: 6272–80.

196. Noss EH, Pai RK, Sellati TJ *et al.* Toll-like receptor 2-dependent inhibition of macrophage class II MHC expression and antigen processing by 19-kDa lipoprotein of *Mycobacterium tuberculosis*. *J Immunol* 2001; 167: 910–18.

197. Pennini ME, Pai RK, Schultz DC *et al. Mycobacterium tuberculosis* 19-kDa lipoprotein inhibits IFN-gamma-induced chromatin remodeling of MHC2TA by TLR2 and MAPK signaling. *J Immunol* 2006; 176: 4323–30.

198. Pai RK, Convery M, Hamilton TA *et al.* Inhibition of IFN-gamma-induced class II transactivator expression by a 19-kDa lipoprotein from *Mycobacterium tuberculosis*: a potential mechanism for immune evasion. *J Immunol* 2003; 171: 175–84.

199. Gehring AJ, Rojas RE, Canaday DH *et al.* The *Mycobacterium tuberculosis* 19-kilodalton lipoprotein inhibits gamma interferon-regulated HLA-DR and Fc gamma R1 on human macrophages through Toll-like receptor 2. *Infect Immun* 2003; 71: 4487–97.

200. Gehring AJ, Dobos KM, Belisle JT *et al. Mycobacterium tuberculosis* LprG (Rv1411c): a novel TLR-2 ligand that inhibits human macrophage class II MHC antigen processing. *J Immunol* 2004; 173: 2660–8.

201. Hanekom WA, Mendillo M, Manca C *et al. Mycobacterium tuberculosis* inhibits maturation of human monocyte-derived dendritic cells in vitro. *J Infect Dis* 2003; 188: 257–66.

202. Geijtenbeek TB, Van Vliet SJ, Koppel EA *et al.* Mycobacteria target DC-SIGN to suppress dendritic cell function. *J Exp Med* 2003; 197: 7–17.

203. Van Kooyk Y, Geijtenbeek TB. DC-SIGN: escape mechanism for pathogens. *Nat Rev Immunol* 2003; 3: 697–709.

204. Manca C, Tsenova L, Barry CE *et al. Mycobacterium tuberculosis* CDC1551 induces a more vigorous host response *in vivo* and *in vitro*, but is not more virulent than other clinical isolates. *J Immunol* 1999; 162: 6740–6.

205. Engele M, Stossel E, Castiglione K *et al.* Induction of TNF in human alveolar macrophages as a potential evasion mechanism of virulent *Mycobacterium tuberculosis*. *J Immunol* 2002; 168: 1328–37.

206. Janulionis E, Sofer C, Schwander SK *et al.* Survival and replication

of clinical *Mycobacterium tuberculosis* isolates in the context of human innate immunity. *Infect Immun* 2005; **73**: 2595–601.

207. Reed MB, Domenech P, Manca C et al. A glycolipid of hypervirulent tuberculosis strains that inhibits the innate immune response. *Nature* 2004; **431**: 84–7.

208. Comstock GW. Tuberculosis in twins: a re-analysis of the Prophit survey. *Am Rev Respir Dis* 1978; **117**: 621–4.

209. Bellamy R, Beyers N, McAdam KP et al. Genetic susceptibility to tuberculosis in Africans: a genome-wide scan. *Proc Nat Acad Sci U S A* 2000; **97**: 8005–9.

210. Amirzargar AA, Yalda A, Hajabolbaghi M et al. The association of HLA-DRB, DQA1, DQB1 alleles and haplotype frequency in Iranian patients with pulmonary tuberculosis. *Int J Tuberc Lung Dis* 2004; **8**: 1017–21.

211. Ravikumar M, Dheenadhayalan V, Rajaram K et al. Associations of HLA-DRB1, DQB1 and DPB1 alleles with pulmonary tuberculosis in south India. *Tuberc Lung Dis* 1999; **79**: 309–17.

212. Goldfeld AE, Delgado JC, Thim S et al. Association of an HLA-DQ allele with clinical tuberculosis. *J Am Med Assoc* 1998; **279**: 226–8.

213. Lopez-Maderuelo D, Arnalich F, Serantes R et al. Interferon-gamma and interleukin-10 gene polymorphisms in pulmonary tuberculosis. *Am J Respir Crit Care Med* 2003; **167**: 970–5.

214. Lio D, Marino V, Serauto A et al. Genotype frequencies of the +874T–>A single nucleotide polymorphism in the first intron of the interferon-gamma gene in a sample of Sicilian patients affected by tuberculosis. *Eur J Immunogenet* 2002; **29**: 371–4.

215. Cervino AC, Lakiss S, Sow O, Hill AV. Allelic association between the NRAMP1 gene and susceptibility to tuberculosis in Guinea-Conakry. *Ann Hum Genet* 2000; **64**: 507–12.

216. Bellamy R, Ruwende C, Corrah T et al. Variations in the NRAMP1 gene and susceptibility to tuberculosis in West Africans. *N Engl J Med* 1998; **338**: 640–4.

217. Soborg C, Andersen AB, Madsen HO et al. Natural resistance-associated macrophage protein 1 polymorphisms are associated with microscopy-positive tuberculosis. *J Infect Dis* 2002; **186**: 517–21.

218. Stein CM, Guwatudde D, Nakakeeto M et al. Heritability analysis of cytokines as intermediate phenotypes of tuberculosis. *J Infect Dis* 2003; **187**: 1679–85.

219. Fenhalls G, Stevens L, Moses L et al. In situ detection of *Mycobacterium tuberculosis* transcripts in human lung granulomas reveals differential gene expression in necrotic lesions. *Infect Immun* 2002; **70**: 6330–8.

220. Selvaraj P, Narayanan PR, Reetha AM. Association of functional mutant homozygotes of the mannose binding protein gene with susceptibility to pulmonary tuberculosis in India. *Tuberc Lung Dis* 1999; **79**: 221–7.

221. El Sahly HM, Reich RA, Dou SJ et al. The effect of mannose binding lectin gene polymorphisms on susceptibility to tuberculosis in different ethnic groups. *Scand J Infect Dis* 2004; **36**: 106–8.

222. Fraser DA, Bulat-Kardum L, Knezevic J et al. Interferon-gamma receptor-1 gene polymorphism in tuberculosis patients from Croatia. *Scand J Immunol* 2003; **57**: 480–4.

223. Ogus AC, Yoldas B, Ozdemir T et al. The Arg753GLn polymorphism of the human toll-like receptor 2 gene in tuberculosis disease. *Eur Respir J* 2004; **23**: 219–23.

224. Ben Ali M, Barbouche MR, Bousnina S et al. Toll-like receptor 2 Arg677Trp polymorphism is associated with susceptibility to tuberculosis in Tunisian patients. *Clin Diagn Lab Immunol* 2004; **11**: 625–6.

225. Bornman L, Campbell SJ, Fielding K et al. Vitamin D receptor polymorphisms and susceptibility to tuberculosis in West Africa: a case–control and family study. *J Infect Dis* 2004; **190**: 1631–41.

226. Wilkinson RJ, Llewelyn M, Toossi Z et al. Influence of vitamin D deficiency and vitamin D receptor polymorphisms on tuberculosis among Gujarati Asians in west London: a case–control study. *Lancet* 2000; **355**: 618–21.

227. Bellamy R, Ruwende C, Corrah T et al. Tuberculosis and chronic hepatitis B virus infection in Africans and variation in the vitamin D receptor gene. *J Infect Dis* 1999; **179**: 721–4.

228. Wilkinson RJ, Patel P, Llewelyn M et al. Influence of polymorphism in the genes for the interleukin (IL)-1 receptor antagonist and IL-1beta on tuberculosis. *J Exp Med* 1999; **189**: 1863–74.

229. Bellamy R, Ruwende C, Corrah T et al. Assessment of the interleukin 1 gene cluster and other candidate gene polymorphisms in host susceptibility to tuberculosis. *Tuberc Lung Dis* 1998; **79**: 83–9.

230. de Jong R, Altare F, Haagen IA et al. Severe mycobacterial and *Salmonella* infections in interleukin-12 receptor-deficient patients. *Science* 1998; **280**: 1435–8.

231. Altare F, Lammas D, Revy P et al. Inherited interleukin 12 deficiency in a child with bacille Calmette–Guérin and *Salmonella enteritidis* disseminated infection. *J Clin Invest* 1998; **102**: 2035–40.

232. Altare F, Durandy A, Lammas D et al. Impairment of mycobacterial immunity in human interleukin-12 receptor deficiency. *Science* 1998; **280**: 1432–5.

233. Dorman SE, Holland SM. Interferon-gamma and interleukin-12 pathway defects and human disease. *Cytokine Growth Factor Rev* 2000; **11**: 321–33.

234. Jouanguy E, Altare F, Lamhamedi S et al. Interferon-gamma-receptor deficiency in an infant with fatal bacille Calmette–Guérin infection. *N Engl J Med* 1996; **335**: 1956–61.

235. Jouanguy E, Lamhamedi-Cherradi S, Lammas D et al. A human IFNGR1 small deletion hotspot associated with dominant susceptibility to mycobacterial infection. *Nat Genet* 1999; **21**: 370–8.

236. Newport MJ, Huxley CM, Huston S et al. A mutation in the interferon-gamma-receptor gene and susceptibility to mycobacterial infection. *N Engl J Med* 1996; **335**: 1941–9.

237. Altare F, Jouanguy E, Lamhamedi-Cherradi S et al. A causative relationship between mutant IFNgR1 alleles and impaired cellular response to IFNgamma in a compound heterozygous child. *Am J Hum Genet* 1998; **62**: 723–6.

238. Holland SM, Dorman SE, Kwon A et al. Abnormal regulation of interferon-gamma, interleukin-12, and tumor necrosis factor-alpha in human interferon-gamma receptor 1 deficiency. *J Infect Dis* 1998; **178**: 1095–104.

239. Selwyn PA, Hartel D, Lewis VA et al. A prospective study of the risk of tuberculosis among intravenous drug users with human immunodeficiency virus infection. *N Engl J Med* 1989; **320**: 545–50.

240. Tuberculosis and AIDS – Connecticut. *MMWR Morb Mortal Wkly Rep* 1987; **36**: 133–5.

241. Sonnenberg P, Murray J, Glynn JR et al. HIV-1 and recurrence, relapse, and reinfection of tuberculosis after cure: a cohort study in South African mineworkers. *Lancet* 2001; **358**: 1687–93.

242. Di Perri G, Cruciani M, Danzi MC et al. Nosocomial epidemic of active tuberculosis among HIV-infected patients. *Lancet* 1989; **2**: 1502–4.

243. Small PM, Schecter GF, Goodman PC et al. Treatment of tuberculosis in patients with advanced human immunodeficiency virus infection. *N Engl J Med* 1991; **324**: 289–94.

244. Lucas SB, Hounnou A, Peacock C et al. The mortality and pathology of HIV infection in a west African city. *AIDS* 1993; **7**: 1569–79.

245. Di Perri G, Cazzadori A, Vento S et al. Comparative histopathological study of pulmonary tuberculosis in human immunodeficiency virus-infected and non-infected patients. *Tuberc Lung Dis* 1996; **77**: 244–9.

246. Toossi Z, Mayanja-Kizza H, Hirsch CS et al. Impact of tuberculosis (TB) on HIV-1 activity in dually infected patients. *Clin Exp Immunol* 2001; **123**: 233–8.

247. Mayanja-Kizza H, Johnson JL, Hirsch CS et al. Macrophage-

activating cytokines in human immununodeficiency virus type 1-infected and -uninfected patients with pulmonary tuberculosis. *J Infect Dis* 2001; **183**: 1805–9.

248. Elliott AM, Hodsdon WS, Kyosiimire J *et al.* Cytokine responses and progression to active tuberculosis in HIV-1-infected Ugandans: a prospective study. *Trans R Soc Trop Med Hyg* 2004; **98**: 660–70.

249. Aandahl EM, Michaelsson J, Moretto WJ *et al.* Human CD4+ CD25+ regulatory T cells control T-cell responses to human immunodeficiency virus and cytomegalovirus antigens. *J Virol* 2004; **78**: 2454–9.

250. Zhang M, Gong J, Iyer DV *et al.* T cell cytokine responses in people with tuberculosis and human immunodeficiency virus infection. *J Clin Invest* 1994; **94**: 2435–42.

251. Wallis RS, Vjecha M, Amir-Tahmasseb M *et al.* Influence of tuberculosis on human immunodeficiency virus (HIV-1): enhanced cytokine expression and elevated beta 2-microglobulin in HIV-1-associated tuberculosis. *J Infect Dis* 1993; **167**: 43–8.

252. Toossi Z, Sierra-Madero JG, Blinkhorn RA *et al.* Enhanced susceptibility of blood monocytes from patients with pulmonary tuberculosis to productive infection with human immunodeficiency virus type 1. *J Exp Med* 1993; **177**: 1511–16.

253. Toossi Z, Xia L, Wu M, Salvekar A. Transcriptional activation of HIV by *Mycobacterium tuberculosis* in human monocytes. *Clin Exp Immunol* 1999; **117**: 324–30.

254. Lederman MM, Georges DL, Kusner DJ *et al.* *Mycobacterium tuberculosis* and its purified protein derivative activate expression of the human immunodeficiency virus. *J Acquir Immune Defic Syndr* 1994; **7**: 727–33.

255. Imperiali FG, Zaninoni A, La Maestra L *et al.* Increased *Mycobacterium tuberculosis* growth in HIV-1-infected human macrophages: role of tumour necrosis factor-alpha. *Clin Exp Immunol* 2001; **123**: 435–42.

256. Kampmann B, Tena-Coki GN, Nicol MP *et al.* Reconstitution of antimycobacterial immune responses in HIV-infected children receiving HAART. *AIDS* 2006; **20**: 1011–18.

257. Kindler V, Sappino AP, Grau GE *et al.* The inducing role of tumor necrosis factor in the development of bactericidal granulomas during BCG infection. *Cell* 1989; **56**: 731–40.

258. Flynn JL, Goldstein MM, Chan J *et al.* Tumor necrosis factor-alpha is required in the protective immune response against *Mycobacterium tuberculosis* in mice. *Immunity* 1995; **2**: 561–72.

259. Zganiacz A, Santosuosso M, Wang J *et al.* TNF-alpha is a critical negative regulator of type 1 immune activation during intracellular bacterial infection. *J Clin Invest* 2004; **113**: 401–13.

260. Smith S, Liggitt D, Jeromsky E *et al.* Local role for tumor necrosis factor alpha in the pulmonary inflammatory response to *Mycobacterium tuberculosis* infection. *Infect Immun* 2002; **70**: 2082–9.

261. Algood HM, Lin PL, Yankura D *et al.* TNF influences chemokine expression of macrophages *in vitro* and that of CD11b+ cells *in vivo* during *Mycobacterium tuberculosis* infection. *J Immunol* 2004; **172**: 6846–57.

262. Mohan VP, Scanga CA, Yu K *et al.* Effects of tumor necrosis factor alpha on host immune response in chronic persistent tuberculosis: possible role for limiting pathology. *Infect Immun* 2001; **69**: 1847–55.

263. Keane J, Gershon S, Wise RP *et al.* Tuberculosis associated with infliximab, a tumor necrosis factor alpha-neutralizing agent. *N Engl J Med* 2001; **345**: 1098–104.

264. Tuberculosis associated with blocking agents against tumor necrosis factor-alpha – California, 2002–2003. *J Am Med Assoc* 2004; **292**: 1676–8.

265. Winthrop KL, Siegel JN. Tuberculosis cases associated with infliximab and etanercept. *Clin Infect Dis* 2004; **39**: 1256–7.

266. Wallis RS, Broder MS, Wong JY *et al.* Granulomatous infectious diseases associated with tumor necrosis factor antagonists. *Clin Infect Dis* 2004; **38**: 1261–5.

267. Keane J. Tumor necrosis factor blockers and reactivation of latent tuberculosis. *Clin Infect Dis* 2004; **39**: 300–2.

268. Mohan AK, Cote TR, Block JA *et al.* Tuberculosis following the use of etanercept, a tumor necrosis factor inhibitor. *Clin Infect Dis* 2004; **39**: 295–9.

269. Saliu OY, Sofer C, Stein DS *et al.* Tumor-necrosis-factor blockers: differential effects on mycobacterial immunity. *J Infect Dis* 2006; **194**: 486–92.

270. Lawn SD, Bekker LG, Miller RF. Immune reconstitution disease associated with mycobacterial infections in HIV-infected individuals receiving antiretrovirals. *Lancet Infect Dis* 2005; **5**: 361–73.

271. Shelburne SA, Visnegarwala F, Darcourt J *et al.* Incidence and risk factors for immune reconstitution inflammatory syndrome during highly active antiretroviral therapy. *AIDS* 2005; **19**: 399–406.

272. Michailidis C, Pozniak AL, Mandalia S *et al.* Clinical characteristics of IRIS syndrome in patients with HIV and tuberculosis. *Antivir Ther* 2005; **10**: 417–22.

273. Breton G, Duval X, Estellat C *et al.* Determinants of immune reconstitution inflammatory syndrome in HIV type 1-infected patients with tuberculosis after initiation of antiretroviral therapy. *Clin Infect Dis* 2004; **39**: 1709–12.

274. Ordway DJ, Costa L, Martins M *et al.* Increased interleukin-4 production by CD8 and gammadelta T cells in health-care workers is associated with the subsequent development of active tuberculosis. *J Infect Dis* 2004; **190**: 756–66.

275. Carcelain G, Debre P, Autran B. Reconstitution of CD4+ T lymphocytes in HIV-infected individuals following antiretroviral therapy. *Curr Opin Immunol* 2001; **13**: 483–8.

276. Lederman MM. Immune restoration and CD4+ T-cell function with antiretroviral therapies. *AIDS* 2001; **15** (Suppl. 2): S11–S15.

277. Hengel RL, Allende MC, Dewar RL *et al.* Increasing CD4+ T cells specific for tuberculosis correlate with improved clinical immunity after highly active antiretroviral therapy. *AIDS Res Hum Retrovir* 2002; **18**: 969–75.

278. Grode L, Seiler P, Baumann S *et al.* Increased vaccine efficacy against tuberculosis of recombinant *Mycobacterium bovis* bacille Calmette–Guérin mutants that secrete listeriolysin. *J Clin Invest* 2005; **115**: 2472–9.

279. Hess J, Miko D, Catic A *et al. Mycobacterium bovis* bacille Calmette–Guérin strains secreting listeriolysin of *Listeria monocytogenes. Proc Natl Acad Sci U S A* 1998; **95**: 5299–304.

280. Horwitz MA, Harth G, Dillon BJ, Maslesa-Galic S. Recombinant bacillus Calmette–Guérin (BCG) vaccines expressing the *Mycobacterium tuberculosis* 30-kDa major secretory protein induce greater protective immunity against tuberculosis than conventional BCG vaccines in a highly susceptible animal model. *Proc Natl Acad Sci U S A* 2000; **97**: 13853–8.

281. Horwitz MA, Harth G, Dillon BJ, Maslesa-Galic S. Enhancing the protective efficacy of *Mycobacterium bovis* BCG vaccination against tuberculosis by boosting with the *Mycobacterium tuberculosis* major secretory protein. *Infect Immun* 2005; **73**: 4676–83.

282. Dietrich J, Aagaard C, Leah R *et al.* Exchanging ESAT6 with TB10.4 in an Ag85B fusion molecule-based tuberculosis subunit vaccine: efficient protection and ESAT6-based sensitive monitoring of vaccine efficacy. *J Immunol* 2005; **174**: 6332–39.

283. Ibanga HB, Brookes RH, Hill PC *et al.* Early clinical trials with a new tuberculosis vaccine, MVA85A, in tuberculosis-endemic countries: issues in study design. *Lancet Infect Dis* 2006; **6**: 522–8.

284. McShane H, Pathan AA, Sander CR *et al.* Boosting BCG with MVA85A: the first candidate subunit vaccine for tuberculosis in clinical trials. *Tuberculosis (Edinb)* 2005; **85**: 47–52.

PART 3

CLINICAL ASPECTS

9

Respiratory tuberculosis

STEPHEN GORDON AND HENRY MWANDUMBA

INTRODUCTION

Tuberculosis is disease caused by infection with mycobacteria from the *Mycobacteria tuberculosis* complex. Nearly one-third of the world's population (1.8 billion from a total of 6.5 billion people) are estimated to be infected with *M. tuberculosis*, but the majority do not develop symptoms of disease.[1] Disease develops in 8–10 million new cases per year, resulting in 2–3 million deaths.[2] *M. tuberculosis* can cause disease in any organ of the body, but infection of the lung is of overarching importance.[3] This is because all of the transmission of infection and the vast majority of the deaths due to tuberculosis occur as a result of pulmonary infection.[4] An understanding of pulmonary tuberculosis, once known as consumption and described by John Bunyan in the seventeenth century as 'the captain of all these men of death',[5] is therefore central to the diagnosis, treatment and prevention of tuberculosis.

DEFINITIONS

Tuberculosis infection is infection with mycobacteria from the *M. tuberculosis* complex comprising *Mycobacterium tuberculosis*, *Mycobacterium bovis*, *Mycobacterium africanum* and *Mycobacterium microti*.[6] Infection does not necessarily lead to disease (discussed below). Environmental mycobacteria may also infect humans, particularly those with damaged lungs or immunodeficiency. These infections may be tissue damaging, particularly in the lung, but are not contagious and are described in detail in Chapter 29, Environmental mycobacteria.

Respiratory tuberculosis is defined as active infection of the lungs, pleural cavity, mediastinal lymph nodes or larynx.[7]

Pulmonary tuberculosis is defined as active infection of the lungs; extrapulmonary tuberculosis is infection of any other organ. Pulmonary infections are critically important because they may be highly contagious as well as being life-threatening to the affected patient. Extrapulmonary infections are less common and are not highly contagious.

Primary disease is active tuberculosis infection in an immunologically naive patient. In endemic areas, primary tuberculosis is found in children,[8] but in areas of low tuberculosis prevalence, primary disease is often seen in adults. Primary disease is often mild or asymptomatic.

Post-primary disease is active tuberculosis infection in patients who have been previously exposed to tuberculosis infection. Post-primary disease forms the bulk of the world's symptomatic infections[1] and is characterized by substantial tissue damage. It can be caused by reactivation of the primary infection or by exogeneous reinfection (a second infection).

A case of tuberculosis is a person infected with *M. tuberculosis*. The case definition varies according to available technology in different regions of the world. In Europe, a 'definite case' is defined as 'a case with culture-confirmed disease caused by *M. tuberculosis* complex'.[7] In the many parts of the world where mycobacterial culture is not possible, other case definitions are employed using identification of mycobacteria in clinical samples with

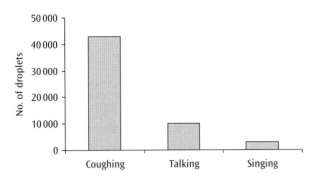

Figure 9.1 Number of droplets produced by various aerosol-generating manoeuvres (reproduced from Loudon RG, Roberts RM. Singing and the dissemination of tuberculosis. *Am Rev Respir Dis* 1968; **98**: 297–300. © American Thoracic Society).

smear microscopy using Ziehl–Neelsen staining.[9] Culture is the gold standard in diagnosis because it allows the accurate exclusion of environmental mycobacteria.

TRANSMISSION OF TUBERCULOSIS

Tuberculosis is a disease of humans typically spread by droplets from person to person.[10] Patients with pulmonary disease generate infective aerosols comprising a large number of infected droplets particularly by coughing, but also by sneezing, singing, talking and breathing[11] (see Figure 9.1).

Droplet size is critical in infection as transmission most often occurs when infected droplets of respirable size (approximately 1 μm diameter) are inspired and retained in the alveoli of a susceptible host. Approximately six mycobacteria are carried by each respirable droplet to the level of the alveolus.[12] Mycobacteria enter alveolar macrophages of the host by active uptake using complement and other receptors.[13–15] The internalized mycobacteria then alter the macrophage phagosome to make that environment less hostile and prevent mycobacterial killing.[16] Mycobacteria then replicate intracellularly and successful mycobacterial replication eventually results in macrophage death, cell rupture and the release of new mycobacteria to set up a focus of pulmonary infection in the alveolus. Alternatively, mycobacteria may impact with tonsillar tissue or laryngeal tissue and set up infection in macrophage cell populations there, but this is normally a complication of pulmonary infection. Laboratory aerosols are hazardous due to the extremely low infective dose required to acquire tuberculosis infection.[12] Parenteral injection of mycobacteria can also result in infection by haematogenous or lymphatic spread of mycobacteria to tissue macrophages, but this is very rare.

RISK FACTORS FOR INFECTION

Risk factors for droplet transmission and hence infection include close contact between a person with tuberculosis

and susceptible others. The likelihood of infection increases with increased duration and intensity of exposure. This association has been clearly demonstrated for crowded housing,[17] but has also been documented in detail during the enforced close proximity of air travel.[18] Droplets are rendered sterile by ultraviolet radiation and so sunshine reduces transmission,[19] as do appropriate protective masks. Unfortunately, these conditions do not pertain in the cramped conditions under which miners[20,21] or prison inmates[22] live and these populations suffer particularly high transmission rates of tuberculosis.

Impaired host immunity

Certain lifestyles predispose exposed people to tuberculosis infection. These include factors that reduce host immunity. Globally, the most important acquired immune deficiency is that related to HIV infection (see Chapter 18, DOTS and DOTS plus, and Chapter 19, The association between HIV and tuberculosis in the developing world).[23] Malnutrition also results in impaired cellular responses to mycobacterial antigens, as well as reduced immunoglobulins and innate immune factors.[24] Excessive alcohol consumption has been shown to acutely impair alveolar macrophage function, as well as producing a fall in immunoglobulin when end-stage liver disease occurs. Exposure to cigarette[25] and other smokes, including cooking smoke,[26] from consumption of biomass fuels (burned organic material) increase the risk of tuberculosis in adults and children. An important environmental risk factor in some communities is the effect of inhaled dust. Silicosis, asbestosis and anthracosis are all associated with increased rates of tuberculosis infection.[27]

Host genetics

Genetics has been shown to have an important role in host defence. There is a critical role for both interleukin 12 (IL-12), interferon gamma (IFN-γ) and tumour necrosis factor (TNF) in the formation and function of the tuberculous granuloma. Families with polymorphisms of either IL-12,[28] IFN-γ,[29] TNF[30] or their receptors have excessive susceptibility to mycobacterial infections (usually detected by excessive susceptibility to bacillus Calmette–Guérin (BCG) disease). At a community level, these families result in an insignificant number of cases of tuberculosis, but careful study of the immune deficiency resulting from their genetic polymorphisms has allowed major advances in our understanding of the pathogenesis of tuberculosis.[31]

Immunosuppressive and immunomodulatory drugs

Immune modulation is a rapidly expanding arm of the therapeutic armamentarium in developed countries. In

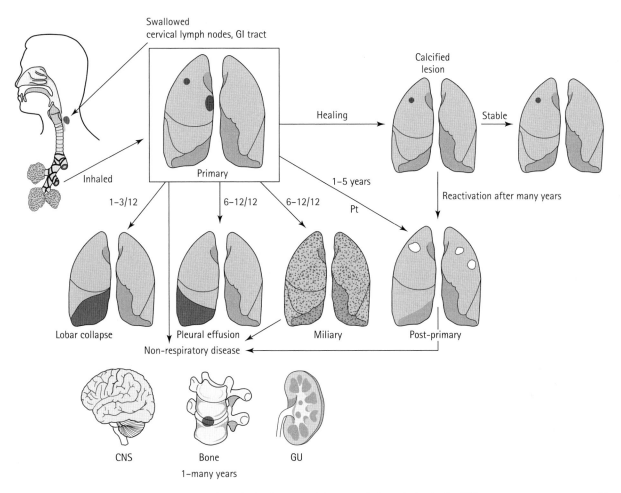

Figure 9.2   Diagram of the development of tuberculosis disease and its spread through the body. CNS, central nervous system; GI, gastrointestinal; GU, genitourinary.

particular, the selective immune deficiency induced by TNF antagonist medication (Infliximab) used for rheumatoid disease and seronegative arthropathies has resulted in exquisite susceptibility to tuberculosis in treated patients.[32] This has led to guidelines suggesting that patients contemplating this treatment should be fully evaluated for latent tuberculosis and treated with 6 months of antituberculous chemotherapy in case of doubt.[33] Similarly, corticosteroids reduce cell-mediated immunity and can result in dramatically increased mycobacterial replication in latently infected patients.[34] Cyclosporin usage has resulted in tuberculosis in 12–20 per cent of Pakistani renal transplant patients.[35]

Close contact with individuals with active tuberculosis

In the UK, the single most important risk factor for acquisition of tuberculosis is contact with a person who has active tuberculosis, particularly sputum smear-positive (open) pulmonary tuberculosis. The most affected groups are those with recent travel to highly endemic areas or con-

tact with family members recently arrived from endemic areas.[36] Among the UK white population, the most affected age group are the elderly as they experienced high exposure early in life and now develop reactivation disease, due to the waning cell-mediated immunity associated with old age.

INFECTION, LATENT INFECTION AND DISEASE IN TUBERCULOSIS

When considering the epidemiology, pathogenesis, diagnosis or treatment of tuberculosis, it is important to bear in mind the distinction between infection and disease (Figure 9.2).[37] Primary infection is frequently asymptomatic and is an immunizing event.[38] There are good data, however, to suggest that in many cases the successful resolution of primary infection, while immunizing, is not sterilizing. Post-mortem studies from populations with high tuberculosis prevalence rates showed that viable mycobacteria could be recovered from 50 per cent of normal lung samples from patients dying of a cause other than tuberculosis.[39] This finding has been recently replicated when polymerase chain reaction (PCR) analysis was applied to normal lung tissue obtained at post-mortem in Ethiopia, Mexico and Norway.[40] Among Ethiopian and Mexican samples, a high percentage of samples from histologically normal lung had positive PCR detection of *M. tuberculosis* DNA. The implication of both the traditional and molecular microbiology results is that surveillance immune functions control primary infection, but without necessarily killing all of the mycobacteria, even outside the classical granuloma and in the absence of any detectable inflammation.[41] One hypothesis to explain this observation is that patrolling antigen-specific T-lymphocytes maintain appropriate local macrophage activation to contain any infection.[42]

Disease, characterized by unchecked mycobacterial replication, tissue damage[43] and concomitant symptoms, occurs when immune surveillance fails.[44] Clearly, disease can occur when primary host defence fails as discussed above, or when a new exogeneous mycobacterial infection that can evade the host immune response occurs. Importantly, however, disease can also occur when the stable immune surveillance of viable bacteria (this state is often called 'latent infection') fails due to immunodeficiency in the host.[45] This type of host immunodeficiency can be congenital or acquired. Acquired immunodeficiency is more common and is associated with malnutrition,[46] old age, HIV infection,[47] cytotoxic and anti-inflammatory medication (discussed further below). Congenital immunodeficiency leading to specific susceptibility to disease by non-tuberculous mycobacteria and *Mycobacterium bovis* BCG is found in families with polymorphism of IL-12, IFN-γ or the receptors for either cytokine,[31] and may be relevant to *M. tuberculosis* infection.

CLINICAL FEATURES OF PRIMARY INFECTION

Epidemiology

Primary infection typically occurs in children in the developing world.[48,49] In the developed world, where the prevalence of tuberculosis is low, primary infection often occurs in elderly people (greater than 65 years of age)[50] and in immunocompromised patients who were not exposed to tuberculosis as children.[51]

Pathogenesis

Primary infection in children and immunocompetent adults is usually contained by appropriate activation of cellular host immunity. Antigen presentation of proteins derived from *M. tuberculosis* antigens by MHC class I and class II mechanisms results in production and activation of antigen-specific T lymphocytes.[52] These lymphocytes surround infected macrophages and activate the macrophages in an IL-12, IFN-γ and TNF-dependent manner. Activated

macrophages and lymphocytes together form the classical histological structure associated with tuberculosis – the granuloma (see Chapter 6, Immunodiagnostic tests, and Chapter 7, Histopathology). Mycobacteria within the granuloma are either killed or contained in a non-replicating state.

Typical clinical outcome

In the vast majority of cases of primary infection, the containment of primary infection by the mechanism described above is asymptomatic.[53] The initial focus of infection becomes infiltrated with lymphocytes and activated macrophages. Ipsilateral hilar lymph nodes (site of antigen presentation) become enlarged. The combination of a peripheral lung infection (85 per cent within 1 cm of the pleural surface) and enlarged lymph nodes is then called a Ghon complex (Figure 9.2). Successful containment of the infection may result in residual scarring of the primary lung infection site and calcification after some years (Ghon focus). The clinical diagnosis of primary infection is therefore made on the basis of an altered skin test and radiological features of lymphadenopathy or middle and lower lobe infiltration.[7,54] Approximately 90 per cent of cases will have hilar or paratracheal lymphadenopathy.[51] Less than one quarter of primary infections occur in the upper lobe, presumably due to the dependent distribution of inhaled particulates.[55]

Progressive primary disease

In a small proportion of cases, this proportion being greater among susceptible adults than among children, primary infection is not immediately contained, and mycobacterial replication continues in the lung. This results in progressive pulmonary pathology, local (respiratory) spread and proliferation outside the respiratory system[54] within 2 years of primary infection.[56]

Progressive primary disease in the lung is characterized by further 'soft' (poorly defined margins) infiltrates seen on the chest x-ray,[57,58] together with symptoms of cough, fever, haemoptysis or weight loss often diagnosed initially as acute pneumonia. The correct diagnosis must be achieved by microscopy and culture of the sputum.[7]

Primary disease may involve the pleura and result in unilateral pleural effusion with seeding of mycobacteria on to the infected pleural surface.[59] Pleural fluid rarely shows mycobacteria on microscopy, but culture is positive in 20 per cent of cases and the culture-positive rate is substantially increased by the addition of pleural biopsy.[55] Modern video-assisted thorascopic surgery (VATS) techiques allow direct visualization of the pleural surface and biopsy of nodules seen. In a study by Sakuraba *et al.*,[60] a combination of pleural fluid and pleural biopsies obtained by VATS successfully diagnosed pleural TB by bacteriological and histological examination in 93.8 per cent of the patients recruited to the study compared with 18.8 per cent of patients in whom pleural TB was diagnosed by bacteriological examination of pleural fluid obtained by thoracocentesis.

Mycobacteria are transported to the hilar lymph nodes both intracellularly in lung macrophages, and free in the lymphatics within 16 hours in experimental animal infections.[61] Lymphatic spread can result in further clinical presentations including lymph node tuberculosis. The cervical lymph nodes are commonly infected (scrofula); the enlarged nodes eventually undergo caseous necrosis and may even rupture on to the skin as cold abscesses.

Haematogenous spread of mycobacteria occurs directly from the primary infection site. This can result in seeding of mycobacteria to the meninges, pleura, abdominal cavity, bones, kidneys, adrenal glands and eyes.[62] The specific features of non-respiratory tuberculosis are discussed in Chapter 10, Non-respiratory tuberculosis.

Tuberculin conversion

When antigen-specific lymphocyte responses develop, the patient becomes reactive to skin testing with mycobacterial proteins (Mantoux and Heaf tests are discussed in more detail in Chapter 5, The diagnosis of tuberculosis). Interferon gamma can also be detected in blood samples challenged with mycobacterial protein in the laboratory (discussed in Chapter 6, Immunodiagnostic tests). This tuberculin conversion typically occurs 3–6 weeks after the initial infection. It must be stressed that the best method of diagnosis is culture of the organism from an infected clinical sample, usually sputum.[7]

Hypersensitivity phenomena

Coincident with the development of tuberculin conversion, patients may develop erythema nodosum (Figure 9.3). These are raised, painful red or brown dermal swellings, often present on the shins or extensor surface of the forearms. They are usually 3–12 cm in diameter and are easily seen in white or brown skin, but difficult to see in black skin. The lesions are caused by perivascular inflammation, probably by an immune complex deposition mechanism rather than due to antigen-specific T lymphocytes. Erythema nodosum is not exclusive to TB and may occur in sarcoidosis, autoimmune diseases, including rheumatoid disease and systemic lupus erythematosus (SLE), connective tissue diseases, streptococcal infection, drug reactions and inflammatory bowel disease.[63]

Another hypersensitivity phenomenon associated with primary disease is phlyctenular conjunctivitis (Figure 9.4). This appears as small grey or yellow nodules on the conjunctiva near the limbus with dilated vessels radiating outwards. The lesions can result in pain, irritation, lacrima-

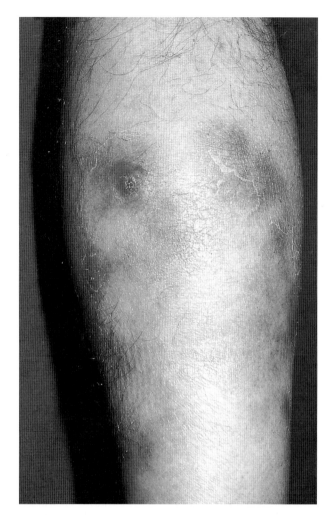

Figure 9.3 View of patient's shins showing erythema nodosum.

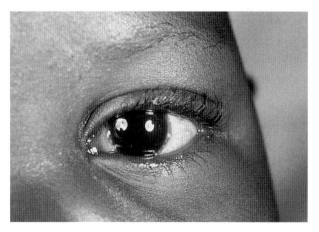

Figure 9.4 Phlyctenular conjunctivitis in an African infant.

tion and photophobia, and may be treated with topical steroids. In chronic cases, ophthalmological advice should be sought as differential diagnoses, including *Chlamydia* co-infection and steroid-dependent corneal inflammation, require alternative management.[64]

Complications of primary disease

Primary tuberculosis may be complicated by collapse of a lobe due to external pressure on the bronchus by enlarged peribronchial lymph nodes. Right middle lobe bronchiectasis as a late sequela of primary tuberculosis is known as Brock's syndrome or middle lobe syndrome and can be successfully managed with surgical resection of the affected lobe.[65]

Pleural effusion may complicate primary disease, particularly in patients with concurrent HIV infection (see Chapter 18, DOTS and DOTS plus). In this case, the pleural seeding with mycobacteria occurs by haematogenous spread and parenchymal lung infection is not usually a feature. Diagnosis may present a problem but standard antituberculous treatment is effective and chest drainage is not usually necessary.

Radiology of primary tuberculosis

Radiologically, primary respiratory tuberculosis can be divided into parenchymal disease, lymphadenopathy, pleural effusion and miliary disease.[66]

Parenchymal lung changes are homogeneous, dense opacities with ill-defined borders. There is a predilection for the right side (more lung) and although cavitation can occur, it is uncommon.[67,68] A lobar distribution with enlargement of the lobe may be seen. Parenchymal changes resolve in 6–24 months after appropriate therapy.

Lymphadenopathy is the defining feature of primary tuberculosis. The radiological appearance is of paratracheal and hilar lymph node enlargement, much better seen on computed tomography (CT) scanning than on chest x-ray. Unilateral hilar or paratracheal enlargement is common, again showing a predilection for the right side.[67] Lymph node enlargement may lead to secondary lobar collapse due to bronchial compression. CT scanning also allows visualization of lymph node involvement of adjacent structures, such as pericardium, large bronchi and the spine.[69]

Pleural effusion in primary tuberculosis often occurs in the absence of radiologically evident parenchymal disease and is more often seen in adults than in children.

Miliary tuberculosis, better termed disseminated tuberculosis, is best seen on CT scanning where multiple opacities of similar size are seen distributed throughout the lung parenchyma. Opacities are typically 2–3 mm in diameter and normal chest x-rays are seen in 50 per cent of cases.

Paradoxical worsening of radiological features is common in the first 3 months of effective therapy for primary tuberculosis.[70] This should not cause alarm or change of therapy provided that the patient is clinically improving. These changes can include the development of new opacities, as well as enlargement of existing ones. True worsening of tuberculosis is characterized by the development of macronodules, while transient paradoxical worsening is characterized by the development of ground glass opacity.

CLINICAL FEATURES OF POST-PRIMARY INFECTION

Epidemiology

Post-primary pulmonary tuberculosis accounts for the majority of adult tuberculosis cases treated worldwide and almost all of the transmission of infection.[1] The global pandemic of HIV infection has resulted in approximately 25 million cases of AIDS in sub-Saharan Africa.[23] In this region, the high-prevalence of tuberculosis has resulted in an exponential increase in the number of HIV/TB cases. Many HIV-infected patients develop reactivation tuberculosis as their native immunity wanes,[71] but careful molecular epidemiological studies (see Chapter 3, Genotyping and its implications for transmission dynamics and tuberculosis control) have shown that an equal number acquire exogenous reinfection due to impaired pulmonary defence (see Chapter 18, DOTS and DOTS plus, and Chapter 19, The association between HIV and tuberculosis in the developing world).[20]

The clinical features of post-primary tuberculosis in immunocompetent adults are the combined result of unchecked mycobacterial replication and a destructive host immune response. In the lung, these combined influences result in tissue necrosis and cavitation. Tuberculous lung cavities contain copious sputum with approximately 1 million mycobacteria per millilitre. Lung inflammation triggers coughing which aerosolizes this sputum and results in the effective droplet infection discussed above. Post-primary tuberculosis in other organs, such as the spine or kidneys, is also characterized by extensive tissue destruction. Whilst this may be catastrophic for the individual, it is of less public health significance as transmission of infection is negligible.

The clinical features of pulmonary and extrapulmonary tuberculosis in HIV-infected adults are different than those in immunocompetent adults due to the relative paucity of the host response. The important differences in clinical presentation, diagnosis and management are presented for developing countries in Chapter 19 and for the developed world in Chapter 20.

Pathogenesis

The characteristic feature of post-primary tuberculosis is the granuloma.[72] This is an organized mass of activated macrophages, antigen-specific lymphocytes and fibroblasts (see Chapter 7, Histopathology, for more detail). High levels of IFN-γ and TNF are produced and extensive tissue destruction with fibrosis results. Many of the clinical symptoms can be explained by the aggressive host response that accompanies active pulmonary infection. Experimental models have shown that immunosuppression can result in decreased tissue destruction and decreased symptoms, but at the price of very high numbers of proliferating mycobacteria. This observation was confirmed by De Cock et al.[73] in a careful clinical observational study of patients with HIV infection and varying degrees of immunosuppression. HIV-infected patients with peripheral blood CD4 lymphocyte counts of 500/μL or more presented with cavitating pulmonary disease typical of patients not infected with HIV. Patients with CD4 counts in the range 200–400 μL presented with lymphatic spread and serous tuberculosis. Immunocompromised patients with CD4 counts of less than 200/μL (a case definition of AIDS) presented with disseminated mycobacterial infection.

Typical clinical features and outcome

Untreated post-primary pulmonary tuberculosis has a mortality of 50 per cent or higher. Fever, weight loss, cough and sputum production are followed by debilitating weakness, breathlessness and haemoptysis as cavitating lung disease destroys the lung. This process was aptly termed 'consumption' when endemic and epidemic tuberculosis caused much suffering in Renaissance and post-Renaissance Europe.[74]

In modern times, the clinical presentation and course of tuberculosis are dependent on the duration of symptoms, the speed of diagnosis and the effectiveness of treatment.[75]

The earliest symptom of tuberculosis and the most common one being present in more than 85 per cent of cases is cough.[76] This is initially a dry, irritating cough which may be worse at night when prone. Fever is also common early in disease, typically worse in the evening and followed at night (at defervescence) by sweating. These features, however, do not distinguish tuberculosis from other acute pulmonary infections.[77] It requires a high index of suspicion to insist on sputum microscopy and culture for mycobacteria at this stage. Many patients do not produce sputum, but a suitable sample can be obtained using chest percussion, sputum induction using nebulized 3 per cent saline (hypertonic saline) or bronchoscopy with lavage.[78]

In established pulmonary tuberculosis, TNF-related weight loss becomes obvious. TNF was called 'cachexin' when first described and indeed patients with tuberculosis can lose up to 50 per cent of their body weight within several months of the onset of disease. Accompanying the weight loss are drenching night sweats of sufficient volume that patients frequently report not only having to change their clothes, but the bed linen as well. In a study associating symptoms and detection of mycobacteria on sputum culture, only weight loss and night sweats were significantly associated with a diagnosis of tuberculosis.[79] Sputum production is more marked in established disease. Sputum can be mucoid, mucopurulent, blood-stained or frank haemoptysis. Blood staining usually alarms the patient and precipitates presentation to hospital.

Fibrosis and lung destruction are a late feature of tuberculosis and shortness of breath is not a frequent early symptom. By the time shortness of breath has become obvious to the patient, extensive lung destruction will have already occurred and the more dramatic and alarming symptom of haemoptysis may have occurred too. Small volumes of haemoptysis are seen with increasing frequency as disease progresses. Large volume haemoptysis is an infrequent complication of lung cavitation or colonization of lung cavities by Aspergillus fumigatus (see below).[80]

Clinical features often provide evidence of successful therapy. In particular, one mark of successful therapy is the reversal of weight loss. Measurable weight gain can occur within a week of starting successful treatment. Fever disappears quickly too; night sweats reduce and stop completely after several weeks of therapy.

Paradoxical responses to treatment

Extensive tuberculosis can produce sufficient debilitation that it becomes an immunosuppressive influence on the host. This effect is relieved shortly after the initiation of successful therapy and can result in paradoxical worsening of the patient's clinical condition. This can be extremely marked in the treatment of tuberculous adenitis in the cervical lymph nodes and can also result in increased pulmonary infiltration with breathlessness. In its most extreme form, immune reconstitution following tuberculosis therapy results in the immune reconstitution inflammatory syndrome (IRIS) in patients infected with both HIV and TB.[81]

Complications of post-primary disease

Post-primary pulmonary tuberculosis may be complicated by extensive lung destruction, pleural disease and by tuberculosis infection outside the lungs (Figure 9.5) (see Case history 1).

LUNG COMPLICATIONS

In the lungs, endobronchial infection, fibrosis and cavitation can result in loss of lung volume, distortion of pulmonary architecture, including mediastinal displacement, traction bronchiectasis and ultimately respiratory failure. Enlarging cavities erode pulmonary vessels and result in haemoptysis – usually small in volume but can be a cause of sudden death.

Endobronchial TB

Evidence of endobronchial infection may be found in up to 40 per cent of cases of pulmonary tuberculosis.[82] Direct

Case history 1

A 27-year-old student from Somalia was admitted to hospital with a 2-month history of cough productive of white sputum, fever, night sweats, dyspnoea on exertion, mild central chest pain and weight loss of 6 kg. One month earlier, she had been diagnosed with a chest infection by her general practitioner and treated with antibiotics, but her symptoms did not improve. She was previously healthy and did not require any medication prior to this illness. The patient was born and grew up in Somalia, but had come to the UK 2 years previously to study. She did not smoke or drink alcohol; she lived alone and had no recent contact with anyone who was known to have active TB.

On examination she was unwell, thin and had a fever of 38.2°C. The chest was clear with normal breath sounds on auscultation. The remainder of the physical examination was unremarkable. Chest radiography and CT scan both showed extensive miliary shadowing in both lungs (Figure 9.5a,b). The haemoglobin was 10.5 g/dL, ESR 96 mm/hour, CRP 45, ALT 46, GGT 69. Other blood tests were normal and an HIV test was negative. Microscopy of sputum smears was positive for acid-fast bacilli. She was started on rifampicin-containing quadruple therapy for TB to which she responded well with significant reduction in cough, night sweats and resolution of fever. She was discharged from hospital 2 weeks later. Sputum culture grew *Mycobacterium tuberculosis* after 4 weeks' incubation. The isolate was susceptible to all first-line anti-TB drugs. Her treatment was adjusted to a triple-drug, rifampicin-containing short-course chemotherapy regimen. She received 6 months of TB treatment and made a full recovery.

Comment

This patient presented with sputum smear-positive pulmonary TB which had disseminated locally.

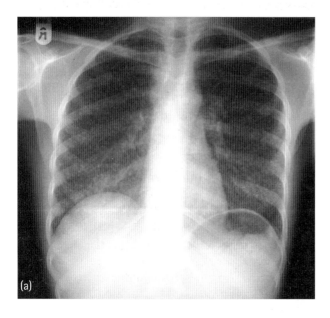

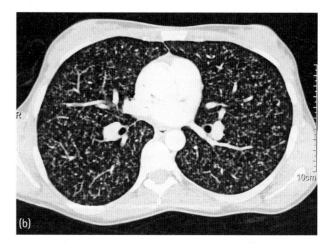

Figure 9.5 Chest x-ray (a) and CT scan (b) from a 27-year-old student with disseminated tuberculosis (see Case History 1). Multiple small opacities (miliary shadowing) are seen in the periphery of the chest x-ray and much more clearly in all areas of the CT scan.

bronchial wall infection with mycobacteria may occur in continuity with a focus of infection such as a cavity or by haematogenous spread. Infected bronchi have thickened walls, reduced luminal diameter and may develop post-stenotic dilatation.

Clinical symptoms of endobronchial tuberculosis are the same as for parenchymal disease with the addition of wheezing. In particular, localized monophonic wheeze may be heard over stenotic bronchial segments and distal pulmonary collapse may also occur.

At bronchoscopy, different endobronchial appearances and biopsy features have led to a classification of endo-

bronchial tuberculosis into actively caseating (oozing pus), oedematous-hyperaemic (swollen airways), fibrostenotic (narrowed distorted airway), tumorous (mass seen occluding airway), granular (looks like granulation tissue), ulcerative and non-specific groups. The granular, ulcerative and non-specific appearances have a good prognosis, but the prognosis is very poor in the other groups, all of which pass a critical point and then progress rapidly to tight bronchial stenosis. Interventional bronchoscopy can be combined with antituberculous chemotherapy – repeated balloon dilatation, stenting and laser treatment have all been used with varying success dependent on case selection and operator skill.[83]

Laryngeal TB

Laryngeal TB is a specific example of endobronchial tuberculosis that presents early with hoarseness of the voice. The diagnosis can be made using sputum or local biopsy and treatment success depends on early intervention with effective antituberculous therapy.

Bronchiectasis and post-primary TB

Bronchiectasis occurs either due to bronchial dilatation at the site of endobronchial tuberculosis or as a secondary phenomenon following parenchymal lung destruction and fibrosis (traction bronchiectasis). Secondary bacterial infection allows a chronic cycle of purulent infection, inflammation and loss of airway function to develop. Frequent sputum microscopy and culture is needed to be sure that persistent, reactivation or new exogenous infection with mycobacteria has not occurred.

Haemoptysis and Rasmussen aneurysm

Blood-stained sputum is common in patients with active tuberculosis due to inflamed airways and erosion of small capillaries. The process of active cavitation may erode larger pulmonary vessels and result in massive haemoptysis. A particular example of this latter process is the Rasmussen aneurysm in which invasion of a peripheral pulmonary artery is followed by fibrinous dilatation of the arterial wall. These mycotic aneurysms are prone to sudden rupture and consequent fatal haemoptysis.[84]

Aspergilloma

Old tuberculous lung cavities may become colonized with *Aspergillus fumigatus*. This occurs in about 11 per cent of cavities[85,86] and may take the form of semi-invasive infection of the cavity wall or form a mobile mycetoma (termed 'aspergilloma'). Aspergilloma is often clinically silent but has a dramatic, mobile radiographic appearance (Figure 9.6). Successful treatment requires aggressive antifungal therapy followed by surgery to remove the cavity. If untreated, aspergillomas may be complicated by massive haemoptysis.

Bronchial artery embolization has been reported as a successful management strategy in acute massive haemoptysis, but this treatment relies on demonstration of an actively bleeding vessel and successful occlusion of that vessel in a timely manner using angiography or CT guidance. The angiographic signs in haemoptysis include hyperplasia of the bronchial artery trunk, bronchopulmonary anastomoses and bronchial artery aneurysms. A risk of the procedure is pulmonary infarction, but this is uncommon due to the anastomoses mentioned. The number of patients successfully treated by bronchial artery embolization is small.

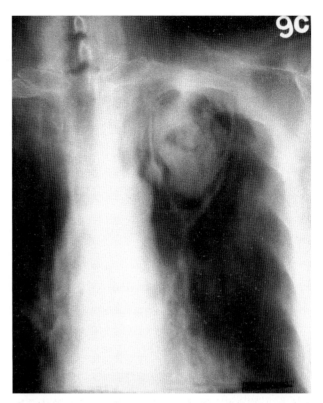

Figure 9.6 Posteroanterior chest x-ray showing an aspergilloma in the left apex.

Tuberculous gangrene

A rare, severe form of post-primary pulmonary tuberculosis results in pulmonary vasculitis in the site of infection and secondary gangrene. This condition is rapidly fatal.[87]

Lung carcinoma and other neoplasia

Lung carcinoma is common in tuberculosis patients due to common risk factors, particularly smoke exposure. Tuberculosis is common in lung carcinoma patients and patients with other malignancy (e.g. Hodgkin's lymphoma and other haematological malignancies) due to the immunosuppression that occurs as a consequence of those diseases. The clinical features of tuberculosis and pulmonary neoplasia are similar and radiological features may be difficult to distinguish, including those on CT scanning (Figure 9.7 and Case history 2).[85,88,89]

PLEURAL COMPLICATIONS

Pneumothorax

Rupture of a tuberculous cavity into the pleura can result in pneumothorax or bronchopleural fistula.[90] The clinical symptoms are of sudden pain and/or shortness of breath.

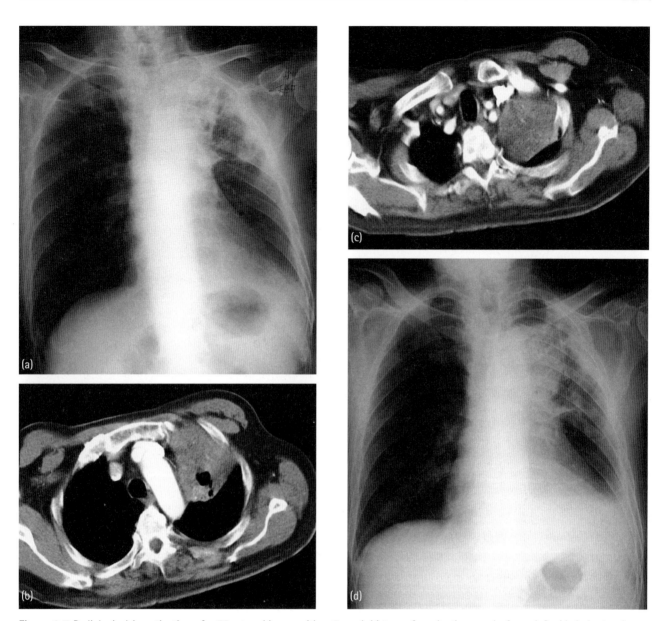

Figure 9.7 Radiological investigation of a 78-year-old man with a 6-week history of productive cough, fever, left-sided chest pain, dyspnoea on exertion and hoarse voice (see Case History 2). Chest x-ray (a) and CT scan (b) showed a soft tissue mass in the left upper lobe which encased the left upper lobe bronchus (c). A chest x-ray performed at the end of TB treatment showed a significant resolution of the initial consolidation seen in the left upper lobe, persistence of the mass (diagnosed as being carcinoid tumour), left upper lobe fibrosis, loss of left lung volume, a left pleural effusion and a large heart shadow (d).

Classical signs of pneumothorax (increased resonance on percussion, decreased breath sounds) can be confirmed by chest x-ray. Pneumothorax may complicate both active infection and healed cavities. Treatment of pneumothorax in either context may be complicated due to the abnormal nature of the damaged underlying lung.

Bronchopleural fistula

Acutely enlarging cavities may also rupture into the pleura resulting in tuberculous pleural effusion or bronchopleural fistula. Bronchopleural fistula was common prior to effective antituberculous chemotherapy being available and pre-sented a major therapeutic challenge. If chest drainage with suction is prolonged and combined with effective antituberculous therapy, the fistula will eventually close.

Pleural effusion and tuberculous empyema

Pleural effusion is common in post-primary tuberculosis and particularly common in HIV-infected patients. In sub-Saharan Africa, tuberculosis is the most common cause of pleural effusion due to the high incidence of patients with HIV/TB.[91] In pleural effusion complicating post-primary disease, parenchymal disease may be seen on 50 per cent of chest x-rays.

Case history 2

A 78-year-old Chinese man who had spent the last 40 years in England presented to the Accident and Emergency Department with a 6-week history of productive cough, fever, left-sided chest pain, dyspnoea on exertion and hoarse voice. He also complained of palpitations, loss of appetite and had lost 4 kg in weight over the 6-week period. He was a lifelong non-smoker.

On examination, he was thin, apyrexial, had finger clubbing and an irregular pulse of 115 beats/minute. Examination of the chest revealed wasting of the left pectoral muscles, reduced chest movement, dull percussion and reduced air entry in the left upper zone anteriorly. The heart sounds were normal and there was no cardiac murmur. The rest of the clinical examination was normal. Chest radiography and CT scan showed a soft tissue mass in the left upper lobe which encased the left upper lobe bronchus. There was collapse/consolidation of the left upper lobe and a left pleural effusion (Figure 9.7a–c). An electrocardiogram (ECG) confirmed atrial fibrillation with fast ventricular response. Sputum smear microscopy was positive for AFB, but cytological examination did not reveal malignant cells. Sputum culture grew *M. tuberculosis* after 6 weeks' incubation. The isolate was susceptible to all first-line anti-TB drugs. He was commenced on standard, rifampicin-containing short-course chemotherapy for TB. Bronchoscopy performed 2 weeks after starting TB treatment confirmed the left upper lobe tumour, which was diagnosed as atypical carcinoid tumour on histological examination of tissue samples. He was referred to the oncology service and started on a course of radiotherapy 6 weeks into TB treatment. He completed 6 months of TB treatment and was sputum smear and culture negative at the end of treatment. A chest x-ray performed at the end of TB treatment showed significant resolution of the initial consolidation seen in the left upper lobe, persistence of the mass, left upper lobe fibrosis, loss of left lung volume, a left pleural effusion and a large heart shadow (Figure 9.7d). An echocardiogram confirmed moderate pericardial effusion. As the patient was still receiving radiotherapy at the end of TB treatment, he continued to receive isoniazid as secondary chemoprophylaxis for TB. His condition progressively deteriorated with extensive intrathoracic spread of the carcinoid tumour. He died 5 months after completing TB treatment.

Comment

This patient presented with two different pathologies which could not be distinguished easily from the clinical history. Despite extensive abnormalities in the left upper lobe, close examination of the initial chest radiograph revealed a possible mass and prompted an early request for a CT scan of the thorax. He was cured of TB at the end of treatment, but required isoniazid chemoprophylaxis to prevent relapse, while he remained immunosuppressed as a result of the radiotherapy.

In post-primary tuberculosis, a subpleural tuberculous cavity ruptures into the pleural space seeding the pleural cavity with mycobacteria, caseating material and high levels of pro-inflammatory mycobacterial antigens, such as arabinogalactan and arabinomannan. Mycobacterial antigens produce an exudative pleural response characterized by high levels of monocytes and IFN-γ producing lymphocytes.[92] Granulomata are produced on the pleural surface and mycobacterial proliferation is inhibited. IL-12 has been shown to be critical in this response as inhibition of IL-12 results in mycobacterial proliferation.

Clinical symptoms of pleural effusion in post-primary tuberculosis include increasing shortness of breath and pain on the affected side. Cough and fever also occur, as in classical post-primary tuberculosis, but the cough is often less pronounced. After several months, weight loss is prominent and there may be accompanying ascites. Clinical detection of a pulmonary effusion is by classical clinical features (decreased resonance, decreased breath sounds), radiological features and needle aspiration to obtain straw-coloured or blood-stained fluid.

Tuberculous empyema refers to thick pus in the pleural cavity that is encased in rind-like thickened pleura. This term may become obsolete as tuberculous pleural effusion can be more accurately defined using microbiological and CT scanning criteria into (1) pure pleural tuberculosis, (2) pure pleural disease with mixed tuberculous/pyogenic infection, (3) pleuroparenchymal tuberculosis and (4) pleuroparenchymal disease with mixed tuberculous/pyogenic infection.[66,89] These cases usually require protracted, appropriate antibiotic therapy and surgical drainage or decortication of the pleural space. The goal of surgery in either case is to obliterate the infected space (see Chapter 16, The surgical management of tuberculosis and its complications).

EXTRAPULMONARY COMPLICATIONS OF POST-PRIMARY DISEASE

A full description of the diagnosis and management of non-respiratory tuberculosis are described in Chapter 10, Non-respiratory tuberculosis. The most common presentations of extrapulmonary tuberculosis are cervical adenitis and pleural effusion (described above). Certain other features of relevance to patients with respiratory tuberculosis are described here.

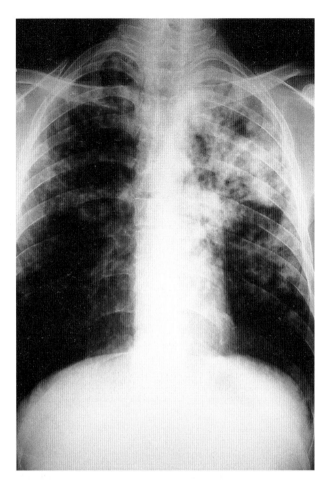

Figure 9.8 Chest x-ray of 40-year-old man showing characteristic changes of post-primary tuberculosis. Soft cavitating lesions in the upper zones, particularly the left.

Pericardial disease may occur by local extension of pulmonary infection. In areas of high HIV seroprevalence, tuberculosis is the most common cause of pericardial effusion and tamponade. In a medical unit with 800–1000 admissions per month, this presentation was seen in four cases per month.[93] The clinical presentation is of breathlessness which is worst on lying down. Classical clinical (paradoxical movement of the jugular venous pressure (JVP), diminished heart sounds), radiological (globular enlarged heart shadow) and electrocardiographic features (swinging axis, small complexes) allow the diagnosis to be made. The fibrinous strands seen in the pericardial fluid using ultrasound at pericardiocentesis allow pericardial effusion due to congestive cardiac failure to be distinguished. The management of pericardial disease with antituberculous chemotherapy should also be accompanied by prednisolone in high dose for the first month to minimize the risk of pericardial fibrosis leading to constrictive pericarditis.

Spinal tuberculosis may be a primary progressive or post-primary condition, complicated eventually by vertebral collapse (Pott's disease of the spine). Vertebral tuberculosis can communicate directly with the pleura and result in tuberculous pleural effusion.

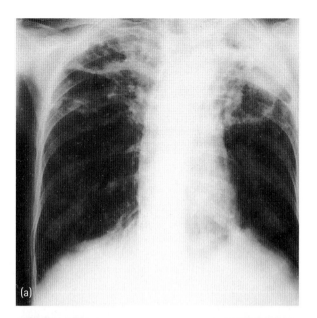

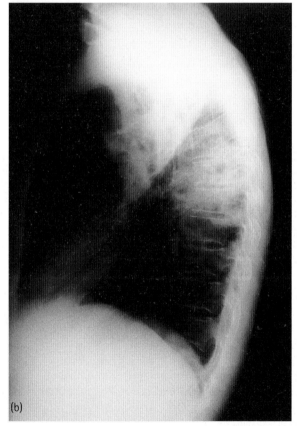

Figure 9.9 Chronic active pulmonary tuberculosis. There is extensive upper lobe fibrosis with tracheal deviation. (a) Posteroanterior view; (b) lateral view showing the posterior nature of the disease.

Poncet's arthropathy is a rarely seen fleeting arthropathy that rapidly responds to antituberculous therapy.[94] Amyloidosis is a very late complication of protracted tuberculosis infection. The typical presentation is with nephritic syndrome.

Radiology of post-primary tuberculosis

Post-primary tuberculosis pathology is characterized by fibrosis and cavitation (Figure 9.8). These are also the predominant radiological features of post-primary tuberculosis,[66] but there is substantial overlap with the radiological appearance of progressive primary tuberculosis.[95]

Parenchymal disease develops from early patchy consolidation in apical lobes (Figure 9.9) or apical segments of the lower lobes to widespread bronchopneumonia leading back to the hilum (Figure 9.10). Unlike primary disease, hilar or paratracheal adenopathy is rare. Healing by fibrosis can lead to lobar collapse, tracheal displacement, compensatory emphysema in adjacent lung and bulla formation.

Cavitation is a common part of the tissue destruction associated with post-primary disease. It is seen in 40–80 per cent of cases of post-primary tuberculosis and gives a high likelihood of infectivity.[96] Cavities vary in wall thickness and may have an air–fluid level. Fungal colonization occurs in 11 per cent of cavities larger than 3 cm diameter.[86] Large mycetomas can be seen on plain chest x-ray (with decubitus films to show movement), but are best imaged by CT scanning.

Endobronchial disease occurs by local invasion of bronchi and is best imaged by CT scanning. Radiological features of endobronchial disease include bronchial stenosis, post-stenotic dilation, persistent lobar collapse and nodular opacities in the parenchyma termed 'tree in bud' opacities.[97] These nodules have a sharp outline and are the result of centrilobular plugging. In later disease, typical features of bronchiectasis supervene.

A tuberculoma is a solid encapsulated mass which may present as a solitary mass on chest x-ray. The mass has a risk of cavitation and spread in 5 per cent of cases.[67] CT scanning shows no enhancement with contrast.

Pleural disease in post-primary disease differs from that in primary disease in that the majority of cases show parenchymal radiological features of tuberculosis. Old tuberculosis may show calcification in both the pleura and parenchyma (Figure 9.11). Pleural disease, including bronchopleural fistulae, are best imaged by CT scanning. Involvement of adjacent structures including osteomyelitis of the ribs can be visualized at the same time.

The radiological appearance of tuberculosis in patients with HIV/TB can be predicted from the immunology. In patients with good immunity, radiological features typical of post-primary tuberculosis are seen. As immunity wanes,

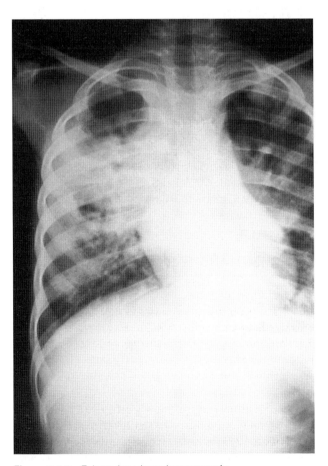

Figure 9.10 Tuberculous bronchopneumonia.

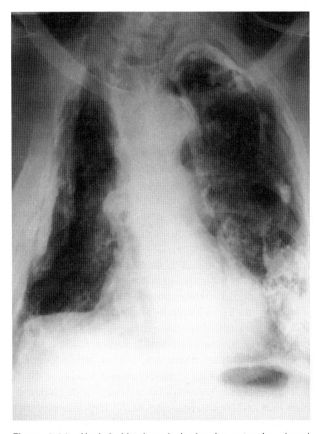

Figure 9.11 Healed old tuberculosis showing extensive pleural and parenchymal calcification.

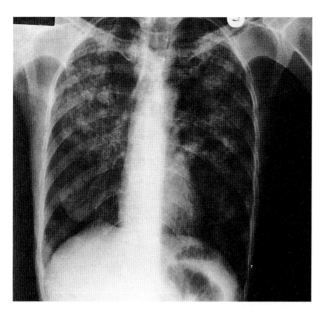

Figure 9.12 Chest x-ray of patient with HIV-seropositive tuberculosis. No clear pattern is present.

the host immune response declines resulting in less fibrosis and cavitation and radiological appearances become more suggestive of primary disease. The typical diagnostic features are lost (Figure 9.12), and in 15 per cent of cases of sputum smear-positive pulmonary tuberculosis, the chest x-ray is normal.[95]

DIAGNOSIS OF TUBERCULOSIS

Microbiology

The diagnosis of tuberculosis is based on microbiological identification of *M. tuberculosis* from appropriate clinical specimens. In the majority of respiratory cases, the first and most important test is the acid and alcohol fast staining of repeated sputum smears using the Ziehl–Neelsen technique. Not only does this test make the diagnosis in a large number of cases, but it also defines the infective population of patients. Ideally the identification of acid-alcohol fast bacilli is followed by culture of the organism and identification of drug sensitivity. This is not possible in many regions of the world. The diagnosis of tuberculosis by microbiological techniques is discussed in detail in Chapter 5, The diagnosis of tuberculosis. PCR techniques are a useful addition in defining nontuberculous mycobacteria (see Chapter 29, Environmental mycobacteria) when potentially contaminated clinical specimens, such as gastric lavage, are found to contain acid-alcohol fast bacilli. PCR techniques are also useful in the rapid diagnosis of drug-resistance genes in mycobacteria isolated from clinical samples. PCR techniques, however, have a high false-negative rate in samples with low numbers of mycobacteria and should not be used as a test of exclusion. This is discussed in Chapter 5, The diagnosis of tuberculosis.

Confirming tuberculosis as the cause of pleural fluid may be difficult.[98] The fluid is usually an exudate by Light's criteria (protein effusion:serum ratio >0.5; LDH >307 IU/mL; LDH effusion:serum ratio >0.6) and is usually negative for mycobacteria on smear microscopy. Pleural fluid is culture positive for mycobacteria in only 20–50 per cent of cases due to the immunological phenomena described above. The additional characteristic features of tuberculous pleural fluid are pH <7.4, white cell count 5000–10 000 cells/μL and less than 5 per cent mesothelial cells, low glucose and raised adenosine deaminase (ADA). In a study from India, ADA levels above 100 IU/L had a sensitivity of 40 per cent and a specificity of 100 per cent,[99] but these findings were not replicated in a study from South Africa.[100] Pleural biopsy is more often diagnostic, particularly if histological features of granulomata are accepted as a basis for a trial of treatment. Blind pleural biopsy with Abram's needle or a guided biopsy as part of a video-assisted-thoroscopy surgical procedure (VATS) may be used (see Chapter 16, The surgical management of tuberculosis and its complications).

Radiology

Radiological features often support a diagnosis of pulmonary tuberculosis, particularly when clinical examination is unremarkable. In other instances, however, atypical x-ray features may suggest alternative diagnoses and it is in these cases that rigorous pursuit of a diagnosis of tuberculosis is important.

Immunology

In cases where sputum microscopy and culture are negative, immunodiagnostic techniques are of value in excluding a diagnosis of tuberculosis in certain cases. These are discussed in detail in Chapter 5, The diagnosis of tuberculosis, Chapter 6, Immunodiagnostic tests, and Chapter 22, Preventive therapy.

TREATMENT AND EARLY TREATMENT DEATH

The treatment of tuberculosis is described in detail in Chapters 12–18. Early diagnosis and effective antituberculous chemotherapy will result in a cure in most cases. Standard short-course chemotherapy for drug-susceptible tuberculosis consists of four drugs (rifampicin, isoniazid, pyrazinamide and ethambutol) for 2 months followed by two drugs (rifampicin and isoniazid) for a further 4 months. In sputum-positive cases, the patient will be rendered non-infectious after 2 weeks of appropriate therapy, although dead mycobacteria may still be visible in the sputum for some weeks after this time. Fixed drug combinations allow simpler prescribing and may increase patient compliance, but are less flexible should side effects become a problem.

In endemic areas, particularly those affected by the HIV/TB epidemic, a significant proportion of TB deaths occurs in the early stages of appropriate treatment. In a study from Malawi, Harries et al.[101] reported that 23 and 26 per cent of sputum smear-positive and sputum smear-negative pulmonary tuberculosis patients, respectively, died within 8 months of starting appropriate antituberculosis treatment. Nearly 40 per cent of these deaths occurred during the first month of treatment. The mechanism of these deaths is the subject of much current research and may relate to late presentation and diagnosis of TB, advanced HIV disease and the release of large quantities of mycobacterial antigens in the early bactericidal phase of treatment.

DIFFERENTIAL DIAGNOSES OF RESPIRATORY TB

Differential diagnoses of pulmonary disease

- Other pulmonary infection
  - Bacteria causing cavitatory disease
    - *Staphylococcus*: usually bilateral cavitation
    - *Klebsiella*: usually unilateral cavitation
    - *Nocardia*
  - Other bacteria
    - Meliodosis (severe necrotizing pneumonia in Far East)
  - In HIV-positive patients
    - *Pneumocystis jiroveci*
    - *Penicillium marneffii* (South East Asia)
    - Cytomegalovirus
    - Kaposi sarcoma (KS) (often found with palatal KS)
  - Other mycobacterial infections (unilateral cavitation in previously damaged lungs)
    - MAIC (*Mycobacterium avium intracellulare* complex)
    - *Mycobacterium malmoense*
    - *Mycobacterium kansasii*
    - *Mycobacterium xenopi*
    - *Mycobacterium chelonei*
  - Viral pneumonia
  - Parasitic diseases
    - Paragonamiasis
    - Hydatid disease
  - Fungal infections (Histoplasma, Coccidiomycosis)
- Malignancy
  - Bronchogenic carcinoma (squamous cell often unilateral apical cavity)
  - Alveolar cell carcinoma
  - Lymphoma
  - Leukaemia (usually solitary lesion)
- Vasculitides
  - Granulomatous disease (Wegener's, polyarteritis nodosa)
  - Rheumatoid nodule
  - Organizing pneumonia (usually multiple lesions)
- Pulmonary infarction (usually mid or lower zones)
- Fibrotic lung disease
- Extrinsic allergic alveolitis
- Sarcoidosis (skin test usually negative)
  - Mild (bilateral hilar lymphadenopathy; primary tuberculosis usually unilateral)
  - Necrotizing (multiple lesions, cavities and histological features of vasculitis)

Differential diagnoses for pleural effusion

- Other infection, including para-pneumonic effusion and empyema
- Metastatic malignancy (especially breast and ovary)
- Bronchogenic carcinoma
- Mesothelioma
- Pulmonary infarction
- Autoimmune disease
- Rheumatoid arthritis
- Congestive cardiac failure (CCF)
- Chylous effusion

Differential diagnosis of miliary disease

- Tuberculosis
- Non-tuberculous infection
  - Nocardiosis
- Fungal infections
  - Histoplasmosis
  - Blastomycosis
  - Coccidiomycosis
  - Cryptococcosis
- Viral infections
- Pneumoconiosis
- Sarcoidosis
- Metastatic carcinoma
- Histiocytosis X
- Amyloidosis
- Alveolar microlithiasis

Differential diagnoses for mediastinal enlargement

- Tuberculosis
- Carcinoma
- Lymphoma
- Sarcoidosis
- Thymoma
- Hamartoma
- Neurofibroma

LEARNING POINTS

- Tuberculosis infection and disease are not the same. One-third of the world population is infected, but the majority do not experience disease.

- Transmission of tuberculosis is person-to-person by droplet infection. Patients with cough and cavitary disease are the most infectious. Close contacts and people with immunodeficiency are at greatest risk of infection.

- Primary disease is when *Mycobacterium tuberculosis* infects an immunologically naive host and immune responses occur for the first time. Often this is asymptomatic but progressive disease can result, particularly in children or adults with immunodeficiency.

- Post-primary disease is when *M. tuberculosis* causes symptoms either by reactivation of primary infection or reinfection with a new strain. Symptoms are due to the combined effect of pathogen replication and host response.

- The diagnosis of tuberculosis is by identification of the organism in sputum or other clinical samples. Radiology and other tests are supportive, but do not make the diagnosis.

- Untreated tuberculosis progresses to cause lung damage and death, but effective treatment results in cure in over 90 per cent of patients.

- Early diagnosis and appropriate treatment are essential for good outcomes.

REFERENCES

1. Dye C. Global epidemiology of tuberculosis. *Lancet* 2006; **367**: 938-40.
2. Frieden TR, Sterling TR, Munsiff SS, Watt CJ, Dye C. Tuberculosis. *Lancet* 2003; **362**: 887-99.
3. Onyebujoh P, Rodriguez W, Mwaba P. Priorities in tuberculosis research. *Lancet* 2006; **367**: 940-2.
4. Raviglione MC. The global plan to stop TB, 2006-2015. *Int J Tuberc Lung Dis* 2006; **10**: 238-9.
5. Bunyan J. *The life and death of Mr Badman*. New York: Russell RH, 1900.
6. Osoba AO. Microbiology of tuberculosis. In: Madkour MM (ed.). *Tuberculosis*, 1st edn. Berlin: Springer-Verlag, 2004: 115-32.
7. National Collaborating Centre for Chronic Conditions. *Tuberculosis: clinical diagnosis and management of tuberculosis, and measures for its prevention and control*. London: Royal College of Physicians, 2006.
8. Mwinga A. Challenges and hope for the diagnosis of tuberculosis in infants and young children. *Lancet* 2005; **365**: 97-8.
9. Harries A, Hargreaves N, Kemp J et al. Diagnosis of tuberculosis in Africa. *Lancet* 2000; **355**: 2256.
10. Mangura BT, Reichman LB. Pulmonary tuberculosis. In: Pennington JE (ed.). *Respiratory infections: diagnosis and management*, 3rd edn. New York: Raven, 1994: 633-53.
11. Loudon RG, Roberts RM. Singing and the dissemination of tuberculosis. *Am Rev Respir Dis* 1968; **98**: 297-300.
12. Nardell EA. Catching droplet nuclei: toward a better understanding of tuberculosis transmission. *Am J Respir Crit Care Med* 2004; **169**: 553-4.
13. Schlesinger LS. Macrophage phagocytosis of virulent but not attenuated strains of *Mycobacterium tuberculosis* is mediated by mannose receptors in addition to complement receptors. *J Immunol* 1993; **150**: 2920-30.
14. Hirsch CS, Ellner JJ, Russell DG, Rich EA. Complement receptor-mediated uptake and tumor necrosis factor-alpha-mediated growth inhibition of *Mycobacterium tuberculosis* by human alveolar macrophages. *J Immunol* 1994; **152**: 743-53.
15. Tailleux L, Schwartz O, Herrmann JL et al. DC-SIGN is the major *Mycobacterium tuberculosis* receptor on human dendritic cells. *J Exp Med* 2003; **197**: 121-7.
16. Mwandumba HC, Russell DG, Nyirenda MH et al. *Mycobacterium tuberculosis* resides in nonacidified vacuoles in endocytically competent alveolar macrophages from patients with tuberculosis and HIV infection. *J Immunol* 2004; **172**: 4592-8.
17. Hill PC, Jackson-Sillah D, Donkor SA et al. Risk factors for pulmonary tuberculosis: a clinic-based case control study in The Gambia. *BMC Public Health* 2006; **6**: 156.
18. Driver CR, Valway SE, Morgan WM et al. Transmission of *Mycobacterium tuberculosis* associated with air travel. *J Am Med Assoc* 1994; **272**: 1031-5.
19. Edwards LB, Tolderlund K. BCG vaccine studies. III. Preliminary report on effect of sunlight and BCG vaccine. *Bull World Health Organ* 1952; **5**: 245-8.
20. Sonnenberg P, Murray J, Glynn JR et al. HIV-1 and recurrence, relapse, and reinfection of tuberculosis after cure: a cohort study in South African mineworkers. *Lancet* 2001; **358**: 1687-93.
21. Corbett EL, Charalambous S, Moloi VM et al. Human immunodeficiency virus and the prevalence of undiagnosed tuberculosis in African gold miners. *Am J Respir Crit Care Med* 2004; **170**: 673-9.
22. Nyangulu DS, Harries AD, Kang'ombe C et al. Tuberculosis in a prison population in Malawi. *Lancet* 1997; **350**: 1284-7.
23. Corbett EL, Marston B, Churchyard GJ, De Cock KM. Tuberculosis in sub-Saharan Africa: opportunities, challenges, and change in the era of antiretroviral treatment. *Lancet* 2006; **367**: 926-37.
24. Cegielski JP, McMurray DN. The relationship between malnutrition and tuberculosis: evidence from studies in humans and experimental animals. *Int J Tuberc Lung Dis* 2004; **8**: 286-98.
25. Arcavi L, Benowitz NL. Cigarette smoking and infection. *Arch Intern Med* 2004; **164**: 2206-16.
26. Perez-Padilla R, Perez-Guzman C, Baez-Saldana R, Torres-Cruz A. Cooking with biomass stoves and tuberculosis: a case control study. *Int J Tuberc Lung Dis* 2001; **5**: 441-7.
27. Ross MH, Murray J. Occupational respiratory disease in mining. *Occup Med (Lond)* 2004; **54**: 304-10.
28. de Jong R, Altare F, Haagen I-A et al. Severe mycobacterial and salmonella infections in interleukin-12 receptor deficient patients. *Science* 1998; **280**: 1435-8.
29. Cooke GS, Campbell SJ, Sillah J et al. Polymorphism within the interferon-gamma/receptor complex is associated with pulmonary tuberculosis. *Am J Respir Crit Care Med* 2006; **174**: 339-43.
30. Selvaraj P, Sriram U, Mathan KS, Reetha AM, Narayanan PR. Tumour necrosis factor alpha (-238 and -308) and beta gene polymorphisms in pulmonary tuberculosis: haplotype analysis with HLA-A, B and DR genes. *Tuberculosis (Edinb)* 2001; **81**: 335-41.
31. Casanova JL, Abel L. The human model: a genetic dissection of immunity to infection in natural conditions. *Nat Rev Immunol* 2004; **4**: 55-66.
32. Keane J, Gershon S, Wise RP et al. Tuberculosis associated with infliximab, a tumor necrosis factor alpha-neutralizing agent. *N Engl J Med* 2001; **345**: 1098-104.
33. Rychly DJ, DiPiro JT. Infections associated with tumor necrosis factor-alpha antagonists. *Pharmacotherapy* 2005; **25**: 1181-92.
34. Mok MY, Lo Y, Chan TM, Wong WS, Lau CS. Tuberculosis in

systemic lupus erythematosus in an endemic area and the role of isoniazid prophylaxis during corticosteroid therapy. *J Rheumatol* 2005; **32**: 609–15.

35. Naqvi A, Rizvi A, Hussain Z *et al.* Developing world perspective of post-transplant tuberculosis: morbidity, mortality, and cost implications. *Transplant Proc* 2001; **33**: 1787–8.

36. Tocque K, Bellis MA, Beeching NJ *et al.* A case–control study of lifestyle risk factors associated with tuberculosis in Liverpool, North-West England. *Eur Respir J* 2001; **18**: 959–64.

37. Rook GA, Dheda K, Zumla A. Immune responses to tuberculosis in developing countries: implications for new vaccines. *Nat Rev Immunol* 2005; **5**: 661–7.

38. Ordway DJ, Costa L, Martins M *et al.* Increased interleukin-4 production by CD8 and gammadelta T cells in health-care workers is associated with the subsequent development of active tuberculosis. *J Infect Dis* 2004; **190**: 756–66.

39. Opie EL, Aronson JD. Tubercle bacilli in latent tuberculous lesions and in lung tissue without tuberculous lesions. *Arch Pathol Lab Med* 1927; **4**: 1–21.

40. Hernandez-Pando R, Jeyanathan M, Mengistu G *et al.* Persistence of DNA from *Mycobacterium tuberculosis* in superficially normal lung tissue during latent infection. *Lancet* 2000; **356**: 2133–8.

41. Scanga CA, Mohan VP, Yu K *et al.* Depletion of CD4(+) T cells causes reactivation of murine persistent tuberculosis despite continued expression of interferon gamma and nitric oxide synthase 2. *J Exp Med* 2000; **192**: 347–58.

42. Serbina NV, Flynn JL. CD8(+) T cells participate in the memory immune response to *Mycobacterium tuberculosis*. *Infect Immun* 2001; **69**: 4320–8.

43. Leemans JC, Thepen T, Weijer S *et al.* Macrophages play a dual role during pulmonary tuberculosis in mice. *J Infect Dis* 2005; **191**: 65–74.

44. Kahnert A, Seiler P, Stein M *et al.* Alternative activation deprives macrophages of a coordinated defense program to *Mycobacterium tuberculosis*. *Eur J Immunol* 2006; **36**: 631–47.

45. Lazarevic V, Nolt D, Flynn JL. Long-term control of *Mycobacterium tuberculosis* infection is mediated by dynamic immune responses. *J Immunol* 2005; **175**: 1107–17.

46. Long R. Tuberculosis and malnutrition. *Int J Tuberc Lung Dis* 2004; **8**: 276–7.

47. Sharma SK, Mohan A, Kadhiravan T. HIV-TB co-infection: epidemiology, diagnosis and management. *Indian J Med Res* 2005; **121**: 550–67.

48. Marais BJ, Gie RP, Schaaf HS *et al.* The spectrum of disease in children treated for tuberculosis in a highly endemic area. *Int J Tuberc Lung Dis* 2006; **10**: 732–8.

49. Beyers JA. The radiological features of primary pulmonary tuberculosis. *S Afr Med J* 1979; **55**: 994–7.

50. Alexander WJ, Avent CK, Bailey WC. Simple primary tuberculosis in an elderly woman. *J Am Geriatr Soc* 1979; **27**: 123–5.

51. Madkour MM. Primary tuberculosis in adults. In: Madkour MM (ed.). *Tuberculosis*, 1st edn. Berlin: Springer, 2004: 265–70.

52. Rook GA, Zumla A. Advances in the immunopathogenesis of pulmonary tuberculosis. *Curr Opin Pulm Med* 2001; **7**: 116–23.

53. Stead WW, Kerby GR, Schlueter DP, Jordahl CW. The clinical spectrum of primary tuberculosis in adults. Confusion with reinfection in the pathogenesis of chronic tuberculosis. *Ann Intern Med* 1968; **68**: 731–45.

54. Khan MA, Kovnat DM, Bachus B *et al.* Clinical and roentgenographic spectrum of pulmonary tuberculosis in the adult. *Am J Med* 1977; **62**: 31–8.

55. Choyke PL, Sostman HD, Curtis AM *et al.* Adult-onset pulmonary tuberculosis. *Radiology* 1983; **148**: 357–62.

56. Kim HC, Goo JM, Kim HB *et al.* Tuberculosis in patients with myelodysplastic syndromes. *Clin Radiol* 2002; **57**: 408–14.

57. Segarra F, Sherman DS, Rodriguez-Aguero J. Lower lung field tuberculosis. *Am Rev Respir Dis* 1963; **87**: 37–40.

58. Hadlock FP, Park SK, Awe RJ, Rivera M. Unusual radiographic findings in adult pulmonary tuberculosis. *AJR Am J Roentgenol* 1980; **134**: 1015–8.

59. Roper WH, Waring JJ. Primary serofibrinous pleural effusion in military personnel. *Am Rev Tuberc* 1955; **71**: 616–34.

60. Sakuraba M, Masuda K, Hebisawa A *et al.* Thoracoscopic pleural biopsy for tuberculous pleurisy under local anesthesia. *Ann Thorac Cardiovasc Surg* 2006; **12**: 245–8.

61. Milburn HJ. Primary tuberculosis. *Curr Opin Pulm Med* 2001; **7**: 133–41.

62. Sharma SK, Mohan A, Sharma A, Mitra DK. Miliary tuberculosis: new insights into an old disease. *Lancet Infect Dis* 2005; **5**: 415–30.

63. Franco-Paredes C, az-Borjon A, Senger MA *et al.* The ever-expanding association between rheumatologic diseases and tuberculosis. *Am J Med* 2006; **119**: 470–7.

64. Doan S, Gabison E, Gatinel D *et al.* Topical cyclosporine A in severe steroid-dependent childhood phlyctenular keratoconjunctivitis. *Am J Ophthalmol* 2006; **141**: 62–6.

65. Ayed AK. Resection of the right middle lobe and lingula in children for middle lobe/lingula syndrome. *Chest* 2004; **125**: 38–42.

66. Al Shahed M, Abd el Bagi M, Madkour MM. Radiology of pulmonary tuberculosis. In: Madkour MM (ed.). *Tuberculosis*, 1st edn. Berlin: Springer, 2004: 359–84.

67. Andreu J, Caceres J, Pallisa E, Martinez-Rodriguez M. Radiological manifestations of pulmonary tuberculosis. *Eur J Radiol* 2004; **51**: 139–49.

68. Wang JY, Hsueh PR, Lee CH *et al.* Recognising tuberculosis in the lower lung field: an age- and sex-matched controlled study. *Int J Tuberc Lung Dis* 2006; **10**: 578–84.

69. Harisinghani MG, McLoud TC, Shepard JA *et al.* Tuberculosis from head to toe. *Radiographics* 2000; **20**: 449–70.

70. Cheng VC, Ho PL, Lee RA et al. Clinical spectrum of paradoxical deterioration during antituberculosis therapy in non-HIV-infected patients. *Eur J Clin Microbiol Infect Dis* 2002; **21**: 803–9.

71. Rook GA, Dheda K, Zumla A. Immune systems in developed and developing countries; implications for the design of vaccines that will work where BCG does not. *Tuberculosis (Edinb)* 2006; **83**: 152–62.

72. Houben EN, Nguyen L, Pieters J. Interaction of pathogenic mycobacteria with the host immune system. *Curr Opin Microbiol* 2006; **9**: 76–85.

73. De Cock KM, Soro B, Coulibaly IM, Lucas SB. Tuberculosis and HIV infection in sub-Saharan Africa. *J Am Med Assoc* 1992; **268**: 1581–7.

74. Chretien J. *Tuberculosis: the illustrated history of a disease*, 1st edn. Bethune: Andre Harle, 1998.

75. Khan K, Campbell A, Wallington T, Gardam M. The impact of physician training and experience on the survival of patients with active tuberculosis. *CMAJ* 2006; **175**: 749–53.

76. English RG, Bachmann MO, Bateman ED *et al.* Diagnostic accuracy of an integrated respiratory guideline in identifying patients with respiratory symptoms requiring screening for pulmonary tuberculosis: a cross-sectional study. *BMC Pulm Med* 2006; **6**: 22.

77. den BS, White NW, van Lill SW *et al.* An evaluation of symptom and chest radiographic screening in tuberculosis prevalence surveys. *Int J Tuberc Lung Dis* 2006; **10**: 876–82.

78. Vargas D, Garcia L, Gilman RH *et al.* Diagnosis of sputum-scarce HIV-associated pulmonary tuberculosis in Lima, Peru. *Lancet* 2005; **365**: 150–2.

79. Wisnivesky JP, Kaplan J, Henschke C *et al.* Evaluation of clinical parameters to predict *Mycobacterium tuberculosis* in inpatients. *Arch Intern Med* 2000; **160**: 2471–6.

80. Buckingham SJ, Hansell DM. Aspergillus in the lung: diverse and coincident forms. *Eur Radiol* 2003; **13**: 1786–800.

81. Orlovic D, Smego RA Jr. Paradoxical tuberculous reactions in HIV-infected patients. *Int J Tuberc Lung Dis* 2001; **5**: 370–5.

82. Chung KS. Endobronchial tuberculosis. In: Madkour MM (ed.). *Tuberculosis*, 1st edn. Berlin: Springer, 2004: 329–48.

83. Shim YS. Endobronchial tuberculosis. *Respirology* 1996; **1**: 95–106.

84. Picard C, Parrot A, Boussaud V *et al.* Massive hemoptysis due to Rasmussen aneurysm: detection with helicoidal CT angiography and successful steel coil embolization. *Intens Care Med* 2003; **29**: 1837–9.

85. Kim HY, Song KS, Goo JM *et al.* Thoracic sequelae and complications of tuberculosis. *Radiographics* 2001; **21**: 839–58.

86. Fraser RS, Muller NL, Colman N, Pare PD. *Diagnosis of diseases of the chest*, 4th edn. Philadelphia: Saunders, 1999.

87. Lopez-Contreras J, Ris J, Domingo P *et al.* Tuberculous pulmonary gangrene: report of a case and review. *Clin Infect Dis* 1994; **18**: 243–5.

88. Tocque K, Convrey RP, Bellis MA *et al.* Elevated mortality following diagnosis with a treatable disease: tuberculosis. *Int J Tuberc Lung Dis* 2005; **9**: 797–802.

89. Lee HY, Goo JM, Lee HJ *et al.* The value of computed tomography for predicting empyema-associated malignancy. *J Comput Assist Tomogr* 2006; **30**: 453–9.

90. Lois M, Noppen M. Bronchopleural fistulas: an overview of the problem with special focus on endoscopic management. *Chest* 2005; **128**: 3955–65.

91. Harries AD, Maher D, Graham SM. *TB/HIV A clinical manual*, 2nd edn. Geneva: World Health Organization, 2004.

92. Okamoto M, Kawabe T, Iwasaki Y *et al.* Evaluation of interferon-gamma, interferon-gamma-inducing cytokines, and interferon-gamma-inducible chemokines in tuberculous pleural effusions. *J Lab Clin Med* 2005; **145**: 88–93.

93. Maher D, Harries AD. Tuberculous pericardial effusion: a prospective clinical study in a low-resource setting – Blantyre, Malawi. *Int J Tuberc Lung Dis* 1997; **1**: 358–64.

94. Kroot EJ, Hazes JM, Colin EM, Dolhain RJ. Poncet's disease: reactive arthritis accompanying tuberculosis. Two case reports and a review of the literature. *Rheumatology (Oxford)* 2007; **46**: 484–9.

95. Geng E, Kreiswirth B, Burzynski J, Schluger NW. Clinical and radiographic correlates of primary and reactivation tuberculosis: a molecular epidemiology study. *J Am Med Assoc* 2005; **293**: 2740–5.

96. Grzybowski S, Barnett GD, Styblo K. Contacts of cases of active pulmonary tuberculosis. *Bull Int Union Tuberc* 1975; **50**: 90–106.

97. Rossi SE, Franquet T, Volpacchio M *et al.* Tree-in-bud pattern at thin-section CT of the lungs: radiologic–pathologic overview. *Radiographics* 2005; **25**: 789–801.

98. Light RW. The undiagnosed pleural effusion. *Clin Chest Med* 2006; **27**: 309–19.

99. Sharma SK, Suresh V, Mohan A *et al.* A prospective study of sensitivity and specificity of adenosine deaminase estimation in the diagnosis of tuberculosis pleural effusion. *Indian J Chest Dis Allied Sci* 2001; **43**: 149–55.

100. Carstens ME, Burgess LJ, Maritz FJ, Taljaard JJ. Isoenzymes of adenosine deaminase in pleural effusions: a diagnostic tool? *Int J Tuberc Lung Dis* 1998; **2**: 831–5.

101. Harries AD, Hargreaves NJ, Gausi F *et al.* High early death rate in tuberculosis patients in Malawi. *Int J Tuberc Lung Dis* 2001; **5**: 1000–5.

10

Non-respiratory tuberculosis

PETER ORMEROD

INTRODUCTION

The number of cases of tuberculosis (TB) in the world was estimated to be 7.9 million cases (95 per cent confidence interval (CI), 6.3–11.1) and 1.8 million (1.4–2.8) deaths per year[1] and rising by at least 1 per cent per annum. Whilst the majority of cases are respiratory, the proportion of cases with non-respiratory disease is rising in both developed and developing countries, but for different reasons. In developed countries, particularly in Europe, but also in the USA,[2] an increasing proportion of cases of TB are occurring in ethnic minority groups which have both a much higher incidence of TB and also a higher proportion of non-respiratory disease. In England and Wales for example in 2005, only 27 per cent of cases were in the white ethnic group, with 73 per cent of cases from non-white ethnic groups and 67 per cent of all cases being foreign born.[3] In England and Wales in the national survey of 1993, the most recent to report detailed sites of disease, 32 per cent of previously untreated cases had non-respiratory disease.[4] There were important ethnic differences with over half of all non-respiratory disease coming from the 3 per cent of the population of South Asian ethnic origin. Only 22 per cent of white cases had non-respiratory disease, compared with 35 per cent of other ethnic groups and 42 per cent of the South Asian cases (Table 10.1). Even within non-pulmonary sites there were ethnic differences. In all ethnic groups, lymph node disease was the most common site, with 38, 47 and 63 per cent of white, South Asian and other ethnic groups respectively, whereas bone/joint TB was proportionately higher in white (15 per cent) and South Asian (14 per cent) cases than in other ethnic groups (8 per cent), and geni-

tourinary cases were higher in white cases (17 per cent) than in South Asian (3.7 per cent) and other ethnic groups (5.6 per cent) (Table 10.1).

The proportion of TB at extrapulmonary sites has not only risen in the United Kingdom, but also in other developed countries. In 1964, only 8 per cent of reported TB in the USA was non-respiratory, which increased to 15 per cent in 1981,[5] 17.5 per cent in 1986[6] and is now higher still.[2] Another country showing rises in the proportion of extrapulmonary TB is Hong Kong, with an increase to 6.6 per cent in 1990 from 1.2 per cent in 1967.[7] While the increase in extrapulmonary TB in developed countries is largely due to immigration from developing, high-prevalence countries, there are changes in epidemiology in developing countries which have over 98 per cent of the world burden.[1]

HIV co-infection particularly in sub-Saharan Africa,[8] but now increasingly in South Asia, alters the clinical pattern of disease, as well as increasing the incidence. Not only are HIV co-infected people much more likely to develop tuberculosis, but particularly extrapulmonary forms which occur in over 50 per cent of such TB-HIV cases.[9] Some sites, such as lymph nodes or the central nervous system, may also be more common in HIV co-infected than in HIV-negative individuals.[10]

Extrapulmonary disease is more difficult to diagnose. In developed countries, where until the last decade numbers of cases were falling and there is a very uneven distribution of disease, reduced clinician experience coupled with atypical or gradual presentations have contributed to delays in diagnosis and treatment leading to further morbidity or even death. In the less-developed world, the problems of

Table 10.1 Sites of disease England and Wales 1993.[4]

	White	Indian subcontinent	Other	Total
No. previously untreated patients	1088	1014	356	2458
Respiratory				
No. of patients[a]	834	612	253	1699
Type of lesions[b] (per cent)				
Pulmonary	778 (93)	484 (79)	219 (87)	1481 (87)
Pleural	59 (7.1)	70 (11)	24 (9.5)	153 (9.0)
Intrathoracic lymph nodes	6 (0.7)	52 (8.5)	13 (5.1)	71 (4.2)
Other	11 (1.3)	34 (5.6)	7 (2.8)	52 (3.1)
Non-respiratory				
No. of patients[a]	241	428	125	794
Type of lesions[b] (per cent)				
Lymph node	91 (38)	201 (47)	79 (63)	371 (47)
Bone and joint	35 (15)	60 (14)	10 (8.0)	105 (13)
Genitourinary tract	41 (17)	16 (3.7)	7 (5.6)	64 (8.1)
Abdomen	16 (6.6)	54 (12.6)	11 (8.8)	81 (10)
Central nervous system	9 (3.7)	19 (4.4)	2 (1.6)	30 (3.8)
Miliary	20 (8.3)	29 (6.8)	8 (6.4)	57 (7.2)
Abscess	8 (3.3)	21 (4.9)	7 (5.6)	36 (4.5)
Other	29 (12)	42 (9.8)	8 (6.4)	79 (9.9)
Site of disease not known	36	27	11	74

[a]23 white patients, 53 Indian subcontinent patients and 33 of other ethnic origin had both respiratory and non-respiratory sites.
[b]Some patients had lesions at more than one site (per cent are of total respiratory or non-respiratory lesions in each ethnic group).

diagnosis are compounded by a lack of diagnostic resources, with few forms of extrapulmonary TB showing acid-fast bacilli on microscopy. Studies on HIV-associated deaths in sub-Saharan Africa show significant levels of extrapulmonary tuberculosis.[11,12] Empirical treatment, or trials of treatment are more often given on clinical and/or radiological grounds without bacteriological and/or histological support or confirmation in such settings.

LYMPH NODE

Over 90 per cent of lymph node tuberculosis is in the cervical lymph nodes with only a small proportion of cases involving axillary, inguinal or chest wall nodes.[13] In England and Wales, it is most frequently seen in South Asian immigrants in whom it accounts for nearly 50 per cent of extrapulmonary disease.[3,4] Lymph node disease also accounts for over 30 per cent of extrapulmonary forms of disease in the USA,[2,14] and 45 per cent in Hong Kong.[7]

Mycobacterium bovis, which formerly accounted for a significant proportion of lymph node disease, is now much less common, *Mycobacterium tuberculosis* being the almost invariable isolate.[15] In young children in developed countries, particularly aged under 5 years of age, lymph node disease caused by opportunist mycobacteria such a *Mycobacterium avium* complex or *Mycobacterium malmoense* can simulate TB histologically. Isolation of such opportunist organisms, confirming a non-tuberculous

aetiology should lead to surgical excision as management, not drug treatment.

The organisms usually reach the lymph node by dissemination during the initial airborne infection in the lung and then later reactivation. Such reactivation occurs, as at other sites, when host defence mechanisms weaken, allowing previously contained disease to reactivate. Primary lymph node disease and lymphatic spread from adjacent sites can also occur. In England and Wales, up to 10 per cent of cervical lymph node disease in the South Asian ethnic group have associated mediastinal lymphadenopathy, suggesting retrograde spread from the mediastinal to the cervical nodes.[3,4] A prospective study of the source of cervical lymph node infection, whilst confirming that one-third had evidence of past or current respiratory tuberculosis consistent with earlier dissemination from a pulmonary source, also showed 6 per cent had nasopharyngeal TB and that cervical lymph nodes were part of the primary complex.[16] In developed countries,[17] the peak incidence of disease is between 20 and 40 years of age, but in high-prevalence countries it is highest in childhood. A deficiency of vitamin D has been invoked to explain the female preponderance of this form of disease in the South Asian ethnic group.[18]

Clinical features

The nodal enlargement in TB is usually painless and gradual, but can occasionally be painful if it is rapid.

Individually, the nodes are firm and discrete, but can later fluctuate as central caseation develops and mat together. The absence of erythema and warmth makes the classical 'cold abscess'. Without treatment, the nodes may proceed to discharge through the skin with resultant sinus formation, superficial ulceration and subsequent scarring. In patients who are immunosuppressed, the presentation can mimic an acute pyogenic abscess, with erythema, and marked local pain and swelling. Constitutional features involving weight loss, fever, malaise and night sweats are seen in only a minority of patients. Evidence of tuberculosis at other sites should be sought. Pulmonary disease or mediastinal lymph node involvement, the latter in ethnic minority groups,[3,4] is most commonly found on x-ray or clinically.

Diagnosis

In resource-poor settings, lymph node tuberculosis is a clinical diagnosis based on typical features, sometimes supported by a strongly positive tuberculin skin test. The diagnosis in its purest form depends on the demonstration of *M. bovis* or *M. tuberculosis* in pus, aspirates or biopsies from the gland. Direct smears from such samples, however, are rarely positive on direct microscopy, as the bacterial load in the nodes is small, the majority of the clinical features not being due to the infection itself, but to the marked immunological response to mycobacterial antigens. Biopsy samples from nodes may show acid-fast bacilli on smears more frequently, but even larger biopsy samples only have a positive culture rate of 50–70 per cent (Figure 10.1).[13,17,19,20]

The histological features on biopsy show a spectrum from a few granulomas with mild reactive hyperplasia

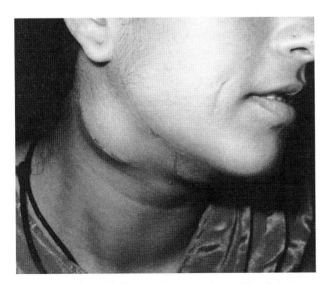

Figure 10.1 Cervical lymphadenopathy in an Asian female present for 3 months: biopsied as no pus on aspiration. Caseating granulomas on histology and *M. tuberculosis* cultured from biopsy material.

through to extensive caseation and necrosis. Lymph node biopsy is sometimes carried out as a diagnostic procedure when TB is not suspected, and when carcinoma or lymphoma is thought more likely. Under such circumstances, the surgeon often fails to send any sample for mycobacterial culture, placing all the sample in formalin. Excision biopsy itself has been shown not to enable shorter durations of treatment or to speed up healing.[13,17] Granulomatous histology, particularly if the granulomas are non-caseating, can be caused by a wide number of pathologies. Fungal infections, brucellosis and sarcoidosis are in the differential diagnosis, and classical 'tuberculous histology' with acid-fast bacilli on microscopy can occur with opportunist mycobacteria. Fine needle aspiration cytology (FNAC), which may be more applicable in resource-poor settings, has been shown to have a high specificity[21] and demonstrates granulomas in 71–83 per cent of cases.[21–24] These findings in addition to a strongly positive tuberculin test are an alternative to surgical intervention.[23]

Treatment

Controlled studies performed from the 1970s to the 1990s have defined the management of lymph node tuberculosis. Following a clinical study in the 1970s which showed 18 months of treatment with either isoniazid/rifampicin or isoniazid/ethambutol supplemented with 2 months' initial streptomycin gave good results,[13] the British Thoracic Society carried out a prospective controlled study comparing 9- and 18-month regimens of isoniazid/rifampicin supplemented with 2 months' initial ethambutol.[17] The 9-month regimen performed just as well both during treatment[17] and during 5 years' follow up where there were no microbiological relapses and good cosmetic results were obtained.[25] Pyrazinamide is better than ethambutol in the initial phase of treatment because it can reach bacteria sequestered inside lymphocytes and macrophages, acts at intracellular pH and is bactericidal rather than bacteriostatic.[26] Therefore, a further study was carried out by the British Thoracic Society[20] comparing two 9-month regimens of isoniazid/rifampicin supplemented by either ethambutol or pyrazinamide for two initial months, and a 6-month regimen of isoniazid/rifampicin supplemented by 2 months initial pyrazinamide. During treatment, all three regimens did not differ in the proportions with residual nodes or in terms of lymph node resolution.[20] Repeat aspiration after commencement of treatment, however, was more common with the ethambutol regimen ($p = 0.005$).[20] During follow up for 30 months from commencement of treatment, there were no differences between the regimens in terms of the proportions with residual glands, development of new glands or sinuses, or enlargement of glands.[27] In the follow-up period, there were nine clinical relapses, but no bacteriological relapse was found in the five cases where material was cultured.[27]

An earlier retrospective clinical series with the 6-month pyrazinamide regimen in fully susceptible organisms had also shown good results.[28] Short-course treatment in Indian children, but with a different regimen of thrice weekly supervised isoniazid/rifampicin/streptomycin/pyrazinamide for 2 months followed by twice weekly outpatient isoniazid/rifampicin for 4 months, had a 97 per cent success rate.[29] Following the third British Thoracic Society trial,[20,27] a six-month regimen with a four-drug initial phase including ethambutol is now recommended as standard treatment in the United Kingdom.[30]

The success of short-course therapy has been shown for fully susceptible organisms,[25,27] but may not apply to organisms with isoniazid or other significant resistance. In the British Thoracic Society studies, isoniazid resistance increased over time from 0/32 in 1977[31] and 0/29 in 1985[17] to 13/108 (12 per cent) in 1992.[20] The 6-month regimen is applicable therefore only to fully susceptible organisms.[27,30]

Modification for isoniazid-resistant organisms with a longer continuation phase of rifampicin/ethambutol is recommended,[30] and clinical studies have shown a good outcome with a 7-month continuation phase.[32]

In all three of the British Lymph Node trials, development of new nodes and enlargement of existing nodes are reported,[13,17,20] as were enlargement of persistent nodes which were residual at the end of treatment and the development of new glands after cessation of treatment.[25,27,31] Physicians who are not experienced in treating lymph node disease are concerned by the persistence of lymphadenopathy at the end of treatment, and particularly by the development of new lymphadenopathy during or after treatment. Treatment is sometimes unnecessarily prolonged or is restarted because of the 'relapse'. Such events of themselves do imply relapse and occur in a significant minority of treated patients. In the second[17] and third studies,[20] 12 per cent and 16–22 per cent, respectively, developed new lymph nodes during treatment. After treatment cessation, similar rates of persistent lymphadenopathy at the end of treatment and development of new nodes of 9 and 11 per cent[25] and 15 and 5 per cent[27] were reported. If biopsied, these nodes are usually negative on culture,[27] and although a clinical 'relapse' may be diagnosed, they are bacteriologically sterile. These phenomena do not indicate an unfavourable outcome and are likely to be immunologically mediated being due to hypersensitivity to tuberculoproteins released perhaps for disrupted macrophages.[17] Short courses of corticosteroids may be used to suppress these phenomena.

Surgical excision or biopsy is not part of the treatment of lymph node disease; those patients with no surgery did just as well as those with intervention.[17,25] A biopsy may need to be carried out as a procedure to both obtain histology and culture material, if aspiration of pus or fine needle aspiration cytology[21–24] is not used. Surgical biopsy is needed for culture material if no pus can be aspirated. Surgical excision is the treatment of choice for opportunist mycobacterial lymphadenopathy.[33–35]

BONE AND JOINT

This form of tuberculosis presents typically 3–5 years after the initial respiratory infection,[36] with the haematogenous spread at that initial infection, which has a predilection for the spine and growing ends of long bones, then lying dormant until clinical disease occurs. In developed countries, bone and joint tuberculosis can make up some 10–15 per cent of sites in both white and ethnic minority cases.[5] Studies, however, show much higher incidences in immigrant groups with, for example, rates of 0.2/100 000 and 16/100 000 in white and South Asian ethnic groups, respectively.[37]

The spine is the most common site of bone and joint TB at approximately 50 per cent of sites.[38,39] The most common initial symptom is back pain which may be present for weeks or months before diagnosis. Local tenderness or slight kyphosis may be present; grosser kyphosis occurs when disease has progressed. More unusual presentations with radicular pain mimicking abdominal conditions can occur.[40] Symptoms, both motor and sensory, involving the legs and sphincters can occur due to spinal cord compression. Paraspinal abscess not uncommonly complicates spinal tuberculosis, which can suggest a paraspinal mass or a psoas abscess, which appears or discharges in the groin. Associated psoas spasm causing hip flexion may be the presenting symptom in some cases.

Diagnosis

Diagnosis can be delayed in low-prevalence groups because of the rarity of the condition (incidence <1:100 000 per annum).[37,41] The spinal infection usually commences in the intravertebral disc and this discitis then spreads along the longitudinal and anterior spinal ligaments (Figure 10.2) to involve the inferior and superior borders of the adjacent vertebrae and the disc space is lost. As disease progresses, there is increasing vertebral destruction leading to angulation and loss of height at that level leading to kyphosis (Figure 10.3). The thoracic and lumbar spines are the usual sites of disease, with the cervical spine less commonly involved. Whilst a single intervertebral space is usually involved, multiple levels can be involved, sometimes with normal vertebrae between.

In developed countries new scanning modalities, computed tomography (CT) and magnetic resonance imaging (MRI), have greatly helped in the diagnosis and assessment of spinal tuberculosis. CT may show involvement before changes can be seen on standard x-rays[42] and often show the extent and associated complications better,[42–44] including psoas and paravertebral abcesses (Figure 10.4). MRI is also useful,[45,46] and the T_2-weighted images may show epidural inflammation.[46] The ability for three-dimensional image reconstruction of MRI images is particularly useful if spinal surgery is being contemplated.[47] Only in a minority of cases is there co-existent pulmonary tuberculosis,[38]

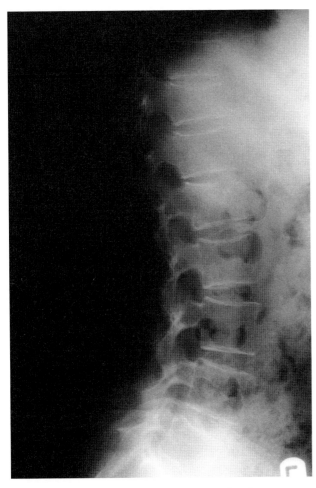

Figure 10.2 Early disease involving the D12/L1 disc space with erosion of the upper anterior surface of L1.

but if this is present with classical spinal x-ray appearances, a clinical diagnosis can be made without biopsy. Open or needle biopsy may be needed to make or confirm a diagnosis of spinal disease. Appropriate cultures may not be taken unless mycobacterial as well as pyogenic infections are considered and both diagnosis and appropriate treatment may then be delayed.[38,41] The main differential diagnoses are metastatic spinal disease and acute pyogenic infection. With metastatic disease, the x-ray features are different with preservation of the disc space but erosion of the vertebral bodies and pedicles, unlike tuberculous or pyogenic infection. Pyogenic infection, e.g. with staphylococci, can mimic tuberculosis, but there are often systemic features, and the onset is more acute and pain more prominent.

Treatment

The relative roles of chemotherapy and surgery in spinal tuberculosis were assessed over a prolonged period by a number of studies by the British Medical Research Council. Before the advent of short-course chemotherapy

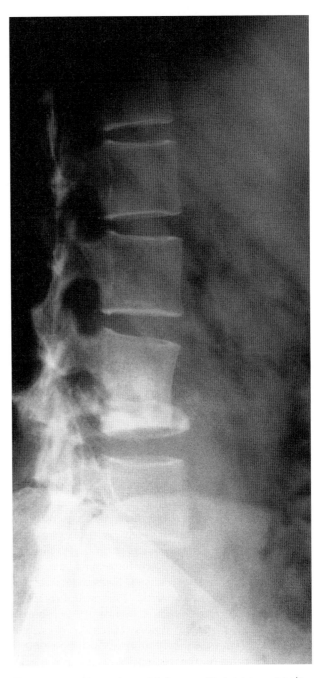

Figure 10.3 More substantial disease with total loss of L4/3 disc space and extensive collapse of L4 vertebral body.

studies were performed in Korea,[48,49] Rhodesia[50] and Hong Kong[51] using isoniazid/para-aminosalicylic acid (PAS) for 18 months. These studies showed over 80 per cent achieving favourable status at 3 years, but also showed no additional benefit from bed rest for the initial 6 months of therapy, plaster jackets, from the addition of streptomycin for the initial 3 months of therapy, or of debridement operations.[48–51]

An operation which involved excision of the spinal focus and creating anterior fusion by bone grafting was developed in Hong Kong, becoming known as the 'Hong

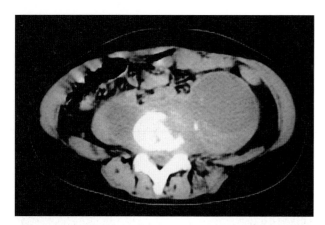

Figure 10.4 Bilateral L > R psoas abscesses related to spinal disease. Presented with left psoas spasm. One litre of pus drained from left by ultrasound-guided aspiration which grew *M. tuberculosis*.

Kong operation'. When used in combination with chemotherapy less residual deformity and more rapid bone fusion were obtained.[52] When patients treated by chemotherapy alone were later compared with those treated by the 'Hong Kong operation', no additional benefit accrued from surgery.[53] These comparisons also showed that a regimen of six or nine months of isoniazid and rifampicin, supplemented by twice weekly streptomycin was highly effective.[54]

Because pyrazinamide is more bactericidal than streptomycin, has good tissue penetration and is only required for the initial 2 months of treatment, 6 months short-course regimens can be recommended for spinal tuberculosis.[30] The advent of MRI scanning is causing some surgeons to advocate a more radical surgical approach,[55,56] particularly in younger children to prevent later deformity.[57] The overall assessment is still that spinal tuberculosis without instability or evidence of spinal cord compression should be treated medically and not have routine anterior spinal fusion.[30,58] Anterior spinal fusion should only be considered for those with spinal instability or evidence of spinal cord compression.[30]

Other bone/joint sites

Whilst spinal sites account for approximately half of all bone disease, any bone or joint can be involved. In developed countries, increasing numbers of cases are seen, with a shift to younger age and in ethnic minority and immigrant groups.[59]

Clinical series in South Asian patients in England show a wide variety of sites (Figure 10.5).[38] Tuberculosis should be included in the differential diagnosis of unusual bone or joint lesions, particularly of an isolated lesion or monoarthritis in an immigrant ethnic group, otherwise there may be substantial delays in making a diagnosis.[38,60] Single[61] and multiple[62] joint presentations are described

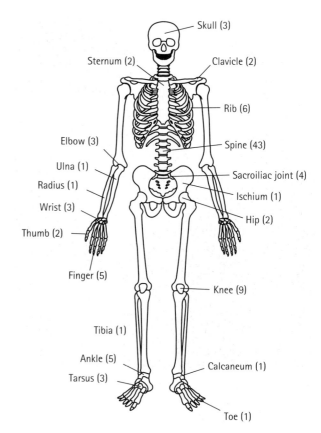

Figure 10.5 Sites of bony tuberculosis in Asian patients updated from Ref. 38. Number of patients for each site in parentheses.

(Figures 10.6–10.8). There are occasional reports of cases with so many sites and of a cystic type that metastatic bone disease is mimicked.[63] Such non-spinal sites seldom require surgical treatment, but surgical intervention to obtain biopsy material for histology and culture is often initially required, either by arthroscopy, e.g. knee or elbow, or by open biopsy.[38,60] A 6-month short-course regimen is also recommended for bone and joint disease at non-spinal sites.[30] Surgery is occasionally required after the completion of antituberculosis drug treatment if there has been substantial joint disease or instability caused by either extensive disease and/or late presentation. Arthrodesis of unstable joints may be required, and replacement of knee and hip joints, sometimes under antituberculosis drug cover, has been carried out.

Combined management of orthopaedic tuberculosis of whatever site is advised,[38] with the physician supervising the antituberculosis drug treatment[30] and the orthopaedic surgeon managing the mechanical aspects of the disease.

GASTROINTESTINAL

This form of tuberculosis is uncommon in the indigenous populations of developed countries. In the United Kingdom in 1993, only 6 per cent of white non-pulmonary

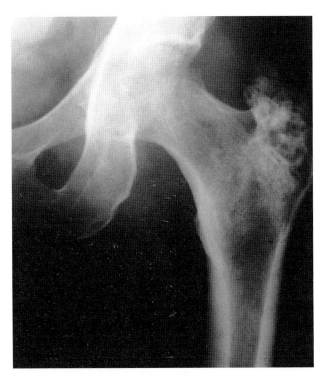

Figure 10.6 Tuberculosis of the left hip and greater trochanter presenting with a sinus over the hip from which *M. tuberculosis* was isolated.

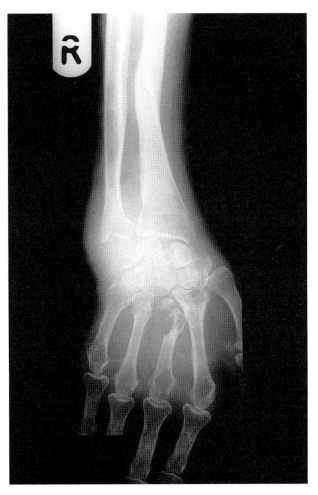

Figure 10.7 Tuberculosis of the right third metacarpal with erosion of the bone.

disease was in the gastrointestinal tract,[4] and in 1983 the rate in the South Asian ethnic group was 50 times that of the white population.[37] In developing countries, gastrointestinal tuberculosis is reported commonly in both HIV-negative and HIV-positive patients. In the pre-HIV era, one-third of all ascites was tuberculous in aetiology,[64] with a proportion of over 40 per cent being reported in Lesotho in 1986.[65] Pulmonary and abdominal tuberculosis have both been shown to contribute significantly to the wasting in HIV-positive persons known as 'slim disease' seen in Africa, with intra-abdominal lymphadenopathy being a significant feature in such cases.[66]

Clinical features and presentation

The gastrointestinal tract can be involved anywhere along its length; however, involvement of the upper gastrointestinal tract or perianal disease are uncommon, the former accounting for only 3 per cent of a 500-patient series of surgically treated patients.[67] Infection in the gastrointestinal tract can be due to either ingestion of bacilli either from swallowed sputum or from infected milk, haematogenous spread or by local extension to the peritoneum from gut or nodes. Gastric and duodenal ulcers are described,[68] which are not distinguishable from peptic ulcers other than by a positive culture for *M. tuberculosis* or finding granulomas on histology. Oesophageal involvement is described, usually presenting as dysphagia, due

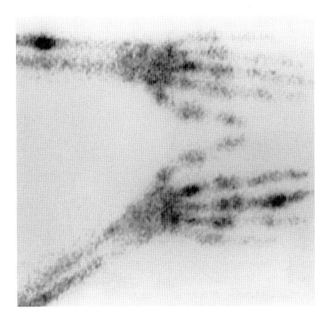

Figure 10.8 Isotope bone scan of a patient with tuberculosis dactylitis of the right third finger showing additional subclinical lesions in the right second metacarpal and left radius.

usually to direct spread from contiguous mediastinal lymph node involvement. At endoscopy, the appearances can simulate ulcerating oesophageal carcinoma.[69,70]

In series in both developing[71] and developed countries[68] approximately one-third present acutely simulating abdominal emergencies and two-thirds present with more gradual onset of symptoms, usually abdominal pain. Of cases with an acute presentation, approximately half have right iliac fossa pain simulating acute appendicitis and the other half have acute intestinal obstruction.[68,72,73] Fever and malaise, abdominal pain and weight loss are the most common described symptoms,[68] being found in 72, 60 and 58 per cent of cases, respectively, in another series.[74] Abdominal distension, usually due to ascites, is described in proportions varying from 10[68] to 65 per cent.[75] The proportion of cases with co-existing respiratory tuberculosis varies from series to series. This proportion has varied from under 30 per cent[68,76] to 36 per cent,[74] 40 per cent[77] and up to nearly 65 per cent in children.[78]

Abdominal tuberculosis has no classical diagnostic signs[79] and the supposed classical 'doughy' abdomen is not reported in some large series.[68] There may be right iliac tenderness simulating appendicitis or a right iliac fossa mass simulating appendix abscess or carcinoma. The ileocaecal area is the most common site of disease, with frequencies between 25 and 80 per cent reported.[68,75,80,81] With bowel involvement, acute or subacute small bowel obstruction is the presentation, with vomiting and abdominal distension, and there may also be a palpable mass.[68,73] The colon distal to the caecum is involved in up to 10 per cent[68,82] and is a cause of gastrointestinal bleeding.[83,84] Tuberculous ischiorectal abscesses[68] and anal margin disease are also described.[85]

Diagnosis

The non-specific presentation in the majority of cases, coupled with the fact that two-thirds have normal chest x-rays, means that tuberculosis is often not suspected in those cases, with inflammatory bowel disease or malignancy thought more likely.[73] Anaemia, either normochromic or hypochromic, a reduced serum albumen (<35 g/L) and raised inflammatory markers, such as erythrocyte sedimentation rate (ESR) or C-reactive protein (CRP), are frequently seen but are non-specific.[68] While the tuberculin skin test is positive in most cases,[68] it can be negative in HIV-positive people, in the undernourished, those immunosuppressed by medication and those with advanced disease.

In common with other serous membrane tuberculosis, the ascitic fluid in abdominal tuberculosis is an exudate (protein >35 g/L), is usually straw coloured, and is a lymphocyte predominant fluid on cytology. Acid-fast bacilli are seldom seen on microscopy of the fluid by either Ziehl–Nielsen or auramine staining,[86,87] and the positive culture rate is under 50 per cent.[68,76] When the chest x-ray

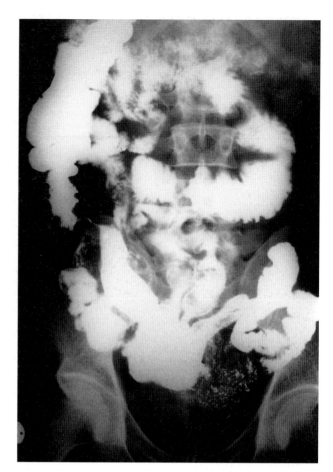

Figure 10.9 *Tuberculosis of the small bowel and caecum. Barium follow-through showing strictures in the ileum and at the ileocaecal junction with an abnormal lower pole of the caecum.*

shows features of pulmonary or other tuberculosis, e.g. mediastinal glands or pleural effusion, then the diagnosis is suggested. Positive bacteriology should be sought from sputum and/or other respiratory samples, e.g. gastric washings in children.

The utility of radiology investigation varies with the type of examination and the type of gastrointestinal disease. Plain abdominal x-rays give little specific help other than to show either ascites or, on an erect film, distended bowel loops confirming bowel obstruction. Barium meal is seldom helpful, but barium studies of the small bowel or barium enema may be. Small bowel studies may show mucosal abnormalities, strictures, 'skip lesions' and fistulas (Figure 10.9). These features, however, are often seen in Crohn's disease and tuberculosis cannot be differentiated from inflammatory bowel disease on radiological features alone. The small bowel barium studies may also show ileocaecal disease as the contrast progresses. Barium enema can also show ileocaecal disease, when vertical passage of the ileum into the colon or shortening of the ascending colon being suggestive of tuberculosis.[72] In the colon, carcinoma is mimicked by annular lesions and strictures or shouldering (Figure 10.10).[68]

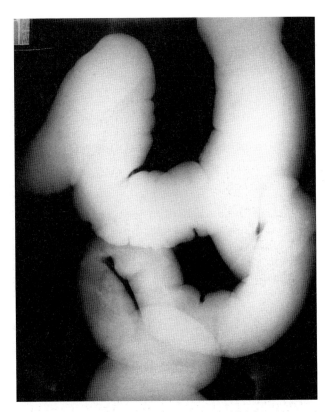

Figure 10.10   Barium enema in a 38-year-old Asian woman with two stone (13 kg) weight loss. Obstruction in the ascending colon is shown mimicking carcinoma. Ileocaecal tuberculosis was resected.

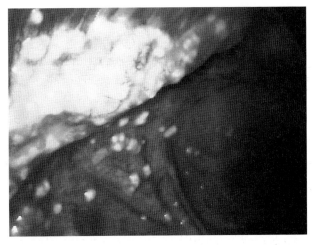

Figure 10.11   Laparoscopic appearances of peritoneal tuberculosis with multiple granulomatous deposits on serosal surfaces. Caseating granulomas seen on histology and positive on culture for *M. tuberculosis.*

Ultrasound and CT or MRI scanning can give suggestive but not diagnostic appearances in both ascites and bowel disease.[88] Ultrasound may show ascites in which there are thin fibrin strands, thickened omentum or retroperitoneal lymphadenopathy, or ileocaecal changes. Ultrasound-guided fine needle biopsy, particularly if there is only retroperitoneal or mesenteric lymphadenopathy, may give cytological evidence of tuberculosis.[89] On CT, the ascitic element is usually of high (15–30 Hounsfield units) density. A variety of features from lymphadenopathy, ascites, bowel wall involvement and mesenteric thickening is described.[90,91]

Irregular soft tissue densities in the omentum or lymph nodes with a well-demarcated central area of low density, which is thought to represent caseation, are very suggestive.[92] With intravenous contrast, these features can be enhanced further, the inflammatory ring becoming more predominant.[93] This feature, however, has also been described in both lymphoma and carcinoma. Bowel thickening with nodularity of the wall is also described[94–96] and all the above features may be seen in combination with bowel loops in a poorly defined mass.[97–99]

A definitive diagnosis required either positive cultures from ascitic fluid or intra-abdominal biopsy material, or classical histological features from biopsy material. Whilst laparotomy will give a definite diagnosis in nearly all cases

if adequate culture and biopsy material is taken, less invasive techniques can be used to avoid full laparotomy. The use of a blind, percutaneous, peritoneal needle biopsy was described by Levine,[96] with few complications and a high yield. Other series, however, have not been able to reproduce this level of results.[99] Other authors before the wider availability of laparoscopy felt that open biopsy was safer because the biopsy under direct vision carried a lower risk of bowel perforation.[100]

Laparoscopy is now the initial biopsy procedure of choice, with good safety, few complications and a very high positive diagnosis rate (Figure 10.11).[81,87,99,100] Laparoscopy has the lowest risk of bowel perforation when there are ascites present. Mini-laparotomy may be preferred when there is either intense plastic peritonitis or ultrasound or CT shows bowel loops adherent to the anterior abdominal wall, which greatly increase the risk of perforation. Colonoscopy can now reach the entire colon and sometimes the ileocaecal valve,[82,101] but adequate specimens are essential. Fine-needle aspiration in addition at colonoscopy may give additional evidence.[102]

If bacteriological cultures are not positive, there can be problems differentiating Crohn's disease and tuberculosis, both of which have granulomatous patterns. In Crohn's disease, the granulomas are more evident in the bowel wall than in lymph nodes associated with the bowel, whereas in tuberculosis the pattern is reversed with more granulomas in the nodes.[103]

Treatment

Abdominal tuberculosis carried a high mortality in the prechemotherapy era.[104,105] Series reporting overall results using short-course chemotherapy show mortalities of 5–7 per cent,[68,106] although some of the mortality was pre-diagnosis. There are no prospective trials of short-course chemotherapy in gastrointestinal tuberculosis, but a 6-month regimen is recommended in the UK.[30] Adjuvant corticosteroids which are of benefit in pericardial disease (see later) and may have a place in pleural disease, are seldom needed and are not advised for routine clinical use.[68] Bowel resection is only required if there is mechanical obstruction and, if carried out, should be by end to end anastomosis rather than by ileo-transverse anastomosis.[68,72,107] Longer-term morbidity seems to be low with modern short-course treatment. In one large series of 103 patients followed for 15 months post-treatment, there was no recurrence of gastrointestinal problems,[68] but 10 per cent of female patients of childbearing age had either primary or secondary infertility after intra-abdominal tuberculosis.[68]

GENITOURINARY

Genitourinary tuberculosis is one of the more common sites of extrapulmonary tuberculosis in white patients in the UK. In 1993, it accounted for 17 per cent of cases in the white ethnic group compared with under 4 per cent in the South Asian ethnic group.[4] An earlier detailed analysis of sites of disease showed rates of genitourinary tuberculosis of 0.4/100 000 and 4/100 000, respectively, in the white and South Asian ethnic groups.[37] At a ratio of 10:1 South Asian:White, this was the lowest ratio for all extrapulmonary sites. This, together with the numerical preponderance of white cases, raised questions as to why genitourinary tuberculosis was under-represented in South Asian patients.[108] The explanation may be that this is an age-related phenomenon in developed countries as the median age of the white cases is over 50 years, whilst the median age of South Asian cases is 29 years. This would fit in with the natural history of renal tuberculosis (see below). The same survey also showed that in white patients renal tract lesions predominated, but female genital disease predominated in the South Asian ethnic group.[37] There are fewer data from resource-poor countries, but a recent West African study showed 9 per cent of pulmonary cases had renal involvement on urine Z–N positivity, and 14 per cent if sterile pyuria and renal histology were added.[109]

Although renal involvement is common in the first few months of primary infection, with M. tuberculosis detected in the urine,[36] showing blood-borne dissemination early in the disease, clinical disease was often over 20 years after primary infection, with the organism lying dormant for that length of time often in the renal parenchyma. The finding of M. bovis in genitourinary isolates,[110,111] in areas where M. bovis has been eradicated from cattle for many years, also supports this natural history. Additional support also comes from reactivation tuberculosis from presumed dormant foci in transplanted kidneys following immunosuppression.[112] Conversely, chronic renal failure

is a risk factor for the development of tuberculosis in many settings.[113–115] The renal failure itself seems to have an immunospuppresive effect as this increase in incidence is seen in patients without immunosuppressant drug therapy.[114,116] The clinical aspects of urological tuberculosis and gynaecological tuberculosis will be discussed separately.

Clinical aspects of urological tuberculosis

Renal tuberculosis is frequently a 'silent' disease which progresses insidiously and can lead to total unilateral renal destruction before diagnosis. Systemic features, such as fever, weight loss and night time sweats, are not common. With progressive disease, dysuria, haematuria, nocturia and pain either in the loin or anteriorly may occur. Younger patients, under 25 years, appear more likely to describe pain as a symptom.[117] Renal tuberculosis may be found during investigation of hypertension,[118] but rarely presents as renal failure due to parenchymal involvement or as obstructive hydronephrosis due to ureteric involvement.[119] Diffuse interstitial nephritis can be caused by tuberculosis,[120] which should not be missed as treatment by antituberculosis drugs supplemented by corticosteroids can improve renal function substantially and prevent progression to renal replacement. This phenomenon has also been described in transplanted kidneys.[121]

Renal disease can lead to ureteric and then bladder involvement by tubercle bacilli being seeded into the urine and implanting distally. Ureteric involvement can cause an irregular stenosis with distal obstructive uropathy, and in extreme cases complete obstruction leading to a tuberculous pyonephrosis. Bladder involvement initially leads to cystitis symptoms with frequency and dysuria, but as bladder wall inflammation with associated fibrosis worsens, bladder capacity reduces and can be greatly diminished, the so-called 'thimble bladder', leading to marked frequency and nocturia due to this tiny bladder capacity. The urine with renal and ureteric disease, but particularly with bladder disease, shows haematuria and proteinuria on dipstick testing, and pus cells on microscopy, but is negative for standard bacterial pathogens on culture. The finding of a sterile pyuria should lead to the routine sending of three early-morning urines for TB culture. The prostate, epididymis and testis are less commonly involved.[122] Although haematogenous spread, and occasionally direct spread from foci in the genital tract, do occur, antegrade spread from the kidney and bladder are thought much more common. Local symptoms of discharge or dysuria can mimic chlamydial or bacterial infections, and in testicular disease a mass may mimic testicular tumour.

The diagnosis of urinary tract tuberculosis still depends heavily on the intravenous pyelogram (IVP) and early-morning urine cultures. The IVP shows a high percentage of abnormalities in renal disease. In early disease, there may just be clubbing or calyceal abnormalities, sometimes with pelviureteric junction narrowing with associated

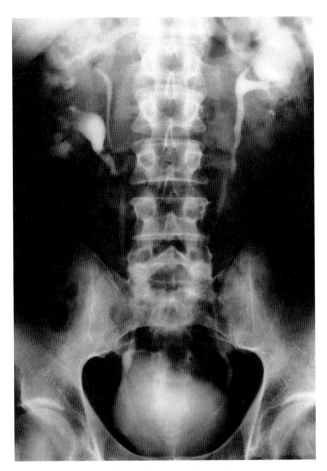

Figure 10.12 Intravenous pyelogram in renal tuberculosis with calyceal clubbing particularly of the lower right kidney. Prostatic calcification is just visible at the bottom of the film. Positive early morning urine culture for *M. tuberculosis*.

pelvic dilatation. The process progresses to pelvic obliteration and on to a small or non-functioning kidney. Calcification in the kidney or other parts of the urinary tract, e.g. prostate, are quite common and an important clue to the diagnosis (Figure 10.12).[123] Ultrasound may show hydronephrosis and/or reduced renal size, but is not specific. CT scanning may show calcification and parenchymal retraction, low parenchymal density and clubbing of the calyces in two-thirds of cases[124] and also pelvic contraction or ureteropelvic fibrosis with or without obstruction.[125] Associated perinephric abscess may occur, which can point either to the loin[126] or to a psoas abscess in the groin. Isotope renography is useful in assessing differential renal function, and by showing delayed excretion may be the first clue to ureteric obstruction. Serial isotope urograms are also helpful in showing whether there is improvement to treatment modalities if significant ureteric stenosis has been shown.

Cultures of urine and tissue, if possible, should be undertaken, particularly if an abscess is found in association with the epididymis or kidney. Urine cultures, best done as early-morning samples on three consecutive mornings, should be carried out on all patients with sus-

pected urological tuberculosis. Microscopy of urine has a low positive microscopy rate, the main yield being on culture. A positive microscopy for acid-fast bacilli on urine should be questioned. False-positive microscopy can be obtained by either the sample being contaminated by *Mycobacterium smegmatis*, a saprophytic mycobacterium found in genital secretions, or laboratory reagents being contaminated by environmental mycobacteria. Molecular amplification tests may have a role in helping confirm a positive organism is tuberculosis, or to suggest the diagnosis,[127–129] but may not work in some 10 per cent of samples because of inhibitors,[128] and are more sensitive if used on concentrates from large urine volumes.[128] Active pulmonary tuberculosis is not commonly associated with urological tuberculosis in developed countries, but this may not be true in other settings.[109] Obviously if the chest x-ray suggests respiratory disease, sputum should be examined for acid-fast bacilli. The diagnosis may also be made from biopsies taken when tuberculosis is not initially expected, and tumour, e.g. testis or kidney, is thought to be the diagnosis.

Management

Surgery may initially be needed to obtain a diagnostic biopsy, but has significant utility in genitourinary tuberculosis. All patients require drug treatment even if all apparent disease has been removed, because of potential foci elsewhere. Controlled trials of short-course chemotherapy are not available for urological tuberculosis, but the short-course six-month regimen is recommended.[30] Rifampicin is an excellent drug for urological tuberculosis because of the very high concentrations achieved in the urine, which can reach 100 times serum levels, comfortably exceeding the required minimum inhibitory concentration (MIC) for *M. tuberculosis*. If the organism is *M. bovis*, a nine-month regimen of rifampicin/isoniazid supplemented by two months' initial ethambutol has to be used. Corticosteroids are advised to prevent progression of ureteric disease,[130] but has not been tested by controlled trial. Benefit of corticosteroids has been shown for tuberculous interstitial nephritis where it improves renal function.[120] Excisional surgery may be needed for a destroyed non-functioning kidney. In one very large series of 1117 patients, 30 per cent had nephrectomies, 17 per cent epididymectomies and 4 per cent orchidectomy, and 7 per cent underwent partial nephrectomy because of tuberculous lesions causing problems such as recurrent infections.[130] In the same series,[130] which was before modern non-invasive interventions, 6 per cent required ureteric implantation, 5 per cent required bladder reconstruction and 2 per cent ureterocolonic transplantation. Ureteric stenosis can be managed by stenting at the upper end or dilatation at the lower end.[131,132] Renal function can be monitored qualitatively and quantitatively by isotope renography, but deterioration in function can be rapid.[133]

Reimplantation or urinary diversion can now be reserved for those cases where other measures fail or are not possible.[134] For those few patients with severe bladder capacity, reduction due to tuberculous cystitis, bladder augmentation by ileal loop attached to the dome of the bladder can improve the bladder capacity by some 300–400 mL.[135] Such procedures are best carried out after the completion of drug treatment.

Gynaecological tuberculosis

Female genital tuberculosis is more common in the South Asian ethnic group[37] and occurs by direct spread from tuberculous peritonitis or by haematogenous spread. As with urological tuberculosis, systemic features are not common unless there is associated abdominal tuberculosis. Infertility, either primary or secondary, is the most common presentation of tubal and endometrial involvement.[136] Most have no associated features; menorrhagia or pelvic pain are reported in 20–25 per cent, but amenorrhoea or post-menopausal bleeding are much less common.[136] The frequency of diagnosis of female genital TB varies with the setting. An incidence of 0.5 per cent of investigated infertility patients is described from Nigeria,[137] but in India over one-third of patients with tubal factors in infertility had tuberculosis.[138] In a further study, patients with active pulmonary tuberculosis were investigated, with 12.3 per cent found to have genital tuberculosis.[139] Endometrial disease may rarely present as congenital tuberculosis in a neonate,[140] although conception with active endometrial disease is uncommon. Vulval disease is also uncommon and may imitate sexually transmitted diseases.[141] In high-prevalence groups, patients are sometimes thought to have ovarian cancer, but in fact have abdominal tuberculosis,[142] a further complication being that high levels of CA125 are described in abdominal/pelvic tuberculosis.[143]

Six months of short-course chemotherapy is advised,[30] although as with urological tuberculosis, this is not based on controlled clinical trials. Whilst active disease is cured bacteriologically, the residual damage, particularly to the Fallopian tubes, leads to high levels of infertility, with low conception rates and even lower live birth rates,[144] with *in vitro* fertilization or other techniques sometimes offering the only hope of conception.

MILIARY TUBERCULOSIS

Miliary tuberculosis occurs when tubercle bacilli are spread acutely through the blood stream. In high-prevalence areas, the majority of cases follow shortly after initial infection, but in low-prevalence areas, the majority of cases are in the elderly, representing reactivation. The lung is always involved, other organs variably so.

Microscopically, the miliary lesions consist of Langhans giant cells, epithelioid cells and lymphocytes, and contain acid-fast bacilli, sometimes with central caseation. In elderly or immunosuppressed patients, non-reactive pathological appearances are decribed with necrotic lesions containing no specific tuberculous features, but teeming with acid-fast bacilli. In such cases, the diagnosis is usually made post mortem.[145] The symptoms are insidious in onset[146] and include anorexia, malaise, fever and weight loss and occur in both the 'acute' and cryptic forms. Miliary tuberculosis accounts for between 6 and 8 per cent of cases of extrapulmonary tuberculosis in England and Wales.[4]

Acute miliary tuberculosis

In addition to the general symptoms, headache from coexistent tuberculous meningitis occurs frequently and should alert the clinician to perform a lumbar puncture. Cough, dyspnoea and haemoptysis are less common symptoms. Physicial signs are few; the chest almost invariably sounds clear on auscultation. Enlargement of the liver, spleen or lymph nodes may be found in a small number of cases.[147] Involvement of the serosal surfaces can lead to the development of small pericardial or pleural effusions or slight ascites. Fundal examination should be carried out to detect choroidal tubercles, which are more commonly seen in children. Skin lesions may also occur in the form of papules, macules and purpuric lesions. These probably represent local vasculitic lesions caused by reaction to mycobacterial antigen. The typical x-ray shows an even distribution of uniform-sized lesions 1–2 mm throughout all zones of the lung (Figure 10.13). Small

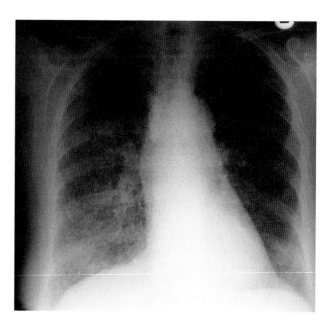

Figure 10.13 Classical miliary tuberculosis in an elderly white female. Calcification of the right paratracheal glands shows this is reactivation disease. Presented as meningitis with positive cerebrospinal fluid cultures.

Table 10.2 Comparison between classical and cryptic forms of miliary tuberculosis (TB).

Feature	Cryptic	Classical acute
Age	Majority over 60 years	Majority under 40 years
TB history or contact	Up to 25%	Up to 33%
Malaise/weight loss	75%	75%
Fever	90%	75%
Choroidal tubercles	Absent	Up to 20%
Meningitis	Rare unless terminal	Up to 20%
Lymphadenopathy	Absent	Up to 20%
Miliary shadowing on x-ray	Rare	Usual except in early stages
Tuberculin test	Usually negative	Usually positive
Pancytopenia/leukaemoid reaction	Common	Rare
Bacteriological confirmation	Urine, sputum, bone marrow	Sputum, cerebrospinal fluid
Biopsy evidence	Liver up to 75%; bone marrow, lymph node	Seldom required

bilateral pleural effusions may also be seen. An unusual variation with reticular shadowing due to lymphatic involvement has been described.[148]

Cryptic miliary tuberculosis

As tuberculosis declines in incidence in the native populations of developed countries, a form of miliary tuberculosis without typical x-ray shadowing, so-called 'cryptic' miliary tuberculosis has been seen more frequently. This is usually seen in patients aged over 60 years,[149] but may be seen in young patients in some immigrant groups. The symptoms are usually insidious, with weight loss, lethargy and intermittent fever.[150] Meningitis and choroidal tubercles are rarely found; mild hepatosplenomegaly may be found but physical signs are usually absent. Because of this, a high index of suspicion is required to reach a diagnosis, and commonly the diagnosis is not made until post mortem.[151] The main differential diagnosis is disseminated carcinoma. Table 10.2 contrasts the features of classical 'acute' and 'cryptic' forms of miliary disease.

Diagnosis

The classical form of the disease is usually easy to diagnose because of the typical x-ray appearances (Figure 10.13), which are only absent in the early stages, but which may be detected earlier on high-resolution CT scanning (Figure 10.14). The tuberculin test is usually positive, and bacteriological confirmation may be obtained from sputum, urine and cerebrospinal fluid (CSF). The detection of the cryptic form rests initially on having clinical suspicion of the diagnosis and then carrying out specific tests or monitoring response to a trial of antituberculosis drugs. Blood dyscrasias are not uncommonly seen in the cryptic form, pancytopenia,[152,153] leukaemoid reactions,[154,155] and other granulocyte abnormalities,[156] have all been reported. Bone

marrow aspiration may yield both granulomata on biopsy and acid-fast bacilli on culture, and should be considered if a blood dyscrasia is present. Liver biopsy has the highest yield of granulomata which have been reported in up to 75 per cent of biopsies. In cases where the patient is unwilling, or where facilities for them do not exist, a clinical trial of antituberculosis drugs should be given. The fever usually responds within 7–10 days, followed by clinical improvement in 4–6 weeks.

Complications

Tuberculous meningitis may complicate miliary tuberculosis and is a manifestation of acute haematogenous spread. It occurs overtly in up to 20 per cent of cases. Lumbar puncture should be performed if there are any

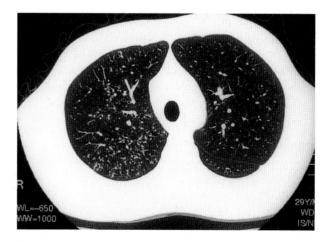

Figure 10.14 High-resolution computed tomography (CT) in a patient with a pyrexia of unknown origin and weight loss whose standard chest x-ray suggested minimal nodularity, particularly in the right upper zone. The high-resolution CT may show early miliary disease more clearly than on plain x-rays. Positive cultures obtained from bronchial washings.

symptoms of meningism or headache. A positive microscopy for acid-fast bacilli from the CSF may be the most rapid way of confirming the clinical diagnosis of miliary tuberculosis. Adult respiratory distress syndrome (ARDS) can, rarely, be the presentation of miliary TB.[157] In such cases, the breathlessness due to the ARDS can be dominant and the classical x-ray appearances obscured by diffuse confluent or ground-glass shadowing.[158,159]

CENTRAL NERVOUS SYSTEM

Although only making up some 5 per cent of notified cases of extrapulmonary disease in developed countries,[4,37] central nervous system tuberculosis has a disproportionate importance because of the significant morbidity and mortality associated with this form of tuberculosis. These are a major cause of death and disability, particularly in developing countries where reduced treatment facilities and availability, and also difficulties in making the diagnosis may also contribute. An increased risk of central nervous system (CNS) disease in HIV-infected individuals is reported, with rates of up to 2/100 in one series.[10]

Whilst the substantial majority of cases are of tuberculous meningitis, intracranial tuberculomata occur sometimes in association or occasionally on their own. Rarely tuberculous extradural abscesses are reported in association with bony lesions involving the skull vault.[38] Meningeal infection is almost always from a distal focus by haematogenous spread, with up to 20 per cent having obvious miliary tuberculosis (Table 10.2). Small subpial tuberculomata develop from this blood-borne spread, from which the tubercle bacilli gain access to the cerebrospinal fluid.[160] CNS infection often provokes an intense inflammatory response. The meninges look to be covered by a grey, thickened exudate, which can be sufficiently intense to occlude foramina, particularly in the posterior fossa. These meningeal changes then lead to an endarteritis obliterans which more often causes focal neurological signs by infarction than do tuberculomata. The meningeal exudate can also extend down the spinal cord on to spinal roots.[160] This inflammatory response is often more the cause of symptoms and signs than the infection itself.

Clinical features

The early symptoms are non-specific, with anorexia, malaise, headache and vomiting. The dominant features in children may be poor feeding, irritability, altered behaviour or drowsiness. These somewhat non-specific features may mean that diagnosis is delayed during this prodromal phase, which can last between 2 weeks and 2 months, particularly if there is no evidence of tuberculosis elsewhere.

This particularly applies to low-prevalence countries and low-prevalence groups, where the rate of CNS tuberculosis can be close to 1 per million per annum.[4,37] The

clinical staging system developed by the British Medical Research Council on the status at diagnosis remains useful.[161] In this classification, with stage I disease there is no disturbance of conciousness or focal neurological signs. Stage II disease is where there is some clouding of conciousness but without coma or delirium, or focal neurological signs and cranial nerve palsies may be present. Stage III is the most advanced when patients are comatose or stuperose, with or without focal neurological disease.

The meningeal inflammation is accompanied by low-grade fever, with some neck stiffness in adults, drowsiness or irritability in children sometimes with neck retraction, and in infants bulging fontanelles. Papilloedema occurs not infrequently, usually without reduced visual acuity, and this may not be accompanied by raised intracranial pressure. Choroidal tubercles may occur occasionally. Cranial nerve palsies occur in a significant proportion. Third and sixth nerve palsies are more common than seventh or eighth nerve palsies. Internuclear ophthalmoplegia or lateral gaze palsies are less common, but of more serious import because of the worsened prognosis with midbrain or brain stem involvement.[162] Other neurological signs can develop depending on the site of endarteritis or infarction; these include cerebellar signs, extrapyramidal movements including choreoathetosis, hemiparesis and monoparesis. Spinal meningeal involvement can lead to absent or reduced deep tendon reflexes. This can be the dominant feature on occasion with a paraplegia with urinary and sphincter involvement.[163] Epilepsy occurs at any of the stages (I–III), but is more common in children.

Diagnosis

This depends substantially on CSF examination, as the tuberculin skin test may be negative particularly in HIV-associated cases, and blood tests give non-specific abnormalities. The diagnosis of CNS tuberculosis is more readily suggested if there is associated tuberculosis elsewhere. This may be miliary tuberculosis (Table 10.2) or changes of pulmonary tuberculosis which have been reported in up to 50 per cent of cases,[163] or other forms of extrapulmonary tuberculosis which are much more common in HIV-positive cases.[164] The CSF pressure is often raised, but lumbar puncture is safe in this form of chronic meningitis and can be carried out even if there is papilloedema. The white cell count in the CSF is usually raised, but is seldom above 500/mm^3, and in the early stages is of a polymorph predominance, but changes as the disease progresses to a lymphocyte-predominant pattern. Diagnosis is further complicated in HIV-positive individuals where TB meningitis can occur with an entirely acellular CSF pattern.[164] The CSF appearance is usually clear, but with an almost invariably raised CSF protein level.[165] The CSF glucose is usually reduced,[166] but can be within the normal range, particularly early in the disease process. In an HIV-negative individual, a completely normal CSF result in protein, glucose and cell count effectively excludes tuberculous meningitis, but in an HIV-positive individual because of poor immune response this may not fully exclude disease, as CSF microscopy-negative but culture-positive disease can be present without other CSF changes.[164] In early disease, particularly if there is a neutrophil leucocytosis, the differential includes a partially treated meningitis if antibiotics have been given. In these circumstances serial lumbar punctures have to be performed if no acid-fast bacilli are seen on microscopy or other organisms on Gram stain, the CSF changes of a partly treated meningitis improving over time, whereas those of TB meningitis do not. The diagnosis is confirmed by the identification of acid-fast bacilli on culture or on microscopy. A thorough search has to be made on microscopy with the positive yield being higher if a larger volume of up to 10 mL of CSF is examined.[167] In areas of high TB prevalence, but with limited facilities, newer tests (see below) to facilitate the diagnosis are not likely to be available. The diagnosis therefore has to be made on clinical features and simple laboratory tests. Under these circumstances, five features were independently predictive of TB meningitis in children.[168] These were a prodromal stage of 7 days or greater, optic atrophy on fundal examination, focal neurological deficit, abnormal movements and CSF leucocytes less than 50 per cent polymorphs.[168] If the clinical diagnosis is felt to be tuberculous meningitis, samples from other sites for TB culture should be considered, particularly if there is evidence of disease elsewhere, e.g. sputum, urine, node aspirates or gastric washings in children. The initiation of treatment, however, should not be delayed.

Because only a minority of cases have a positive microscopy for acid-fast bacilli and cultures may take several weeks to give a positive result, a number of other tests have been used to try and obtain early confirmation of the diagnosis. However, these are seldom available in resource-poor settings because of expense and the technical resources needed. CSF adenosine deaminase (ADA) has been looked at and a level of >15 U/L strongly supports tuberculous meningitis,[169] but this chemical has not been found useful by other authors.[170] Molecular techniques, usually polymerase chain reaction (PCR) to amplify mycobacterial DNA fragments have been more widely studied in TB meningitis.[170–172] In these studies, the sensitivity of the tests is in the order of 60–75 per cent and specificity 90–95 per cent.[170,173]

There are, however, problems with false-positive results, with 6 per cent positive results for non-TB controls resported.[172] False-negative results for cases with positive CSF cultures may also be obtained, because of the presence of inhibitors in the CSF which can affect the results.[170,174] If the clinical picture and CSF features are consistent with TB meningitis, without other causes found, then treatment is indicated irrespective of other tests because of the consequences of delayed diagnosis on outcome (see below).[30]

CNS imaging

CT scanning in CNS tuberculosis is useful in both providing supportive evidence for the diagnosis,[175–178] and should therefore be carried out at diagnosis, and if there is deterioration if this resource is available. With the wider availability of CT scanning, it is clear that a significant proportion of cases have small granulomas which are often asymptomatic.[177] The other abnormalities seen are infarctions and hydrocephalus.[175,176,178] Ventricular dilatation and infarcts may be more common in HIV-positive patients.[179] The development of tuberculomata during treatment[177,180,181] and the paradoxical enlargement of those present at diagnosis is now well recognized (Figures 10.15 and 10.16).[177,182] The great majority of such lesions resolve without problems. Surgery is only needed in a small number of cases,[183] but may be required if a vital structure, e.g. the optic chiasm, is prejudiced.[184] Tuberculomas usually regress when monitored sequentially, at a slower rate initially but then more rapidly, with authors recommending at least a 2-month trial of TB therapy before considering surgical exploration.[185]

Hydrocephalus is well demonstrated on CT scanning, which can be either communicating or non-communicating.[186] Early drainage of hydrocephalus is required,[187–189] such drainage improving outcome against those not drained.[190] Surgery for drainage may be required if an intracranial[191] or an extradural abscess forms.

MRI is a more recent development applied to TB meningitis. The meningeal enhancement can often be shown in T_1-weighted images after gadolinium, with ring or nodular enhancing lesions in post-contrast T_1 images.[192] Such lesions are hypointense on T_2-weighted images.[192] MRI appearances may be useful in distinguishing TB from pyogenic, viral and fungal meningoencephalitis.[192] The finding of one or more solid rim or homogeneously enhancing nodules smaller than 2 cm had a sensitivity of 86 per cent, a specificity of 90 per cent and an accuracy of 88 per cent, respectively.[193]

Medical treatment

The penetration of drugs into the CSF depends on whether the blood–brain barrier is intact and partly on their protein binding. Isoniazid penetrates very well, reaching many times the MIC even when the blood–brain barrier is intact.[194,195] Rifampicin penetrates poorly[196–198] and its penetration may well be related to inflammation.[199] Pyrazinamide penetrates well[200,201] and reaches the MIC needed independent of the stage or activity of the disease.[202,203] Streptomycin penetrates adequately only when the blood–brain barrier is defective.[194] Ethambutol penetrates the CSF poorly, except where there is inflammation.[204–206] Ethionamide, however, has good CSF penetration which is independent of inflammation.[207,208]

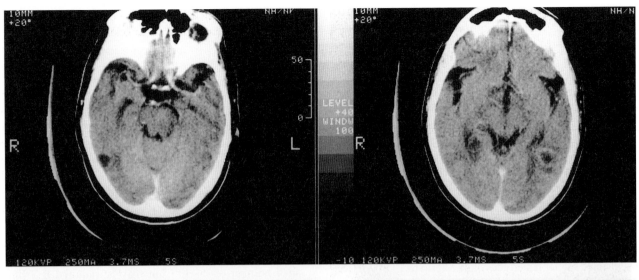

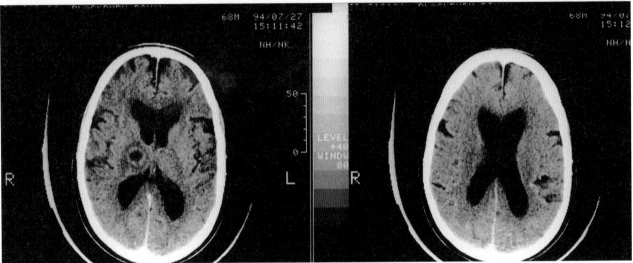

Figure 10.15 Computed tomography scans showing multiple tuberculomata, particularly in the left parietal and right periventricular areas, developing during treatment of tuberculosis meningitis. Mild hydrocephalus also present.

Antituberculosis drug treatment should be commenced as soon as possible. Unless CSF microscopy if positive for acid-fast bacilli, it may take several weeks to confirm the diagnosis by positive culture. Isoniazid, rifampicin and pyrazinamide should be given for the first 2 months, supplemented by a fourth drug. Of the drugs available, streptomycin, ethambutol and ethionamide each have advantages and disadvantages. Ethionamide has the better CSF penetration and is preferred in South Africa,[209] but is potentially teratogenic and should be avoided in pregnancy.

Streptomycin is used in Hong Kong for the first 2 months when CSF penetration is better, but requires intramuscular administration; intrathecal administration is no longer advised. Streptomycin also needs to be avoided in pregnancy because of potential ototoxicity to the fetus. Ethambutol can be used, but has to be avoided in comatose patients because visual acuity cannot be tested. In comatose patients, drugs other than streptomycin should be administered by nasogastric tube.[30]

The optimum duration of therapy is debated. Some authors recommend 12 months treatment, but up to 18 months for stage III disease and between 18–24 months for tuberculomata.[210] The British NICE Guidelines[30] and the American Thoracic Society[211] recommended 12 months' total treatment; 9 months of treatment[212] and 6-month regimens,[213,214] sometimes with high-dose treatment in children,[215] however, have given good results. Although there have been no controlled trials of 6 months versus 12 months of treatment in TB meningitis, one meta-analysis suggests that 6 months of treatment is as good as longer treatment for fully susceptible bacteria.[216] However, an analysis of studies for the British NICE guidelines[30] showed many were methodologically flawed and that there was not sufficient evidence to recommend any shorter duration than a 12-month regimen.

The use of corticosteroids as an adjunct to antituberculosis treatment in TB meningitis is debated. Their use has been shown to improve the outcome in stage II and III

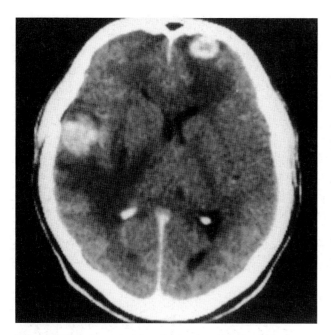

Figure 10.16 Frontal and parietal tuberculomata with associated oedema in a patient presenting with altered behaviour and fever. Positive culture from cerebrospinal fluid. Resolved on standard treatment with dexamethasone.

disease[217] and in a random prospective trial in children with TB meningitis,[218] and is supported by early reviews.[219] A Cochrane review[220] has technical limitations, but showed reduced deaths and residual disability. A well-conducted randomized controlled trial from Vietman showed benefit in a reduced death rate, but no reduction in disability.[221]

Prognosis

TB meningitis remains a serious form of tuberculosis with a severe outcome in terms of death or morbidity in many parts of the world. In a Turkish series, from the mid-1980s to the mid-1990s, 44 per cent died and only 31 per cent made a full recovery;[222] 57 per cent died in a large Egyptian series[223] and 69 per cent died in South Africa independent of HIV status.[164] Outcome is better in developed countries, but even there in a major paediatric teaching centre 13 per cent died and 47 per cent had permanent neurological sequelae.[224] Outcome at various stages has been examined. The 3-month outcome was determined by stage of TB meningitis, age, focal weakness, cranial nerve palsies and hydrocephalus using the Barthel index in one study.[225] Outcome at 6 and 12 months again using the Barthel index depended on stage at presentation, Glasgow Coma Scale and brain infarction.[226] A study in Chinese children showed by multivariate analysis that age and stage at presentation were the only significant factors.[165] This same study showed that recovery occurred in 96, 78 and 21 per cent, respectively, with stage I, II or III disease. All studies show that outcome is significantly linked to stage at diag-

nosis, emphasizing the importance of early diagnosis, and treatment, if there is clinical suspicion of the diagnosis.

SKIN

Skin involvement occurs in a small percentage of cases and can arise through a number of mechanisms. The most common is scrofuloderma, which is direct involvement of the skin from underlying structures, and is usually from underlying disease of lymph node, bone or urogenital tract.[126,227] The skin can be involved by primary inoculation, by blood-borne spread, and the tuberculides are thought to be mainly immunological reactions to tuberculosis elsewhere in the body.

Primary infection in the skin can be seen, often in children, where minor skin trauma allows material from a usually sputum smear-positive family member to inoculate. A primary lesion develops at the site of inoculation, typically a limb, which then ulcerates, and with regional lymphadenopathy forms a primary complex. This has also been described following needle-stick injury from HIV-positive patients.[228] The other forms of cutaneous tuberculosis with inoculation as a presumed mechanism, but now in an already tuberculin-sensitized individual, are verrucosa cutis, a warty form and verruca necrogenita, which is more painful and acute. Those in potential contact with tuberculous material such as post-mortem workers or pathologists, and those with potential contact with *M. bovis*, butchers, abbatoir workers and veterinary surgeons, are at risk.

Skin involvement in the acute haematogenous form of miliary disease is described, with usually extensive, multiple, small papular lesions from which acid-fast bacilli can sometimes be cultured. With the advent of HIV disease, this form may be more common and has been described in patients,[229] and in combination with *M. avium-intracellulare* infection.[230]

Lupus vulgaris is another common form of skin tuberculosis (Figure 10.17).[231,232] This is a slowly progressive form, more common in older patients, over periods ranging from months to many years. The lesions are dull red or violaceous, with the extremities, face and head being the most common sites. There is sometimes an active psoriaform edge of active disease and residual scarring with 'tissue-paper' skin where the past infection has been. If deeper tissues, such as cartilage in ears and nose become involved, substantial deformity can result (hence the name 'lupus vulgaris') and the disease is occasionally complicated by squamous carcinoma.

The tuberculides, which were thought to be forms of tuberculosis without direct skin involvement, have a number of presentations. Erythema nodosum associated with tuberculosis is usually seen shortly after the initial infection and the tuberculin skin test is strongly positive as it is associated with tuberculin conversion.[36] Erythema induratum (Bazin's disease), papular and papulonecrotic

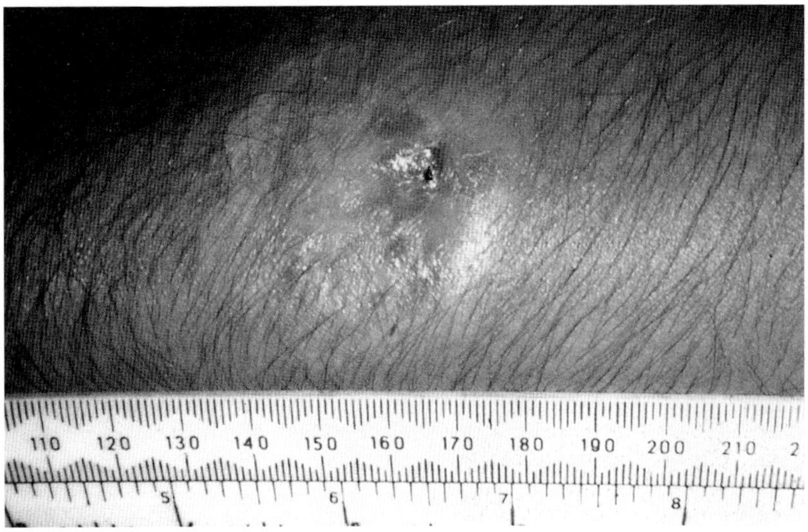

Figure 10.17 Lupus vulgaris on the forearm. Granulomas on punch skin biopsy and strongly positive tuberculin test. Resolved on short-course chemotherapy.

tuberculosis, and other forms of panniculitis, where perivascular inflammation of venules, arterioles, but sometimes also fat and subcutaneous tissues, are described. *M. tuberculosis* was rarely cultured from such skin lesions. The tuberculin skin test is usually positive and there is sometimes evidence of tuberculosis elsewhere in the body. The tuberculides used to be considered an immunological response to tuberculous infection elsewhere in the body. The advent of molecular tests, particularly PCR, has led to some re-evaluation. Using these tests, mycobacterial DNA can be identified in a significant proportion of these lesions, so they could be an immunological response to microscopic amounts of tuberculosis proteins in the skin.[233–235] Skin tuberculosis responds well to 6-month short-course chemotherapy.[126]

PERICARDIUM

This is an uncommon form of tuberculosis in developed countries, making up only some 1 per cent of cases in England and Wales,[34] and only slightly above this in the USA.[236] In developed countries, the proportion of cases of pericardial disease (acute pericarditis, constrictive pericarditis or tamponade)[237,238] due to tuberculosis overall is some 4–7 per cent. In developing countries, and in sub-Saharan Africa in particular,[239] it is an important cause of congestive heart failure.

The bacilli usually reach the pericardium by direct extension from adjacent mediastinal glands, but this can occasionally be haematogenous, e.g. in miliary disease. Acute pericarditis can be seen, thought to be mediated by an immune response to tuberculoproteins. When chronic pericarditis or constriction are present, the pathology is granulomatous, which can then progress to fibrosis and then calcification at a later date. The pericardium is the major site of cardiac involvement, but post-mortem studies do show involvement, but to a lesser degree, of both the myocardium and the endocardium.[240]

Clinical features

Symptoms, as with other forms of tuberculosis, begin insidiously with fever, malaise, sweats, cough, retrosternal discomfort, weight loss and tachycardia. The median age of occurrence is between the third and fifth decades.[241] The signs depend on the type of disease. With an effusion, the major signs are oedema, pulsus paradoxus, low blood pressure with a narrow pulse pressure and a raised venous pressure. If the effusion is sufficiently large to cause tamponade, oedema and pulsus paradoxus are prominent, and if there is tamponade then dyspnoea is a major feature. As with other forms of chronic pericarditis, the electrocardiogram shows generalized T-wave changes and is of low voltage. The cardiac outline is enlarged in over 80 per cent on chest x-ray, and associated pleural effusions occur in over 50 per cent.[238]

The pericarditis can progress to constriction in a time period varying between several weeks to several years after onset. In Africa and Asia, constrictive pericarditis is commonly caused by tuberculosis, with over 60 per cent of cases in one Indian series.[242] With constrictive pericarditis oedema, abdominal distension and dyspnoea are prominent features. Pulsus paradoxus is present, with quiet heart sounds and a venous pressure which rises with inspiration (Kussmaul's sign). Apparent cardiac enlargement is seen in over 50 per cent of cases.[243]

Diagnosis

This should be suspected in patients with pericardial effusion or signs of tamponade and fever, especially if from a high-incidence ethnic group. In addition to an enlarged heart shadow, the chest x-ray may show pericardial calcification in constrictive pericarditis, and associated pulmonary tuberculosis is described in up to 30 per cent of cases.[243,244] In those with evidence of pulmonary tuberculosis, sputum smear and culture should be performed. In

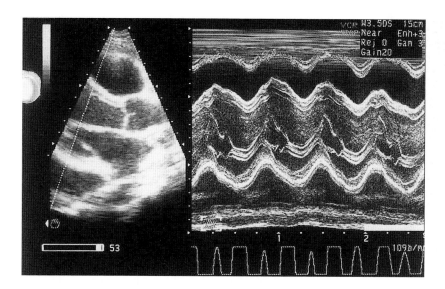

Figure 10.18 Echocardiogram of tuberculosis pericarditis showing a significant effusion. Sometimes fibrin strands can be seen in the fluid. Lymphocyte-predominant exudate on aspiration.

keeping with other forms of serous membrane tuberculosis, the tuberculin test is positive in 80–100 per cent of cases.[238] In resource-rich settings, the best way of confirming an effusion and its extent is by echocardiography (Figure 10.18). Pericardial thickening or amorphous debris within the pericardial space may be shown in addition to fluid. Radiological techniques, such as nuclear magnetic resonance or computer tomographic scanning, have also been used to demonstrate pericardial thickening and/or fluid.[245] Pericardiocentesis may be needed for both diagnosis and relief of symptoms. This can be done from either the subxiphisternal or apical directions. It is best done under echocardiogram control if at all possible, particularly with the apical approach. The fluid is an exudate (protein >35 g/L), and is usually lymphocyte-predominant on cytology, although the cells differential can be polymorph-predominant in early disease. Definitive diagnosis comes from either demonstrating acid-fast bacilli in the fluid or finding granulomatous histology on biopsy. Microscopy-positive rates of up to 40 per cent are described, and in the Transkei study 59 per cent were culture positive.[244] Pericardial biopsy usually requires thoracotomy with positive results in up to 70 per cent.[244] Nonsurgical methods of pericardial biopsy are described, using x-ray control, with some modest initial success.[246] Newer molecular methods, such as PCR, may have a role, but the sensitivity may be less than standard culture, there may be false-positive tests, and this technology is not available where most of the cases occur.[247]

Treatment

This divides into medical and surgical. The studies from Transkei[244,248] showed that short-course chemotherapy with isoniazid/rifampicin for 6 months supplemented in this case by streptomycin and pyrazinamide for an initial 3 months worked for both constriction and effusion. The place of additional corticosteroids was also addressed in

these studies. In patients with effusion, the requirement for open drainage and repeated pericardiocentesis was reduced, as was the death rate (4 versus 14 per cent).[244] In constrictive pericarditis, when given as an initial dose of 30–60 mg/day tapering over 11 weeks, the improvement in the active treatment group was more rapid, fewer needed pericardectomy, and the death rate was reduced (4 versus 11 per cent).[248] These studies have been reported at 10 years on an intention-to-treat basis and confirm these significant findings.[249] Corticosteroids should therefore be given in a tapering dose over the first 2–3 months of treatment.[30]

There are conflicting views on the need for surgery. On the one hand, an active policy of pericardial window procedures with pericardectomy if thickening is present has been advocated;[250] others have advocated a more conservative approach since little constrictive pericarditis was found on follow up of medically treated patients.[251] Since adjuvant corticosteroid therapy is clearly of benefit,[244,248] then surgery should be reserved for those with late presentations of constriction or calcification, or those who have life-threatening tamponade at any stage,[238–239] or who fail to respond to the initial 6–8 weeks of medical treatment and have a raised venous pressure.

OTHER SITES

Adrenal

Tuberculosis is now an uncommon cause of hypoadrenalism in developed countries, with autoimmune adrenalitis now being the cause in the majority of cases.[252] Adrenal tuberculosis is more common in developing countries, but is seldom an isolated site,[253] and is often associated with other extrapulmonary tuberculosis, but which may be undiagnosed until autopsy.[254] Rifampicin, which is included in all short-course chemotherapy regimens, can unmask subclinical adrenal involvement, causing adrenal

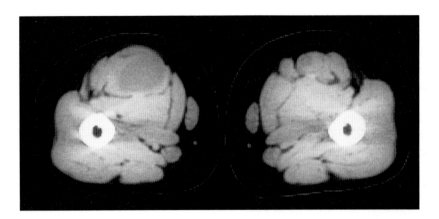

Figure 10.19 Cold tuberculosis abscess of the left hamstring muscles without underlying bone disease. Collection shown on computed tomography and aspirated. Grew *M. tuberculosis* resistant to isoniazid on culture.

crisis some 2–4 weeks after the commencement of treatment.[255] As a potent inducer of hepatic microsomal enzymes, the plasma half-life of corticosteroids is significantly reduced by rifampicin.[256] Adrenal crisis may thus be precipitated in those people just producing sufficient cortisol under maximum stress to maintain minimum blood levels. This phenomenon is offered as an explanation for unexplained deaths soon after starting antituberculosis medication.[257]

Liver

The liver is usually involved as part of miliary disease (Table 10.2), which can be diagnosed on liver biopsy and usually is a diffuse infiltrative process.[258] The miliary involvement of the liver can produce a 'bright' appearance on ultrasound,[259] which however is non-specific. Nodular forms of liver involvement are described which can mimic either cirrhosis or carcinoma,[260] and present as either portal hypertension[261] or gastric varices.[262] The diagnosis depends on finding granulomas and acid-fast bacilli on biopsy, so if tuberculosis is suspected the liver should routinely be cultured. Localized tuberculous abscesses are described,[263] but these cannot be distinguished from amoebic or pyogenic abscesses on their CT or ultrasound appearances.[264,265] Sometimes, multiple small abscesses occur which can give a psuedotumour appearance.[266]

Pancreas

Pancreatic involvement is seen either as part of miliary disease, but occasionally as a pancreatic mass with weight loss and fever in a young adult.[267] It should, therefore, be in the differential diagnosis in a young adult in a high-prevalence setting.

Soft tissue abscesses

Isolated cold abscesses can be found in soft tissue or in muscles without evidence of underlying bone or other

structural disease.[268,269] A 'cold' abscess in a high-prevalence setting, or in high-prevalence groups in low-prevalence countries, should raise the strong possibility of tuberculosis, and aspirate should be sent for TB microscopy and culture (Figure 10.19).

CONCLUSION

The wide diversity of sites, types and presentations of non-respiratory tuberculosis continue to present a challenge to clinicians. Clinical awareness needs to be maintained so that delays in diagnosis and performing appropriate investigations do not increase morbidity and mortality. The management of the drug treatment of non-pulmonary forms of tuberculosis should only be by physicians experienced in tuberculosis treatment.[30] Surgical aspects, either for diagnosis or as part of treatment, should be managed as part of a team approach to the patient.

LEARNING POINTS

- Surveys from England and Wales show that whereas 22 per cent of white patients have a non-respiratory site, 42 per cent of those from the Indian subcontinent do.
- Many countries other than the UK have shown an increase in non-respiratory presentations in the last decade.
- HIV infection plays a large part in the increase in non-respiratory disease.
- Ninety per cent or peripheral lymph node disease occurs in the cervical nodes.
- Constitutional symptoms are uncommon in lymph node disease at the time of presentation.
- About a third of patients have evidence of previous or current respiratory disease.
- Fine needle aspiration for histology and culture has a high specificity for diagnosis.
- A 6-month regimen of isoniazid, rifampicin with pyrazinamide for the first 2 months has been shown to be as effective as a 9-month regimen.

- Surgical excision should be used for lymphadenopathy caused by environmental mycobacteria.
- Involvement of the spine occurs in about 50 per cent of bone and joint sites.
- The standard 6-month regimen (2HRZE/4HR) is effective in bone and joint disease. Surgical intervention is not usually required, except in cases of gross deformity.
- One-third of patients presenting with a gastroenterological site present as an acute abdomen, while in two-thirds the onset is insidious.
- There have been no randomized trials for the treatment of abdominal tuberculosis, but a 6-month regimen is recommended.
- Genitourinary disease accounts for 17 per cent of non-respiratory cases among white patients, but only 4 per cent in the Indian subcontinent ethnic group in the UK.
- Clinical genitourinary disease may occur over 20 years after the primary infection.
- Diagnosis is made from culture of the urine. Smear-positive urine is very uncommon.
- The 6-month regimen is recommended for genitourinary tuberculosis.
- HIV infection causes increased risk of central nervous system tuberculosis.
- In an HIV-negative patient, a normal CSF protein, glucose and cell count effectively excludes tuberculous meningitis.
- Five features are independently predictive of meningeal tuberculosis in children: a prodromal stage of over 6 days, optic atrophy, focal neurological deficit, abnormal movements and a CSF leucocytosis less than 50 per cent polymorphs.
- There may be paradoxical enlargement of CNS granulomata on treatment causing a worsening of symptoms.
- In the treatment of CNS tuberculosis four drugs should be given initially, isoniazid, rifampicin, pyrazinamide and streptomycin which is preferred to ethambutol. The two-drug continuation phase is normally continued for 10 months. Streptomycin should be avoided in pregnancy.
- Steroids are thought to improve outcomes in stages II and III.
- A negative CNS culture does not necessarily exclude CNS tuberculosis.
- Steroids have been shown to be of benefit in pericardial disease.
- Most cases of non-respiratory tuberculosis are best managed jointly between a specialist in the area diseased and a physician experienced in the use of antituberculosis drugs.

REFERENCES

1. Dye C, Scheele S, Dolin P et al. Consensus statement: Global burden of tuberculosis: estimated incidence, prevalence and mortality by country. World Health Organisation Global Surveillance and Monitoring Project. J Am Med Assoc 1999; 282: 677–86.
2. Talbot EA, Moore M, McCray E, Binkin NJ. Tuberculosis among foreign-born persons in the United States, 1993-98. J Am Med Assoc 2000; 284: 2894–900.
3. Health Protection Agency. Tuberculosis in England and Wales. London: HPA, 2005.
4. Kumar D, Watson JM, Charlett A et al. Tuberculosis in England and Wales in 1993: results of a national survey. Thorax 1997; 52: 1060–7.
5. Weir MR, Thornton GF. Extrapulmonary tuberculosis. Am J Med 1985; 79: 467–8.
6. Pitchenik AE, Fertel D, Bloch AB. Pulmonary effects of AIDS: mycobacterial disease – epidemiology, diagnosis, treatment and prevention. Clin Chest Med 1988; 9: 425–41.
7. Chest Service, Medical and Health Department. Annual report, 1990. Hong Kong: Hong Kong Government, 1990.
8. Corbett EL, Steketee RW, Kuile FO et al. HIV-1/AIDS and the control of other infectious diseases in Africa. Lancet 2002; 359: 2177–87.
9. Pitchenik AE, Cole C, Russell BW et al. Tuberculosis, atypical mycobacteriosis and acquired immunodeficiency syndrome among Haitian and non-Haitian patients in South Florida. Ann Int Med 1984; 101: 641–5.
10. Berenguer J, Santiago M, Laguna F et al. Tuberculous meningitis in patients infected with the human immunodeficiency virus. N Engl J Med1992; 326: 668–72.
11. Rana FS, Hawken MP, Mwachari C et al. Autopsy study of HIV-1 positive and HIV-1 negative adult medical patients in Nairobi, Kenya. J Acquir Immune Defic Syndr 2000; 24: 23–9.
12. Harries AD, Hargreaves JN, Kemp J et al. Deaths from tuberculosis in sub-Saharan African Countries with a high prevalence of HIV-1. Lancet 2001; 375: 1519–23.
13. Campbell IA, Dyson AJ. Lymph node tuberculosis: a comparison of various methods of treatment. Tubercle 1977; 58: 171–9.
14. Mehta JB, Dutt A, Harvill L, Mathews KM. Epidemiology of extrapulmonary tuberculosis. Chest 1991; 99: 1134–38.
15. Alvarez S, McCabe WR. Extrapulmonary tuberculosis revisited: a review of experience at Boston City Hospital and other hospitals. Medicine 1984; 63: 25–53.
16. Lau SK, Kwan S, Lee J, Wei WR. Source of tubercle bacilli in cervical lymph nodes: a prospective study. J Laryngol Otol 1991; 105: 558–61.
17. British Thoracic Society Research Committee. Short course chemotherapy for tuberculosis of lymph nodes: a controlled trial. Br Med J 1985; 290: 1106–108.
18. Finch PJ, Millard FJC, Maxwell JD. Risk of tuberculosis in immigrant Asians: culturally acquired immunodeficiency. Thorax 1991: 46: 1–5.
19. Huhti E, Brander E, Ploheimo S, Sutinen S. Tuberculosis of cervical lymph nodes: a clinical, pathological and bacteriological study. Tubercle 1975: 56: 27–36.
20. British Thoracic Society Research Committee. Six-months versus nine-months chemotherapy for tuberculosis of lymph nodes: preliminary results. Respir Med 1992; 86: 15–19.
21. Lau SK, Wei WI, Hau C, Engzell UC. Efficacy of fine needle aspiration cytology in the diagnosis of tuberculosis cervical lymphadenopathy. J Laryngol Otol: 1990; 104: 24–7.
22. Lau SK, Wei WI, Kwan S, Engzell UC. Fine needle aspiration biopsy of tuberculosis cervical lymphadenopathy. Aust NZ J Surg 1988; 58: 947–50.
23. Lau SK, Wei WI, Kwan S, Yew WW. Combined use of fine-needle aspiration cytologic examination and tuberculin skin test in the

23. diagnosis of cervical tuberculous lymphadenitis: a prospective study. *Arch Otolaryngol Head Neck Surg* 1991; **117**: 87–90.
24. Shaha A, Webber C, Marti J. Fine needle aspiration in the diagnosis of cervical lymphadenopathy. *Am J Surg* 1986; **152**: 420–3.
25. British Thoracic Society Research Committee. Short course chemotherapy for lymph node tuberculosis: final report at 5 years. *Br J Dis Chest* 1988; **82**: 282–4.
26. Jindani A, Aber VR, Edwards EA, Mitchison DA. The early bactericidal activity of drugs in patients with pulmonary tuberculosis. *Am Rev Resp Dis* 1980; **121**: 139–48.
27. British Thoracic Society Research Committee. Six-months versus nine-months chemotherapy for tuberculosis of lymph nodes: final results. *Respir Med* 1993; **87**: 621–3.
28. McCarthy OR, Rudd RM. Six-months chemotherapy for lymph node tuberculosis. *Respir Med* 1989; **89**: 425–7.
29. Jawahar MS, Sivasubramanian S, Vijayan VK et al. Short-course chemotherapy for tuberculous lymphadenitis in children. *Br Med J* 1990; **301**: 359–61.
30. The National Collaborating Centre for Chronic Conditions. *Tuberculosis: Clinical diagnosis and management of tuberculosis, and measures for its prevention and control.* London: Royal College of Physicians of London, 2006, ISBN 1 86016 227 0.
31. Campbell IA, Dyson AJ. Lymph node tuberculosis: a comparison of treatments 18 months after completion of chemotherapy. *Tubercle* 1979; **60**: 95–8.
32. Ormerod LP, Horsfield N, Green RM. Can a nine-month regimen be used to treat isoniazid resistant tuberculosis diagnosed after standard treatment is started? *J Infection* 2001; **42**: 1–3.
33. Prissick FH, Masson AM. Cervical lymphadenitis in children caused by chromogenic mycobacteria. *Can Med Assoc J* 1956; **75**: 798–803.
34. McKellar A. Diagnosis and management of atypical mycobacterial lymphadenitis in children. *J Paediatr Surg* 1976: **11**: 85–9.
35. White MP, Bangash H, Goel KM et al. Non-tuberculous mycobacterial lymphadenitis. *Arch Dis Child* 1986; **61**: 368–71.
36. Walgren A. The timetable of tuberculosis. *Tubercle* 1948; **29**: 245–51.
37. Medical Research Council Tuberculosis and Chest Diseases Unit. National survey of tuberculosis notifications in England and Wales in 1983: characteristics of disease. *Tubercle* 1987; **68**: 19–32.
38. Hodgson SP, Ormerod LP. Ten year experience with bone and joint tuberculosis in Blackburn 1978–87. *J Roy Coll Surg Edin* 1990; **35**: 259–62.
39. Davies PDO, Humphries MJ, Byfield SP et al. Bone and joint tuberculosis in a national survey in England and Wales in 1978/9. *J Bone Joint Surg* 1984; **66**: 326–30.
40. Humphries MJ, Sister Gabriel M, Lee YK. Spinal tuberculosis presenting as abdominal symptoms – a report of two cases. *Tubercle* 1986; **67**: 303–307.
41. Walker GF. Failure of early recognition of skeletal tuberculosis. *Br Med J* 1986; **i**: 682.
42. Gorse GJ, Pais JM, Kurske JA et al. Tuberculous spondylitis: a report of six cases and a review of the literature. *Medicine* 1983; **62**: 178–93.
43. Ip M, Chen NK, So SY et al. Unusual rib destruction in pleuropulmonary tuberculosis. *Chest* 1989; **95**: 242–44.
44. Lin-Greenberg A, Cholankeril J. Vertebral arch destruction in tuberculosis: CT features. *J Comput Assist Tomogr* 1990; **14**: 462–65.
45. Bell GR, Stearns KL, Bonutti PM, Boumphrey FR. MRI diagnosis of tuberculous vertebral osteomyelitis. *Spine* 1990; **15**: 462–65.
46. Smith DF, Smith FW, Douglas JG. Tuberculous radiculopathy: the value of magnetic resonance imaging of the neck. *Tubercle* 1989; **70**: 213–16.
47. Angtuaco EGC, McConnell JR, Chadock WM, Flannigan S. Magnetic resonance imaging of spinal epidural sepsis. *Am J Roentgen* 1987; **42**: 1249–53
48. Medical Research Council Working Party on Tuberculosis of the Spine. A controlled trial of ambulant outpatient treatment and inpatient rest in bed in the management of tuberculosis of the spine in young Korean patients on standard chemotherapy. A study in Masan, Korea. *J Bone Joint Surg* 1973; **55**: 678–97.
49. Medical Research Council Working Party on Tuberculosis of the Spine. A controlled trial of plaster-of-Paris jackets in the management of ambulant outpatient treatment of tuberculosis of the spine in children on standard chemotherapy: a study in Pusan, Korea. *Tubercle* 1973; **54**: 261–82.
50. Medical Research Council Working Party on Tuberculosis of the Spine. A controlled trial of debridement and ambulatory treatment in the management of tuberculosis of the spine on standard chemotherapy. A study in Bulawayo, Rhodesia. *J Trop Med Hyg* 1974; **77**: 72–92.
51. Medical Research Council Working Party on Tuberculosis of the Spine. A controlled trial of anterior spinal fusion and debridement in the surgical management of tuberculosis of the spine in patients on standard chemotherapy: a study in Hong Kong. *Br J Surg* 1974; **61**: 853–66.
52. Medical Research Council Working Party on Tuberculosis of the Spine. A 10-year assessment of a controlled trial comparing debridement and anterior spinal fusion in the management of tuberculosis of the spine in patients on standard therapy in Hong Kong. *J Bone Joint Surg* 1982; **64**: 393–8.
53. Medical Research Council Working Party on Tuberculosis of the Spine. A ten-year assessment of controlled trials of inpatient and outpatient treatment and of plaster-of-Paris jackets for tuberculosis of the spine in children on standard chemotherapy: studies in Masan and Pusan. *J Bone Joint Surg* 1985; **67**: 103–10.
54. Medical Research Council Working Party on Tuberculosis of the Spine. A controlled trial of six-month and nine-month regimens of chemotherapy in patients undergoing radical surgery for tuberculosis of the Spine in Hong Kong. *Tubercle* 1986; **67**: 243–59.
55. Narlawar RS, Shah JR, Mahesh K et al. Isolated tuberculosis of the posterior elements of spine: magnetic resonance imaging findings in 33 patients. *Spine* 2002; **27**: 275–81.
56. Mehta JS, Bhojraj SY. A classification based on the selection of surgical strategies. *J Bone Joint Surg Br* 2001; **83**: 859–63.
57. Rajasekaran S, Shanmugasundraram TK, Prabhakar R et al. Tuberculous lesions of the lumbosacral region. A 15 year follow-up of patients treated with ambulant chemotherapy. *Spine* 1998; **23**: 1163–7.
58. Moon MS. Tuberculosis of the spine. Controversies and a new challenge. *Spine* 1997; **22**: 1791–7.
59. Houshian S, Poulsen S, Riegels-Nielsen P. Bone and joint tuberculosis in Denmark: increase due to immigration. *Acta Orthop Scand* 2000; **71**: 312–15.
60. Rasool MN. Osseous manifestations of tuberculosis in children. *J Pedatr Orthop* 2001; **21**: 749–55.
61. Parkinson RW, Hodgson SP, Noble J. Tuberculosis of the elbow: a report of 5 cases. *J Bone Joint Surg* 1990; **72**: 523–4.
62. Valdazo JP, Perez-Ruiz F, Albarracin A et al. Tuberculous arthritis: Report of a case with multiple joint involvement and periarticular tuberculous abscesses. *J Rheumatol* 1988; **17**: 399–401.
63. Ormerod LP, Grundy M, Rahman MA. Multiple tuberculous bone lesions simulating metastatic disease. *Tubercle* 1989; **70**: 305–307.
64. Nwokolo C. Ascites in Africa. *Dr Med J* 1961; **i**: 33.
65. Menzies RI, Alasen H, Fitzgerald JM, Mohapeola RG. Tuberculous peritonitis in Lesotho. *Tubercle* 1986; **67**: 47–54.
66. Lucas SB, De Kock KM, Hounnou A et al. Contribution of tuberculosis slim disease in Africa. *Br Med J* 1994; **308**: 1531–3.
67. Mukherjee P, Singal AK. Intestinal tuberculosis: 500 operated cases. *Proc Assoc Surg East Africa* 1979; **2**: 70–5.
68. Klimach OE, Ormerod LP. Gastrointestinal tuberculosis: a retrospective review of 109 cases in a district general hospital. *Quart J Med* 1985; **56**: 569–78.

69. deMas R, Lombeck G, Rieman JF. Tuberculosis of the oesophagus masquerading as an ulcerated tumour. *Endoscopy* 1986; **18**: 153–5.

70. Gupta SP, Arora A, Bhargava DK. An unusual presentation of oesophageal tuberculosis. *Tuberc Lung Dis* 1992; **73**: 174–6.

71. Khan MR, Khan IR, Pal KM. Diagnostic issues in abdominal tuberculosis. *J Pak Med Assoc* 2001; **51**: 138–42.

72. Addison NV. Abdominal tuberculosis – a disease revived. *Ann Roy Coll Surg Engl* 1983; **65**: 103–11.

73. Lambrianides AL, Ackroyd N, Shorey B. Abdominal tuberculosis. *Br J Surg* 1980; **67**: 887–9.

74. Sherman S, Rohwedder JJ, Ravikrishnan KP, Weg JG. Tuberculous enteritis and peritonitis – report of 36 general hospital cases. *Arch Intern Med* 1980; **140**: 506–508.

75. Bastani B, Shariatzadeh MR, Dehdashti F. Tuberculous peritonitis and a review of the literature. *Quart J Med* 1985; **56**: 549–57.

76. Muneef MA, Memish Z, Mahmoud SA *et al.* Tuberculosis in the belly: a review of forty-six cases involving the gastrointestinal tract and peritoneum. *Scand J Gastroenterol* 2001; **36**: 528–32.

77. Thoreau N, Fain O, Bahmet P *et al.* Peritoneal tuberculosis: 27 cases in the suburbs of north-east Paris. *Int J Tuberc Lung Dis* 2002; **6**: 253–8.

78. Saczek KB, Schaaf HS, Voss M, Cotton MF, Moore SW. Diagnostic dilemmas in abdominal tuberculosis in children. *Pediatr Surg Int* 2001; **17**: 111–15.

79. Shukla HS, Hughes LE. Abdominal tuberculosis in the 1970's: a continuing problem. *Br J Surg* 1978; **65**: 403–405.

80. Gilinsky NH, Marks IN, Kottler RE. Abdominal tuberculosis. A 10-year review. *S Afr Med J* 1983; **64**: 849–57.

81. Das Pritam, Shukla HS. Clinical diagnosis of abdominal tuberculosis. *Br J Surg* 1976; **63**: 941–6.

82. Naga MI, Okasha HH, Ismail Z *et al.* Endoscopic diagnosis in colon tuberculosis. *Gastrointest Endosc* 2001; **53**: 789–93.

83. Anand AC, Patnaik PK, Bhalla VP. Massive lower intestinal bleeding – a decade of experience. *Trop Gastroenterol* 2001; **22**: 131–4.

84. Pozniak AL, Dalton-Clarke HJ. Colonic tuberculosis presenting as massive rectal bleeding. *Tubercle* 1985; **66**: 295–9.

85. Kraemer M, Gill SS, Seow-Choen F. Tuberculous anal sepsis: report of clinical features in 20 cases. *Dis Colon Rectum* 2000; **43**: 1589–91.

86. Rodriguez de Lope C, San Miguel Joglar G, Pons Romero F. Laparoscopic diagnosis of tuberculous ascites. *Endoscopy* 1982; **14**: 178–9.

87. Sochocky S. Tuberculous peritonitis. A review of 100 cases. *Am Rev Resp Dis* 1967; **95**: 398–401.

88. Akhan O, Pringot J. Imaging in abdominal tuberculosis. *Eur Radiol* 2002; **12**: 312–23.

89. Gupta S, Rajak CL, Sood BP *et al.* Sonographically guided fine needle aspiration biopsy of abdominal lymph nodes: experience in 102 patients. *J Ultrasound Med* 1999; **18**: 135–9.

90. Andronikou S, Welam CJ, Kader E. The CT features of abdominal tuberculosis in children. *Pediatr Radiol* 2002; **32**: 75–81.

91. Zissin R, Gayer G, Chowers M *et al.* Computerized tomography findings in abdominal tuberculosis: report of 19 cases. *Isr Med Assoc J* 2001; **3**: 414–8.

92. Hanson RD. Turner TB. Tuberculous peritonitis: CT appearance. *Am J Radiol* 1985; **144**: 931–2.

93. Hulnick DH, Megibow AJ, Naidich DP *et al.* Abdominal tuberculosis – a CT evaluation. *Radiology* 1985; **157**: 199–204.

94. Denath FM. Abdominal tuberculosis in children: CT findings. *Gastrointestinal Radiol* 1990; **15**: 303–306.

95. Epstein BM, Mann JH. CT of abdominal tuberculosis. *Am J Radiol* 1982; **139**: 861–6.

96. Levine H. Needle biopsy of the peritoneum in exudative ascites. *Arch Intern Med* 1967; **120**: 542–5.

97. Singh MM, Bhargava AN, Jain KP, Tuberculous peritonitis: an evaluation of pathogenic mechanisms, diagnostic problems and therapeutic measures. *N Engl J Med* 1969; **281**: 1091–6.

98. Shukla HS, Naitrani YP, Bhatia S *et al.* Peritoneal biopsy for diagnosis of abdominal tuberculosis. *Postgrad Med J* 1982; **58**: 226–8.

99. Jorge JD. Peritoneal tuberculosis. *Endoscopy* 1984; **16**: 10–12.

100. Manohar A, Simjee AE, Haffejee AA. Symptoms and investigative findings in 145 patients with tuberculous peritonitis diagnosed by peritoneoscopy and biopsy over a five year period. *Gut* 1990; **31**: 1130–2.

101. Kalvaria I, Kottler RE, Marks IN. The role of colonoscopy in the diagnosis of tuberculosis. *J Clin Gastroenterol* 1988; **10**: 516–23.

102. Kochhar RJ, Rajwanshi A, Goenka MK *et al.* Colonoscopic fine needle aspiration cytology in the diagnosis of ileo-caecal tuberculosis. *Am J Gastroenterol* 1991; **86**: 102–104.

103. Yandon HD, Prakash A. Pathology of intestinal tuberculosis and its distinction from Crohns disease. *Gut* 1972; **13**: 260–9.

104. Abrams JS, Holden WD. Tuberculosis of the gastrointestinal tract. *Arch Surg* 1964; **89**: 282–93.

105. Dineen P, Homan WP, Grafe WR. Tuberculous peritonitis: 43 years experience in diagnosis and treatment. *Ann Surg* 1976; **84**: 717–23.

106. McMillen MA, Arnold SD. Tuberculous peritonitis associated with alcoholic liver disease. *N Y State J Med* 1979; **79**: 922–4.

107. Byrom HB, Mann CV. Clinical features and surgical management of ileocaecal tuberculosis. *Proc Roy Soc Med* 1969; **62**: 1230–33.

108. Chijoke A. Current views on the epidemiology of renal tuberculosis. *West Afr J Med* 2001; **20**: 217–9.

109. Ormerod LP. Why does genitourinary tuberculosis occur less often than expected in ISC ethnic patients. *J Infect* 1993; **27**: 27–32.

110. Stoller JK. Late recurrence of *Mycobacterium bovis* genitourinary tuberculosis: case report and a review of the literature. *J Urol* 1985; **134**: 565–6.

111. Yaqoob M, Goldsmith HJ, Ahmad R. Bovine genitourinary tuberculosis revisited. *Quart J Med* 1990; **74**: 105–109.

112. Lichtenstein IH, MacGregor RR. Mycobacterial infections in renal transplant recipients: report of 5 cases and a review of the literature. *Rev Infect Dis* 1983; **5**: 216–26.

113. Al-Shohaib S. Tuberculosis in chronic renal failure in Jeddah. *J Infect* 2000; **40**: 150–3.

114. Lui SL, Tang S, Li FK *et al.* Tuberculosis infection in Chinese patients undergoing continuous ambulatory peritoneal dialysis. *Am J Kidney Dis* 2001; **38**: 1055–60.

115. Moore DAJ, Lightstone E, Javid B, Friedland JS. High rates of tuberculosis in end stage renal failure: the impact of international migration. *Emerg Inf Dis* 2002; **8**: 77–8.

116. Quantrill SJ, Woodhead MA, Bell CE *et al.* Peritoneal tuberculosis in patients receiving continuous ambulatory peritoneal dialysis. *Nephrol Dial Transplant* 2001; **16**: 1024–7.

117. Ferrie BG, Rundle JSH. Genitourinary tuberculosis in patients under 25 years of age. *Urology* 1985; **25**: 576–8.

118. Datta SK. Renal tuberculosis presenting as hypertension. *J Assoc Phys India* 1987; **35**: 798–9.

119. Benn JJ, Scoble JE, Thomas AC, Eastwood JB. Cryptogenic tuberculosis presenting as a preventable cause of end-stage renal failure. *Am J Nephrol* 1988; **8**: 306–308.

120. Morgan SH, Eastwood JB, Baker LRI. Tuberculous interstitial nephritis – the tip of an iceberg? *Tubercle* 1990; **71**: 5–6.

121. al-Sulaiman MH, Dhar JM, al-Hasani MK *et al.* Tuberculous interstitial nephritis after kidney transplantation. *Transplantation* 1990; **50**: 162–4.

122. Gorse GJ, Belshe RB. Male genital tuberculosis: a review of the literature with instructive case reports. *Rev Infect Dis* 1985; **7**: 511–14.

123. Dolev E, Bass A, Nossinowitz N. Frequent occurrence of renal calculi in tuberculous kidneys in Israel. *Urology* 1985; **26**: 544–5.

124. Okawaza N, Sekiya T, Tada S. Computed tomographic features of renal tuberculosis. *Radiat Med* 1985; **3**: 209–13.

125. Goldman SM, Fishman EK, Hartman DS. Computed tomography of renal tuberculosis and its pathological correlates. *J Comput Assist Tomogr* 1985; **9**: 771–6.

126. Yates VM, Ormerod LP. Cutaneous tuberculosis in Blackburn District UK: a 15 year prospective series 1981-95. *Br J Dermatol* 1997; **137**: 483-9.

127. Fontana D, Pozzi E, Porpiglia F et al. Rapid identification of *Mycobacterium tuberculosis* complex on urine samples by Gen-Probe amplification test. *Urol Res* 1997; **25**: 391-4.

128. van-Vollenhoven P, Heyns CF, de Beer PM et al. Polymerase chain reaction in the diagnosis of urinary tract tuberculosis. *Urol Res* 1996; **24**: 107-11.

129. Hemal AK, Gupta NP, Rajeev TP et al. Polymerase chain reaction in clinically suspected genitourinary tuberculosis: comparison with intravenous urography, bladder biopsy, and urine acid fast bacilli culture. *Urology* 2000; **56**: 570-4.

130. Gow JG, Barbosa S. Genitourinary tuberculosis. A study of 1117 cases over a period of 34 years. *Br J Urol* 1984; **56**: 449-55.

131. Ravery V, de-la-Taille A, Hoffman P et al. Balloon catheter dilatation in the treatment of ureteral and ureteroenteric stricture. *J Endourol* 1998; **12**: 335-40.

132. Ramanathan R, Kumar A, Kapoor R, Bhandari M. Relief of urinary tract obstruction in tuberculosis to improve renal function. An analysis of predictive factors. *Br J Urol* 1998; **81**: 199-205.

133. Psihramis KE, Donahoe PK. Primary genitourinary tuberculosis: rapid progression and tissue destruction during treatment. *J Urol* 1986; **135**: 1033-6.

134. Osborn DE, Rao NJ, Blacklock NJ. Tuberculous stricture of the ureter. A new method of intubated ureterostomy. *Br J Urol* 1986; **58**: 103-104.

135. Hemal AK, Aron M. Orthoptic neobladder in management of tubercular thimble bladders: initial experience and long term results. *Urology* 1999; **53**: 298-301.

136. Sutherland AM. Gynaecological tuberculosis; analysis of a personal series of 710 cases. *Aust NZ J Obstet Gynaecol* 1985; **25**: 203-207.

137. Adewole IF, Babarinsa IA, Akang EE, Thompson MO. The value of routine endometrial biopsy in gynaecological practice in Nigeria. *West Afr Med J* 1997; **16**: 242-5.

138. Parikh FR, Nadkarni SG, Kamat SA et al. Genital tuberculosis – a major pelvic factor causing infertility in Indian women. *Fertil Steril* 1997; **67**: 497-500.

139. Aka N, Vural EZ. Evaluation of patients with active pulmonary tuberculosis for genital involvement. *J Obstet Gynaecol Res* 1997; **23**: 337-40.

140. Lee LH, LeVea CM, Graman PS. Congenital tuberculosis in a neonatal intensive care unit: case report, epidemiological investigation, and management of exposures. *Clin Infect Dis* 1998; **27**: 474-7.

141. Sardana K, Koranne RV, Sharma RC, Mahajan S. Tuberculosis of the vulva masquerading as a sexually transmitted disease. *J Dermatol* 2001; **28**: 505-507.

142. Geisler JP, Crook DE, Geisler HE et al. The great imitator: miliary peritoneal tuberculosis mimicking stage III ovarian carcinoma. *Eur J Gynaecol Oncol* 2000; **21**: 115-16

143. Sheth SS. Elevated CA 125 in advanced abdominal or pelvic tuberculosis. *Int J Gynaecol Obstet* 1996; **52**: 167-71.

144. Tripathy SN, Tripathy SN. Infertility and pregnancy outcome in female genital tuberculosis. *Int J Gynaecol Obstet* 2002; **76**: 159-63.

145. Bobrowitz ID. Active tuberculosis undiagnosed until autopsy. *Am J Med* 1982; **72**: 650-8.

146. Monie RDH, Hunter AM, Rocchiccioli KMS et al. Retrospective survey of the management of miliary tuberculosis in South and West Wales 1976-78. *Thorax* 1983; **38**: 369-73.

147. Sahn SA, Neff TA. Miliary tuberculosis. *Am J Med* 1968; **56**: 495-505.

148. Price M. Lymphangitis reticularis tuberculosa. *Tubercle* 1968; **49**: 377-84.

149. Proudfoot AT, Akhtar AJ, Douglas AC, Horne NW. Miliary tuberculosis in adults. *Br Med J* 1969; ii: 273-7.

150. Proudfoot AT. Cryptic disseminated tuberculosis. *Br J Hosp Med* 1971; **5**: 773-80.

151. Grieco MH, Chmel H. Acute disseminated tuberculosis as a diagnostic problem. *Am Rev Resp Dis* 1974; **109**: 554-60.

152. Medd WE, Hayhoe FGJ. Tuberculous miliary necrosis with pancytopenia. *Quart J Med* 1955; **24**: 351-64.

153. Cooper W. Pancytopenia associated with disseminated tuberculosis. *Ann Intern Med* 1959; **50**: 1497-501.

154. Hughes JT, Johnstone RM, Scott AC, Stewart PD. Leukaemoid reactions in disseminated tuberculosis. *J Clin Pathol* 1959; **12**: 307-11.

155. Twomey JJ, Leavell BS. Leukaemoid reactions to tuberculosis. *Arch Intern Med* 1965; **116**: 21-8.

156. Oswald NC. Acute tuberculosis and granulocytic disorders. *Br Med J* 1963; ii: 1489-96.

157. So SY, Yu D. The adult respiratory distress syndrome associated with miliary tuberculosis. *Tubercle* 1981; **62**: 49-53.

158. Heap MJ, Bion JF, Hunter KR. Miliary tuberculosis and the adult respiratory distress syndrome. *Respir Med* 1989; **83**: 153-6.

159. Dyer RA, Chappell WA, Potgeiter PD. Adult respiratory distress syndrome associated with miliary tuberculosis. *Crit Care Med* 1985; **13**: 12-15.

160. Rich AR, McCordock HA. The pathogenesis of tuberculous meningitis. *Bull Johns Hopkins Hosp* 1933; **52**: 5-37.

161. Medical Research Council Streptomycin in Tuberculosis Trials Committee. Streptomycin treatment in tuberculous meningitis. *Lancet* 1948; i: 582-97.

162. Teoh R, Humphries MJ, Chan JCN et al. Internuclear opthalmoplegia in tuberculous meningitis. *Tubercle* 1989; **70**: 61-4.

163. Wadia NH, Dastur DK. Spinal meningitis with radiculomyelopathy. Part I: clinical and radiological features. *J Neurol Sci* 1969; **8**; 239-60.

164. Karstaedt AS, Valtchanova S, Barriere R, Crewe-Brown HH. Tuberculous meningitis in South African urban adults. *Q J Med* 1998; **91**: 743-7.

165. Humphries MJ, Teoh R, Lau J, Gabriel M. Factors of prognostic significance in Chinese children with tuberculous meningitis. *Tubercle* 1990; **71**: 161-8.

166. Jeren T, Beus I. Characteristics of cerebrospinal fluid in tuberculous meningitis. *Acta Cytol* 1982; **26**: 678-80.

167. Kennedy DH, Fallon RJ. Tuberculous meningitis. *J Am Med Assoc* 1979; **241**: 264-8.

168. Kumar R, Singh SN, Kohli N. A diagnostic rule in tuberculous meningitis. *Arch Dis Child* 1999; **81**: 221-4.

169. Gambir IS, Mehta M, Singh DS, Khanna HD. Evaluation of CSF-adenosine deaminase activity in tubercular meningitis. *J Assoc Phys India* 1999; **47**: 192-4.

170. Caws M, Wilson SM, Clough C, Drobniewski F. Role of IS*6110*-targeted PCR, culture, biochemical, clinical and immunological criteria for diagnosis of tuberculous meningitis. *J Clin Microbiol* 2000; **38**: 3150-5.

171. Bonington A, Strang JI, Klapper PE et al. TB PCR in the early diagnosis of tuberculous meningitis: evaluation of the Roche semi-automated COBAS Ampiclor MTB test with reference to the manual Ampiclor MTB PCR test. *Tuber Lung Dis* 2000; **80**: 191-6.

172. Seth P, Ahuja GK, Bhanu NV et al. Evaluation of polymerase chain reaction for rapid diagnosis of clinically suspected tuberculous meningitis. *Tuberc Lung Dis* 1996; **77**: 353-7.

173. Bonington A, Strang JI, Klapper PE, et al. Use of Roche AMPICLOR *Mycobacterium tuberculosis* PCR in early diagnosis of tuberculous meningitis. *J Clin Microbiol* 1998; **36**: 1251-4.

174. Melzer M, Brown TJ, Flood J et al. False negative polymerase chain reaction on cerebrospinal fluid samples in tuberculous meningitis established by culture. *J Neurol Neurosurg Psychiatry* 1999; **67**: 249-50.

175. Teoh R, Humphries MJ, Hoare RD, O'Mahoney G. Clinical correlation of CT changes in 64 Chinese patients with tuberculous meningitis. *J Neurol* 1989; **236**: 48-51.

176. Kingsley DPE, Hendrickse WA, Kendall BE et al. Tuberculous

meningitis: role of CT scan in management and prognosis. *J Neurol Neurosurg Psychol* 1987; **50**: 30–6.

177. Ravenscroft A, Schoeman JF, Donald PR. Tuberculous granulomas in childhood tuberculous meningitis: radiological features and course. *J Trop Pediatr* 2001; **47**: 5–12.

178. Ozates M, Kemaloglu S, Gurkan F et al. CT of the brain in tuberculous meningitis. A review of 289 patients. *Acta Radiol* 2000; **41**: 13–17.

179. Schutte CM. Clinical, cerebrospinal fluid and pathological findings and outcomes in HIV-positive and HIV-negative patients with tuberculous meningitis. *Infection* 2001; **29**: 213–17.

180. Teoh R, Humphries MJ, O'Mahoney G. Symptomatic intracranial tuberculoma developing during treatment of tuberculosis: a report of 10 cases and review of the literature. *Q J Med* 1987; **241**; 449–60.

181. Lees AJ, MacLeod AF, Marshall J. Cerebral tuberculomas developing during treatment of tuberculous meningitis. *Lancet* 1980; **i**: 1208–11.

182. Chambers T, Hendrickse WA, Record C et al. Paradoxical expansion of intracranial tuberculomas during treatment. *Lancet* 1984; **ii**: 181–4.

183. Tandon PN, Bhargava S. Effect of medical treatment on intracranial tuberculoma – a CT study. *Tubercle* 1985; **66**: 85–97.

184. Teoh R, Poon W, Humphries MJ, O'Mahoney G. Suprasellar tuberculoma developing during treatment of tuberculous meningitis requiring urgent surgical decompression. *J Neurol* 1988; **235**: 321–2.

185. Awada A, Daif AK, Pirani M et al. Evolution of brain tuberculomas under standard antituberculous treatment. *J Neurol Sci* 1998; **156**: 47–52.

186. Schoeman JF, Laubscher JA, Donald PR. Serial lumbar CSF pressure measurements and cranial computed tomographic findings in childhood tuberculous meningitis. *Childs Nerv Syst* 2000; **16**: 203–208.

187. Bullock MR, Welchman JM. Diagnostic and prognostic features of tuberculous meningitis on CT scanning. *J Neurol Neurosurg Psychol* 1982; **45**: 1098–101.

188. Roy TK, Sircar PK, Chandar V. Peritoneal-ventricular shunt in the management of tuberculous meningitis. *Indian J Paediatr* 1979; **16**; 1023–7.

189. Palur R, Rajshekar V, Chandy MJ et al. Shunt surgery for hydrocephalus in tuberculous meningitis: a long term follow up study. *J Neurosurg* 1991; **74**: 64–9.

190. Peacock WJ, Deeny JE. Improving the outcome of tuberculous meningitis in childhood. *S Afr Med J* 1984; **66**: 597–8.

191. Tang ESC, Chau A, Fong D, Humphries MJ. The treatment of multiple intracranial abscesses: a case report. *J Neurol* 1991; **238**: 183–5.

192. Tayfun C, Ucoz T, Tasar M et al. Diagnostic value of MRI in tuberculous meningitis. *Eur Radiol* 1996; **6**: 380–6.

193. Pui MH, Memon WA. Magnetic resonance imaging findings in tuberculous meningoencephalitis. *Can Assoc Radiol J* 2001; **52**: 43–9.

194. Ellard GA, Humphries MJ, Allen BW. Penetration of isoniazid, rifampicin and streptomycin into the cerebrospinal fluid and the treatment of tuberculous meningitis. *Am Rev Resp Dis* 1993; **148**: 650–5.

195. Fletcher AP. CSF isoniazid levels in tuberculous meningitis. *Lancet* 1953; **ii**: 694–7.

196. D'Olivera JJ. Cerebrospinal fluid concentrations of rifampicin in meningeal tuberculosis. *Am Rev Resp Dis* 1972; **105**: 432–7.

197. Forgan-Smith R, Ellard GA, Newton D, Mitchison DA. Pyrazinamide and other drugs in tuberculous meningitis. *Lancet* 1973; **ii**: 374.

198. Kaojarern S, Supmonchai K, Phuapradit P et al. Effect of steroids on cerebrospinal fluid penetration of antituberculosis drugs in tuberculous meningitis. *Clin Pharmacol Ther* 1991; **49**: 6–12.

199. Woo J, Humphries MJ, Chan K, O'Mahoney G, Teoh R. Cerebrospinal fluid and serum levels of pyrazinamide and

rifampicin in patients with tuberculous meningitis. *Curr Ther Res* 1987; **42**: 235–42.

200. Ellard GA, Humphries MJ, Gabriel M, Teoh R. The penetration of pyrazinamide into the cerebrospinal fluid in patients with tuberculous meningitis. *Br Med J* 1987; **294**: 284–5.

201. Donald PR, Seifart H. Cerebrospinal fluid pyrazinamide concentrations in children with tuberculous meningitis. *Paediatr Infect Dis* 1988; **7**: 469–71.

202. Stottmeier KD, Beam RE, Kubica GP. Determination of drug susceptibility of mycobacteria to pyrazinamide in 7H10 agar. *Am Rev Resp Dis* 1967; **96**: 1072–5.

203. Carlone NA, Acocella G, Cuffini AN, Forno-Pizzoglio M. Killing of macrophage-ingested mycobacteria by rifampicin, pyrazinamide, pyrazinoic acid alone and in combination. *Am Rev Resp Dis* 1985; **132**: 1274–7.

204. Gundert-Remy U, Lett M, Weber E. Concentration of ethambutol in cerebrospinal fluid in man as a function of non-protein-bound fraction in serum. *J Clin Pharmacol* 1964; **6**: 133–6.

205. Borrowitz ID. Ethambutol in tuberculous meningitis. *Chest* 1972; **61**: 629–32.

206. Place VA, Pyle MM, de la Huerga J. Ethambutol in tuberculous meningitis. *Am Rev Resp Dis* 1969; **99**: 783–5.

207. Hughes IE, Smith HV, Kane PO. Ethionamide and its passage into the cerebrospinal fluid in man. *Lancet* 1962; **i**: 616–17.

208. Donald PR, Seifart HI. Cerebrospinal fluid concentrations of ethionamide in children with tuberculous meningitis. *J Paediatr* 1989; **115**: 383–6.

209. Donald PR, Schoeman JF, Kennedy A. Hepatic toxicity during chemotherapy for severe tuberculous meningitis. *Am J Dis Child* 1987; **141**: 741–3.

210. Humphries MJ. The management of tuberculous meningitis. *Thorax* 1992; **47**: 577–81.

211. American Thoracic Society. Treatment of tuberculosis and tuberculous infection in adults and children. *Am J Respir Care Med* 1994; **149**: 1359–74.

212. Acharya VN, Kudva BT, Retnam VJ, Mehta PJ. Adult tuberculous meningitis: comparative study of different chemotherapeutic regimens. *J Assoc Phys India* 1985; **33**: 583–5.

213. Phuapradit P, Vejjajiva A. Treatment of tuberculous meningitis: the role of short course chemotherapy. *Q J Med* 1987; **239**: 249–58.

214. Jacobs RF, Sunakorn P, Chotitayasunonah T et al. Intensive short course chemotherapy for tuberculous meningitis. *Pediatr Infect Dis* 1992; **11**: 194–8.

215. Donald PR, Schoeman JF, Van-Zyl LE et al. Intensive short course chemotherapy in the management of tuberculous meningitis. *Int J Tuberc Lung Dis* 1998; **2**: 704–11.

216. van-Loenhout-Rooyackers JH, Keyser A, Laheij RJ et al. Tuberculous meningitis: is a 6 month treatment regimen sufficient. *Int J Tuberc Lung Dis* 2001; **5**: 1028–35.

217. Shaw PP, Wang SM, Tung SG et al. Clinical analysis of 445 adult cases of tuberculous meningitis. *Chin J Tuberc Respir Dis* 1984; **3**; 131–2.

218. Schoeman JF, Van-Zyl LE, Laubscger JA, Donald PR. Effect of corticosteroids on intracranial pressure, computed tomographic findings and clinical outcome in young children with tuberculous meningitis. *Pediatrics* 1997; **99**: 226–31.

219. Horne NW. A critical evaluation of corticosteroids in tuberculosis. *Adv Tuberc Res* 1966; **15**: 1–54.

220. Prasad K, Volmink J, Menon GR. Steroids for treating tuberculous meningitis. *Cochrane Database Syst Rev* 2000; CD002244.

221. Thwaites GE, Hguyen HD, Hoang TQ et al. Dexamethasone for the treatment of tuberculous meningitis in adolescents and adults. *N Engl J Med* 1994; **351**: 1741–51.

222. Hosoglu S, Ayaz C, Geyik MF et al. Tuberculous meningitis in adults: an eleven year review. *Int J Tuberc Lung Dis* 1998; **2**: 553–7.

223. Girgis NI, Sultan Y, Farid Z et al. Tuberculous meningitis. Ababassia Fever Hospital, Naval Medical Research Unit No 3,

Cairo, Egypt from 1976 to 1996. *Am J Trop Med Hyg* 1998; **58**: 28–34.

224. Farinha NJ, Razali KA, Holzel H *et al.* Tuberculosis of the central nervous system in children: a 20 year survey. *J Infect* 2000; **41**: 61–8.

225. Misra UK, Kalita J, Srivastava M, Mandal SK. Prognosis in tuberculous meningitis: a multivariate analysis. *J Neurol Sci* 1996; **137**: 57–61.

226. Kalita J, Misra UK. Outcome in tuberculous meningitis at 6 and 12 months: a multiple regression analysis. *Int J Tuberc Lung Dis* 1999; **3**: 261–5.

227. Kumar B, Rai R, Kaur I *et al.* Childhood cutaneous tuberculosis: a study over 25 years from northern India. *Int J Dermatol* 2001; **40**: 26–32.

228. Kramer F, Sasse SA, Simms JC, Leedom JM. Primary cutaneous tuberculosis after a needle stick injury from a patient with AIDS and undiagnosed tuberculosis. *Ann Intern Med* 1993; **119**: 594–5.

229. Stack RJ, Bickley LK, Coppel IG. Miliary tuberculosis presenting as skin lesions in a patient with the acquired immunodeficiency syndrome. *J Am Acad Dermatol* 1990; **23**: 1031–5.

230. Lombardo PC, Weitzman I. Isolation of *Mycobacterium tuberculosis* and *M. avium* complex from the same skin lesions in AIDS. *N Engl J Med* 1990; **323**: 916–17.

231. Kumar B, Muralidhar S. Cutaneous tuberculosis: a twenty-year prospective study. *Int J Tuberc Lung Dis* 1999; **3**: 494–500.

232. Ramesh V, Misra RS, Beena KR, Mukherjee A. A study of cutaneous tuberculosis in children. *Pediatr Dermatol* 1999; **16**: 264–9.

233. Jordan HF, Schneider JW, Schaaf HS *et al.* Papulonecrotic tuberculid in children. A report of eight patients. *Am J Dermatopathol* 1996; **18**: 172–85.

234. Tan SH, Tan HH, Sun YJ, Goh CL. Clinical utility of polymerase chain reaction in the detection of *Mycobacterium tuberculosis* in different types of cutaneous tuberculosis and tuberculids. *Ann Acad Med Singapore* 2001; **30**: 3–10.

235. Margall N, Balsega E, Coll P *et al.* Detection of *Mycobacterium tuberculosis* complex DNA by the polymerase chain reaction for rapid diagnosis of cutaneous tuberculosis. *Br J Dermatol* 1996; **135**: 231–6.

236. Larrieu AJ, Tyers GF, Williams EH, Derrick JR. Recent experience with tuberculous pericarditis. *Ann Thorac Surg* 1980; **29**: 464–8.

237. Lorell BH, Braunwald E. Pericradial disease: tuberculous pericarditis. In: Braunwald E (ed.). *Heart disease – a textbook of cardiovascular medicine*, 3rd edn. Philadelphia: WB Saunders, 1988: 1509–11.

238. Fowler NO. Tuberculous pericarditis. *J Am Med Assoc* 1991; **266**: 99–103.

239. Strang JIG. Tuberculous pericarditis in Transkei. *Clin Cardiol* 1984; **7**: 667–70.

240. Dave T, Narula JP, Chopra P. Myocardial and endocardial involvement in tuberculous constrictive pericarditis. *Int J Cardiol* 1990; **28**: 245–51.

241. Rooney JJ, Crocco JA, Lyons HA. Tuberculous pericarditis. *Ann Intern Med* 1970; **72**: 73–8.

242. Bashi VV, John S, Ravindakumar H *et al.* Early and late results of pericardectomy in 118 cases of constrictive pericarditis. *Thorax* 1988; **43**: 637–41.

243. Sagrosta-Sauleda J, Permanyer-Miralda G, Soler-Soler J. Tuberculous pericarditis: ten-year experience with a prospective protocol for diagnosis and treatment. *J Am Coll Cardiol* 1988: **11**: 724–8.

244. Strang JIG, Kakaza HHS, Gibson DG *et al.* Controlled trial of complete open drainage and prednisolone in the treatment of tuberculous pericardial effusion in Transkei. *Lancet* 1988; ii: 759–63.

245. Pohost GM, O'Rourke RA (eds). *Principles and practice of cardiovascular imaging.* Boston: Little Brown, 1991: 457.

246. Endrys J, Simo M, Shafie MZ *et al.* New non-surgical technique for multiple pericardial biopsies. *Cathet Cardiovasc Diagn* 1988; **15**: 92–4.

247. Cegielski JP, Devlin BH, Morris AJ *et al.* Comparison of PCR, culture, and histopathology for diagnosis of tuberculous pericarditis. *J Clin Microbiol* 1997; **35**: 3254–7.

248. Strang JIG, Kakaza HHS, Gibson DG, Girling DJ, Nunn AJ, Fox W. Controlled trial of prednisolone as adjuvant in treatment of tuberculous constrictive pericarditis in Transkei. *Lancet* 1987; ii: 1418–22.

249. Strang JIG. Management of tuberculous constrictive pericarditis and tuberculous pericardial effusion in Transkei: results at 10 years follow-up. *Q J Med* 2004; **97**: 525–35.

250. Quale JM, Lipshick GY, Heurich AE. Management of tuberculous pericarditis. *Ann Thorac Surg* 1987; **43**: 653–5.

251. Long R, Younes M, Patton N, Hershfield E. Tuberculous pericarditis: long term outcome in patients who received medical treatment alone. *Am Heart J* 1989; **117**: 1133–9.

252. Willis AC, Vince FP. The prevalence of Addisons disease in Coventry, UK. *Postgrad Med J* 1997; **73**: 286–8.

253. Llewelyn M, Adler M, Steer K, Pasvol G. Acute adrenal insufficiency precipitated by isolated involvement of the adrenal gland by tuberculosis. *J Infect* 1999; **39**; 244–5.

254. Lam KY, Lo CY. A critical examination of adrenal tuberculosis and a 28-year autopsy experience of active tuberculosis. *Clin Endocrinol* 2001; **54**: 633–9.

255. Wilkins EGL, Hnizdo E, Cope A. Addisonian crisis induced by treatment with rifampicin. *Tubercle* 1989; **70**: 69–73.

256. McAllister WAC, Thompson FJ, Al-Habet S *et al.* Adverse effects of rifampicin on prednisolone deposition. *Thorax* 1982; **37**: 792.

257. Ellis ME, Webb AK. Cause of death in patients admitted to hospital with pulmonary tuberculosis. *Lancet* 1983; I; 665–7.

258. Essop AR, Posen JA, Hodgkinson JH, Segal I. Tuberculous hepatitis: a clinical review of 96 cases. *Q J Med* 1984; **212**: 465–77.

259. Andrew WK, Thomas RG, Gollach BL. Miliary tuberculosis of the liver – another cause of 'bright liver' on ultrasound examination. *S Afr Med J* 1982; **62**: 808–809.

260. Nagai H, Shimizu S, Kawamoto H *et al.* A case of solitary tuberculosis of the liver. *Jpn J Med* 1989; **28**: 251–5.

261. Gibson JA. Granulomatous liver disease and portal hypertension. *Proc Roy Soc Med* 1973; **66**; 502–503.

262. Sheen-Chen SM, Chou FF, Tai DI, Eng HL. Hepatic tuberculosis: a rare cause of bleeding gastric varices. *Tubercle* 1990; **71**: 225–7.

263. Rahmatulla RH, al-Mofleh IA, al-Rashed RS *et al.* Tuberculous liver abscess: a case report and a review of the literature. *Eur J Gastroenterol Hepatol* 2001; **13**: 437–40.

264. Spiegel CT, Tuazon CU. Tuberculous liver abscess. *Tubercle* 1984; **65**: 127–31.

265. Epstein BM, Liebowitz CB. Ultrasonographic and computed tomographic appearance of focal tuberculosis of the liver. A case report. *S Afr Med J* 1987; **71**: 461–2.

266. Denath FM. Abdominal tuberculosis in children: CT findings. *Gastrointest Radiol* 1990; **15**: 303–306.

267. Demir K, Kaymakoglu S, Besisik F *et al.* Solitary pancreatic tuberculosis in immunocompetent patients mimicking pancreatic carcinoma. *J Gastroenterol Hepatol* 2001; **16**: 1071–4.

268. Ergin F, Arslan H, Bilezikci B, Agildere AM, Ozdemir N. Primary tuberculosis of the gluteal muscle of a patient with chronic renal failure. A rare presentation. *Nephron* 2001; **89**: 463–6.

269. Trikha V, Gupta V. Isolated tuberculous abscess in biceps brachii muscle of a young male. *J Infect* 2002; **44**: 265–6.

11

Tuberculosis in childhood

DELANE SHINGADIA

INTRODUCTION

Mycobacterium tuberculosis (MTB) is the most prevalent infection in the world with an estimated 8.8 million new cases globally in 2005, 7.4 million of which are in Asia and sub-Saharan Africa. A total of 1.6 million people died of tuberculosis (TB), including 195 000 patients infected with HIV.[1]

The TB incidence rate has been falling or stable in five out of six World Health Organization (WHO) regions, but growing at 1.0 per cent per year globally. The South-East Asian region has the largest total number of people with TB cases, with three countries (India, Indonesia and Bangladesh) accounting for the majority of cases. However, the incidence has been rising more quickly in sub-Saharan African countries, particularly in those countries with higher HIV prevalence rates. While incidence rates in Western Europe have fallen since 1980, many Eastern European countries have shown increasing rates during the 1990s, which peaked around 2001 and have since fallen.[2]

EPIDEMIOLOGY

The WHO suggested that in 1989 there were 1.3 million annual cases of TB in children less than 15 years of age and 450 000 deaths.[3] However, these figures are likely to be inaccurate due to the many difficulties in estimating the burden of TB in children. In particular, there is some difficulty in establishing a definitive diagnosis of TB in children because of lower positive microscopy rates (less than 5 per cent of children are microscopy smear-posi-

tive), more extrapulmonary disease in young children, the lack of standard case definition and the lower public health priority given to childhood TB compared to that of adult TB. In many resource-limited countries, surveillance data are often unreliable due to poor diagnostic facilities and reporting systems.[4] For purposes of reporting to the WHO, TB cases in general are defined as those that are sputum smear-positive for acid-fast bacilli. This means that more than 80 per cent of children with TB will not be recorded in most national tuberculosis registers. The proportion of TB cases in individual countries that occur in children is highly variable. In low-prevalence countries, this may be <5 per cent, whereas in some high-prevalence countries it is estimated to be four times this figure. It has been suggested that in developing countries, where a large proportion of the population consists of children, as incidences of smear-positive adults increase in a community, the case load of children increases exponentially with the highest reported childhood case load being 39 per cent of the total case load.[5]

Most of the accurate paediatric data come from low-prevalence countries such as the USA and Western Europe. In the USA, the national rates of TB in children 0–14 years have been falling from 3.1/100 000 in 1992 to 1.5/100 000 in 2001 with a constant 6 per cent of total cases occurring in children. Case rates are the highest for ethnic minority groups. Caucasian children <5 years have a rate of 0.5 per 100 000, compared with Hispanic, Black and Asian/Pacific Island children whose rates are 7.0, 6.2 and 6.5, respectively. Similarly, in low-prevalence countries in Europe, such as the UK, notification rates for TB have also declined over the last 20 years.[6] Rates in children and young people overall have remained relatively constant over the last 5 years.[7] However, TB notifications have increased substantially in metropolitan centres, such as London, which accounts for 40 per cent of national cases. Some areas have recorded rates of >40 cases/100 000 notifications in children.[8] The proportion of Black African children with TB in 1998 (44 per cent) has increased substantially from 1993 (23 per cent), whereas the proportion of paediatric cases from the Indian subcontinent (ISC) has fallen (21 per cent in 1998 compared with 50 per cent in 1993). Similar patterns have been reported in other low-prevalence countries in Europe, such as Sweden and Denmark.[9,10]

Accurate data from high-prevalence countries are less readily available. The proportion of childhood TB to the total cases in South Africa is estimated to be 20 per cent.[5] In the Western Cape Province of South Africa (overall TB incidence estimated 1149 cases/100 000 notifications), 39 per cent of the case load was due to children younger than 14 years of age.[11] In Botswana, 12 per cent of all reported TB occurred among children <15 years of age in 2000, although these accounted for only 2 per cent of all smear-positive cases. In Malawi, the largest increases in cases in Blantyre from 1985 to 1995 occurred among children aged 1–5 years.[12] Since sub-Saharan Africa also has the highest burden of HIV infection, this will no doubt have a major impact on TB epidemiology in this region. It is has been estimated that based on contact with smear-positive adults 700 000–800 000 children would develop TB disease over 5 years.[13]

There have been several factors that have been associated with the resurgence of TB in children in different parts of the world. Increased travel and migration, particularly from high- to low-incidence countries, have resulted in increases in childhood TB. In North America and Europe, high-risk groups include immigrants, where higher rates of disease are observed in those born overseas compared with low rates in the non-immigrant population.[14–20] Immigrant children born in high-prevalence countries who migrate to low-prevalence countries are at much higher risk of developing TB. Furthermore, children of immigrants will have higher rates of TB than non-immigrant children, presumably because of higher rates of TB within those communities. Socioeconomic risk factors, such as poverty and crowding, continue to be associated with a greater risk of children developing both latent infection and active TB.[21] In South Africa, a significant correlation was found between TB case notification rates in childhood and crowding, economic status and parental education.[11] Similarly, the overall risk of TB was linked to deprivation, population density and ethnicity in the UK.[22] The HIV pandemic has had a profound effect on the incidence of TB, particularly in sub-Saharan Africa, where up to a quarter of the population are HIV infected. HIV is known to greatly increase the annual risk of progression from TB infection to active TB and is thought to be one of the principal causes of the resurgence of TB in this region. The average annual case rates for TB after 1985 have increased approximately twice as fast in countries with high versus low or intermediate

HIV seropositivity rates.[23] In children, the association between HIV and TB infection is not as well characterized, with co-infection rates of 11–64 per cent.[24] In Brazil, the numbers of children with TB with HIV co-infection increased from 23.5 to 31.4 per cent.[25] Similarly, high rates have been noted in South Africa, where in one study almost half of children under 12 years of age with culture-proven pulmonary TB were also HIV infected.[26] Despite the high rates of co-infection with HIV and TB in these children, it is still unclear whether HIV-infected children are more vulnerable to TB infection or more likely to progress to disease than HIV-negative children. An important risk factor for TB in HIV-infected children is that they are more likely to be a close contact of a smear-positive adult than HIV-uninfected children. Because TB is the most common opportunistic infection in HIV-infected adults in the developing world, children in this setting are more likely to be exposed to TB irrespective of their HIV status. The difficulty of diagnosing TB in children, coupled with the difficulty of diagnosing HIV-associated pulmonary infections in children, may have important confounding effects on assessing the epidemiology of TB and TB-HIV co-infection in children. Drug-resistant TB is of great importance worldwide as it reflects on TB control in the population. However, there are limited data available on drug-resistant TB in children because of difficulties in confirming TB in children, especially due to lower rates of microbiological identification from paediatric samples. Often the diagnosis of drug-resistant TB will be made on the basis of confirmation of drug resistance in the adult index case. Children most often have primary resistance which has been transmitted to them by an adult with new or retreatment-resistant TB.[27] A large South African study, conducted between 1994 and 1998 in TB culture-positive children, found 5.6 per cent had isoniazid (INH) resistance and 1 per cent had multidrug resistance (MDR) (defined as resistance to both isoniazid and rifampicin).[28] These results were essentially the same as surveillance data from adults with TB during the same time period, of 3.9 per cent INH resistance and 1.1 per cent MDR. In the UK, the rate of INH resistance in paediatric cases is 6.5 per cent and that for MDR-TB is 0.5 per cent, again similar to the rates in adults of 6.4 and 1.2 per cent, respectively.[7]

NATURAL HISTORY OF TUBERCULOSIS IN CHILDREN

The natural history of TB has traditionally been divided into 'infection' and 'disease'. Following initial exposure to an infectious individual, inhalation of an aerosolized particle containing tubercle bacilli results in infection in the lung. The initial encounter with the bacilli results in a series of immunological events, particularly a cell-mediated immune response, resulting in the formation of a subpleural granuloma (called the Gohn focus) with accompanying regional mediastinal lymphadenitis (called the primary or Gohn complex). In most children, the primary complex resolves spontaneously with residual calcification or scarring at the site of the Gohn focus. However, in some children, particularly infants, the primary complex may result in progressive and persistent lymphadenopathy, which may compress the surrounding structures, such as the bronchi.[29] Inability to control infection within the primary parenchymal infiltrate results in the development of a caseating lesion, known as 'progressive primary tuberculosis'. Invasion and rupture into surrounding structures, such as pleural or pericardial spaces, will result in disease at those sites. Erosion of caseating lesions into intrathoracic vessels can result in haematogenous dissemination within the lung and also extrathoracic anatomic sites. The most common manifestation of this is miliary tuberculosis (MT), which involves the lungs, as well as liver and spleen. MT usually occurs as an early complication of primary infection and usually affects infants and young children. In the majority of children, initial infection is successfully controlled and the primary complex resolves without the development of any symptoms. Persistence of bacilli within the lung (called latent TB infection or LTBI) and subsequent reactivation at a later stage occurs in 3–5 per cent of individuals following infection (called 'post-primary tuberculosis'). Older children and adults will develop reactivation pulmonary disease which typically follows infection acquired after 7 years of age and commonly occurs at the time of puberty.[30] Post-primary TB is characterized by extensive pulmonary infiltration and cavitation, especially of the upper lobe of the lung, which are usually found on chest x-ray. Compared with progressive primary disease, post-primary disease is characterized by large numbers of bacilli within the pulmonary cavities, resulting in higher yields on microbiological testing of samples (see below).

Progressive primary tuberculosis with haematogenous dissemination and subsequent spread to extrathoracic sites results in extrapulmonary TB. Extrapulmonary disease is more common in children than adults, occurring in approximately 25 per cent of infants and young children <4 years age.[31] Superficial lymphadenitis is the most common form of extrapulmonary TB in children, typically involving the supraclavicular, anterior cervical, tonsillar and submandibular nodes. Without treatment, cold abscess and chronic sinus formation may occur. Central nervous system disease, especially TB meningitis, is the most serious complication of TB in children and occurs in about 4 per cent of children with TB.[32] The overall mortality has been reported to be 13 per cent, with approximately half of survivors developing permanent neurological sequelae.[33] Tuberculomas infection of the central nervous system may occur and are usually characterized by solitary brain lesions, sometimes occurring after commencement of antituberculous treatment. Musculoskeletal disease primarily involves weight-bearing bones and joints, particularly the vertebrae (called Pott's disease).[34] Other less common extrapulmonary manifestations of TB include gastrointestinal or renal disease. Renal disease is particularly rare in children mainly because the long incubation following haematogenous dissemination will mean that disease will often not develop until adulthood.

CLINICAL FEATURES

It is important to distinguish TB infection (also referred to as LTBI) from TB disease as discussed above. In both, there is evidence of TB infection (either by tuberculin skin testing or by a blood-based immunological assay), but in latent infection the clinical, radiological or microbiological evidence of disease is lacking. The majority of children (>50 per cent) with TB disease will be asymptomatic. Of those who develop symptoms, most will have pulmonary manifestations, while 25–35 per cent of children will have extrapulmonary symptoms.[35] Systemic complaints, such as fever, night sweats, anorexia and decreased activity, occur less often. The most common symptoms at presentation in children with TB disease are cough in the preceding 3 months, persistent fatigue and weight loss.[36]

Intrathoracic disease

PULMONARY DISEASE

Following infection, the primary complex is characterized by a lung parenchymal infiltrate, commonly subpleural, and regional lymph node enlargement. Most children are asymptomatic at this stage and the infiltrate and lymphadenopathy will resolve spontaneously in the majority of cases. In some children, particularly infants, the lymph nodes continue to enlarge causing pressure effects on surrounding structures, such as the trachea and bronchi, which may result in partial or complete bronchial obstruction. This obstruction may result in wheeze as a presenting symptom or in some instances after commencement of antituberculous therapy. Endobronchial disease may also occur when encroaching, enlarged lymph nodes erode into the bronchi with extrusion of caseous material into the bronchial lumen.[37] The clinical presentation may be insidious or acute. The right middle lobe syndrome may result due to chronic lobar atelectasis secondary to post-inflammatory bronchial stenosis.[38] In general, the most common pulmonary symptoms of primary infection, if any, include non-productive cough and mild dyspnoea. There may be few clinical signs on examination; however, some infants and young children may have localized wheezing or decreased breath sounds accompanied by increased respiratory rate or respiratory distress. Older children and adolescents are more likely to develop adult-type reactivation disease.[39,40] Most of these children will present with the classic symptoms of fever, malaise, weight loss, night sweats, productive cough, chest pain and haemoptysis. Again there may be very few or no clinical signs on physical examination.

PLEURAL DISEASE

Pleural involvement may occur in reaction to release of a few mycobacteria into the pleural space from a subpleural focus. This may result in clinically significant pleural effusions, which are often unilateral. Pleural fluid is typically yellow in colour with elevated protein and white blood cells. Microscopy and culture yields from pleural fluid are often low; however, pleural biopsy will demonstrate caseating granulomas in the majority of cases. Clinical symptoms include fever, chest pain and reduced air entry on the side of the effusion.

CARDIAC DISEASE

Pericarditis is the most common cardiac manifestation of TB occurring in 1–4 per cent of children.[41] Pericardial fluid is serofibrinous or slightly haemorrhagic. Clinical symptoms may be non-specific, including low-grade fever, malaise and weight loss; chest pain is unusual in children. Auscultation of the cardiovascular system may reveal a pericardial friction rub or reduced heart sounds.

Extrapulmonary disease

Lymphohaematogenous spread following primary complex formation occurs more commonly in children and results in disseminated TB, including miliary TB, and extrapulmonary TB. Extrapulmonary TB includes peripheral lymphadenopathy (65 per cent), TB meningitis (10–15 per cent), bone and joint disease (4 per cent) and miliary TB (5 per cent).[42]

PERIPHERAL LYMPHADENOPATHY

Local spread from primary infection in the lungs results in peripheral tuberculous lymphadenopathy, particularly in the supraclavicular and paratracheal regions. Lymphohaematogenous spread may result in more distant lymph node involvement. Peripheral TB lymphadenopathy commonly presents as slowly enlarging, firm, nontender lymph nodes with no overlying skin discoloration. There are often no systemic symptoms, such as fever or weight loss. With time, the enlarged lymph nodes become fluctuant and may discharge with sinus formation. The lymph nodes most often involved are in the anterior or posterior cervical and supraclavicular regions.

MILIARY TUBERCULOSIS

Miliary TB is the most common form of disseminated disease and usually occurs early after the infection, within the first 2–6 months and may represent uncontrolled primary infection in children. The median age at presentation is 10.5 months, with about half of cases occurring in those younger than 1 year. The clinical manifestations of miliary TB are protean with involvement of the lungs, spleen and bone marrow. The presenting symptoms are often non-specific: cough (72 per cent); fever (61 per cent); loss of appetite and weight (40 per cent); and diarrhoea and vomiting (33 per cent). The main presenting signs are hepatomegaly (82 per cent), splenomegaly (54 per cent), lymphadenopathy (46 per cent) and pyrexia (39 per cent).[43] Like adults with miliary TB, children are usually smear-negative. With progressive pulmonary disease, respiratory distress, hypoxia and pneumothorax/pneumomediastinum may occur. Signs or symptoms of meningitis or peritonitis are found in 20–40 per cent of patients with advanced disease. Choroid tubercles occur in 13–87 per cent of patients and are highly specific for TB.

CENTRAL NERVOUS SYSTEM TUBERCULOSIS

Involvement of the central nervous system, particularly meningitis, is among the more common manifestations of extrapulmonary disease.[33,44–47] Tuberculous meningitis is the most serious complication in children and is almost invariably fatal without treatment. The brain stem is the most common focus with cranial nerve involvement (III, VI and VII).[48] The clinical progression of tuberculous meningitis may be rapid or gradual. Rapid progression tends to occur more often in infants who may experience symptoms for only several days before the onset of acute hydrocephalus, seizures or cerebral oedema.

Signs and symptoms may evolve and progress over time. Early disease is characterized by non-specific symptoms, such as fever, headache, irritability and malaise, and usually lasts several weeks. There are few to no clinical signs and at this stage there is no reduction in consciousness. Infants may experience delay or loss of developmental milestones. Progression of disease is characterized by drowsiness and lethargy. Clinical signs are those of meningitis (including nuchal rigidity and positive Kernig's or Brudzinski's signs), cranial nerve palsies, vomiting and seizures. This clinical picture usually correlates with the development of hydrocephalus and increased intracranial pressure. Advanced disease is usually characterized by stupor or coma, often accompanied by gross paresis (hemiplegia or paraplegia), hypertension and decerebrate posturing. Paresis most commonly reflects ischaemic infarction from vasculitis, although it may be exacerbated by hydrocephalus. The prognosis of tuberculous meningitis correlates most closely with the clinical stage of illness at the time antituberculosis chemotherapy begins.[49] The majority of patients in the earlier stages of disease have an excellent outcome, whereas most patients in the advanced stage will have permanent disabilities, including blindness, deafness, paraplegia and mental retardation.[50]

In children with TB meningitis (TBM), 40–80 per cent will have abnormal chest x-rays, including hilar adenopathy (33 per cent), infiltrates (33 per cent), miliary pattern (20 per cent) and pleural effusions (1 per cent).[51] Cranial CT scans of the patients presenting with TBM showed hydrocephalus in 80–90 per cent and basilar enhancement in over 90 per cent of cases. MTB may be cultured or identified by acid-fast stain from cerebrospinal fluid (CSF) or brain tissue from 63 per cent of children. New tuberculoma may develop during treatment.[33]

OTHER EXTRAPULMONARY TUBERCULOSIS

Skeletal TB is a late complication of lymphohaematogenous spread and usually presents many years following primary infection. The most common sites of involvement are the weight-bearing bones and joints, such as the vertebral column (40–50 per cent), hip, knee and elbow. Vertebral TB may be very insidious, often presenting with referred pain, abnormal posturing or paravertebral abscess formation.

Other extrapulmonary sites of TB are generally very rare in children, particularly genitourinary disease which occurs many years after primary infection and hence unlikely to occur in the paediatric age group.

CONGENITAL TUBERCULOSIS

TB in the newborn may arise as a result of infection *in utero*, typically through the transplacental route. There is high morbidity and mortality experienced at this age. The signs are often non-specific, with tachypnoea, hepatosplenomegaly and prolonged jaundice being the most common.

DIAGNOSIS

Microscopy and culture

Microscopic examination of clinical samples for identification of tubercle bacilli using acid-fast staining techniques, such as the Ziehl–Neelsen (ZN) stain, has been a standard tool for the diagnosis of TB. Acid-fast smears of sputum have become the cornerstone of TB diagnosis in many countries and in some settings the only test used to diagnose TB. Microscopic examination can detect 60–70 per cent of culture-positive samples with a lower limit of detection of 5×10^3 organisms/mL. Detection is increased by collection of multiple samples and concentration of samples (cumulative proportion positive for three smears for concentrated specimens were 74, 83 and 91 per cent and for direct smears were 57, 76 and 81 per cent).[52] Detection will depend on numbers of bacilli in the sample and therefore also the type of disease (i.e. progressive primary disease versus post-primary disease). Newer fluorochrome stains, such as auramine and rhodamine, appear to have higher detection when compared with the ZN stain.[53] These tests are generally easy to perform, cheap and give rapid results. However, young children and infants may be unable to produce sputum and, when they do, microscopic examination is often negative because they have progressive primary disease. Early-morning gastric

aspirate samples are often collected from young infants unable to expectorate by aspiration of overnight gastric contents via a nasogastric tube. This takes advantage of the fact that infants and young children will often swallow respiratory secretions, which are pooled in the stomach overnight and which can be collected prior to ingestion of food in the morning. The yield from microscopy of gastric aspirate samples in children with proven pulmonary TB is less than 20 per cent, compared with 75 per cent in adults.[54] In a study of Haitian children, the sensitivity, specificity and positive predictive value of fluorescence microscopy of gastric washings compared with culture were 58, 95 and 81 per cent, respectively.[55]

The rates of detection on microscopy from other extrapulmonary samples, such as cerebrospinal fluid, are even lower, mainly because of the paucibacillary nature of disease at these sites.

Culture of gastric aspirates has provided a more useful method of diagnosis in children with suspected pulmonary tuberculosis where this testing is available. Three consecutive morning gastric aspirates yield positive cultures in 30–50 per cent of cases and may be as high as 70 per cent in infants.[56] The culture yield from other body fluids or tissues from children with extrapulmonary tuberculosis is usually less than 50 per cent due to lower numbers of mycobacteria at these sites of disease.[57] A recent study from South Africa has shown that culture yields in children with intrathoracic disease manifestations (excluding uncomplicated lymph node disease) were as high as 77 per cent compared with those with uncomplicated lymph node disease alone, where the yield was only 35 per cent.[58]

The role of bronchoscopy in the diagnosis of pulmonary TB in children remains controversial. Cultures from broncho-alveolar lavage fluid in children with suspected pulmonary TB have a low yield and do not aid bacteriologic confirmation.[59] Comparison of culture yields from a single bronchoscopic sample were lower than for three gastric aspirates.[60] Bronchoscopy may, however, play a useful role in the diagnosis of certain forms of TB, such as endobronchial tuberculosis or bronchial obstruction, especially if transbronchial biopsy is performed.[61] Bronchoscopy may also be useful in excluding other causative agents, such as opportunistic infections, particularly in immunocompromised children and children with HIV where the radiological findings might be similar.

Sputum induction with nebulized hypertonic (5 per cent) saline has recently been used to obtain sputum from young infants and children in resource-limited settings. A single induced sputum sample has been shown to be equivalent to three consecutive early-morning gastric aspirates with little difference in the HIV status of the child.[62] Although this procedure was well tolerated in most children, including infants, there are concerns regarding the infection control aspects, particularly with immunocompromised individuals and resistant TB.[63]

The string test is a novel approach that has recently been evaluated in adults for its ability to retrieve *M. tuberculosis* from the upper gastrointestinal tract. This test was developed for the diagnosis of enteric parasites, such as *Giardia lamblia*. In a study of HIV-positive adults in Peru, the string test was shown to be safe and effective for retrieval of useful clinical specimens for diagnosis of pulmonary TB, and was at least as sensitive as sputum induction.[64] A recent study in children as young as 4 years showed that the string test is well tolerated; however, there are no published data on bacteriologic yield in children compared with other sample collection methods.[65] Further studies are needed to evaluate the utility of this test, particularly in young children where sputum samples may be difficult to obtain.

Tuberculin skin test

Tuberculin was developed in the early part of the twentieth century as a treatment for TB, but subsequently as a test of sensitivity to mycobacterial infection. In essence, tuberculin contains tuberculoproteins and is available in solubilized form as purified protein derivative (PPD). The tuberculin skin test (TST) relies on an individual's delayed-type hypersensitivity reaction to these tuberculoproteins following infection, past or present. A positive TST reaction is therefore regarded as a hallmark of primary infection with *M. tuberculosis*. In most children, tuberculin reactivity becomes apparent within 3–6 weeks after initial infection, but occasionally can take up to 3 months. Tuberculin reactivity due to *M. tuberculosis* infection usually remains positive for the life time of the individual, even after treatment.[66]

TST suffers from both poor sensitivity (false-negative results) and specificity (false-positive results). The TST has the lowest sensitivity in younger children. Up to 10 per cent of otherwise normal children with culture-proven tuberculosis do not react to tuberculin initially.[57] Most of these children will become reactive during treatment, suggesting that tuberculosis disease may itself contribute to immunosuppression. False-negative TST may also occur in children with severe tuberculosis disease, those with debilitating or immunosuppressive illnesses, malnutrition or other severe infections. The rate of false-negative TST in children with TB who are infected with HIV is unknown, but it is certainly higher than 10 per cent and is dependent on the degree of immunosuppression, particularly the CD4 count.

False-positive TST results may also occur. Bacille Calmette–Guérin (BCG) is a vaccine derived from an attenuated strain of *Mycobacterium bovis* and because of antigenic similarities with *M. tuberculosis* may transiently cause a reactive TST. However, most children who received BCG as infants will have a non-reactive TST at 5 years of age.[67] A recent meta-analysis suggests that the effect of BCG on TST measurements was less after 15 years, and induration greater than 15 mm was more likely to be due to tuberculosis infection than BCG.[68] Among older children or adolescents who receive BCG, most

develop a reactive TST initially; however, by 10–15 years post vaccination, the majority will have lost tuberculin reactivity.[69] Recent studies have shown that BCG vaccination had little impact on the interpretation of TST in children being tested as part of a contact investigation.[70] Another reason for false-positive TST is that of infection or exposure to non-tuberculous mycobacteria (also called environmental mycobacteria). This phenomenon may arise through antigenic cross-reactivity with tuberculin.[71] Skin reactivity can also be boosted, probably through antigenic stimulation, by serial testing with TST in many children and adults who received BCG.[72]

Radiology

Chest x-ray imaging has been an important tool in the diagnosis of pulmonary tuberculosis. Chest x-ray changes will depend on the type and stage of disease. Primary complex and progressive primary disease (most often seen in household contacts of smear-positive adults) will result in intrathoracic lymphadenopathy (hilar or mediastinal) (Figure 11.1). Following resolution and containment of the primary complex, a subpleural area of fibrosis or calcification may be visible on chest x-ray. Endobronchial disease may occur with progressive primary disease and is characterized by multiple small, acinar shadows in the lower lobes indicating bronchogenic spread. Other radiological features of progressive primary disease include segmental hyperinflation, atelectasis, alveolar consolidation, pleural effusion/empyema and, rarely, a focal mass. Miliary TB following haematogenous dissemination is characterized by fine bilateral reticular shadowing, described as a 'snowstorm' appearance (Figure 11.2). Cavitary disease is relatively rare in young children, but is more common in adolescents (Figure 11.3), who may develop adult-type post-primary disease and are hence more likely to be infectious.[73] Reactivation disease characteristically shows upper lobe infiltrates and/or cavitation on chest x-ray.

Newer radiological investigations, such as computed tomography (CT) and high-resolution CT has been useful in demonstrating early pulmonary disease, such as cavitation, often in the absence of any abnormality on chest x-ray (Figure 11.4). CT imaging is also better than chest x-ray in demonstrating bronchial involvement, such as bronchial compression and bronchiectasis. CT imaging may also be useful in detecting intrathoracic hilar lymphadenopathy including in those with normal chest x-rays.[74–76] There is, however, interobserver variability in the detection of mediastinal and hilar lymph nodes on CT in children with suspected pulmonary tuberculosis and diagnostic accuracy might be improved by refining radiological criteria for lymphadenopathy.[77]

CT imaging has also been used for evaluation of pericardial effusions which when associated with mediastinal lymphadenoapthy and a positive TST are strongly suggestive of tuberculous disease.[78] Central nervous system

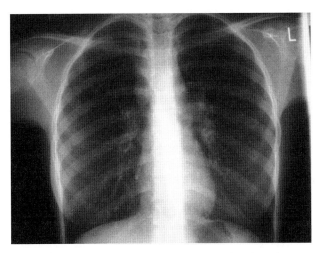

Figure 11.1 Chest x-ray showing intrathoracic tuberculous lymphadenopathy.

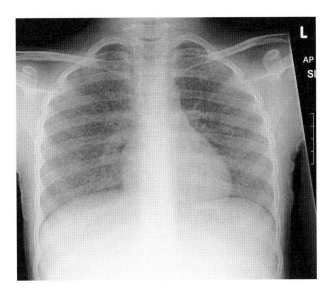

Figure 11.2 Chest x-ray showing bilateral reticular shadowing or 'snowstorm' appearance of miliary tuberculosis.

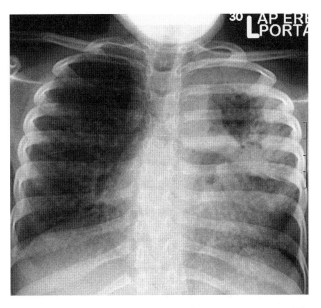

Figure 11.3 Chest x-ray showing post-primary adult-type left upper lobe consolidation and cavitation.

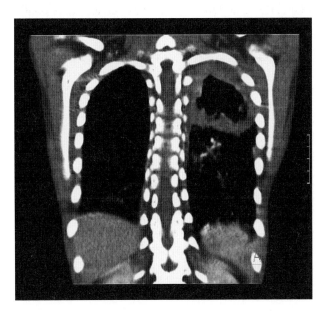

Figure 11.4 Computed tomography scan of the chest showing left upper lobe cavitation.

disease, such as tuberculous meningitis or tuberculoma, may also be identified on CT imaging. TB meningitis is characterized by basilar meningeal enhancement (Figure 11.5).

Magnetic resonance imaging (MRI) has been found to be useful for musculoskeletal and soft tissue tuberculosis, particularly involving bones and joints.[79] Figure 11.6 shows a Pott's fracture of the spine, which was identified on MRI scan.

Diagnostic approaches in childhood tuberculosis

The diagnosis of tuberculosis in children is based mainly on a combination of history of contact with an adult infectious case, clinical signs and symptoms, and investigations mentioned above, particularly chest radiograph and tuberculin skin testing. However, symptoms may often be non-specific with over half of children being asymptomatic with early disease.[73] A positive history of contact with a case of tuberculosis, especially if the source case was a parent or other member of the household who was also bacteriologically positive, has been strongly associated with disease in a child.[80] These epidemiological, clinical and diagnostic parameters have been used to devise simple, cheap and reliable tests to enable accurate diagnosis of TB in children, especially in low-income countries. Several diagnostic approaches exist and most are grouped broadly into four families based on point scoring systems,

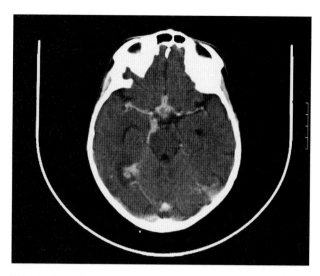

Figure 11.5 Computed tomography scan of the head showing basal enhancement consistent with tuberculous meningitis.

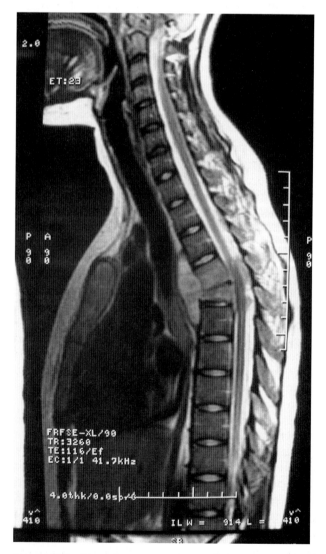

Figure 11.6 Magnetic resonance image of the spine showing Pott's fracture.

diagnostic classifications, diagnostic algorithms or combinations of these.[81] Most of these diagnostic approaches have not been standardized, making comparison difficult, and few have been properly validated.[81] Some diagnostic approaches have been modified for populations where HIV is prevalent; however, only one diagnostic approach has been specifically designed to diagnose TB in such a population.[12] In a high HIV-prevalent population, clinical scoring systems have been found to have low specificity (25 per cent), resulting in overdiagnosis of TB.[82] A recent prospective, community-based study from South Africa has suggested that combining symptoms of a persistent non-remitting cough of >2 weeks' duration, documented failure to thrive (in the preceding 3 months) and fatigue provided reasonable diagnostic accuracy in HIV-uninfected children (sensitivity, 82.3 per cent; specificity, 90.2 per cent; positive predictive value, 82.3 per cent).[83] However, this symptom-based approach offered little diagnostic value in HIV-infected children diagnosed with pulmonary TB. Further studies are therefore needed to develop standardized diagnostic approaches that are relevant to developing countries with limited resources with a high burden of TB, malnutrition and HIV/AIDS.

Immunodiagnosis

The underlying principles and methodology surrounding immunodiagnostic tests are more extensively discussed in Chapter 6, Immunodiagnostic tests. As outlined above, the TST suffers from poor specificity and sensitivity, particularly in immunocompromised individuals. New immunodiagnostic tests (ELISPOT and QUANTIFERON) have been the developed based on *in vitro* T cell-based interferon-γ assays utilizing antigens more specific to *M. tuberculosis*. At present, there are limited data regarding the performance of this test in children, particularly <5 years of age. In a large school outbreak in the UK, ELISPOT testing improved sensitivity when compared with TST and showed better correlation with degree of exposure to an active case of TB.[84] A study in South African children showed that sensitivity of ELISPOT was 83 per cent, significantly higher than the 63 per cent sensitivity of TST. The sensitivity of the TST fell significantly in children younger than 3 years (51 per cent), with HIV co-infection (36 per cent) or with malnutrition (44 per cent), while sensitivity of ELISPOT was unaffected in these groups.[85]

In a study of 979 Turkish children who were household contacts of adults with sputum smear-positive TB, previous BCG vaccination was more likely to be associated with a positive TST but negative ELISPOT assay. Risk factors associated with positive TST and ELIPSOT included the number of TB cases in the household, being a first-degree relative of a TB case and increasing age. Interestingly, BCG-vaccinated children had a lower odds ratio (0.60) for TB infection compared with non-vaccinated children, suggesting some protection from BCG against TB infection.[86]

However, a study from the Gambia of children who were TB contacts showed similar rates of positive TST and ELISPOT (32.5 and 32.3 per cent, respectively) with overall agreement between the two tests of 83 per cent. Interestingly, previous BCG did not seem to have any impact on either of the tests. The ELISPOT assay did appear to be less sensitive in this study.[87]

Connell et al.[88] used the QuantiFERON assay to test 106 children with a risk of latent TB infection or TB disease. There was poor correlation between the QuantiFERON test and TST for the diagnosis of latent infection. The QuantiFERON assay appeared to have lower sensitivity than TST and also yielded inconclusive results in 17 per cent of children due to failure of positive or negative controls.

Current evidence suggests that interferon-γ assays have the potential to become useful diagnostic tools in clinical and public-health settings. Studies in different populations suggest that these tests have greater specificity (>90 per cent) compared with TST, although sensitivity may be equivalent or less, especially for latent infection. The accuracy and reliability of these studies in diagnosing both TB infection and TB disease in infants and children need to be established. Furthermore, there are limited data from specific populations, particularly children and immunosuppressed individuals. Nevertheless, new guidelines have incorporated interferon-γ testing as an alternative and/or adjunct to TST.[89] However, the cost-effectiveness and utility of these tests, especially in certain population groups, remains unclear.

TREATMENT

Treatment of children can be divided broadly into treatment of TB infection and treatment of TB disease. As mentioned above, the distinction between these different categories may be unclear in some patients, particularly young children.

Several controlled and observational trials of 6-month therapy in children with pulmonary TB caused by organisms known or presumed to be susceptible to the first-line drugs have been published.[90–97] Although 6 months of therapy with INH and rifampicin has been shown to be effective for treatment of hilar adenopathy and pulmonary TB, a three-drug regimen (isoniazid, rifampicin and pyrazinamide) has been shown to have success rates of greater than 95 per cent and low adverse reaction rates. In general, extrapulmonary TB in children can be treated with the same regimen as pulmonary disease. However, there are no data from children and extrapolations have been made from studies in adults. Meningitis and disseminated TB, however, may not be adequately treated with 6 months' duration and longer treatment durations of 9–12 months are recommended. The optimal treatment of TB in children and adolescents with HIV infection is unknown. Drug interactions and overlapping toxicities make treatment of HIV and TB co-infection complex. Furthermore, an immune reconstitution inflammatory syndrome has been described in individuals with TB and HIV co-infection after commencing antiretroviral therapy. Treatment durations of at last 9 months have been suggested.[98]

Treatment schedules, policies and drug doses as advocated by a number of national and international bodies often differ. Tables 11.1 and 11.2 compare drug regimens and dosages recommended by authorities in the UK, USA and by the World Health Organization (WHO).[98–100] Traditionally, antituberculous regimens have included bactericidal and bacteriostatic drugs that have required treatment for long periods, between 18 and 24 months. More recently, multidrug regimens have been used with more rapid microbiological cure rates that allow shorter durations of therapy (short-course chemotherapy). Isoniazid, rifampicin and pyrazinamide are mainstays of antituberculous therapy. Other agents often used in children, include streptomycin and ethambutol.

Adverse reactions to antituberculosis therapy occur in children on antituberculosis therapy, but generally the drugs are well tolerated. Gastrointestinal reactions, such as nausea, vomiting and abdominal pain are common, particularly in the first few weeks of therapy. In most cases, these reactions can be managed symptomatically. Isoniazid and rifampicin may both be hepatotoxic, causing elevation of serum aminotransferase levels (significant if three or more times the upper limit of normal). These hepatotoxic abnormalities are rarely severe in children and modest increases in aminotransferases generally resolve spontaneously. All drugs used in treating TB can cause

Table 11.1 Recommended dosages of first-line standard antituberculous drugs for children.[98–100]

Drug	British Thoracic Society		American Thoracic Society		World Health Organization	
	Daily	Intermittent	Daily	Intermittent	Daily	Intermittent
Isoniazid	5–10 mg/kg	15 mg/kg 3 times weekly	10–15 mg/kg	20–30 mg/kg twice weekly	5 mg/kg	10 mg/kg 3 times weekly
Rifampicin	10 mg/kg	15 mg/kg 3 times weekly	10–20 mg/kg	10–20 mg/kg twice weekly	10 mg/kg	10 mg/kg 3 times weekly
Pyrazinamide	35 mg/kg	50 mg/kg 3 times weekly	20–40 mg/kg	50 mg/kg twice weekly	25 mg/kg	35 mg/kg 3 times weekly
Ethambutol	15 mg/kg	30 mg/kg 3 times weekly	15–25 mg/kg	50 mg/kg twice weekly	15 mg/kg	30 mg/kg 3 times weekly

Table 11.2   Recommended treatment schedules for tuberculosis disease in children.[89,98,100]

	National Institute for Health and Clinical Excellence (UK)	American Thoracic Society	World Health Organization
Hilar adenopathy	2 months of RHZE then 4 months of RH	2 months of RHZ(E[a]) then 4 months of RH	2 months of RHZ then 4 months of RH
Pulmonary tuberculosis	2 months of RHZE then 4 months of RH	2 months of RHZ(E[a]) then 4 months of RH	2 months of RHZE then 4 months of RH
Extrapulmonary tuberculosis	2 months of RHZE then 4 months of RH	2 months of RHZ(E[a]) then 4 months RH	2 months of RHZE then 4 months of RH
TB meningitis	2 months of RHZE then 10 months of RH	2 months of RHZE then 9–12 months of RH	2 months of RHZS then 4 months of RH
HIV	2 months of RHZE then 4–7 months of RH	2 months of RHZ then 7 months of RH	2 months of RHZE then 4 months of HR or 6 months of HE

[a]If resistance is suspected.
E, ethambutol; H, isoniazid; R, rifampicin; S, streptomycin; Z, pyrazinamide.

skin rash, which is usually minor and may be managed symptomatically. Isoniazid has also been associated with symptomatic pyridoxine deficiency, particularly in severely malnourished children. Supplemental pyridoxine is indicated in these malnourished children, as well as in breast-feeding infants (dose 5 mg in infants from birth to 1 month, 5–10 mg in infants and children less than 12 years, and 10 mg in children 12–18 years). Pyrazinamide is generally well tolerated in children and rarely causes hepatic dysfunction. Ethambutol has been associated with retrobulbar neuritis, which presents with blurred vision, central scotoma and colour blindness. Trebucq[101] reviewed the literature regarding recommendations for ethambutol use in children and concluded that ethambutol was safe in children greater than 5 years of age at a dose of 15 mg/kg/day and also in younger children without undue fear of side effects. It is often appropriate to obtain a base-line ophthalmological assessment in younger children before starting ethambutol therapy. This should be repeated after 1–2 months.

Compliance is a major determinant of the success of drug treatment – compliance of the physician in prescribing the optimum appropriate regimen and monitoring it, and compliance of the patient in taking the medication as prescribed. Compliance in children is further compounded by the fact that children may have difficulties in taking medications, many of which are not specifically packaged or produced in paediatric formulations. Difficulties with taste, consistency of formulations and gastrointestinal toxicity may be important factors in children that may dramatically affect treatment compliance.

MULTIDRUG-RESISTANT TUBERCULOSIS

Single, multiple and multidrug resistance is increasing worldwide. Isoniazid resistance has been found in 6.8–7.2 per cent of isolates in children less than 15 years old in England and Wales from 1995 to 1999. Multidrug resistance (defined as resistance to both isoniazid and rifampicin) over the same period was 0.5–0.7 per cent. Higher levels of resistance occur in ethnic minority groups, especially those from the Indian subcontinent and sub-Saharan Africa. As children have lower rates of tuberculosis isolation, multidrug-resistant (MDR) TB is often initially only identified in the adult index case or in other contacts. Recently, extensively drug-resistant TB (XDR-TB) has been reported in a number of countries.[102,103] XDR-TB is defined as resistance to at least isoniazid and rifampicin, plus additional resistance to at least three of the six classes of second-line drugs used to treat MDR-TB. XDR-TB is of particular concern among HIV-infected or immunocompromised individuals. The greatest concern is that XDR-TB leaves some patients virtually untreatable with the currently available drugs. To date, XDR-TB has not been reported in children, but paediatric infection is probably inevitable in high-incidence populations, which often have high rates of HIV co-infection.

Treatment of patients with drug-resistant TB should only be carried out by specialists with appropriate experience in the management of such cases. The most common isolated drug resistance is to isoniazid. It is particularly important to add ethambutol as a fourth agent where isoniazid resistance is suspected, or in those patients at higher risk of resistance. Treatment should be continued for 9–12 months, initially with rifampicin, pyrazinamide and ethambutol for 2 months followed by rifampicin and ethambutol for the complete duration of therapy. Isolated drug resistance to other first-line drugs is unusual and appropriate therapy must begin based on recommended guidelines.[99] Rifampicin resistance most commonly occurs in conjunction with isoniazid resistance (called MDR-TB). Treatment should be carried out by a specialist with substantial experience in managing complex resistant cases, and only in hospitals with appropriate isolation facilities. Such treatment should also be monitored closely not only for drug toxicity, but more importantly to ensure compliance. Treatment will in most cases involve five or more drugs and for durations of at least 2 years. Several alternative antituberculosis drugs may need to be used, although the efficacy of these drugs has not been evaluated in children. The drugs that have been used previously include aminoglycosides (streptomycin, amikacin, capreomycin, kanamycin), ethionamide/prothionamide, cycloserine, quinolones (ciprofloxacin, ofloxacin), rifabutin, macrolides (azithromycin, clarithromycin) and para-amino salicylic acid.

Corticosteroids

Corticosteroids have been found to be beneficial in situations where the host response to *M. tuberculosis* contributes to significant tissue damage. Corticosteroids have been shown to significantly decrease mortality and long-term neurological sequelae in patients with TB meningitis.[104,105] Children with bronchial obstruction due to enlarged lymph nodes may also benefit from corticosteroid therapy.[106] Corticosteroids may also be of benefit in extensive pulmonary TB, pericardial effusion and pleural effusion. A dose of 1–2 mg/kg (maximum of 60 mg) for 4–6 weeks is recommended, followed by a period of weaning doses.

LATENT TUBERCULOSIS INFECTION

The rationale for treating LTBI is the significant risk of progression to TB disease in untreated infection, especially in children. The risk is greatest in younger children (<5 years of age), but the exact age-related risk is difficult to ascertain from the available data, which are historical and include studies of both adults and children. Treatment of LTBI is highly effective in reducing the risk of TB disease, especially in children, where efficacy is well over 90 per cent.

Various regimens have been suggested for LTBI treatment, but most have not been subjected to randomized controlled trials in children. Six months of isoniazid therapy is the standard prophylactic therapy and the current recommendation for LTBI in many countries.[107] Alternative regimens for treatment of LTBI have been used in children. Isoniazid and rifampicin for 3 months is well tolerated and generally more acceptable to children and families.[108] A meta-analysis in adults showed that this combination was equally as efficacious as 6 months' isoniazid monotherapy.[109] Rifampicin monotherapy for 4 months is also used, but infrequently in children.[110] In adults with silicosis, who have a high risk of disease progression from LTBI, 3 months of rifampicin was as efficacious as 6 months of isoniazid,[111] but there are no studies in children. Data, again only

from adults, indicate that the combination of rifampicin and pyrazinamide potentially causes fatal hepatotoxicity and is best avoided.[112,113]

LEARNING POINTS

- Childhood TB is caused by droplet infection from adults and therefore reflects the prevalence of sputum smear-positive tuberculosis in the community.
- Morbidity and mortality is highest in young children, who tend to develop the most severe forms of disease, such as miliary and meningitis.
- Between 90 and 95 per cent of TB in children is non-infectious.
- The risk of infection leading to disease is 10–30 per cent and progression is usually in the 3–12 months following infection.
- HIV considerably increases the risk of infection progressing to disease.
- Following infection, bacterial dissemination occurs for 6–8 weeks, at which point the tuberculin test becomes positive.
- Infection incurs a lifelong risk of disease, but primary infection survived gives 60–80 per cent protection against later disease.
- Only 10 per cent of childhood cases are confirmed by culture.
- Symptoms and signs of pulmonary disease are dominated by hilar and paratracheal lymph node enlargement and consequent obstruction of neighbouring bronchi.
- Treatment is the same as for adult disease, the dose of medication being adjusted by weight.
- In 1989, it was estimated that there were 1.3 million annual cases of TB in children aged under 15 years. This may be an inaccurate estimate, as paediatric TB is difficult to diagnose.
- Extrapulmonary TB is more common in children being 25 per cent of all cases in the <4 years of age. Superficial lymphadenopathy is the most common form.

REFERENCES

1. World Health Organization. *Global tuberculosis control: surveillance, planning, financing: WHO report 2007.* Geneva: World Health Organization, 2007.
2. World Health Organization. *Global tuberculosis control: surveillance, planning, financing. WHO report 2005.* Geneva: World Health Organization, 2005.
3. World Health Organization. *Expanded program on immunization. Update 1989.* Geneva: World Health Organization, 1989.
4. Hershfield E. Tuberculosis in children: guidelines for diagnosis, prevention and management (a statement of the scientific committees of the IUATLD). *Bull World Health Organ* 1991; 66: 61–7.

5. Donald P. Childhood tuberculosis: out of control? *Curr Opin Pulm Med* 2002; **8**: 178–82.
6. World Health Organization. *Global tuberculosis control*. Geneva: World Health Organization, 2003.
7. Public Health Laboratory Service. *Tuberculosis surveillance in England and Wales*. London: Public Health Laboratory Service, 2001.
8. Atkinson P, Taylor H, Sharland M, Maguire H. Resurgence of paediatric tuberculosis in London. *Arch Dis Child* 2002; **86**: 264–5.
9. Eriksson M, Bennet R, Danielsson N. Clinical manifestations and epidemiology of childhood tuberculosis in Stockholm 1976–95. *Scand J Infect Dis* 1997; **29**: 569–72.
10. Rosenfeldt V, Paerregaard A, Fuursted K *et al.* Childhood tuberculosis in a Scandinavian metropolitan area 1984–93. *Scand J Infect Dis* 1998; **30**: 53–7.
11. van Rie A, Byers N, Gie R *et al.* Childhood tuberculosis in an urban population in South Africa; burden and risk factors. *Arch Dis Child* 1999; **80**: 433–7.
12. Kiwanuka J, Graham S, Coulter J *et al.* Diagnosis of pulmonary tuberculosis in children in an HIV-endemic area, Malawi. *Ann Trop Paediatr* 2001; **21**: 5–14.
13. Chakraborty A. Problem of tuberculosis among children in the community: situation analysis in the perspective of tuberculosis in India. *Ind J Tuberc* 1999; **46**: 91–103.
14. Centers for Disease Control. *Reported tuberculosis in the United States 2001*. Atlanta, GA: CDC, 2002.
15. Nunn A, Darbyshire J, Fox W *et al.* Changes in the annual tuberculosis notification rates between 1978/79 and 1983 for the population of Indian subcontinent ethnic origin residents in England. *J Epidemiol Community Health* 1986; **40**: 357–63.
16. Yang Z, deHaas P, Wachmann C *et al.* Molecular epidemiology of tuberculosis in Denmark in 1992. *J Clin Microbiol* 1995; **33**: 2077–81.
17. Rose A, Watson J, Graham C *et al.* Tuberculosis at the end of the 20th century in England and Wales: results of a national survey in 1998. *Thorax* 2001; **56**: 173–9.
18. Surinder S, Hawker J, Ali S. The epidemiology of tuberculosis by ethnic group in Birmingham and its implications for future trends in tuerculosis in the UK. *Ethn Health* 1997; **2**: 147–53.
19. Long R, Sutherland K, Kunimoto D *et al.* The epidemiology of tuberculosis among foreign-born persons in Alberta, Canada 1989–1998: identification of high-hrisk groups. *Int J Tuberc Lung Dis* 2002; **6**: 615–21.
20. Dahle U, Sandven P, Heldal E, Caugant D. Molecular epidemiology of Mycobacterium tuberculosis in Norway. *J Clin Microbiol* 2001; **39**: 1802–7.
21. Drucker E, Alcabes P, Bosworth W, Sckell B. Childhood tuberculosis in the Bronx, New York. *Lancet* 1994; **343**: 1482–5.
22. Parslow R, El-Shimy N, Cundall D, McKinney P. Tuberculosis, deprivation and ethnicity in Leeds, UK, 1982–97. *Arch Dis Child* 2001; **84**: 109–13.
23. Cantwell M, Binkin N. Impact of HIV on tuberculosis in sub-Saharan Africa: a regional perspective. *Int J Tuberc Lung Dis* 1997; **1**: 205–14.
24. Coovadia H, Jeena P, Wilkinson D. Childhood human immunodeficiency virus and TB co-infections: reconciling conflicting data. *Int J Tuberc Lung Dis* 1998; **2**: 844–51.
25. Alves R, Ledo A, Cunha A, Sant'anna C. Tuberculosis and HIV co-infection in children under 15 years of age in Rio de Janeiro, Brazil. *Int J Tuberc Lung Dis* 2003; **7**: 198–9.
26. Jeena P, Pillay P, Pillay T, Coovadia H. Impact of HIV-1 co-infection on presentation and hospital-related mortality in children with culture proven pulmonary tuberculosis in Durban, South Africa. *Int J Tuberc Lung Dis* 2002; **6**: 672–8.
27. Steiner P, Rao M. Drug-resistant tuberculosis in children. *Semin Pediatr Infect Dis* 1993; **4**: 275–82.
28. Schaaf H, Gie R, Beyers N. Primary drug-resistant tuberculosis in children. *Int J Tuberc Lung Dis* 2000; **4**: 1149–55.
29. Daly J, Brown D, Lincoln E. Endobronchial tuberculosis in children. *Dis Chest* 1952; **22**: 380.
30. Lincoln E, Gilbert L, Morales S. Chronic pulmonary tuberculosis in individuals with known previous tuberculosis. *Dis Chest* 1960; **38**: 473.
31. Jacobs R, Starke J. Tuberculosis in children. *Med Clin North Am* 1993; **77**: 1335–51.
32. Kumar D, Watson J, Charlett A. Tuberculosis in England and Wales in 1993: results of a national survey. *Thorax* 1997; **52**: 1060–67.
33. Farinha N, Razali K, Holzel H, Morgan G, Novelli V. Tuberculosis of the central nervous system in children: a 20-year survey. *J Infect* 2000; **41**: 61–8.
34. Janssens J, deHaller R. Spinal tuberculosis in a developed country. *Clin Orthop Relat Res* 1990; **256**: 67–75.
35. Ussery X, Valway S, McKenna M. Epidemiology of tuberculosis among children in the United States. *Pediatr Infect Dis J* 1996; **15**: 697–704.
36. Marais BJ, Gie RP, Obihara CC *et al.* Well-defined symptoms are of value in the diagnosis of childhood pulmonary tuberculosis. *Arch Dis Child* 2005; **90**: 1162–5.
37. Prada Arias M, Jardon Bahia J, Rodriguez Barca P *et al.* Endobronchial tuberculous granuloma in children. *Eur J Pediatr Surg* 2006; **16**: 265–8.
38. Gupta P, Gupta G, Agarwal D. Middle lobe syndrome due to tuberculous etiology: a series of 12 cases. *Indian J Tuberc* 2006; **53**: 104–108.
39. Harris V, Dida F, Lander S. Cavitary tuberculosis in children. *J Pediatr* 1977; **90**: 660–1.
40. Nemir R, Krasinski K. Tuberculosis in children and adolescents in the 1980s. *Pediatr Infect Dis J* 1988; **7**: 375–9.
41. Boyd G. Tuberculous pericarditis in children. *AMA Am J Dis Child* 1953; **86**: 293–300.
42. Smith K. Tuberculosis in children. *Curr Probl Pediatr* 2001; **31**: 1–30.
43. Hussey G, Chisholm T, Kibel M. Miliary tuberculosis in children: review of 94 cases. *Pediatr Infect Dis J* 1991; **10**: 832–6.
44. Udani P, Parekh U, Dastur D. Neurological and related syndromes in CNS tuberculosis: clinical features and pathogenesis. *J Neurosurg Sci* 1971; **14**: 341–57.
45. Waecker N, Conner J. Central nervous system tuberculosis in children: a review of 30 cases. *Pediatr Infect Dis J* 1990; **9**: 539.
46. Starke J. Tuberculosis of the central nervous system in children. *Semin Pediatr Neurol* 1999; **6**: 318–31.
47. Idriss Z, Sinno A, Kronfol N. Tuberculous meningitis in childhood: 43 cases. *AMA Am J Dis Child* 1976; **130**: 364.
48. Rich A, McCordock H. The pathogenesis of tuberculous meningitis. *Bull Johns Hopkins Hosp* 1933; **52**: 43–9.
49. Humphries M, Teoh R, Lau J. Factors of prognostic significance in Chinese children with tuberculous meningitis. *Tubercle* 1990; **71**: 161–8.
50. Doerr C, Starke J, Ong L. Clinical and public health aspects of tuberculous meningitis in children. *J Pediatr* 1995; **127**: 27–33.
51. Yaramis A, Gurkan F, Elevli M *et al.* Central nervous system tuberculosis in children: a review of 214 cases. *Pediatrics* 1998; **102**: E49.
52. Peterson E, Nakasone A, Platon-DeLeon J, Jang Y. Comparison of direct and concentrated acid-fast smears to identify specimens culture positive for *Mycobacterium* spp. *J Clin Microbiol* 1999; **11**: 3564–8.
53. Ba F, Rieder H. A comparison of fluorescence microscopy with the Ziehl–Neelsen technique in the examination of sputum for acid-fast bacilli. *Int J Tuberc Lung Dis* 1999; **3**: 1101–5.
54. Strumpf I, Tsang A, Syre J. Reevaluation of sputum staining for the diagnosis of pulmonary tuberculosis. *Am Rev Respir Dis* 1979; **119**: 599–602.
55. Laven G. Diagnosis of tuberculosis in children using fluorescence microscopic examination of gastric washings. *Am Rev Respir Dis* 1977; **115**: 743–9.

56. Vallejo J, Ong L, Starke J. Clinical features, diagnosis and treatment of tuberculosis in infants. *Pediatrics* 1994; **94**: 1–7.

57. Starke J, Taylor-Watts K. Tuberculosis in the pediatric population of Houston, Texas. *Pediatrics* 1989; **84**: 28–35.

58. Marais B, Hesseling A, Schaaf H *et al*. The bacteriologic yield in children with intrathoracic tuberculosis. *Clin Infect Dis* 2006; **42**: e69–71.

59. Bibi H, Mosheyev A, Shoseyov D *et al*. Should bronchoscopy be performed in the evaluation of suspected pediatric pulmonary tuberculosis? *Chest* 2002; **122**: 1604–8.

60. Abadco D, Steiner P. Gastric lavage is better than bronchoalveolar lavage for isolation of *Mycobacterium tuberculosis* in childhood tuberculosis. *Pediatr Infect Dis J* 1993; **11**: 735–8.

61. deBlic J, Azevedo I, Burren C *et al*. The value of flexible bronchoscopy in childhood pulmonary tuberculosis. *Chest* 1991; **100**: 688–92.

62. Zar H, Tannenbaum E, Apolles P *et al*. Sputum induction for the diagnosis of pulmonary tuberculosis in infants and young children in an urban setting in South Africa. *Arch Dis Child* 2000; **82**: 305–308.

63. Zar H, Hanslo D, Apolles P *et al*. Induced sputum versus gastric lavage for microbiological confirmation if pulmonary tuberculosis in infants and young children: a prospective study. *Lancet* 2005; **365**: 130–34.

64. Vargas D, Garcia L, Gilman R *et al*. Diagnosis of sputum-scarce HIV-associated pulmonary tuberculosis in Lima, Peru. *Lancet* 2005; **365**: 150–52.

65. Chow F, Espiritu N, Gilman R *et al*. La cuerda dulce – a tolerability and acceptability study of a novel approach to specimen collection for diagnosis of paediatric pulmonary tuberculosis. *BMC Infect Dis* 2006; **6**: 67.

66. Hsu K. Tuberculin reaction in children treated with isoniazid. *AMA Am J Dis Child* 1983; **137**: 1090–92.

67. Lifschitz M. The value of the tuberculin skin test as a screening test for tuberculosis among BCG-vaccinated children. *Pediatrics* 1965; **36**: 624–7.

68. Wang L, Turner M, Elwood R *et al*. A meta-analysis of the effect of bacille Calmette–Guérin vaccination on tuberculin skin test measurements. *Thorax* 2002; **57**: 804–809.

69. Menzies R, Vissandjee B. Effect of bacille Calmette–Guérin vaccination on tuberculin reactivity. *Am Rev Respir Dis* 1992; **141**: 621–5.

70. Almeida L, Barbieri M, Da Paixao A, Cuevas L. Use of purified protein derivative to assess the risk of infection in children in close contact with adults in a population with high Calmette–Guérin bacillus coverage. *Pediatr Infect Dis J* 2001; **20**: 1061–5.

71. Larsson L, Bentzon M, Lind A *et al*. Sensitivity to senstins and tuberculin in Swedish Children. Part 5: A study of school children in an inland rural area. *Tuberc Lung Dis* 1993; **74**: 371–6.

72. Sepulveda R, Burr C, Ferrer X, Sorensen R. Booster effect of tuberculin testing in healthy 6-year-old school children vaccinated with bacille Calmette–Guérin at birth in Santiago, Chile. *Pediatr Infect Dis J* 1988; **7**: 578–82.

73. Khan E, Starke J. Diagnosis of tuberculosis in children: increased need for better methods. *Emerg Infect Dis* 1995; **1**: 115–23.

74. Delacourt C, Mani T, Bonnerot V. Computed tomography with normal chest radiograph in tuberculous infection. *Arch Dis Child* 1993; **69**: 430–32.

75. Uzum K, Karahan O, Dogan S *et al*. Chest radiography and thoracic computed tomography findings in children who have family members with active pulmonary tuberculosis. *Eur J Radiol* 2003; **48**: 258–62.

76. Andronikou S, Joseph E, Lucas S *et al*. CT scanning for the detection of tuberculous mediastinal and hilar lymphadenopathy in children. *Pediatr Radiol* 2004; **34**: 232–6.

77. Swingler G, Du Toit G, Andronikou S *et al*. Diangostic accuracy of chest radiography in detecting mediastinal lymphadenopathy in suspected pulmonary tuberculosis. *Arch Dis Child* 2005; **90**: 1153–6.

78. Cherian G, Uthaman B, Salama A *et al*. Tuberculous pericardial effusion: features, tamponade and computed tomography. *Angiology* 2004; **55**: 431–40.

79. De Backer A, Mortele K, Vanhoenacker F, Parizel P. Imaging of extraspinal musculoskeletal tuberculosis. *Eur J Radiol* 2006; **57**: 119–30.

80. Fourie P, Becker P, Festenstein F *et al*. Procedures for developing a simple scoring method based on unsophisticated criteria for screening children for tuberculosis. *Int J Tuberc Lung Dis* 1998; **2**: 116–23.

81. Hesseling A, Schaaf H, Gie R *et al*. A critical review of diagnostic approaches used in the diagnosis of childhood tuberculosis. *Int J Tuberc Lung Dis* 2002; **6**: 1038–45.

82. Van Rheenen P. The use of the paediatric tuberculosis score chart in an HIV-endemic area. *Trop Med Int Health* 2002; **7**: 435–41.

83. Marais B, Gie RP, Hesseling AC *et al*. A refined symptom-based approach to diagnose pulmonary tuberculosis in children. *Pediatrics* 2006; **118**: 1350–9.

84. Ewer K, Deeks J, Alvarez L. Comparison of T-cell-based assay with tuberculin skin test for diagnosis of *Mycobacterium tuberculosis* infection in a school tuberculosis outbreak. *Lancet* 2003; **361**: 1168–73.

85. Liebeschuetz S, Bamber S, Ewer K *et al*. Diagnosis of tuberculosis in South African children with a T-cell-based assay: a prospective cohort study. *Lancet* 2004; **364**: 2196–203.

86. Soysal A, Millington K, Bakir M *et al*. Effect of BCG vaccination on risk of *Mycobacterium tuberculosis* infection in children with household tuberculosis contact: a prospective community-based study. *Lancet* 2005; **366**: 1443–51.

87. Hill C, Brookes R, Adetifa I *et al*. Comparison of enzyme-linked immunospot assay and tuberculin skin test in healthy children exposed to *Mycobacterium tuberculosis*. *Pediatrics* 2006; **117**: 1542–8.

88. Connel T, Curtis N, Ranganathan S, Buttery J. Performance of a whole blood interferon gamma assay for detecting latent infection with *Mycobacterium tuberculosis* in children. *Thorax* 2006; **61**: 616–20.

89. National Institute of Clinical Excellence. *Tuberculosis: Clinical diagnosis and management of tuberculosis, and measures for its prevention and control*. London: Royal College of Physicians of London, 2006.

90. te Water Naude J, Donald P, Hussey G *et al*. Twice weekly vs. daily chemotherapy for childhood tuberculosis. *Pediatr Infect Dis J* 2000; **19**: 405–10.

91. Tsakalidis D, Pratsidou P, Hitoglou-Makedou A *et al*. Intensive short course chemotherapy for treatment of Greek children with tuberculosis. *Pediatr Infect Dis J* 1992; **11**: 1036–42.

92. Biddulph J. Short course chemotherapy for childhood tuberculosis. *Pediatr Infect Dis J* 1990; **9**: 794–801.

93. Jacobs R, Abernathy R. The treatment of tuberculosis in children. *Pediatr Infect Dis J* 1985; **4**: 513–7.

94. Varudkar B. Short course chemotherapy for tuberculosis in children. *Indian J Pediatr* 1985; **52**: 593–7.

95. Al-Dossary F, Ong L, Correa A, Starke J. Treatment of childhood tuberculosis using a 6-month, directly observed regimen with only 2 weeks of daily therapy. *Pediatr Infect Dis J* 2002; **21**: 91–7.

96. Kumar L, Dhand R, Singhi P *et al*. A randomized trial of fully intermittent vs daily followed by intermittent short course chemotherapy for childhood tuberculosis. *Pediatr Infect Dis J* 1990; **9**: 802–806.

97. Reis F, Bedran M, Moura J *et al*. Six-month isoniazid–rifampicin treatment for pulmonary tuberculosis in children. *Am Rev Respir Dis* 1990; **142**: 996–9.

98. Pickering L (ed.). *Red book: Report of the Committee on Infectious Diseases*, 25th edn. Elk Grove Village: American Academy of Pediatrics, 2000.

99. British Thoracic Society. Chemotherapy and management of tuberculosis in the United Kingdom: recommendations 1998. *Thorax* 1998; **53**: 536–48.

100. World Health Organization. *Treatment of tuberculosis: guidelines for national programmes*, 5th edn. Geneva: World Health Organization, 1997.

101. Trebucq A. Should ethambutol be recommended for routine treatment of tuberculosis in children? A review of the literature. *Int J Tuberc Lung Dis* 1997; **1**: 12–15.

102. Gandhi N, Moll A, Sturm A *et al*. Extensively drug-resistant tuberculosis as a cause of death in patients co-infected with tuberculosis and HIV in a rural area of South Africa. *Lancet* 2006; **368**: 1575–80.

103. Masjedi M, Farnia P, Sorooch S *et al*. Extensively drug-resistant tuberculosis: 2 years of surveillance in Iran. *Clin Infect Dis* 2006; **43**: 841–7.

104. Girgis N, Farid Z, Kilpatrick M. Dexamethasone as an adjunct to treatment of tuberculous meningitis. *Pediatr Infect Dis J* 1991; **10**: 179.

105. Schoeman J, Van Zyl L, Laubscher J, Donald P. Effect of corticosteroids on intracranial pressure, computed tomographic findings, and clinical outcome with tuberculous meningitis. *Pediatrics* 1997; **99**: 226–31.

106. Nemir R, Cordova J, Vaziri F. Prednisone as an adjunct in the chemotherapy of lymph node-bronchial tuberculosis in childhood: a double-blinded study. *Am Rev Respir Dis* 1967; **95**: 402.

107. World Health Organization. Efficacy of various durations of isoniazid preventive therapy for tuberculosis: five years of follow-up in the IUAT trial. International Union Against Tuberculosis Committee on Prophylaxis. *Bull World Health Organ* 1982; **60**: 555–64.

108. Ormerod L. Rifampicin and isoniazid prophylactic chemotherapy for tuberculosis. *Arch Dis Child* 1998; **78**: 169–71.

109. Ena J, Valls V. Short-course therapy with rifampin plus isoniazid, compared with standard therapy with isoniazid, for latent tuberculosis infection: a meta-analysis. *Clin Infect Dis* 2005; **40**: 670–76.

110. Reichman LB, Lardizabal A, Hayden CH. Considering the role of four months of rifampin in the treatment of latent tuberculosis infection. *Am J Resp Crit Care Med* 2004; **170**: 832–5.

111. Medical Research Council. A double-blind placebo-controlled clinical trial of three antituberculosis chemoprophylaxis regimens in patients with silicosis in Hong Kong. Hong Kong Chest Service/Tuberculosis Research Centre, Madras/British Medical Research Council. *Am Rev Respir Dis* 1992; **145**: 36–41.

112. Ijaz K, Jereb JA, Lambert LA *et al*. Severe or fatal liver injury in 50 patients in the United States taking rifampin and pyrazinamide for latent tuberculosis infection. *Clin Infect Dis* 2006; **42**: 346–55.

113. McElroy PD, Ijaz K, Lambert LA *et al*. National survey to measure rates of liver injury, hospitalization, and death associated with rifampin and pyrazinamide for latent tuberculosis infection. *Clin Infect Dis* 2005; **41**: 1125–33.

TREEATMENT

12

Clinical pharmacology of the antituberculosis drugs

CHARLES A PELOQUIN

INTRODUCTION

The antituberculosis drugs include those that are used only for mycobacterial infections: isoniazid, pyrazinamide, ethambutol, para-aminosalicylic acid, capreomycin, viomycin, ethionamide, clofazimine, and thiacetazone. Other tuberculosis (TB) drugs have potentially broader application, including rifamycins (rifampicin, rifabutin, rifapentine), aminoglycosides (streptomycin, amikacin, kanamycin), fluoroquinolones (ciprofloxacin, levofloxacin, moxifloxacin, gatifloxacin), and earlier in its development, cycloserine. A few other agents, including some β-lactam antibiotics, currently have undefined roles in the management of TB. Well-designed, prospective TB treatment studies are lacking for many of these agents against TB. Therefore, some treatment recommendations, especially those for multidrug-resistant TB (MDR-TB), reflect accumulated anecdotal experience.

Excepting the treatment of latent infection, the treatment of TB requires combination chemotherapy. This prevents the emergence of the naturally occurring drug-resistant mutants that are present inside most patients. Since these organisms carry mutations that generally are specific for a single agent, multidrug treatment provides cross-coverage against these various mutations. This approach to multidrug TB treatment differs from that seen for bacterial infections. In the latter case, drug combinations are often selected based on complementary or potentially

synergistic, mechanisms of action. For example, ampicillin and gentamicin are used together against enterococci, while piperacillin and tobramycin are used together against *Pseudomonas aeruginosa*. These represent combinations of cell wall active agents (β-lactams) and intracellular poisons (aminoglycosides), which have been shown to enhance each other's activity against several pathogens. In contrast, when most TB treatment regimens were developed, investigators had little idea of how the TB drugs worked. Regimens were developed empirically and the best regimen among the available alternatives became the standard treatment, at least for a while. Given this history of incremental improvement, it is likely that we have not optimized TB treatment. We simply continue to use the best of what has been tested to date.

Pharmacodynamics (PD) is the study of the relationships between the concentrations of drugs and the effects that they produce. Much PD work has been undertaken for the antibacterial agents, while far less has been done for the antituberculosis drugs. Using *in vitro* models, the maximum plasma concentration (C_{max}), the duration of drug exposure (TIME) and the integral of the concentration-versus-time curve, or area under the curve (AUC), can be varied relative to the minimal inhibitory concentration (MIC), while holding the other parameters constant.[1,2] These studies can determine which parameter has the greatest influence on the elimination of log-phase growth bacteria. Calculations can be made for the relationships

C_{max}/MIC, TIME > MIC and AUC/MIC. For Gram-positive and Gram-negative infections, the efficacy of the intracellular poisons, such as the fluoroquinolones, aminoglycosides and rifamycins, depend upon maximizing the AUC/MIC and the C_{max}/MIC ratios. Rephrasing, the AUC/MIC ratio usually is the most important parameter, but for any given AUC/MIC ratio, one must maximize the C_{max}/MIC to derive full benefit from these intracellular poisons. High C_{max}/MIC ratios improve bacterial killing and limit both adaptive resistance (temporary refractoriness) and the selection of drug-resistant subpopulations. For the cell wall active agents, such as the penicillins and the cephalosporins, TIME > MIC should be maximized.[1,2]

These relationships are well described for bacteria during logarithmic-phase growth. Similar conditions prevail for most tubercle bacilli early in the treatment of TB, when the disease process is largely extracellular. How these relationships apply to intracellular *Mycobacterium tuberculosis*, or organisms in the poorly understood 'latent' and 'persisting' states, is not known. In general, organisms that are multiplying very slowly, or only intermittently, are less susceptible to drugs. AUC/MIC and C_{max}/MIC likely remain the most important parameters for the TB drugs with intracellular targets, including the fluoroquinolones, aminoglycosides and rifamycins, at least early in treatment. For cycloserine, which has a mechanism of action that parallels that of penicillin, TIME > MIC likely is the most important parameter.[3] For the other agents that affect steps leading up to cell wall construction, such as isoniazid, ethionamide and ethambutol, an argument can be made either way. The AUC/MIC ratio will always show some correlation with activity, since it reflects both the C_{max}/MIC ratio and a time component. Therefore, in the absence of concrete data, the initial guess regarding PD should be focused on maximizing the AUC/MIC ratio. Only continued research using *in vitro* and *in vivo* methods can define the key PD parameters for the TB drugs.[2]

The terms 'bacteriostatic' and 'bactericidal' have specific meanings when bacteria are discussed. However, these terms have had various meanings during the history of TB treatment and their meanings have varied with the test conditions studied. For TB, perhaps the best use of bacteriostatic and bactericidal is limited to *in vitro* studies.[4] Laboratory end points can be defined clearly and demonstrated reproducibly. In humans, the situation is far more complex and the end points often are elusive. An apparent lack of clinical signs and symptoms does not mean that all tubercle bacilli have been killed.

The terms 'early bactericidal activity' (EBA) and 'sterilizing activity' have emerged to describe complex *in vivo* phenomenon. The EBA refers to the ability of a drug to rapidly decrease the number of viable mycobacteria in the sputum of a TB patient, and typically is measured during the first 2 days of treatment.[5,6] 'Extended EBA' looks at the clearance of organisms over days 2–5 of treatment. Isoniazid consistently has shown the largest EBA. In contrast, sterilizing activity reflects the ability of a drug to kill off the 'persisters', so that patients remain smear and culture negative after the end of treatment. From clinical trials, it appears that the rifamycins have the most potent sterilizing activity. Various models have been proposed, describing different TB subpopulations that may reside within a TB patient.[5] Although useful for teaching purposes, these models cannot be applied directly in the clinical management of a TB patient, since there is no way to measure the number of organisms in each of the proposed states inside a live patient.

ISONIAZID

Isoniazid (INH) is one of the two most important TB drugs, along with rifampicin. It is exceptionally active against *M. tuberculosis*, and has the most profound EBA of the TB drugs.

Structure and activity

INH is a synthetic agent and its pyridine nucleus and carboxylic acid hydrizide side chain both are key structural features.[7–9] INH is a pro-drug, activated within *M. tuberculosis* by the enzyme, katG.[10–12] INH-derived reactive intermediates that form adducts with NAD+ (nicotinamide adenine dinucleotide) and NADP+ (phosphate form), leading to a blockade of mycolic acid synthesis.[12] The *katG* gene encodes for mycobacterial catalase peroxidase and organisms lacking this gene do not synthesize catalase or peroxidase, and generally show INH resistance. InhA, an enoyl acyl carrier protein reductase, appears to be the primary target for the INH-NAD product described above.[13] Resistance occurs at a rate of about 1 in 10^7 organisms.

INH has an MIC against *M. tuberculosis* of 0.01–0.25 µg/mL.[8,9,14] *Mycobacterium kansasii* and *Mycobacterium xenopi* are also susceptible to INH, but most other non-tuberculous mycobacteria (NTM) are resistant. INH is considered bactericidal, with minimal bactericidal concentrations (MBCs) close to its MIC. *In vitro*, INH's maximum bactericidal effect is seen around 1 µg/mL.[14] With long periods of exposure, INH can produce a prolonged post-antibiotic effect (PAE), lasting up to 5 days.[15] However, in humans, INH is relatively short-lived, so the clinical relevance of this finding is not clear. In animal models, INH-resistant isolates may show reduced virulence, but the clinical relevance of this observation also remains debatable.[14] INH appears to lack clinically significant cross-resistance with the other TB drugs.

Pharmacokinetics

INH is not stable in blood left at room temperature, so PK studies must provide for rapid centrifugation, harvesting of plasma and prompt freezing. INH shows good absorption from the gastrointestinal (GI) tract and from intramuscular (i.m.) injection sites.[16] Food, including high-fat food, reduces oral absorption, so INH is best given on an empty stomach.[17] INH reacts with reducing sugars, thus limiting the choices of sweeteners for oral solutions to non-reducing sugars, such as sorbitol.[7] Antacids have demonstrated variable affects on INH's absorption.[17] The time of maximum plasma concentrations (T_{max}) ranges from 0.5 to 2 hours after oral doses.[17] C_{max} of 3–5 µg/mL typically are achieved after 300 mg doses and 9–15 µg/mL after 900 mg doses. The C_{max} may be somewhat lower in fast acetylators, due to greater first-pass metabolism. The absorption of INH is unaffected by formulation with other TB drugs in combination products.[18]

INH is widely distributed into most body tissues and fluids, with a volume of distribution (V_d) of roughly 0.7 L/kg.[16,17] It has low protein binding (~10 per cent), and penetrates the cerebrospinal fluid (CSF), even in the absence of inflammation (20–100 per cent of plasma concentrations).[18,19] INH crosses the placenta and is excreted in human breast milk. INH enters macrophages and displays intracellular activity against M. tuberculosis.[14]

INH is extensively metabolized, especially in the liver, to a number of inactive compounds, mostly by acetylation and dehydrazination.[14,16,19] N-acetyl transferase 2 (NAT2) forms acetyl-INH, which is further metabolized to mono- and diacetylhydrazine. Slow acetylation, an autosomal recessive trait, is the result of a relative NAT2 deficiency. Rapid acetylators can be heterozygous or homozygous for the trait. Approximately 50 per cent of white people and black people are slow acetylators, while 80–90 per cent of Asians and Eskimos are rapid acetylators.[19,20] Acetylator status does not correlate with treatment efficacy when INH is given at least twice a week. However, rapid acetylators receiving once-weekly INH-containing regimens have poorer outcomes.[20,21] Clinical trials do not show a good correlation between acetylator status and the risk of hepatotoxicity. The plasma half-life ($t_{1/2}$) of INH ranges from 1 to 1.8 hours in most rapid acetylators and from 3 to 4 hours in most slow acetylators.[16] Over 80 per cent of INH is excreted in the urine in 24 hours as unchanged drug or metabolites.

Dosing

For adults, the once-daily (q.d.) dose of INH is 3–5 mg/kg up to 300 mg.[22] INH twice-weekly (b.i.w.) doses are 15 mg/kg, up to 900 mg, using directly observed therapy (DOT). Oral doses should be given 1 hour before or 2 hours after a meal. When required, it is possible to administer the i.m. preparation intravenously (i.v.) as a short (5–10 minute) infusion on INH in normal saline.[23] The American Thoracic Society (ATS)/Centers for Disease Control and Prevention (CDC)/Infectious Disease Society of America (IDSA) recommend a dose of 10–20 mg/kg/day up to 300 mg q.d. for children.[22] INH should be administered with pyridoxine (10–20 mg of vitamin B_6) in high-risk patients, such as preg-

nant women, the malnourished, alcoholics, cancer patients and those predisposed to peripheral neuritis.

Malabsorption of INH clearly has been linked to failure, relapse and the selection of rifamycin-resistant TB.[24,25] Therapeutic drug monitoring (TDM) can be used to adjust doses in patients at risk of poor drug absorption, those who are critically ill and those who are not responding to treatment as expected.[1,2] Plasma INH concentrations are drawn at 2 and 6 hours post dose. The C_{max} values listed above are generally achieved by 2 hours post dose, while the 6-hour concentration allows one to distinguish between delayed and malabsorption. Assuming a T_{max} of ≤2 hours, one also can calculate the elimination $t_{1/2}$ and determine acetylator status from these two values.

INH dosing generally does not require adjustment in patients with renal impairment.[19] INH should be administered after dialysis to avoid premature removal of the drug.[26] It should be used cautiously in patients with hepatic disease. INH has been used safely in pregnant women.[22] As with any drug, consider waiting until the second trimester before starting treatment.

Adverse effects

Subclinical hepatitis occurs in up to 10 per cent of patients on INH.[16,18,22,27] A clinical picture similar to viral hepatitis may develop, with anorexia, nausea, vomiting, abdominal pain and weight loss. Laboratory changes include elevations in plasma AST, ALT and occasionally bilirubin. The hepatitis is independent of INH plasma concentrations. Risk factors include age >35 years, chronic alcohol intake, pre-existing hepatic disease and concurrent hepatotoxic agents.[22,27] Hepatitis in combination with rifampicin is additive, but not synergistic.[27,28] INH should be stopped immediately, allowing time for the liver enzymes to return to baseline and for any clinical symptoms to resolve before carefully reintroducing the drug.

INH-induced rheumatic complications (arthralgias) have been reported and it is known to cause drug-induced lupus syndrome.[16,18] INH forms hydrazones that prevent the conversion of pyridoxine to its active form, pyridoxal phosphate, leading to neuropathies. Slow acetylators appear to be at a greater risk and it is more common with q.d. INH doses of 8 mg/kg or more.[16] INH, especially in overdose situations, causes central nervous system (CNS) effects, including psychosis, delirium, euphoria, somnolence, coma, seizures and possibly death.[22,29] Intravenous pyridoxine is given in doses equal to the ingested INH dose to counteract the effects.

Drug interactions

INH can inhibit cytochrome P450 enzymes, including CYP2C19, CYP3A and CYP2E1.[16,30,31] Other drugs affected include phenytoin and carbamazepine, and plasma concentrations of these drugs should be monitored carefully.[16,18] INH can also induce CYP2E1. Acetaminophen toxicity has been reported in patients on inhibition by INH. Histaminase inhibition of INH has led to reports of histamine reactions in patients ingesting skipjack tuna and other fish. Coagulation (international normalized ratio, or INR) should be checked in patients concurrently receiving warfarin, as conflicting reports suggest there might be an interaction (see Table 12.1).

RIFAMPICIN

Rifampicin (RIF) (also known as rifampicin) is derived from natural rifamycin products first isolated in Italy.[18,32] Several other rifamycins, including rifabutin and rifapentine, share a common structure, with alterations present in selected substituents. These changes especially affect the PK and drug interaction profiles of the drugs.[32,33] RIF is the key antituberculosis drug, allowing for 'short-course' regimens of 6–9 months, due to its excellent sterilizing activity.[15,33]

Structure and activity

RIF is bactericidal against *M. tuberculosis* and several other mycobacterial species, including *Mycobacterium bovis* and *M. kansasii*.[4,32] Its *in vitro* bactericidal activity is concentration dependent.[14] Mouse models have also shown that RIF's activity is strongly dose dependent.[34,35] RIF shows excellent sterilizing activity *in vivo* against semi-dormant *M. tuberculosis*, possibly due to its rapid onset of action.[14] Most, but not all, investigators have shown a relatively short PAE against *M. tuberculosis*. The current field of investigation is focused on finding the maximally effective dose, balanced against any potential toxicity. Studies to date are encouraging in regards to RIF doses of 900 or 1200 mg given daily, and more studies are planned.[36–41]

RIF inhibits DNA-dependent RNA polymerase, blocking transcription.[8,9,11,32] RIF resistance results from single amino acid substitutions in the β-subunit of RNA polymerase.[11] This alters the binding of RIF, with the degree of resistance depending upon the location and nature of the amino acid substitution. The mutations leading to this resistance occur at a rate of about 1 in 10^8.[10,11] Higher doses of RIF as monotherapy do not prevent the emergence of resistance.[14] *In vitro*, subinhibitory concentrations enhance the selection of resistant organisms.

Pharmacokinetics

Oral RIF doses of 600 mg produce C_{max} values of 8–24 µg/mL about 2 hours post dose.[1,19,42] Food decreases the C_{max} by 36 per cent and the AUC to a lesser degree.[42] Because of its concentration-dependent effects, RIF should be given on an empty stomach. Antacids and ranitidine have little effect on the absorption of RIF.[33,42] Combination

products with INH (Rifamate®, Aventis, Bridgewater, NJ, USA), or INH plus pyrazinamide (Rifater®, Aventis) have been formulated to prevent selective drug ingestion by patients. The absorption of INH and pyrazinamide (PZA) are not affected by these combined formulations, but RIF's absorption is reduced by the presence of PZA. To compensate, the typical dose of Rifater contains 720 mg of RIF instead of the typical 600 mg dose.

Delayed and/or reduced RIF absorption has been observed in certain patients, including those with diabetes mellitus, cystic fibrosis, HIV or previous GI surgery.[1,2,33,42–45] In some cases, drug malabsorption has been associated with clinical failure and acquired drug resistance.[2,33] Clearly, not all patients with these conditions malabsorb RIF, but it is wise to observe these patients closely for a delayed response to treatment. Some clinicians elect to perform TDM early in the course of treatment to head off such problems.[1,2] Given these periodic absorption issues and the clearly demonstrated concentration-dependent killing of RIF, a good case for higher initial doses can be made.[39] Tantalizing data regarding the efficacy and apparent safety of high-dose RIF are accumulating, and the next step appears to be a large phase II clinical trial.[36–41] Provided that concentration-related toxicity does not emerge, considerably higher doses of RIF may offer the best potential to reduce the duration of treatment for TB.

RIF is widely distributed in the body, with a V_d around 0.7 L/kg, similar to INH's. Unlike INH, RIF has variable CSF penetration that generally is better with inflamed meninges.[19] Protein binding is about 85 per cent. RIF is extensively metabolized by intestinal and hepatic esterases, and has a $t_{1/2}$ of 2–4 hours.[46,47] Its main metabolite is 25-desacetyl-RIF, which retains much of RIF's activity. RIF and its metabolites are largely excreted in the bile and eliminated in the faeces. About 10 per cent of the dose is excreted in the urine as unchanged drug.[19,33] Auto-induction of RIF clearance is characterized by a decrease in AUCs and terminal half-lives of RIF and its 25-desacetyl metabolite.[33] Steady-state usually is achieved after 6 days, at least with the 600 mg dose.

Dosing

The usual adult and paediatric dose of RIF is 10–20 mg/kg, up to 600 mg orally q.d.[22,33] Oral doses should be given 1 hour before or 2 hours after a meal. RIF may also be given intravenously over 30 minutes when required.[18,32] Unlike other TB drugs, the dose of RIF is not increased to accommodate thrice- or twice-weekly regimens.[22,32] When TDM is performed, concentrations are drawn at 2 and 6 hours post dose, as described for INH.[1,2]

Because RIF is predominantly cleared by the liver, dosage adjustment is not necessary in renal impairment.[19] It should be used with caution in the face of hepatic failure, although there is no standardized approach.[19,27] RIF generally has been used safely in pregnant women.[19,22,32] RIF does cross the human placenta and on rare occasions, fetal malformations have occurred.[18,19] The use of RIF in pregnancy should be reserved for cases where it is clearly indicated.

Adverse effects

RIF use leads to a small risk of hepatotoxicity and this risk is additive to that of INH.[18,19,29,27,32] Risk factors include advanced age, alcohol consumption, diabetes and concomitant hepatotoxic agents. Other adverse effects associated with intermittent RIF dosing include the 'flu-like' syndrome, which generally occurs after 3 months of treatment with doses of 900–1800 mg given once or twice weekly.[22,32] More severe effects, including thrombocytopenia, haemolytic anemia and acute renal failure, also may occur, and these require permanent discontinuation of RIF.[18,29,32] These reactions appear to be immunologically related, as they are associated with the presence of RIF-dependent IgM or IgG antibodies. RIF has variable effects on cellular and humoral immunity. Suppression of *in vitro* lymphocyte responses in cells collected from TB patients have been reported, but clinically evident immunosuppression has not been demonstrated.[32,48]

Drug interactions

RIF is a profound inducer of CYP3A4 and other hepatic P450 enzymes.[32,49,50] However, RIF is not a substrate for these enzymes, so other agents, such as HIV protease inhibitors, do not affect RIF's clearance.[19,32,33] Extensive lists of drugs affected by the co-administration of RIF have been published.[33,49,50] A simple rule of thumb is that most hepatically metabolized drugs will have shorter half-lives in the presence of RIF, especially if they are substrates for CYP3A4, and to a lesser degree, 2C9, 2C19 and 2D6. Enzyme activity and the pharmacodynamic effects of the affected drug generally return to baseline levels within 2 weeks after discontinuing RIF therapy.[33,49,50]

RIFABUTIN

Rifabutin (RBN) retains RIF's activity against *M. tuberculosis* and appears to have superior activity against *M. avium* complex.[51–53] RBN's primary advantage in the treatment of TB is its reduced induction of hepatic metabolism, roughly 40 per cent of that seen with RIF.[33,50] This allows for combinations of TB and anti-HIV drugs that are not possible with RIF-containing regimens.[51,54,55]

Pharmacokinetics and dosing

RBN 300 mg doses produce C_{max} values around 0.3–0.9 µg/mL 3–4 hours post dose, far lower than RIF or

rifapentine.[1,33,50] Food has only slight effects on its absorption.[56] Didanosine formulations that contains antacids do not effect RBN absorption, and RBN appears to have more predictable absorption among HIV-infected patients than does RIF.[33,50] RBN has a large V_d of 8–9 L/kg, which explains the low plasma concentrations. CSF penetration is variable, 30–70 per cent, while protein binding is 70–80 per cent. Recent clinical trials clearly show that poor absorption of RBN is associated with failure, relapse and the selection of rifamycin resistance.[25] Given that and given the fact that various doses are recommended in HIV-positive patients, depending on co-administered drugs, a case can be made for RBN TDM (for more information, see www.cdc.gov/nchstp/tb/tb_hiv_drugs/toc).

RBN undergoes extensive intestinal and hepatic metabolism, with major metabolites being de-acetylated and hydroxylated RBN.[33,50] Over 20 metabolites have been found, with 25-desacetyl-RBN as the primary, microbiologically active metabolite.[57,58] Less than 10 per cent of a RBN dose is excreted in urine as unchanged drug. The elimination $t_{1/2}$ is 32–67 hours.[59] Like RIF, RBN induces its own gut and hepatic metabolism. Unlike RIF, CYP3A is the major isozyme that transforms RBN to its oxidative metabolites in human enterocytes and liver microsomes, and CYP3A also catalyses oxidation of 25-O-desacetyl-RBN.[33,50] As noted above, RIF is not a substrate for this enzyme.

Adverse effects

RBN differs somewhat from RIF and rifapentine (RPNT) in its adverse effect profile. RBN can show concentration-related toxicity, typically when administered with CPY3A4 inhibitors. These inhibitors increase RBN and dramatically increase 25-O-desacetyl RBN concentrations, leading to arthralgias, anterior uveitis, skin discoloration and leucopenia.[18,32] Given that too much RBN (and metabolite) leads to toxicity and too little leads to clinical failure and drug resistance, this author recommends TDM for RBN.

Drug interactions

Most drug interactions that involve RIF also involve RBN, but to a lesser degree (about 40 per cent).[32,33,49,50] Induction of metabolic enzymes, particularly CYP3A, is the reason for most interactions. Like RIF, RBN also induces CYP1A2, CYP2D6, the phase II enzymes glucuronosyltransferase and sulfotransferase, and the efflux transporter P-glycoprotein.[33,49,50] After stopping RBN, enzyme activity returns to baseline levels in about 2 weeks.[33,49,50]

RBN induces and is metabolized by CYP3A. As a result, the macrolide antibiotics, azole antifungal drugs and the HIV-1 protease inhibitors have complex bidirectional interactions with RBN.[33,49,50,55,56] The CYP3A-inducing effect of RBN results in decreased concentrations of the macrolides and protease inhibitors, sometimes to levels that substantially decrease their antimicrobial activity.[33,50] Conversely, as CYP3A inhibitors, the macrolides (excepting azithromycin) and protease inhibitors increase the concentrations of RBN and 25-O-desacetyl-RBN, and can cause RBN toxicity.[33,49,50] The enzyme inducer efavirenz requires the use of increased doses of RBN, typically 600 mg[22,32,33] (for more information, see www.cdc.gov). Various treatment studies for HIV-infected TB patients, designed to overcome these complex drug interactions, are under way. Because it is almost impossible to predict drug concentrations in patients receiving three or more interacting drugs, TDM is a reasonable tool to apply in such situations. Blood samples can be collected at 3–4 hours and 7 hours post dose to assess the peak concentration, and to detect delayed absorption.[1,2,60]

RIFAPENTINE

RPNT is the cyclopentyl derivative of RIF, with the same mechanism of action and a similar toxicity profile overall.[32,61–64] The major focus recently for RPNT is to find the correct dose and frequency to maximize its effect. Like RIF and RBN, RPNT shows concentration-dependent killing.[32] Also like RIF, regimens that include MOXI and exclude INH appear to be more active in the mouse model.[65] The United States Public Health Service (USPHS) TB trial 29 will include dose escalation of RPNT (milligram dose, as well as number of doses per week) in order to determine the best balance between efficacy and toxicity, should the latter be seen.

Pharmacokinetics and dosing

The current approved dose of RPNT is 600 mg once weekly, but that is likely to change to 900 or 1200 mg given two, three or more times per week. Clinical studies currently are in the design stage. RPNT has a long plasma half-life (14–18 hours compared to 2–3 hours for RIF), although its $t_{1/2}$ is shorter than that or RBN.[32,33] RPNT is more slowly absorbed that RIF or RBN (T_{max} about 5 hours) and its C_{max} of 8–30 µg/mL is somewhat higher than RIF's when both are dosed at 600 mg.[33,66,67] Unlike RIF, a high-fat meal increases the C_{max} and AUC of RPNT by 50 per cent; other foods have varying effects on RPNT absorption.[33] The absorption of RPNT is reduced by about 20 per cent in HIV-infected patients compared with healthy adults when both are tested in the fasted state.[68] Protein binding is very high, about 97 per cent; few data are available regarding CSF penetration. RPNT is similar to RIF in its metabolic pathway, being metabolized by esterases. The metabolite 25-desacetyl-RPNT retains much of the activity of RPNT. RPNT has little effect on its own metabolism and biliary secretion, unlike RIF and RBN.[69]

Adverse effects and drug interactions

RPNT is very similar to RIF regarding drug interactions and adverse effects. Given its structural similarity, this comes as no surprise. RPNT is about 85 per cent as potent as RIF in inducing CYP3A.[33,49,50] Therefore, RPNT does not offer any advantage in sparing the drug interactions, unlike RBN, which is significantly less potent an enzyme inducer. However, because both RPNT and RIF are not substrates for CYP enzymes, they are not the objects of drug interactions, as is the case with RBN.

PYRAZINAMIDE

PZA initially was used at daily doses approaching 50 mg/kg and this led to unacceptable rates of hepatotoxicity.[70] After years on the shelf, PZA was rediscovered for clinical use as the third most important TB drug, after INH and RIF. PZA contributes important sterilizing activity to the treatment regimens during the first 2 months of therapy. It is also used for longer durations in the face of resistance to INH or RIF.

Structure and activity

PZA is a synthetic agent with a molecular weight (MW) of 123.[71] Morphazinamide is the N-morpholinomethyl derivative of PZA and is similar in most ways to the parent drug. PZA has useful activity only against *M. tuberculosis* and *Mycobacterium africanum*. *M. bovis* and the other mycobacteria are naturally resistant.[4] Understanding the mechanism of action has been problematic. Pyrazinoic acid appears to be the active moiety, although it is only the pyrazinoic acid created within tubercle bacilli that appears to be active, since the organisms do not appear to take up significant amounts of the acid from their surroundings.[4,72–74] Some reports have suggested that PZA acts against fatty acid synthesis, as does 5-chloro-PZA, by inhibiting fatty acid synthase I (FAS-I) and this debate continues.[75,76] It may be that the accumulation of inorganic acids within the organisms produces a stress that they cannot withstand.[72–74] Mutations in the *pncA* gene are associated with PZA resistance.[77]

Pharmacokinetics

Of all the TB drugs, oral PZA is the most reliably absorbed. T_{max} is at 1–2 hours and concentrations generally increase linearly with dose over the clinically applicable range.[1,19,78–80] Most C_{max} values fall between 20 and 60 µg/mL, but occasionally go as high as 90 µg/mL. The lower range is associated with 25 mg/kg q.d. doses and the higher end is associated with 50 mg/kg b.i.w. doses. PZA has a V_d of about 0.6 L/kg and its protein binding data are not available. CSF penetration is good: 50–100 per cent of plasma concentrations. PZA is metabolized to pyrazinoic acid and 5-OH-pyrazinoic acid, which do not appear to contribute to the activity. The $t_{1/2}$ is about 9 hours. PZA is generally well absorbed in adults, but a recent report suggests this may not be so in children with HIV.[44,81,82]

Dosing

In the USA, PZA is generally given as 25 mg/kg q.d., or 50 mg/kg b.i.w. Doses in other nations may vary somewhat. Although PZA is metabolized, the metabolites can accumulate in patients with renal failure. Because the relative contribution of the parent drug versus the metabolites to the adverse effect profile of PZA is not known, it appears prudent to reduce the frequency of PZA dosing in such patients to a maximum of three times weekly.[26] The effect of advanced liver dysfunction on PZA disposition is not known. TDM would be advisable for such patients.[1,2,19]

Adverse effects

The main toxicities of PZA are GI upset and arthralgias.[18,29,71] PZA routinely causes an increase in plasma uric acid concentrations, but not frank gout. In fact, normal uric acid concentrations during treatment with PZA generally indicate non-compliance. Hepatotoxicity is the most important PZA-associated toxicity.[29,70] High daily doses dramatically increase the incidence of this toxicity and they are no longer used. PZA has been associated with an unexpected number of severe liver injuries when used daily with RIF for the treatment of latent infection.[83] Because the true incidence is not known, currently it is not possible to say if this rate is particularly high. When given b.i.w, PZA plus RIF apparently has not caused significant liver injury, based upon available reports.[84]

Drug interactions

PZA is not associated with significant drug interactions. When co-formulated with RIF and INH, the absorption of RIF is decreased by about 13 per cent. This is overcome by the somewhat higher RIF dose used in Rifater.

ETHAMBUTOL

In the USA, ethambutol (EMB) is generally used as part of the initial treatment regimen for TB until susceptibility data are known.[22] Once full susceptibility is confirmed, EMB is not required. If the organisms prove to be INH- or RIF-resistant, EMB is usually continued for the duration of treatment.[85]

Structure and activity

EMB has a unique synthetic structure and was specifically designed for treating TB.[18,86] Only the dextro-isomer of the chiral compound is used clinically and it is only active against mycobacteria. *M. tuberculosis*, *M. bovis*, *M. kansasii*, *M. intracellulare* and *M. avium* all are inhibited by EMB. The MIC for TB is 0.5–2.0 µg/mL, depending upon media, and its effects are not apparent for about 24 hours. Under clinical conditions, EMB is probably bacteriostatic, although higher concentrations may kill TB.

Work on determining the mechanism of action and the genetic basis for EMB resistance have produced results. EMB inhibits arabinotransferases involved in the biosynthetic pathway of the mycobacterial cell wall.[87] Arabinotransferase is involved in the polymerization of arabinofuranose, required for synthesis of arabinogalactan (AG), a structural component of mycobacterial cell wall.[88] Ethambutol also has an inhibitory effect on the polymerization of arabinofuranose into lipoarabinomannan (LAM), but this occurs more slowly, requiring longer exposure to the drug. Mutations in the *embB* region, specifically codon 306, appear to be the most common source of EMB resistance.[89]

Pharmacokinetics

More recent studies have shown that EMB absorption following oral doses is variable.[1,19,43,44,90] Peak concentrations of 2–6 µg/ml occur 2–3 hours after oral doses *embB* in patients with normal absorption.[90] Unfortunately, some patients do not absorb EMB normally.[43,44,91–93] Food does not reduce absorption significantly, although antacids should be avoided within 2 hours of EMB dosing.[90] The V_d is large, over 3 L/kg, while protein binding is less than 30 per cent.[19] CSF penetration is variable and often poor (5 per cent), although it is occasionally higher. Since EMB is a fairly weak drug to begin with, it should not be considered a mainstay for TB meningitis.[19] EMB is cleared both renally and hepatically, so patients should be dosed cautiously should they have end-organ damage.[19,26] It shows a biphasic decline in plasma concentrations, with an apparent $t_{1/2}$ of 3–4 hours if a one-compartment model is used. A slower elimination phase becomes apparent 10–12 hours after doses, which may represent release from tissues or red blood cells. This secondary $t_{1/2}$ is 10–15 hours.[19,90]

Dosing

EMB is dosed at 15–25 mg/kg q.d. or 50 mg/kg b.i.w.[22] Most clinicians begin with the higher q.d. doses for at least the first 2 months, since EMB is a relatively weak antituberculosis drug. The frequency of dosing should be reduced to three times weekly in patients with poor renal function.[26,90]

Adverse effects

Optic neuritis, specifically retrobulbar neuropathy, is the most important EMB toxicity.[18,29,86] It is uncommon with standard q.d. doses when given to otherwise healthy individuals. However, some patients with pre-existing ocular problems, such as those resulting from diabetes, may be at greater risk of toxicity. Patients should be tested routinely for visual acuity (Snellen charts) and red–green colour discrimination (Ishihara colour plates) at baseline and throughout treatment.[22] Daily doses of 30 mg/kg or more increase the likelihood of this toxicity, as does the administration of standard q.d. doses (15–25 mg/kg) to patients with impaired renal function.[29,86] Should the toxicity develop, the drug should be stopped promptly. When this is done, gradual improvement in vision generally is achieved.

Other adverse reactions include elevations in plasma uric acid, and uncommonly, cholestatic jaundice, interstitial nephritis, thrombocytopenia, neutropenia and skin reactions.[29,86] It is possible to desensitize patients to EMB.[94]

Drug interactions

EMB should not be given with antacids and presumably sucralphate, iron or other drugs or supplements containing di- or trivalent cations.[90] EMB does not have other significant drug interactions.

PARA–AMINOSALICYLIC ACID

Para-aminosalicylic acid (PAS) was unseated as a first-line TB drug by EMB, because the latter was better tolerated.[95] Because of limited use, most TB isolates remain susceptible to PAS, making it a valuable drug against MDR-TB.

Structure and activity

PAS is a synthetic agent, resulting from the work of Lehmann in Sweden during the 1940s. It is a structural analogue of aminobenzoic acid.[95] Most structural changes eliminate its activity against TB.[95] PAS is active against *M. tuberculosis* and *M. bovis,* with concentrations of 0.5–2.0 µg/mL producing roughly 90 per cent inhibition of cultures.[4,12,96] PAS is not bactericidal, does not display a PAE, and appears to work primarily if not exclusively against extracellular TB.[8,9] Its mechanism of action is not clearly known, but may involve iron transfer.[95] Other theories hold that PAS has activity against the folic acid pathway or mycobactin synthesis. In general, PAS does not show cross-resistance with other TB drugs.

Pharmacokinetics

PAS and its sodium salt are well absorbed from the GI tract.[18,97–99] A C_{max} of 70–80 µg/mL is achieved within 1–2 hours of a 4 g dose.[18,70] Single doses of sustained-release PAS granules (Paser®, Jacobus Pharmaceuticals, Princeton, NJ, USA) produce a C_{max} of 15–20 µg/mL 4–6 hours post dose, with somewhat higher concentrations seen with chronic dosing.[97,98,100] PAS is widely distributed, especially to the kidney, lung and liver, but CSF penetration may be variable and low (10–50 per cent).[19] Plasma protein binding is 50–70 per cent and the $t_{1/2}$ of PAS is about 45–60 minutes.[95] The V_d is about 1.5 L/kg. PAS is rapidly metabolized in the gastrointestinal tract and liver to N-acetyl-PAS and p-aminosalicyluric acid. The metabolites are not active.[8,9,95] Most of a dose is recovered in the urine as metabolites.

Dosing

The typical PAS dose is 4 g, three times daily.[22] Because the granules produce sustained inhibitory concentrations, 4 g twice daily (b.i.d.) appears to be an acceptable alternative.[97,98] The usual paediatric dose is 50 mg/kg three times daily, up to a total of 12 g/day.[22] The granules are best absorbed with food, but the granules themselves should not be chewed.[100] For TDM purposes, a 4- to 6-hour sample approaches T_{max}, with concentrations of 20–60 µg/mL considered normal for the granules.[1,2,97,98]

Historically, PAS was thought to exacerbate uraemic symptoms and possibly acidosis in renal failure patients, although there are no data showing this.[101] Therefore, it is reasonable to use PAS in these patients if indicated. The PAS $t_{1/2}$ is not prolonged in renal disease, but N-acetyl-PAS is retained significantly longer.[102] Since it is not clear if PAS or the metabolite is most associated with adverse reactions, caution is advised.[19,95] Haemodialysis removes both PAS and N-acetyl-PAS.[101] Since PAS can cause hepatotoxicity, it should be used with caution in patients with hepatic impairment.[18,29,95] PAS has been used safely in pregnant women, although a complete safety profile has not been established.[22,95] As a general precaution, it should be avoided in the first trimester of pregnancy if possible.

Adverse effects

Gastrointestinal disturbances from PAS are the most common adverse effects.[29,95] With the older dosage forms nausea, vomiting, abdominal pain and diarrhoea were very common. The new Paser® granules have offered significant relief from the nausea, vomiting and abdominal pain; however, diarrhoea remains a significant problem.[95,97,98] This diarrhoea is usually self-limited, with symptoms improving after the first 1–2 weeks of therapy. It is also important to note that the empty granules will appear in the stool.[95]

Various types of malabsorption have been reported with PAS, including steatorrhoea.[18,95]

Other reported forms of malabsorption include that of vitamin B_{12}, folate, xylose and iron.[95] Megaloblastic anaemia has not been reported. Hypersensitivity reactions, often with fever, conjunctivitis and rash, may occur.[18,95] Less common manifestations include vasculitis, arthralgias, eosinophilia, leucopenia, thrombocytopenia, hepatitis and a lymphoma-like syndrome consisting of lymphadenopathy, rash and hepatomegaly.[95] Desensitization to PAS hypersensitivity is not recommended, and with hepatitis, the drug should be discontinued permanently. Early recognition of the initial symptoms is important, as PAS-induced hepatitis may be fatal.

PAS does not have known effects on host immunity.[95] It may cause a positive direct Coombs' test and patients with glucose-6-phosphate dehydrogenase deficiency may experience haemolytic anaemia.[18] PAS-induced haemolytic anaemia has been reported to cause acute renal failure. PAS is known to produce goitre, with or without myxoedema, and appears to be more common with concurrent use of ethionamide.[95] This can be prevented or treated with thyroxine. Sodium overload was a problem with the sodium-PAS tablets.

Drug interactions

There are few, if any, significant PK interactions with current dosage forms of PAS.

CYCLOSERINE

Structure and activity

Cycloserine (CS), specifically D-cycloserine, is a natural product of *Streptomyces orchidaceus* and *Streptomyces garyphalus*.[3,7] It has a molecular weight of 102, it is soluble in water and it is stable in alkaline, but not acidic or neutral solutions. Terizidone is formed by the reaction of two CS molecules with terephthalaldehyde and it has similar antibacterial activity.[103]

Cycloserine's MIC against *M. tuberculosis* range from 6.2 to 25 µg/mL, depending on the media, pH and the presence of D-alanine, which inhibits the drug's activity.[3,4,8,9] It has similar activity against *M. kansasii*, *M. intracellulare* and *M. avium*.[3] CS is generally bacteriostatic and the onset of action appears to be relatively slow *in vitro*.[14] Sustained concentrations above the MIC are required for effect *in vitro*, as CS possesses little if any PAE.[3,4] CS disrupts D-alanine incorporation into peptidoglycan during bacterial cell wall synthesis, similar but not identical to the action of β-lactams.[8,9,14,96] CS targets the peptidoglycan biosynthetic enzymes D-alanine racemase (Alr) and D-alanine: D-alanine ligase (Ddl).[104] The activity of CS has been significantly enhanced *in vitro* in combination with other small alanine antagonists, such as beta-chloro-D-alanine, but there are no published *in vivo* results following up on this observation.[105] Because of limited use, CS-resis-

tant isolates of *M. tuberculosis* are uncommon and cross-resistance has not been demonstrated.[3]

Pharmacokinetics

CS is well absorbed after oral doses, with a T_{max} of 2–3 hours.[1,3,19,103,106,107] Doses of 250–500 mg produce C_{max} of 20–35 µg/mL about 1–2 hours post dose. Food reduces and delays the drug's absorption.[107] CS appears to have very low protein binding and penetrates the CSF with concentrations that are 54–79 per cent of plasma concentrations.[3] About 30–90 per cent of a dose appears in the urine within 24 hours.[19,107] Cycloserine's $t_{1/2}$ ranges from 8 to 25 hours, depending on renal function, with most patients in the range of 10–12 hours.[19,107] Probenecid does not alter its renal elimination, so tubular secretion appears not to be an important excretory route.[20]

Dosing

The usual CS dose ranges from 250 to 1000 mg per day, typically given as 250–500 mg every 12 hours.[1,2,19,22] Higher doses appear to produce greater CNS toxicity. Most patients should be started on 250 mg doses q.d. or b.i.d. and gradually increased over several days to 750 or 1000 mg total, divided b.i.d. TDM can be very helpful in minimizing CNS effects. A 2-hour sample approaches C_{max} and a 6-hour sample can be used to rule out late absorption.[1,2,19]

Paediatric doses are generally 10–20 mg/kg/day (maximum 1000 mg) in two equally divided doses. Plasma concentrations should be monitored, as experience in this population is limited.[3]

Therapeutic drug monitoring of CS is highly recommended for patients with renal dysfunction.[1,22,101] The goal appears to be maintaining concentrations above the MIC, and in renal failure, this probably can be done with daily doses of 250–500 mg.[107] Some patients may require less frequent dosing.[101] CS should be given after haemodialysis, because it is removed into the dialysate.[101] Dosage adjustment for patients in hepatic failure should be unnecessary. CS has been used safely in pregnant women, although it should be used only when necessary.[3,18,22,108] As with most drugs, CS should be avoided during the first trimester if possible.

Adverse effects

The main adverse effect of CS is CNS toxicity.[3,18,95] Effects include hyper-excitability, dizziness, lethargy, depression, anxiety, confusion, memory loss and, very rarely, focal or grand mal seizures.[3,109–111] Effects may be worse with elevated plasma CS concentrations (>35 µg/mL), although lethargy and difficulty concentrating are often seen at normal concentrations. CS does not have known effects on host immunity. Pyridoxine is given at 50–60 mg q.d. in an attempt to reduce the CNS effects of CS, although the efficacy of this practice is not clear.[3,112,113] Other rare side effects reported include GI disturbances rash, drug fever and cardiac arrhythmias.[3,19,95]

Drug interactions

PK interactions are not described for CS. However, increased neurological symptoms may be seen when fluoroquinolones or INH are given with cycloserine.[3]

ETHIONAMIDE

Ethionamide (ETA) is a singularly unpleasant drug to take, as most patients will experience some GI intolerance.[114] In addition, it is perhaps the weakest of the TB drugs, so it is reserved for cases when there is nothing else.[7,18,114]

Structure and activity

ETA (2-ethylisothionicotinamide, 2-ethyl-4-pyridinecarbothioamide), a thioamide, was first synthesized in 1956.[114] Prothionamide, the n-propyl derivative of ETA, is very similar to ETA in most regards. ETA shares structural features with INH and, to a degree, thiacetazone.[114] The free carbothionamide group, also found in thiacetazone, is essential for activity.[8,9] ETA's pyridine ring is also found in INH. ETA's mechanism of action may overlap with those of INH and with thiacetazone, disrupting mycolic acid synthesis.[8,9,14,20] ETA is active against extra- and intracellular mycobacteria in monocytes.[114]

ETA is useful only against mycobacteria, including M. tuberculosis, M. avium and M. leprae.[4,8,9] The MICs versus M. tuberculosis in 7H12 broth range from 0.3 to 1.2 µg/mL, and in 7H11 agar 2.5–10 µg/mL.[4] ETA may suffer 50 per cent loss under in vitro testing conditions.[14] The MBC/MIC ratios are 2–4, putting cidal concentrations beyond the range of clinically achievable concentrations for most patients.[4,14,114] PAE also does not appear to be clinically achievable. In vitro, activity appears best when concentrations remain above the MIC.[14]

Considerable effort has been made recently to define the mechanisms of action and resistance to ETA. Both INH and ETA are pro-drugs, requiring activation by mycobacterial cell processes prior to inhibition of mycolic acid synthesis.[115,116] The gene ethA, through the production of the flavin-containing monooxygenase EtaA, appears responsible for activation of ETA. ETA activity is further influenced by the gene inhA, which is also associated with INH resistance.[116,117] This appears to explain the partial cross-resistance between ETA and INH. Agents that might modulate this system could enhance the activity of ETA or could be potent TB drugs in and of themselves.

Pharmacokinetics

ETA is not stable in blood left at room temperature, so pharmacokinetic studies must provide for rapid centrifugation, harvesting of plasma and prompt freezing. Oral absorption appears to be nearly complete.[118–121] T_{max} following single 500 mg oral doses is 1.5–2.5 hours, although this can be more variable. C_{max} is 1.5–3.0 µg/mL, occasionally as high as 5.0 µg/mL.[120,121] ETA suppositories have an AUC 57 per cent of that seen with oral doses.[85] ETA is distributed widely throughout the body and 10–30 per cent is protein bound.[114] CSF concentrations can approach those found in the plasma. ETA readily crosses the placenta.[114] It is metabolized by sulphoxidation, desulphuration and deamination, followed by methylation.[118,119] The sulphoxide metabolite has similar activity to the parent compound and interconversion between the two compounds occurs in humans.[114,118,119] The plasma concentrations of the metabolite are slightly lower than ETA's. Little drug is excreted in the urine. ETA's $t_{1/2}$ ranges from 1.5 to 3.0 hours.[120,121]

Dosing

The usual ETA dose is 250–1000 mg per day, generally as 250–500 mg every 12 hours.[1,22,114] Higher doses are rarely tolerated. Most patients should be started on 250 mg doses q.d. or b.i.d. and gradually increased over several days to 750 or 1000 mg total, divided b.i.d. Paediatric doses are 15–20 mg/kg/day.[22] Doses greater than 500 mg at one time are usually not tolerated. Plasma ETA concentrations can be drawn at 2 and 6 hours post dose, and the target range is 1–5 µg/mL.[1] No dosage adjustment is necessary in renal impairment.[19] Severe hepatic impairment might reduce ETA's clearance and TDM is recommended.[1,19] ETA can cause premature delivery, congenital deformities and Down syndrome, so it should be avoided in pregnant women if at all possible.[18,19]

Adverse effects

GI intolerance, including nausea or vomiting, is the main problem with ETA.[114,122] ETA suppositories, alone or combined with smaller oral doses, might help some patients to continue treatment. Hepatotoxicity occasionally occurs with ETA and ETA may be associated with CNS and visual disturbances, and with peripheral neuritis.[114] True cause and effect relationships remain elusive. Like PAS, ETA can cause goitre, with or without hypothyroidism, and using the two drugs together makes this likely. Gynaecomastia, alopecia, impotence, menorrhagia, photodermatitis, acne and arthritis complete the list of complaints with ETA.[114] ETA does not directly affect host immunity.

Drug interactions

PK interactions have not been described for ETA.

AMINOGLYCOSIDES AND POLYPEPTIDES

Structure and activity

The aminoglycosides used for TB include amikacin (AK), kanamycin (KM) and streptomycin (SM).[1,19,123] In SM, the aminocyclitol ring is streptidine; in AK and KM, it is 2-deoxystreptamine.[22] Aminoglycosides irreversibly bind to the 30S ribosomal subunit in susceptible aerobic organisms, leading to the termination of protein synthesis.[123,124] Additional mechanisms may be involved. Typical MICs for *M. tuberculosis* are 1–2 µg/mL in liquid media and 10–20 µg/mL in solid media.[4] Single-step mutations lead to resistance against KM and AK, independent of the mutations for SM resistance, and independent of those for capreomycin (CM) and viomycin (VM) resistance.[123]

CM and VM are polypeptides.[7] CM and VM appear to inhibit the translocation of peptidyl-tRNA and the initiation of protein synthesis.[8,9,96] Unlike the aminoglycosides, CM and VM apparently do not cause misreading. Typical agar MICs for CM are in the range of 15–20 µg/mL.[4] Resistance mechanisms are not well described.

SM deserves special mention as one of the first two TB drugs along with PAS. Although PAS may have been used in humans first, SM was the first TB drug with published efficacy against human TB. In that regard, it was heralded as a true miracle drug, alongside penicillin and the first sulpha drugs. In recent years, only zidovudine (AZT) has received such notoriety, when AZT became the first anti-HIV drug. Further, most of the relevant lessons regarding TB chemotherapy are found in the early literature for SM. SM proved that a single drug was insufficient treatment against active TB disease. Initially, combined with PAS and later combined with PAS and INH, durable cures of TB were first achieved with SM-containing regimens. Treatment interruptions due to SM-related toxicities and the difficulties of giving long-term treatments by i.m. injection, first came to light with SM. These valuable early lessons remain relevant to modern chemotherapy of TB. SM is over 60 years old, yet it remains an important first-line agent. SM is used as an alternative to EMB as the fourth drug in the empiric treatment of newly diagnosed TB. It has the advantage of the 'tether' of injectable therapy, in which the patient must return to the clinic for frequent follow up. Of course, this is a two-edged sword, with some patients chaffing under these repeated and often uncomfortable injections. In addition, injectable therapy is a serious concern in resource-poor nations. The reuse of needles is highly undesirable, particularly in areas with high incidences of hepatitis B and HIV infections. SM is also a first choice for many cases of MDR-TB, provided that the isolate remains susceptible to SM.

Pharmacokinetics

In general, all of these drugs have similar PK.[19] Intramuscular injections generally are absorbed over 30–90 minutes and i.v. infusions in 100 mL of 5 per cent dextrose in water or normal saline can be given over 30 minutes.[125,126] The V_d is roughly 0.25–0.30 L/kg and plasma protein binding is low.[123] They are eliminated by glomerular filtration and no metabolites have been identified.[18] The typical elimination half-lives are 2–4 hours and renal clearances parallel the creatinine clearance.[123]

Dosing

Doses (adult and paediatric) are typically 12–15 mg/kg five to seven times weekly, or 20–27 mg/kg two to three times weekly.[1,22] Daily doses produce C_{max} of 35–45 µg/mL and b.i.w. doses produce C_{max} of 65–80 µg/mL.[1,19,126] These C_{max} values are back-calculated to the end of the infusion using linear regression upon two post-infusion concentrations.

Adverse effects

Vestibular, auditory and renal toxicities are the most important.[18,19,22,127] True differences in the incidences of these toxicities across the agents appear to be small.[123,127] Plasma creatinine concentrations may increase due to reversible non-oliguric acute tubular necrosis. Renal cation wasting may also occur.[19,124] Periodic monitoring (every 2–4 weeks) of the plasma blood urea nitrogen, creatinine, calcium, potassium and magnesium should be considered. Vestibular changes may be noted on physical examination and may occur with or without tinnitus or auditory changes.[123] The latter is best detected by monthly audiograms for those patients requiring prolonged treatment. Less common toxicities include eosinophilia, skin rashes and drug fever.[18] CM does not cross-sensitize with the aminoglycosides. Aminoglycosides and polypeptides can potentiate other nephrotoxins, such as amphotericin B or the neuromuscular blocking agents.[124]

Drug interactions

PK interactions for the aminoglycosides and polypeptides appear to be limited primarily to situations where concurrent medications reduce the patients' renal function, leading to their accumulation, or the converse.

FLUOROQUINOLONES

Structure and activity

Ciprofloxacin (CIP), ofloxacin (OFL), levofloxacin (LEVO, the optical S-(–) isomer of the racemic mixture OFL), gatifloxacin (GATI) and moxifloxacin (MOXI) are the most active fluoroquinolones against *M. tuberculosis*.[4,128–130] Because LEVO is an isomer of OFL, LEVO will be listed primarily throughout this section. The fluoroquinolones inhibit DNA gyrase.[131,132] They are bactericidal against *M. tuberculosis*, with MBC/MIC ratios generally between 2 and 4.[132,133] CIP and OFL inhibit *M. tuberculosis* at concentrations of 0.5 to 2.0 µg/mL, and LEVO is twice as active as OFL. GATI and MOXI are roughly one doubling dilution more potent *in vitro*. Point mutations in DNA gyrase lead to resistance and cross-resistance among these drugs is common.[123,131]

Pharmacokinetics

Currently, LEVO and MOXI are the class members most commonly used for TB, with use varying by institution and by country. Oral absorption for LEVO exceeds 90 per cent.[123,131] Its T_{max} is 1–2 hours post dose and its V_d range is about 1.5 L/kg. Oral absorption for MOXI exceeds 85 per cent.[131] Its T_{max} is about 2 hours post dose and its V_d is about 2.7 L/kg. For most fluoroquinolones, intracellular concentrations usually exceed those in the plasma, and this might be desirable for addressing a portion of the mycobacterial population. Concentrations of OFL in inflamed meninges are 40–90 per cent of concomitant plasma concentrations; LEVO's penetration may be somewhat lower than the racemic mixture based on available data. Fluoroquinolones cross the placenta and penetrate into breast milk. LEVO and MOXI are moderately bound to plasma proteins, 25 and 50 per cent, respectively.[131]

LEVO is primarily excreted unchanged in the urine, while MOXI primarily is eliminated by non-renal mechanisms (80 per cent).[131] The elimination half-life of MOXI is about two times longer than LEVO's (6 versus 12 hours).[123] At our institution, we use large daily doses of LEVO to maximize the C_{max} to MIC ratio.[1,2,134]

Dosing and drug interactions

Many centres use LEVO doses 750–1000 mg once daily, while most use MOXI 400 mg once daily. Comparable paediatric doses would be roughly 10 mg/kg for LEVO and 5 mg/kg for MOXI, although the drugs are currently not approved for either paediatric use or for TB.[22,123] Food modestly reduces C_{max} but not AUC; however, concomitant ingestion of dairy products or drugs containing di- or trivalent cations should be avoided.[18,123,131] Dose adjustment in renal insufficiency is recommended, but is probably unnec-

essary in patients with hepatic impairment. Fluoroquinolones are not recommended in pregnant or lactating women, or in children, unless absolutely necessary.

Adverse effects

GI and CNS adverse effects are the most common.[18,131,134] These agents should be used with caution in patients with prior history of seizure.[123,131] QT interval prolongation generally is not a concern at the doses listed above for LEVO and MOXI.[131,135] GATI does appear more prone to causing hyper- and hypoglycaemia.[136] Concomitant administration with antacids, sulcralphate and multivitamins containing minerals should be avoided or at least spaced by 4 to 6 hours.[18,131] Drug interactions are not a major problem with either LEVO or MOXI, although RIF does reduce the AUC of MOXI by about 27 per cent.[137]

Recent advances in TB

Recent studies have provided additional insight into the use of fluoroquinolones for TB. First, in the mouse model, substituting MOXI for INH seems to enhance the regimen, leading to more rapid sterilization. Presumably, this is a class effect and reflects both the sterilizing activity of the fluoroquinolones, and some antagonistic effect of INH.[65] Hence, USPHS TB trial 27 compared MOXI to EMB to test for long-term safety and trial 28 currently compares the standard regimen of RIF, PZA and EMB with either INH or MOXI.[138] Second, an EBA study has shown comparable activity across GATI 400 mg, MOXI 400 mg and LEVO 1000 mg, with the latter being slightly more active at that dose.[139] Since LEVO apparently can be used at the higher dose without the risk of QT interval prolongation, it remains a viable alternative to MOXI when the latter is not available. Human clinical trials continue, primarily with MOXI and GATI, to confirm the roles of these drugs in the treatment of TB.

CLOFAZIMINE

Structure and activity

Clofazimine (CF) is a riminophenazine derivative originally synthesized in 1957.[18,123] Capsules contain micronized drug suspended in an oil-wax base. CF may inhibit replication by binding selectively to mycobacterial DNA at the guanine base.[140] CF appears bactericidal against *M. tuberculosis in vitro*, compared to its bacteriostatic activity against other mycobacteria. CF MICs ranged from 0.06 to 2.0 µg/mL when tested in 7H9 BACTEC.[141] CF's intracellular activity against *M. tuberculosis* is reported to be good and cross-resistance with other TB drugs has not been described.

Table 12.1 Tuberculosis drug interactions.

Drug X	Drug Y			
	Y increases X concentrations	Y decreases X concentrations	X increases Y concentrations	X decreases Y concentrations
Aminoglycosides[a]	None (except drug-induced renal failure)	None	None	None
Cycloserine	None (except drug-induced renal failure)	None	None	None
Ethambutol	None (except drug-induced renal failure)	Antacids	None	None
Ethionamide	None	None	(INH)	None
Fluoroquinolones[b]	None	Antacids Sulcralphate Iron and other di- and trivalent cations	Theophylline (ciprofloxacin only)	None
Isoniazid	± prednisolone	± antacids	Carbamazepine Phenytoin ± diazepam ± warfarin	Enflurane
PAS	None	None	None	None
Pyrazinamide	None	Allopurinol	(Probenecid)	None
Rifamycins[c] (most hepatically metabolized drugs can display lower concentrations when administered concurrently with rifamycins)	Rifabutin only: Clarithromycin Fluconazole Itraconazole See Table 12.2	Rifabutin only: Efavirenz Possibly nevirapine Possibly phenyotin Voriconazole	None See Table 12.2	RIF > RPNT > RBN Antidepressants β-blockers Benzodiazepines Clarithromycin Calcium channel blockers Contraceptives (oral) Enalapril Fluvastatin Glucocorticoids Immunosuppressants Itraconazole Opiods Sulphonylureas Verapamil Voriconazole Warfarin See Table 12.2

[a]Streptomycin, amikacin, kanamycin, and the polypeptides capreomycin and viomycin.
[b]Ciprofloxacin, ofloxacin, levofloxacin, gatifloxacin, moxifloxacin.
[c]Rifampicin > rifapentine (85%) > rifabutin (40%).
See also references under individual drugs.
INH, isoniazid; PAS, para-aminosalicylic acid; RBN, rifabutin; RIF, rifampicin; RPNT, rifapentine.

Pharmacokinetics and dosing

Oral bioavailability of the microcrystalline formulation of CF is approximately 70 per cent and is increased by high-fat meals.[18,123,142] The T_{max} is variable, 2–12 hours, and multiple daily oral doses produce C_{max} of 0.5–2.0 μg/mL. CF is widely distributed, especially into adipose, skin and the reticuloendothelial system. Crystal deposition has been reported in virtually all organs. CF is excreted into breast milk and is found in placental tissues, but not in the CSF.[18,19] The elimination of CF is bi-exponential, with $t_{1/2}$ of about 7 days initially and about 70 days from the tissue sites. Very little is known about its metabolism. CF is unaffected by haemodialysis; the effect of hepatic dysfunction on CF is unknown.[19,101] The usual dosage of CF for MDR-TB is 50–200 mg once daily. Paediatric doses are not clearly established, but can be estimated at 2–3 mg/kg.[123]

Table 12.2 HIV Rx and rifamycin interactions.

HIV Rx that inhibit CYP3A	Rifabutin on Rx % decrease in AUC	Rx on Rifabutin % increase in AUC	Rifampicin on Rx % decrease in AUC	Rx on Rifampicin % increase in AUC
Amprenavir	Unchanged	193	82	NR
Atazanavir	Unchanged	250	67[a]	160
Darunavir[b]	Expected decrease	Expected increase	Expected decrease	Expected no change
Delavirdine	80	100	95	Unchanged
Indinavir	32	204	89	NR
Lopinavir/ritonavir	Unchanged	303	75	NR
Nelfinavir	32	207	82	NR
Ritonavir	Unchanged	430	35	Unchanged
Saquinavir	43	NR	84	NR
Tipranavir	Unchanged	190	Expected decrease[b]	NR

HIV Rx that induce CYP3A	Rifabutin on Rx % decrease in AUC	Rx on Rifabutin % decrease in AUC	Rifampicin on Rx % decrease in AUC	Rx on Rifampicin % increase in AUC
Efavirenz	10	38	22	Unchanged
Nevirapine	Unchanged	Unchanged	37 to 58	NR

AUC, area under the curve; NR, not reported.
See also references in rifamycin sections.
More details are available at www.cdc.gov/nchstp/tb.
[a]Determined with boosted atazanavir (300 mg plus ritonavir 100 mg) reduced by rifampicin.
[b]Expected larger decrease with unboosted atazanavir (expected based on known pathways of clearance; data not published.

Adverse effects and drug interactions

CF causes a dose-related red-brown or bronze discoloration of body tissues and fluid that usually appears within 1–4 weeks and lasts 6–12 months after CF is discontinued.[123] Hyperpigmentation may also affect the conjunctiva and cornea. Dry skin is common.[18] CF can cause serious GI problems due to crystal deposition. Drug interactions appear to be rare.

OTHER DRUGS

Amoxicillin-clavulanic acid has been used for MDR-TB, although its role remains uncertain.[123] The macrolides clarithromycin and azithromycin have very limited activity against *M. tuberculosis* and are better options for *M. avium* infections.[123] Finally, thiacetazone is an inexpensive but weak drug against TB. It remains an option for desperate cases of MDR-TB. Its use is limited by severe rashes that are more prevalent in HIV-positive patients.[123]

NEW DRUGS

In contrast to the previous edition of this chapter, there is now something to write about regarding new TB drugs.[143,144] The interested reader is directed to these references and to on-line sources such as PubMed

(www.pubmed.gov) to search for the latest articles on the following compounds. While several are very interesting, as with all new chemical entities, the road to becoming an approved and marketed drug is a long and difficult one, with considerable attrition along the way. Since it is not yet known if any of these drugs will make it into clinical practice, only brief introductions will be provided here.

As noted above, MOXI appears to be the furthest along. Although not really 'new', it is being studied intensively as a potential component of first-line treatment. The diarylquinoline R207910 (now known as TMC207) is chemically related to the malaria drug chloroquine, and has entered clinical phase II testing for TB.[143–146] It is equally active against drug-sensitive and drug-resistant strains of *M. tuberculosis*, with an MIC of about 0.03 μg/mL, and it is active against many other types of mycobacteria. Plasma concentrations of TMC207 are significantly reduced by concurrent use of RIF. The initial focus for this drug will likely be on MDR-TB.

PA-824 is a nitroimidazopyran being advanced by the TB Alliance.[143,144,147] It has an MIC of 0.015–0.25 μg/mL, similar to that of isoniazid.[143] While PA-824 may not add significantly to the current standard regimen, PA-824, PZA and MOXI would provide a very potent regimen for MDR-TB.[148] It will soon be entering clinical phase II testing for TB.[149]

PA-824's chemical cousin, OPC-67683 is a newly synthesized nitro-dihydroimidazo-oxazole from Otsuka Pharmaceutical Company (Tokyo, Japan).[143,144,150] The compound has an MIC against *M. tuberculosis* from 0.006 to 0.024 µg/mL and has shown promising activity in the mouse model.[143] It is in clinical phase II testing for TB.[151]

A pyrrole derivative, LL3858, is currently in development for tuberculosis by Lupin (Mumbai, India).[143,144] It appears to be active *in vitro* and in animal models against TB. Currently, there are no publications on PubMed regarding this compound, so apparently no data have been subjected to peer review so far. Other pyrrole derivatives are at earlier stages of development.[152]

N-adamantan-2-yl-*N*-(3,7-dimethylocta-2,6-dienyl)-ethane-1,2-diamine (SQ109) was derived from ethambutol, but appears to have a unique mechanism of action against the mycobacterial cell wall.[143,144] It has an MIC

Case history

LH is a 37-year-old white male with a history of intravenous drug and cocaine abuse. He presents with cough, weight loss and fatigue. Medical evaluation provides the diagnosis of pulmonary TB, accompanied by cervical lymphadenopathy. He is begun on a TB regimen consisting of isoniazid, rifampin, pyrazinamide and ethambutol pending susceptibility data.

Four days into treatment, his HIV blood test has been reported to be positive and consideration is made for initiating anti-HIV drug treatment. The consulting HIV specialist prefers the regimen of atazanavir, tenofovir and emtricitabine. Discussion focuses on how to combine the TB drug regimen with the HIV drug regimen.

Considerations are:

1   Patient reliability with the TB drug regimen has not been established. The TB specialist recommends directly observed treatment (DOT) and the HIV specialist concurs. She also enquires if the same service can provide DOT for the HIV drugs.
2   Rifampicin generally should not be given with a protease inhibitor-containing regimen, because of its potent enzyme-inducing properties. Although rifampicin plus ritonavir may be acceptable, rifampicin-atazanavir is not.[38,39] Discussion includes the potential for switching rifampicin to rifabutin.
3   The physicians have read about paradoxical reactions, in which the TB patient worsens with the introduction of anti-HIV medications.[103] One of the physicians has seen a patient hospitalized with severe respiratory compromise under such circumstances. Combined with the first point above, unknown patient reliability, the decision is made to defer HIV treatment for now. Although the precise period to wait is not known and likely varies by patient, the decision is made to continue DOT TB treatment for 2 months prior to starting HIV treatment.

The patient continues on the four-drug TB regimen. By day 7, he experiences arthralgias and his serum uric acid is noted to be 7.2 mg%. The patient is counselled that this is likely the result of pyrazinamide and that this is not a serious condition, although it is quite annoying. Three weeks into treatment, the patient continues to have intermittent fevers and weight has not changed since the time of diagnosis. The TB specialist had read that some HIV-infected patients have poor drug absorption, including TB drug absorption.[1] He decides to check the serum concentrations of the TB drugs.

Blood is collected 2 and 6 hours after a daily DOT treatment. LH complains that this is a major hassle and the DOT staff provide him with lunch money so that he can eat and stay near the clinic for the additional time. One week later (treatment week 4), all the results for the serum concentrations are available:

- isoniazid 2 hours = 1.21 µg/mL, 6 hours = 0.47 µg/mL (normal 2 hours 3–5, and at least 2 µg/mL);
- rifampicin 2 hours = 3.28 µg/mL, 6 hours = 1.45 µg/mL (normal 2 hours 8–24, and at least 6 µg/mL);
- ethambutol 2 hours = 1.22 µg/mL, 6 hours = 2.01 µg/mL (normal 2 hours 2–6 µg/mL);
- pyrazinamide 2 hours = 31.55 µg/mL, 6 hours = 25.89 µg/mL (normal 2 hours 20–60 µg/mL, depending on dose).

The INH and RIF concentrations are low, while the EMB shows delayed absorption, with a concentration at the low end of the range at 6 hours. It is possible that a higher EMB peak was achieved between the two blood draws. The PZA concentrations are normal. The patient remains on daily doses five times weekly. INH is increased to 600 mg daily and RIF to 900 mg daily. The EMB and PZA doses are not changed. One week later (week 5), susceptibility data show that all drugs are active against the patient's isolate, so the EMB is stopped. Two weeks later (week 7), repeat INH and RIF concentrations are in the low end of the normal range. The fevers have stopped and the patient has gained 1.2 kg. Because the patient was slow to respond, the TB specialist extends the duration of PZA a total of 8 weeks from the time LH began to respond to treatment (weeks 5–12). Despite some concerns on the part of the HIV specialist, the two agree that they will try to control the TB first. After week 12, the patient is switched to INH 900 mg three times weekly and rifabutin 300 mg three times weekly, and PZA is stopped. After two doses of this regimen, the HIV drugs are started. The patient is counselled about worsening of TB symptoms, but he does not experience any.

against *M. tuberculosis* of 0.16–0.63 μg/mL and appears to be bactericidal.[143] Early PK and animal model data have been published.[153,154] Like TMC207, it is likely that Sequella (Rockville, MD, USA) will pursue an indication for MDR-TB.[155] This drug has entered clinical phase I testing.[155]

LEARNING POINTS

- The treatment of TB requires a combination of drugs to prevent the emergence of drug resistance.
- We may not yet have optimized treatment with the drugs we have. We are simply using them in the best way we have found so far.
- Bactericidal and bacteriostatic drugs in the treatment of TB are imprecise terms when referring to response *in vivo*.
- The terms early bacterial activity referring to the ability of a drug to render the sputum smear negative and sterilizing activity, referring to the ability of a drug to kill off persistent organisms, are more helpful.
- Isoniazid and rifampicin are metabolized in the liver. They are additive in their effects causing the adverse effect of hepatitis and this is not dose related.
- Pyrazinamide is only useful against *M. tuberculosis* and *M. africanum*. The other mycobacteria of the *M. tuberculosis* complex are totally resistant to it.
- As ethambutol is renally excreted, it should be used with care where renal function is reduced.
- Second-line drugs such as cycloserine, ethionamide and the aminoglycosides are less effective in the treatment of tuberculosis than first-line drugs and are much more likely to cause adverse events.

REFERENCES

1. Peloquin CA. Therapeutic drug monitoring in the treatment of tuberculosis. *Drugs* 2002; **62**: 2169–83.
2. Peloquin CA. Pharmacological issues in the treatment of tuberculosis. *Ann NY Acad Sci* 2001; **953**: 157–64.
3. Peloquin CA. Cycloserine. In: Yu VL, Edwards G, McKinnon PS, Peloquin C, Morse GD (eds). *Antimicrobial chemotherapy and vaccines*, 2nd edn, Vol. II: Antimicrobial agents. Pittsburgh, PA: Esun Technologies, LLC, 2005: 517–22.
4. Heifets LB. Drug susceptibility tests in the management of chemotherapy of tuberculosis. In: Heifets LB (ed.). *Drug susceptibility in the chemotherapy of mycobacterial infections*. Boca Raton, FL: CRC Press, 1991: 89–122.
5. Mitchison DA. Basic mechanisms of chemotherapy. *Chest* 1979; **76** (Suppl.): 771–81.
6. O'Brien RJ. Studies of the early bactericidal activity of new drugs for tuberculosis: a help or a hindrance to antituberculosis drug development? *Am J Respir Crit Care Med* 2002; **166**: 3–4.
7. Offe HA. Historical introduction and chemical characteristics of antituberculosis drugs. In: Bartmann K (ed.). *Antituberculosis drugs*. Berlin: Springer-Verlag, 1988: 1–30.
8. Verbist L. Mode of action of antituberculous drugs (Part I). *Medicon Int* 1974; **3**: 11–23.
9. Verbist L. Mode of action of antituberculous drugs (Parts II). *Medicon Int* 1974; **3**: 3–17.
10. Blanchard JS. Molecular mechanisms of drug resistance in *Mycobacterium tuberculosis. Annu Rev Biochem* 1996; **65**: 215–39.
11. Somoskovi A, Parsons LM, Salfinger M. The molecular basis of resistance to isoniazid, rifampin, and pyrazinamide in *Mycobacterium tuberculosis. Respir Res* 2001; **2**: 164–8.
12. Timmins GS, Deretic V. Mechanism of action of isoniazid. *Mol Microbiol* 2006; **62**: 1220–27.
13. Vilcheze C, Wang F, Arai M *et al*. Transfer of a point mutation in *Mycobacterium tuberculosis* inhA resolves the target of isoniazid. *Nat Med* 2006; **12**: 1027–9.
14. Trnka L, Mison P, Bartmann K, Otten H. Experimental evaluation of efficacy. In: Bartmann K (ed.). *Antituberculosis drugs*. Berlin: Springer Verlag, 1988: 31–232.
15. Awaness AM, Mitchison DA. Cumulative effects of pulsed exposures of *Mycobacterium tuberculosis* to isoniazid. *Tubercle* 1973; **54**: 153–8.
16. Burman WJ, Peloquin CA. Isoniazid. In: Yu VL, Edwards G, McKinnon PS, Peloquin C, Morse GD (eds). *Antimicrobial chemotherapy and vaccines*, 2nd edn. Volume II: Antimicrobial agents. Pittsburgh, PA: Esun Technologies, LLC, 2005: 539–50.
17. Peloquin CA, Namdar R, Dodge AA, Nix DE. Pharmacokinetics of isoniazid under fasting conditions, with food, and with antacids. *Int J Tuberc Lung Dis* 1999; **3**: 703–10.
18. McEvoy GK (ed.). *AHFS drug information*. Bethesda, MD: American Society of Health-Systems Pharmacists, 2006.
19. Peloquin CA. Antituberculosis drugs: pharmacokinetics. In: Heifets LB (ed.). *Drug susceptibility in the chemotherapy of mycobacterial infections*. Boca Raton, FL: CRC Press, 1991: 89–122.
20. Iwainsky H. Mode of action, biotransformation and pharmacokinetics of antituberculosis drugs in animals and man. In: Bartmann K (ed.). *Antituberculosis drugs*. Berlin: Springer Verlag, 1988: 399–553.
21. Ellard GA, Gammon PT. Acetylator phenotyping of tuberculosis patients using matrix isoniazid or sulphadimidine and its prognostic significance for treatment with several intermittent isoniazid-containing regimens. *Br J Clin Pharmacol* 1977; **4**: 5–14.
22. American Thoracic Society. Treatment of tuberculosis and tuberculosis infection in adults and children. *Am J Respir Crit Care Med* 2003; **167**: 603–62.
23. Crabbe SJ. Intravenous isoniazid. *P & T* 1990; **15**: 1483–4.
24. Weiner M, Burman W, Vernon A *et al*. and the Tuberculosis Trials Consortium. Low isoniazid concentration associated with outcome of tuberculosis treatment with once-weekly isoniazid and rifapentine. *Am J Respir Crit Care Med* 2003; **167**: 1341–7.
25. Weiner M, Benator D, Burman W *et al*. and the Tuberculosis Trials Consortium. Association between acquired rifamycin resistance and the pharmacokinetics of rifabutin and isoniazid among patients with HIV and tuberculosis. *Clin Infect Dis* 2005; **40**: 1481–91.
26. Malone RS, Fish DN, Spiegel DM *et al*. The effect of hemodialysis on isoniazid, rifampin, pyrazinamide, and ethambutol. *Am J Respir Crit Care Med* 1999; **159**: 1580–4.
27. Saukkonen JJ, Bernardo J, Cohn D et al. Hepatotoxicity of anti-tuberculosis therapy (HATT). *Am J Respir Crit Care Med* 2006; **174**: 935–52.
28. Steel MA, Burk RF, DesPrez RM. Toxic hepatitis with isoniazid and rifampin A meta-analysis. *Chest* 1991; **99**: 465–71.
29. Girling DJ. Adverse effects of antituberculosis drugs. *Drugs* 1982; **23**: 56–74.
30. Zand R, Nelson SD, Slattery JT *et al*. Inhibition and induction of

cytochrome P4502E1-catalyzed oxidation by isoniazid in humans. *Clin Pharmacol Ther* 1993; **54**: 142–9.

31. Desta Z, Soukhova NV, Flockhart DA. Inhibition of cytochrome P450 (CYP450) isoforms by isoniazid: potent inhibition of CYP2C19 and CYP3A. *Antimicrob Agents Chemother* 2001; **45**: 382–92.

32. Peloquin CA, Vernon A. Antimycobacterial agents: rifamycins for mycobacterial infections. In: Yu VL, Edwards G, McKinnon PS, Peloquin C, Morse GD (eds). *Antimicrobial chemotherapy and vaccines*, 2nd edn. Vol. II: Antimicrobial agents. Pittsburgh, PA: Esun Technologies, LLC, 2005: 383–402.

33. Burman WJ, Gallicano K, Peloquin CA. Comparative pharmacokinetics and pharmacodynamics of the rifamycin antibiotics. *Clin Pharmacokinet* 2001; **40**: 327–41.

34. Verbist L. Rifampicin activity *in vitro* and in established tuberculosis in mice. *Acta Tuberc Pneumol Belg* 1969; **3–4**: 397–412.

35. Jayaram R, Gaonkar S, Kaur P *et al.* Pharmacokinetics-pharmacodynamics of RIF in an aerosol infection model of tuberculosis. *Antimicrob Agents Chemother* 2003; **47**: 2118–24.

36. Kreis B, Pretet S, Birenbaum J *et al.* Two three-month treatment regimens for pulmonary tuberculosis. *Bull Int Un Tuberc* 1976; **51**: 71–5.

37. Bertrand A. Traitement antibiotique de la brucellose. *Presse Med* 1994; **23**: 1128–31.

38. Acocella G, Bertrand A, Beytout J *et al.* Comparison of three different regimens in the treatment of acute brucellosis: a multicenter multinational study. *J Antimicrob Chemother* 1989; **23**: 433–9.

39. Peloquin C. What is the right dose of rifampin? *Int J Tuberc Lung Dis* 2003; **7**: 3–5.

40. Ruslami R, Nijland H, Aarnoutse R *et al.* Evaluation of high-versus standard-dose rifampin in Indonesian patients with pulmonary tuberculosis. *Antimicrob Agents Chemother* 2006; **50**: 822–3.

41. Diacon AH, Patientia RF, Venter A *et al.* The early bactericidal activity of high dose rifampin in patiens with sputum smear-positive pulmonary tuberculosis. *Antimicrob Agents Chemother* 2007; **51**: 2994–6.

42. Peloquin CA, Namdar R, Singleton MD, Nix DE. Pharmacokinetics of rifampin under fasting conditions, with food, and with antacids. *Chest* 1999; **115**: 12–18.

43. Perlman DC, Segal Y, Rosenkranz S *et al.* for the ACTG 309 Team. The clinical pharmacokinetics of pyrazinamide in HIV-infected persons with tuberculosis. *Clin Infect Dis* 2004; **38**: 556–64.

44. Tappero JW, Bradford WZ, Agerton TB *et al.* Serum concentrations of antimycobacterial drugs in patients with pulmonary tuberculosis in Botswana. *Clin Infect Dis* 2005; **41**: 461–9.

45. Nijland HM, Ruslami R, Stalenhoef JE *et al.* Exposure to rifampicin is strongly reduced in patients with tuberculosis and type 2 diabetes. *Clin Infect Dis* 2006; **43**: 848–54.

46. Iatsimirskaia E, Tulebaev S, Storozhuk E *et al.* Metabolism of rifabutin in human enterocyte and liver microsomes: kinetic parameters, identification of enzyme systems, and drug interactions with macrolides and antifungal agents. *Clin Pharmacol Ther* 1997; **61**: 554–62.

47. Jamis-Dow CA, Katki AG, Collins JM *et al.* Rifampin and rifabutin and their metabolism by human liver esterases. *Xenobiotica* 1997; **27**: 1015–24.

48. Humber DP, Nsanzumuhire H, Aluoch JA *et al.* Controlled double-blind study of the effect of rifampin on humoral and cellular immune responses in patients with pulmonary tuberculosis and in tuberculosis contacts. *Am Rev Respir Dis* 1980; **122**: 425–36.

49. Namdar R, Ebert S, Peloquin CA. Drugs for tuberculosis. In: Piscitelli SC, Rodvold KA (eds). *Drug interactions in infectious diseases*, 2nd edn. Totowa, NJ: Humana Press, 2006: 191–214.

50. Burman WJ, Gallicano K, Peloquin C. Therapeutic implications of drug interactions in the treatment of HIV-related tuberculosis. *Clin Infect Dis* 1999; **28**: 419–30.

51. Heifets LB, Iseman MD. Determination of *in vitro* susceptibility of mycobacteria to ansamycin. *Am Rev Respir Dis* 1985; **132**: 710–11.

52. Schwander S, Rusch-Gerdes S, Mateega A *et al.* A pilot study of antituberculosis combinations comparing rifabutin with rifampicin in the treatment of HIV-1 associated tuberculosis: a single-blind randomized evaluation in Ugandan patients with HIV-1 infection and pulmonary tuberculosis. *Tuberc Lung Dis* 1995; **76**: 210–18.

53. McGregor MM, Olliaro P, Wolmarans L *et al.* Efficacy and safety of rifabutin in the treatment of patients with newly diagnosed pulmonary tuberculosis. *Am J Respir Crit Care Med* 1996; **154**: 1462–7.

54. Centers for Disease Control and Prevention. Prevention and treatment of tuberculosis among patients infected with human immunodeficiency virus: principles of therapy and revised recommendations. *MMWR Morb Mortal Wkly Rep* 1998; **47**: 1–58.

55. Centers for Disease Control and Prevention. Updated guidelines for the use of rifabutin or rifampin for the treatment and prevention of tuberculosis among HIV-infected patients taking protease inhibitors or non-nucleoside reverse transcriptase inhibitors. *MMWR Morb Mortal Wkly Rep* 2000; **49**: 185–9.

56. Narang PK, Lewis RC, Bianchine JR. Rifabutin absorption in humans: relative bioavailability and food effect. *Clin Pharmacol Ther* 1992; **52**: 335–41.

57. Cocchiara G, Strolin BM, Vicario GP *et al.* Urinary metabolites of rifabutin, a new antimycobacterial agent, in human volunteers. *Xenobiotica* 1989; **19**: 769–80.

58. Utkin I, Koudriakova T, Thompson T *et al.* Isolation and identification of major urinary metabolites of rifabutin in rats and humans. *Drug Metab Dispos* 1997; **25**: 963–9.

59. Brogden RN, Fitton A. Rifabutin: a review of its antimicrobial activity, pharmacokinetic properties and therapeutic efficacy. *Drugs* 1994; **47**: 983–1009.

60. Peloquin CA. Tuberculosis drug serum levels (letter). *Clin Infect Dis* 2001; **33**: 584–5.

61. Chan SL, Yew WW, Porter JHD *et al.* Comparison of Chinese and Western rifapentines and improvement by prior taking of various meals. *Int J Antimicrob Agents* 1994; **3**: 267–74.

62. Acocella G. Clinical pharmacokinetics of rifampicin. *Clin Pharmacokinet* 1978; **3**: 108–27.

63. Tam CM, Chan SL, Lam CW *et al.* Rifapentine and isoniazid in the continuation phase of treating pulmonary tuberculosis: initial report. *Am J Respir Crit Care Med* 1998; **157**: 726–33.

64. Tuberculosis Trials Consortium. Rifapentine and isoniazid once a week versus rifampin and isoniazid twice a week for the treatment of drug-susceptible pulmonary tuberculosis in HIV-negative pateints: a randomized clinical trial. *Lancet* 2002; **360**: 528–34.

65. Rosenthal IM, Williams K, Tyagi S *et al.* Potent twice-weekly rifapentine-containing regimens in murine tuberculosis. *Am J Respir Crit Care Med* 2006; **174**: 94–101.

66. Keung AC, Reith K, Eller MG *et al.* Enzyme induction observed in healthy volunteers after repeated administration of rifapentine and its lack of effect on steady-state rifapentine pharmacokinetics: Part I. *Int J Tuberc Lung Dis* 1999; **3**: 426–36.

67. Keung AC, Eller MG, McKenzie KA *et al.* Single and multiple dose pharmacokinetics of rifapentine in man: Part II. *Int J Tuberc Lung Dis* 1999; **3**: 437–44.

68. Keung ACF, Owens RC, Eller MG *et al.* Pharmacokinetics of rifapentine in subjects seropositive for the human immunodeficiency virus: a phase I study. *Antimicrob Agents Chemother* 1999; **43**: 1230–3.

69. Strolin Benedetti M, Dostert P. Induction and autoinduction properties of rifamycin derivatives: a review of animal and human studies. *Environ Health Perspect* 1994; **102** (Suppl. 9): 101–5.

70. McDermott W, Ormond L, Muschenheim C et al. Pyrazinamide-isoniazid in tuberculosis. Am Rev Tuberc 1954; 69: 319–33.

71. Heifets LB. Antimycobacterial agents: pyrazinamide. In: Yu VL, Edwards G, McKinnon PS, Peloquin C, Morse GD (eds). Antimicrobial chemotherapy and vaccines, 2nd edn. Vol. II: Antimicrobial agents. Pittsburgh, PA: Esun Technologies, LLC, 2005: 559–69.

72. Boshoff HI, Mizrahi V, Barry CE. Effects of pyrazinamide on fatty acid synthesis by whole mycobacterial cells and purified fatty acid synthase I. J Bacteriol 2002; 184: 2167–72.

73. Zhang Y, Wade MM, Scorpio A et al. Mode of action of pyrazinamide: disruption of Mycobacterium tuberculosis membrane transport and energetics by pyrazinoic acid. J Antimicrob Chemother 2003; 52: 790–5.

74. Zhang Y, Mitchison D. The curious characteristics of pyrazinamide: a review. Int J Tuberc Lung Dis 2003; 7: 6–21.

75. Zimhony O, Cox JS, Welch JT et al. Pyrazinamide inhibits the eukaryotic-like fatty acid synthetase I (FASI) of Mycobacterium tuberculosis. Nat Med 2000; 6: 1043–7.

76. Zimhony O, Vilcheze C, Arai M et al. Pyrazinoic acid and its n-propyl ester inhibit fatty acid synthase i in replicating tubercle bacilli. Antimicrob Agents Chemother 2007; 51: 752–4.

77. Somoskovi A, Dormandy J, Parsons LM et al. Sequencing of the pncA gene in members of the Mycobacterium tuberculosis complex has important diagnostic applications: identification of a species-specific pncA mutation in Mycobacterium canettii, and the reliable and rapid predictor of pyrazinamide resistance. J Clin Microbiol 2007; 45: 595–9.

78. Peloquin CA, Jaresko GS, Yong CL et al. Population pharmacokinetic modeling of isoniazid, rifampin, and pyrazinamide. Antimicrob Agents Chemother 1997; 41: 2670–9.

79. Peloquin CA, Bulpitt AE, Jaresko GS et al. Pharmacokinetics of pyrazinamide under fasting conditions, with food, and with antacids. Pharmacotherapy 1998; 18: 1205–11.

80. Zhu M, Starke JR, Burman WJ et al. Population pharmacokinetic modeling of pyrazinamide in children and adults with tuberculosis. Pharmacotherapy 2002; 22: 686–95.

81. Perlman DC, Segal Y, Rosenkranz S et al. for the ACTG 309 Team. The clinical pharmacokinetics of pyrazinamide in HIV-infected persons with tuberculosis. Clin Infect Dis 2004; 38: 556–64.

82. Graham SM, Bell DJ, Nyirongo S et al. Low levels of pyrazinamide and ethambutol in children with tuberculosis and impact of age, nutritional status, and human immunodeficiency virus infection. Antimicrob Agents Chemother 2006; 50: 407–13.

83. US Centers for Disease Control and Prevention. Update: fatal and sever liver injuries associated with rifampin and pyrazinamide for latent tuberculosis infection, and revisions in American Thoracic Society/CDC recommendations – United States. MMWR Morb Mortal Wkly Rep 2001; 50: 733–5.

84. Chaisson RE, Armstrong J, Stafford J, Golub J. Safety and tolerability of intermittent rifampin/pyrazinamide for the treatment oflatent tuberculosis infection in prisoners. J Am Med Assoc 2002; 288: 165–6.

85. Iseman MD. Treatment of multidrug-resistant tuberculosis. New Engl J Med 1993; 329: 784–91.

86. Lewis ML. Antimycobacterial agents: ethambutol. In: Yu VL, Edwards G, McKinnon PS, Peloquin C, Morse GD (eds). Antimicrobial chemotherapy and vaccines, 2nd edn. Vol. II: Antimicrobial agents. Pittsburgh, PA: Esun Technologies, LLC, 2005: 523–31.

87. McNeil MR, Brennan PJ. Structure, function and biogenesis of the cell envelope of mycobacteria in relation to bacterial physiology, pathogenesis and drug resistance: some thoughts and possibilities arising from recent structural information. Res Microbiol 1991; 142: 451–63.

88. Mikusova K, Slayden RA, Besra GS, Brennan PJ. Biogenesis of the mycobacterial cell wall and the site of action of ethambutol. Antimicrob Agents Chemother 1995; 39: 2484–9.

89. Srivastava S, Garg A, Ayyagari A et al. Nucleotide polymorphism associated with ethambutol resistance in clinical isolates of Mycobacterium tuberculosis. Curr Microbiol 2006; 53: 401–405.

90. Peloquin CA, Bulpitt AE, Jaresko GS et al. Pharmacokinetics of ethambutol under fasting conditions, with food, and with antacids. Antimicrob Agents Chemother 1999; 43: 568–72.

91. Graham SM, Bell DJ, Nyirongo S et al. Low levels of pyrazinamide and ethambutol in children with tuberculosis and impact of age, nutritional status, and human immunodeficiency virus infection. Antimicrob Agents Chemother 2006; 50: 407–13.

92. McIlleron H, Wash P, Burger A et al. Determinants of rifampin, isoniazid, pyrazinamide, and ethambutol pharmacokinetics in a cohort of tuberculosis patients. Antimicrob Agents Chemother 2006; 50: 1170–7.

93. Donald PR, Maher D, Maritz JS, Qazi S. Ethambutol dosage for the treatment of children: literature review and recommendations. Int J Tuberc Lung Dis 2006; 10: 1318–30.

94. Matz J, Borish LC, Routes JM, Rosenwasser LJ. Oral desensitization to rifampin and ethambutol in mycobacterial disease. Am J Respir Crit Care Med 1994; 149: 815–17.

95. Peloquin CA. Para-aminosalicylic acid. In: Yu VL, Edwards G, McKinnon PS, Peloquin C, Morse GD (eds). Antimicrobial chemotherapy and vaccines, 2nd edn. Vol. II: Antimicrobial agents. Pittsburgh, PA: Esun Technologies, LLC, 2005: 551–8.

96. Winder FG. Mode of action of the antimycobacterial agents and associated aspects of the molecular biology of the mycobacteria. In: Ratledge C, Stanford J (eds). The biology of mycobacteria. Vol 1. Physiology, identification, and classification. London: Academic Press, 1982: 353–438.

97. Peloquin CA, Henshaw TL, Huitt GA et al. Pharmacokinetic evaluation of p-aminosalicylic acid granules. Pharmacotherapy 1994; 14: 40–46 (correction: Pharmacotherapy 1994; 14: P-2).

98. Peloquin CA, Berning SE, Huitt GA et al. Once-daily and twice-daily dosing of p-aminosalicylic acid (PAS) granules. Am J Respir Crit Care Med 1999; 159: 932–4.

99. Way EL, Smith PK, Howie DL et al. The absorption, distribution, excretion and fate of para-aminosalicylic acid. J Pharmacol Exp Ther 1948; 93: 368–82.

100. Peloquin CA, Zhu M, Adam RD et al. Pharmacokinetics of p-aminosalicylate under fasting conditions, with orange juice, food, and antacids. Ann Pharmacother 2001; 35: 1332–38.

101. Malone RS, Fish DN, Spiegel DM et al. The effect of hemodialysis on cycloserine, ethionamide, para-aminosalicylate, and clofazimine. Chest 1999; 116: 984–90.

102. Held H, Fried F. Elimination of para-aminosalicylic acid in patients with liver disease and renal insufficiency. Chemotherapy 1977; 23: 405–415.

103. Morton RF, McKenna MH, Charles E. Studies on the absorption, diffusion, and excretion of cycloserine in man. Antibiot Ann 1955-6; 169–71.

104. Feng Z, Barletta RG. Role of Mycobacterium smegmatis D-alaninie: D-alanine ligase and D-alanine racemase in the mechanism of action and resistance of the peptidoglycan inhibitor D-cycloserine. Antimicrob Agents Chemother 2003; 47: 283–91.

105. David S. Synergic activity of D-cycloserine and β-chloro-D-alanine against Mycobacterium tuberculosis. J Antimicrob Chemother 2001; 47: 203–206.

106. Nair KGS, Epstein IG, Baron H, Mulinos MG. Absorption, distribution and excretion of cycloserine in man. Antibiot Ann 1955-6: 136–9.

107. Zhu M, Nix DE, Adam RD et al. Pharmacokinetics of cycloserine under fasting conditions, with orange juice, food, and antacids. Pharmacotherapy 2001; 21: 891–7.

108. Hamadeh MA, Glassroth J. Tuberculosis and pregnancy. Chest 1992; 101: 1114–20.

109. Aceto JN, Covert DF. Observations on cycloserine-isoniazid in pulmonary tuberculosis. Antibiot Med Clin Ther 1960; 7: 705–12.

110. Anderson RC, Worth HM, Welles JS et al. Pharmacology and toxicology of cycloserine. *Antibiot Chemother* 1956; **6**: 360–8.

111. Baroni V, Foddai G, Lukinovig N, Pontiggia P. Clinical evalutation of intolerance to cycloserine. *Scand J Resp Dis Suppl* 1970; **71**: 217–19.

112. Bucco T, Meligrana G, DeLuca V. Neurotoxic effects of cycloserine therapy in pulmonary tuberculosis of adolescents and young adults. *Scand J Resp Dis Suppl* 1970; **71**: 259–65.

113. Riska N. Tolerance to cycloserine. *Scand J Resp Dis Suppl* 1970; **71**: 209–14.

114. Namdar R, Peloquin CA. Ethionamide. In: Yu VL, Edwards G, McKinnon PS, Peloquin C, Morse GD (eds). *Antimicrobial chemotherapy and vaccines*, 2nd edn. Vol. II: Antimicrobial agents. Pittsburgh, PA: Esun Technologies, LLC, 2005: 533–8.

115. Vilcheze C, Weisbrod TR, Chen B et al. Altered NADH/NAD+ ratio mediates coresistance to isoniazid and ethionamide in *Mycobacteria*. *Antimicrob Agents Chemother* 2005; **49**: 708–20.

116. Hanoulle X, Wieruszeski JM, Rousselot-Pailley P et al. Selective intracellular accumulation of the ajor metabolite isued from the activation of the prodrug ethionamide in mycobacteria. *J Antimicrob Chemother* 2006; **58**: 768–72.

117. Morlock GP, Metchock B, Sikes D et al. ethA, inhA, and katG loci of ethionamide-resistant clinical *Mycobacterium tuberculosis* isolates. *Antimicrob Agents Chemother* 2003; **47**: 3799–805.

118. Jenner PJ, Ellard GA, Gruer PJK, Aber VR. A comparison of the blood levels and urinary excretion or ethionamide and prothionamide in man. *J Antimicrob Chemother* 1984; **13**: 267–77.

119. Jenner PJ, Smith SE. Plasma levels of ethionamide and prothionamide in a volunteer following intravenous and oral dosages. *Lepr Rev* 1987; **58**: 31–7.

120. Peloquin CA, James GT, McCarthy EA, Goble M. Pharmacokinetics of ethionamide suppositories. *Pharmacotherapy* 1991; **11**: 359–63.

121. Auclair B, Nix DE, Adam RD et al. Pharmacokinetics of ethionamide under fasting conditions, with orange juice, food, and antacids. *Antimicrob Agents Chemother* 2001; **45**: 810–14.

122. Fox W, Robinson DK, Tall R et al. A study of acute intolerance to ethionamide, including a comparison with prothionamide, and of the influence of a vitamin B-complex additive in prophylaxis. *Tubercle* 1969; **50**: 125–43.

123. Peloquin CA, Auclair B. Pharmacology of the second-line antituberculosis drugs. In: Portaels F, Bastian I (eds). *MDR Mycobacterium tuberculosis*. Dordrecht: Kluwer Academic, 2000: 163–74.

124. Quintiliani R, Nicolau DP, Potoski BA. Aminoglycosides. In: Yu VL, Edwards G, McKinnon PS, Peloquin C, Morse GD (eds). *Antimicrobial chemotherapy and vaccines*, 2nd edn. Vol. II: Antimicrobial agents. Pittsburgh, PA: Esun Technologies, LLC, 2005: 21–44.

125. Peloquin CA, Berning SE. Comment: Intravenous streptomycin (letter). *Ann Pharmacother* 1993; **27**: 1546–7.

126. Zhu M, Burman WJ, Jaresko GS et al. Population pharmacokinetics of intravenous and intramuscular streptomycin in patients with tuberculosis. *Pharmacotherapy* 2001; **21**: 1037–45.

127. Peloquin CA, Berning SE, Nitta AT et al. Aminoglycoside toxicity: daily versus thrice-weekly dosing for treatment of mycobacterial diseases. *Clin Infect Dis* 2004; **38**: 1538–44.

128. Berning SE. The role of fluoroquinolones in tuberculosis today. *Drugs* 2001; **61**: 9–18.

129. Alvirez-Freites EJ, Carter JL, Cynamon MH. In vitro and in vivo activities of gatifloxacin against *Mycobacterium tuberculosis*. *Antimicrob Agents Chemother* 2002; **46**: 1022–45.

130. Lounis N, Bentoucha A, Truffot-Pernot C et al. Effectiveness of once-weekly rifapentine and moxifloxacin regimens against *Mycobacterium tuberculosis* in mice. *Antimicrob Agents Chemother* 2001; **45**: 3482–6.

131. Davis SL, Neuhauser MM, McKinnon PS. Quinolones. In: Yu VL, Edwards G, McKinnon PS, Peloquin C, Morse GD (eds). *Antimicrobial chemotherapy and vaccines*, 2nd edn. Vol. II:

Antimicrobial agents. Pittsburgh, PA: Esun Technologies, LLC, 2005: 337–66.

132. Garcia-Rodriguez JA, Gomez Garcia AC. In-vitro activities of quinolones against mycobacteria. *J Antimicrob Chemother* 1993; **32**: 797–808.

133. Rastogi N, Goh KS. In vitro activity of the new difluorinated quinolones sparfloxacin (AT-4140) against *Mycobacterium tuberculosis* compared with activities of ofloxacin and ciprofloxacin. *Antimicrob Agents Chemother* 1991; **35**: 1933–6.

134. Berning SE, Madsen L, Iseman MD, Peloquin CA. Long-term safety of ofloxacin and ciprofloxacin in the treatment of mycobacterial infections. *Am J Respir Crit Care Med* 1995; **151**: 2006–2009.

135. Owens RC. Risk assessment for antimicrobial agent-induced QTc interval prolongation and torsades de pointes. *Pharmacotherapy* 2001; **21**: 301–19.

136. Owens RC Jr. Fluoroquinolone-associated dysglycemias: a tale of two toxicities. *Pharmacotherapy* 2005; **25**: 1291–5.

137. Weiner M, Burman W, Luo CC et al. for the TBTC. The effects of rifampin and human multidrug resistance gene polymorphism on serum concentrations of moxifloxacin. *American Thoracic Society International Conference*, 19–24 May 2006, San Diego, CA (Abstr. 667).

138. Burman WJ, Goldberg S, Johnson JL et al. Moxifloxacin versus ethambutol in the first 2 months of treatment for pulmonary tuberculosis. *Am J Respir Crit Care Med* 2006; **174**: 331–8.

139. Johnson JL, Hadad DJ, Boom WH et al. Early and extended early bactericidal activity of levofloxacin, gatifloxacin and moxifloxacin in pulmonary tuberculosis. *Int J Tuber Lung Dis* 2006; **10**: 605–12.

140. Arbiser JL, Moschella SL. Clofazimine: A review of its medical uses and mechanisms of action. *J Am Acad Dermatol* 1995; **32**: 241–7.

141. Reddy VM, Nadaahur G, Daneluzzi D et al. Antituberculosis activities of clofazimine and its new analogs B4154 and B4157. *Antimicrob Agents Chemother* 1996; **40**: 633–6.

142. Nix DE, Zhu M, Adam RD et al. Pharmacokinetics of clofazimine under fasting conditions, with orange juice, food, and antacids. *Tuberculosis* 2004; **84**: 365–73.

143. O'Brien RJ, Spigelman M. New drugs for tuberculosis: current status and future prospects. *Clin Chest Med* 2005; **26**: 327–430.

144. Spigelman M, Gillespie S. Tuberculosis drug development pipeline: progress and hope. *Lancet* 2006; **367**: 945–7.

145. McNeeley D. Diarylquinoline TMC207. *The Second Annual Open Forum on Key Issues in TB Drug Development*, London, UK, 12–13 December 2006.

146. Andries K, Verhasselt P, Guillemont J et al. A diarylquinoline drug active on the ATP synthase of *Mycobacterium tuberculosis*. *Science* 2005; **307**: 223–27.

147. Stover CK, Warrener P, VanDevanter DR et al. A small-molecule nitroimidazopyran drug candidate for the treatment of tuberculosis. *Nature* 2000; **405**: 962–6.

148. Nuermberger E, Rosenthal I, Tyagi S et al. Combination chemotherapy with the nitroimidazopyran PA-824 and first-line drugs in a murine model of tuberculosis. *Antimicrob Agents Chemother* 2006; **50**: 2621–5.

149. Lorenzi M. Nitroimidazo-oxazine PA-824. *The Second Annual Open Forum on Key Issues in TB Drug Development*, London, UK, 12–13 December 2006.

150. Matsumoto M, Hashizume H, Tomishige T et al. OPC-67683, a nitro-dihydro-imidazooxazole derivative with promising action against tuberculosis in vitro and in mice. *PLoS Med* 2006; **3**: e466, 2131–44.

151. Hittel N. Nitrodihydro-imidazooxazole derivative OPC-67683. *The Second Annual Open Forum on Key Issues in TB Drug Development*, London, UK, 12–13 December 2006.

152. Biava M, Porretta GC, Poce G et al. Antimycobacterial agents. Novel diarylpyrrole derivatives of BM212 endowed with high activity toward *Mycobacterium tuberculosis* and low cytotoxicity. *J Med Chem* 2006; **49**: 4946–52.

153. Jia L, Noker PE, Coward L *et al*. Interspecies pharmacokinetics and *in vitro* metabolism of SQ109. *Br J Pharmacol* 2006; **147**: 476–85.

154. Chen P, Gearhart J, Protopopova M *et al*. Synergistic interactions of SQ109, a new ethylene diamine, with front-line antitubercular drugs *in vitro. J Antimicrob Chemother* 2006; **58**: 332–37.

155. Nacy C. Diamine SQ109. *The Second Annual Open Forum on Key Issues in TB Drug Development*, London, UK, 12–13 December 2006.

13

Chemotherapy including drug-resistant therapy and future developments

WING WAI YEW

INTRODUCTION

Chemotherapy for tuberculosis was possible only after the discovery of streptomycin in 1944. Improvement in clinical state, sputum bacteriology and radiography occurred after 2–3 months of treatment with the drug. These good responses were, however, short lasting. Subsequently, bacillary resistance to streptomycin developed after the monotherapy resulting in disease deterioration again.[1] A few years later, it was found that combined therapy of streptomycin and para-aminosalicylic acid prevented drug resistance from developing and achieved better results.[2] The introduction of isoniazid as a drug in the combination regimen for treating tuberculosis formed the basis of primary chemotherapy in the 1950s to 1960s.[3] The standard regimen then comprised streptomycin, isoniazid and para-aminosalicylic acid for a few months followed by the last two drugs up to a total period of 18 months. Para-aminosalicylic acid could be replaced by ethambutol or thiacetazone depending on their availability and acceptability in the community.

Besides relating to adverse drug reactions, patients often gave up prematurely or took drugs irregularly when they became symptom free after a few weeks to months of therapy. This brought about treatment failure and development of drug resistance. In the early 1960s, the experience in Madras and Hong Kong obtained from collaborative studies between the British Medical Research Council and relevant health-care authorities demonstrated the effectiveness and efficacy of ambulatory treatment.[4] Prolonged hospitalization in sanatoria became unnecessary. Fully supervised chemotherapy (later also known as directly observed therapy or DOT), in the form of streptomycin and isoniazid given on an intermittent basis twice a week in the continuation phase, after the initial few months of the daily triple-drug therapy referred to earlier, was utilized. For patients who failed on this standard regimen, second-line drugs that included pyrazinamide, ethionamide and cycloserine were given for 6 months, followed by 12–18 months of combination therapy with the first two drugs. In 1965, rifampicin was discovered. In the 1970s, short-course chemotherapy was introduced for the treatment of tuberculosis.[5]

BIOLOGICAL CHARACTERISTICS OF *MYCOBACTERIUM TUBERCULOSIS* AND THE SCIENTIFIC BASIS OF SHORT-COURSE CHEMOTHERAPY

Mycobacterium tuberculosis, the causative organism of tuberculosis, is a slow-growing bacterium and it can also enter a phase of dormancy which is drug refractory. A patient with tuberculosis can basically harbour four populations of organisms. The first population is the actively growing extracellular organisms which are usually present in abundance within aerated cavities. The second population

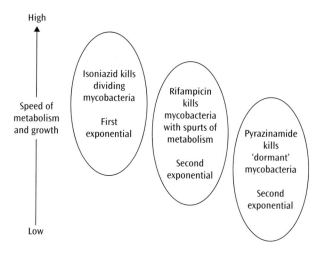

Figure 13.1 Actions of antituberculosis drugs regarding the hypothetical mycobacterial populations. Adapted with permission from Mitchison DA, *Am J Respir Crit Care Med* 2005; 171: 699–706.

consists of slow intermittently growing organisms in an unstable part of the lesion. The third population includes organisms surviving in a low environmental pH which can occur in inflammatory lesions or within phagolysosomes of macrophages. The last population refers to the completely dormant organisms surviving under anaerobic conditions. The three major actions of antituberculosis drugs[6] are (1) bactericidal action, defined as their ability to kill actively growing bacilli rapidly, (2) sterilizing action, defined as their capacity to kill the semi-dormant organisms and (3) prevention of emergence of resistance. Isoniazid is the most potent bactericidal drug. Rifampicin is also important as such. Rifampicin and pyrazinamide are the most important drugs for sterilizing the tuberculous lesions and preventing disease relapse (see Figure 13.1). Resistance to an antituberculosis drug is due to spontaneous chromosomal mutation at a frequency of 10^{-6} to 10^{-8} bacterial replications.[7] As mutations resulting in drug resistance are unlinked, the probability of resistance to all three drugs[8] used simultaneously becomes 10^{-18} to 10^{-20}. Thus, the chance of drug resistance is practically nil when three effective drugs are used in combination for the treatment of tuberculosis. Among the first-line antituberculosis drugs, isoniazid and rifampicin are most effective in preventing the emergence of resistance.[6] Streptomycin, ethambutol and pyrazinamide are less so. Thiacetazone and para-aminosalicylic acid are the least effective for such a purpose.

AIMS OF CHEMOTHERAPY

The aims of drug treatment of tuberculosis are:

- to cure the patients of tuberculosis by the shortest duration of drug administration, preferably with minimum interference with their living;

- to prevent death from tuberculosis or late effects of disease;
- to prevent relapse of disease;
- to prevent emergence of drug resistance;
- to reduce transmission of tuberculosis to people within or outside the community.

TREATMENT OF SMEAR-POSITIVE PULMONARY TUBERCULOSIS

In the past few decades, a number of effective drug regimens have been found, largely through clinical trials, for treating patients with newly diagnosed smear-positive pulmonary tuberculosis. These regimens are summarized in Table 13.1.[9–19] Most regimens are given for 6 months, this currently being the shortest duration of treatment required. Regimens that do not contain pyrazinamide in the initial intensive phase must be given for longer than 6 months. The relapse rates during 6–30 months after stopping treatment are generally <5 per cent. In countries or communities with a high level of initial resistance to isoniazid (≥4 per cent),[16] as in most Asian countries, a four-drug regimen (for 2 months) followed by two drugs used together (for 4 months) is advisable. This is the standard regimen recommended by the World Health Organization and International Union Against Tuberculosis and Lung Disease (WHO/IUATLD) today.[20] Although the relapse rates on 5-year follow up appeared similar for 1SHRZ/5H$_3$R$_3$ and 2SHRZ/4H$_3$R$_3$ (see Table 13.1 for explanation of abbreviations), the inferior sputum culture negativity rate at 2 months for the former regimen[10] led to its being discarded from routine use. Furthermore, the administration of pyrazinamide beyond 2 months has not been shown to be of advantage.[21,22] However, for individual cases with extensive disease and slow sputum bacteriological conversion to negative, prolongation of the administration of pyrazinamide ± streptomycin/ethambutol beyond 2 months may be acceptable. Prolongation of the total duration of treatment can also be considered on a case-by-case basis.[23] Indeed, presence of cavity and positive sputum culture after 2 months of treatment have been found to be associated with an increased risk of failure/relapse,[24,25] and thus may justify prolongation of the 6-month therapy to a total of 9 months.[26] The 8-month regimen 2SHRZ/6HT or 6HE combined with hospitalization in the first 2 months has been proven to be very effective in controlled clinical trials and programme settings in Africa.[15] In confirmed or suspected HIV-infected patients, ethambutol should be used in place of thiacetazone in light of possibly severe cutaneous reaction to the latter drug.[27] There is indication that thiacetazone should be dropped from the antituberculosis regimens in the developing countries, many of which are experiencing rising HIV infection rates.[28] A recent study has also found that the 8-month regimen gave inferior performance when compared to the standard 6-month short-course regimen with

Table 13.1 Drug regimens for the treatment of new cases of smear-positive pulmonary tuberculosis.

Regimen	Ref.
Standard 6-month regimen	
2 EHRZ/4 HR	9
2 SHRZ/4 HR	
Variants of standard 6-month regimen when directly observed, intermittent chemotherapy can be organized	
2 EHRZ/4 H_3R_3	
2 SHRZ/4 H_3R_3	10
2 $E_3H_3R_3Z_3$/4 H_3R_3	
2 $S_3H_3R_3Z_3$/4 H_3R_3	11,12
0.5 SHRZ/1.5 $S_2H_2R_2Z_2$/4 H_2R_2	13
2 SHRZ/4 H_2R_2	14
Alternative less active regimens of longer durations	
1. With a highly active initial four-drug phase	
2 SHRZ/6 HT	15
2 EHRZ/6 HT	
2 SHRZ/6 HE	
2 EHRZ/6 HE	
2 SHRZ/6 $S_2H_2Z_2$	16
2. With a less active or no initial phase	
2 SHR/7 HR	17
2 EHR/7 HR	18
9 HR	19

S, streptomycin; E, ethambutol; H, isoniazid; R, rifampicin; Z, pyrazinamide; T, thiacetazone; X, daily; X_3, three times a week; X_2, twice a week.

rifampicin included throughout.[29] Regimens based almost entirely on isoniazid and rifampicin[17–19] are only good for pansusceptible tuberculosis with perhaps limited bacillary load, and has to be given for 9 months (namely 2HRE/7HR or 9HR). These regimens are usually not applicable to patients in Asian countries, except those who cannot tolerate pyrazinamide. Intermittent regimens comprising two drugs in the continuation phase, following an intensive phase of four drugs given on a daily basis, have been proven to be highly effective (2SHRZ/4H_3R_3 or 2SHRZ/4H_2R_2).[10,23] The WHO, however, does not generally recommend twice-weekly regimens because of the higher risk of treatment failure when missing doses occur.[20] Data from China (including Hong Kong) on 2$S_3H_3R_3Z_3$/4H_3R_3 also have shown the high efficacy of such a regimen in both study and programme settings.[11,12] Intermittent short-course regimens that are administered three times per week have largely equivalent efficacy to daily regimens. In addition, they have lower cost, greater feasibility for ambulatory administration under supervised settings and possibly lower drug toxicity. However, a more recent analysis has cast concerns on the efficacy of the three times weekly 6-month regimen in suppressing disease relapse in the presence of cavitation.[30]

Rifapentine, a long-acting cyclopentyl rifamycin, has been shown to yield rather encouraging activity, when given with isoniazid in a once-weekly dosing schedule, during the continuation treatment phase of pulmonary tuberculosis among HIV-uninfected subjects, though a failure/relapse rate of around 10 per cent still sounds high.[24,25] Such scheduling, while facilitating supervised treatment, does not appear suitable for HIV-infected patients with tuberculosis because of unfavourable treatment outcome and risk of emergence of rifamycin resistance.[31] A prospective, randomized, double-blind study on the tolerability of rifapentine 600, 900 and 1200 mg plus isoniazid in the continuation phase of antituberculosis treatment has suggested that rifapentine 900 mg once-weekly dosing appears to be safe and well tolerated.[32] Thus, further exploration of the optimal dosing and scheduling of rifapentine, perhaps alongside new agents such as moxifloxacin, a potent 8-methoxy-fluoroquinolone, might be warranted.[33,34]

For treatment of smear-positive relapse cases of pulmonary tuberculosis, as well as retreatment after interruption, an 8-month regimen has been recommended by the WHO/IUATLD, namely 2SHRZE/1HRZE/5HRE or 5$H_3R_3E_3$.[20] Bacillary drug susceptibilities *in vitro* can help to guide modification of this regimen as required.

The use of fixed-dose drug combination (FDC) tablets comprising two to three and even four drugs can enhance ease of prescription for physicians, reducing inadvertent medication errors, simplifying drug procurement and supply, and treatment adherence by patients.[35] When used properly, FDC tablets should decrease the risk of development of multidrug-resistant tuberculosis (MDR-TB), i.e. tuberculosis caused by bacillary strains resistant to at least isoniazid and rifampicin *in vitro*.[36] While FDC tablets by self-administered therapy can constitute an alternative to DOT when the latter cannot be practised, the delivery of DOT using FDC tablets should be recommended as there is still a potential risk of emergence of drug resistance when these FDC tablets are taken irregularly.[37] The main concern in using FDC tablets is the quality and bioavailability of its component drugs, especially rifampicin.[38] In 1994, the IUATLD and WHO issued a joint statement advising that only FDC of proven good quality should be used in the treatment of tuberculosis.[39] The majority of studies found no significant difference between FDC tablets and single drugs regarding sputum smear conversion rates and frequency of side effects and relapses.[40] Some studies, however, produced controversial results. The Singapore study, in particular, found higher relapse rates at 2 and 5 years of follow up in patients who received FDC.[41] Furthermore, the WHO has recently made a recommendation for some FDC tablets to be included in the list of essential drugs.[42]

DOTS

Drug-resistant tuberculosis usually results from poor patient adherence and other aspects in failure of implementation of an effectively functioning tuberculosis

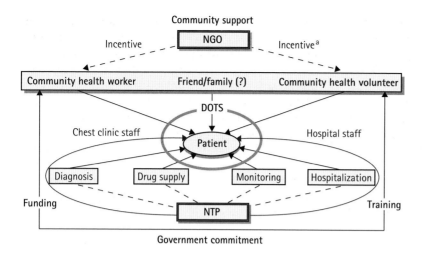

Figure 13.2 Complementary roles of the government and the community in delivery of DOTS. [a]Can be non-monetary. NGO, non-governmental organization; NTP, National Tuberculosis Programme.

control programme.[43] Although some patient characteristics, such as homelessness, alcohol or substance abuse, behavioural problems, mental retardation and lack of social or family support are more commonly associated with non-adherence to therapy, it is generally difficult to identify poorly adherent patients because the underlying reasons for such behaviour are not only multifaceted and complex, but range from characteristics of the individual patients to qualities of the societal and economic environment.[44] DOT was in fact shown to be highly efficacious in ensuring patient adherence by experience gained in Madras and Hong Kong many decades ago. In order to facilitate the delivery of DOT, other concomitant strategic interventions must be incorporated. Short-course chemotherapy has been shown to be the most important component. In 1993, the WHO officially announced the new global strategy for tuberculosis control known as DOTS.[45] The DOTS strategy is clearly more than DOT (directly observed therapy) alone. The five key components include:[46] (1) a network of trained health-care or community workers to administer DOT, (2) properly equipped laboratories with personnel trained to perform sputum microscopy diagnosis for tuberculosis, (3) a reliable supply of high-quality drugs (preferably at no cost to patients), (4) an accurate record keeping and cohort analysis system for monitoring case findings, treatment and outcomes, and (5) sustained political commitment and funding. Figure 13.2 depicts the complementary roles of the National Tuberculosis Programme and community participation in the organization of DOTS. This would be of great relevance in countries with limited resources. To reiterate, the DOTS strategy should be viewed as a comprehensive service or an integral part thereof, which possesses ingredients also inclusive of enablers, incentives, education and holistic care that are conducive to the success of the treatment programme. Regarding holistic care, resolution of social disadvantage particularly poverty is of paramount importance. Figure 13.3 shows the devastating

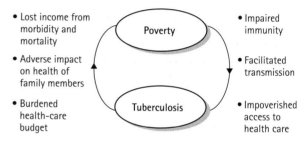

Figure 13.3 The important link between poverty and tuberculosis.

link between poverty and tuberculosis. Poverty predisposes to the development of this disease and tuberculosis perpetuates poverty. In addition, a higher prevalence of multidrug resistance was found to be associated with a lower gross national product (GNP) per capita income,[47] thus further negatively impacting the control of disease in many poor communities and countries. In summary, with the use of DOTS, the treatment success of tuberculosis can be maximized and the chance of development of drug resistance markedly curtailed.[43,46] Indeed, this strategy should be regarded as the most cost-effective intervention in the control of tuberculosis.

TREATMENT OF SMEAR–NEGATIVE PULMONARY TUBERCULOSIS

In many countries, nearly 50 per cent of patients are diagnosed as having active pulmonary tuberculosis on clinical and radiographic grounds, without immediate bacteriological confirmation. In the first smear-negative study in Hong Kong,[48] it was subsequently found that 36 per cent of these patients had one or more initial sputum cultures positive for *M. tuberculosis*. When patients were observed until the appearance of radiographic and/or bacteriological evidence for active disease, 57 per cent of this control (selective chemotherapy) group of patients required treatment within 60 months. When smear-negative, culture-positive patients (even with drug-susceptible disease) were treated with 2–3 months of daily streptomycin, isoniazid, rifampicin and pyrazinamide, relapses occurred in 32 and 13 per cent, respectively, over 60 months of follow up. The corresponding relapse rates for culture-negative patients for the two durations of therapy were 11 and 7 per cent, respectively. In the second smear-negative study in Hong Kong,[49] which again included 35 per cent of subjects with sputum cultures initially positive for *M. tuberculosis*, all patients were treated with streptomycin, isoniazid, rifampicin and pyrazinamide, daily or three times per week, for 3–4 months for those initially culture negative, and 4–6 months for those who were culture positive. Over 60 months, the combined relapse rates for culture-negative

patients who had 3 and 4 months of treatment were 7 and 4 per cent, respectively. The relapse rate for the 4-month regimen was 2 per cent in patients with initially drug-susceptible organisms and 8 per cent in patients with initial organisms resistant to isoniazid, streptomycin or both. There was no significant difference between the relapse rates among patients allocated 4- and 6-month regimens of the same four drugs.

However, the WHO recommends the use of 6-month regimens – daily isoniazid, rifampicin and pyrazinamide for 2 months followed by daily or three times per week isoniazid and rifampicin for another 4 months in the treatment of new smear-negative pulmonary tuberculosis.[20] For patients living in countries with high levels of initial resistance to isoniazid and/or having extensive radiographic disease, or who are HIV-infected, adding ethambutol to the regimen in the initial 2 months should be considered.

Case history

Multidrug-resistant TB

A 76-year-old male chronic smoker presented at the chest clinic in December 1994 for treatment of smear-positive pulmonary tuberculosis. He gave a history of previous treatment of tuberculosis by private practitioners about 20 years ago for uncertain duration with drugs on a self-administered basis. Due to his poor ambulatory status, he was again given drugs by the clinic staff to take at home with adequate counselling of the importance of good adherence. The treatment regimen used then included daily isoniazid, rifampicin and pyrazinamide. In February 1995, ethambutol was added with the knowledge of pretreatment bacillary resistance to isoniazid *in vitro*. Subsequently, ethambutol was further replaced by ofloxacin because of subjective deterioration of visual acuity of the patient. However, sputum stayed positive for acid-fast bacilli on direct microscopy after a total of 6 months of treatment from December 1994. Sputum culture in March

1995 subsequently grew *M. tuberculosis* resistant to isoniazid and rifampicin *in vitro*. Chest x-ray then showed bilateral upper lobe cavitary disease amidst fibrocalcific lesions (Figure 13.4). He was therefore treated from June 1995 onwards with streptomycin, ethambutol alongside second-line drugs that included ofloxacin, ethionamide and cycloserine for 6 months, followed by the four oral drugs for another 6 months. Sputum culture conversion to negativity was achieved after 4 months of such second-line drug treatment. Chemotherapy was finally stopped in the middle of 1996 after 1 year of directly observed treatment in hospital (for poor physical and socioeconomic conditions). Afterwards, he died of carcinoma of lung in 2000 with no evidence of relapse of tuberculosis radiographically and bacteriologically.

Comment

This case illustrates vividly that poor adherence during antituberculosis therapy can result in the progressive development of acquired drug resistance eventually leading to MDR-TB. For a retreatment case, the use of just rifampicin, isoniazid and pyrazinamide in combination should not be advocated. Directly observed therapy with second-line drugs is mandatory in achieving success in the management of MDR-TB.

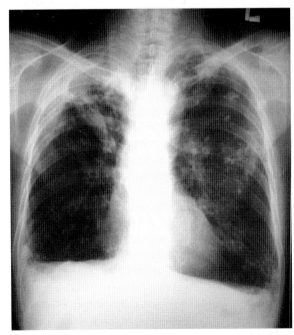

Figure 13.4   Chest x-ray of the patient with multidrug-resistant tuberculosis before administration of second-line drugs.

TREATMENT OF MONORESISTANT PULMONARY TB

For patients who are subsequently known to harbour organisms resistant to streptomycin, there would obviously be no unfavourable sequelae using the conventional short-course regimens just described for treatment of new cases. For patients with isoniazid-resistant tuberculosis, one of the following approaches can be adopted:

- continuation of rifampicin, ethambutol and pyrazinamide for another 10 months or rifampicin plus ethambutol for 12 months after having administered rifampicin, isoniazid, ethambutol and pyrazinamide for 2 months before drug susceptibility testing results are known,[50,51] or
- no modification of the initially administered four-drug regimen is made and all drugs are given for a total of 6 months.[52]

Reducing the regimen components from four to two drugs after 2 months, as in the management of drug-susceptible tuberculosis, is also acceptable for the purposes of the programme, except that the relapse rate is somewhat higher, i.e. 10 versus 3 per cent.[22] When patients are already known to have isoniazid-resistant disease at the commencement of therapy, a 9-month regimen comprising streptomycin, rifampicin, pyrazinamide and ethambutol for 2 months, followed by rifampicin and ethambutol for 7 months, has also been shown to be effective.[53] On the other hand, for patients with isolated rifampicin-resistant tuberculosis, which is rare in clinical practice, especially among HIV-uninfected subjects, the recommendation has been made to treat patients with isoniazid, pyrazinamide and ethambutol for 18–24 months.[54] Some authorities feel that the duration of treatment can be shortened to 9–12 months by the addition of a fluoroquinolone to this three-drug regimen.[26]

DRUG TREATMENT OF MULTIDRUG-RESISTANT PULMONARY TB

The WHO/IUATLD global project on antituberculosis drug resistance surveillance[55] has found that drug resistance was indeed a widespread phenomenon. Data obtained from a number of countries worldwide between 1999 and 2002 have revealed the following statistics.[55] For patients with newly diagnosed tuberculosis, the frequency of resistance to at least one drug ranged from 0 to 57.1 per cent (median, 10.2 per cent). The median prevalence of MDR-TB among new cases was 1.1 per cent (range, 0 to 14.2 per cent). For patients with previous treatment, the frequency of resistance to at least one drug ranged from 0 to 82.1 per cent (median, 18.4 per cent). The prevalence of MDR-TB among previously treated cases ranged from 0 to 58.3 per cent (median, 7.0 per cent).

Although DOTS is highly effective in the management of drug-susceptible tuberculosis, it is not sufficient for controlling established MDR-TB.[56] Short-course chemotherapy including standardized retreatment regimens is unlikely to cure most patients with MDR-TB and can cause an 'amplifier effect' by creating additional drug resistance when empiric treatment courses have been repeatedly administered. The treatment success rates of patients with MDR-TB are much lower when compared with those from patients with drug-susceptible disease, namely 56 to 80 per cent versus ≥90 per cent.[57–61] Also, the standard retreatment short-course chemotherapy regimen (US\$ 30–35 (£15–17)) is about 50 per cent more costly than a first-line conventional short-course regimen (US\$ 20 (£9)), and the cheapest reserve regimen comprising second-line and new antimycobacterial drugs is at least 100 times more costly (US\$ 2000 (£980)).

On the basis of the available data, the WHO has recommended a three-part response to the global threat of MDR-TB,[62] namely the widespread implementation of DOTS as the cornerstone of good tuberculosis control, improved drug susceptibility testing and surveillance, and the careful introduction of second-line drugs after a sound evaluation of cost, effectiveness and feasibility. This new initiative known as DOTS-Plus[56] is currently coordinated by the WHO in partnership with many agencies and institutions worldwide. Thus, for established MDR-TB, effective treatment should be alternative-specific and perhaps ideally individualized regimens. It appears that the most important determinant in the guidance of formulating a drug regimen for MDR-TB is the patient's current drug susceptibility pattern in vitro.[58,61,63] It has been shown that patients given appropriate drugs based on susceptibility testing in vitro had better outcomes.[60,64] One practical obstacle to the usefulness of conventional drug susceptibility testing to guide treatment regimen modification/design is the prolonged turnaround time. Rapid drug susceptibility testing broth systems based on non-radiometric or radiometric techniques have enabled improvement in this aspect,[63,65] but these are more costly than the conventional ones. Newer phenotypic or genotypic technology advances would help in further accelerating the delineation of drug resistance.[65] Furthermore, the methodology of assessing drug susceptibilities for many second-line drugs is not yet totally standardized and therefore there can be an observed discrepancy in microbiological response of the patient and results of the drug susceptibility tests in vitro.[60] More work needs to be done in the relevant area.[66] The fluoroquinolones are, however, new antimycobacterial drugs that have consistent activities in vitro, often independent of culture medium, inoculum size and method of assessment.[61]

A patient with MDR-TB should receive a regimen comprising at least five of these second-line drugs for the initial months, followed by three to four drugs subsequently. One regimen recommended by the WHO consists of treatment with ethambutol, ethionamide/prothionamide, ofloxacin/ciprofloxacin, pyrazinamide and aminoglycoside – for 6 months, with the first three or four drugs being administered for at least a further 18 months.[67] In fact, in a recent large-scale trial in Peru, 55 per cent of compliant patients given a similar regimen, namely kanamycin, ciprofloxacin, pyrazinamide, ethambutol and ethionamide, after failure of the standard retreatment short-course regimen that comprised streptomycin, rifampicin, isoniazid, ethambutol and pyrazinamide could be cured.[68] Indeed, ofloxacin-containing multidrug regimens gave rather impressive cure rates of about 80 per cent in MDR-TB cohorts in several reports.[57,59–61] Preliminary data from three reports have also suggested that levofloxacin possibly has somewhat better efficacy than ofloxacin in the treatment of MDR-TB.[61,69,70] Among the agents used in the multidrug regimens, the fluoroquinolones are most likely the pivotal drugs with a major contribution to the efficacy of the regimens. In a retrospective analysis of patients with MDR-TB treated with ofloxacin/levofloxacin together with similar accompanying drugs that principally included aminoglycosides, ethionamide/prothionamide, cycloserine, pyrazinamide and ethambutol, resistance to ofloxacin *in vitro* was found to be a significant variable independently associated with adverse treatment outcomes.[61] Apart from the fluoroquinolone's efficacy *in vivo* resulting from good bactericidal and sterilizing activities,[71] though the latter is still apparently inferior to that of pyrazinamide especially in tuberculosis patients co-infected with HIV,[72] ofloxacin/ levofloxacin also has the following favourable therapeutic characteristics: high peak serum drug concentration: MIC ratio, good tissue penetration particularly into the lungs and good tolerance by patients during long-term administration even at high dosages.[61,69,73,74] The good tolerance is therapeutically beneficial and sets some fluoroquinolones aside from most second-line antituberculosis agents. However, interactive toxicities of ofloxacin with cycloserine can be of genuine concern.[75]

The good patient tolerance of fluoroquinolones is not a class effect. Sparfloxacin, for example, has better antituberculosis activity than ofloxacin/levofloxacin.[76,77] However, the significant phototoxicity and potential cardiotoxicity have jeopardized its further role in the clinical management of MDR-TB.[78–80] By the same token, new fluoroquinolones with good antimycobacterial activities like moxifloxacin,[81] DU-6859a[82] and gatifloxacin[83] might share a similar fate unless their safety profiles on long-term use can be established in the future. Experience regarding moxifloxacin has accumulated rather favourably.[84,85] The optimum duration of therapy for patients with MDR-TB is currently unclear. While a number of authorities, including the WHO, have recommended a total duration of at least 18 months after smear conversion, even for HIV-negative patients,[67] there is some preliminary evidence that at least a proportion of immunocompetent patients who managed to achieve sustained sputum culture conversion early in the treatment course could be adequately treated with 12 months of fluoroquinolone-containing regimens.[61] It does appear, however, that patients who are immunocompromised (including those with diabetes mellitus and silicosis), or have extensive radiographic evidence of disease (particularly with cavities), extensive drug resistance *in vitro*, delayed sputum culture conversion (i.e. after more than 3 months of chemotherapy) or extrapulmonary involvement should receive longer than 12 months of therapy. In formulating the optimum duration of therapy for MDR-TB, the key factors to be considered include the number of active agents, as well as their bactericidal capacity, dosage, cost and toxicity, alongside the anticipated patient adherence.[61,86]

Finally, fluoroquinolones must be used with great vigilance in the management of MDR-TB to prevent emergence of cross-resistance among members of this important class of drugs.[57,77] This has been reported in some communities,[87,88] and might have a negative impact on the potential usefulness of emerging members of this drug class with greater antimycobacterial activities. Furthermore, the widespread use of fluoroquinolones in the treatment of various types of community-acquired infections can pose a threat in escalating resistance of *M. tuberculosis* against fluoroquinolones.[89,90]

In September 2006, the WHO expressed concern regarding the emergence of virulent drug-resistant tuberculosis referred to as 'extensively drug-resistant' or 'extremely drug-resistant' tuberculosis (XDR-TB). This term was first used earlier in 2006, following a joint survey (2000–2004) by the WHO and US Centers for Disease Control and Prevention. Initially, it was defined as the bacillary resistance to ≥3 classes of second-line drugs, in addition to dual resistance to rifampicin and isoniazid (with or without concomitant resistance to other first-line agents). Subsequently, it has been revised by the WHO Global Task Force on XDR-TB to stand for bacillary resistance to any fluoroquinolone, and at least one of three injectable drugs (capreomycin, kanamycin and amikacin), on top of the standard definition of MDR-TB. At the moment, while XDR-TB has been identified in all regions of the world, its frequency was found to be highest in countries which belonged to the former Soviet Union and Asia. Given the underlying HIV epidemic, XDR-TB might also have a significant impact on mortality in Africa. Thus, urgent attention globally should be focused on this form of 'emerging' tuberculosis with potentially devastating consequences.

SURGICAL TREATMENT OF MULTIDRUG-RESISTANT PULMONARY TB

There are three basic selection criteria for adjunctive surgical treatment of patients with MDR-TB.[91] First, profound drug resistance *in vitro* is present, leading to a high probability of failure or relapse with medical therapy alone. Second, the disease is sufficiently localized so that its great preponderance could be resected with expectation of adequate post-operative cardiopulmonary capacity. Third, there is sufficient drug activity to suppress the mycobacterial burden to facilitate healing of the bronchial stump. Patients must receive chemotherapy prior to surgery for a minimum duration of 3 months. If possible, patients

Table 13.2 Worldwide experience on surgical treatment of multidrug-resistant tuberculosis.

Investigator	Patient No.	Success rate	Operative mortality rate	Postoperative complication rate
Treasure et al.[93]	19	89%	0%	9%
van Leuven et al.[94]	62	75%	2%	23%
Sung et al.[95]	27	96%	0%	26%
Pomerantz et al.[96]	172	98%	3%	12%
Chiang et al.[97]	27	92%	4%	11%
Park et al.[98]	49	94%	0%	16%
Takeda et al.[99]	26	89%	3%	14%
Shiraishi et al.[100]	87	93%	0%	8%
Kir et al.[101]	79	95%	3%	5%

Reproduced from Yew WW, Chiu SW. In: Schlossberg D (ed.). *Tuberculosis and non-tuberculous mycobacterial infections*, 5th edn. New York: McGraw-Hill Co, 2006, with the permission of the McGraw-Hill Companies.

should achieve sputum culture conversion to negativity before surgery.[91,92] Unfortunately, this may not always occur. In some reports, sputum culture conversion only occurred after surgery together with prolonged duration of medical therapy afterwards. Ventilation/perfusion scan, pulmonary function test and computed tomography of the chest are important investigations for preoperative assessment.[92] In patients with suspected pulmonary arterial hypertension, it may be necessary to perform right heart catheterization. Bronchoscopy may be required for patients with suspected bronchostenosis. The nutritional status of the patient should be optimized to improve outcome. In experienced hands, the operative outcome is often rewarding (see Table 13.2). The cure rate was very often noted to reach ≥90 per cent when combined medical and surgical modalities were applied in treating selected MDR-TB patients.[93–101] In a recently published large-scale series that involved 205 patients with MDR-TB, surgical resection and fluoroquinolone therapy were associated with improved microbiological and clinical outcomes after adjusting for other variables.[102] The improvement was statistically significant for surgery, and among older patients for fluoroquinolone therapy. Furthermore, a recently published analysis on the prognostic factors for surgical resection in patients with MDR-TB has revealed low patient body mass index (<18.5 kg/m^2) and bacillary resistance to ofloxacin as adverse ones, in addition to the presence of cavitation beyond the range of surgical resection.[103] Complications of surgery include respiratory failure, bronchopleural fistulae, infections and other problems of the wound, bleeding, pneumonia and recurrent laryngeal nerve injury (see also Chapter 16, The surgical management of tuberculosis and its complications).

IMMUNOTHERAPY OF MULTIDRUG-RESISTANT PULMONARY TB

In humans, cell-mediated immunological protective response is based on macrophage activation and granu-loma formation that require the cytokines, especially interferon-gamma (IFN-γ) and tumour necrosis factor. IFN-γ was shown to have efficacy in lowering bacillary load in patients with MDR-TB and non-tuberculous mycobacteriosis in anecdotal reports.[104,105] Adjunctive immunotherapy with low-dose recombinant human interleukin-2 was also found to stimulate immune activation and may enhance the antimicrobial response in MDR-TB.[106] Aerosolized IFN-α treatment was shown in a study to reduce the sputum culture colony counts of patients with MDR-TB.[107] Preliminary data concerning the use of heat-killed *Mycobacterium vaccae* (NCTC 11659) in patients with MDR-TB in several centres in different continents have suggested possible efficacy.[108,109] A randomized clinical trial of this form of immunotherapy in MDR-TB patients appears warranted. It is clear that the current data on the role of immunotherapy in MDR-TB are limited and further evaluation of this modality of therapy is required.

SUMMARY OF MANAGEMENT PLAN OF MULTIDRUG-RESISTANT PULMONARY TB

A proposed plan is depicted in Figure 13.5. The crucial elements for its prevention are shown at the highest level.

DOSAGES AND ADVERSE REACTIONS OF ANTITUBERCULOSIS DRUGS

The usual dosages of the drugs used in conventional short-course chemotherapy and therapy of MDR-TB are shown in Table 13.3. The important adverse reactions to these antituberculosis drugs are listed in Table 13.4. Although 25–60 per cent of a large number of patients in studies undertaken in Hong Kong reported at least one type of reaction,[21,22,49] most of these were mild and required no modification of treatment regimens. The most common

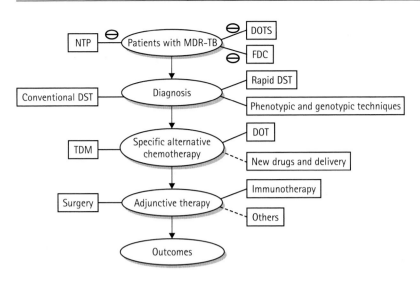

Figure 13.5 Strategies in the management of multidrug-resistant tuberculosis. DOT, directly observed therapy; DST, drug susceptibility testing; FDC, fixed-dose combination drugs; NTP, national tuberculosis programme; TDM, therapeutic drug monitoring.

Table 13.3   Usual dosages of antituberculosis drugs.

Drug	Daily dosage			Intermittent dosage		
	Adults and children (mg/kg)	Adults		Adults and children (mg/kg)	Adults	
		Weight (kg)	Dosage		Weight (kg)	Dosage
Drugs commonly used in conventional therapy[a]						
Isoniazid	5	–	300 mg	10 three times/week	–	–
				15 twice/week	–	–
Rifampicin	10	<50	450 mg	10–12 three times/week	–	600 mg
		≥50	600 mg	10–12 twice/week	–	600 mg
Streptomycin	12–15	<50	500 mg	12–15 three times or twice/week	<50	500 mg
		≥50	750 mg		≥50	750 mg
Pyrazinamide	20–30	<50	1.0–1.5 g	30–40 three times/week	<50	2.0 g
		≥50	1.5–2.0 g		≥50	2.5 g
				40–60 twice/week	<50	2.5–3.0 g
					≥50	3.0–3.5 g
Ethambutol	15	–		30 three times/week	–	–
				45 twice/week		
Thiacetazone	2.5	–	150 mg	–	–	–
Rifater		per 10 kg	1 tablet			
(R120H50Z300)		>50 kg	5 tablets			
Drugs commonly used in therapy for MDR-TB[b]						
Amikacin	15		750 mg	three to five times/week		
Kanamycin	15		750 mg	three to five times/week		
Capreomycin	15		750 mg	three to five times/week		
Ofloxacin			600–800 mg			
Levofloxacin			500–600 mg			
Ciprofloxacin			750–1500 mg			
Ethionamide	15 (adults)	<50	500 mg			
Prothionamide	15 (adults)	≥50	750 mg			
Cycloserine	15 (adults)	<50	500 mg			
		≥50	750 mg			
Para-aminosalicylic acid	2 g/10 kg	<50	8–10 g			
		≥50	10–12 g			

[a]Some authorities recommend higher dosages of isoniazid, rifampicin, and streptomycin, for children.
[b]Drugs for treatment of multidrug-resistant tuberculosis (MDR-TB) may require split dosing to meet tolerance; other reserve drugs of uncertain efficacy include rifabutin, amoxicillin-clavulanate and clofazimine.

Table 13.4   Adverse reactions to antituberculosis drugs.

Drug	Reactions		
	Common	**Uncommon**	**Rare**
Drugs commonly used in conventional therapy			
Isoniazid		Hepatitis Cutaneous hypersensitivity Peripheral neuropathy	Giddiness Convulsion Optic neuritis Mental symptoms Haemolytic anaemia Aplastic anaemia Lupoid reactions Arthralgia Gynaecomastia
Rifampicin		Hepatitis Cutaneous hypersensitivity Gastrointestinal reactions Thrombocytopenic purpura Febrile reaction 'Flu syndrome'	Shortness of breath Shock Haemolytic anaemia Acute renal failure
Pyrazinamide	Anorexia Nausea Flushing Photosensitization	Hepatitis Vomiting Arthralgia Cutaneous reactions	Sideroblastic anaemia Gout
Ethambutol		Retrobulbar neuritis Arthralgia	Hepatitis Cutaneous reactions Peripheral neuropathy
Streptomycin	Cutaneous hypersensitivity Giddiness Numbness Tinnitus	Vertigo Ataxia Deafness	Renal damage Aplastic anaemia
Thiacetazone	Gastrointestinal reactions Cutaneous hypersensitivity Vertigo Conjunctivitis	Hepatitis Erythema multiforme Exfoliative dermatitis Haemolytic anaemia	Agranulocytosis
Drugs commonly used in therapy for MDR-TB			
Amikacin Kanamycin Capreomycin	Ototoxicity: hearing damage, vestibular disturbance Nephrotoxicity: deranged renal function tests	Clinical renal failure	
Ofloxacin Ciprofloxacin	Gastrointestinal reactions Insomnia	Anxiety Dizziness Headache Tremor	Convulsion Haemolysis
Ethionamide Prothionamide	Gastrointestinal reactions	Hepatitis Peripheral neuropathy	Convulsion Mental symptoms Impotence Gynaecomastia
Cycloserine	Dizziness Headache Depression Memory loss	Psychosis Convulsion	Sideroblastic anaemia
Para-aminosalicylic acid	Gastrointestinal reactions	Hepatitis Drug fever	Hypothyroidism Haematological reactions

MDR-TB, multidrug-resistant tuberculosis.

reactions were gastrointestinal and cutaneous in nature.[21,22] Adverse reactions mostly tended to occur in the first 3 months of treatment. Only ≤10 per cent of patients had treatment interrupted for 1 week or longer and ≤8 per cent of patients had one or more drugs (more frequently streptomycin and pyrazinamide) terminated. Peripheral neuropathy caused by isoniazid can be prevented by an adequate intake of pyridoxine (vitamin B$_6$). Patients groups with dietary deficiency and/or predisposition to neuropathy are particularly at risk. Arthralgia can occur during pyrazinamide administration. It is less likely to occur during intermittent than during daily administration and is usually mild and self-limited. It responds well to symptomatic treatment. If a serious reaction, such as haematological, circulatory or renal in type, occurs after administration of rifampicin, the drug should be withdrawn and never given again.

Rifampicin is a powerful enzyme inducer acting on the cytochrome P450 family, and may therefore cause reduction in serum concentration of other drugs that the patient may be taking. This is of particular importance for women using oral contraceptives. They should be warned that rifampicin may reduce the efficacy of the pill so that alternative methods of contraception should be used. Rifampicin also reduces the serum concentration of corticosteroid so that the dose should be approximately doubled during rifampicin administration. Other important agents interacting significantly with rifampicin include anticoagulants, anticonvulsants, anti-infectives, cardiovasculo-therapeutics, immunosuppressants, psychotropics, sulphonylureas and theophylline.[110]

When a significant cutaneous reaction resulting from drug hypersensitivity (allergy) occurs, all chemotherapy must be stopped until the reaction has subsided. Reintroduction of drugs should follow the suggested protocol (Table 13.5). The rationale of drug challenge is to identify the drug responsible for the reaction. The purpose of starting with a small challenge dose is that if reaction indeed occurs, it will not be as severe as a full dose. The dose is gradually increased over 3 days. There is no evidence that this challenge process invites the development of drug resistance. If the initial cutaneous reaction was rather severe, smaller initial challenge doses (approximately one-tenth of the doses shown for day 1) should be given. If a reaction occurs with the first challenge dose, it is known that the patient is hypersensitive to that drug. When starting to desensitize, it is usually safe to begin with one-tenth of the normal dose. Then the dose is increased by one-tenth each day. If the patient has a mild reaction to a dose, the same dose (instead of a higher dose) is given next day. If there is no reaction, the dose should be increased again by one-tenth each day. If the reaction is severe (which is unusual), a lower dose is used and then increased more gradually. If a reaction occurs with the second challenge dose as shown in Table 13.5, desensitization can be started with the first challenge dose and then the dose is increased by the amount equal to the first

Table 13.5 A suggested protocol for reintroducing antituberculosis drugs after subsidence of the cutaneous reaction.

Sequence of reintroduction	Challenge doses		
	Day 1	Day 2	Day 3
Isoniazid	50 mg	300 mg	300 mg
Rifampicin	75 mg	300 mg	Full dose
Pyrazinamide	250 mg	1 g	Full dose
Ethambutol	100 mg	500 mg	Full dose
Streptomycin	125 mg	500 mg	Full dose

challenge dose each day. Some patients may need antihistamines or steroids to control the severe reaction. For very severe drug reactions requiring high-dose corticosteroid therapy, desensitization should not be attempted. Desensitization is a tedious process and should be undergone in specialized centres. It is important to remember that the desensitization process can be associated with the risk of development of drug resistance. If other effective drugs are available, it is easier to substitute another drug for the one that has caused the reaction, except when the tuberculosis is severe and the incriminated drug(s) is the most potent/crucial one(s). Desensitization can be dangerous for HIV-infected patients and is therefore not recommended.[20]

On the whole, second-line drug regimens are more toxic and difficult to tolerate. In a study on patients with MDR-TB in Hong Kong,[61] about 40 per cent of them experienced adverse reactions of varying severity. However, only half of these patients required modification of their drug regimens.[61] Yet in a recently reported series of MDR-TB patients in Turkey, about 70 per cent of cases experienced side effects to these drugs and 55.5 per cent required treatment modification.[86] Fortunately, with timely and appropriate management, the success rate of treatment (77.6 per cent) was not markedly compromised.

TREATMENT OF PULMONARY TB IN SPECIAL SETTINGS

Pregnancy and lactation

Rifampicin, isoniazid, ethambutol and pyrazinamide are still commonly used in many parts of the world for treating tuberculosis during pregnancy, although the manufacturers of rifampicin advise caution. Pyridoxine administration is often recommended for pregnant women receiving isoniazid. Streptomycin should be avoided because of ototoxicity to the fetus.[20,23,40,51] The safety profiles of the second-line drugs and fluoroquinolones have not been ascertained. Thus, these drugs should also be generally avoided during pregnancy. The taking of antituberculosis drugs is not an absolute contraindication to breastfeeding.[20,23,40,51] Only small subtherapeutic amounts of drugs are secreted into the milk. If there is concern, the mother may take her medications directly after breastfeeding and then use a bottle for the next feed.[111] The interested reader can also refer to the guidelines published by WHO for greater detail.[112]

Elderly people

The treatment of tuberculosis in geriatric patients does not basically differ from that in the younger population. However, due regard should be paid to the physiological, psychological and social changes, as well as the increased prevalence of co-morbidity that may be associated with ageing. As the risk of hepatotoxicity is higher,[113] especially in those who are malnourished, some individualized dosage reduction of the drugs used in short-course regimens may appear warranted. Pyridoxine supplement should also be considered for those with poor nutritional intake or at increased risk of neuropathy. When the drug susceptibility pattern of the bacilli recovered from culture is known to be favourable, use of rifampicin and isoniazid together may prove sufficient for disease with limited bacillary load.[114] A total treatment duration of 9 months is required when only these two drugs are co-administered. Use of ethambutol can be problematic in some elderly patients with poor baseline visual function and/or difficulty in assessing visual acuity.

Liver impairment

Transient changes in bilirubin and alanine transaminase levels are relatively common during antituberculosis chemotherapy and may not signify true hepatotoxicity. However, drug-induced hepatotoxicity during administration of standard short-course antituberculosis treatment has been well documented, and deaths due to fulminant liver necrosis (though rare) have been reported.[115] Data also suggest that liver transplantation might be a viable option for treating such patients with severe liver failure and dismal prognosis.[116]

Patients with underlying liver diseases, particularly related to alcohol,[113,117] hepatitis B,[117,118] hepatitis C[117,119] and HIV,[119] appear to be more prone to develop drug-induced liver dysfunction or toxicity. The relative risk, compared with the general population, for patients with these chronic viral hepatitides in developing such liver toxicity is about three. Other possible predisposing factors include old age and malnourishment. Chronic hepatitis B is endemic in many South East Asian countries. In Hong Kong, for example, the rate reaches 10 per cent of the overall population.[120] Hepatitis C infection is also gaining importance in some Asian countries, such as Japan and Thailand.[121,122] Furthermore, HIV infection is surging in Asia.[123]

Although it is somewhat controversial whether routine monitoring of liver function tests is required in patients receiving antituberculosis drugs, those at risk should be managed with distinct vigilance both clinically and biochemically. When the tuberculous disease is mild or has improved markedly when drug-induced hepatitis develops, one can wait until the liver chemistry has normalized before retrial of the conventional antituberculosis drugs by gradual reinstitution. Although it is apparent that coadministration of rifampicin and isoniazid confers additive and even synergistic potential of liver toxicity,[124] whenever possible, isoniazid and rifampicin should be included in the final regimen so that treatment duration is not unduly prolonged. The use of streptomycin, ethambutol and isoniazid followed by isoniazid and ethambutol may be an alternative regimen. It is important to note that toxicity due to isoniazid alone can occur. The contribution of pyrazinamide to development of liver toxicity appeared controversial in earlier reports.[125,126] However, later studies or analyses, especially recent ones, have been more in favour of the drug's potential hepatotoxicity, among the various components of a short-course antituberculosis drug regimen.[127–132]

In the face of extensive disease when delay in therapy might be detrimental to the patient's health, ofloxacin can be used together with streptomycin and ethambutol as an interim regimen for treatment.[133] This has been found to be safe and efficacious for the majority of such patients. One randomized clinical trial has also shown that an ofloxacin-based regimen appeared safe in patients with chronic liver disease. The hepatotoxic potential of a combination of isoniazid and rifampicin was found to be greater than that of isoniazid, ofloxacin and pyrazinamide.[134] Incorporation of ofloxacin as a component of a definitive regimen should only be considered when the patient is unable to tolerate the co-administration of rifampicin and isoniazid. The optimum dosage of ofloxacin is unknown at present. The fluoroquinolone dosage should probably be tailored to age, body weight, renal function, extent of disease and the number of accompanying drugs. The optimum duration of use of ofloxacin together with ethambutol, plus either rifampicin or isoniazid, as a definitive chemotherapeutic regimen is also currently unknown.

Renal impairment

The development of antituberculosis therapy-related renal impairment necessitates the withdrawal of the drug(s). Examples include streptomycin and rifampicin. In general, isoniazid, rifampicin and pyrazinamide can be used in normal doses in the face of renal impairment, the last three times weekly.[20,40,51] In severe renal impairment, the dosage of isoniazid should be reduced to 200 mg once daily and pyridoxine supplementation is needed to prevent the development of peripheral neuropathy. Streptomycin and aminoglycosides should be avoided,[20,40,51] or must have dosages adjusted in the presence of renal impairment. Ethambutol is also predominantly removed by the kidney. Dosage reduction is also mandatory.[20,40,51] In patients with creatinine clearances of 50–100 mL per minute, ethambutol at 25 mg/kg three times per week can be given; for patients with creatinine clearances of 30–50 mL per minute, the same dose should be given twice a week. With lower creatinine clearance (10–30 mL per minute), a dose of 15 mg/kg at 48-hour intervals has been suggested. Therapeutic drug monitoring of streptomycin and ethambutol concentrations in serum may help to optimize therapy and minimize toxicity. Ofloxacin and ciprofloxacin are also dependent on renal clearance, and dosage reduction in the presence of renal impairment must be made accordingly.

Isoniazid has previously been shown to be significantly removed by haemodialysis,[135] but a recent study showed that the median isoniazid recovery in the dialysate was only 9.2 per cent, suggesting that hepatic metabolism remains the primary mechanism of clearing isoniazid.[136] Rifampicin is not significantly removed by haemodialysis.[135–137] Both of the above drugs may be given in their usual daily dosage.[136,138] The primary metabolite of pyrazinamide, pyrazinoic acid, has been shown to accumulate in patients with renal failure. Haemodialysis removal of pyrazinamide is significant.[136] It is still not clear whether dose reduction or spacing is more advisable for patients on haemodialysis and receiving pyrazinamide.[136,137] A dosage of 25–30 mg/kg three times per week has been recommended by some authorities,[136] whereas 40 mg/kg three times per week has been recommended by others.[138] It has been suggested that ethambutol can still be given at a dosage of 15 mg/kg three times per week in patients on regular haemodialysis.[40,136] Regarding the timing of administration of drugs, some authorities have recommended dosing 6–24 hours prior to haemodialysis,[138] while others have recommended post-dialysis treatment.[136,137]

Silicosis

It is recognized that silicotic patients are at risk of developing active pulmonary tuberculosis and are more difficult to treat because of impaired function of the alveolar macrophages, as well as impeded penetration of drugs into the fibrotic disease sites. In Hong Kong, a rocky island of granite and a place where the building industry prospers, silicosis is a common disease, and at one time 40 per cent of silicotic patients were found to suffer from active pulmonary tuberculosis. A study on such patients[139] showed that with a regimen of $H_3R_3Z_3S_3$, ethambutol being added in the first 3 months if there was a history of previous chemotherapy, treatment for 6 months is not adequate. A relapse rate of 22 per cent over 3 years and 33 per cent over 5 years occurred, compared with only 7 per cent over 3 years in patients treated for 8 months. The study also

showed slower conversion of sputum in the silicotic patients than in the non-silicotic ones even when the same four- or five-drug regimens were given. Only 80 per cent of the group studied had negative sputum culture at 2 months after treatment. One major problem is that about 20 per cent of patients experienced adverse reactions to this intensive regimen, with intolerance largely to streptomycin and pyrazinamide. A prospective study for silico-tuberculosis undertaken in Taiwan showed that a 9-month regimen comprising HRZS for 2 months followed by HR for 7 months yielded a success rate of 95 per cent and relapse rate of 5 per cent after 18–40 months of follow up.[140] This latter regimen was better tolerated when compared with the Hong Kong regimen.

HIV co-infection

For HIV-infected patients with drug-susceptible tuberculosis, the standard 6-month regimen results in good sputum bacteriological conversion and a low rate of treatment failure. However, the relapse rate of tuberculosis is higher than that in HIV-negative patients. Prolongation of therapy to 12 months resulted in lower relapse rate, but no significant impact on survival.[141] The most recent guidelines of the Centers for Disease Control and Prevention (CDC) recommend the minimum duration of treatment to be 6 months, but that if the clinical or bacteriological response is slow, treatment should be offered for a total period of 9 months, or for at least 4 months after achievement of culture negativity.[142]

Combination regimens of highly active antiretroviral drugs have improved the prognosis of HIV-infected patients, but have complicated the management of those with concomitant tuberculosis. Interactions between rifamycins (rifampicin > rifabutin) with HIV protease inhibitors/non-nucleoside reverse transcriptase inhibitors are complex and adjustment of drug dosages is very often required.[143] To circumvent this, the CDC also lists a non-rifamycin-containing regimen as a possible alternative, namely the administration of isoniazid, pyrazinamide and streptomycin for 9 months with ethambutol for the first 2 months.[142] However, there are a number of concerns with this latter strategy, especially regarding its inferior efficacy and the need to utilize prolonged duration of parenteral streptomycin therapy.

ROLE OF CORTICOSTEROIDS AS ADJUNCTIVE TREATMENT IN TB

Apart from replacement therapy in patients who develop Addison's disease secondary to tuberculous adrenalitis,[144] corticosteroids have been found to be useful as adjunctive therapy in some clinical settings of tuberculosis.[145] Two controlled trials using prednisolone have demonstrated benefit in active fibrino-effusive tuberculous pericarditis in terms of survival, resolution of clinical symptoms and the need for repeat pericardiocentesis.[146,147] Adjunctive prednisone given at high dose to 10 patients in the initial month followed by gradual tapering off also brought about dramatic resolution of pericardial effusion within 1 week.[148] In a relatively recent double-blind randomized placebo-controlled trial of adjunctive prednisolone in the treatment of effusive tuberculous pericarditis in HIV-seropositive patients, a pronounced reduction of mortality was also observed.[149] Data from trials of varying degrees of rigour have shown that corticosteroids as an adjunct in the management of tuberculous meningitis (stages 2 and 3) offered an advantage over antituberculosis chemotherapy alone for survival, frequency of sequelae or both.[150–152] A recent randomized double-blind placebo-controlled trial in Vietnam has shown that dexamethasone therapy improved survival but did not prevent severe disability in tuberculous meningitis.[153] Change in intracranial pressure or incidence of basal ganglia infarction were not significantly affected.[152] However, as many existing reports are limited in patient population size or study design, further controlled studies would appear beneficial. While one double-blind, placebo-controlled, randomized study has demonstrated that adjunctive corticosteroid led to resolution of clinical symptoms and resorption of pleural effusion more quickly,[154] another study not only revealed no such benefit but also similar pleural sequelae among the steroid and non-steroid groups.[155] There appears to be inadequate evidence currently to know whether steroids are effective in tuberculous pleural effusion. The efficacy of adjunctive corticosteroid in endobronchial tuberculosis in adults has been found to be equivocal.[156,157] Preliminary retrospective data have also suggested that corticosteroid administration combined with antituberculosis treatment could reduce the frequency of morbidity and mortality in patients with peritoneal tuberculosis.[158] Two studies, including one randomized controlled trial, have shown that adjunctive corticosteroid therapy could be beneficial in causing defervescence, improvement in serum albumin, body weight gain and even radiographic clearing more rapidly in patients with pulmonary tuberculosis associated with significant toxic (immunological) reactions.[159,160] Corticosteroids can also be used to suppress severe drug-related hypersensitivity reactions.[161] Paradoxical response to antituberculosis drugs has been reported to respond to corticosteroid therapy.[162] Such response, presumably due to immunological awakening, has been reported to be more common among tuberculosis and HIV co-infected patients following initiation of highly active antiretroviral therapy.[163] Indeed, corticosteroid treatment was reported to result in a favourable response in some HIV-infected patients with disseminated tuberculosis.[164] However, there has been some concern about the relative risks and benefits of administration of corticosteroids in HIV-positive patients and more controlled studies are still needed.[165,166] Evaluation of the use of inhaled corticosteroids in this patient population might be warranted.[167]

LEARNING POINTS

- The main aims of antituberculosis chemotherapy are:
  - to cure the patient in the shortest possible time;
  - to prevent death or late effects from disease;
  - to prevent relapse;
  - to prevent emergence of drug resistance;
  - to protect the community from infection.
- Isoniazid is the most potent bactericidal drug currently available.
- Rifampicin is the most commonly available rifamycin with effective sterilizing activity.
- A 6-month drug regimen comprising rifampicin and isoniazid, supplemented by pyrazinamide plus ethambutol/streptomycin in the first 2 months provides the cornerstone chemotherapy for newly diagnosed smear-positive cases of pulmonary tuberculosis.
- Retreatment smear-positive cases of pulmonary tuberculosis require drug therapy which is at least 8 months in duration.
- Patients with radiographically active pulmonary tuberculosis and negative sputum smear for acid-fast bacilli also warrant chemotherapy.
- DOTS for pulmonary tuberculosis is the best way to ensure high treatment success and to prevent development of drug resistance.
- Established multidrug-resistant pulmonary tuberculosis requires supervised treatment (DOT) with alternative-specific chemotherapy using second-line (reserve) drugs that are generally more expensive and/or toxic.
- Regular liver function monitoring during antituberculosis treatment may be unnecessary providing the patient has been well informed of the symptoms of hepatotoxicity. However, those subjects at increased risks of drug-induced liver dysfunction should be monitored both biochemically and clinically.
- Administration of highly active antiretroviral therapy for HIV infection concomitantly in patients receiving antituberculosis treatment generally results in complex drug interactions that require special management and care.

REFERENCES

1. Medical Research Council. A Medical Research Council Investigation. Streptomycin treatment of pulmonary tuberculosis. *Br Med J* 1948; ii: 769–82.
2. Medical Research Council. A Medical Research Council Investigation. Treatment of pulmonary tuberculosis with

streptomycin and para-aminosalicylic acid. *Br Med J* 1950; ii: 1073–85.

3. Medical Research Council. Various combinations of isoniazid with streptomycin or with PAS in the treatment of pulmonary tuberculosis. Seventh report to the Medical Research Council by their Tuberculosis Chemotherapy Trials Committee. *Br Med J* 1955; i: 434–45.

4. Bayer R, Wilkinson D. Directly observed therapy for tuberculosis: History of an idea. *Lancet* 1995; **345**: 1545–8.

5. Fox W, Mitchison DA. Short-course chemotherapy for pulmonary tuberculosis. *Am Rev Respir Dis* 1975; **111**: 845–8.

6. Mitchison D. Basic mechanisms of chemotherapy. *Chest* 1979; **76** (Suppl.): 771–81.

7. David HL. Drug resistance in *Mycobacterium tuberculosis* and other mycobacteria. *Clin Chest Med* 1980; **1**: 227–30.

8. Iseman MD, Madsen LA. Drug-resistant tuberculosis. *Clin Chest Med* 1989; **10**: 341–53.

9. British Thoracic Society. A controlled trial of 6-months' chemotherapy in pulmonary tuberculosis. Final report: Results during the 36-months after the end of chemotherapy and beyond. *Br J Dis Chest* 1984; **78**: 330–6.

10. Singapore Tuberculosis Service/British Medical Research Council. Five-year follow-up of a clinical trial of three 6-month regimens of chemotherapy given intermittently in the continuation phase in the treatment of pulmonary tuberculosis. *Am Rev Respir Dis* 1988; **137**: 1147–50.

11. China Tuberculosis Control Collaboration. Results of directly observed short-course chemotherapy in 112,842 Chinese patients with smear-positive tuberculosis. *Lancet* 1996; **347**: 358–62.

12. Tam CM, Chan SL, Lam CW et al. Rifapentine and isoniazid in the continuation phase of treating pulmonary tuberculosis: Initial report. *Am J Respir Crit Care Med* 1998; **157**: 1726–33.

13. Cohn DL, Catlin BJ, Peterson KL et al. A 62-dose, 6-month therapy for pulmonary and extrapulmonary tuberculosis: a twice-weekly, directly observed and cost effective regimen. *Ann Intern Med* 1990; **112**: 407–15.

14. Snider DE Jr, Graczyk J, Bek E, Rogowski J. Supervised 6-month treatment of newly diagnosed pulmonary tuberculosis using isoniazid, rifampin, and pyrazinamide with and without streptomycin. *Am Rev Respir Dis* 1984; **130**: 1091–4.

15. Third East African/British Medical Research Council Study. Controlled clinical trial of four short-course regimens of chemotherapy for two durations in the treatment of pulmonary tuberculosis. Second Report. *Tubercle* 1980; **61**: 59–69.

16. Hong Kong Chest Service/British Medical Research Council Study. Controlled trial of 6-month and 8-month regimens in the treatment of pulmonary tuberculosis. The results up to 24 months. *Tubercle* 1979; **60**: 201–10.

17. British Thoracic and Tuberculosis Association. Short-course chemotherapy in pulmonary tuberculosis: a controlled trial by the British Thoracic and Tuberculosis Association. *Lancet* 1976; ii: 1102–4.

18. Slutkin G, Schecter GF, Hopewelll PC. The results of 9-month isoniazid-rifampin therapy for pulmonary tuberculosis under program conditions in San Francisco. *Am Rev Respir Dis* 1988; **138**: 1622–4.

19. Combs D, O'Brien R, Geiter L. USPHS tuberculosis short-course chemotherapy trial 21: effectiveness, toxicity and acceptability – the report of final results. *Ann Intern Med* 1990; **112**: 397–406.

20. World Health Organization. Treatment of tuberculosis: Guidelines for national programmes, 2nd edn. Geneva: WHO, 1997.

21. Hong Kong Chest Service/British Medical Research Council. Second report: controlled trial of four three-times weekly regimens and a daily regimen all given for 6 months for pulmonary tuberculosis. The results up to 24 months. *Tubercle* 1982; **63**: 89–98.

22. Hong Kong Chest Service/British Medical Research Council. Controlled trial of 2, 4 and 6 months of pyrazinamide in 6-month three-times weekly regimens for smear-positive pulmonary tuberculosis, including an assessment of a combined preparation of isoniazid, rifampin and pyrazinamide. Results at 30 months. *Am Rev Respir Dis* 1991; **143**: 700–6.

23. American Thoracic Society/Centers for Disease Control and Prevention. Treatment of tuberculosis and tuberculosis infection in adults and children. *Am J Respir Crit Care Med* 1994; **149**: 1359–74.

24. Tam CM, Chan SL, Kam KM et al. Rifapentine and isoniazid in the continuation phase of a 6-month regimen. Final report at 5 years: prognostic value of various measures. *Int J Tuberc Lung Dis* 2002; **6**: 3–10.

25. Benator D, Bhattacharya M, Bozeman L et al. The Tuberculosis Trials Consortium. Rifapentine and isoniazid once a week versus rifampicin and isoniazid twice a week for treatment of drug-susceptible pulmonary tuberculosis in HIV-negative patients: a randomized clinical trial. *Lancet* 2002; **360**: 528–34.

26. American Thoracic Society/Centers for Disease Control and Prevention/Infectious Diseases Society of America. Treatment of tuberculosis. *Am J Respir Crit Care Med* 2003; **167**: 603–62.

27. Ipuge YA, Rieder HL, Enarson DA. Adverse cutaneous reactions to thiacetazone for tuberculosis treatment in Tazania. *Lancet* 1995; **346**: 657–60.

28. Elliott AM, Foster SD. Thiacetazone: time to call a halt? Considerations on the use of thiacetazone in African populations with a high prevalence of human immunodeficiency virus infection. *Tuber Lung Dis* 1996; **77**: 27–9.

29. Jindani A, Nunn AJ, Enarson DA. Two 8-month regimens of chemotherapy for treatment of newly diagnosed pulmonary tuberculosis: international multicentre randomised trial. *Lancet* 2004; **364**: 1244–51.

30. Chang KC, Leung CC, Yew WW et al. A nested case–control study on treatment-related risk factors for early relapse of tuberculosis. *Am J Respir Crit Care Med* 2004; **170**: 1124–30.

31. Vernon AA, Burman W, Benator D et al. Tuberculosis Trials Consortium. Acquired rifamycin monoresistance in patients with HIV-related tuberculosis treated with once-weekly rifapentine and isoniazid. *Lancet* 1999; **353**: 1843–7.

32. Bock NN, Sterling TR, Hamilton CD et al. The Tuberculosis Trials Consortium, Centers for Disease Control and Prevention. A prospective, randomized double-blind study of the tolerability of rifapentine 600, 900, 1200 mg plus isoniazid in the continuation phase of tuberculosis treatment. *Am J Respir Crit Care Med* 2002; **165**: 1526–30.

33. Rosenthal IM, Williams K, Tyagi S et al. Weekly moxifloxacin and rifapentine is more active than the Denver regimen in murine tuberculosis. *Am J Respir Crit Care Med* 2005; **172**: 1457–62.

34. Rosenthal IM, Williams K, Tyagi S et al. Potent twice-weekly rifapentine-containing regimens in murine tuberculosis. *Am J Respir Crit Care Med* 2006; **174**: 94–101.

35. Sbarbaro J, Blomberg B, Chaulet P. Fixed-dose combination formulations for tuberculosis treatment. *Int J Tuberc Lung Dis* 1999; **3**: S286–8.

36. Moulding T, Dutt AK, Reichman LB. Fixed-dose combinations of antituberculosis medications to prevent drug resistance. *Ann Intern Med* 1995; **122**: 951–4.

37. Mitchison DA. How drug resistance emerges as a result of poor compliance during short course chemotherapy for tuberculosis. *Int J Tuber Lung Dis* 1998; **2**: 10–15.

38. Fox W. Drug combinations and the bioavailability of rifampicin. *Tubercle* 1990; **71**: 241–5.

39. A Joint Statement of the International Union Against Tuberculosis and Lung Disease/World Health Organization. The promise and reality of fixed dose combinations with rifampicin. *Tuber Lung Dis* 1994; **75**: 180–1.

40. ERS, WHO, IUATLD (Europe Region) Task Force. Tuberculosis management in Europe: Recommendations of a task force of the European Respiratory Society, the World Health Organization and

the International Union against Tuberculosis and Lung Disease (Europe Region). *Eur Respir J* 1999; **14**: 978–92.

41. Teo SK. Assessment of a combined preparation of isoniazid, rifampicin and pyrazinamide (Rifater®) in the initial phase of chemotherapy in three 6-month regimens for smear-positive pulmonary tuberculosis: a five-year follow-up report. *Int J Tuberc Lung Dis* 1999; **3**: 120–32.

42. Blomberg B, Spinaci S, Fourie B, Laing R. The rationale for recommending fixed-dose combination tablets for treatment of tuberculosis. *Bull World Health Organ* 2001; **79**: 61–8.

43. Yew WW. Directly observed therapy, short-course: The best way to prevent multidrug-resistant tuberculosis. *Chemotherapy* 1999; **45** (Suppl. 2): S26–33.

44. Sumartojo E. When tuberculosis treatment fails. A social behavioral account of patient adherence. *Am Rev Respir Dis* 1993; **147**: 1311–20.

45. World Health Organization Global Tuberculosis Programme. *Global tuberculosis control.* WHO/GTB/97.225. Geneva: WHO 1997.

46. Kochi A. *Is DOTS the health breakthrough of the 1990s?* World Health Forum. Geneva: WHO 1997; **18**: 225–47.

47. World Health Organization. *Anti-tuberculosis drug resistance in the world.* Report No. 2 Prevalence and trends. The WHO/IUATLD Global Project on Anti-tuberculosis Drug Resistance Surveillance. WHO/CDS/TB/2000.278. Geneva: WHO, 2000.

48. Hong Kong Chest Service/Tuberculosis Research Centre, Madras/British Medical Research Council. A controlled trial of 2-month, 3-month and 12-month regimens of chemotherapy for sputum-smear-negative pulmonary tuberculosis: Results at 60 months. *Am Rev Respir Dis* 1984; **130**: 23–8.

49. Hong Kong Chest Service/Tuberculosis Research Centre, Madras/British Medical Research Council. A controlled trial of 3-month, 4-month and 6-month regimens of chemotherapy for sputum-smear-negative pulmonary tuberculosis. Results at 5 years. *Am Rev Respir Dis* 1989; **139**: 871–6.

50. Davidson PT. Drug resistance and the selection of therapy for tuberculosis. *Am Rev Respir Dis* 1987; **136**: 255–7.

51. Joint Tuberculosis Committee of the British Thoracic Society. Chemotherapy and management of tuberculosis in the United Kingdom: recommendations 1998. *Thorax* 1998; **53**: 536–48.

52. Hong Kong Chest Service/British Medical Research Council. Five-year follow-up of a controlled trial of five 6-month regimens of chemotherapy for pulmonary tuberculosis. *Am Rev Respir Dis* 1987; **136**: 1339–42.

53. Babu Swai O, Aluoch JA, Githui WA et al. Controlled clinical trial of a regimen of two durations for the treatment of isoniazid resistant pulmonary tuberculosis. *Tubercle* 1988; **69**: 5–14.

54. Barnes PF, Bloch AB, Davidson PT, Snider DE Jr. Tuberculosis in patients with human immunodeficiency virus infection. *N Engl J Med* 1991; **324**: 1644–50.

55. World Health Organization. *Anti-tuberculosis drug resistance in the world.* Report No. 3. The WHO/IUATLD Global Project on Anti-tuberculosis Drug Resistance Surveillance 1999–2002. WHO/HTM/TB/2004.343. Geneva: WHO, 2004.

56. Farmer P, Kim JY. Community based approaches to the control of multidrug resistant tuberculosis: introducing 'DOTS-plus'. *Br Med J* 1998; **317**: 671–4.

57. Yew WW, Kwan SY, Ma WK et al. In-vitro activity of ofloxacin against *Mycobacterium tuberculosis* and its clinical efficacy in multiply resistant pulmonary tuberculosis. *J Antimicrob Chemother* 1990; **26**: 227–36.

58. Goble M, Iseman MD, Madsen LA et al. Treatment of 171 patients with pulmonary tuberculosis resistant to isoniazid and rifampin. *N Engl J Med* 1993; **328**: 527–32.

59. Telzak EE, Sepkowitz K, Alpert P et al. Multidrug-resistant tuberculosis in patients without HIV infection. *N Engl J Med* 1995; **333**: 907–11.

60. Park SK, Kim CT, Song SD. Outcome of chemotherapy in 107 patients with pulmonary tuberculosis resistant to isoniazid and rifampin. *Int J Tuberc Lung Dis* 1998; **2**: 877–84.

61. Yew WW, Chan CK, Chau CH et al. Outcomes of patients with multidrug-resistant pulmonary tuberculosis treated with ofloxacin/levofloxacin-containing regimens. *Chest* 2000; **117**: 744–51.

62. Dye C, Williams BG, Espinal MA, Raviglione MC. Erasing the world's slow stain: strategies to beat multidrug-resistant tuberculosis. *Science* 2002; **295**: 2042–6.

63. Crofton J, Chaulet P, Maher D. *Guidelines for the management of drug-resistant tuberculosis.* WHO/TB/96.210 (rev 1). Geneva: World Health Organization, 1997.

64. Park MM, Davis AL, Schluger NW et al. Outcome of MDR-TB patients 1983–1993: Prolonged survival with appropriate therapy. *Am J Respir Crit Care Med* 1996; **153**: 317–24.

65. Heifets LB, Cangelosi GA. Drug susceptibility testing of *Mycobacterium tuberculosis*: a neglected problem at the turn of the century. *Int J Tuberc Lung Dis* 1999; **3**: 564–81.

66. World Health Organization. *Guidelines for drug susceptibility testing for second-line anti-tuberculosis drugs for DOTS-Plus.* WHO/CDS/TB/2001.288. Geneva: WHO, 2001.

67. World Health Organization. *Treatment of tuberculosis. Guidelines for national programmes,* 3rd edn. WHO/CDS/TB/2003.313, 2003.

68. Suarez PG, Floyd K, Portocarrero J et al. Feasibility and cost-effectiveness of standardised second-line drug treatment for chronic tuberculosis patients: a national cohort study in Peru. *Lancet* 2002; **359**: 1980–9.

69. Telzak EE, Chirgwin KD, Nelson ET et al. Predictors for multidrug-resistant tuberculosis among HIV-infected patients and response to specific drug regimens. *Int J Tuberc Lung Dis* 1999; **3**: 337–43.

70. Yew WW, Chan CK, Leung CC et al. Comparative roles of levofloxacin and ofloxacin in the treatment of multidrug-resistant tuberculosis: preliminary results of a retrospective study from Hong Kong. *Chest* 2003; **124**: 1476–81.

71. Kennedy N, Fox R, Kisyombe GM et al. Early bactericidal and sterilizing activities of ciprofloxacin in pulmonary tuberculosis. *Am Rev Respir Dis* 1993; **148**: 1547–51.

72. Kennedy N, Berger L, Curram J et al. Randomized controlled trial of a drug regimen that includes ciprofloxacin for the treatment of pulmonary tuberculosis. *Clin Infect Dis* 1996; **22**: 827–33.

73. Berning SE, Madsen L, Iseman MD, Peloquin CA. Long-term safety of ofloxacin and ciprofloxacin in the treatment of mycobacterial infections. *Am J Respir Crit Care Med* 1995; **151**: 2006–9.

74. Kennedy N, Fox R, Uiso L et al. Safety profile of ciprofloxacin during long-term therapy for pulmonary tuberculosis. *J Antimicrob Chemother* 1993; **32**: 897–902.

75. Yew WW, Wong CF, Wong PC et al. Adverse neurological reactions in patients with multidrug-resistant tuberculosis after co-administration of cycloserine and ofloxacin. *Clin Infect Dis* 1993; **17**: 288–9.

76. Rastogi N, Goh KS. In vitro activity of the new difluorinated quinolone sparfloxacin, against *Mycobacterium tuberculosis* compared with activities of ofloxacin and ciprofloxacin. *Antimicrob Agents Chemother* 1991; **35**: 1933–6.

77. Yew WW, Piddock LJ, Li MS et al. In-vitro activity of quinolones and macrolides against mycobacteria. *J Antimicrob Chemother* 1994; **34**: 343–51.

78. Lubasch A, Erbes R, Mauch H, Lode H. Sparfloxacin in the treatment of drug-resistant tuberculosis or intolerance of first line therapy. *Eur Respir J* 2001; **17**: 641–6.

79. Jaillon P, Morganroth J, Brumpt I, Talbot G. Overview of electrocardiographic and cardiovascular safety data for sparfloxacin. Sparfloxacin Safety Group. *J Antimicrob Chemother* 1996; **37** (Suppl. A): 161S–7S.

80. Singla R, Gupta S, Gupta R, Arora VK. Efficacy and safety of sparfloxacin in combination with kanamycin and ethionamide in multidrug-resistant pulmonary tuberculosis: preliminary results. *Int J Tuberc Lung Dis* 2001; **5**: 559–63.

81. Miyazaki E, Miyazaki M, Chen JM et al. Moxifloxacin (BAY12-8039), a new 8-methoxyquinolone, is active in a mouse model of tuberculosis. *Antimicrob Agents Chemother* 1999; **43**: 85–9.

82. Saito H, Tomioka H, Sato K, Dekio S. *In vitro* and *in vivo*

antimycobacterial activities of a new quinolone DU-6859a. *Antimicrob Agents Chemother* 1994; **38**: 2877–82.

83. Fung-Tomc J, Minassian B, Kolek B *et al. In vitro* antibacterial spectrum of a new broad-spectrum 8-methoxyfluoroquinolone, gatifloxacin. *J Antimicrob Chemother* 2000; **45**: 437–46.

84. Valerio G, Bracciale P, Manisco V *et al.* Long-term tolerance and effectiveness of moxifloxacin therapy for tuberculosis: preliminary results. *J Chemother* 2003; **15**: 66–70.

85. Burman WJ, Goldberg S, Johnson JL *et al.* Moxifloxacin versus ethambutol in the first two months of treatment for pulmonary tuberculosis. *Am J Respir Crit Care Med* 2006; **174**: 331–8.

86. Torun T, Gungor G, Ozmen I *et al.* Side effects associated with the treatment of multidrug-resistant tuberculosis. *Int J Tuberc Lung Dis* 2005; **9**: 1373–7.

87. Sullivan EA, Kreiswirth BN, Palumbo L *et al.* Emergence of fluoroquinolone-resistant tuberculosis in New York City. *Lancet* 1995; **345**: 1148–50.

88. Perlman DC, El Sadr WM, Heifets LB *et al.* Susceptibility to levofloxacin of *Mycobacterium tuberculosis* isolates from patients with HIV-related tuberculosis and characterization of a strain with levofloxacin monoresistance. *AIDS* 1997; **11**: 1473–8.

89. Grimaldo ER, Tupasi TE, Rivera AB *et al.* Increased resistance to ciprofloxacin and ofloxacin multidrug-resistant mycobacterium tuberculosis isolates from patients seen at a tertiary hospital in the Philippines. *Int J Tuberc Lung Dis* 2001; **5**: 546–50.

90. Ginsburg AS, Hooper N, Parrish N *et al.* Fluoroquinolone resistance in patients with newly diagnosed tuberculosis. *Clin Infect Dis* 2003; **37**: 1448–52.

91. Iseman MD, Madsen L, Goble M, Pomerantz M. Surgical intervention in the treatment of pulmonary disease caused by drug-resistant *Mycobacterium tuberculosis. Am Rev Respir Dis* 1990; **141**: 623–5.

92. Pomerantz M, Brown JM. Surgery in the treatment of multidrug-resistant tuberculosis. *Clin Chest Med* 1997; **18**: 123–30.

93. Treasure RL, Seaworth BJ. Current role of surgery in *Mycobacterium tuberculosis. Ann Thorac Surg* 1995; **59**: 1405–7.

94. van Leuven M, De Groot M, Shean KP *et al.* Pulmonary resection as an adjunct in the treatment of multiple drug-resistant tuberculosis. *Ann Thorac Surg* 1997; **63**: 1368–72.

95. Sung SW, Kang CH, Kim YT *et al.* Surgery increased the chance of cure in multidrug-resistant pulmonary tuberculosis. *Eur J Cardiothorac Surg* 1999; **16**: 187–93.

96. Pomerantz BJ, Cleveland JC Jr, Olson HK, Pomerantz M. Pulmonary resection for multidrug-resistant tuberculosis. *J Thorac Cardiovasc Surg* 2001; **121**: 448–53.

97. Chiang CY, Yu MC, Bai KJ *et al.* Pulmonary resection in the treatment of patients with pulmonary multidrug-resistant tuberculosis in Taiwan. *Int J Tuberc Lung Dis* 2001; **5**: 272–7.

98. Park SK, Lee CM, Heu JP, Song SD. A retrospective study for the outcome of pulmonary resection in 49 patients with multidrug-resistant tuberculosis. *Int J Tuberc Lung Dis* 2002; **6**: 143–9.

99. Takeda S, Maeda H, Hayakawa M *et al.* Current surgical intervention for preliminary tuberculosis. *Ann Thorac Surg* 2005; **79**: 959–63.

100. Shiraishi Y, Nakajima Y, Katsuragi N *et al.* Resectional surgery combined with chemotherapy remains the treatment of choice for multidrug-resistant tuberculosis. *J Thorac Cardiovasc Surg* 2004; **128**: 523–8.

101. Kir A, Inci I, Torun T *et al.* Adjuvant resectional surgery improves cure rates in multidrug-resistant tuberculosis. *J Thorac Cardiovasc Surg* 2006; **131**: 693–6.

102. Chan ED, Laurel V, Strand MJ *et al.* Treatment and outcome analysis of 205 patients with multidrug-resistant tuberculosis. *Am J Respir Crit Care Med* 2004; **169**: 1103–9.

103. Kim HJ, Kang CH, Kim YT *et al.* Prognostic factors for surgical resection in patients with multidrug-resistant tuberculosis. *Eur Respir J* 2006; **28**: 576–80.

104. Condos R, Rom WN, Schluger NW. Treatment of multidrug-resistant pulmonary tuberculosis with interferon-γ via aerosol. *Lancet* 1997; **349**: 1513–15.

105. Holland SM, Eisenstein EM, Kuhns DB *et al.* Treatment of refractory disseminated nontuberculous mycobacterial infection with interferon-gamma: a preliminary report. *N Engl J Med* 1994; **330**: 1348–55.

106. Johnson BJ, Bekker LG, Rickman R *et al.* rhuIL-2 adjunctive therapy in multidrug resistant tuberculosis: a comparison of two treatment regimens and placebo. *Tuber Lung Dis* 1997; **78**: 195–203.

107. Giosue S, Casarini M, Ameglio F *et al.* Aerosolized interferon-alpha treatment in patients with multidrug-resistant pulmonary tuberculosis. *Eur Cytokine Netw* 2000; **11**: 99–104.

108. Stanford JL, Stanford CA, Grange JM *et al.* Does immunotherapy with heat-killed *Mycobacterium vaccae* offer hope for the treatment of multidrug-resistant pulmonary tuberculosis? *Respir Med* 2001; **95**: 444–7.

109. Stanford J, Stanford C, Grange J. Immunotherapy with *Mycobacterium vaccae* in the treatment of tuberculosis. *Front Biosci* 2004; **9**: 1701–19.

110. Yew WW. Clinically significant interactions with drugs used in the treatment of tuberculosis. *Drug Saf* 2002; **25**: 111–33.

111. Hamadeh M, Glassroth J. Tuberculosis and pregnancy. *Chest* 1992; **101**: 1114–20.

112. World Health Organization (Division of Child Health Development). Breastfeeding and maternal tuberculosis. 1998; **23**: 1–4 (www.who.int/child-adolescent-health/New_Publications/NUTRITION/Breastfeeding_Tub.pdf).

113. Pande JN, Singh SPN, Khilnani GC *et al.* Risk factors for hepatotoxicity from antituberculosis drugs: a case–control study. *Thorax* 1996; **51**: 132–6.

114. Stead WW. Tuberculosis among elderly persons, as observed among nursing home residents. *Int J Tuberc Lung Dis* 1998; **2**: S64–S70.

115. Whittington RM. Fatal hepatotoxicity of antitubercular chemotherapy. *Lancet* 1991; **338**: 1083–4.

116. Mitchell I, Wendon J, Fitt S, Williams R. Antituberculous therapy and acute liver failure. *Lancet* 1995; **345**: 555–6.

117. Fernandez-Villar A, Sopena B, Fernandez-Villar J *et al.* The influence of risk factors on the severity of anti-tuberculosis drug-induced hepatoxocity. *Int J Tuberc Lung Dis* 2004; **8**: 1499–505.

118. Wong WM, Wu PC, Yuen MF *et al.* Antituberculosis drug-related liver dysfunction in chronic hepatitis B infection. *Hepatology* 2000; **31**: 201–6.

119. Ungo JR, Jones D, Ashkin D *et al.* Antituberculosis drug-induced hepatotoxicity: The role of hepatitis C virus and the human immunodeficiency virus. *Am J Respir Crit Care Med* 1998; **157**: 1871–6.

120. Yeoh EK, Chang WK, Kwan JPW. Epidemiology of viral hepatitis B infection in Hong Kong. In: Lam SK, Lai CL, Yeoh EK (eds). *Viral hepatitis B infection: vaccine and control.* Singapore: World Scientific, 1984: 33–41.

121. Moriya T, Koyama T, Tanaka J, Mishiro S, Yoshizawa H. Epidemiology of hepatitis C virus in Japan. *Intervirology* 1999; **42**: 153–8.

122. Songsivilai S, Jinathongthai S, Wongsena W *et al.* High prevalence of hepatitis C infection among blood donors in northeastern Thailand. *Am J Trop Med Hyg* 1997; **57**: 66–9.

123. Dye C, Scheele S, Dolin P *et al.* Consensus statement. *Global burden of tuberculosis: Estimated incidence, prevalence and mortality by country.* WHO Global Surveillance and Monitoring Project. *J Am Med Assoc* 1999; **282**: 677–86.

124. Steele MA, Burk RF, DesPrez RM. Toxic hepatitis with isoniazid and rifampin. A meta-analysis. *Chest* 1991; **99**: 465–71.

125. Girling DJ. Adverse effects of antituberculosis drugs. *Drugs* 1982; **23**: 56–74.

126. Parthasarathy R, Sarma GR, Janardhanam B *et al.* Hepatic toxicity in South Indian patients during treatment of tuberculosis with

short-course regimens containing isoniazid, rifampicin and pyrazinamide. *Tubercle* 1986; **67**: 99–108.

127. Singh J, Arora A, Garg PK *et al.* Antituberculosis treatment-induced hepatotoxicity: role of predictive factors. *Postgrad Med J* 1995; **71**: 359–62.

128. Durand F, Bernuau J, Pessayre D *et al.* Deleterious influence of pyrazinamide on the outcome of patients with fulminant or subfulminant liver failure during antituberculous treatment including isoniazid. *Hepatology* 1995; **21**: 929–32.

129. Schaberg T, Rebhan K, Lode H. Risk factors for side-effects of isoniazid, rifampin and pyrazinamide in patients hospitalized for pulmonary tuberculosis. *Eur Respir J* 1996; **9**: 2026–30.

130. Tahaoglu K, Ataç G, Sevim T *et al.* The management of antituberculosis drug-induced hepatotoxicity. *Int J Tuberc Lung Dis* 2001; **5**: 65–9.

131. Teleman MD, Chee CBE, Earnest A, Wang YT. Hepatotoxicity of tuberculosis chemotherapy under general programme conditions in Singapore. *Int J Tuberc Lung Dis* 2002; **6**: 699–705.

132. Yee D, Valiquette C, Pelletier M *et al.* Incidence of serious side effects from first-line antituberculosis drugs among patients treated for active tuberculosis. *Am J Respir Crit Care Med* 2003; **167**: 1472–7.

133. Yew WW, Lee J, Wong PC, Kwan SYL. Tolerance of ofloxacin in treatment of pulmonary tuberculosis in presence of hepatic dysfunction. *Int J Clin Pharm Res* 1992; **XII**: 173–8.

134. Saigal S, Agarwal SR, Nandeesh HP, Sarin SK. Safety of an ofloxacin-based antitubercular regimen for the treatment of tuberculosis in patients with underlying chronic liver disease: a preliminary report. *J Gastroenterol Hepatol* 2001; **16**: 1028–32.

135. Andrew OT, Schoenfeld PY, Hopewell PC, Humphreys MH. Tuberculosis in patients with end-stage renal disease. *Am J Med* 1980; **68**: 59–65.

136. Malone RS, Fish DN, Spiegel DM *et al.* The effect of hemodialysis on isoniazid, rifampin, pyrazinamide and ethambutol. *Am J Respir Crit Care Med* 1999; **159**: 1580–4.

137. Swan SK, Bennett WM. Use of drugs in patients with renal failure. In: Schrier RW, Gottschalk CW (eds). *Diseases of the kidney*, 6th edn. Vol. 3. New York: Little Brown, 1997: 2968–3011.

138. Ellard GA. Chemotherapy of tuberculosis for patients with renal impairment. *Nephron* 1993; **64**: 169–81.

139. Hong Kong Chest Service/Tuberculosis Research Centre, Madras/British Medical Research Council. A controlled clinical comparison of 6 and 8 months of antituberculosis chemotherapy in the treatment of patients with silicotuberculosis in Hong Kong. *Am Rev Respir Dis* 1991; **143**: 262–7.

140. Lin TP, Suo J, Lee CN *et al.* Short-course chemotherapy of pulmonary tuberculosis in pneumoconiotic patients. *Am Rev Respir Dis* 1987; **136**: 808–10.

141. Perriens JH, St Louis ME, Mukadi YB *et al.* Pulmonary tuberculosis in HIV-infected patients in Zaire: a controlled trial of treatment for either 6 or 12 months. *N Engl J Med* 1995; **332**: 779–84.

142. Centers for Disease Control and Prevention. Prevention and treatment of tuberculosis among patients infected with human immunodeficiency virus: principles of therapy and revised recommendations. *MMWR Morb Mortal Wkly Rep* 1998; **47** (RR-20): 1–58.

143. Centers for Disease Control and Prevention. Updated guidelines for the use of rifabutin or rifampin for the treatment and prevention of tuberculosis among HIV-infected patients taking protease inhibitors or non-nucleoside reverse transcriptase inhibitors. *MMWR Morb Mortal Wkly Rep* 2000; **49**: 185–9.

144. Dedon JF, Courtney DL, Holmes FF. Addison's disease from tuberculosis in a centenarian. *J Am Geriatr Soc* 1992; **40**: 618–19.

145. Dooley DP, Carpenter JL, Rademacher S. Adjunctive corticosteroid therapy for tuberculosis: a critical reappraisal of the literature. *Clin Infect Dis* 1997; **25**: 872–87.

146. Strang JI, Kakaza HH, Gibson DG *et al.* Controlled trial of prednisolone as adjuvant in treatment of tuberculous constrictive pericarditis in Transkei. *Lancet* 1987; **ii**: 1418–22.

147. Strang JI, Kakaza HH, Gibson DG *et al.* Controlled clinical trial of complete open surgical drainage and of prednisolone in treatment of tuberculous pericardial effusion in Transkei. *Lancet* 1988; **ii**: 759–64.

148. Strang JIG. Rapid resolution of tuberculous pericardial effusions with high dose prednisone and anti-tuberculous drugs. *J Infect* 1994; **28**: 251–4.

149. Hakim JG, Ternouth I, Mushangi E *et al.* Double blind randomized placebo controlled trial of adjunctive prednisolone in the treatment of effusive tuberculous pericarditis in HIV seropositive patients. *Heart* 2000; **84**: 183–8.

150. Girgis NI, Farid Z, Kilpatrick ME *et al.* Dexamethasone adjunctive treatment for tuberculous meningitis. *Pediatr Infect Dis J* 1991; **10**: 179–83.

151. Humphries M. The management of tuberculous meningitis. *Thorax* 1992; **47**: 577–81.

152. Schoeman JF, Van Zyl LE, Laubscher JA, Donald PR. Effect of corticosteroids on intracranial pressure, computed tomographic findings and clinical outcome in young children with tuberculous meningitis. *Pediatrics* 1997; **99**: 226–31.

153. Thwaites GE, Nguyen DB, Nguyen HD *et al.* Dexamethasone for the treatment of tuberculosis meningitis in adolescents and adults. *N Engl J Med* 2004; **351**: 1741–51.

154. Lee C-H, Wang W-J, Lan R-S *et al.* Corticosteroids in the treatment of tuberculous pleurisy. *Chest* 1988; **94**: 1256–9.

155. Galarza I, Canete C, Granados A *et al.* Randomised trial of corticosteroids in the treatment of tuberculous pleurisy. *Thorax* 1995; **50**: 1305–7.

156. Ip MS, So SY, Lam WK, Mok CK. Endobronchial tuberculosis revisited. *Chest* 1986; **89**: 727–30.

157. Chan HS, Sun A, Hoheisel GB. Endobronchial tuberculosis – is corticosteroid treatment useful? A report of 8 cases and review of the literature. *Postgrad Med J* 1990; **66**: 822–6.

158. Alrajhi AA, Halim MA, Al-Hokrail A *et al.* Corticosteroid treatment of peritoneal tuberculosis. *Clin Infect Dis* 1998; **27**: 52–6.

159. Muthuswamy P, Hu TC, Carasso B *et al.* Prednisone as adjunctive therapy in the management of pulmonary tuberculosis: report of 12 cases and review of the literature. *Chest* 1995; **107**: 1621–30.

160. Bilaceroglu S, Perim K, Buyuksirin M, Celikten E. Prednisolone: a beneficial and safe adjunct to antituberculosis treatment? A randomized controlled trial. *Int J Tuberc Lung Dis* 1999; **3**: 47–54.

161. Morris H, Muckerjee J, Akhtar S *et al.* Use of corticosteroids to suppress drug toxicity in complicated tuberculosis. *J Infect* 1999; **39**: 237–40.

162. Bukharie H. Paradoxical response to anti-tuberculous drugs: resolution with corticosteroid therapy. *Scand J Infect Dis* 2000; **32**: 96–7.

163. Narita M, Ashkin D, Hollender ES, Pitchenik AE. Paradoxical worsening of tuberculosis following anti-retroviral therapy in patients with AIDS. *Am J Respir Crit Care Med* 1998; **158**: 157–61.

164. Masud T, Kemp E. Corticosteroid in treatment of disseminated tuberculosis in patient with HIV infection. *Br Med J* 1988; **296**: 464–5.

165. Mayanja-Kizza H, Jones-Lopez E, Okwera A *et al.* Uganda–Case Western Research Collaboration. Immunoadjuvant prednisolone therapy for HIV-associated tuberculosis: a phase 2 clinical trial in Uganda. *J Infect Dis* 2005; **191**: 856–65.

166. Elliott AM, Luzze H, Quigley MA *et al.* A randomized double-blind, placebo-controlled trial of the use of prednisolone as an adjunct to treatment in HIV-associated pleural tuberculosis. *J Infect Dis* 2004; **190**: 869–78.

167. Yew WW, Lee J, Chau CH. Role of inhaled budesonide in the treatment of tuberculous pyrexia. *Chest* 2000; **118**: 567.

14

New developments in treatment

QIJIANG CHENG, WILLIAM R BISHAI AND ERIC L NUERMBERGER

THE NEED FOR NEW ANTITUBERCULOSIS DRUGS

As espoused in the World Health Organization's Stop TB Strategy, control of tuberculosis (TB) requires political commitment and funding, high-quality diagnostic laboratory facilities, highly effective, standardized treatment regimens and the infrastructure to provide supervised therapy. In the most highly developed countries, these elements came together in the 1950s after the introduction of streptomycin, para-aminosalicylic acid and isoniazid. Although 18–24 months of treatment was required to assure success, the morbidity and mortality from TB dropped precipitously in the developed world over the next 25 years before the advent of modern short-course therapy. In the United States, TB incidence rates are again declining and are currently at historic lows.[1] However, in many parts of the developing world, TB remains the single greatest killer among bacterial diseases, driven largely by inadequate public health infrastructure and other limited resources that compromise diagnosis and implementation of supervised treatment. In sub-Saharan Africa in particular, the situation is greatly exacerbated by the extraordinarily high incidence of TB-HIV co-infection.

Current TB treatment consists of a regimen of four antibiotics that must be taken for 6–9 months. Daily drug administration likely provides the most effective therapy.[2] Although this regimen can cure virtually all patients with drug-susceptible pulmonary tuberculosis, it remains lengthy and complex and commonly leads to poor adherence, default and treatment failure or relapse under field conditions.[3] Supervised treatment programmes can overcome these obstacles, but are resource-intensive and therefore difficult to implement in the developing world. It is widely believed that shorter and/or simpler regimens will facilitate the implementation of supervised therapy, increase treatment completion rates, enhance TB control efforts and prevent the emergence of drug resistance. The development of such regimens will require new antituberculosis agents with improved sterilizing activity to reduce the duration of therapy and/or longer elimination half-lives to allow more effective intermittent treatment regimens. Ideally, such new agents would also have novel mechanisms of action to be effective against bacterial strains that are resistant to available first-line drugs and would not have drug–drug interactions with HIV protease inhibitors and non-nucleoside reverse transcriptase inhibitors to reduce the complexity of managing TB-HIV co-infection.

Nearly 40 years since the introduction of rifampicin in the late 1960s, there are again new classes of drugs in the pipeline for TB. At present, there are eight agents from six distinct classes in clinical stages of development. These drugs include existing drugs approved for use in other bacterial infections (fluoroquinolones and oxazolidones) and the long-acting rifamycin derivative, rifapentine, that is approved for use in TB, but is under study again to determine whether it can be employed more effectively. The remaining compounds are new chemical entities that have been identified primarily through whole-cell-based screening methods, but their subsequent development has been greatly facilitated by recent methodological advances in mycobacterial genetics.[1,4–8] These promising new drug candidates and their structures and targets are shown in Table 14.1. Other compounds in earlier stages of development are outside the scope of this review, but have been reviewed recently.[9,10]

Table 14.1 Promising new drug candidates and their structures and targets.

Molecular structure	Drug	Class	Sponsor(s)[a]	Mechanism of action	Target	Development stage
	Moxifloxacin	Fluoroquinolone	Bayer, GATB, CDC, NIH, FDA	Inhibition of DNA synthesis	DNA gyrase	Phase II/III
	Gatifloxacin	Fluoroquinolone	OFLOTUB consortium,[b] NIH	Inhibition of DNA synthesis	DNA gyrase	Phase II/III
	Rifapentine	Rifamycin	Sanofi-aventis, CDC, NIH	Inhibition of RNA synthesis	DNA dependent RNA polymerase	Phase II (thrice weekly, daily therapy)
	TMC207	Diarylquinoline	Tibotec	Inhibition of ATP synthesis and membrane potential	F1F0 proton ATP synthase	Phase II
	PA824	Nitroimidazo-oxazine	GATB	Inhibition of protein and cell wall lipid synthesis	Unknown	Phase I
	OPC-67683	Nitroimidazo-oxazole	Otsuka	Inhibition of protein and cell wall lipid synthesis	Unknown	Phase II
	SQ109	Diethylamine	Sequella	Inhibition of cell wall synthesis	Unknown	Phase II
	LL-3858	Pyrrole	Lupin	Unknown	Unknown	Phase I
	Linezolid and others	Oxazolidinone	NIH, Pfizer	Inhibition of protein synthesis	Ribosomal initiation complex	Lead optimization

[a]GATB, Global Alliance for TB Drug Development; CDC, US Centers for Disease Control and Prevention TB Trials Consortium; NIH, US National Institutes of Health; FDA, US Food and Drug Administration.
[b]Lupin Ltd, NIH National Institute of Allergy and Infectious Diseases TB Research Unit, TB Research Centre (Chennai), World Health Organization Special Programme for Research and Training in Tropical Diseases.

FLUOROQUINOLONES: MOXIFLOXACIN AND GATIFLOXACIN

The fluoroquinolones represent the first new antibiotic class to be considered for first-line usage against TB since the introduction of rifampicin in 1968. Their excellent oral bioavailability, bactericidal action, lack of cross-resistance with existing TB drugs and favourable safety and tolerability profile have made them the most important second-line drugs for treating patients with multidrug-resistant (MDR)-TB. Several retrospective studies have demonstrated that patients with MDR-TB who receive a fluoroquinolone as part of their treatment have higher rates of cure and survival than patients who do not receive a fluoroquinolone.[11–14]

Efforts by the pharmaceutical industry to improve the activity of fluoroquinolones against *Streptococcus pneumoniae* for treatment of respiratory tract infections have fortuitously also improved activity of these drugs against *Mycobacterium tuberculosis*. Earlier fluoroquinolones, such

Table 14.2 Comparative pharmacokinetics and pharmacodynamics of fluoroquinolones after a single oral dose in humans[a]

Drug	Pharmacokinetics			Pharmacodynamics		
	Dose (mg/kg)	C_{max} (µg/ml)	AUC (µg/h/ml)	MIC_{90} (µg/ml)	C_{max}/MIC_{90}	AUC/MIC_{90}
Ciprofloxacin	500 (8.3)	2.4	11.6	1.0	2.4	11.6
Ofloxacin	400 (6.6)	3	24	2.0	1.5	12
Levofloxacin	500 (8.3)	6.2	45	1.0	6.2	45
Levofloxacin[b]	1000 (16.6)	9.4	108	1.0	9.4	108
Gatifloxacin	400 (6.6)	3.4	30	0.5	6.8	60
Moxifloxacin	400 (6.6)	4.3	39	0.5	8.6	78

[a]Adapted from Lubasch et al.[80]
[b]Adapted from Fish et al.[81]

as ciprofloxacin and ofloxacin, have largely bacteriostatic activity against *M. tuberculosis* at conventional doses,[15] while newer fluoroquinolones, such as levofloxacin (LEV), gatifloxacin (GAT) and moxifloxacin (MXF), have bactericidal activity. The 8-methoxy-fluoroquinolones, GAT and MXF, have the most potent activity against *M. tuberculosis*, including non-replicating rifampin-tolerant persisters, in *in vitro* models.[16] At conventional doses, MXF and GAT also have the most favourable pharmacodynamic profiles for the treatment of TB.[17] Table 14.2 shows the pharmacokinetics and pharmacodynamics of various fluoroquinolones after a single oral dose in humans. According to the ratio of AUC_{24}/MIC_{90}, which is predictive of bactericidal activity against other pathogens, MXF and GAT should have the most potent antituberculosis activity among the fluoroquinolones at conventional doses. Although it is less potent than MXF or GAT, LEV appears to be well tolerated at 1000 mg daily, a dose that is predicted to be at least as active as MXF and GAT. A recent clinical trial to assess the early bactericidal activity (EBA) of these fluoroquinolones reinforces this pharmacodynamic argument. Over the first 7 days of monotherapy of smear-positive cavitary TB, LEV at 1000 mg daily was at least as active as GAT and MXF at 400 mg daily.[18] The activity of GAT and MXF was inferior to that of isoniazid (INH) during the first 2 days of treatment, but the activity of all fluoroquinolones was greater than that of INH between days 2 and 7. Although GAT is being evaluated in an ongoing phase II/III clinical trial, problems related to its effects on glucose homeostasis may prevent its future use. However, there is no *a priori* reason that MXF or LEV 1000 mg could not be used in its place.

Recent experimental data suggest that newer fluoroquinolones may play a role in potent new regimens that may permit the duration of treatment for active TB to be shortened, including MDR-TB, or that are effective against latent TB infection caused by MDR strains. MXF has been examined most intensively. In murine models using drug doses that are deemed equipotent to conventional human doses, MXF has the greatest activity among the fluoroquinolones tested to date (excluding GAT) and is as active against *M. tuberculosis* as INH.[19–24] These comparisons in

the murine model are reinforced by observations that the EBA of MXF during the first 2 days of therapy approaches that of INH, while between days 2 and 7, it exceeds that of INH.[18,25,26]

To determine whether MXF has a place in first-line treatment regimens, MXF was added or substituted for individual components of the standard regimen of rifampicin (RMP), INH and pyrazinamide (PZA) in long-term experiments in the murine model.[27,28] Remarkably, while addition of MXF to the standard regimen had a modest impact on bactericidal activity, substitution of MXF for INH dramatically improved activity. All mice treated with 4 months of RMP + MXF + PZA were cured, whereas 6 months of RMP + INH + PZA was necessary to achieve similar results.[28] These promising studies raise hopes that MXF might replace INH in the current short-course regimen and shorten the duration of TB therapy in humans to 4 months or less. The effect of substituting MXF for INH in the standard RMP + INH + PZA + ethambutol (EMB) regimen is currently being evaluated in two phase II clinical trials with primary efficacy end points related to sputum conversion over the initial 2 months of therapy.

A recent clinical trial investigating the substitution of MXF for EMB in combination with RMP + INH + PZA during the 2-month initial phase of therapy demonstrated a modestly more rapid sputum conversion in the MXF-treated patients, although similar proportions of patients were culture negative in both groups after 2 months of treatment.[29] Thus far, MXF has been well tolerated, although the number of patients treated beyond 2 months is limited.[30,31] A phase III trial is currently under way to determine whether an abbreviated regimen consisting of 2 months of RMP + INH + PZA + GAT followed by 2 months of RMP + INH + GAT is not inferior to 2 months of RMP + INH + PZA + EMB followed by 4 months of RMP + INH.

The fluoroquinolones are broad-spectrum antibiotics that inhibit bacterial topoisomerases, enzymes that are essential for efficient DNA replication. While most bacteria have two topoisomerase enzymes, *M. tuberculosis* has only one, DNA gyrase, encoded by *gyrA* and *gyrB*.[15] Fluoroquinolone resistance occurs via mutations in a conserved 320-bp region of *gyrA*. Resistance occurs spontaneously at a frequency of 2×10^{-6} to 1×10^{-8},[32–34] and reduces susceptibility to all fluoroquinolones.[35] Because of increasing use of fluoroquinolones for drug-resistant TB, as well as inadvertent usage for drug-susceptible TB that is misdiagnosed as bacterial pneumonia, fluoroquinolone resistance is emerging in *M. tuberculosis*. Selection of fluoroquinolone-resistant *M. tuberculosis* has occurred after less than 2 weeks of fluoroquinolone monotherapy,[36] raising concerns that widespread use of fluoroquinolones for treatment of other bacterial infections might undermine the potential clinical utility of the class for TB. Among 1852 isolates collected in 1995–2001 from the United States and Canada, 1.8 per cent were ciprofloxacin-resistant, most of them among MDR-TB isolates.[37] However, a concurrent study from a high-incidence TB area in the Philippines found that 27 per cent of all *M. tuberculosis* isolates and 51 per cent of MDR strains were fluoroquinolone resistant. Moreover, a four- to five-fold increase in fluoroquinolone resistance was noted for 1995–2000 compared with 1989–94, while resistance to the first-line drugs was not significantly different.[38] These findings suggest that the consequences of widespread fluoroquinolone use may be more serious in high-prevalence areas and raise concerns that the availability of fluoroquinolones for other indications may undermine the utility of fluoroquinolones for TB treatment.

RIFAMYCIN DERIVATIVES: RIFAPENTINE

RMP is considered the cornerstone of modern short-course TB therapy since its introduction permitted the duration of treatment to be shortened from 18–24 to 9 months. Its ability to sterilize tuberculous lesions of the persisting and otherwise drug-tolerant bacilli that remain viable despite intensive combination chemotherapy ('sterilizing activity') likely stems from its high-affinity binding to, and rapid inhibition of, the bacterial DNA-dependent RNA polymerase.

In the search for a widely spaced intermittent treatment to simplify supervised TB therapy, a number of rifamycin derivatives with much longer serum half-lives than that of RMP (2–4 hours) have been evaluated, including rifabutin (RBT), rifalazil (RLZ) and rifapentine (RPT). However, trials investigating twice-weekly RBT-based regimens or once-weekly RPT-based regimens have had disappointing results, due to acquired rifamycin resistance in patients with advanced HIV disease[39,40] and, in the case of once-weekly RPT, suboptimal efficacy in HIV-negative patients at high risk of relapse.[41] RBT is now used primarily as a substitute for RMP in patients who cannot use the latter drug because of drug–drug interactions or intolerance.[42] Use of RLZ was associated with the occurrence of a flu-like syndrome at 50 mg per day and limited activity at lower doses.[3,43] Because its side effects are considered prohibitive, RLZ is no longer under investigation for TB.

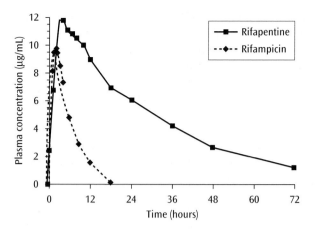

Figure 14.1 Rifampicin and rifapentine pharmacokinetics following a 600 mg dose in normal adults (from Ref. 3).

RPT was approved in 1998 for the treatment of TB as part of a once-weekly continuation phase regimen, but this regimen has seen little use because it is not recommended in patients with advanced HIV infection, cavitary TB or positive sputum cultures after the initial 2 months of treatment.[44] Interest is increasing, however, in the use of RPT in more frequently administered regimens, because RPT has greater *in vitro* activity than RMP, with four-fold lower MIC values[45–47] and a longer half-life of 14–18 hours which permits more sustained rifamycin exposure with intermittent dosing.[3]

Recent observational studies suggest that intermittent treatment with RMP-based short-course therapy is not as effective as daily therapy, particularly in patients at high risk for relapse.[2,48–50] Because RPT provides greater rifamycin exposure (as measured by free drug AUC/MIC) than RMP when administered at the same dose and frequency (Figure 14.1), Rosenthal *et al.*[51] set out to determine, in the murine model, the impact of substituting RPT for RMP in the largely twice-weekly regimens used for directly observed therapy in the USA. While a twice-weekly RMP-based regimen yielded significantly lower bactericidal activity than daily drug administration, the twice-weekly RPT-based regimen (15 mg/kg, equipotent to 900 mg in humans) resulted in activity that was as good as the daily RMP-based regimen. Moreover, a twice-weekly RPT-based regimen of 20 mg/kg (equipotent to 1200 mg in humans) showed greater activity than that of the daily RMP-based regimen.

Because low levels of isoniazid and rapid isoniazid acetylation were associated with relapse and selection of rifamycin-resistant mutants in patients receiving once-weekly RPT plus INH, it has been suggested that a more effective companion drug might improve once-weekly treatment regimens.[52] Because MXF has a half-life of 9–12 hours which approaches that of RPT and because substitution of MXF for INH substantially improves the activity of the RMP + INH + PZA regimen in the murine model,[28] MXF was also examined as a companion drug. Twice-weekly regimens in which RPT 15 or 20 mg/kg was combined with MXF instead of INH had even greater activity. Mice treated for 4 months with predominantly twice-weekly regimens based on RPT 15 mg/kg were free of relapse, whereas 6 months of treatment with the standard daily regimen were required to prevent relapse among all mice. These data raise the exciting prospect that twice- or thrice-weekly regimens based on RPT at 15 or 20 mg/kg may be significantly more active than daily RMP-based regimens and may permit intermittent regimens that are shorter than 6 months.

In this regard, the registration trial performed by the sponsor to obtain regulatory approval showed that twice-weekly administration of RPT at 10 mg/kg for 2 months was safe and well tolerated. A subsequent trial examined the pharmacokinetics, safety and tolerability of escalating RPT doses, from 600 to 1200 mg, administered once weekly with INH during the continuation phase of therapy in HIV-negative patients with TB. All regimens were well tolerated and only one patient receiving 1200 mg stopped treatment because of a possible drug-related adverse event.[53] Another clinical study has shown that RPT 900 mg/INH 900 mg once-weekly for 3 months may provide effective and better tolerated treatment for LTBI (latent tuberculosis infection), with efficacy comparable to that of 2 months of daily RMP and PZA.[54] Overall, the results suggest that 600 mg of RPT twice weekly and 900–1200 mg of RPT once weekly are safe and well tolerated. It will be important to determine the safety and efficacy of administering 900–1200 mg of RPT twice or thrice weekly, as this could form the basis for new treatment regimens that are shorter than the current 6-month course.

TMC207, A DIARYLQUINOLINE

The diarylquinolines are a newly identified class of compounds with antimycobacterial properties. Structurally and mechanistically, they differ from the fluoroquinolones and other quinolines. The most active diarylquinoline is TMC207 (also called R207910), which has specific activity against mycobacteria, with a remarkably broad spectrum of activity within the genus. Against M. tuberculosis, the MIC is 0.03 to 0.12 μg/mL and rivals that of INH.

TMC207 acts through a novel mechanism: inhibition of the mycobacterial F1F0 proton ATP synthase, an essential enzyme of M. tuberculosis.[55] Resistant mutants are selected at a frequency of 5×10^{-8} in vitro and harbour mutations in the atpE gene. Importantly, there is no evidence of cross-resistance with existing TB drugs.

TMC207 displays time-dependent bactericidal activity both in vitro and in vivo. In the murine model, 25 mg/kg of TMC207 daily for 1 or 2 months is more active than conventional doses of INH or RMP and at least as active as the first-line combination regimen, RMP + INH + PZA. Substitution of TMC207 for any of the three first-line

drugs significantly increases potency. The synergistic activity with PZA is particularly impressive, consistent with the observation that N,N'-dicyclohexylcarbodiimide – which inhibits the same chain of the F0 moiety of F1F0 ATPase as TMC207 – has synergy with PZA against M. tuberculosis.[56] Long-term studies in the murine model are needed to assess the ability of TMC207-containing regimens to prevent relapse and confirm the sterilizing activity of TMC207 in combination with both first- and second-line agents and its potential to shorten the duration of therapy.

Importantly, pharmacokinetic studies in humans have shown TMC207 to be well absorbed after oral administration, with linear kinetics up to the highest dose tested (700 mg), although steady state is not reached before 14 days of treatment. Daily doses of 100–400 mg are well tolerated after administration for up to 2 weeks and appear to provide drug exposure that is at least similar to that obtained with 25 mg/kg/day in the mouse.[55]

To determine the EBA of TMC207, patients with smear-positive pulmonary TB were treated for 7 days with INH 300 mg, RMP 600 mg, or TMC207 at 25, 100 or 400 mg. Unlike INH and RMP, TMC207 had no effect on viable bacterial counts in sputum until after the fourth day of treatment and then only at doses of 100 and 400 mg. The daily fall in sputum bacterial burden observed with TMC207 400 mg from day 4 onwards looked similar to that observed with INH or RMP from day 1 onwards. While these results might appear discouraging, they may reflect the time required for TMC207 to attain steady-state concentrations, as well as its time-dependent activity.[57] In addition, the magnitude of a drug's EBA may have no bearing on its potential to sterilize the lung of persistent bacilli and therefore shorten the duration of treatment.

Because of its potent activity against M. tuberculosis, its distinct mechanism of action, and its impressive activity at what appear to be human-equipotent dosages in the murine model, TMC207 is a particularly promising new drug candidate. One drawback is a drug–drug interaction with RMP that reduces the bioavailability of TMC207 by 50 per cent upon co-administration.

NITROIMIDAZOLE DERIVATIVES: PA-824 AND OPC-67683

Two nitroimidazole derivatives have recently advanced to human testing for the treatment of TB. The nitroimidazo-oxazine PA-824 was identified as the most active compound from a library of 328 3-substituted nitroimidazopyran derivatives of lead compound CGI-17341, using a novel murine model.[58,59] Importantly, it does not appear to have the mutagenic potential of the parent compound. In 2002, the Global Alliance for TB Drug Development licensed PA-824 and related nitroimidazole compounds from Chiron (Emeryville, CA, USA) for further development as antituberculosis drugs.

PA-824 has three key characteristics: (1) a unique mechanism of action, (2) a narrow spectrum of activity and (3) no cross-resistance with current antituberculosis drugs.[59] Like metronidazole, PA-824 is a pro-drug, requiring nitroreductive activation by a bacterial F420-dependent mechanism. The active moiety or moieties appear to inhibit the synthesis of proteins and cell wall lipids through an unknown mechanism.[59] Resistance to PA-824 arises spontaneously at a frequency of approximately 1×10^{-6}, similar to that observed for INH, implying a low barrier to emergence of resistance.[59] Most mutants selected in vitro have mutations in Rv0407 (which encodes the glucose-6-phosphate dehydrogenase, FGD1, responsible for reduction of F420), others have mutations in Rv3261 and/or Rv3262 (which encode FbiA and FbiB, respectively, and are necessary for synthesis of F420) or in Rv3547, which encodes a conserved hypothetical protein with no known function.[59–61]

PA-824 has a narrow spectrum of activity that is limited to the M. tuberculosis complex. Against M. tuberculosis, including MDR-TB isolates, the MIC is 0.015–0.25 µg/mL, indicating a lack of cross-resistance with current antituberculosis agents.[59,62] PA-824 has bactericidal activity against replicating and static M. tuberculosis.[59,62]

In murine models, PA-824 has dose-dependent bactericidal activity during the initial phase of treatment that, at 100 mg/kg/day, approaches that of INH. In a murine model of the continuation phase of therapy, the activity of 100 mg/kg of PA-824 approached that of RMP and INH in combination, which indicates significant activity against non-replicating persistent bacilli,[63] and suggests good sterilizing activity. Compared with the standard regimen of RMP + INH + PZA, substitution of PA-824 for INH led to significantly lower lung bacterial counts after 2 months of treatment and more rapid culture conversion. However, there was no difference in the proportion of mice relapsing after 6 months of therapy.[64] No other PA-824-containing regimen tested was superior to the standard regimen on any assessment. Therefore, the potential role for PA-824 in a treatment-shortening regimen that includes two or more current first-line drugs remains unclear. In the murine model, PA-824 also combines well with MXF and PZA, suggesting that PA-824 or other nitroimidazole derivatives may represent an important building block for novel regimens that are active against MDR-TB and/or circumvent the drug interactions that plague the rifamycins. PA-824 is currently in phase I clinical testing. If it proves to be safe and well tolerated, additional preclinical studies are needed to evaluate PA-824 at the human equipotent dosage in order to better define its potential contribution to therapy. A better understanding of the pharmacodynamics of PA-824's antituberculosis activity would also contribute to the clinical development of this and other nitroimidazole derivatives.

OPC-67683 is a nitroimidazo-oxazole that has advanced to phase II testing. It appears to have a mechanism of action like that of PA-824, but is as much as 20 times more potent.[65] Cross-resistance between PA-824 and OPC-67683 is anticipated. As described for PA-824, preliminary data from the murine model suggest that substitution of OPC-67683 for INH in the standard regimen of RMP + INH + PZA results in greater bactericidal activity and more rapid culture conversion.[65]

SQ109, A DIETHYLAMINE

SQ109 is an investigational new drug candidate that was identified from a library of over 60 000 combinatorial compounds, based on a 1,2-ethylenediamine pharmacophore from ethambutol. However, only the diamine nucleus remains and studies to date suggest that SQ109 should not necessarily be considered a second-generation EMB analogue.

Although its mechanism of action involves cell wall inhibition, the specific target of SQ109 remains unknown. In vitro, it has an MIC range of 0.11–0.64 µg/mL against M. tuberculosis, including strains resistant to INH, RMP or EMB.[66] It inhibits growth of M. tuberculosis in macrophages to a similar extent as INH and to a greater extent than EMB.[66,67] In vitro, at sub-MIC concentrations, SQ109 demonstrates synergy with RMP and INH and additive activity with streptomycin, but neutral effects with EMB and PZA. Some synergy between SQ109 and RMP is also evident against RMP-resistant strains.[68]

SQ109 has demonstrated activity in murine models, where it is at least four times as potent as EMB, as 25 mg/kg of SQ109 and 100 mg/kg of EMB have similar effects.[66] Substitution of SQ109 for EMB enhances the activity of the standard four-drug 2-month initial regimen of RMP + INH + PZA + EMB.[69] The activity of SQ109 in the mouse is particularly remarkable, given the low serum concentrations. This is presumably because the drug has a rapid tissue distribution that results in sustained concentrations in lungs and spleen that exceed the MIC.[67]

In summary, although it was synthesized as an EMB derivative, SQ109 may differ from EMB in its mechanism of action, pharmacokinetics and pharmacodynamics. It is currently in phase I testing. Provided it is safe and well tolerated, it will be important to assess its ability to prevent relapse in animal models and to accelerate sputum culture conversion in human clinical trials.

LL-3858, A PYRROLE

Pyrrole derivatives have demonstrated activity against M. tuberculosis in vitro.[3] Recently, a substituted pyrrole derivative, LL-3858, has advanced to phase I testing for TB. Preliminary data suggest that LL-3858 has potent in vitro activity, with an MIC range of 0.06–0.5 µg/mL against M. tuberculosis, including MDR strains.[70] Monotherapy in a murine model of TB yielded bactericidal activity at doses well below the toxic threshold. Moreover, addition of LL-

3858 significantly enhanced the sterilizing activity of the standard INH + RMP + PZA regimen.[70] Further news on this compound is eagerly awaited.

OXAZOLIDINONES

The oxazolidinones are a new class of synthetic antibiotics with broad activity against Gram-positive bacteria and mycobacteria through a unique mechanism of ribosomal protein synthesis inhibition. Other positive attributes include high oral bioavailability and lack of cross-resistance with existing antibiotics. Linezolid is the first oxazolidinone to be used clinically, although it is not approved for use in TB. Its MIC for *M. tuberculosis* is 0.125–1 µg/mL, with an MIC_{50} of 0.5 µg/mL and an MIC_{90} of 1 µg/mL.[71–73] Previous pharmacokinetic work suggests that 100 mg/kg of oral linezolid in mice is equivalent to 600 mg orally in humans.[74–77] Administration of 50 mg/kg of linezolid daily to infected mice, beginning the day after intravenous infection, failed to prevent growth of *M. tuberculosis*.[73] However, 100 mg/kg once daily appeared to be bacteriostatic or weakly bactericidal, causing approximately 1–1.5 log reduction in bacterial counts over 28 days in another study.[72] These results are supported by anecdotal reports that 600 mg of linezolid orally twice daily in salvage regimens for MDR-TB has been associated with sputum culture conversion and cure, albeit with frequent dose- or treatment-limiting side effects such as anaemia, thrombocytopenia and peripheral or optic neuropathy.[78,79]

Linezolid is not the most potent oxazolidinone against *M. tuberculosis*. In the mouse model, PNU-100480 was more active than linezolid and, at 100 mg/kg daily, had activity similar to that of INH 25 mg/kg or RMP 20 mg/kg.[72] Importantly, the activity could be considered bactericidal because just 28 days of therapy produced a >2 $\log_{10}$ reduction in bacterial counts. While PNU-100480 provided no additive activity when combined with INH, it had a modest additive effect with RMP (approximately a 0.5 log reduction in bacterial number). This effect is supported by *in vitro* studies and may be more significant if PNU-100480 is combined with a lower, more clinically relevant dose of RMP of 10 mg/kg.

Together these results suggest that the oxazolidinones could contribute to treatment of drug-susceptible and MDR-TB. Although PNU-100480 has yet to be developed for clinical use, ongoing efforts to produce analogues with more potent and selective antituberculosis activity and less toxicity could be rewarding.

CONCLUSIONS

For the first time in 40 years, several new drugs with promising attributes have entered the clinical development pipeline for the treatment of TB. With good fortune, one or more of these agents will fulfil or exceed its potential demonstrated in animal models and provide a new cornerstone for the treatment of TB. Additional candidates are percolating up through discovery and preclinical development programmes. Despite the apparent robustness of this portfolio, many challenges must be overcome before any of these new drugs contributes meaningfully to control of TB. Beyond bringing a new drug to market, defining the most appropriate use of new agents and assuring the availability and reliability of the best new regimens in the areas that need them most will require an unprecedented level of cooperation between drug sponsors, those who conduct clinical trials, funding agencies and national treatment programmes.

LEARNING POINTS

- The main objectives of TB drug development are to shorten the current 6- to 9-month duration of treatment for active TB and the current 3- to 9-month duration of treatment for latent TB infection, improve the treatment of MDR-TB and to reduce the potential for drug–drug interactions with antiretroviral agents.

- Desirable characteristics of new TB drugs include unique mechanisms of action, improved potency against dormant tubercle bacilli, longer elimination half-lives, no cross-resistance with existing drugs and few interactions with antiretroviral agents.

- Newer fluoroquinolones have potent bactericidal activity against *M. tuberculosis* and have demonstrated the potential to shorten the duration of treatment. However, resistance to fluoroquinolones has occurred as a result of inappropriate use and selective pressure, especially in areas where the incidence of TB is high.

- Rifapentine has more potent *in vitro* activity than rifampicin and a longer half-life of 14–18 hours. Although it is currently approved for once-weekly administration at 600 mg in the continuation phase of treatment, regimens employing more frequent administration, sometimes with higher doses, may have the potential to shorten the duration of treatment.

- For the first time in 40 years, several novel drug candidates from new antibiotic classes are in clinical testing for TB. Each of these compounds has some potential to shorten the duration of treatment in animal models of TB and has no cross-resistance with current antituberculosis drugs.

- The diarylquinoline TMC207 has a distinct mechanism of action, is more active than INH or RMP in the murine model and has excellent synergistic activity with PZA. However, RMP reduces its bioavailability.

> - The nitroimidazole derivative, PA-824, has a unique mechanism of action and a narrow spectrum of activity limited to the *M. tuberculosis* complex. Studies of the continuation phase of therapy in murine models suggest that it has significant sterilizing activity. OPC-67683 has a mechanism of action similar to that of PA-824, but is more potent.
> - The diethylamine SQ109 and the pyrrole LL-3858 also have promising antituberculosis activity, but less information is available about these agents than about TMC207 and PA-824.

REFERENCES

1. Corbett EL, Watt CJ, Walker N et al. The growing burden of tuberculosis: global trends and interactions with the HIV epidemic. *Arch Intern Med* 2003; **163**: 1009–21.
2. Chang KC, Leung CC, Yew WW et al. Dosing schedules of 6-month regimens and relapse for pulmonary tuberculosis. *Am J Respir Crit Care Med* 2006; **174**: 1153–8.
3. O'Brien RJ, Spigelman M. New drugs for tuberculosis: current status and future prospects. *Clin Chest Med* 2005; **26**: 327–40, vii.
4. Cole ST, Brosch R, Parkhill J et al. Deciphering the biology of *Mycobacterium tuberculosis* from the complete genome sequence. *Nature* 1998; **393**: 537–44.
5. Jacobs WR Jr, Kalpana GV, Cirillo JD et al. Genetic systems for mycobacteria. *Methods Enzymol* 1991; **204**: 537–55.
6. Mollenkopf HJ, Mattow J, Schaible UE et al. Mycobacterial proteomes. *Methods Enzymol* 2002; **358**: 242–56.
7. Sassetti CM, Rubin EJ. Genetic requirements for mycobacterial survival during infection. *Proc Natl Acad Sci U S A* 2003; **100**: 12989–94.
8. Lamichhane G, Tyagi S, Bishai WR. Designer arrays for defined mutant analysis to detect genes essential for survival of *Mycobacterium tuberculosis* in mouse lungs. *Infect Immun* 2005; **73**: 2533–40.
9. Ballell L, Field RA, Duncan K, Young RJ. New small-molecule synthetic antimycobacterials. *Antimicrob Agents Chemother* 2005; **49**: 2153–63.
10. Tomioka H. Current status of some antituberculosis drugs and the development of new antituberculous agents with special reference to their *in vitro* and *in vivo* antimicrobial activities. *Curr Pharm Des* 2006; **12**: 4047–70.
11. Chiang CY, Enarson DJ, Yu MC et al. Outcome of pulmonary multidrug-resistant tuberculosis: a 6-yr follow-up study. *Eur Respir J* 2006; **28**: 980–5.
12. Yew WW, Chan CK, Chau CH et al. Outcomes of patients with multidrug-resistant pulmonary tuberculosis treated with ofloxacin/levofloxacin-containing regimens. *Chest* 2000; **117**: 744–51.
13. Tahaoglu K, Törün T, Sevim T et al. The treatment of multidrug-resistant tuberculosis in Turkey. *N Engl J Med* 2001; **345**: 170–4.
14. Chan ED, Laurel V, Strand MJ et al. Treatment and outcome analysis of 205 patients with multidrug-resistant tuberculosis. *Am J Respir Crit Care Med* 2004; **169**: 1103–9.
15. Aubry A, Pan XS, Fisher LM et al. *Mycobacterium tuberculosis* DNA gyrase: interaction with quinolones and correlation with antimycobacterial drug activity. *Antimicrob Agents Chemother* 2004; **48**: 1281–8.
16. Hu Y, Coates AR, Mitchison DA. Sterilizing activities of fluoroquinolones against rifampin-tolerant populations of *Mycobacterium tuberculosis*. *Antimicrob Agents Chemother* 2003; **47**: 653–7.
17. Nuermberger E, Grosset J. Pharmacokinetic and pharmacodynamic issues in the treatment of mycobacterial infections. *Eur J Clin Microbiol Infect Dis* 2004; **23**: 243–55.
18. Johnson JL, Hadad DJ, Boom WH et al. Early and extended early bactericidal activity of levofloxacin, gatifloxacin and moxifloxacin in pulmonary tuberculosis. *Int J Tuberc Lung Dis* 2006; **10**: 605–12.
19. Miyazaki E, Miyazaki M, Chen JM et al. Moxifloxacin (BAY12-8039), a new 8-methoxyquinolone, is active in a mouse model of tuberculosis. *Antimicrob Agents Chemother* 1999; **43**: 85–9.
20. Ji B, Lounis N, Maslo C et al. *In vitro* and *in vivo* activities of moxifloxacin and clinafloxacin against *Mycobacterium tuberculosis*. *Antimicrob Agents Chemother* 1998; **42**: 2066–9.
21. Lounis N, Bentoucha A, Truffot-Pernot C et al. Effectiveness of once-weekly rifapentine and moxifloxacin regimens against *Mycobacterium tuberculosis* in mice. *Antimicrob Agents Chemother* 2001; **45**: 3482–6.
22. Yoshimatsu T, Nuermberger E, Tyagi S et al. Bactericidal activity of increasing daily and weekly doses of moxifloxacin in murine tuberculosis. *Antimicrob Agents Chemother* 2002; **46**: 1875–9.
23. Alvirez-Freites EJ, Carter JL, Cynamon MH. *In vitro* and *in vivo* activities of gatifloxacin against *Mycobacterium tuberculosis*. *Antimicrob Agents Chemother* 2002; **46**: 1022–5.
24. Lenaerts AJ, Gruppo V, Brooks JV, Orme IM. Rapid *in vivo* screening of experimental drugs for tuberculosis using gamma interferon gene-disrupted mice. *Antimicrob Agents Chemother* 2003; **47**: 783–5.
25. Gosling RD, Uiso LO, Sam NE et al. The bactericidal activity of moxifloxacin in patients with pulmonary tuberculosis. *Am J Respir Crit Care Med* 2003; **168**: 1342–5.
26. Pletz MW, De Roux A, Roth A et al. Early bactericidal activity of moxifloxacin in treatment of pulmonary tuberculosis: a prospective, randomized study. *Antimicrob Agents Chemother* 2004; **48**: 780–2.
27. Nuermberger EL, Yoshimatsu T, Tyagi S et al. Moxifloxacin-containing regimen greatly reduces time to culture conversion in murine tuberculosis. *Am J Respir Crit Care Med* 2004; **169**: 421–6.
28. Nuermberger EL, Yoshimatsu T, Tyagi S et al. Moxifloxacin-containing regimens of reduced duration produce a stable cure in murine tuberculosis. *Am J Respir Crit Care Med* 2004; **170**: 1131–4.
29. Burman WJ, Goldberg S, Johnson JL et al. Moxifloxacin versus ethambutol in the first 2 months of treatment for pulmonary tuberculosis. *Am J Respir Crit Care Med* 2006; **174**: 331–8.
30. Codecasa LR, Ferrara G, Ferrarese M et al. Long-term moxifloxacin in complicated tuberculosis patients with adverse reactions or resistance to first line drugs. *Respir Med* 2006; **100**: 1566–72.
31. Valerio G, Bracciale P, Manisco V et al. Long-term tolerance and effectiveness of moxifloxacin therapy for tuberculosis: preliminary results. *J Chemother* 2003; **15**: 66–70.
32. Jacobs MR. Activity of quinolones against mycobacteria. *Drugs* 1999; **58** (Suppl. 2): 19–22.
33. Alangaden GJ, Manavathu EK, Vakulenko SB et al. Characterization of fluoroquinolone-resistant mutant strains of *Mycobacterium tuberculosis* selected in the laboratory and isolated from patients. *Antimicrob Agents Chemother* 1995; **39**: 1700–3.
34. Williams KJ, Chan R, Piddock LJ. gyrA of ofloxacin-resistant clinical isolates of *Mycobacterium tuberculosis* from Hong Kong. *J Antimicrob Chemother* 1996; **37**: 1032–4.
35. Rastogi N, Ross BC, Dwyer B et al. Emergence during unsuccessful chemotherapy of multiple drug resistance in a strain of *Mycobacterium tuberculosis*. *Eur J Clin Microbiol Infect Dis* 1992; **11**: 901–7.
36. Ginsburg AS, Woolwine SC, Hooper N et al. The rapid development of fluoroquinolone resistance in *M. tuberculosis*. *N Engl J Med* 2003; **349**: 1977–8.
37. Bozeman L, Burman W, Metchock B et al. Tuberculosis Trials

Consortium. Fluoroquinolone susceptibility among *Mycobacterium tuberculosis* isolates from the United States and Canada. *Clin Infect Dis* 2005; **40**: 386–91.

38. Grimaldo ER, Tupasi TE, Rivera AB *et al*. Increased resistance to ciprofloxacin and ofloxacin in multidrug-resistant *Mycobacterium tuberculosis* isolates from patients seen at a tertiary hospital in the Philippines. *Int J Tuberc Lung Dis* 2001; **5**: 546–50.

39. Vernon A, Burman W, Benator D *et al*. Acquired rifamycin monoresistance in patients with HIV-related tuberculosis treated with once-weekly rifapentine and isoniazid. Tuberculosis Trials Consortium. *Lancet* 1999; **353**: 1843–7.

40. Centers for Disease Control and Prevention (CDC). Acquired rifamycin resistance in persons with advanced HIV disease being treated for active tuberculosis with intermittent rifamycin-based regimens. *MMWR Morb Mortal Wkly Rep* 2002; **51**: 214–5.

41. Benator D, Battacharya M, Bozeman L *et al*. Rifapentine and isoniazid once a week versus rifampicin and isoniazid twice a week for treatment of drug-susceptible pulmonary tuberculosis in HIV-negative patients: a randomised clinical trial. *Lancet* 2002; **360**: 528–34.

42. Center for Disease Control and Prevention (CDC). Updated guidelines for the use of rifabutin or rifampin for the treatment and prevention of tuberculosis among HIV-infected patients taking protease inhibitors or nonnucleoside reverse transcriptase inhibitors. *MMWR Morb Mortal Wkly Rep* 2000; **49**: 185–9.

43. Dietze R, Teixeira L, Rocha LM *et al*. Safety and bactericidal activity of rifalazil in patients with pulmonary tuberculosis. *Antimicrob Agents Chemother* 2001; **45**: 1972–6.

44. Blumberg HM, Burman WJ, Chaisson RE *et al*. American Thoracic Society/Centers for Disease Control and Prevention/Infectious Diseases Society of America: treatment of tuberculosis. *Am J Respir Crit Care Med* 2003; **167**: 603–62.

45. Dickinson JM, Mitchison DA. *In vitro* properties of rifapentine (MDL473) relevant to its use in intermittent chemotherapy of tuberculosis. *Tubercle* 1987; **68**: 113–8.

46. Heifets LB, Lindholm-Levy PJ, Flory MA. Bactericidal activity *in vitro* of various rifamycins against *Mycobacterium avium* and *Mycobacterium tuberculosis*. *Am Rev Respir Dis* 1990; **141**: 626–30.

47. Bemer-Melchior P, Bryskier A, Drugeon HB. Comparison of the *in vitro* activities of rifapentine and rifampicin against *Mycobacterium tuberculosis* complex. *J Antimicrob Chemother* 2000; **46**: 571–6.

48. Hong Kong Chest Service/British Medical Research Council. Five-year follow-up of a controlled trial of five 6-month regimens of chemotherapy for pulmonary tuberculosis. *Am Rev Respir Dis* 1987; **136**: 1339–42.

49. Chang KC, Leung CC, Yew WW *et al*. A nested case-control study on treatment-related risk factors for early relapse of tuberculosis. *Am J Respir Crit Care Med* 2004; **170**: 1124–30.

50. Li J, Munsiff SS, Driver CR, Sackoff J. Relapse and acquired rifampin resistance in HIV-infected patients with tuberculosis treated with rifampin- or rifabutin-based regimens in New York City, 1997–2000. *Clin Infect Dis* 2005; **41**: 83–91.

51. Rosenthal IM, Williams K, Tyagi A *et al*. Potent twice-weekly rifapentine-containing regimens in murine tuberculosis. *Am J Respir Crit Care Med* 2006; **174**: 94–101.

52. Weiner M, Burman W, Vernon A *et al*. Low isoniazid concentrations and outcome of tuberculosis treatment with once-weekly isoniazid and rifapentine. *Am J Respir Crit Care Med* 2003; **167**: 1341–7.

53. Bock NN, Sterling TR, Hamilton CD *et al*. A prospective, randomized, double-blind study of the tolerability of rifapentine 600, 900, and 1,200 mg plus isoniazid in the continuation phase of tuberculosis treatment. *Am J Respir Crit Care Med* 2002; **165**: 1526–30.

54. Schechter M, Zajdenverg R, Falco G *et al*. Weekly rifapentine/isoniazid or daily rifampin/pyrazinamide for latent tuberculosis in household contacts. *Am J Respir Crit Care Med* 2006; **173**: 922–6.

55. Andries K, Verhasselt P, Guillemont J *et al*. A diarylquinoline drug active on the ATP synthase of *Mycobacterium tuberculosis*. *Science* 2005; **307**: 223–7.

56. Zhang Y, Wade MM, Scorpio A *et al*. Mode of action of pyrazinamide: disruption of *Mycobacterium tuberculosis* membrane transport and energetics by pyrazinoic acid. *J Antimicrob Chemother* 2003; **52**: 790–5.

57. Diacon AH, McNeeley DF, Kerstens R *et al*. Early bactericidal activity , tolerabilibty, and pharmacokinetics of the investigational diarylquinoline TMC207. 37th World Conference International Union of TB and Lung Disease, Paris, 2006.

58. Ashtekar DR, Costa-Perira R, Nagrajan K *et al*. In vitro and in vivo activities of the nitroimidazole CGI 17341 against *Mycobacterium tuberculosis*. *Antimicrob Agents Chemother* 1993; **37**: 183–6.

59. Stover CK, Warrener P, VanDevanter DR *et al*. A small-molecule nitroimidazopyran drug candidate for the treatment of tuberculosis. *Nature* 2000; **405**: 962–6.

60. Choi KP, Bair TB, Bae YM, Daniels L. Use of transposon Tn5367 mutagenesis and a nitroimidazopyran-based selection system to demonstrate a requirement for fbiA and fbiB in coenzyme F(420) biosynthesis by *Mycobacterium bovis* BCG. *J Bacteriol* 2001; **183**: 7058–66.

61. Manjunatha UH, Boshoff H, Dowd CS *et al*. Identification of a nitroimidazo-oxazine-specific protein involved in PA-824 resistance in *Mycobacterium tuberculosis*. *Proc Natl Acad Sci U S A* 2006; **103**: 431–6.

62. Lenaerts AJ, Gruppo V, Marietta KS *et al*. Preclinical testing of the nitroimidazopyran PA-824 for activity against *Mycobacterium tuberculosis* in a series of *in vitro* and *in vivo* models. *Antimicrob Agents Chemother* 2005; **49**: 2294–301.

63. Tyagi S, Nuermberger E, Yoshimatsu T *et al*. Bactericidal activity of the nitroimidazopyran PA-824 in a murine model of tuberculosis. *Antimicrob Agents Chemother* 2005; **49**: 2289–93.

64. Nuermberger E, Rosenthal I, Tyagi S *et al*. Combination chemotherapy with the nitroimidazopyran PA-824 and first-line drugs in a murine model of tuberculosis. *Antimicrob Agents Chemother* 2006; **50**: 2621–5.

65. Matsumoto M, Hashizume H, Tomishige T *et al*. OPC-67683, a nitro-dihydro-imidazooxazole derivative with promising action against tuberculosis in vitro and in mice. *PLoS Med* 2006; **3**: e466.

66. Protopopova M, Hanrahan C, Nikonenko B *et al*. Identification of a new antitubercular drug candidate, SQ109, from a combinatorial library of 1,2-ethylenediamines. *J Antimicrob Chemother* 2005; **56**: 968–74.

67. Jia L, Tomaszewski JE, Hanrahan C *et al*. Pharmacodynamics and pharmacokinetics of SQ109, a new diamine-based antitubercular drug. *Br J Pharmacol* 2005; **144**: 80–7.

68. Chen P, Gearhart J, Protopopova M *et al*. Synergistic interactions of SQ109, a new ethylene diamine, with front-line antitubercular drugs *in vitro*. *J Antimicrob Chemother* 2006; **58**: 332–7.

69. Nikonenko BV, Protopopova M, Samala R *et al*. Drug therapy of experimental TB: improved outcome by combining SQ109, a new diamine antibiotic with existing TB drugs. *Antimicrob Agents Chemother* 2006; **51**: 1563–5.

70. Arora S. Eradication of *Mycobacterium tuberculosis* infection in 2 months with LL-3858: a preclinical study. *Int J Tuberc Lung Dis* 2004; **8** (Suppl. 1): S29.

71. Alcalá L, Ruiz-Serrano MJ, Pérez-Fernández Turégano C *et al*. In vitro activities of linezolid against clinical isolates of *Mycobacterium tuberculosis* that are susceptible or resistant to first-line antituberculous drugs. *Antimicrob Agents Chemother* 2003; **47**: 416–7.

72. Cynamon MH, Klemens SP, Sharpe CA, Chase S. Activities of several novel oxazolidinones against *Mycobacterium tuberculosis* in a murine model. *Antimicrob Agents Chemother* 1999; **43**: 1189–91.

73. Fattorini L, Tan D, Iona E *et al.* Activities of moxifloxacin alone and in combination with other antimicrobial agents against multidrug-resistant *Mycobacterium tuberculosis* infection in BALB/c mice. *Antimicrob Agents Chemother* 2003; **47**: 360–2.

74. Andes D, van Ogtrob NL, Peng J, Craig WA. *In vivo* pharmacodynamics of a new oxazolidinone (linezolid). *Antimicrob Agents Chemother* 2002; **46**: 3484–9.

75. Gee T, Ellis R, Marshall G *et al.* Pharmacokinetics and tissue penetration of linezolid following multiple oral doses. *Antimicrob Agents Chemother* 2001; **45**: 1843–6.

76. Slatter JG, Adams LA, Bush EC *et al.* Pharmacokinetics, toxicokinetics, distribution, metabolism and excretion of linezolid in mouse, rat and dog. *Xenobiotica* 2002; **32**: 907–24.

77. Stalker DJ, Jungbluth GL, Hopkins NK Batts DH. Pharmacokinetics and tolerance of single- and multiple-dose oral or intravenous linezolid, an oxazolidinone antibiotic, in healthy volunteers. *J Antimicrob Chemother* 2003; **51**: 1239–46.

78. Fortún J, Martín-Dávila P, Navas E *et al.* Linezolid for the treatment of multidrug-resistant tuberculosis. *J Antimicrob Chemother* 2005; **56**: 180–5.

79. von der Lippe B, Sandven P, Brubakk O. Efficacy and safety of linezolid in multidrug resistant tuberculosis (MDR-TB) – a report of ten cases. *J Infect* 2006; **52**: 92–6.

80. Lubasch A, Keller I, Borner K *et al.* Comparative pharmacokinetics of ciprofloxacin, gatifloxacin, grepafloxacin, levofloxacin, trovafloxacin, and moxifloxacin after single oral administration in healthy volunteers. *Antimicrob Agents Chemother* 2000; **44**: 2600–603.

81. Fish DN, Chow AT. The clinical pharmacokinetics of levofloxacin. *Clin Pharmacokinet* 1997; **32**: 101–19.

15

International standards for tuberculosis care: integrating tuberculosis care and control

PHILIP C HOPEWELL, ELIZABETH L FAIR AND MADHUKAR PAI

INTRODUCTION

Provision of care to patients with or suspected of having tuberculosis is the key element in the public health response to tuberculosis and is the cornerstone of tuberculosis control. Only by prompt and accurate diagnoses and effective treatment can the spread of tuberculosis be minimized and the development of drug resistance halted, thereby enabling the disease to be controlled. Substandard care will result in poor patient outcomes, continued infectiousness with transmission of *Mycobacterium tuberculosis* to others, and generation and propagation of drug resistance, all leading to ineffective disease control.

Reports describing the emergence of tuberculosis caused by *M. tuberculosis* that is resistant not only to isoniazid and rifampicin, the definition of multiple drug resistance (MDR), but also to the fluoroquinolones and at least one of the second-line injectable agents (kanamycin, amikacin, capreomycin), designated extensively drug-resistant (XDR) tuberculosis, have gained a good deal of recent attention.[1–3] The emergence of XDR tuberculosis is alarming but not unexpected as the root cause of the problem is poor tuberculosis management practices which are an internationally acknowledged problem.

PRINCIPLES OF TUBERCULOSIS CARE AND THE INTERNATIONAL STANDARDS FOR TUBERCULOSIS CARE

The basic principles of care for people with, or suspected of having, tuberculosis are the same worldwide: a diagnosis should be established promptly and accurately. Standardized treatment regimens of proven efficacy should be used, together with appropriate treatment support and supervision to assure successful completion of the prescribed regimen. The response to treatment should be monitored and the essential public health responsibilities must be carried out. As an approach to improving the care of patients with tuberculosis, these principles have been utilized as the foundation for a set of evidence-based standards, the International Standards for Tuberculosis Care (ISTC).[4,5] Since its release in 2006, the ISTC has been endorsed by more than 40 international and national organizations, including the World Health Organization (WHO), the Stop TB Partnership, the International Union against Tuberculosis and Lung Disease (IUATLD), the US Centers for Disease Control and Prevention, the International Council of Nurses and the World Care Council, a patient organization. In addition, the ISTC has been endorsed by a number of the world's medical professional societies of both general physicians and specialists in respiratory medicine, infectious diseases and other areas, and a number of national tuberculosis control programmes. This broad range of endorsers is indicative of wide acceptance of the approach to patient care described in the ISTC.

The purpose of the ISTC is to describe a widely endorsed level of care that all practitioners, public and private, should seek to achieve in managing patients who have, or are suspected of having, tuberculosis. The ISTC is not intended to replace either WHO or local guidelines and was written to accommodate local differences in practice. The main target audience for the ISTC is the broad group of health-care professionals who provide diagnostic and treatment services for tuberculosis outside government tuberculosis programmes. It is anticipated that the ISTC will be used as a tool to unify approaches to tuberculosis care between public (at least government tuberculosis control programmes) and private providers. Although the standards themselves should not be modified, clearly there will need to be local approaches to their use and implementation. For example, in a number of countries, professional medical societies are very influential and can serve as a conduit through which the standards can be disseminated. Moreover, professional societies can serve to exert peer pressure both on their members and, when necessary, on government programmes to adhere to the ISTC. Another anticipated use of the ISTC is to serve as a focus of curricula for medical, nursing and allied health students, as well as for in-service education.

The ISTC was developed by a 28 member steering committee that, during a period of 15 months, examined existing evidence and, for some topics, commissioned systematic reviews. The result was agreement on a group of 17 standards: six addressing diagnosis, nine addressing treatment and two addressing public health responsibilities. Perhaps as its main message, the document emphasizes that any clinician who provides services for tuberculosis is assuming an important public health function. It is evident that care of the quality specified in the ISTC could have prevented the emergence of XDR tuberculosis.[2]

RATIONALE FOR USE OF THE ISTC IN THE PRIVATE AND PUBLIC SECTORS

Studies of the performance of the private sector in diagnosing and treating tuberculosis conducted in several different parts of the world suggest that poor quality care is common.[6–15] Clinicians, in particular those who work in the private health-care sector, often deviate from standard, internationally recommended, tuberculosis management practices.[13,15] These deviations include under-utilization of sputum smear microscopy for diagnosis, generally associated with over-reliance on radiography and use of unproven diagnostic tests. In addition, non-recommended drug regimens with incorrect combinations of drugs and mistakes in both drug dosage and duration of treatment, and failure to supervise and assure adherence to treatment are common.[7–15]

Full, effective engagement of all care providers through various forms of public–private and public–public partnerships is an important component of both the WHO's expanded Stop TB strategy for tuberculosis control[16] and the *Global plan to stop TB, 2006–2015.*[17] Although there have been several approaches developed for involvement of the private sector (as well as for government-employed providers who are not affiliated with a tuberculosis control programme), there has been no generally agreed upon set of standards describing the essential actions that should be

taken by all practitioners in providing tuberculosis services to ensure the quality of these services. The ISTC is intended to fill this gap. To be effective in this role, it is essential that the ISTC be a living document that will undergo regular review and revision as new information emerges.

SCOPE OF PATIENTS TO WHOM ISTC APPLIES

The ISTC applies to patients of all ages, including those with smear-positive, smear-negative and extrapulmonary tuberculosis, tuberculosis caused by drug-resistant *M. tuberculosis* complex organisms and tuberculosis combined with HIV infection. For all forms of tuberculosis, a high standard of care is essential to restore the health of individuals, to prevent the disease in their families and others with whom they come into contact, and to protect the health of communities.[6] The ISTC focuses on the contribution that good clinical care of individual patients with, or suspected of having, tuberculosis makes to population-based tuberculosis control. An integrated approach emphasizing both individual patient care and public health principles of disease control is essential to reduce the human suffering and economic losses from tuberculosis.

Clearly, there are many elements that are necessary for tuberculosis care and control to be optimally effective. These include patient and community awareness, engagement and mobilization, access to care, availability of quality-assured laboratories, appropriate information systems and adequate primary services and health systems in general.[16] Although these elements are of considerable importance, they are beyond the scope of the ISTC, but are addressed in a number of other documents, particularly by the new Global Stop TB Strategy.[16]

ISTC STANDARDS FOR DIAGNOSIS

Standard 1

All people with otherwise unexplained productive cough lasting 2–3 weeks or more should be evaluated for tuberculosis.

The most common symptom of pulmonary tuberculosis is persistent productive cough, commonly accompanied by systemic symptoms, such as fever, night sweats and weight loss. In a WHO survey of primary health-care services of nine low- and middle-income countries, respiratory complaints, including cough, constituted an average of 18.4 per cent of symptoms that prompted a visit to a health centre for people older than 5 years of age. Of this group, 5 per cent of patients were categorized as possibly having tuberculosis because of the presence of an unexplained cough for more than 2–3 weeks.[18] Other studies have shown that 4–10 per cent of adults attending outpatient health facilities in developing countries may have a persistent cough of more than 2–3 weeks' duration.[19] This percentage varies somewhat depending on whether there is active questioning concerning the presence of cough.

Data from India, Algeria and Chile generally show that the percentage of patients with positive sputum smears increases with increasing duration of cough from 1–2 weeks, increasing to 3–4 and >4 weeks.[20] However, in these studies even patients with shorter duration of cough had an appreciable prevalence of tuberculosis. A more recent assessment from India demonstrated that by using a threshold of ≥2 weeks to prompt collection of sputum specimens the number of patients with suspected tuberculosis increased by 61 per cent, but, more importantly, the number of tuberculosis cases identified increased by 46 per cent compared with a threshold of >3 weeks.[21] The results also suggested that actively enquiring as to the presence of cough in all adult clinic attendees may increase the yield of cases.[21]

Choosing a threshold of 2–3 weeks is an obvious compromise. In countries with a low prevalence of tuberculosis, it is likely that cough of this duration will be due to conditions other than tuberculosis. Conversely, in high-prevalence countries, tuberculosis will be one of the leading diagnoses to consider, together with other conditions, such as asthma, bronchitis and bronchiectasis, that are common in many areas. Unfortunately, several studies suggest that, commonly, patients with subacute or chronic respiratory symptoms receive an inadequate evaluation for tuberculosis.[7,9–12,15,22]

Standard 2

All patients (adults, adolescents and children who are capable of producing sputum) suspected of having pulmonary tuberculosis should have at least two and, preferably, three sputum specimens obtained for microscopic examination. When possible at least one early-morning specimen should be obtained.

A diagnosis of tuberculosis can only be confirmed by culturing *M. tuberculosis* complex (or under appropriate circumstances, identifying specific nucleic acid sequences in a clinical specimen) from any suspected site of disease. In practice, however, there are many resource-limited settings in which culture is not currently feasible. Fortunately, microscopic examination of stained sputum is feasible in nearly all settings and the diagnosis of tuberculosis can be strongly inferred by finding acid-fast bacilli by microscopic examination. In nearly all clinical circumstances in high-prevalence areas, finding acid-fast bacilli in stained sputum is highly specific and, thus, is the equivalent of a confirmed diagnosis.

Failure to perform a proper diagnostic evaluation before initiating treatment potentially exposes the patient to the risks of unnecessary or wrong treatment with no benefit. Moreover, such an approach may delay accurate

diagnosis and proper treatment. This standard applies to adults, adolescents and children. With proper instruction and supervision many children 5 years of age and older can generate a specimen. Thus, age alone is not sufficient justification for failing to attempt to obtain a sputum specimen from a child or adolescent.

The optimum number of sputum specimens to establish a diagnosis has been examined in a number of studies. Current international tuberculosis guidelines recommend the microscopic examination of three sputum specimens for acid-fast bacilli in the evaluation of people suspected of having pulmonary tuberculosis. As part of the process for developing the ISTC, a rigorous systematic review of studies that quantified the diagnostic yield of each of three sputum specimens was conducted.[23] By searching multiple databases and sources, a total of 37 eligible studies were identified. The incremental yield in smear-positive results (in studies using all smear-positive cases as the denominator) and the increase in sensitivity (in studies that used all culture-positive cases as the denominator) of the third specimen were the main outcomes of interest. Although heterogeneity in study methods and results presented challenges for data synthesis, subgroup analyses suggest that the average incremental yield and/or the increase in sensitivity of the second specimen was 11–12 per cent and ranged between 2 and 5 per cent for the third specimen. Reducing the recommended number of specimens examined from three to two (particularly to two specimens collected on the same day) could increase laboratory efficiency and improve services.

A re-analysis of data from a study involving 42 laboratories in four high-burden countries demonstrated similar results: the incremental yield from a third sequential smear ranged from 0.7 to 7.2 per cent.[24]

The timing of specimen collection is also important. The yield appears to be greatest from early-morning (overnight) specimens.[25–28] Thus, at least one specimen should be obtained from an early-morning collection.

A variety of methods have been used to improve the performance of sputum smear microscopy. In general the sensitivity of microscopy (as compared with culture) is higher with concentration by centrifugation and/or sedimentation (usually after pretreatment with chemicals such as bleach, sodium hydroxide or *N*-acetyl cysteine sodium hydroxide) or both, as compared to direct smear microscopy. As part of developing the ISTC, a systematic review of 83 studies describing the effects of various physical and/or chemical methods for concentrating and processing sputum prior to microscopy was conducted.[29] The review demonstrated that concentration resulted in a higher sensitivity (15–20 per cent increase) and smear-positivity rate when compared with direct smears. Although there are demonstrable advantages to concentration of sputum, there are also disadvantages. Centrifugation is more complex, requires electrical power and may be associated with increased infection risk to laboratory personnel. Consequently, it is not clear that the advantages offset the disadvantages in low-resource settings.

A systematic review of 45 studies in which the performance of direct sputum smear microscopy with fluorescence staining was compared with Ziehl–Neelsen (ZN) staining using culture as the gold standard showed that fluorescence microscopy was on average about 10 per cent more sensitive than conventional light microscopy and has comparable specificity.[30] The combination of increased sensitivity with little or no loss of specificity makes fluorescence microscopy a more accurate test, although the increased cost and complexity might make it less applicable in many areas. For this reason, fluorescence staining is probably best used in centres with specifically trained and proficient microscopists, in which a large number of specimens are processed daily and in which there is an appropriate quality assurance programme.

Standard 3

For all patients (adults, adolescents and children) suspected of having extrapulmonary tuberculosis, appropriate specimens from the suspected sites of involvement should be obtained for microscopy and, where facilities and resources are available, for culture and histopathological examination.

Because appropriate specimens may be difficult to obtain from extrapulmonary sites and the number of bacilli is generally low, bacteriological confirmation of extrapulmonary tuberculosis is often more difficult than for pulmonary tuberculosis. Given the low yield of microscopy, both culture and histopathological examination of tissue specimens, such as may be obtained by needle biopsy of lymph nodes, are important. In addition to the collection of specimens from the sites of suspected tuberculosis, sputum should be examined and a chest film obtained, especially in patients with HIV infection, in whom there is an appreciable frequency of subclinical pulmonary tuberculosis.[31]

Standard 4

All people with chest radiographic findings suggestive of tuberculosis should have sputum specimens submitted for microbiological examination.

Chest radiography is a sensitive but non-specific test to detect tuberculosis.[32] Radiographic examination of the thorax or other suspected sites of involvement may be useful to identify people for further evaluation; however, a diagnosis of tuberculosis cannot be established by radiography alone. Reliance on the chest radiograph as the only diagnostic test for tuberculosis will result in both overdiagnosis of tuberculosis and missed diagnoses of tuberculosis and other diseases. In a study from India in which 2229 outpatients were examined by photofluorography, 227 were classified as having tuberculosis by radiographic criteria.[33,34] Of the 227, 81 (36 per cent) had negative sputum cultures, whereas of the remaining 2002 patients 31 (1.5 per cent) had positive cultures. Looking at these results in terms of the sensitivity of chest radiography 32 (20 per cent) of 162 culture-positive cases would have been missed by radiography.

Chest radiography is useful to evaluate people who have negative sputum smears to attempt to find evidence for pulmonary tuberculosis and to identify other abnormalities that may be responsible for the symptoms. With regard to tuberculosis, radiographic examination is most useful when applied as part of a systematic approach in the evaluation of people whose symptoms and/or findings suggest tuberculosis, but who have negative sputum smears (see Standard 5, below).

Standard 5

The diagnosis of sputum smear-negative pulmonary tuberculosis should be based on the following criteria: at least three negative sputum smears (including at least one early-morning specimen); chest radiography findings consistent with tuberculosis; and lack of response to a trial of broad-spectrum antimicrobial agents. (NOTE: Because the fluoroquinolones are active against M. tuberculosis *complex and, thus, may cause transient improvement in people with tuberculosis, they should be avoided). For such patients, if facilities for culture are available, sputum cultures should be obtained. In people with known or suspected HIV infection the diagnostic evaluation should be expedited.*

Given the non-specific nature of the symptoms of tuberculosis and the multiplicity of other diseases that could be the cause of the patient's illness, it is important that a rigorous approach be taken in diagnosing tuberculosis in a patient in whom at least three adequate sputum smears are negative. Because patients with HIV infection and tuberculosis frequently have negative sputum smears and because of the broad differential diagnosis in this group, such a systematic approach is crucial. It is important, however, to balance the need for a systematic approach with the need for prompt treatment in a patient with an illness that is progressing rapidly. A presumptive diagnosis of tuberculosis when the illness has another cause will delay correct diagnosis and treatment, whereas underdiagnosis will lead to more severe consequences of tuberculosis, as well as ongoing transmission of *M. tuberculosis*.

A number of algorithms have been developed as a means to diagnose smear-negative tuberculosis. Although none of the algorithms has been adequately validated under field conditions, they generally provide a useful framework for systematizing the approach to diagnosis.[35,36] Of particular concern, however, is the lack of evidence on which to base approaches to the diagnosis of smear-negative tuberculosis in people with HIV infection. There are several pitfalls in using algorithms. First, strict adherence to the sequential steps of the algorithm may delay appropriate treatment in patients with an illness that is worsening rapidly. Second, several studies have shown that patients with tuberculosis may respond, at least transiently, to empiric broad-spectrum antimicrobial treatment, a frequent element of diagnostic algorithms.[37–40] Obviously such a response will lead one to delay a diagnosis of tuberculosis. Fluoroquinolones, in particular, are bactericidal for *M. tuberculosis* complex. Empiric fluoroquinolone monotherapy for respiratory tract infections has been associated with delays in initiation of appropriate antituberculosis therapy and acquired resistance to the fluoroquinolones.[41] Third, the approach outlined in an algorithm may be quite costly to patients and deter them from continuing with the diagnostic evaluation.

Although sputum microscopy is the first bacteriological diagnostic test of choice, where resources permit and adequate, quality-assured laboratory facilities are available, culture should be included in the evaluation of patients suspected of having tuberculosis, but who have negative sputum smears. Properly done, culture increases diagnostic sensitivity which should result in earlier case detection.[42,43] The disadvantages of culture are its cost, technical complexity and the time required to obtain a result, thereby imposing a diagnostic delay if there is less reliance on sputum smear microscopy. In addition, ongoing quality assessment is essential for culture results to be credible. Such quality assurance measures are not widely available in most low-resource settings.

Nucleic acid amplification tests (NAATs), although widely distributed, do not offer major advantages over culture at this time. Although a positive result can be obtained more quickly than with any of the culture methods, the NAATs are not sufficiently sensitive for a negative result to exclude tuberculosis.[44–50] In addition, NAATs are not of proven value in identifying *M. tuberculosis* in specimens from extrapulmonary sites of disease.[45–47,49] Other approaches to establishing a diagnosis of tuberculosis, such as serological tests, are not of proven value and should not be used in routine practice at this time.[44,50–52]

Since the ISTC was released the Stop TB Department at WHO has published a set of guidelines focused on the diagnosis of tuberculosis in people with known HIV infection or in areas of high HIV prevalence.[53] The reader is referred to these recommendations for more specific guidance in addressing smear-negative tuberculosis in people with HIV infection.

Standard 6

The diagnosis of intrathoracic (i.e. pulmonary, pleural and mediastinal or hilar lymph node) tuberculosis in symptomatic children with negative sputum smears should be based on the finding of chest radiographic abnormalities consistent with tuberculosis, and either a history of exposure to an infectious case or evidence of tuberculosis infection (positive tuber-

culin skin test or interferon-γ release assay). For such patients, if facilities for culture are available, sputum specimens should be obtained (by expectoration, gastric washings or induced sputum) for culture.

Compared with adults, sputum smears from children are more likely to be negative and cultures of sputum or other specimens, radiographic examination of the chest and tests to detect tuberculous infection (generally, a tuberculin skin test) are of relatively greater importance. Because many children less than 5 years of age do not cough and produce sputum effectively, culture of gastric washings or induced sputum has a higher yield than spontaneous sputum.[54]

Several recent reviews have examined the effectiveness of various diagnostic tools, scoring systems and algorithms to diagnose tuberculosis in children.[54–58] Many of these approaches lack standardization and validation, and, thus, are of limited applicability. The Integrated Management of Childhood Illness (IMCI) programme of WHO which is widely used in first-level facilities in low- and middle-income countries provides a list of clinical features suggestive of tuberculosis.[59] A systematic approach to assessing all the available diagnostic evidence is particularly important where HIV infection is common because HIV infection compounds the diagnostic difficulties.[55,60]

Since publication of the ISTC, the Childhood Tuberculosis Subgroup of the Stop TB Partnership has published more detailed recommendations concerning the diagnostic approach to children suspected of having tuberculosis.[61]

ISTC STANDARDS FOR TREATMENT

Standard 7

Any practitioner treating a patient for tuberculosis is assuming an important public health responsibility. To fulfill this responsibility, the practitioner must not only prescribe an appropriate regimen, but also be capable of assessing the adherence of the patient to the regimen and addressing poor adherence when it occurs. By so doing, the provider will be able to ensure adherence to the regimen until treatment is completed.

The main interventions to prevent the spread of tuberculosis are the detection of patients with infectious tuberculosis and providing them with effective treatment to ensure a rapid and lasting cure. Consequently, treatment for tuberculosis is not only a matter of individual health, it is also a matter of public health. For this reason, all providers who undertake to treat an individual patient with tuberculosis must have the knowledge to prescribe a standard treatment regimen and the means to assess adherence to the regimen and address poor adherence to ensure that treatment is completed.[62] National tuberculosis programmes commonly possess approaches and tools to ensure adherence with treatment and, when properly organized, can offer these to non-programme providers. Failure of a provider to ensure adherence could be equated with, for example, failure to ensure that a child receives the full set of immunizations.

Standard 8

All patients (including those with HIV infection) who have not been treated previously should receive an internationally accepted first-line treatment regimen using drugs of known bioavailability. The initial phase should consist of 2 months of isoniazid, rifampicin, pyrazinamide and ethambutol. (Ethambutol may be omitted in the initial phase of treatment for adults and children who have negative sputum smears, do not have extensive pulmonary tuberculosis or severe forms of extrapulmonary disease and who are known to be HIV negative.)

The preferred continuation phase consists of isoniazid and rifampicin given for 4 months. Isoniazid and ethambutol given for 6 months is an alternative continuation phase regimen that may be used when adherence cannot be assessed but is associated with a higher rate of failure and relapse, especially in patients with HIV infection.

The doses of antituberculosis drugs used should conform to international recommendations. Fixed dose combinations of two (isoniazid and rifampicin), three (isoniazid, rifampicin and pyrazinamide) and four (isoniazid, rifampicin, pyrazinamide and ethambutol) drugs are highly recommended, especially when medication ingestion is not observed.

A large number of well-designed clinical trials have provided the evidence base for this standard and several sets of treatment recommendations based on these studies have been written in the past few years.[62–64] All these data indicate that a rifampicin-containing regimen is the backbone of antituberculosis chemotherapy and is highly effective in treating tuberculosis caused by drug-susceptible *M. tuberculosis*. It is also clear from these studies that the minimum duration of treatment for smear and/or culture-positive tuberculosis is 6 months. For the 6-month treatment duration to be maximally effective, the regimen must include pyrazinamide during the initial 2-month phase and rifampicin, together with isoniazid, must be included throughout the full 6 months. There are several variations in the frequency of drug administration that have been shown to produce acceptable results.[62–64]

Two systematic reviews of regimens of less than 6 months have found that shorter durations of treatment have an unacceptably high rate of relapse.[65,66] Thus, the current international standard for smear- or culture-positive tuberculosis is a regimen administered for a minimum duration of 6 months.[62,64]

Although the 6-month regimen is the preferred option, an alternative continuation phase regimen, consisting of isoniazid and ethambutol given for 6 months, making the total duration of treatment 8 months, may also be used. It

should be recognized, however, that this regimen, presumably because of the shorter duration of rifampicin administration, is associated with a higher rate of failure and relapse, especially in patients with HIV infection.[67–69] Nevertheless the 8-month regimen may be used when adherence to treatment throughout the continuation phase cannot be assessed.[64] The rationale for this approach is that if the patient is non-adherent, the emergence of resistance to rifampicin will be minimized. A retrospective review of the outcomes of treatment of tuberculosis in patients with HIV infection shows that tuberculosis relapse is minimized by the use of a regimen containing rifampicin throughout a 6-month course.[67] However, the patient's HIV stage, the need for and availability of anti-retroviral drugs, and the quality of treatment supervision/support must be considered in choosing an appropriate continuation phase of therapy.

Intermittent administration of antituberculosis drugs enables supervision to be provided more efficiently and economically with no reduction in efficacy. The evidence on effectiveness of intermittent regimens was reviewed recently.[70,71] These reviews, based on several trials,[72–77] suggest that antituberculosis treatment may be given intermittently three times a week throughout the full course of therapy or twice weekly in the continuation phase without apparent loss of effectiveness. However, the WHO and the IUATLD do not recommend the use of twice-weekly intermittent regimens because of the potentially greater consequences of missing one of the two doses.[63,64,78] The evidence on drug dosages and safety and the biological basis for dosage recommendations have been extensively reviewed elsewhere.[62–64,78–80]

Treatment of tuberculosis in special clinical situations such as the presence of liver disease, renal disease, pregnancy and HIV infection may require modification of the standard regimen or alterations in dosage or frequency of drug administration. Guidelines for these situations can be found elsewhere.[62,64]

Although there is no evidence that fixed-dose combinations (FDCs) are superior to individual drugs, expert opinion suggests that they minimize inadvertent monotherapy and may decrease the frequency of acquired drug resistance and medication errors.[62,64] FDCs also reduce the number of tablets to be consumed and may thereby increase patient adherence to recommended treatment regimens.[81,82]

Standard 9

To foster and assess adherence, a patient-centred approach to administration of drug treatment, based on the patient's needs and mutual respect between the patient and the provider, should be developed for all patients. Supervision and support should be gender-sensitive and age-specific and should draw on the full range of recommended interventions and available support services, including patient counselling and education. A central element of the patient-centred strategy is the use of measures to assess and promote adherence to the treatment regimen and to address poor adherence when it occurs. These measures should be tailored to the individual patient's circumstances and be mutually acceptable to the patient and the provider. Such measures may include direct observation of medication ingestion (directly observed therapy (DOT)) by a treatment supporter who is acceptable and accountable to the patient and to the health system.

The approach described in the standard is designed to encourage and facilitate a positive partnership between providers and patients, working together to improve adherence. Assuming an appropriate drug regimen is prescribed, adherence to treatment is the critical factor in determining treatment success.[83] This partnership between patients and providers is embodied in the Patients' Charter for Tuberculosis Care (available at www.worldcarecouncil.org) developed as a companion to the ISTC. Achieving adherence is not an easy task, either for the patient or the provider. Yet, failure to complete treatment for tuberculosis leads to prolonged infectivity, poor outcomes and drug resistance.[84]

Adherence is a multidimensional phenomenon determined by the interplay of five categories of factors: health system, socioeconomic, therapy-related, condition-related and patient-related.[83] Despite evidence to the contrary, there is a widespread tendency to focus on patient-related factors as the main cause of poor adherence.[83] Less attention is paid to provider and health system-related factors. Sociological and behavioural research during the past 40 years has shown that patients need to be supported, not blamed.[83] Several studies have evaluated various interventions to improve adherence to tuberculosis therapy. There are a number of reviews that examine the evidence on the effectiveness of these interventions.[62,83,85–91]

Among the interventions evaluated, DOT has generated the most debate and controversy. A key component of the global DOTS strategy, now widely recommended as the most effective strategy for controlling tuberculosis worldwide, is the administration of a standardized, rifampicin-based regimen using case management interventions that are appropriate to the individual and the circumstances.[62,64,92] These interventions should include DOT as one of a range of measures to promote and assess adherence to treatment.

The main advantage of DOT is that the treatment is carried out entirely under close supervision.[88] This provides both an accurate assessment of the degree of adherence and greater assurance that the medications have actually been ingested. When a second individual observes a patient swallowing medications, there is greater certainty that the patient is actually receiving the prescribed medications. This approach, therefore, results in a high cure rate and a reduction in the risk of drug resistance. Also, because there is close contact between the patient and the treatment supporter, adverse drug effects and other complications can be identified quickly and managed appropriately.[88] Moreover, such case management can also serve to identify and assist

in addressing the myriad other problems experienced by patients with tuberculosis such as undernutrition, poor housing and loss of income, to name a few.

In a Cochrane systematic review that synthesized the evidence from six controlled trials comparing DOT with self-administered therapy,[85,86] the authors found that patients allocated to DOT and those allocated to self-administered therapy had similar cure rates (RR 1.06, 95 per cent CI 0.98, 1.14) and rates of cure plus treatment completion (RR 1.06; 95 per cent CI 1.00, 1.13). They concluded that direct observation of medication ingestion did not improve outcomes.[85,86]

In contrast, other reviews have found DOT to be associated with high cure and treatment completion rates.[62,64,87,88,93] Also, programmatic studies on the effectiveness of the DOTS strategy have shown high rates of treatment success in several countries.[83] It is likely that these inconsistencies across reviews are due to the fact that primary studies are often unable to separate the effect of DOT alone from the overall DOTS strategy.[83,90] In a retrospective review of programmatic results, the highest rates of success were achieved with 'enhanced DOT' which consisted of 'supervised swallowing' plus social supports, incentives, and enablers as part of a larger programme to encourage adherence to treatment.[87] Such complex interventions are not easily evaluated within the conventional randomized controlled trial framework.[83]

Interventions other than DOT have also shown promise.[91,83] For example, interventions that used incentives, peer assistance, repeated motivation of patients, and staff training and motivation all have been shown to improve adherence significantly.[91] In addition, adherence may be enhanced by provision of more comprehensive primary care, as described in the Integrated Management of Adolescent and Adult Illness,[94–96] as well as by provision of specialized services, such as opiate substitution for injection drug users.

Interventions that target adherence must be tailored or customized to the particular situation and cultural context of a given patient.[83] Such an approach must be developed in concert with the patient to achieve optimum adherence. This patient-centred, individualized approach to treatment support is now a core element of all tuberculosis care and control efforts. It is important to note that treatment support measures, and not just the treatment regimen itself, must be individualized to suit the unique needs of the patient.

Standard 10

All patients should be monitored for response to therapy, best judged in patients with pulmonary tuberculosis by follow-up sputum microscopy (two specimens) at least at the time of completion of the initial phase of treatment (2 months), at 5 months and at the end of treatment. Patients who have positive smears during the fifth month of treatment should be considered as treatment failures and have therapy modified appropriately (see standards 14 and 15). In patients with extrapulmonary tuberculosis and in children, the response to treatment is best assessed clinically. Follow-up radiographic examinations are usually unnecessary and may be misleading.

Patient monitoring is necessary to evaluate the response of the disease to treatment and to identify adverse drug reactions. To judge response of pulmonary tuberculosis to treatment, the most expeditious method is sputum smear microscopy. Ideally, where quality-assured laboratories are available, sputum cultures, as well as smears, should be performed for monitoring.

Having a positive sputum smear at completion of 5 months of treatment defines treatment failure, indicating the need for determination of drug susceptibility and initiation of a retreatment regimen.[92,97,98] Radiographic assessments, although used commonly, have been shown to be unreliable for evaluating response to treatment.[99] Similarly, clinical assessment can be unreliable and misleading in the monitoring of patients with pulmonary tuberculosis.[99] In patients with extrapulmonary tuberculosis and in children, clinical evaluations may be the only available means of assessing the response to treatment.

Standard 11

A written record of all medications given, bacteriologic response, and adverse reactions should be maintained for all patients.

A recording and reporting system enables targeted, individualized follow up to identify patients who are failing therapy.[100] It also helps in facilitating continuity of care, particularly in settings where the same practitioner might not see the patient during every visit. A good record of medications given, results of investigations such as smears, cultures and chest radiographs, and progress notes on clinical improvement, adverse events and adherence will provide for more uniform monitoring and ensure a high standard of care.

Records are important to provide continuity when patients move from one care provider to another and enable tracing of patients who miss appointments. In patients who default and then return for treatment, and patients who relapse after treatment completion, it is critical to review previous records in order to assess the likelihood of drug resistance. Lastly, management of complicated cases (e.g. multidrug-resistant tuberculosis) is not possible without an adequate record of previous care. It should be noted that, wherever patient records are concerned, care must be taken to ensure confidentiality of the information.

Standard 12

In areas with a high-prevalence of HIV infection in the general population where tuberculosis and HIV infection are

likely to co-exist, *HIV counselling and testing is indicated for all tuberculosis patients as part of their routine management. In areas with lower prevalence rates of HIV, HIV counselling and testing is indicated for tuberculosis patients with symptoms and/or signs of HIV-related conditions, and in tuberculosis patients having a history suggestive of high risk of HIV exposure.*

Infection with HIV changes the clinical manifestations of tuberculosis.[60,101,102] In comparison with non-HIV-infected patients, patients with HIV infection who have pulmonary tuberculosis have a lower likelihood of having acid-fast bacilli detected by sputum smear microscopy.[60,101,102] Moreover, the chest radiographic features are atypical and the proportion of extrapulmonary tuberculosis is greater in patients with advanced HIV infection compared with those who do not have HIV infection. Consequently, knowledge of a person's HIV status would influence the approach to a diagnostic evaluation for tuberculosis. For this reason it is important, particularly in areas in which there is a high-prevalence of HIV infection, that the history and physical examination include a search for indicators that suggest the presence of HIV infection.[60,103,104]

Even though in low HIV prevalence countries, few tuberculosis patients will be HIV-infected, the connection is sufficiently strong and the impact on the patient sufficiently great that the test should always be considered in managing individual patients, especially among groups in which the prevalence of HIV is higher, such as injecting drug users. In countries having a high-prevalence of HIV infection, the yield of positive results will be high and, again, the impact of a positive result on the patient will be great. Thus, the indication for HIV testing is strong; co-infected patients may benefit by access to antiretroviral therapy as HIV treatment programmes expand or through administration of cotrimoxazole for prevention of opportunistic infections, even when antiretroviral drugs are not available locally.[60,105,106]

Standard 13

All patients with tuberculosis and HIV infection should be evaluated to determine if antiretroviral therapy is indicated during the course of treatment for tuberculosis. Appropriate arrangements for access to antiretroviral drugs should be made for patients who meet indications for treatment. Given the complexity of co-administration of antituberculosis treatment and antiretroviral therapy, consultation with a physician who is expert in this area is recommended before initiation of concurrent treatment for tuberculosis and HIV infection, regardless of which disease appeared first. However, initiation of treatment for tuberculosis should not be delayed. Patients with tuberculosis and HIV infection should also receive cotrimoxazole as prophylaxis for other infections.

All patients with tuberculosis and HIV infection either currently are, or will be, candidates for antiretroviral therapy. Antiretroviral therapy results in remarkable reductions in morbidity and mortality in HIV-infected people and may improve the outcomes of treatment for tuberculosis. Highly active antiretroviral therapy (HAART) is the internationally accepted standard of care for people with advanced HIV infection.

In patients with HIV-related tuberculosis, treating tuberculosis is the first priority. In the setting of advanced HIV infection, untreated tuberculosis can progress rapidly to death. However, antiretroviral treatment may be life-saving for patients with advanced HIV infection. Consequently, concurrent treatment may be necessary in patients with advanced HIV disease (e.g. CD4$^+$ count <200/μL). It should be emphasized, however, that treatment for tuberculosis should not be interrupted in order to initiate antiretroviral therapy, and, in patients who do not have advanced HIV infection, it may be safer to defer antiretroviral treatment until at least the completion of the initial phase of tuberculosis treatment.[60]

There are a number of problems associated with concomitant therapy for tuberculosis and HIV infection. These include overlapping drug toxicity profiles, drug–drug interactions (especially with rifamycins and protease inhibitors), potential problems with adherence to multiple medications and immune reconstitution reactions.[60,62] Consequently, consultation with an expert in HIV management is needed in deciding when to start antiretroviral drugs, the agents to use, the plan for monitoring adverse reactions and response to both therapies. Patients with tuberculosis and HIV infection should also receive cotrimoxazole as prophylaxis for other infections. Several studies have demonstrated the benefits of cotrimoxazole prophylaxis and this intervention is currently recommended by the WHO as part of the TB-HIV management package.[60,106–112]

drugs and lack of appropriate supervision to prevent erratic drug intake.[113]

The strongest factor associated with drug resistance is previous antituberculosis treatment.[113,114] In previously treated patients, the odds of any resistance are at least four-fold higher and that of MDR at least 10-fold higher than in new (untreated) patients.[114] Patients with chronic tuberculosis (sputum-positive after retreatment) and those who fail treatment (sputum-positive after 5 months of treatment) are at highest risk of having MDR tuberculosis, especially if rifampicin was used throughout the course of treatment.[98,114] People, especially children and HIV-infected individuals, who are in close contact with confirmed MDR tuberculosis patients are also at high risk of being infected with MDR strains. In some closed settings, prisoners, people staying in homeless shelters and certain categories of immigrants and migrants are at increased risk of MDR tuberculosis.[113–118]

Drug susceptibility testing (DST) to the first-line antituberculosis drugs should be performed in specialized reference laboratories that participate in an ongoing, rigorous quality assurance programme. DST for first-line drugs is currently recommended for all patients with a history of previous antituberculosis treatment: patients who have failed treatment, especially those who have failed a standardized retreatment regimen, and chronic cases are the highest priority.[113] Patients who develop tuberculosis and are known to have been in close contact with people known to have MDR tuberculosis also should have DST performed on an initial isolate. Although HIV infection has not been conclusively shown to be an independent risk factor for drug resistance, MDR tuberculosis outbreaks in HIV settings and high mortality rates in people with MDR tuberculosis and HIV infection justify routine DST in all HIV-infected tuberculosis patients, resources permitting.[113]

Standard 14

An assessment of the likelihood of drug resistance, based on history of prior treatment, exposure to a possible source case having drug-resistant organisms, and the community prevalence of drug resistance, should be obtained for all patients. Patients who fail treatment and chronic cases should always be assessed for possible drug resistance. For patients in whom drug resistance is considered to be likely, culture and drug susceptibility testing for isoniazid, rifampicin and ethambutol should be performed promptly.

Drug resistance is largely man-made and is a consequence of suboptimal regimens and treatment interruptions. Clinical errors that commonly lead to the emergence of drug resistance include failure to provide effective treatment support and assurance of adherence, failure to recognize and address patient non-adherence, inadequate drug regimens, adding a single new drug to a failing regimen and failure to recognize existing drug resistance.[113] Programmatic causes of drug resistance include drug shortages, administration of poor-quality

Standard 15

Patients with tuberculosis caused by drug-resistant (especially MDR) organisms should be treated with specialized regimens containing second-line antituberculosis drugs. At least four drugs to which the organisms are known or presumed to be susceptible should be used and treatment should be given for at least 18 months. Patient-centred measures are required to ensure adherence. Consultation with a provider experienced in treatment of patients with MDR tuberculosis should be obtained.

Current recommendations for treatment of MDR tuberculosis are based on observational studies, general microbiological and therapeutic principles, extrapolation from available evidence from pilot MDR tuberculosis treatment projects and expert opinion.[113,119,120] Three strategic options for treatment of MDR tuberculosis are currently recommended by WHO. These are standardized regimens, empiric regimens and individualized treatment regimens.[113] The choice among these should be based on availability of second-line drugs and DST for first- and second-line drugs, local drug resistance patterns, and the history of use of second-line drugs.

BASIC PRINCIPLES

Basic principles involved in the design of any regimen include the use of at least four drugs with either certain or highly likely effectiveness, drug administration at least 6 days a week, drug dosage determined by patient weight, the use of an injectable agent (an aminoglycoside or capreomycin) for at least 6 months, treatment duration of 18–24 months and DOT throughout the treatment course.

STANDARDIZED TREATMENT

Standardized treatment regimens are based on representative drug-resistance surveillance data or on the history of drug usage in the country. Based on these assessments, regimens can be designed that will have a high likelihood of success. Advantages include less dependency on highly technical laboratories, less reliance on highly specialized clinical expertise required to interpret DST results, simplified drug ordering and easier operational implementation. A standardized approach is useful in settings where second-line drugs have not been used extensively and where resistance levels to these drugs are consequently low or absent.

EMPIRIC TREATMENT

Empiric treatment regimens are commonly used in specific groups of patients while the DST results are pending. Unfortunately, most of the available DST methods have a turnaround time of several months. Empiric regimens are strongly recommended to avoid clinical deterioration and to prevent transmission of MDR strains of *M. tuberculosis* to contacts while awaiting the DST results.[113] Once the results of DST are known, an empiric regimen may be changed to an individualized regimen. Ongoing global efforts to address the problem of MDR tuberculosis will likely result in broader access to laboratories performing DST and a faster return of results.

INDIVIDUALIZED TREATMENT

Individualized treatment regimens (based on DST profiles and previous drug history of individual patients, or on local patterns of drug utilization) have the advantage of avoiding toxic and expensive drugs to which the MDR strain is resistant. However, an individualized approach requires access to substantial human, financial and technical capacity. DST for second-line drugs are notoriously difficult to perform.[121] Also, laboratory proficiency testing results are not yet available for second-line drugs; as a result little can be said about the reliability of DST for these drugs.[114,121] Clinicians treating MDR tuberculosis

patients must be aware of these limitations and interpret DST results with this in mind. MDR tuberculosis treatment is a complex health intervention and medical practitioners are strongly advised to consult colleagues experienced in the management of these patients.

Since publication of the ISTC, the WHO and the Stop TB Partnership have published the Global MDR-TB and XDR-TB Response Plan, and this plan provides additional information on approaches to controlling the XDR-TB problem.[122]

ISTC STANDARDS FOR PUBLIC HEALTH RESPONSIBILITIES

Standard 16

All providers of care for patients with tuberculosis should ensure that people (especially children under 5 years of age and people with HIV infection) who are in close contact with patients who have infectious tuberculosis are evaluated and managed in line with international recommendations. Children under 5 years of age and people with HIV infection who have been in contact with an infectious case should be evaluated for both latent infection with M. tuberculosis *and for active tuberculosis.*

Close contacts of patients with tuberculosis are at high risk for acquiring the infection; thus, contact investigation is an important activity, to find both people with previously undetected tuberculosis and people who are candidates for treatment of latent tuberculosis infection.[123,124] The potential yield of contact investigation in high- and low-incidence settings has been reviewed previously.[123,124] In low-incidence settings (e.g. United States), it has been found that, on average, 5–10 contacts are identified for each incident tuberculosis case. Of these, about 30 per cent are found to have latent tuberculosis infection, and another 1–4 per cent have active truberculosis.[123,125,126] A recent systematic review of 41 studies describing household contact investigations in high-incidence settings showed that, on average, 4.5 per cent (95 per cent CI 4.3–4.8 per cent) of the contacts were found to have active tuberculosis, both bacteriologically confirmed and clinical/radiological diagnoses.[127] Of these 2.3 per cent (95 per cent CI 2.3–2.5 per cent) were confirmed by microscopy or culture.[128] An average of 51.4 per cent (95 per cent CI 50.6–52.2 per cent) of contacts evaluated had latent tuberculosis infection. The median number of household contacts that were evaluated to find one case of active tuberculosis was 19.[127] The median number of contacts evaluated in order to find one person with latent tuberculosis infection was two.[127] Evidence from this review suggests that contact investigation in high-incidence settings is a high-yield strategy for case finding.

Among close contacts, there are certain subgroups that are particularly at high risk for acquiring the infection with *M. tuberculosis* and progressing rapidly to active disease –

children and people with HIV infection. Children (particularly those under the age of 5 years) are a vulnerable group because of the high likelihood of progressing from latent infection to active disease. Children are also more likely to develop disseminated and serious forms of tuberculosis. In the systematic review cited above, the yield for active tuberculosis among children who were named as contacts of new cases was 8.5 per cent (95 per cent CI 7.4–9.7 per cent). In the studies reviewed, there were insufficient data to determine the yield of active tuberculosis for people with HIV infection; however, clearly such people constitute a high-risk group.

Standard 17

All providers must report both new and retreatment tuberculosis cases and their treatment outcomes to local public health authorities, in conformance with applicable legal requirements and policies.

Reporting tuberculosis cases to the local tuberculosis control programme is an essential public health function, and in many countries is legally mandated. An effective reporting system enables a determination of the overall effectiveness of tuberculosis control programmes, of resource needs and of the true distribution and dynamics of the disease within the population as a whole, not just the population served by the government tuberculosis control programme. A system of recording and reporting information on tuberculosis cases and their treatment outcomes is one of the key elements of the DOTS strategy.[100] The recording and reporting system allows for targeted, individualized follow up to help patients who are not making adequate progress (i.e. failing therapy).[100] The system also allows for evaluation of the performance of the practitioner, the hospital or institution, local health system and the country as a whole. Although reporting to public health authorities is essential, it is also essential that patient confidentiality be maintained. Thus, reporting must follow predefined channels using standard procedures that guarantee that only authorized people see the information.

CONCLUSION

It should be apparent to the reader that the ISTC presents no new information. It does, however, provide a new way to present old information. It is hoped that the new presentation with its sound evidence base, extensive input from a diverse group of interested people and broad endorsement by public and private sectors alike will serve to bring a higher standard of quality to the care of people with tuberculosis, regardless of their source of care.

As we face the new threat of XDR tuberculosis, it is imperative to revisit the cornerstones of tuberculosis care.

Without diligent attention to these fundamentals we may see further creation and spread of XDR organisms. Unquestionably, new drugs and new diagnostic tests are needed, but currently and even after they become available, it will continue to be imperative to adhere to the essential standards of tuberculosis care as described in the ISTC. By so doing, patients will be cured, transmission will be minimized and XDR tuberculosis will be prevented.

LEARNING POINTS

- Prompt diagnosis and treatment of patients with tuberculosis minimizes spread and halts development of resistance.
- Emergence of drug resistance, particularly extreme drug resistance, is caused by poor tuberculosis management practices.
- The purpose of the International Standards for Tuberculosis Care is to describe agreed levels of care for TB patients by all practitioners.
- The principal target audience is health professional managing TB outside government TB programmes.
- The ISTC is not intended to replace national and other guidelines.
- Local approaches will be needed to adapt the standards to facilitate their implementation.
- Professional bodies can exert pressure on members and governments to adhere to standards.
- The standards have been drawn up by wide agreement of health professionals because of poor medical practice in managing tuberculosis across much of the world.
- The intention is to apply standards for the management of
  - symptoms;
  - sputum examination;
  - facilities to diagnose extrapulmonary TB;
  - radiology;
  - diagnosis of pulmonary disease;
  - diagnosis of extrapulmonary disease;
  - treatment adherence;
  - aspects of treatment length and drug quality;
  - patient centrality, including directly observed therapy (DOT);
  - monitoring of response to treatment;
  - recording of medication use and outcome;
  - HIV testing;
  - use of concomitant treatment with antiretroviral drugs, as required;
  - assessment for drug resistance;
  - use of specialized treatment for drug resistance;
  - contact tracing;
  - national and local reporting.

REFERENCES

1. Gandhi NR, Moll A, Sturm AW *et al*. Extensively drug-resistant tuberculosis as a cause of death in patients co-infected with tuberculosis and HIV in a rural area of South Africa. *Lancet* 2006; **368**: 1575–80.

2. The tuberculosis X factor. *Lancet Infect Dis* 2006; **6**: 679.

3. Raviglione M. XDR-TB: entering the post-antibiotic era? *Int J Tuberc Lung Dis* 2006; **10**: 1185–7.

4. Tuberculosis Coalition for Technical Assistance. *International standards for tuberculosis care (ISTC)*. The Hague: Tuberculosis Coalition for Technical Assistance, 2006: 1–56.

5. Hopewell PC, Pai M, Maher D, Uplekar M, Raviglione MC. International standards for tuberculosis care. *Lancet Infect Dis* 2006; **6**: 710–25.

6. Hopewell PC, Pai M. Tuberculosis, vulnerability, and access to quality care. *J Am Med Assoc* 2005; **293**: 2790–3.

7. Lonnroth K, Thuong LM, Linh PD, Diwan VK. Delay and discontinuity – a survey of TB patients' search of a diagnosis in a diversified health care system. *Int J Tuberc Lung Dis* 1999; **3**: 992–1000.

8. Olle-Goig JE, Cullity JE, Vargas R. A survey of prescribing patterns for tuberculosis treatment amongst doctors in a Bolivian city. *Int J Tuberc Lung Dis* 1999; **3**: 74–8.

9. Prasad R, Nautiyal RG, Mukherji PK *et al*. Diagnostic evaluation of pulmonary tuberculosis: what do doctors of modern medicine do in India? *Int J Tuberc Lung Dis* 2003; **7**: 52–7.

10. Shah SK, Sadiq H, Khalil M *et al*. Do private doctors follow national guidelines for managing pulmonary tuberculosis in Pakistan? *East Mediterr Health J* 2003; **9**: 776–88.

11. Singla N, Sharma PP, Singla R, Jain RC. Survey of knowledge, attitudes and practices for tuberculosis among general practitioners in Delhi, India. *Int J Tuberc Lung Dis* 1998; **2**: 384–9.

12. Suleiman BA, Houssein AI, Mehta F, Hinderaker SG. Do doctors in north-western Somalia follow the national guidelines for tuberculosis management? *East Mediterr Health J* 2003; **9**: 789–95.

13. Uplekar M, Pathania V, Raviglione M. Private practitioners and public health: weak links in tuberculosis control. *Lancet* 2001; **358**: 912–6.

14. Uplekar MW, Shepard DS. Treatment of tuberculosis by private general practitioners in India. *Tubercle* 1991; **72**: 284–90.

15. World Health Organization. *Involving private practitioners in tuberculosis control: issues, interventions and emerging policy framework*. Geneva: World Health Organization, 2001: 1–81.

16. Raviglione MC, Uplekar MW. WHO's new Stop TB Strategy. *Lancet* 2006; **367**: 952–5.

17. Stop TB Partnership and World Health Organization. *The global plan to stop TB 2006–2015*. Geneva: World Health Organization, 2006.

18. World Health Organization. *Respiratory care in primary care services: a survey in 9 countries*. Geneva: World Health Organization, 2004.

19. Luelmo F. What is the role of sputum microscopy in patients attending health facilities? In: Frieden TR (ed.). *Toman's tuberculosis. Case detection, treatment and monitoring*, 2nd edn. Geneva: World Health Organization, 2004: 7–10.

20. Organizacion Panamericana de la Salud. *Control de tuberculosis en America Latina: Manual de normas y procedimientos para programas Integrados*. Washington, DC: Organizacion Panamericana de la Salud, 1979.

21. Santha T, Garg R, Subramani R *et al*. Comparison of cough of 2 and 3 weeks to improve detection of smear-positive tuberculosis cases among out-patients in India. *Int J Tuberc Lung Dis* 2005; **9**: 61–8.

22. Khan J, Malik A, Hussain H *et al*. Tuberculosis diagnosis and treatment practices of private physicians in Karachi, Pakistan. *East Mediterr Health J* 2003; **9**: 769–75.

23. Mase SR, Ramsay A, Ng V *et al*. Yield of serial sputum specimen examinations in the diagnosis of pulmonary tuberculosis: a systematic review. *Int J Tuberc Lung Dis* 2007; **11**: 485–95.

24. Rieder HL, Chiang CY, Rusen ID. A method to determine the utility of the third diagnostic and the second follow-up sputum smear examinations to diagnose tuberculosis cases and failures. *Int J Tuberc Lung Dis* 2005; **9**: 384–91.

25. Mase S, Ng V, Henry MC *et al*. Yield of serial sputum smear examinations in the evaluation of pulmonary tuberculosis: a systematic review (unpublished report). Geneva: Special Programme for Research and Training in Tropical Diseases (TDR), World Health Organization, and Foundation for Innovative New Diagnostics (FIND). 2005.

26. Gopi PG, Subramani R, Selvakumar N *et al*. Smear examination of two specimens for diagnosis of pulmonary tuberculosis in Tiruvallur District, south India. *Int J Tuberc Lung Dis* 2004; **8**: 824–8.

27. Van Deun A, Salim AH, Cooreman E *et al*. Optimal tuberculosis case detection by direct sputum smear microscopy: how much better is more? *Int J Tuberc Lung Dis* 2002; **6**: 222–30.

28. Sarin R, Mukerjee S, Singla N, Sharma PP. Diagnosis of tuberculosis under RNTCP: examination of two or three sputum specimens. *Indian J Tuberc* 2001: 13–16.

29. Steingart KR, Ng V, Henry M *et al*. Sputum processing methods to improve the sensitivity of smear microscopy for tuberculosis: a systematic review. *Lancet Infect Dis* 2006; **6**: 664–74.

30. Steingart KR, Henry M, Ng V *et al*. Fluorescence versus conventional sputum smear microscopy for tuberculosis: a systematic review. *Lancet Infect Dis* 2006; **6**: 570–81.

31. Mtei L, Matee M, Herfort O *et al*. High rates of clinical and subclinical tuberculosis among HIV-infected ambulatory subjects in Tanzania. *Clin Infect Dis* 2005; **40**: 1500–7.

32. Koppaka R, Bock N. How reliable is chest radiography? In: Frieden TR (ed.). *Toman's tuberculosis. Case detection, treatment and monitoring*, 2nd edn. Geneva: World Health Organization, 2004: 51–60.

33. Harries A. What are the relative merits of chest radiography and sputum examination (smear microscopy and culture) in case detection among new outpatients with prolonged chest symptoms? In: Frieden TR (ed.). *Toman's tuberculosis. Case detection, treatment and monitoring*, 2nd edn. Geneva: World Health Organization, 2004: 61–5.

34. Nagpaul DR, Naganathan N, Prakash M. Diagnostic photofluorography and sputum microscopy in tuberculosis case findings. Proceedings of the 9th Eastern Region Tuberculosis Conference and 29th National Conference on Tuberculosis and Chest Diseases, Delhi, 1974.

35. Colebunders R, Bastian I. A review of the diagnosis and treatment of smear-negative pulmonary tuberculosis. *Int J Tuberc Lung Dis* 2000; **4**: 97–107.

36. Siddiqi K, Lambert ML, Walley J. Clinical diagnosis of smear-negative pulmonary tuberculosis in low-income countries: the current evidence. *Lancet Infect Dis* 2003; **3**: 288–96.

37. Bah B, Massari V, Sow O *et al*. Useful clues to the presence of smear-negative pulmonary tuberculosis in a West African city. *Int J Tuberc Lung Dis* 2002; **6**: 592–8.

38. Oyewo TA, Talbot EA, Moeti TL. Non-response to antibiotics predicts tuberculosis in AFB-smear-negative TB suspects, Botswana, 1997–1999. *Int J Tuberc Lung Dis* 2001; **5** (Suppl. 1): S126 (Abstr.).

39. Somi GR, O'Brien RJ, Mfinanga GS, Ipuge YA. Evaluation of the MycoDot test in patients with suspected tuberculosis in a field setting in Tanzania. *Int J Tuberc Lung Dis* 1999; **3**: 231–8.

40. Wilkinson D, De Cock KM, Sturm AW. Diagnosing tuberculosis in a resource-poor setting: the value of a trial of antibiotics. *Trans R Soc Trop Med Hyg* 1997; **91**: 422–4.

41. Sterling TR. The WHO/IUATLD diagnostic algorithm for tuberculosis and empiric fluoroquinolone use: potential pitfalls. *Int J Tuberc Lung Dis* 2004; **8**: 1396–400.

42. van Deun A. What is the role of mycobacterial culture in diagnosis and case finding? In: Frieden TR (ed.). *Toman's tuberculosis. Case detection, treatment and monitoring*, 2nd edn. Geneva: World Health Organization, 2004: 35–43.

43. Kim TC, Blackman RS, Heatwole KM *et al*. Acid-fast bacilli in sputum smears of patients with pulmonary tuberculosis. Prevalence and significance of negative smears pretreatment and positive smears post-treatment. *Am Rev Respir Dis* 1984; **129**: 264–8.

44. Menzies D. What is the current and potential role of diagnostic tests other than sputum microscopy and culture? In: Frieden TR (ed.). *Toman's tuberculosis. Case detection, treatment and monitoring*, 2nd edn. Geneva: World Health Organization, 2004: 87–91.

45. Pai M. The accuracy and reliability of nucleic acid amplification tests in the diagnosis of tuberculosis. *Natl Med J India* 2004; **17**: 233–6.

46. Pai M, Flores LL, Hubbard A, Riley LW, Colford JM Jr. Nucleic acid amplification tests in the diagnosis of tuberculous pleuritis: a systematic review and meta-analysis. *BMC Infect Dis* 2004; **4**: 6.

47. Pai M, Flores LL, Pai N *et al*. Diagnostic accuracy of nucleic acid amplification tests for tuberculous meningitis: a systematic review and meta-analysis. *Lancet Infect Dis* 2003; **3**: 633–43.

48. Flores LL, Pai M, Colford JM Jr, Riley LW. In-house nucleic acid amplification tests for the detection of *Mycobacterium tuberculosis* in sputum specimens: meta-analysis and meta-regression. *BMC Microbiol* 2005; **5**: 55.

49. Nahid P, Pai M, Hopewell PC. Advances in the diagnosis and treatment of tuberculosis. *Proc Am Thorac Soc* 2006; **3**: 103–10.

50. Pai M, Kalantri S, Dheda K. New tools and emerging technologies for the diagnosis of tuberculosis: Part 2. Active tuberculosis and drug resistance. *Expert Rev Mol Diagn* 2006; **6**: 423–32.

51. Steingart KR, Henry M, Laal S *et al*. Commercial serological antibody detection tests for the diagnosis of pulmonary tuberculosis: a systematic review. *PLoS Med* 2007; **4**: e202.

52. Steingart KR, Henry M, Laal S *et al*. A systematic review of commercial serological antibody detection tests for the diagnosis of extrapulmonary tuberculosis. *Thorax* 2007; **62**: 911–18.

53. World Health Organization. *Improving the diagnosis and treatment of smear-negative pulmonary and extrapulmonary tuberculosis among adults and adolescents*. Geneva: World Health Organization, 2007.

54. Shingadia D, Novelli V. Diagnosis and treatment of tuberculosis in children. *Lancet Infect Dis* 2003; **3**: 624–32.

55. Gie RP, Beyers N, Schaaf HS, Goussard P. The challenge of diagnosing tuberculosis in children: a perspective from a high incidence area. *Paediatr Respir Rev* 2004; **5** (Suppl A): S147–9.

56. Hesseling AC, Schaaf HS, Gie RP *et al*. A critical review of diagnostic approaches used in the diagnosis of childhood tuberculosis. *Int J Tuberc Lung Dis* 2002; **6**: 1038–45.

57. Nelson LJ, Wells CD. Tuberculosis in children: considerations for children from developing countries. *Semin Pediatr Infect Dis* 2004; **15**: 150–54.

58. Marais BJ, Gie RP, Schaaf HS *et al*. Childhood pulmonary tuberculosis: old wisdom and new challenges. *Am J Respir Crit Care Med* 2006; **173**: 1078–90.

59. World Health Organization. *Management of the child with a serious infection or severe malnutrition: guidelines for care at the first-referral level in developing countries*. Geneva: World Health Organization, 2000.

60. World Health Organization. *TB/HIV: A clinical manual*. Geneva: World Health Organization, 2004.

61. World Health Organization. *Guidance for national tuberculosis programmes on the management of tuberculosis in children*. Geneva: WHO, 2006.

62. American Thoracic Society/Centers for Disease Control and Prevention/Infectious Diseases Society of America. Treatment of tuberculosis. *Am J Respir Crit Care Med* 2003; **167**: 603–62.

63. Enarson DA, Rieder HL, Arnadottir T, Trebucq A. *Management of tuberculosis. A guide for low income countries*, 5th edn. Paris: International Union Against Tuberculosis and Lung Disease, 2000.

64. World Health Organization. *Treatment of tuberculosis. Guidelines for national programmes*. Geneva: World Health Organization, 2003.

65. Gelband H. Regimens of less than six months for treating tuberculosis. *Cochrane Database Syst Rev* 2000: CD001362.

66. Santha T. What is the optimum duration of treatment? In: Frieden TR (ed.). *Toman's tuberculosis. Case detection, treatment and monitoring*, 2nd edn. Geneva: World Health Organization, 2004: 144–51.

67. Korenromp EL, Scano F, Williams BG *et al*. Effects of human immunodeficiency virus infection on recurrence of tuberculosis after rifampin-based treatment: an analytical review. *Clin Infect Dis* 2003; **37**: 101–12.

68. Jindani A, Nunn AJ, Enarson DA. Two 8-month regimens of chemotherapy for treatment of newly diagnosed pulmonary tuberculosis: international multicentre randomised trial. *Lancet* 2004; **364**: 1244–51.

69. Okwera A, Johnson JL, Luzze H *et al*. Comparison of intermittent continuous phase ethambutol with two rifampicin containing regimens in human immunodeficiency virus (HIV) infected adults with pulmonary tuberculosis in Kampala, Uganda. *Int J Tuberc Lung Dis* 2006; **10**: 39–445.

70. Mitchison DA. Antimicrobial therapy for tuberculosis: justification for currently recommended treatment regimens. *Semin Respir Crit Care Med* 2004; **25**: 307–15.

71. Frieden TR. What is intermittent treatment and what is the scientific basis for intermittency? In: Frieden TR (ed.). *Toman's tuberculosis. Case detection, treatment and monitoring*, 2nd edn. Geneva: World Health Organization, 2004: 130–38.

72. Hong Kong Chest Service/British Medical Research Council. Controlled trial of 4 three-times-weekly regimens and a daily regimen all given for 6 months for pulmonary tuberculosis. Second report: the results up to 24 months. *Tubercle* 1982; **63**: 89–98.

73. Hong Kong Chest Service/British Medical Research Council. Controlled trial of 2, 4, and 6 months of pyrazinamide in 6-month, three-times-weekly regimens for smear-positive pulmonary tuberculosis, including an assessment of a combined preparation of isoniazid, rifampin, and pyrazinamide. Results at 30 months. *Am Rev Respir Dis* 1991; **143**: 700–706.

74. Tuberculosis Research Centre. Low rate of emergence of drug resistance in sputum positive patients treated with short course chemotherapy. *Int J Tuberc Lung Dis* 2001; **5**: 40–5.

75. Bechan S, Connolly C, Short GM *et al*. Directly observed therapy for tuberculosis given twice weekly in the workplace in urban South Africa. *Trans R Soc Trop Med Hyg* 1997; **91**: 704–707.

76. Caminero JA, Pavon JM, Rodriguez de Castro F *et al*. Evaluation of a directly observed six months fully intermittent treatment regimen for tuberculosis in patients suspected of poor compliance. *Thorax* 1996; **51**: 1130–33.

77. Cao JP, Zhang LY, Zhu JQ, Chin DP. Two-year follow-up of directly-observed intermittent regimens for smear-positive pulmonary tuberculosis in China. *Int J Tuberc Lung Dis* 1998; **2**: 360–64.

78. Rieder HL. What is the evidence for tuberculosis drug dosage recommendations? In: Frieden TR (ed.). *Toman's tuberculosis. Case detection, treatment and monitoring*, 2nd edn. Geneva: World Health Organization, 2004: 141–3.

79. Rieder HL. What is the dosage of drugs in daily and intermittent regimens? In: Frieden TR (ed.). *Toman's tuberculosis. Case detection, treatment and monitoring*, 2nd edn. Geneva: World Health Organization, 2004: 139–40.

80. World Health Organization. *Ethambutol efficacy and toxicity. Literature review and recommendations for daily and intermittent dosage in children*. Geneva: World Health Organization, 2006.

81. Blomberg B, Spinaci S, Fourie B, Laing R. The rationale for recommending fixed-dose combination tablets for treatment of tuberculosis. *Bull World Health Organ* 2001; **79**: 61–8.

82. Panchagnula R, Agrawal S, Ashokraj Y et al. Fixed dose combinations for tuberculosis: Lessons learned from clinical, formulation and regulatory perspective. Methods Find Exp Clin Pharmacol 2004; 26: 703–21.

83. World Health Organization. Adherence to long-term therapies. Evidence for action. Geneva: World Health Organization, 2003.

84. Mitchison DA. How drug resistance emerges as a result of poor compliance during short course chemotherapy for tuberculosis. Int J Tuberc Lung Dis 1998; 2: 10–15.

85. Volmink J, Garner P. Directly observed therapy for treating tuberculosis. Cochrane Database Syst Rev 2003: CD003343.

86. Volmink J, Matchaba P, Garner P. Directly observed therapy and treatment adherence. Lancet 2000; 355: 1345–50.

87. Chaulk CP, Kazandjian VA. Directly observed therapy for treatment completion of pulmonary tuberculosis: Consensus Statement of the Public Health Tuberculosis Guidelines Panel. J Am Med Assoc 1998; 279: 943–8.

88. Sbarbaro J. What are the advantages of direct observation of treatment? In: Frieden TR (ed.). Toman's tuberculosis. Case detection, treatment and monitoring, 2nd edn. Geneva: World Health Organization, 2004: 183–4.

89. Sbarbaro J. How frequently do patients stop taking treatment prematurely? In: Frieden TR (ed.). Toman's tuberculosis. Case detection, treatment and monitoring, 2nd edn. Geneva: World Health Organization, 2004: 181–2.

90. Pope DS, Chaisson RE. TB treatment: as simple as DOT? Int J Tuberc Lung Dis 2003; 7: 611–5.

91. Gordon AL. Interventions other than direct observation of therapy to improve adherence of tuberculosis patients: a systematic review. University of California, Berkeley, Master's thesis, Spring 2005.

92. WHO/IUATLD/KNCV. Revised international definitions in tuberculosis control. Int J Tuberc Lung Dis 2001; 5: 213–15.

93. Frieden TR. Can tuberculosis be controlled? Int J Epidemiol 2002; 31: 894–9.

94. World Health Organization. Integrated management of adolescent and adult illness (IMAI): Acute care. Geneva: World Health Organization, 2004.

95. World Health Organization. Integrated management of adolescent and adult illness (IMAI): Chronic HIV care with ARV therapy. Geneva: World Health Organization, 2004.

96. World Health Organization. Integrated management of adolescent and adult illness (IMAI): General principles of good chronic care. Geneva: World Health Organization, 2004.

97. Espinal MA, Kim SJ, Suarez PG et al. Standard short-course chemotherapy for drug-resistant tuberculosis: treatment outcomes in 6 countries. J Am Med Assoc 2000; 283: 2537–45.

98. Becerra MC, Freeman J, Bayona J et al. Using treatment failure under effective directly observed short-course chemotherapy programs to identify patients with multidrug-resistant tuberculosis. Int J Tuberc Lung Dis 2000; 4: 108–14.

99. Santha T. How can the progress of treatment be monitored? In: Frieden TR (ed.). Toman's tuberculosis. Case detection, treatment and monitoring, 2nd edn. Geneva: World Health Organization, 2004: 250–2.

100. Maher D, Raviglione MC. Why is a recording and reporting system needed, and what system is recommended? In: Frieden TR (ed.). Toman's tuberculosis. Case detection, treatment and monitoring, 2nd edn. Geneva: World Health Organization, 2004: 270–3.

101. Bock N, Reichman LB. Tuberculosis and HIV/AIDS: epidemiological and clinical aspects (world perspective). Semin Respir Crit Care Med 2004; 25: 337–44.

102. Maher D, Harries A, Getahun H. Tuberculosis and HIV interaction in sub-Saharan Africa: impact on patients and programmes; implications for policies. Trop Med Int Health 2005; 10: 734–42.

103. World Health Organization. Scaling up antiretroviral therapy in resource-limited settings. Guidelines for a public health approach. Geneva: World Health Organization, 2002.

104. World Health Organization. Scaling up antiretroviral therapy in resource-limited settings. Treatment guidelines for a public health approach. Geneva: World Health Organization, 2004.

105. UNAIDS/WHO. UNAIDS/WHO policy statement on HIV testing. Geneva: UNAIDS, 2004: 1–3.

106. Nunn P, Williams B, Floyd K, Dye C, Elzinga G, Raviglione M. Tuberculosis control in the era of HIV. Nat Rev Immunol 2005; 5: 819–26.

107. Chimzizi R, Gausi F, Bwanali A et al. Voluntary counselling, HIV testing and adjunctive cotrimoxazole are associated with improved TB treatment outcomes under routine conditions in Thyolo district, Malawi. Int J Tuberc Lung Dis 2004; 8: 579–85.

108. Chimzizi RB, Harries AD, Manda E, Khonyongwa A, Salaniponi FM. Counselling, HIV testing and adjunctive cotrimoxazole for TB patients in Malawi: from research to routine implementation. Int J Tuberc Lung Dis 2004; 8: 938–44.

109. Grimwade K, Sturm AW, Nunn AJ, Mbatha D, Zungu D, Gilks CF. Effectiveness of cotrimoxazole prophylaxis on mortality in adults with tuberculosis in rural South Africa. AIDS 2005; 19: 163–8.

110. Mwaungulu FB, Floyd S, Crampin AC et al. Cotrimoxazole prophylaxis reduces mortality in human immunodeficiency virus-positive tuberculosis patients in Karonga District, Malawi. Bull World Health Organ 2004; 82: 354–63.

111. Zachariah R, Spielmann MP, Chinji C et al. Voluntary counselling, HIV testing and adjunctive cotrimoxazole reduces mortality in tuberculosis patients in Thyolo, Malawi. AIDS 2003; 17: 1053–61.

112. Zachariah R, Spielmann MP, Harries AD et al. Cotrimoxazole prophylaxis in HIV-infected individuals after completing anti-tuberculosis treatment in Thyolo, Malawi. Int J Tuberc Lung Dis 2002; 6: 1046–50.

113. World Health Organization. Guidelines for the programmatic management of drug-resistant tuberculosis. Geneva: World Health Organization, 2006.

114. World Health Organization. Anti-tuberculosis drug resistance in the world. Third Report. The WHO/IUATLD Project on Anti-tuberculosis Drug Resistance Surveillance. Geneva: World Health Organization, 2004.

115. Coninx R, Mathieu C, Debacker M et al. First-line tuberculosis therapy and drug-resistant Mycobacterium tuberculosis in prisons. Lancet 1999; 353: 969–73.

116. Edlin BR, Tokars JI, Grieco MH et al. An outbreak of multidrug-resistant tuberculosis among hospitalized patients with the acquired immunodeficiency syndrome. N Engl J Med 1992; 326: 1514–21.

117. Fischl MA, Uttamchandani RB, Daikos GL et al. An outbreak of tuberculosis caused by multiple-drug-resistant tubercle bacilli among patients with HIV infection. Ann Intern Med 1992; 117: 177–83.

118. Schaaf HS, Van Rie A, Gie RP et al. Transmission of multidrug-resistant tuberculosis. Pediatr Infect Dis J 2000; 19: 695–9.

119. Caminero JA. Management of multidrug-resistant tuberculosis and patients in retreatment. Eur Respir J 2005; 25: 928–36.

120. Mukherjee JS, Rich ML, Socci AR et al. Programmes and principles in treatment of multidrug-resistant tuberculosis. Lancet 2004; 363: 474–81.

121. Kim SJ. Drug-susceptibility testing in tuberculosis: methods and reliability of results. Eur Respir J 2005; 25: 564–9.

122. World Health Organization. The global MDR-TB and XDR-TB response plan 2007–2008 (WHO/HTM/TB). Geneva: World Health Organization, 2007.

123. Etkind SC, Veen J. Contact follow-up in high and low-prevalence countries. In: Reichman LB, Hershfield ES (eds). Tuberculosis: a comprehensive international approach, 2nd edn. New York: Marcel Dekker, 2000: 377–99.

124. Rieder HL. Contacts of tuberculosis patients in high-incidence countries. Int J Tuberc Lung Dis 2003; 7 (Suppl. 3): S333–6.

125. Mohle-Boetani JC, Flood J. Contact investigations and the continued commitment to control tuberculosis (editorial). *J Am Med Assoc* 2002; **287**: 1040.

126. Reichler MR, Reves R, Bur S *et al.* Evaluation of investigations conducted to detect and prevent transmission of tuberculosis. *J Am Med Assoc* 2002; **287**: 991–5.

127. Morrison JL, Pai M, Hopewell P. Yield of tuberculosis contact investigations within households in high incidence countries: a systematic review. Infectious Diseases Society of America (IDSA) 43rd Annual Meeting 2005, San Francisco, 6–9 October 2005, Abstr. 239.

128. Morrison JPM, Hopewell PC. Tuberculosis and latent tuberculosis infection in close contacts of persons with pulmonary tuberculosis: A systematic review and meta analysis of yield of contact investigation in low and middle income countries. *Lancet Infect Dis* 2007 (in press).

16

The surgical management of tuberculosis and its complications

PETER GOLDSTRAW

INTRODUCTION

The techniques of pulmonary resection in use today were developed to deal with the persisting problem of tuberculosis (TB) in the 1930s, 1940s and 1950s. In addition, collapse therapy led to the development of thoracoplasty, still of value in rare circumstances today,[1] thoracoscopy, now refined by the development of video-assisted technology, and plombage, which has evolved into techniques of space reduction, such as myoplasty and omentoplasty. As the incidence of tuberculosis declined in developed countries, these techniques were left as a valuable legacy and were available to deal with the next epidemic – lung cancer and the chronic infective complications that resulted from this surgery. Today, however, the management of tuberculosis and its sequelae, is benefiting from the subsequent development of techniques such as mediastinoscopy, video-assisted thoracic surgery (VATS) and myoplasty. This cross-pollination has provided the modern thoracic surgeon with a broad range of procedures to deal with the continued threat of tuberculosis in Western countries, the rising incidence of multidrug-resistant organisms and the continued epidemic of tuberculosis in underdeveloped countries. The thoracic surgeon still has an important role, supporting the respiratory physician, in the diagnosis and management of difficult cases.

DIAGNOSIS

The sputum-negative patient may present with mediastinal lymphadenopathy, a pleural effusion or a pulmonary nodule, requiring biopsy to exclude other conditions, especially sarcoidosis, carcinoma and lymphoma, and to obtain tissue for culture and sensitivity. Whilst the chest radiograph may clearly demonstrate lymphadenopathy, a computed tomographic (CT) scan will often be requested to confirm that lymph nodes within reach of biopsy techniques are enlarged, to help in the choice of the appropriate technique (Figure 16.1), to identify any pulmonary focus and to clarify the relationship of vital structures which present a hazard at surgery. The surgeon has several biopsy techniques from which to choose the one that will most reliably establish the diagnosis, and if more than one is possible will choose on the basis of familiarity, the equipment available and cosmetic considerations (Figure 16.2).

Cervical mediastinoscopy

Cervical mediastinoscopy is undertaken under general anaesthesia using a 2- to 3-cm incision midway between the suprasternal notch and the thyroid cartilage. Although a safe and relatively minor procedure, considerable experience is needed to avoid damage to the recurrent laryngeal nerves and major blood vessels in this crowded anatomical region.[2] The development of video-assisted mediastinoscopy has been of considerable benefit in training surgeons to navigate safely through this region.[3] The view of the surgeon is enhanced, the assistant can take part in the procedure and each case is a teaching experience (Figure 16.3). Mediastinoscopy allows access to, and biopsy from, the nodes in the superior mediastinum that lie on either side of the trachea, in the pretracheal position and at the main carina (Figure 16.4). Nodes in the upper

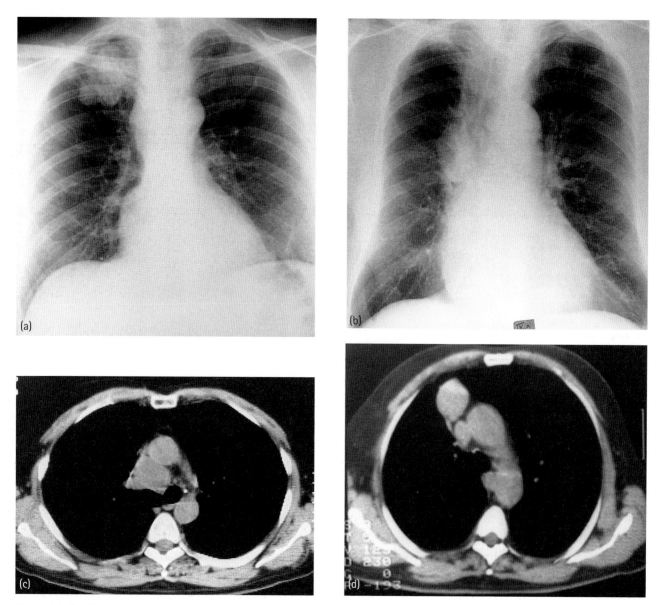

Figure 16.1   While postero-anterior chest x-rays can show that there is a mediastinal abnormality, a computed tomographic (CT) scan is necessary to show the precise site and route for biopsy. The chest film in (a) shows mediastinal widening in a patient with lung cancer, similar in appearance to the mediastinum in (b) of a patient subsequently shown to have a thymoma. The CT films in (c) and (d) clearly show that the abnormality in (a) would be accessible to cervical mediastinoscopy, while that in (b) could not be reached by this route, and requires right anterior mediastinotomy.

pole of the right hilum may be reached, but caution is necessary to avoid damage to the azygos vein and the branch of the pulmonary artery to the upper lobe. Biopsy material, as in all these techniques, will be sent for culture in addition to histological examination, and as sarcoidosis is an ever-present possibility, biopsies should be taken from several nodal stations to avoid the pitfall of detecting only the granulomatous response in a lymph node adjacent to malignancy. In fit patients, mediastinoscopy can be undertaken as a day case[4] or discharge planned after an overnight stay. A post-operative chest radiograph should be taken to ensure that the pleura has not been breached with a resultant pneumothorax.

Anterior mediastinotomy

Anterior mediastinotomy is undertaken under general anaesthesia utilizing a 3–5 cm incision through the intercostal interspace over the area to be biopsied,[2] most commonly the second intercostal space on the left or right (Figure 16.2). Resection of the costal cartilage is unnecessary and results in an ugly sulcus beneath the scar which is prone to haematoma and infection. In any event, the scar is cosmetically less acceptable, particularly for younger women and those who are heavy breasted. This approach provides safe access to nodes in the anterior mediastinum and those outside the aortic arch (Figure 16.4). Digital

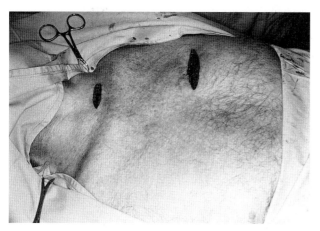

Figure 16.2 The incisions used to explore the mediastinum surgically. The patient's chin is to the left, the clavicles are visible, as is the right nipple. The upper incision at the root of the neck provides access for cervical mediastinoscopy, the longer incision on the left chest wall is for anterior mediastinotomy. The cosmetic result of the former is very satisfactory as the scar is in the skin crease. The latter results in a visible scar that is less satisfactory.

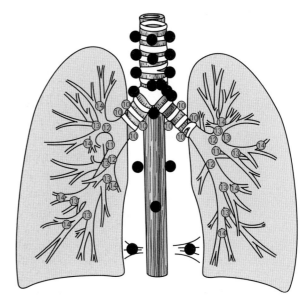

Figure 16.4 A nodal chart used to describe node positions. Those nodes in stations 1–4 in the paratracheal areas, stations 1 and 3 in the pretracheal area and station 7 at the main carina are accessible to cervical mediastinoscopy. Stations 5 and 6 lying beneath the aortic arch and over the ascending aorta are only accessible by anterior mediastinotomy.

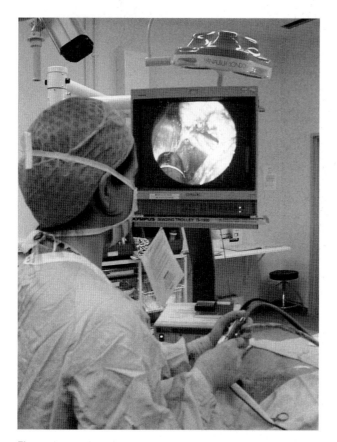

Figure 16.3 A patient undergoing cervical video-mediastinoscopy. The instrument is inserted beneath the pretracheal fascia and dissection proceeds to the main carina. The surgeon and assistant view the field on the monitor allowing both to participate in the operation. The view is magnified and structures are more clearly seen than with conventional mediastinoscopy.

examination through the interspace will identify a safe target that can be incised to provide a large biopsy. The use of the diathermy should be reserved for haemostasis after a representative biopsy has been secured and one should avoid the temptation to biopsy vascular nodes using the diathermy, as this will result in material of little value to the histopathologist. The pleura is often entered when undertaking biopsy through the right side, but this is of little consequence if the breach is recognized and air evacuated before closing the wound using a temporary drain through the incision. A post-operative chest radiograph is mandatory. Most patients will wish to stay overnight before discharge.

Video-assisted thoracoscopy

VATS can be undertaken with a single 2-cm access port under local anaesthesia with the patient breathing spontaneously. However, better access is afforded with greater comfort for the patient and surgeon if general anaesthesia and single-lung ventilation is used, and this is mandatory if more complex procedures are contemplated involving several access ports. Although VATS can be used to access mediastinal lymph nodes that lie in a suitable location, these are usually accessible with greater ease and less equipment using one of the previous techniques. VATS is of value when biopsy of the pleura (Figure 16.5) or lung is needed.

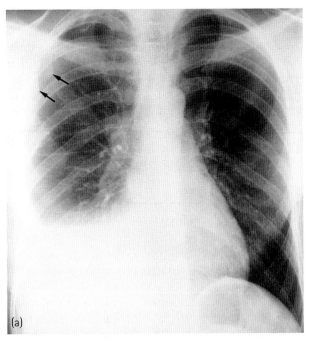

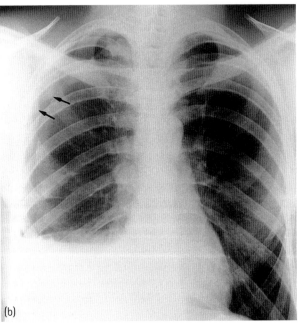

Figure 16.5 The chest x-ray (a) of a patient presenting with a right pleural effusion. The underlying pleural nodules (arrowed) are easier to see on a second radiograph taken after aspiration had resulted in an inadvertent pneumothorax (b). Biopsy by video-thoracoscopy showed the presence of necrotizing granulomata and acid-fast bacilli.

Thoracotomy and pulmonary resection

Thoracotomy and pulmonary resection will on occasions prove the only technique that will allow a firm diagnosis and exclude covert malignancy.[5] Lung lesions greater than 3 cm in diameter cannot be safely excised using VATS techniques, and where the lung abnormalities are larger or

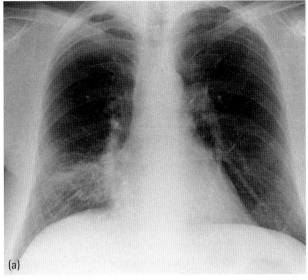

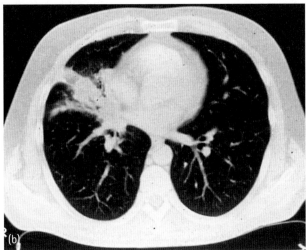

Figure 16.6 The postero-anterior chest x-ray (a) and computed tomographic film (b) of a middle-aged smoker with haemoptysis. The extensive consolidation required exploratory thoracotomy and middle lobectomy to establish a diagnosis of tuberculosis and to exclude an underlying neoplasm.

confluent, thoracotomy is necessary to fully explore the chest (Figure 16.6). The surgeon will wish to avoid taking biopsies from the periphery of such consolidated areas as this may miss an underlying neoplasm, and must ensure for the patient a full and reliable assessment. Progressive dissection, with frequent frozen-section biopsies, is necessary to encircle the abnormality. Often during such a dissection, the true pathology becomes apparent with a diagnosis of malignancy or clear proof of tuberculosis, but if the biopsy reports are of non-specific inflammation, the surgeon will feel that lobectomy is necessary. It is unsure whether resection in these circumstances speeds resolution of the infective process, but it is certainly preferable to failing to resect a potentially curable cancer. Of course, if tuberculosis is established subsequently or seems probable on macroscopic examination of the resection specimen, conventional drug treatment should be started immediately, ahead of culture results.

Lung cancer can occur in conjunction with active tuberculosis, or follow years after exposure or effective therapy if the patient is a smoker (Figure 16.7). The supervising clinician needs to be aware of this possibility if radiological progression is observed despite 'adequate' therapy or if 'reactivation' is suggested by the development of a new opacity. Many such patients are too frail, or have insufficient pulmonary reserve to tolerate resection, but needle biopsy is warranted and effective non-surgical therapy should not be withheld. The fear of reactivation of dormant tuberculous infection by chemotherapy or radiotherapy makes the use of prophylactic antituberculous therapy justified in such circumstances.

MANAGEMENT

'Resistant' tuberculosis

Occasionally, organisms which are sensitive to drug therapy, if sequestered within lung cavities, may not be eradicated by 'adequate' drug therapy (Figure 16.8). The surgeon may complete sterilization in such cases by resecting the cavity. For such major surgery, the patient should be in a good nutritional state with adequate lung function to withstand resection, and should have had a course of appropriate antituberculous chemotherapy for at least 3 months. In practice, in the undernourished subjects who are likely to require such surgery, a considerable period of in-patient preparation will be required to optimize their condition with nutritional support and intensive physiotherapy.[6,7] The surgeon will wish to document the full extent of the lung disease before surgery, to see the size and extent of the cavity, to visualize any additional cavities, to anticipate the probable extent of resection and assess the degree to which fibrosis involves adjacent lung segments. In former times, bronchography was extremely useful in this respect, but has now been superseded by CT scanning. Resection in these circumstances is technically demanding.[7-9] The pleural space and fissural planes are usually obliterated by chronic inflammation and hard, adherent nodes surround the hilar structures. The surgeon's attempts to be conservative will be made difficult by such problems and the surrounding fibrosis that usually extends into lung parenchyma beyond the area of the cavity. Careful and technically taxing dissection is necessary. Despite meticulous haemostasis, blood transfusion is invariably required.[10] The surgeon must make every attempt to preserve lung tissue that is judged to be recoverable. This will on occasions present the clinician with the additional problem posed by a small lung remnant failing to fill the hemithorax. The combination of a small residual lung, fibrotic or emphysematous lung parenchyma with a persistent air-leak and the consequent need for prolonged drainage is a recipe for the development of a chronic space infection. The surgeon will wish to avoid this and if this scenario seems probable, will add a space reduction procedure to the operation, either immediately or after a period of drainage has established the maximal expansion to which the residual lung is capable and defined the extent of chest cavity reduction which is required.[5,11] There are a

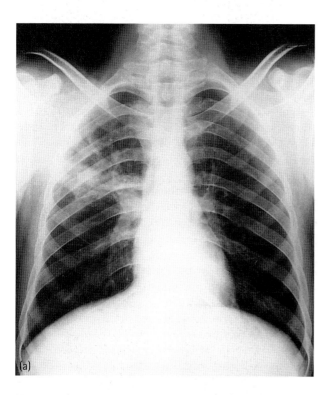

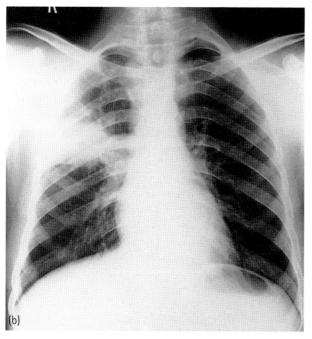

Figure 16.7 The chest x-ray (a) of a patient sputum positive for tuberculosis. During treatment with appropriate antibiotics a second x-ray (b) showed the opacity to have progressed. At thoracotomy, a carcinoma was confirmed and resected.

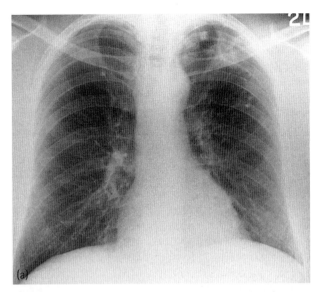

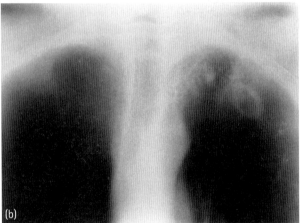

Figure 16.8 The postero-anterior chest x-ray (a) and tomograms (b) of a patient with 'resistant' TB. Bacteriological clearance was obtained by excision of the upper division of the left upper lobe.

number of such techniques available to the surgeon. A 'trimming' thoracoplasty is an old and well-tried operation.[12] This involves the subperiosteal resection of the

upper ribs sufficient to reduce the chest cavity to the size that will accommodate the residual lung. The first rib is removed from the sternum to the neck, protecting the neurovascular structures at the apex, and usually two to four other ribs, from the head of the rib forwards over a sufficient arc of the rib. The anterior extent of the resection of these ribs is progressively tailored to leave the new apex of the chest cavity configured to the shape of the remaining lung segments (Figure 16.9). In this context, it is not usually necessary to resect the transverse processes of the vertebrae. The removal of up to three ribs has little cosmetic impact, although physiotherapy is necessary to preserve posture and good shoulder movement, but more than this is probably now unacceptable (Figure 16.10) as other techniques are available. A pleural tent can be fashioned by extrapleural mobilization over the apex. This produces a haematoma above the tent and will reduce intrapleural volume without irreversibly compressing the lung parenchyma. Unfortunately, in this context, the pleura is usually damaged during dissection and is not available for this technique. The diaphragm may be temporarily paralysed by cryoablation of the phrenic nerve immediately above its insertion, allowing the diaphragm to rise to obliterate any residual space. Unfortunately, this development of the phrenic crush procedure may not prove adequate if the diaphragmatic position is fixed by chronic inflammation and fibrosis. A myoplastic rotation flap provides healthy tissue to help fill the hemithorax. If the services of an expert reconstructive surgeon are to hand, the ipsilateral latissimus dorsi, the pectoralis major and the serratus anterior, separately or in combination, can be mobilized on their vascular pedicle and transposed into the chest cavity through a short rib resection at an appropriate level. Whilst such techniques are technically demanding and require some anticipation on the part of the thoracic surgeon, they provide a good cosmetic result with rapid recovery.[13] In practice, a limited 'trimming' thoracoplasty combined with a myoplastic flap provides good space reduction with a satisfactory cosmetic result, even if only the basal segments of the lower lobe can be preserved.

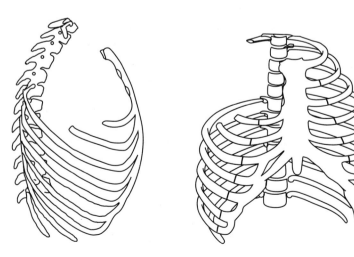

Figure 16.9 A diagram to illustrate the skeletal resection associated with a five-rib thoracoplasty. In this case, the majority of the first rib has been resected, the whole of ribs 2 and 3, with the transverse processes, and tailored resection of ribs 4 and 5 with the transverse processes.

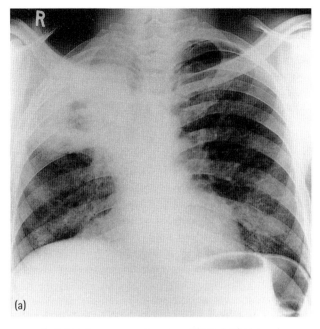

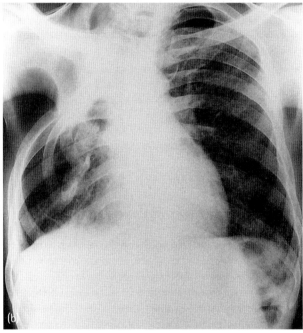

Figure 16.10   The chest x-ray (a) of a patient with extensive cavitation due to tuberculosis, presenting with life-threatening haemoptysis. Emergency surgery was successful (b), but entailed resection of the right upper lobe, the apical segment of the lower lobe and a trimming, five-rib thoracoplasty (note the first rib was left on this occasion).

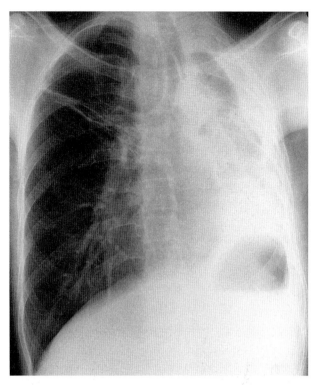

Figure 16.11   The chest x-ray of a patient with 'resistant' TB with extensive destruction of the left lung and minimal disease on the right. Pleuropneumonectomy was performed after 3 months of drug therapy and resulted in sputum conversion.

morbidity remains high, around 30 per cent, chiefly through the development of infective problems often linked with bronchopleural fistula (BPF).

Antituberculous chemotherapy should be continued post-operatively, modified by bacteriological information from the resection specimen. Most authors suggest at least a further 6 months of drug therapy, although others recommend 12 months.[5]

Multidrug-resistant tuberculosis

Mycobacteria resistant to one or more first-line drugs are now increasingly being encountered in developed countries. Although they are mercifully uncommon in Northern Europe,[15] they present the most common indication for surgery in tuberculosis in North America.[11,16] Prolonged medical therapy is important in the selection and preparation of patients for surgery and ideally sputum conversion should be obtained before operation.[11,16] Patients who do not become sputum negative and those with residual cavities or destroyed lung parenchyma should undergo surgery, as long as their disease can be encompassed by resection (Figure 16.11). Those who have widespread, bilateral parenchymal disease are not suitable (Figure 16.12). The risks of BPF makes the addition of a

Sadly, pneumonectomy will still prove necessary on occasions when all function has been lost on one side and the other lung is normal or the site of minimal disease (Figure 16.11). In such circumstances, it is usual to undertake pleuropneumonectomy as this facilitates dissection and ensures the clearance of any infected collections within the pleural space. Whilst the mortality of this formidable operation is now less than 10 per cent,[6,8,14] the myoplastic flap to cover the bronchial stump justified, at least in those undergoing pneumonectomy[11] and some authors would add this routinely to any patient undergoing pulmonary resection for multidrug-resistant TB

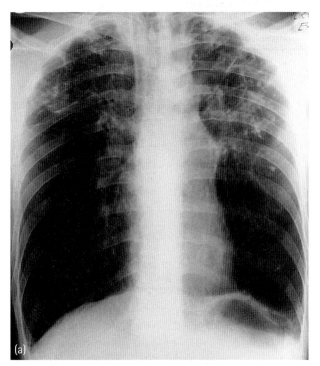

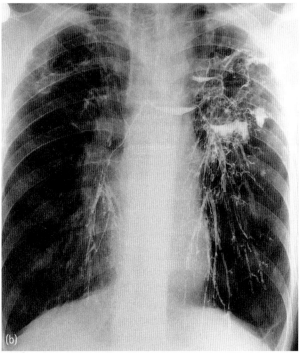

Figure 16.12 (a) The postero-anterior x-ray of a patient with 'resistant' TB referred for surgery. The bronchogram (b) shows that the extent of cavitation would have required bilateral resections, involving upper lobectomy on the right, upper lobectomy and apical sementectomy with trimming thoracoplasty on the left, which was judged too extensive for this patient's fitness.

(MDR-TB).[16] Drugs are continued post-operatively for a prolonged period, but many patients will default despite careful supervision. Prolonged disease control will be achieved with surgery and drug therapy in up to 90 per cent of this difficult population,[11] an improvement on the high relapse rate seen with medical therapy alone.[17]

Surgery for the complications of TB

A tuberculous effusion will resolve with drug therapy unless complicated by pyogenic infection, or the development of a BPF, resulting in an empyema. Such septic complications usually occur during the acute illness, but if resolution is incomplete, the presence of a persisting loculus may lead to empyema many years after successful eradication of the tuberculous infection. The treatment of such a complication, whatever the time course, follows the general principles of any empyema: drainage followed by definitive therapy. Aspiration should be performed to confirm the diagnosis and identify the organism. Occasionally, mycobacteria will be found if the original infection was not treated adequately, but usually pyogenic bacteria are responsible. An intercostal drain may be necessary if the patient is toxic and unwell, but in most cases drainage will be surgical, by rib resection at the most dependent point of the empyema. If this site is not obvious on lateral and postero-anterior chest radiographs, a small volume of heavy radio-opaque contrast material will demonstrate the optimal point for drainage on subsequent erect, lateral and postero-anterior chest x-rays. At the time of drainage, the surgeon will evacuate all fibrin debris and, if there is no clinical or radiographic evidence to suggest a BPF, will irrigate the cavity to clean the space. Such debridement can be facilitated by VAT[18] and at times this may amount to video-assisted decortication.[19] Adequate open drainage, given time, will lead to the slow re-expansion of the underlying lung, as long as the lung has fully recovered from the tuberculous infection (Figure 16.13). In frail, debilitated individuals, the clinician may persist with drainage in the hope that resolution occurs or their condition improves sufficiently to allow other options to be considered. Fenestration, the creation of a skin-lined window or Eloesser flap,[20] facilitates prolonged drainage without the logistical problems associated with tube drainage. Definitive surgical treatment will speed re-expansion and resolution of the chronic infection, but is dependent upon the fitness of the patient and the state of the lung as assessed by CT scanning (see above). Decortication can be difficult if the visceral cortex is calcified, as may be the case in empyemata that occur many years after the tuberculous infection, and this situation is akin to the problems associated with collapse therapy (see below). If the cortex can be removed, the lung will re-expand if the parenchyma is healthy. If bronchiectasis is present in a segment, lobe or the whole lung, pulmonary resection should be combined with decortication. If the residual lung is too small to fill

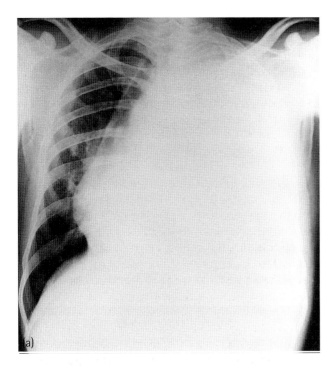

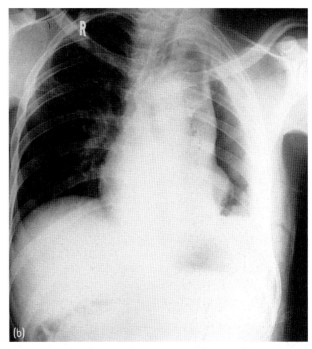

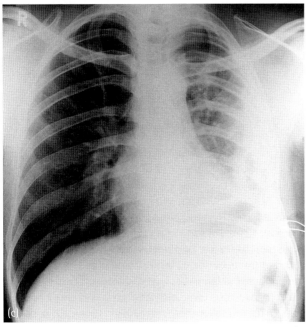

Figure 16.13 The presentation x-ray (a) of a patient with a large, post-tuberculous left empyema. After rib resection and drainage (b), the mediastinum has moved centrally, but a large space remains on the left. (c) After 3 months the space has all but resolved with re-expansion of the left lung. Such recovery suggests that the lung has not suffered severe damage from the tuberculous infection. After a further 6 weeks, a sinogram showed no residual space and the drain was removed.

the hemithorax, due to extensive resection or parenchymal fibrosis, one of the space-filling techniques described above will be added to decortication, unless pneumonectomy has proven necessary. Given the bilateral nature of the lung damage that is often present, the surgeon will strive to preserve any functioning lung tissue on the side of the empyema.

The severity of symptoms may make surgery necessary for some of the other complications of tuberculosis.[7] A persistent cough, productive of large quantities of purulent sputum, may result from bronchiectasis, destroyed lung parenchyma or be due to a persistent cavity. Post-tuberculous bronchiectasis usually results in progressive loss of the lung parenchyma subserved by the affected bronchi and

associated atelectasis (Figure 16.14). Resection of such grossly diseased and functionless lung tissue has little impact on residual lung function. Therefore, if the bronchiectatic segments can be encompassed by pulmonary resection, even if this entails bilateral thoracotomies, surgery offers good symptomatic relief (Figure 16.15). The severity of such disease in each lobe or segment correlates well with the contribution it is making to the patient's symptoms. On occasions therefore, it may be justified to remove a grossly diseased lobe, even if areas of minor damage are left in the ipsilateral or contralateral lung. This can be a difficult decision for the surgeon, but in properly selected cases, significant, if incomplete, relief of symptoms can be expected.

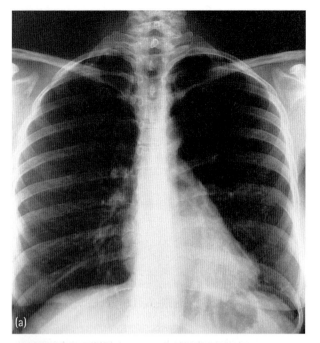

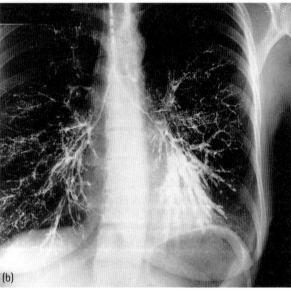

Figure 16.14 The chest x-ray (a) of a patient with collapse of the left lower lobe following tuberculosis. Persistent sputum production was resolved after a bronchogram (b) showed complete bronchiectasis of the left lower lobe, sparing of any other segments, and left lower lobectomy successfully relieved the symptoms.

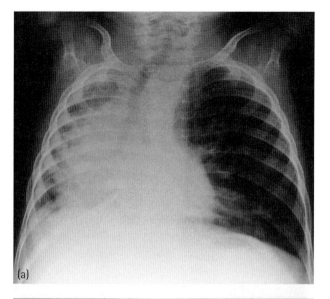

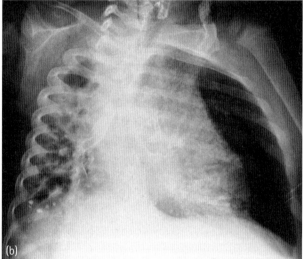

Figure 16.15 The chest x-ray (a) of a 3-year-old child following tuberculosis left with severe cough with sputum production and failure to thrive. The bronchogram (b) shows total destruction of the right lung and left lower lobe bronchiectasis. He successfully underwent right pneumonectomy and left lower lobectomy, with relief of symptoms and no change in exercise capacity.

Haemoptysis may be small and repeated or dramatic and life threatening, and may result from an area of bronchiectasis or destroyed lung, or an uncomplicated cavity. Haemoptysis is much more common and far more problematical when the cavity has been colonized by a fungal ball. Whilst CT scanning is valuable to demonstrate the presence of fungal colonization of a small cavity (Figure 16.16),[21] this is usually obvious on the chest radiograph with large cavities (Figure 16.17). Cough is then also more persistent and especially debilitating when the

patient is supine at night. The technical problems associated with resection for tuberculosis, described previously, are even greater in these circumstances, and surgery is only indicated if symptoms are severe. In many patients, the extent of the disease and their poor health will make such surgery excessively hazardous. Certainly a much greater level of fitness is required than would be needed if undertaking the relatively straightforward resection of a cancer. The surgeon should strive to be conservative, using space reduction techniques where appropriate. The mortality remains high, usually in the region of 10 per cent,[5,22] although others have found it as high as 30 per cent.[23] In

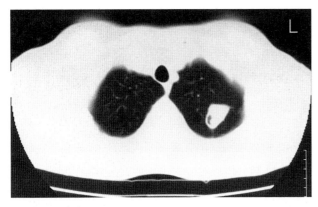

Figure 16.16 The computed tomographic scan of an apical mass showing the typical appearances of a fungal ball, allaying suspicions of a neoplasm.

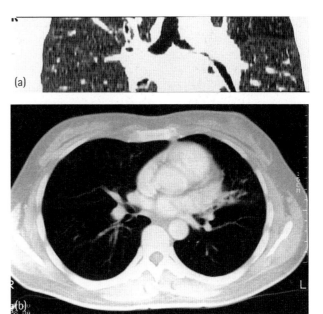

Figure 16.18 A spiral computed tomographic reconstruction (a) of a patient who suffered tuberculous endobronchial infection, showing stenosis of the termination of the left main bronchus. The scan (b) also confirmed damage to the left upper lobe by obstruction with subsequent bronchiectasis. Bronchoplastic resection of the main bronchus with upper lobectomy restored function to the lower lobe and prevented progressive loss of the whole lung.

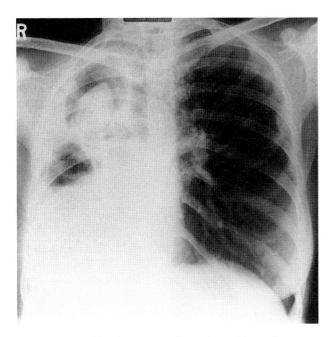

Figure 16.17 The chest x-ray of a patient with total destruction of the right lung following tuberculosis. The largest cavity has been colonized by a large fungal ball. Repeated haemoptysis required pleuropneumonectomy.

the emergency setting, preparation is denied and the risks are even greater. It is not surprising therefore that bronchial embolization is appealing to patient and doctors alike. Although some radiologists, with diligence and persistence, have managed good results,[24] these are often short-lived, although still of value in permitting surgery to be delayed for more thorough assessment. Surgery, however, is justified in this taxing situation as the risk of further fatal bleeding with medical therapy offsets the appeal of conservative management.[25,26]

If fungal balls are present bilaterally, the associated widespread parenchymal disease will leave few patients with sufficient respiratory reserve to tolerate complex, bilateral resections. If the radiologist can identify the

bronchial vessel responsible for the haemorrhage this should be embolized. If not, then all large bronchial vessels will have to be embolized on both sides, taking care to avoid any important spinal branches. Success in such circumstances is lower, but one has little option in such dire situations. The risk of bleeding seems related to the size of the cavity, not the fungal ball.[25] Therefore, if the cavity on one side is considerably larger than on the other side, and if the patient is fit for unilateral surgery, then the clinician may be forced to undertake the speculative resection of the dominant lesion in the hope of salvaging the patient. In patients in whom embolization has failed repeatedly, and who are unfit for conventional surgery, the surgeon may have to resort to unconventional techniques. Injecting antifungal agents, such as brilliant green, natamycin and 'Polish paste', into the cavity, bronchoscopically or percutaneously has been advocated,[27] but the results are unconvincing. We have tried cavernostomy, combined with evacuation of the fungal ball and oversewing of the bleeding vessel, usually a major branch of the pulmonary artery or a side hole in the main vessel itself, with little success. Cavernostomy in the elective situation is successful at relieving cough and less dramatic bleeding, and the cavity may remain radiologically free of colonization for a few years. Transposing a myoplastic flap into the cavity seems to be beneficial even if the flap fails to fill all the interstices of the cavity. Perhaps the muscle with its blood supply exudes cytokines that prevent further colonization. Colleagues in Brazil (personal communication) tell of long-term success where cavernostomy is prolonged by the creation of a skin-lined fenestrum into the cavity.

Endobronchial tuberculosis can result in bronchial stenosis and subsequent destruction of the subserved lung parenchyma. If medical therapy with the addition of steroids does not lead to resolution, early recourse to surgery is necessary to preserve lung function.[28,29] Conservative surgery is often possible and bronchoplastic repair will conserve some or all of the lung parenchyma (Figure 16.18).

Surgery for the late sequelae of collapse therapy

We are often haunted by our successes. Patients who had cavitating tuberculosis in the 1940s and early 1950s and were salvaged from this dismal situation by 'novel' collapse procedures, may return in their twilight years with the late, infective complications of induced pneumothorax, extrapleural pneumothorax, plombage (Figure 16.19) or an inadequate thoracoplasty. The responsible clinician, and even the patient themselves, may overlook the distant history. Indeed, many of the doctors treating such patients would not have been born at the time of the initial treatment. As a consequence, it is not unusual for such problems to be undiagnosed for many months, or dismissed as chest infections or simple empyemata. Once considered, the diagnosis is not difficult and CT scanning will confirm the situation (Figure 16.20). The intrathoracic space will be seen on serial chest x-rays to have enlarged (Figure 16.21) or to have developed a fluid level (Figure 16.22). The infective agent is usually a pyogenic organism, such as *Staphylococcus aureus*, but myobacterium TB may be present and requires additional drug therapy. Surgical management is complex and further complicated by the age and frailty of many patients. Initial drainage should be

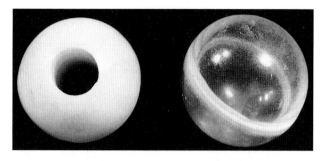

Figure 16.19 Plombage was previously undertaken to facilitate 'collapse therapy', using materials such as 'polystan balls' (left) and 'lucite balls' (right).

performed surgically. Any foreign material is removed from the plomb, which is not difficult if polystan or lucite balls had been used, but can be more troublesome if shredded plastic had been inserted without an envelope (Figure 16.21). Subsequent management, and its timing, will depend upon the level of fitness achieved following drainage, and the patient's attitude to long-term drainage. If they are sufficiently fit to be offered a permanent solution, most will opt for surgery, despite the obvious risks. If the underlying lung is of reasonable volume and CT suggests it is has recovered well from the initial infection and years of collapse, decortication may be attempted. Usually, however, this alone will prove inadequate. The lung may fail to fill the hemithorax or surgical trauma will leave an excessive air-leak. Space obliteration by myoplasty and/or omentoplasty is often necessary, often combined with a 'trimming' thoracoplasty that reduces the cavity to be filled and allows access for the muscle flap. The omentum is particularly well suited to this situation because of its ability to 'mop up' infection and adhere to the underlying lung. A pedicled, rotation flap of omentum may not reach the apex of the chest cavity (Figure 16.23). The addition of a myoplastic flap, based on pectoralis major or serratus anterior, may serve to fill this part of the cavity or the tech-

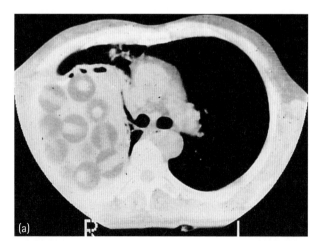

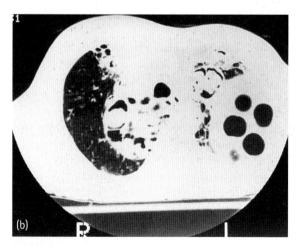

Figure 16.20 Computed tomographic cuts showing the characteristic appearances of 'polystan balls' (a) and 'lucite balls' (b). In addition, this patient also had extensive cavitation and fungal colonization.

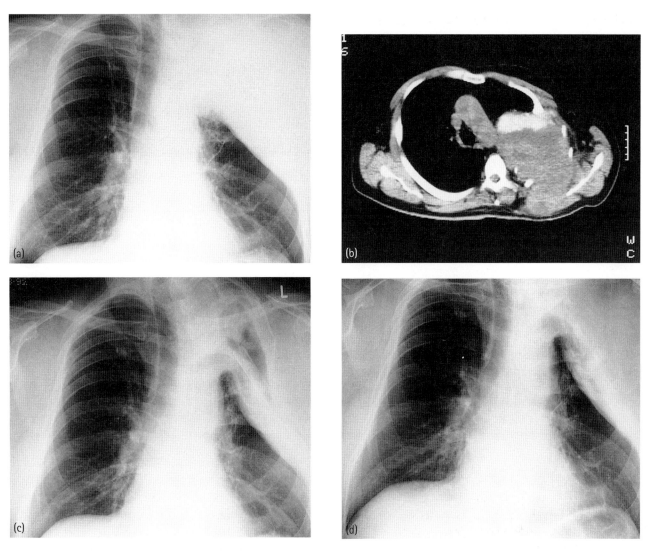

Figure 16.21 The chest x-ray (a) of a patient presenting with chest wall pain and a mass 40 years after plombage for tuberculosis. A sarcoma was suspected, but the computed tomography scan (b) shows the underlying plombage expanding through the chest wall. After the evacuation of the shredded plastic plombage material, drainage shows the size of the residual cavity (c). Six months later, the patient accepted surgery to obliterate the space by trimming thoracoplasty and omental transfer, with complete resolution (d).

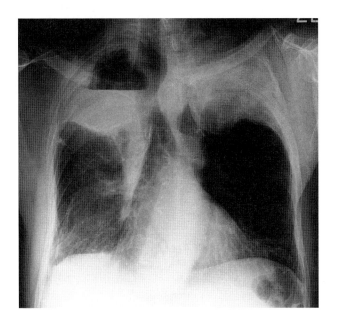

Figure 16.22 The chest x-ray of a patient presenting with fever, cough and haemoptysis 35 years after right extrapleural pneumothorax and right-sided plombage. The fluid level indicates the infection is within the right space.

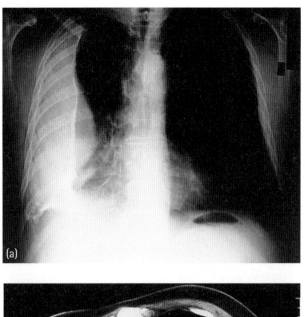

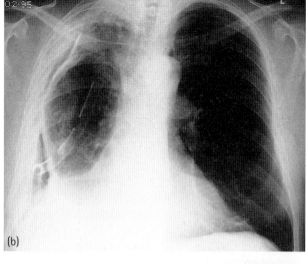

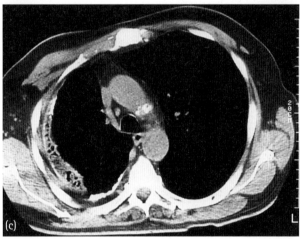

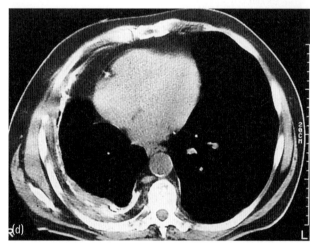

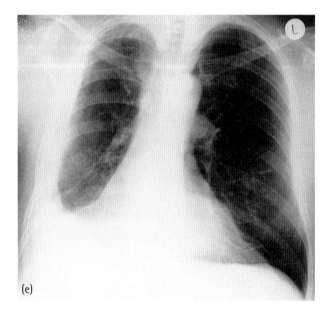

Figure 16.23 The chest x-ray of a patient with right chest pain many years after 'collapse therapy' for tuberculosis. The presence of the wound and the extensive pleural calcification should have alerted the physician to the underlying cause. The patient neglected to mention the history and malignancy was suspected. Eventually, rather inadequate drainage was performed by a surgeon (b) who attempted pleurodesis! The computed tomographic cuts (c,d), clearly show the residual space and heavily calcified visceral and parietal cortex. The patient was reluctant to accept surgery and persisted with drainage for 1 year. The chest x-ray (e) after corrective surgery shows the space obliterated by decortication, omental transfer and a myoplastic flap to the apex of the space.

nically more demanding technique of a free graft of omentum may be necessary, using microsurgical re-anastamosis of the vascular pedicle of the omentum to a suitable artery and vein in the thorax, usually the internal mammary ves-

sels.[13] A shallow, infected pneumothorax cavity may be treated by a localized, Schede type of thoracoplasty[12] with little functional or cosmetic result (Figure 16.24). More extensive thoracoplasty operations of this type are compli-

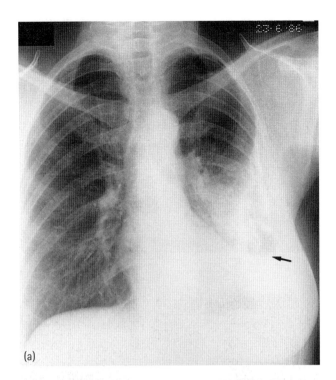

(a)

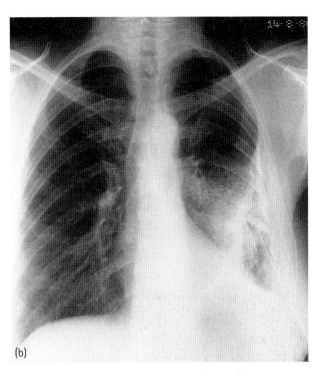

(b)

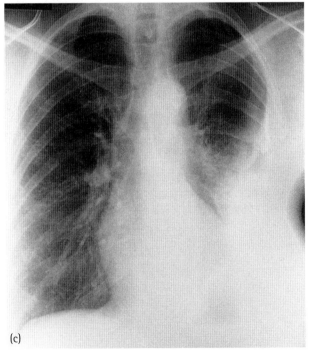

(c)

Figure 16.24 The chest x-ray (a) of a female with persistent fever and cough many years after an artificial pneumothorax for tuberculosis, showing a fluid level (arrow) in the space. After drainage (b), acid-fast bacilli were recovered and the symptoms were relieved. After appropriate drug therapy for 3 months, the space was obliterated by a localized, 'Schede-type' thoracoplasty with acceptable cosmetic results and long-term relief.

cated by the subsequent onset of respiratory failure as a consequence of denervation of the accessory, abdominal muscles of respiration. Revision of the original thoracoplasty may eradicate the residual space (Figure 16.25). If the patient is unfit for definitive surgery, then the options are limited. Long-term drainage requires domiciliary nursing care and the patient may prefer a fenestrum or Eloesser flap procedure.[20] The best quality of life may be afforded by leaving nature alone, and the patient with an intermittent discharging sinus.

Diagnostic procedures for tuberculosis, such as mediastinoscopy and VATS can be performed virtually without risk if the patient is reasonably fit and the surgeon experienced with such techniques,[2] but the risks increase as the procedure becomes more invasive and resection becomes necessary. In such circumstances, considerable experience is necessary to select and prepare the patient, and to choose the appropriate technique from the wide range of options available. Whilst lesser resections can be performed with an operative mortality less than 5 per cent,[5,7]

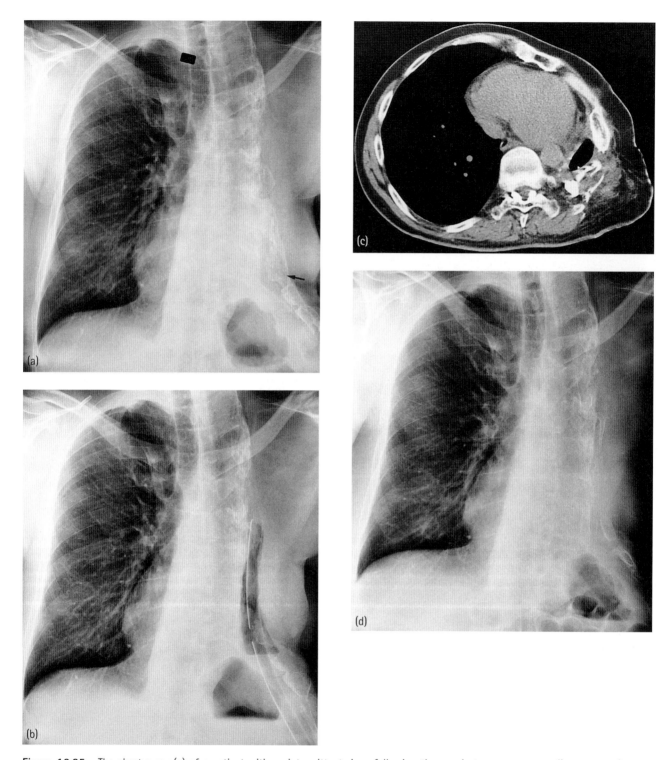

Figure 16.25 The chest x-ray (a) of a patient with an intermittent sinus following thoracoplasty many years earlier, a space is seen (arrow) at the left base beneath the thoracoplasty. After drainage (b), the extent of the cavity is seen, better demonstrated on computed tomographic scan (c). Revision of the thoracoplasty (d) dealt with the problem with no additional deformity.

if operating for the severe complications, such as fungal infection especially with massive haemoptysis, or if pneumonectomy proves necessary, expert surgery is needed to keep the mortality around 10 per cent.[5,8,22] Such surgery is technically challenging, but worthwhile in the desperate situation faced by such patients.

LEARNING POINTS

- The techniques of pulmonary resection used today were developed to deal with the problem of tuberculosis in the 1930s, 1940s and 1950s.
- Today, tuberculosis is benefiting from new surgical techniques such as video-mediastinoscopy, video-assisted thoracic surgery and myoplasty.
- Computed tomographic scan is often useful to help the surgeon plan the operation whether diagnostic or curative or palliative.
- Thoracotomy and pulmonary resection may provide the only sure diagnostic method.
- Lobectomy or even pneumonectomy may be needed if so much lung tissue is damaged at the end of medical treatment that the remainder forms only a potential hazard for suppurative infections.
- Surgery may be an essential part of the therapy for drug-resistant tuberculosis where a large cavity remains. The patient should preferably be rendered smear negative before surgery is carried out, but this is not essential.
- Drainage and later debridement of an empyema may be necessary.
- Surgery for persistent bleeding, such as from an aspergilloma, contained in a cavity may be justified but embolization of the affected segment of lung is preferable if it can be done.
- Surgery may be necessary to preserve the integrity of a main bronchus following endobronchial tuberculosis.
- Novel collapse procedures, such as plombage used in the 1940s or 1950s, may cause infection later in life. Surgical drainage and even excision may be required. Following this, decortication may be attempted, but if the lung is too small to fill the thoracic cavity myoplasty or omentoplasty may be necessary.
- Patients undergoing surgery for tuberculosis or its complications are often malnourished and surgery therefore poses a hazard. As much time as possible should be spent in preparing the patient for surgery.

REFERENCES

1. Peppas G, Molnar TF, Jeyasingham K, Kirk AB. Thoracoplasty in the context of current surgical practice. *Ann Thorac Surg* 1993; **56**: 903–909.
2. Goldstraw P. Mediastinal exploration by mediastinoscopy and mediastinotomy. *Br J Dis Chest* 1988; **82**: 111–20.
3. Mouroux J, Venissac N, Alifano M. Combined video-assisted mediastinoscopy and video-assisted thoracoscopy in the management of lung cancer. *Ann Thorac Surg* 2001; **72**: 1698–704.
4. Cybulsky IJ, Bennett WF. Mediastinoscopy as a routine outpatient procedure. *Ann Thorac Surg* 1994; **58**: 176–8.
5. Mouroux J, Maalouf J, Padovani B *et al.* Surgical management of pleuropulmonary tuberculosis. *J Thorac Cardiovasc Surg* 1996; **111**: 662–70.
6. Conlan AA, Lukanich JM, Shutz J, Hurwitz SS. Elective pneumonectomy for benign lung disease: modern-day mortality and morbidity. *J Thorac Cardiovasc Surg* 1995; **110**: 1118–24.
7. Rizzi A, Rocco G, Robustellini M *et al.* Results of surgical management of tuberculosis: experience in 206 patients undergoing operation. *Ann Thorac Surg* 1995; **59**: 896–900.
8. Reed CE. Pneumonectomy for chronic infection: fraught with danger? *Ann Thorac Surg* 1995; **59**: 408–11.
9. Goldstraw P. Surgery for pulmonary tuberculosis. *Surgery* 1987; **145**: 1071–82.
10. Griffiths EM, Kaplan DK, Goldstraw P, Burman JF. Review of blood transfusion practices in thoracic surgery. *Ann Thorac Surg* 1994; **57**: 736–9.
11. Treasure RL, Seaworth BJ. Current role of surgery in *Mycobacterium tuberculosis*. *Ann Thorac Surg* 1995; **59**: 1405–407.
12. Langston HT. Thoracoplasty: the how and the why. *Ann Thorac Surg* 1991; **52**: 1351–3.
13. al-Kattan KM, Breach NM, Kaplan DK, Goldstraw P. Soft-tissue reconstruction in thoracic surgery. *Ann Thorac Surg* 1995; **60**: 1372–5.
14. al-Kattan KM, Goldstraw P. Completion pneumonectomy: indications and outcome. *J Thorac Cardiovasc Surg* 1995; **110**: 1125–9.
15. Medical Research Council Cardiothoracic Epidemiology Group. National survey of notifications of tuberculosis in England and Wales in 1988. *Thorax* 1992; **47**: 770–5.
16. Pomerantz M, Madsen L, Goble M, Iseman M. Surgical management of resistant *Mycobacterial tuberculosis* and other mycobacterial pulmonary infections. *Ann Thorac Surg* 1991; **52**: 1108–12.
17. Goble M, Iseman MD, Madsen LA *et al.* Treatment of 171 patients with pulmonary tuberculosis resistant to isoniazid and rifampin. *N Engl J Med* 1993; **328**: 527–32.
18. Lawrence DR, Ohri SK, Moxon RE, Fountain SW. Thoracoscopic debridement of empyema thoracis. *Ann Thorac Surg* 1997; **64**: 1448–50.
19. Ferguson MK. Thoracoscopy for empyema, bronchopleural fistula, and chylothorax. *Ann Thorac Surg* 1993; **56**: 644–5.
20. Eloesser L. An operation for tuberculous empyema. *Surg Gynaecol Obstet* 1935; **60**: 1096.
21. Roberts CM, Citron KM, Strickland BS. Intrathoracic aspergilloma: role of CT in diagnosis and treatment. *Radiology* 1987; **165**: 123–8.
22. Massard G, Roeslin N, Wihlm J-M *et al.* Pleuropulmonary aspergilloma: clinical spectrum and results of surgical treatment. *Ann Thorac Surg* 1992; **54**: 1159–64.
23. Daly RC, Pairolero PC, Piehler JM *et al.* Pulmonary aspergillomas. Results of surgical treatment. *J Thorac Cardiovasc Surg* 1986; **92**: 981–8.
24. Remy J, Arnaud A, Fardou H *et al.* Treatment of hemoptysis by embolization of bronchial arteries. *Radiology* 1977; **122**: 33–7.
25. Jewkes J, Kay PH, Paneth M, Citron KM. Pulmonary aspergilloma: analysis of prognosis in relation to haemoptysis and survey of treatment. *Thorax* 1983; **38**: 572–8.
26. Knott-Craig CJ, Oostuizen JG, Rossouw G *et al.* Management and prognosis of massive hemoptysis: recent experience with 120 patients. *J Thorac Cardiovasc Surg* 1993; **105**: 394–7.
27. Henderson AH, Pearson JEG. Treatment of bronchopulmonary aspergillosis with observations on the use of natamycin. *Thorax* 1968; **23**: 519–23.
28. Watanabe Y, Shimizu J, Oda M *et al.* Results in 104 patients undergoing bronchoplastic procedures for bronchial lesions. *Ann Thorac Surg* 1990; **50**: 607–14.
29. Frist WH, Mathisen DJ, Hilgenberg AD, Grillo HC. Bronchial sleeve resection with and without pulmonary resection. *J Thorac Cardiovasc Surg* 1987; **93**: 350–57.

17

Directly observed therapy and other aspects of management of tuberculosis care

S BERTEL SQUIRE

INTRODUCTION AND DEFINITIONS: THE DISTINCTION BETWEEN DOT AND DOTS

In 1993 the World Health Organization (WHO) declared tuberculosis (TB) a global health emergency.[1] Vigorous promotion of DOTS as the recommended five-point strategy for controlling the disease began at around that time and has continued since.

In 1994, DOTS was described by WHO as a policy package which included the following five elements:[2]

Direct microscopy of sputum smears. Case detection through predominantly passive case finding and primarily by microscopy examination.
Observation of therapy. Administration of standardized short-course chemotherapy to … all confirmed sputum smear-positive cases of TB under proper case management which ensures patient compliance by supervised administration of the recommended short-course chemotherapy.
Therapeutic monitoring. Establishment and maintenance of a monitoring system to be used both for programme supervision and evaluation.
Short-course chemotherapy. Establishment of a system of regular drug supply of all essential antituberculosis drugs.
Political commitment. Government commitment to a TB programme aiming at nationwide coverage, as a permanent health system, integrated into the existing health structure with technical leadership from a central unit.

'DOTS!' was intended as a term to denote the full five-component control strategy as indicated above. However, the word 'DOTS' was also used as an acrostic for directly observed therapy, short-course. Many therefore interpreted DOTS purely as direct observation of therapy (DOT or supervised swallowing), placing undue emphasis on the supervised administration of TB drugs within the strategy.[3]

This chapter traces the origins of DOT and explores its role and effectiveness within a decade of experience within DOTS. It goes on to use a poverty analysis of DOT to understand crucial issues in access to TB diagnosis and to examine the role of DOT in the new Global Strategy to Stop TB which was launched in 2006.

ORIGINS OF DOT

Early experience with supervised therapy in Madras, Hong Kong and London

With the introduction of effective chemotherapy for TB in the 1940s and 1950s, treatment of the disease was literally transformed. There was no longer any need to institutionalize patients for long periods, and ambulatory chemotherapy was shown to be as effective as chemotherapy given in hospital, without placing contacts at increased risk of infection.[4,5] However, this transformation of practice brought with it the issue of how to promote adherence to therapy.

Wallace Fox outlined this issue when he wrote: 'Irregularity [had] been a problem throughout the course of treatments'.[6] He concluded, at a very early stage in the history of tuberculosis chemotherapy, that self-administration of therapy was highly problematic. In rather chaotic surroundings in Madras, a system of supervised therapy was developed that, despite requiring clinic attendance 6 days each week to receive a streptomycin injection, achieved very high levels of adherence among large numbers of patients over a short period of time.[7] Was this innovation site- and person-specific, or could it be replicated elsewhere?

In Hong Kong, Moodie[8] instituted ambulatory supervised therapy several years before the trials in Madras and was able to show considerable success: 70 per cent of patients completed a treatment regimen lasting almost 2 years. As in Madras, daily streptomycin injections were administered in clinics. Later, both Moodie and Fox changed to oral regimens, often given intermittently.[9] Success was attributed to strict organization of services that were structured to be as convenient for patients as possible.

In London, Stradling and Poole[10] also developed a system of clinic-based supervised therapy, with considerable success. Like Fox, they also recognized that daily therapy could be inconvenient for patients and clinic staff, and as such therapy itself might inhibit adherence. These practitioners, working in different parts of the world, worked to the principle that a simple system of treatment that could be applied to all patients was required.

Supervised therapy in the USA from 1960s onwards

A different approach was adopted in the USA in the 1960s. Moulding,[11] for example, working in Denver, stated that supervised therapy was 'unnecessary' and a 'diversion of resources'. Others felt the same way. They concluded that most patients could be relied upon to self-administer therapy and that supervised therapy was only required for 'problem patients'.[9] Sbarbaro[12] tried to change this thinking, extending the problem of adherence to therapy beyond a narrow group of 'problem patients' and demonstrated that supervised therapy was cost-effective.

Despite Sbarbaro's efforts, policy in the USA in the 1980s remained centred on self-administration of therapy as the norm, with DOT as the exception and reserved for difficult patients.[13,14] The main reasons that DOT was not the standard of care in the USA at this time were the perceived cost of DOT and the perceived infringement of human rights.[9] However, by the late 1980s and early 1990s the tide was turning in favour of universal DOT. In settings as diverse as Denver, Baltimore and Mississippi, DOT programmes that had started as small initiatives had grown to cover entire cities and states. These programmes were simple and inexpensive. Most were run without additional federal funds, implying that cost was not the overriding reason for resistance to widespread DOT; rather the important consideration of individual autonomy informed the political climate of the day. The political climate changed radically as the number of cases increased, multidrug resistance emerged and spread, and nosocomial outbreaks in hospitals affected health workers. DOT became the standard of care almost overnight and significant federal funds were made available to implement it.[15] The Advisory Council for the Elimination of Tuberculosis believed that, as it was not possible to predict who would fail to complete treatment, all patients should receive DOT.

Thus, from apparently humble beginnings in Madras and Hong Kong, the concept of supervising treatment for tuberculosis became the standard of care in arguably the most influential part of the developed world.

THE EVOLUTION OF DOT AS CENTRAL TO THE DOTS STRATEGY

Between the early days of DOT in Madras and Hong Kong and the enthusiastic uptake of DOT as the standard of care in the USA in the face of the emergence of drug resistance, DOT became one part of the five-point DOTS strategy that was developed by the International Union Against Tuberculosis and Lung Disease (the Union). Through its pioneering work under the guidance of Karel Styblo in Malawi, Tanzania and Mozambique, the Union advocated an approach based on initial hospitalization to ensure adherence followed by a period of self-administered therapy with treatment collected from clinics monthly. These model programmes also elaborated the all-important other elements of the DOTS strategy, particularly the in-built system of programme monitoring and evaluation. That this model of care worked at the time is beyond doubt. The model programmes achieved high cure rates and, as a result of their rigorously collected datasets, were able to demonstrate remarkable cost-effectiveness in the late 1980s.[16] DOT in these programmes was practised as part of the hospitalized intensive phase of therapy. So, if hospital-based DOT for the intensive phase of therapy only was so effective, even in three of the poorest countries in the world, why did the policy shift towards community-based DOT and what are the implications?

There are several reasons why control strategies in developing countries moved away from hospitalization. First, there was the pre-existing evidence from Madras that community-based treatment could be achieved (see above). The second reason for the shift in strategy was the staggering increase in TB caseload reported from many sub-Saharan African countries in association with the HIV

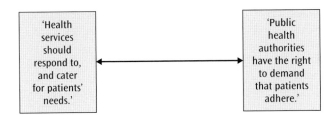

Figure 17.1 The spectrum of opinion underlying prevailing views about treatment adherence.

pandemic. There were simply not enough beds available for the number of patients presenting. The third reason for the change was intimately related to the first: cost. Treatment of TB is itself one of the most cost-effective health interventions available,[16,17] but delivery of that treatment is expensive if it is dependent on hospitalization. This is true both for the patient and for the health system.[18] The fourth reason for dispensing with hospital-based care for the intensive phase of therapy was the increasing recognition that it was cruel, costly and disruptive to patients and their families, especially in very overcrowded, poorly resourced wards. Finally, and most recently, was the concern that hospitalization would promote nosocomial transmission of TB in crowded settings, especially where infectious TB patients were accommodated in crowded wards along with other susceptible patients and health workers – particularly if HIV-infected.

Overall, therefore, DOT was not developed specifically and solely as a means of promoting adherence to therapy. It evolved as a central part of a series of pragmatic approaches to the challenge of delivering effective TB control in a variety of contexts, and under a changing set of political parameters. From an initial health system-driven substitute for hospitalization, DOT was adapted to meet the needs of patients, presaging the spectrum of opinion that now exists around DOT (see Figure 17.1). Despite the apparent disparity in wealth between the health systems of, for example, the USA and Mozambique, patients with TB at both ends of this spectrum of national wealth tend to be poor and to face barriers in adhering to treatment.

REFLECTIONS ON THE EFFECTIVENESS OF DOT AS A MEANS OF PROMOTING ADHERENCE TO TB TREATMENT

As soon as DOT was established as central to the DOTS strategy, questions were raised about the strength of the evidence for its effectiveness as a means of promoting adherence. Experience of DOT had built up as part of the evolution of TB case management described above. There was an accumulation of data on positive cure and treatment completion rates in cohorts of patients who had undergone DOT. The problem was that DOT was always part of the whole package of TB treatment delivery, including various combinations of the following:

1 Interventions aimed at preventing default:
   - *Social support*: e.g. housing or subsistence benefits.
   - *Staff motivation and supervision*: this includes training aimed at improving how providers care for people with TB.
   - *Prompts and reminders*: these are to help patients to keep appointments.
   - *Health education*: provision of information about TB and the importance of completing treatment.
   - *Incentives and reimbursements*: provision of money, or cash in kind (including food tokens) to reimburse expenses of attending health services, or to improve the attractiveness of repeat and sustained attendances with the health service.
   - *Contracts*: written and/or verbal agreements to return for appointments and treatment.
   - *Peer assistance*: lay people from the same social group helping individuals with TB to sustain their contact with the health service by prompting or accompanying them.
2 Interventions to be used once default occurs:
   - *Defaulter action*: a variety of actions (e.g. visiting patients in their homes, sending letters or phone messages, etc.) taken when patients fail to return for appointments, medicines or prescriptions.
   - *Strong public health legislation*: e.g. legal requirements for notification and recourse to incarceration for patients who persistently default from treatment.[19,20]

It was never clear, therefore, whether DOT alone was the crucial element in promoting good treatment outcomes. Randomized controlled trials (RCTs) comparing self-administered (i.e. unobserved) dosing with direct observation provided by a competent health-care worker were set up, with the intention of controlling for the effects of features of health-care delivery other than DOT. Since then, several RCTs have been completed and the results have been synthesized in a Cochrane Systematic Review.[21] Ten trials with 3985 participants met the inclusion criteria. As illustrated in Figure 17.2, the conclusions of this meta-analysis were that there was no statistically significant difference between DOT and self-administration of treatment for the number of people who were cured or completed treatment. Stratification by the location of DOT (home or at a clinic) suggested a possible small effect favouring home-based DOT.

These findings have been met with hostility and distrust among many individuals who have contributed enormously to the development and delivery of modern TB control.[22] Some of this has been a reaction to the 'lumping together' of different kinds of treatment observer (health-care worker, family member or community volunteer). However, the major objection has been that these trials have been conducted within weak TB control systems which achieved poor treatment outcomes amongst both the observed and the unobserved trial participants. In the words of two observers, 'these ... trials do confirm that

Analysis 02.02.   Comparison 02 Direct observation versus self administration: stratified by location of direct observation, Outcome 02 Cure or completion of treatment

Review: Directly observed therapy for treating tuberculosis

Comparison: 02 Direct observation versus self administration: stratified by location of direct observation

Outcome: 02 Cure or completion of treatment

Study	DOT n/N	self n/N	Relative Risk (Fixed) 95% CI	Weight (%)	Relative Risk (Fixed) 95% CI
01 Direct observation at home					
Kamolratanakul 1999	347/414	320/422		66.5	1.11 [1.03, 1.18]
Walley 2001	176/269	105/162		27.5	1.01 [0.88, 1.16]
Zwarenstein 1998	40/54	26/44		6.0	1.25 [0.94, 1.68]
Subtotal (95% CI)	737	628		100.0	1.09 [1.02, 1.16]

Total events: 563 (DOT), 451 (self)

Test for heterogeneity chi-square = 2.17 df = 2 p = 0.34 I^2 = 7.6%

Test for overall efect z=2.64 p=0.008

02 Direct observation at clinic					
Walley 2001	40/66	105/162		48.4	0.94 [0.75, 1.17]
Zwarenstein 1998	60/111	63/105		51.6	0.90 [0.71, 1.14]
Subtotal (95% CI)	177	267		100.0	0.92 [0.78, 1.08]

Total events: 100 (DOT), 168 (self)

Test for heterogeneity chi-square = 0.05 df = 1 p = 0.82 I^2 = 0.0%

Test for overall efect z = 1.04 p = 0.3

0.5 0.7   1   1.5   2
Favours self   Favours DOT

Figure 17.2   Meta-analysis of 10 trials with 3985 participants. From Ref. 21.

direct observation of treatment can, as with any health initiative relying on human effort, be implemented ineffectively'.[9]

HOW DOES DOT MEASURE UP AGAINST OTHER INTERVENTIONS AIMED AT PROMOTING ADHERENCE TO TREATMENT? THE IMPORTANCE OF QUALITATIVE WORK AND PERSPECTIVES FROM PATIENTS

In addition to scepticism about the manner and context in which the RCTs have been conducted, there has also been concern that RCTs are not the best way to test the effectiveness of a complex intervention which is so dependent on the human element within the social and cultural context. Those holding this view have tended to use qualitative research approaches to gain in-depth understanding of the factors considered important by patients, caregivers and health-care providers in contributing to TB medication adherence. Of utmost importance in these studies has been elucidation of patients' perspectives; until this moment in the development of TB control paradigms, the most powerful influences have come from health-care providers and policy-makers. Munro *et al.*[23] have recently published a systematic review of available qualitative studies in order to help develop a comprehensive and holistic understanding of barriers to, and facilitators of, treatment adherence. They found 44 articles that met the prespecified inclusion criteria and identified eight major themes across the studies:

1   organization of treatment and care;
2   interpretation of illness and wellness;
3   the financial burden of treatment;

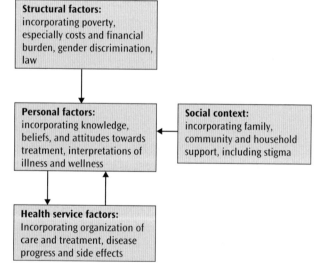

Note:

↑ ↓ suggest a bidirectional relationship between factors. For example, health service interventions directed at patients are likely to influence patient adherence behaviour through the filter of 'personal factors.' Similarly, patients' interactions with health services are likely to be influenced by their knowledge, attitudes, and beliefs about treatment as well as their interpretations of illness and wellness.

Figure 17.3   Four major factors interact to affect patient adherence to tuberculosis treatment. From Ref. 23.

4   knowledge, attitudes and beliefs about treatment;
5   law and immigration;
6   personal characteristics and adherence behaviour;
7   side effects;
8   family, community and household support.

Their interpretation of the themes produced a line-of-argument synthesis describing how four major factors interact to affect adherence to TB treatment as illustrated in Figure 17.3.

The same authors argue that the perspectives of the community of TB experts are arrayed along a spectrum. At one end of the spectrum, the prevailing attitude is that the health service should be delivered in such a way as to respond to, and cater for, people's needs. At the other end of the spectrum, the prevailing view is that public health authorities have the right to demand adherence: there is a public health imperative that infectious, smear-positive patients should complete their treatment in order to minimize the risks of infecting others (see Figure 17.1). Towards the left of the spectrum, poor adherence is seen as a result of failures in the health system and the manner in which health services are delivered. At the right hand end of the spectrum, poor adherence is perceived as the fault of patients who 'don't know, don't care and don't understand why they need to complete treatment'.[10] Maximizing adherence probably requires finding the right path between these extremes. To help find this path, it is instructive to see how Munro et al.[23] have mapped different interventions to promote adherence to therapy against the barriers to completion as derived from the systematic review of qualitative literature (see Table 17.1).

This thoughtful analysis clarifies several important issues. First, most of the documented interventions are aimed at addressing barriers associated with the health service and the individual. Those addressing barriers within the health service do not, on the whole, aim to increase the responsiveness of the service. They are framed in the predominant view that the problems with adherence lie with the patients. Second, few of the interventions address barriers in the social and family category and few have been developed as a result of participatory research with patients, their families and the communities in which they live.

This mapping of barriers against interventions to adherence does not provide a final resolution to the debate about DOT and adherence, but it does clearly point to the way forward. Interventions that address three of the factors identified (health system, social and family, and personal) already exist and must be developed further, especially those addressing social and family issues. What of the fourth set of factors: structural (including poverty, gender discrimination and the law)? These take the debate about TB control beyond a discussion of adherence to therapy and into an analysis of the extent to which TB control addresses not only the needs of patients, but also the needs of those who most often need TB care the most, namely the poor.

DOT, POVERTY AND TB CONTROL

The terms 'poverty' or 'poor' in this context refer to a range of disadvantages (not just income poverty), including a lack of material well-being, of infrastructure, and of power and voice.

Compared with the general population, poor and vulnerable groups are at greater biological risk both of infection with *Mycobacterium tuberculosis* (MTB) and breakdown of latent infection to disease.[24] A variety of factors contribute to this risk including increased aerosol transmission in overcrowded and poorly ventilated living or working conditions,[25] poor nutrition[26] and interaction with other diseases (such as HIV and AIDS). While important, the biological risks of TB that are associated with poverty are not the main issue for this analysis. In recent years, there has been a growing recognition not only that the risk of developing TB is greater among the poor, but that the converse relationship is also important. TB itself diminishes the livelihoods of affected individuals both through the lost productivity associated with chronic ill health and through the direct and indirect costs incurred by patients in their pathway to diagnosis, treatment and cure.[27,28] The concept of a pathway to TB cure is illustrated in Figure 17.4 in an adaptation of a model used by Uplekar at al.[29] This illustrates two concepts. First, the majority of TB cases arising in the community are poor. Second, the poor face barriers which affect them more than they affect the non-poor as they proceed along the pathway to cure. The result is that poorer patients tend to 'drop out' at all stages of the pathway to cure, while non-poor patients tend to follow the pathway through to a successful conclusion. The extent of the 'drop out' illustrated for each stage of the pathway is hypothetical, but recent work using gender as a proxy for poverty supports the overall shape of the curve.[30] It is important to note that adherence, as discussed so far in this chapter, is only one step along the whole pathway towards cure.

Although the pathway is illustrated as a smooth, linear process in order to convey the concept of differential poor/non-poor 'drop out', it is clear that the pathway followed by most patients is more complex. Most patient pathways are characterized by delays at each stage and by repeated visits to multiple care providers within each stage. These delays and repeated visits are costly to patients and can serve to increase the slope of the 'drop-out' rate at each stage.

Poverty, therefore, will tend to sharpen the angle of the slope of the drop-out rate, while pro-poor measures in the delivery of TB control will tend to flatten the slope. TB control that is delivered in a manner that takes account of the needs of the poor will, therefore, improve the effectiveness of TB control: more patients will be diagnosed and cured and taken out of the pool of infectious cases that drive transmission. In addition, pro-poor TB control, therefore, has the potential to reduce poverty by reducing the costs and delays experienced by patients as they move along the pathway to cure. With respect to DOT, the imperative of requiring clinic-based supervision of treatment has led to documented instances when the poor have been systematically excluded from TB care. Researchers observed that health workers used informal 'eligibility criteria' for enrolment with the DOTS programme. Patients considered to be

Table 17.1 Barriers to treatment completion as derived from a systematic review of qualitative literature and mapped on to interventions to promote adherence.

Intervention[a]	Barriers to treatment completion,[b] ranking of importance of intervention[c] and mechanism of action		
	Health system[d]	Social and family[e]	Personal[f]
Staff training	+++, Intervention improves quality of health care	–	–
Cash reimbursement	+++, Intervention increases access by reducing transport costs	++, Intervention reduces financial burden	–
Delivery of DOT by health worker	+++, Intervention provides medicine and offers supervision of patient taking medicine	–	–
Delivery of DOT by community health worker or family member	+++, Intervention provides medicine and offers supervision of patient	++, Intervention influences social and family groups	+, Intervention challenges beliefs and educates patients
Provide peer support	–	++, Intervention influences social and family groups	–
Health education provided by doctor	–	–	+++, Intervention improves knowledge
Health education provided by a nurse	–	–	+++, Intervention improves knowledge
Impose sanctions	–	–	+++, Intervention acts as an extrinsic negative force to alter behaviour
Take defaulter action (actions taken by health workers when patients do not attend for treatment)	–	–	+++, Intervention acts by modifying behaviour
Use prompts to encourage attendance for treatment	–	–	+++, Intervention acts by modifying behaviour
Use contacts to encourage adherence to treatment	–	–	+++, Intervention acts by modifying behaviour

From Garner P, Smith H, Munro S, Volmink J. *Bull World Health Organ* 2007; 85: 404–406.
DOT, directly observed treatment.
[a]Interventions identified from *Clinical Evidence.*[5]
[b]Barriers identified in unpublished systematic review of the qualitative literature on patients' experiences of adherence to tuberculosis treatment.
[c]Main target to be addressed is noted as +++, secondary target denoted as ++; possible target denoted as +. Issues that are generally not a target denoted as –.
[d]Barriers associated with health systems may include lack of access to a health facility, availability of service, length of waiting times, condition of clinic, length of treatment or relationship between provider and patient.
[e]Barriers associated with social and family characteristics may include the sex of the patient, poverty and the financial burden of treatment, the influence of peers, the influence of family and community members and social stigma.
[f]Barriers associated with personal characteristics may include a lack of motivation, lack of knowledge about the requirements of treatment, the patient's perception of disease, the patient's beliefs, attitudes and interpretations of illness and other personal characteristics.

potential defaulters were disqualified from short-course chemotherapy under DOT. Examples of patients' characteristics considered to indicate potential defaulting were social marginalization, low level of integration in the city, absolute poverty, past irregular treatment, itinerant labouring and some types of wage labouring which required regular trips out of the area.[31] In this instance, slavishly following the dogma around DOT and the need to hit the high cure-rate target combined to encourage health-care providers to select patients more likely to adhere. Could it be that the high cure rates reported in DOTS programmes around the world are not only attributable to the promotion of adherence *per se*, but the preselection, through the lengthy and costly diagnostic process,[28] of patients who were more likely to be compliant? The achievement of reaching the global treatment-success rate target of 85 per cent, while failing to meet the global case detection rate target of 70 per cent, would seem to support this possibil-

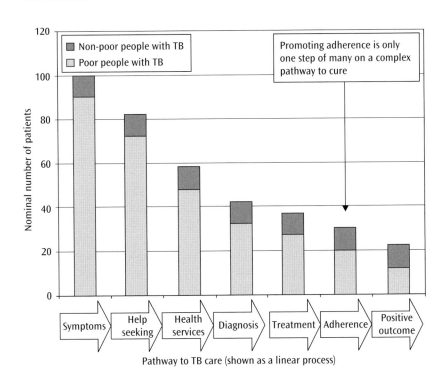

Figure 17.4 A conceptual framework for understanding the relationship between poverty and TB control and the place of action of DOT and other measures to promote adherence to treatment.

Pathway to TB care (shown as a linear process)

Box 17.1: Addressing poverty in tuberculosis control: six practical steps (From Ref. 32)

1 Establish the profile of poor and vulnerable groups.
  - government or other data;
  - locally done surveys.
2 Assess poverty-related barriers to accessing of tuberculosis services
  - economic barriers;
  - geographic barriers;
  - social and cultural barriers;
  - health-system barriers.
3 Take action to overcome barriers to access.
  - *Economic barriers*: integrate services within primary-care provision, encourage pro-poor public–private mix DOTS, promote tuberculosis control in workplaces, improve coverage of smear microscopy networks, avoid user fees, provide free smear microscopy and other diagnostic services.
  - *Geographical barriers*: extend diagnostic and treatment services to remote regions, provide free transport to patients from such regions, promote community-based care.
  - *Social and cultural barriers*: engage former patients and support groups to advocate for services and encourage community mobilization.
  - *Health-system barriers*: engage in health service decentralization to ensure capacity strengthening in less well-served areas and by establishing tuberculosis control as a district-level priority.

4 Work with groups that need special consideration.
  - refugee communities, asylum seekers, economic migrants, displaced populations;
  - pockets of deprivation in wealthier countries; ethnic minorities, homeless people;
  - injecting drug users;
  - prison populations.
5 Harness resources for pro-poor services.
  - Global Fund to Fight AIDS, TB and Malaria, poverty reduction strategies;
  - technologies to enhance efficiency and effectiveness of services.
6 Assess pro-poor performance of tuberculosis control.
  - harness human and other resources through alliances with partners, such as universities;
  - include socioeconomic variables in routine data collection;
  - include tuberculosis-related questions in district health surveys;
  - undertake periodic studies of care-seeking, diagnostic delay and use of DOTS;
  - do qualitative assessments among community members and patients about who benefits from tuberculosis services (including linked services for HIV) and who does not.

---

ity. Clearly, the promotion of adherence among those who start TB treatment is vital, but it has to be implemented in the context of getting all patients, including the poor and 'difficult' on to treatment.

The WHO has recently published a guide for TB control programmes outlining six steps to help them address poverty in TB control (see Box 17.1).[32] These steps refer to 'access to tuberculosis services'. In this context, 'access' refers to the whole process of accessing treatment for TB and taking it through to cure, not just to the steps between onset of symptoms and achieving a diagnosis (see Figure 17.4). These six steps have also been taken up into the Global Plan to Stop TB,[33] which has a special focus on the needs of the poor and vulnerable, in line with TB control activities being set within the Millennium Development Goals.[34]

THE FUTURE OF DOT – FROM DOTS TO THE 2006 GLOBAL STRATEGY TO STOP TB AND BEYOND

It is instructive to reflect on the subtle changes to the description and place of DOT within the internationally advocated strategy for TB control. In 1994, it was characterized in terms of 'supervised administration' of therapy within the five elements of the DOTS package (see also above). By 2006, within the new Global Strategy to Stop TB, the five elements of DOTS are subsumed within a single element of the new six-point strategy (see Box 17.2) and the DOT element is no longer described in terms of supervision or direct observation, but as 'patient support'. There is a distinct sense that the pendulum of global opinion is swinging from a position on the right towards the middle of the spectrum described above (see Figure 17.1, page 289). This is appropriate and timely, and may herald the development of a series of new interventions to promote adherence to treatment, which particularly address the needs of the poor.

Two important new instruments in the world of TB control can help in guiding both patients and providers towards a sensible and effective middle path. These are the International Standards for TB Care[35] and the Patients Charter for TB Care.[33] Both have been developed through a process of careful consultation across the Global Stop TB Partnership by separate groups; predominantly clinicians and health-care providers for the former, and patient activists and advocates for the latter. There was considerable interaction between the two groups in the process of the tandem formulation. Selected extracts from both are relevant to this discussion of the promotion of adherence to treatment within TB control and are summarized in Box 17.3.

Currently in the world of TB control, there is great and justifiable concern around the emergence of both multidrug- and extremely drug-resistant TB (MDR- and XDR-TB). One of the most important safeguards against the rise of these forms of TB is clearly adherence to therapy and it is important that this is promoted as effectively and safely as possible. Experience to date suggests that this will be possible, provided we take careful note both of the pragmatic experience built up within TB control programmes and embrace the growing evidence base around new and innovative approaches. It is important that the threat of MDR- and XDR-TB does not trigger a swing back too far to the right of the spectrum towards a model of adherence based on coercion and control. It is vital that we do all we can to help patients make the active choice to start and complete treatment and achieve cure. While the call in the Global Strategy to Stop TB is to help all patients in this respect, it is important to prioritize. On the whole, the better-off will face fewer barriers to making the right choices in TB control. The real priority is for services to address the needs of the poor. This means both prioritizing adherence promotion models for the poorer nations of the world and for the poorer sections of society within those nations.

Box 17.2: Components of the strategy and implementation approaches[33]

1 Pursue high-quality DOTS expansion and enhancement:
  - political commitment with increased and sustained financing;
  - case detection through quality-assured bacteriology;
  - standardized treatment, with supervision and patient support;
  - an effective drug supply and management system;
  - monitoring and evaluation system, and impact measurement.
2 Address TB/HIV, MDR-TB and other challenges:
  - implement collaborative TB/HIV activities;
  - prevent and control MDR-TB;
  - address prisoners, refugees and other high-risk groups and situations.
3 Contribute to health system strengthening:
  - actively participate in efforts to improve systemwide

policy, human resources, financing, management, service delivery and information systems;
  - share innovation that strengthen systems, including the Practical Approach to Lung Health (PAL);
  - adapt innovations from other fields.
4 Engage all care providers:
  - public–public and public–private mix (PPM) approaches;
  - International Standards for Tuberculosis Care (ISTC).
5 Empower people with TB and communities:
  - advocacy, communication and social mobilization;
  - community participation in TB care;
  - Patients' Charter for Tuberculosis Care.
6 Enable and promote research:
  - programme-based operational research;
  - research to develop new diagnostics, drugs and vaccines.

Box 17.3: Extracts from the International Standards for TB Care and the Patients Charter for TB Care which are relevant to the promotion of adherence to treatment within TB control

International standards for TB care[35]

Standard 7. Any practitioner treating a patient for tuberculosis is assuming an important public-health responsibility. To fulfil this responsibility the practitioner must not only prescribe an appropriate regimen, but also be capable of assessing the adherence of the patient to the regimen and addressing poor adherence when it occurs. By so doing the provider will be able to ensure adherence to the regimen until treatment is completed.

Standard 9. To foster and assess adherence, a patient-centred approach to administration of drug treatment, based on the patient's needs and mutual respect between the patient and the provider should be developed for all patients. Supervision and support should be gender-sensitive and age-specific and should draw on the full range of recommended interventions and available support services, including patient counselling and education. A central element of the patient-centred strategy is the use of measures to assess and promote adherence to the treatment regimen and to address poor adherence when it occurs. These measures should be tailored to the individual patient's circumstances and be mutually acceptable to the patient and the provider. Such measures may include direct observation of medication ingestion (directly observed therapy) by a treatment supporter who is acceptable and accountable to the patient and to the health system.

Standard 17. All providers must report both new and retreatment cases and their treatment outcomes to local public-health authorities, in conformance with applicable legal requirements and policies.

Patients' charter for TB care[33]

Patients' rights
1 Care
   - The right to free and equitable access to TB care, from diagnosis to completion of treatment regardless of resources, race, gender, age, language, legal status, religious beliefs, sexual orientation, culture or health status.

- The right to receive medical advice and treatment fully meets the new International Standards for TB Care, centring on patients' needs.
2 Dignity
   - The right to be treated with respect and dignity, including the delivery of services, without stigma, prejudice or discrimination by health-care providers and authorities.
3 Information
   - The right to information about the availability of health-care services for TB, and the responsibilities, engagements and direct or indirect costs involved.
   - The right to receive a timely, concise and clear description of the medical condition, with diagnosis, prognosis and treatment proposed, with communication of common risks and appropriate alternatives.
   - The right to know the names and dosages of any medications or interventions to be prescribed, its normal actions and potential side effects and its possible impact on other conditions or treatments.
4 Security
   - The right to nutritional security or food supplements if needed to meet treatment

Patients' responsibilities
1 Share information
   - The responsibility to provide as much information as possible to health-care providers about present health, past illnesses, any allergies and any other relevant details.
   - The responsibility to provide information to health-care providers about contacts with immediate family, friends and others who may be vulnerable to TB or who may have been infected.
2 Follow treatment
   - The responsibility to follow the prescribed and agreed treatment regimen and to conscientiously comply with the instructions given to protect the patient's health and that of others.
   - The responsibility to inform health-care providers of any difficulties or problems in following if any part of the treatment is not clearly understood.

LEARNING POINTS

- The definition of DOTS is:
  - direct microscopy of sputum smears requiring good quality microscopy;
  - observation of therapy by supervised administration;
  - therapeutic monitoring by carefully recording all aspects of diagnosis and treatment;
  - short-course chemotherapy requiring a regular supply of good quality drugs;
  - government commitment.

- From the 1950s, it was apparent that self-administration of drugs raised problems of completion so that clinic-based supervision of therapy was implemented in some places.
- By the 1980s, DOT was not accepted as the norm because of the possible infringement of human rights.
- Model DOTS programmes were developed in Africa in the 1970s. There were a number of reasons why hospital-based therapy could not be sustained in the 1990s:
  - community-based therapy could be made to work;

- there were too few hospital beds;
- hospital care was costly for patients and health systems;
- admitting a patient to hospital was socially disruptive;
- there was a threat of nosocomial infection.
- Implementation of DOT often includes additional interventions such as social support.
- Several randomized controlled trials have shown no benefit for DOT. However, these had been set up in relatively weak health-care systems where DOT would fail anyway. Also RTCs may not be the best way of testing complex interventions.
- DOT may not take into account various factors influencing adherence:
  - structural factors, such as poverty;
  - personal factors, such as belief systems;
  - the social context, such as the family;
  - health-service structures.
- The association of TB and poverty complicates control of the disease. Making good quality TB services more accessible to poor patients will be likely to improve control. Some DOTS programmes may exclude the poor.
- Important new tools have been published to aid world TB control:
  - International Standards for Tuberculosis Care (see Chapter 15);
  - Patient Charter for TB care.

REFERENCES

1. World Health Organization. *TB: a global emergency.* WHO report on the TB epidemic. Tuberculosis Programme. Geneva: World Health Organization, 1994: A.71 (WHO/TB/94.177).
2. World Health Organization. *Framework for effective TB control.* Tuberculosis Programme. Geneva: World Health Organization, 1994 (WHO/TB/94.179).
3. Macq JC, Theobald S, Dick J, Dembele M. An exploration of the concept of directly observed treatment (DOT) for tuberculosis patients: from a uniform to a customised approach. *Int J Tuberc Lung Dis* 2003; 7: 103–9.
4. Tuberculosis Chemotherapy Centre, Madras. A concurrent comparison of home and sanatorium treatment of pulmonary tuberculosis in South India. *Bull World Health Organ* 1959; 21: 51–144.
5. Tuberculosis Chemotherapy Centre, Madras. Intermittent treatment of tuberculosis. A concurrent comparison of twice-weekly isoniazid and daily isoniazid plus *p*-aminosalicylic acid in domiciliary treatment. *Lancet* 1963; i: 1078–80.
6. Fox W. The problem of self-administration of drugs with particular reference to pulmonary tuberculosis. *Tubercle* 1958; 39: 269–74.
7. Fox W. Self-administration of medicaments: a review of published work and a study of the problems. *Bull Int Union Tuberc Lung Dis* 1962; 32: 307–31.
8. Moodie AS. Mass ambulatory chemotherapy in the treatment of tuberculosis in a predominantly urban community. *Ann Rev Respir Dis* 1967; 95: 384–7.
9. Bayer R, Wilkinson D. Directly observed therapy for tuberculosis: history of an idea. *Lancet* 1995; 345: 1545–8.
10. Stradling P, Poole G. Towards foolproof chemotherapy for tuberculosis. *Tubercle* 1963; 44: 71–5.
11. Moulding T. New responsibilities for health departments and public health nurses in tuberculosis – keeping the outpatient on therapy. *Am J Publ Health* 1966; 56: 416–27.
12. Sbarbaro JA. All patients should receive directly observed therapy in tuberculosis. *Am Rev Respir Dis* 1988; 1382: 1075–6.
13. American Thoracic Society. Guidelines for short-course tuberculosis chemotherapy. *Am Rev Respir Dis* 1980; 212: 611–14.
14. American Thoracic Society. Standard therapy for tuberculosis. *Chest* 1985; 87: 177–240.
15. Advisory Council for the Elimination of Tuberculosis. Initial therapy for tuberculosis in the era of multidrug resistance: recommendations of the Advisory Council for the Elimination of Tuberculosis. *MMWR Morbid Mortal Wkly Rep* 1993; 42: RR/7.
16. Murray CJ, DeJonghe E, Chum HJ et al. Cost effectiveness of chemotherapy for pulmonary tuberculosis in three sub-Saharan African countries, *Lancet* 1991; 338: 1305–8.
17. Murray CJL, Styblo K, Rouillon A. Tuberculosis in developing countries: burden, intervention and cost. *Bull Int Union Tuberc Lung Dis* 1990; 65: 6–24.
18. Floyd K, Wilkinson D, Gilks C. Comparison of cost effectiveness of directly observed treatment (DOT) and conventionally delivered treatment for tuberculosis: experience from rural South Africa. *Br Med J* 1997; 315: 1407–11.
19. American Thoracic Society/Centers for Disease Control and Prevention. Control of tuberculosis in the United States. *Am Rev Respir Dis* 1992; 146: 1623–33.
20. Volmink J, Matchaba P, Garner P. Directly observed therapy and treatment adherence. *Lancet* 2000; 355: 1345–50.
21. Volmink J, Garner P. Directly observed therapy for treating tuberculosis. *Cochrane Database Syst Rev* 2006; CD003343.
22. Frieden TR, Sbarbaro JA. Promoting adherence to treatment for tuberculosis: the importance of direct observation. *Bull World Health Organ* 2007; 85: 407–409.
23. Munro SA, Lewin SA, Smith H et al. Patient adherence to tuberculosis treatment: A systematic review of qualitative research. *PLoS Med* 2007; 4: e238.
24. Cantwell MF, McKenna MT, McCray E, Onorato IM. Tuberculosis and race/ethnicity in the United States: impact of socioeconomic status. *Am J Respir Crit Care Med* 1998; 157: 1016–20.
25. Antunes JL, Waldman EA. The impact of AIDS, immigration and housing overcrowding on tuberculosis deaths in Sao Paulo, Brazil, 1994–1998. *Soc Sci Med* 2001; 52: 1071–80.
26. Cuevas LE, Almeida LM, Mazunder P et al. Effect of zinc on the tuberculin response of children exposed to adults with smear-positive tuberculosis. *Ann Trop Paediatr* 2002; 22: 313–19.
27. Nhlema-Simwaka B, Benson T, Kishindo P et al. Developing socio-economic measures to monitor access to tuberculosis services in urban Lilongwe, Malawi. *Int J Tuberc Lung Dis* 2007; 11: 65–71.
28. Kemp JR, Mann G, Nhlema-Simwaka B et al. Can Malawi's poor afford free TB services? Patient and household costs associated with a tuberculosis diagnosis in Lilongwe. *Bull World Health Organ* 2007; 85: 580–5.
29. Uplekar MW, Rangan S, Weiss MG et al. Attention to gender issues in tuberculosis control. *Int J Tuberc Lung Dis* 2001; 5: 220–4.
30. Kemp JR, Theobald SJ, Makwiza I et al. Where are the missing women? The impact of HIV on gender and TB and its implications for TB control in Malawi. *Int J Tuberc Lung Dis* 2008 (submitted).
31. Singh V, Jaiswal A, Porter JD et al. TB control, poverty, and vulnerability in Delhi, India. *Trop Med Int Health* 2002; 7: 693–700.

32. World Health Organization. *Addressing poverty in TB control. Options for national TB control programmes.* Geneva: World Health Organization, 2005 (WHO/HTM/TB/2005.352).
33. www.stoptb.org/globalplan. Accessed August 2007.
34. www.un.org/millenniumgoals. Accessed August 2007.
35. Hopewell P, Pai M, Maher D *et al.* International standards for tuberculosis care. *Lancet Infect Dis* 2006; **6**: 710–25.

18

DOTS and DOTS-Plus

SONYA SHIN, JAIME BAYONA AND PAUL FARMER

INTRODUCTION

Tuberculosis (TB) remains one of the world's leading infectious causes of adult deaths, most of which are due not to multidrug-resistant (MDR) strains, but to lack of access to effective treatment for drug-susceptible disease.[1] The past few decades have taught us that good TB control is affordable even in the poor countries in which the disease takes its greatest control. As described elsewhere in this volume (see Chapter 17, Directly observed therapy and other aspects of management of tuberculosis care), sound DOTS-based TB programmes will also prevent or significantly delay the emergence of drug-resistant strains of *Mycobacterium tuberculosis*. A great many data suggest, however, that MDR-TB is emerging as an increasingly important cause of morbidity and death. In the USA, Europe and Latin America, highly resistant strains of TB have caused explosive institutional outbreaks in hospitals, prisons and homeless shelters, with high case fatality rates among immunosuppressed people, as well as high rates of transmission to other patients, caregivers and family members.[2–8] A recent nosocomial outbreak of highly drug-resistant TB among HIV-positive patients demonstrated the devastating impact of drug-resistant disease and its predilection for vulnerable populations.[9] In a rural area in KwaZulu Natal, South Africa, 53 HIV-positive patients were found to be infected with MDR-TB that was resistant to almost all effective drugs; this condition is now termed extensively drug-resistant tuberculosis (XDR-TB).[10] All but one of these patients died, with a median survival time of merely 16 days from the time of diagnosis. Outbreak

investigation confirmed nosocomial transmission as the most likely form of spread. The alarming emergence of XDR-TB is shaping the public health debate around MDR-TB control, as discussed later in this chapter.

While nosocomial and institutional outbreaks provide dramatic examples of MDR-TB transmission and resulting morbidity, MDR-TB (including XDR-TB) is predominantly a community-acquired disease. Population surveys from many countries have revealed MDR-TB to be present in every site studied; community-acquired disease is an emerging problem in several MDR-TB 'hot spots'.[11,12] In fact, the total global burden of MDR-TB in 2004 was estimated at almost 425 000 individuals or 4.3 per cent of all TB cases, with a yearly incidence of 181 400 cases among previously treated cases alone.[13] In settings in which large numbers of prevalent MDR cases may already be documented, universal standardized short-course chemotherapy will not yield the same high cure rates achieved in settings where pan-susceptible disease is the rule.[14] Indeed, some patients will respond to such regimens by failing treatment and also acquiring additional resistance in the process.

This chapter seeks to describe an investigation into a community outbreak in an urban squatter settlement in Peru. The outbreak is revealing for a number of reasons. First, it was brought to light through a 'transnational case': infection acquired in one country was diagnosed in another. Second, the Lima outbreak informs our understanding of the dynamics of such epidemics, since it is occurring not in a country with poor TB control practices but rather in one cited as having one of the world's best

Case history 1

A 50-year-old US citizen working in northern Lima as a relief worker returned to a Boston teaching hospital with a 2-month history of chronic enteropathy, fever and cough. He was found to be HIV-positive, with a CD4 count of less than 50, an erythrocyte sedimentation rate of 68 and marked anaemia. Acid-fast bacilli were present in sputum and stool. Although the initial diagnosis was HIV-associated systemic infection with atypical mycobacteria, the patient's chest x-ray showed scattered granulomas in both lungs (Figure 18.1). Sputum samples were sent to the Massachusetts State Laboratory Institute (MSLI) and the patient was admitted to a common room. Following consultation with the infectious disease service, he was moved to a room meeting requirements for respiratory precautions. The patient was placed on an empiric antituberculous regimen consisting of rifampicin (RIF), isoniazid (INH), ethambutol (ETH) and pyrazinamide (PZA). In contrast to most patients with HIV-associated tuberculosis, however, he did not respond to therapy.[15-17] The patient died of sepsis syndrome within 2 weeks of his presentation. His sputum and blood cultures grew not atypical mycobacteria, but rather *M. tuberculosis*. Drug-susceptibility testing (DST) revealed that the patient had died of disseminated TB resistant to all the first-line drugs.

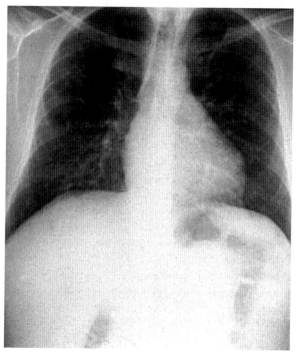

Figure 18.1   Chest x-ray, 'transnational case'.

DOTS programmes. We begin by presenting the alleged 'index case' – not the first case, but rather the first one acknowledged.

Tuberculosis is relatively rare in Massachusetts, which is blessed with a robust TB control infrastructure. When confronted with a case of active pulmonary disease, public health authorities usually conduct active case finding. Contacts are evaluated for active disease or latent TB infection. In this instance, TB control authorities were faced with a lethal and highly resistant strain that had been acquired elsewhere. At the time, there were no provisions for transnational contact tracing; there were no provisions for any sort of formal transnational work. Yet in Massachusetts, 77.4 per cent of all TB cases are diagnosed in the foreign-born, making 'transnational thinking' appropriate to this era of unequal TB risks.[18,19] In fact, active case finding did occur subsequent to documentation of this case. The spread of drug-resistant strains of *M. tuberculosis*, even if it calls for local solutions, constitutes a global problem.

THE EPIDEMIOLOGY OF TB IN NORTHERN LIMA, PERU

In 1996, a Boston-based non-profit organization, Partners In Health (PIH), helped to found Socios En

Salud (SES), a non-governmental organization based in the Peruvian slum in which the relief worker had been living. Upon news of his cause of death, SES began searching for other cases of active MDR-TB. Peru, as noted, has one of the world's most successful TB control programmes, due in large part to its successful implementation of DOTS on a national scale.[20] Directly observed short-course chemotherapy is highly effective in the treatment of drug-susceptible TB. However, since short-course chemotherapy is based on RIF and INH, patients sick from strains resistant to those two medications are unlikely to respond to DOTS-based therapies. In fact, despite both international and national claims that MDR-TB was not a problem in Peru, numerous indicators, in addition to the sentinel case of transnational spread, suggested otherwise.

SES had already conducted an extensive survey of households in the shantytowns of northern Lima, the area where the relief worker had been based. As the SES health workers went door-to-door, conducting interviews in the dirt-floor shacks dotting the dusty hills north of the city, anecdotal stories began to surface. People spoke of *cronicos*, patients who suffered from TB for years and *familias tebeceanas* in which four, five or more family members had died or were dying of TB. Significantly, health centre employees confirmed these anecdotes and also the growing fears of those conducting the survey.

Nurses in the clinics and regional health posts reported that many of the *cronicos* were religiously adherent to the DOTS-based regimens, and, for those who failed initial therapy, to the internationally recommended retreatment regimens. It seemed, then, that both the dead and the dying were patients who had failed to recover from TB despite receiving high-quality directly observed therapy, often for years.

This survey prompted further collaboration with 43 health centres and the regional hospital serving three of the northern Lima districts. Beginning in September 1996, all known 'treatment failures' – defined as any patient who remained persistently smear-positive at the completion of any treatment regimen – were referred to SES. Health workers then sought out these patients in their homes, where they were interviewed and screened for active disease. These individuals were asked to submit at least one sputum specimen for culture and drug susceptibility testing; the latter was conducted at the MSLI.

Between September 1996 and March 1998, 173 patients identified to be 'treatment failures' were referred for evaluation and submitted sputum specimens. Of this group, 92.4 per cent (160) were found to have culture-positive pulmonary TB. Of these, an overwhelming proportion – 94 per cent, or 150/160 – were found to have active MDR-TB. From this sampling, we estimated a regional prevalence of 19.8 active MDR-TB cases per 100 000 – at least three times the official estimate of national MDR-TB prevalence.[21] In fact, the proportion of the reported cases of MDR-TB (7.6 per cent) placed this area among the global MDR-TB 'hot spots', as defined in the population-based surveys cited above.

Even more disturbing was the degree of drug resistance within this cohort of 150 MDR-TB patients. Only 9.3 per cent (14) of these patients had isolates that demonstrated resistance to *only* INH and RIF, while 16.7 per cent had isolates demonstrating resistance to 3 of the 10 antituberculous drugs tested. Of these patients, 136 (90.7 per cent) had isolates demonstrating resistance to at least 3 of the 10 antituberculous drugs tested; 111 (74.0 per cent) to at least 4 drugs; 66 (44.0 per cent) to at least 5 drugs; 36 (24.0 per cent) to at least 6 drugs; 18 (12 per cent) to at least 7 drugs; 6 (4 per cent) to at least 8 drugs; and 3 patients (2.0 per cent) had isolates demonstrating resistance to at least 9 of the 10 drugs tested.

Resistance to second-line antituberculous drugs (kanamycin (KM), capreomycin (CM), cycloserine (CS), ciprofloxacin (CPX) or ethionamide (THA)) was found in 56 (37.3 per cent) of the 150 patients. Of particular clinical relevance was our finding that 60 (40 per cent) of these patients had isolates demonstrating resistance to at least INH, RIF, EMB and PZA, the drugs constituting the first-line empiric regimens used to treat TB in this setting. Furthermore, 44 (29.3 per cent) of the 150 patients had isolates demonstrating resistance to at least INH, RIF, EMB, PZA and streptomycin (SM), which constitutes the first empiric retreatment regimen used in this setting.

Thus, most patients were sick with strains resistant to five drugs; some patients were resistant to as many as nine drugs. Subsequent samples have revealed strains of *M. tuberculosis* resistant to 12 drugs.[22]

Another critical finding of this preliminary work was the geographic variation in patterns of multidrug resistance of these 150 patients when compared with results of a 1995 national sample. In an ostensibly representative national sample of 109 MDR-TB patients, 45 per cent of isolates demonstrated resistance to only INH and RIF, while 16.5 per cent of isolates demonstrated four-drug resistance (INH, RIF, EMB, SM). The isolates obtained from the 150 northern Lima patients, however, revealed that the majority (53.3 per cent) were resistant to all four drugs; only 17.3 per cent of these MDR-TB patients had isolates resistant only to INH and RIF.

As SES sought to uncover the magnitude of the epidemic in northern Lima, similar outbreaks were being identified elsewhere in the world. Whether in the slums of northern Lima or in another of the MDR-TB 'hot spots' described in various World Health Organization (WHO) surveys, it became increasingly difficult to argue that treating drug-susceptible disease alone would lead to the elimination of MDR-TB. This is simply not the case, even in countries – such as Peru – with sound DOTS programmes. While DOTS remains an effective strategy to prevent the emergence of drug resistance, the efficacy of short-course chemotherapy is diminished in areas where drug-resistant tuberculosis has already emerged. Ironically, in 1997, as the WHO announced that 'TB is being defeated by [Peru's] model DOTS programme',[23] the SES team was uncovering hundreds of prevalent and incident cases of MDR-TB in the northern reaches of Lima.

THE COSTS OF NOT TREATING MDR-TB

What was the impact of untreated MDR-TB in this community, and why were such cases appearing in a setting boasting one of the best TB control programmes in the world? Such questions have not been addressed in the scholarly literature, which to date has focused on the economic burden of untreated TB. In northern Lima, however, a very different set of questions emerged from careful study of local epidemiology: What is the epidemiological impact of treating pan-susceptible strains effectively, but leaving infectious drug-resistant strains untreated? What is the cost of nosocomial and intra-household transmission? What is the cost of 'the amplifier effect', which leads to higher-grade resistance rather than suppression or cure? What is the cost to staff morale when patients with MDR-TB are given directly observed doses of a regimen based on precisely those drugs to which other infecting strains are resistant? What is the cost to public trust in TB control programmes when patients receive serial courses of drugs that cannot cure them? Finally, what is the cost, in human terms, of untreated MDR-TB?

Case history 2

As subtle as her initial symptoms may have been, Blanca Pérez had little doubt about what was coming when, in July 1995, she began having fever, chills and a productive cough. Blanca and her husband, Andrés, both then 22 years old, were living in her mother's house with Blanca's six siblings, two of whom were being treated for active TB. Blanca was the fifth in her family to be diagnosed with the disease. Of her nine siblings, two had already died of TB.

It started in 1987, when Blanca's older sister Sonya was diagnosed with TB. Sonya received numerous treatments, which were unsuccessful despite her 'religious' compliance. Given her adherent, directly observed treatment, it is highly likely that Sonya had primary drug resistance – that is, she had been infected initially with a drug-resistant strain, which is why her treatments failed. She remained smear-positive for years, living in a small house in the hills of northern Lima with her mother, nine siblings and a changing cast of partners and children.

It was not long before others in the household became ill. Pablo, the family's only son, was diagnosed with TB in 1990. Pablo was a teenager at the time but was already the main breadwinner in the family. He worked as a street vendor, making a pre-dawn ride to Lima's central market to collect old limes from the trash and then returning to sell them at the local market. Responsible for feeding his siblings, Pablo often missed his medications on days when he was unable to leave work. For years, he was in and out of treatment and was considered a classic 'problem patient' by the health centre.

As the disease destroyed more and more of his lungs, Pablo became increasingly short of breath. Eventually, he was unable to work. In late November 1994, Pablo was referred to a pulmonologist, who told him that if he wanted to be cured, he would have to buy several 'strong' TB medications that were not available through the Ministry of Health. Pablo never had a chance to follow the pulmonologist's advice. He died the following day, still receiving first-line antituberculous drugs.

In 1991, Sonya's husband, Raúl, was also diagnosed with TB. Sonya continued to have positive smears throughout her directly observed therapy, but her illness was not recognized as MDR-TB until 1993; Raúl's resistance was not confirmed until mid-1996. Sonya and Raúl made heroic efforts to buy the same second-line drugs that had been prescribed to Pablo, but they could only do so intermittently, since their work as street vendors could scarcely feed them and their daughter. Both remained smear-positive for years and Sonya was intermittently hospitalized for life-threatening episodes of haemoptysis.

Luisa, another Pérez sister, was also diagnosed with TB in 1991. She followed the same pattern of unsuccessful treatment and retreatment as her siblings. After she saw Pablo die, Luisa gave up hope and refused any further treatment. She died 1 year after Pablo, in November 1995.

Rosa, another sister, was diagnosed with TB in the first months of 1995. While receiving her antituberculous treatment, she became pregnant but miscarried. Since completing her treatment, Rosa has been symptom-free. Blanca's mother was also treated for TB around that time, without relapse to date.

Given this history, Blanca had little doubt that she had TB when her cough began in July 1995. Initially, however, she did not seek either diagnosis or treatment. A month after her symptoms began, Blanca had an episode of massive haemoptysis. Blanca's sisters rushed her to the local health post, where her sputum was found to be abundantly positive for the tubercle bacillus. In spite of her known MDR-TB contacts, Blanca began receiving first-line treatment through the Peruvian National Tuberculosis Programme (NTP) protocol.

As previously mentioned, in patients with fully susceptible TB, directly observed therapy with the four standard first-line drugs leads to rapid response within a few weeks. A month into treatment, Blanca's symptoms had failed to improve. Her chest x-ray looked worse and her sputum smear remained positive.

The local health workers who gave Blanca her daily medications suspected drug resistance and sent a sputum sample for culture and DST. In January 1996, Blanca's drug sensitivity results finally revealed that her TB strain was, like that of her sister, resistant to INH and RIF. Despite these laboratory results, and to the dismay of the health workers who saw her each day, the health authorities told Blanca that she must complete the DOTS regimen, even though at that point it consisted of only two drugs – the exact two drugs to which she had confirmed resistance.

A month later, Blanca reached the end of the 6-month regimen, but her sputum continued to show abundant tubercle bacilli. She was wracked by fevers and coughs and had experienced life-threatening haemoptysis; she weighed less than 40 kg. In keeping with the rules of Peru's NTP, Blanca was evaluated by a programme pulmonologist, who placed her on an approved retreatment regimen which contained only first-line drugs. In addition, this physician prescribed two second-line drugs, CPX and THA, explaining that if she could obtain these drugs, her treatment would be even stronger. Blanca recognized the names of these drugs, which had also been prescribed for Sonya, Raúl and Pablo. Since these drugs were not part of the standard public health programme's regimen, the only way to obtain the medications – at a cost of $200 (£98) a month – would be to buy them herself. This sum was well in excess of her entire family's monthly income.

Blanca's symptoms improved on the retreatment regimen, but she remained smear-positive and quickly worsened after treatment was completed. Without further treatment options, she spent the next 2 months bed-ridden, losing weight and coughing blood – the classic picture of galloping consumption.

When things seemed as if they could not get worse, Blanca's husband fell ill. Andrés worked as a street vendor, selling books and he had assumed all the cooking and housekeeping chores during his wife's illness. Given his multiple MDR-TB contacts, Andrés was reluctant to begin standard therapy with the drugs to which his wife, sisters-in-law and brother-in-law had been resistant. However, he, too, was pulled into the official protocol and remained smear-positive for most of his treatment.

In October, Blanca's 19-year-old sister, Ana, was diagnosed with TB. She was in the first trimester of her first pregnancy. She was the sixth Pérez child to fall ill with TB.

Around the same time, things began to look up for the Pérez family: Blanca, Sonya and Raúl began receiving treatment with drugs to which their isolates had demonstrated susceptibility. These drugs, along with nutritional support and daily visits from a community health worker, were provided by SES. By mid-November, Blanca's sputum test was negative for the first time since her initial diagnosis. Raúl and Sonya were also soon smear-negative.

Meanwhile, despite his contact history, Andrés was not permitted to start MDR-TB therapy until he completed first-line treatment as an 'official' treatment failure. In fact, even when DST revealed that Andrés had resistant disease, his providers insisted he continue with DOTS as per protocol. Frustrated with this absurd management, Andrés refused to take his medications. He was forced to sign a statement acknowledging that he was 'abandoning treatment'. For this reason alone, Andrés will never figure in the national data as a case of primary MDR-TB. Instead, he will be mislabelled, as were all the members of the Pérez family, as having acquired MDR-TB through erratic compliance: they were 'problem patients'. Andrés, as well as Ana, ultimately initiated appropriate individualized therapy with SES.

This case has been adapted from Farmer et al.[24]

A study of household clustering of MDR-TB provides instructive insight into some of the forces that are shaping the MDR-TB epidemic in Lima.[25,26]

Families in which eight young adults are sick or dead from MDR-TB are not unheard of in Peru (Figure 18.2). Within this particular family, restriction fragment length polymorphism (RFLP) analysis and careful clinical history suggest intra-household spread of a single strain of *M. tuberculosis*. That is, these are *intra-household epidemics* in which family members are passing drug-resistant strains to each other. To date, no effective prophylaxis exists for MDR-TB contacts with latent TB infection. In effect, the only means of preventing transmission is treatment. And yet, until recently, conventional wisdom argued that MDR-TB disease is too costly to treat.[27]

Faced with the growing recognition of a sizeable outbreak of MDR-TB, SES was challenged not only to procure funds for treatment, but to bring about a shift in the attitudes of local TB programme officials, as well as global TB experts. This challenge proved far more difficult than anticipated. Despite convincing documentation of a significant epidemic of drug-resistant TB in Lima's northern cone, SES met significant resistance in attempting to broaden the DOTS framework beyond its exclusive

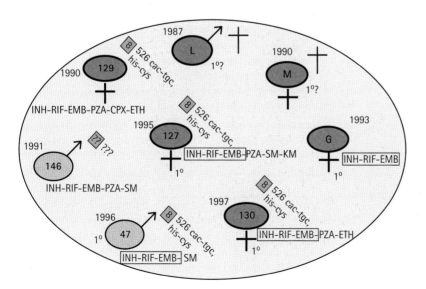

Figure 18.2 Family cluster of MDR-TB. Restriction fragment length polymorphism (RFLP) analysis of four of these isolates confirms clustering (cluster 8) and sequencing for *rpoB* mutations demonstrates the same mutation (His 526) responsible for rifampicin resistance. CPX, ciprofloxacin; EMB, ethambutol; ETH, ethionamide; INH, isoniazid; KM, kanamycin; PZA, pyrazinamide; RIF, riampicin; SM, streptomycin.

reliance on short-course chemotherapy and was castigated for even suggesting that an epidemic existed at all. The hostile reaction stemmed in part from the underlying implication that the Peruvian TB programme not only failed to prevent the emergence of MDR-TB, but that its successful DOTS programme was in fact contributing to the generation of increasingly resistant strains. For some patients, the DOTS programme, despite its managerial success, was a clinical failure.

Consider again the case of Blanca, who probably contracted MDR-TB from one of her siblings. It is highly likely that the isolate collected 3 months into her first treatment regimen reflects primary resistance, given her excellent adherence to directly observed therapy. Standard short-course chemotherapy consists of 2 months of INH, RIF, EMB and PZA followed by 4 months of INH and RIF. Therefore, Blanca essentially received 2 months of EMB and PZA, followed by 4 months of placebo – in fact, worse than placebo, given the potential for drug toxicity. Not only did this regimen fail to cure her, but it provided enough selection pressure to leave her sick with a strain resistant to five drugs instead of two.

In short, DOTS may prove ineffective in controlling MDR-TB once resistant strains have emerged, and the process of cycling failing patients through inadequate therapy results in even worse outcomes than no intervention at all. This phenomenon, the amplifier effect of short-course chemotherapy (Figure 18.3),[28] selects for further resistance as patients infected with drug-resistant strains are treated with inadequate therapy. This represents iatrogenic amplification of drug resistance. Most patients who fail short-course chemotherapy then receive the internationally recommended retreatment regimen, which consists of the same four drugs plus streptomycin. Since streptomycin monotherapy is unlikely to cure active TB, the infecting strain acquires additional resistance to this drug. This is the likely reason why 67 per cent of our patients in Lima were sick with strains resistant to all five first-line drugs. They have failed repeated courses of empiric therapy that were bound to fail.

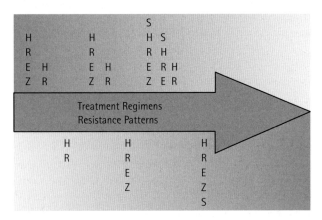

Figure 18.3   The amplifier effect of short-course chemotherapy. E, ethambutol; H, isoniazid; R, rifampicin; S, streptomycin; Z, pyrazinamide (from Farmer et al.[28])

From both epidemiological and clinical standpoints, the effects can be devastating. In this local epidemic, the amplifier effect of short-course chemotherapy was the critical determinant of outcomes and of costs, both in human lives and in dollars. In the case of the Pérez family, eight adults had MDR-TB or were dead from it. Many became too sick to work and, after recovery, had difficulty finding employment. Through serial courses of empiric regimens, these individuals remained infectious and sick for years. In short, the cost of not treating MDR-TB is far higher than imagined, especially when ineffective retreatment regimens follow directly observed short-course chemotherapy. Careful review of the literature suggests that there was no evidence to indicate that such retreatment regimens would cure many patients who had failed DOTS. Rather, these regimens were held to be 'cost-effective'. Since they were ineffective and often led to the amplifier effect even as they eroded total confidence in the NTP, the true cost of ineffective therapy for MDR-TB has yet to be calculated.

INTRODUCING DOTS-PLUS: COMMUNITY-BASED TREATMENT OF MDR-TB

Given that there exist only six or seven highly effective antituberculosis drugs, SES was faced, even from a purely clinical standpoint, with an extraordinary treatment challenge. (Drugs cidal against *M. tuberculosis* include INH, RIF, PZA, ETH, SM (and other aminoglycosides as a class), CM and the fluoroquinolones. Other drugs are weakly cidal or mycobacteriostatic.) It may be true that, for some patients, there is no effective chemotherapy. However, for patients sick with strains resistant to four or five drugs – those deemed 'untreatable' because of the high cost of second-line drugs – it was clear from the outset that much could be done if second-line drugs were made available. In order to do so, however, it was necessary to develop 'DOTS without the S', since short-course chemotherapy was ineffective for these patients.

Ultimately, SES did gain the cooperation of the local Ministry of Health and acquired the funds needed to begin treating a cohort of patients, most of whom were resistant to all first-line drugs and had been sick for several years. Chest x-rays showed extensive parenchymal destruction. The patients received individualized treatment regimens based on their drug resistance patterns, typically a regimen based on an injectable, a fluoroquinolone, cycloserine, para-aminosalicylic acid (PAS) and other agents depending on DST results and the degree of parenchymal destruction. These regimens were designed using a hierarchical algorithm of drug classes based on the bactericidal or static properties of drugs known to be effective against *M. tuberculosis*. If the isolate was susceptible to fewer than five first- or second-line drugs, the regimen was 'reinforced' with drugs that have demonstrated *in vitro* efficacy against *M. tuberculosis*. In addition, additional drugs were often included in the regimen if there existed the possibility of amplification to a drug during the time after the culture was collected and its results obtained. Any first-line drugs to which the infecting strain was deemed susceptible were also included in the regimen, at maximum doses. The injectable agent (aminoglycoside or capreomycin) was ideally administered for 6 months after culture conversion. Treatment was generally continued for 18–24 months after the time of culture conversion. Each dose of treatment was given as directly observed therapy throughout the course of treatment. (These clinical strategies have been described in detail elsewhere.[29,30])

In addition to the clinical complexities of treating these patients, there also existed substantial political and logistical hurdles. At the outset of this novel project, SES received little encouragement from the local and international public health community. SES was constantly reminded that these patients were 'untreatable';[31] that they would not comply with therapy; that there would be too many side effects; that they would quickly abandon treatment.

SES intended to prove otherwise. First, SES trained a group of young people, mostly volunteers, to work as community health workers. The team struggled to build a fragile coalition involving Peru's NTP, local public health facilities, and a supranational reference laboratory, the MSLI. The treatment cohort's mean age was 29 years and most had children; the majority were eager to begin a regimen that held the promise of cure. Indeed, some were loath to stop any of the drugs, even when recommended by their doctors. In contrast to the grim predictions, the patients tolerated their treatment regimens, including daily intramuscular injections and bothersome but minor side effects that occurred much less frequently than reported in the literature[32] and which SES managed mostly in the community. Accustomed to years of bad news from microscopists, these patients were especially pleased to be declared smear-negative month after month. Of the initial 66 patients who completed at least 4 months of therapy, 82 per cent were cured according to the most stringent criteria (culture rather than smear microscopy).[33]

This community-based project eventually succeeded in introducing evidence-based medicine into a Peruvian slum, relying heavily on local resources and also on the basic planks of the DOTS strategy. For these reasons, we named this treatment strategy 'DOTS-Plus'.[34] Initially, however, the project was not embraced beyond the boundaries of the slum. The WHO had gone on record saying that only DOTS was needed and that 'other treatment strategies are also actually causing multidrug-resistant tuberculosis, and may be doing more harm than good'.[23]

TREATMENT OF MDR-TB IN RESOURCE-POOR SETTINGS: THE PUBLIC HEALTH DEBATE AND REVIEW OF THE EVIDENCE

Given the fact that DOTS-Plus could be implemented in a Latin American slum, why was there so much resistance to replicating this programme elsewhere?[35] Those opposed to

MDR-TB treatment in resource-poor settings have cited three major arguments: first, that MDR-TB is less transmissible than drug-susceptible disease and therefore will not contribute significantly to the TB epidemic in the long run; second, that MDR-TB is too expensive to treat in developing countries; and, finally, that treatment of MDR-TB may have adverse consequences on TB control by drawing resources away from pan-susceptible cases and/or by selecting for even more highly drug-resistant strains. Below we review each of these arguments and the evidence to date.

IS MDR-TB LESS TRANSMISSIBLE THAN PAN-SUSCEPTIBLE STRAINS?

Whether MDR-TB strains are less infectious and less virulent than pan-susceptible strains remains a contentious debate. Supporters of this view argue that spread of primary MDR strains is not a significant threat because mutations causing drug resistance result in diminished fitness (less transmissibility and/or less virulence) of the organism and thus render drug-resistant strains less transmissible than drug-susceptible ones.[36,37] For this reason, some experts and policy-makers have argued that DOTS programmes will be adequate for preventing the spread of MDR-TB.[1,38,39]

The origins of this debate can be found early in the chemotherapeutic era. By 1950, for example, it was observed that strains of tuberculosis resistant to INH and/or SM grew less robustly *in vitro* and had attenuated infectiousness in animal models.[40] More recently, mutations of the *KatG* gene (a virulence gene for mycobacteria) have been found to confer resistance to INH, associated with diminished virulence *in vitro*.[41] Animal models have also demonstrated diminished virulence in strains with *KatG* mutation-associated INH resistance.[42]

However, Billington et al.[43] have shown that certain mutations in the *rpoB* gene conferring resistance to RIF are not always associated with reduced fitness. Furthermore, they suggest that many organisms, including *M. tuberculosis*, which may be initially less virulent due to resistance mutations may then undergo compensatory mutations that restore or even enhance baseline fitness. Among mutations associated with INH resistance, mutations at the 315 position of the *KatG* gene may have little or no fitness cost.[44] Accumulating *in vitro* data suggest that the relative fitness associated with drug resistance mutations is highly variable.[45,46] Furthermore, the clinical significance of reduced fitness associated with mutations conferring drug resistance is unclear, given evidence that further adaptation of the organism occurs within the host to compensate for any fitness deficit. Gillespie et al.[47] observed that isogenic strains obtained in a hospital outbreak had variable fitness phenotypes when obtained from different patients, as demonstrated by growth velocity. Similarly, Gagneux et al.[48] have found that clinical isolates with acquired drug resistance due to prolonged treatment often have no fitness defects, despite the high frequency of a fitness cost associated with mutations *in vitro*.

Clustering studies based on molecular epidemiology have also been used to investigate the issue of relative fitness; results from such studies also support *in vitro* observations that drug-resistant strains demonstrate a wide range of fitness phenotypes.[49] The approach to clustering studies has been to use RFLP analysis using the IS6110 genotype of strains, as well as other genotyping methods, to identify clusters of homology. The presence of clustering is used to infer recent transmission of related strains. van Soolingen et al.,[50] one of the earliest groups to apply molecular epidemiology to study TB transmission, initially argued that strains resistant to INH were less transmissible based on a survey of strains assayed in the Netherlands; in this study, strains resistant to INH were less likely to be in a cluster than INH-susceptible strains. However, the same group later investigated the virulence of *katG* gene mutations among *M. tuberculosis* isolates and found that INH-resistant strains possessing the mutation at amino acid position 315 in the *katG* gene were equally likely to be clustered as INH-susceptible strains.[51] Subsequent studies support this observation that strains possessing *katG315* mutations are as transmissible as INH-susceptible strains.[52,53]

The clinical relevance of drug-resistant strains that do not have reduced relative fitness is manifested in the emergence of such strains in population and outbreak surveys. The Beijing strain possesses the *katG315* and *rpoB531* mutations and has been associated with numerous MDR-TB epidemics worldwide, although fitness variations have been observed even among strains within the Beijing family.[54] Reports from numerous developing countries indicate a predominance of the Beijing strain and its association with clustering, thus suggesting that these strains are associated with high rates of recent transmission.[55–58] The Beijing strain was also associated with more advanced disease in a Russian survey, suggesting that the strain could potentially be associated with more aggressive disease progression.[59]

Another method to determine the relative transmissibility of drug-resistant strains has been through prospective cohort studies comparing rates of infection among contacts of MDR and non-MDR index cases. Snider et al.[60] found that young household contacts were equally likely to be infected (defined as a positive PPD at the time of index case diagnosis) by drug-resistant and drug-susceptible index cases. Similarly, Teixeira et al.[61] have shown in a Brazilian cohort that rates of positive PPDs among household contacts of MDR versus drug-susceptible cases were not significantly different; in addition, active cases of TB among household contacts were observed with equal frequency (4 per cent). In a similar study of intrahousehold transmission in Argentina, Palmero et al.[62] found no difference between rates of infection and disease incidence among household contacts of susceptible versus MDR-TB index cases.

In conclusion, although there is *in vitro* evidence that mutations conferring drug resistance are associated with a fitness cost to *M. tuberculosis*, there are also *in vitro*, *in vivo* and epidemiological data to suggest that strains undergo compensatory adaptations to overcome fitness deficits. Furthermore, the relative fitness of drug-resistant strains is highly variable. Given the lack of evidence to support the decreased transmissibility of MDR strains, it stands to reason that MDR-TB transmission will continue in the absence of efforts to control both drug-susceptible and drug-resistant disease. Several groups have used mathematical models to show that, even if MDR strains are less transmissible than pan-susceptible strains, MDR-TB transmission will continue and threaten TB control.[63,64] In the absence of effective treatment for drug-resistant cases, increasing DOTS coverage might in fact perversely lead to a rise in the proportion of drug-resistant cases.[65]

IS MDR-TB TOO COSTLY TO TREAT?

Critics have long noted that MDR-TB is too expensive to treat in developing countries. In order to respond to this claim, the international TB community was forced to ask why treatment of MDR-TB is so expensive, given that the indicated medications have long been off-patent.

Consider CM, manufactured by only one company. On a certain day in 1997, a gram of CM cost $29.90 (£14.70) at the Brigham and Women's Hospital in Boston, $21 (£10) in Peru and $8.80 (£4.30) in Europe. One has to ask hard questions about why an off-patent drug made by the same company would be priced so differently in different countries.

Working with colleagues at Médecins Sans Frontières and the WHO, Partners In Health launched a campaign to lower the prices of second-line antituberculous drugs. It became apparent that certain pharmaceutical companies did not want a TB indication to be found for their drugs: if a certain medication proved effective against *M. tuberculosis*, it could be declared a public-health resource[66] and made 'available within the context of functioning health systems at all times in adequate amounts, in the appropriate dosage forms, with assured quality and adequate information, and at a price the individual and the community can afford'.[67] Ultimately, the international coalition was successful in placing second-line antituberculous agents on the WHO's Essential Drugs List, thus leading to substantial decreases in pricing (Figure 18.4).[68]

In the context of dropping drug prices, the argument shifted from claims that MDR-TB was too costly to treat to claims that it was not cost-effective to treat.[69–71] However, a growing body of literature supports the contention that treating MDR-TB is indeed cost-effective.

First, empiric data from a number of MDR-TB treatment programmes have argued that their programmes have been cost-effective. In Peru, in addition to the individualized treatment efforts described above, the Peruvian

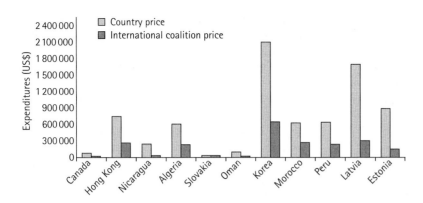

Figure 18.4 Potential savings to countries, based on expenditures (in US$) reported by national TB programmes from 1998 to 2000 using country-specific prices and projected expenditures if international coalition prices were available from that country during the same time period (from Gupta et al.[68]).

NTP also implemented a standardized regimen including second-line drugs in 1997. Despite its suboptimal performance (with cure rates of 48 per cent in the initial cohort), the regimen was deemed cost-effective, making up only 8 per cent of the NTP budget.[72] Another early DOT-Plus project in the Philippines achieved cure rates of 61 per cent in its first cohort; the average cost per patient was less than $3500 (£1723), with a mean cost of $242 (£119) per disability-adjusted life-year (DALY). In Tomsk Oblast, Russia, cure rates rose from 17 to 76 per cent with the implementation of DOTS-Plus; the cost per DALY was $319 (£157).[73]

Modelling studies provide further evidence that treatment of MDR-TB is cost-effective.[74,75] For instance, Resch et al.[76] developed a dynamic state-transition model of TB which took into account the impact of transmission due to untreated, infectious cases. The authors found that retreatment strategies for MDR-TB with regimens that included second-line drugs were highly cost-effective over a wide range of assumptions. Much of the benefit of treating MDR-TB with second-line regimens was due to the impact of reducing ongoing MDR-TB transmission.

IS DOTS-PLUS EFFECTIVE?

As drug costs have declined and pilot MDR-TB projects have demonstrated favourable treatment outcomes, there has been growing acknowledgement of the need to address MDR-TB. The WHO's revision of the Stop TB strategy[77] included MDR-TB treatment as a component of its strategic plan. However, it is unclear if MDR-TB treatment programmes will be truly effective within the context of the broader goal of TB control.

One concern is that efforts to treat MDR-TB, a complex and costly endeavour even with recent advances, will detract attention and resources from the larger TB treatment programmes.[78,79] Sterling et al.[80] argued, for example, that if DOTS-Plus decreased the effectiveness of DOTS by as little as 5 per cent, overall mortality would increase by 16 per cent. Yet that is not what happened in New York City, where an outbreak of MDR-TB led to a massive investment in TB control. Resources were poured into the TB control infrastructure – appropriately, in our view. Although

MDR-TB is no longer incident in New York City, it still receives robust funding for its public TB programme.[81,*]

The idea that MDR-TB treatment might detract from overall TB control is even more pertinent in resource-poor settings, where DOTS infrastructure may be weaker and resources more limited. Several DOTS-Plus programmes have shown, however, that the integration of MDR-TB treatment into DOTS programmes has not weakened the overall programmes. In some cases, in fact, concerted efforts to establish integrated programmes have actually strengthened overall TB programming. For instance, an MDR-TB treatment programme was established in Latvia in 1997 shortly after the DOTS strategy was implemented. Integrated efforts resulted in an increase in cure rates from 60 per cent in 1996 to 78 per cent in 2003. Cure rates rose among both MDR-TB and newly diagnosed patients and the number of MDR-TB patients starting treatment each year declined by more than half.[82]

Based on this and other examples, many involved in advocacy for DOTS-Plus programmes have argued that new resources must be brought to TB control in general and that the threat of MDR-TB can galvanize previously untapped public and private resources.[29] Such has been the case in Tomsk Oblast, Russia, where efforts to improve MDR-TB treatment led to social support programmes, strengthened coordination between the civilian and prison health sectors, and an influx of resources to build laboratory and information system infrastructure, all of which benefited the overall TB programme.[83]

Others have argued that MDR-TB treatment will promote the development of pan-resistant strains by expanding access to second-line drugs in resource-poor settings. However, it is abundantly clear that highly resistant strains already existed in the Peruvian community described

---

*See also: Frieden T, Fujiwara E, Washko R et al. Tuberculosis in New York City: Turning the tide. *N Engl J Med* 1995; **333**: 229–33. For a critical commentary on the relative contribution of DOTS, see Farmer PE and Nardell E. Nihilism and pragmatism in tuberculosis control. *Am J Public Health* 1998; **88**: 4–5 and Bayer R, Stayton C, Desvarieux M et al. Directly observed therapy and treatment completion for tuberculosis in the United States: Is universal supervised therapy necessary? *Am J Public Health* 1998; **88**: 1052–8.

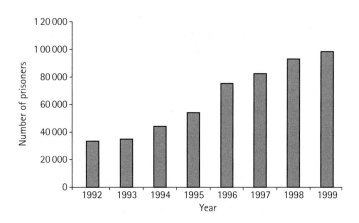

Figure 18.5   Prison prevalence of active pulmonary tuberculosis, Russian Federation, 1992–1999. Source: GUIN, 1999 (unpublished data).

above before the launch of MDR-TB treatment. As noted in the case of Blanca, CPX and THA were already available on the open market. Desperate patients and their families were buying these medications *ad hoc* upon the advice of pulmonologists, some of them advisors for the NTP. The intervention of SES reintegrated these patients into the NTP in order to ensure appropriate and complete treatment instead of the sporadic, inadequate, empiric regimens designed by private physicians.

REPLICATING DOTS–PLUS: OVERCOMING IMPLEMENTATION CHALLENGES

The international public health community now recognizes the need to address MDR-TB in areas of high incidence. SES was able to offer Peru and other resource-poor countries a model of community-based MDR-TB treatment. The DOTS-Plus model was integrated into a DOTS infrastructure and yielded outcomes comparable to those achieved in resource-rich settings. Over the past couple of years, brisk debate has given way to consensus: DOTS remains our best hope of preventing the emergence of resistance to antituberculous drugs but will not suffice once drug resistance is established in a population (for a review of the debate, see Refs 29, 37, 84, 85).

Two final case studies merit discussion. First, Russia offers a dramatic example of the evolution of an uncontrolled MDR-TB epidemic (Figure 18.5). Drug-susceptibility testing revealed that a majority of Siberian prisoners with active TB have strains that are resistant to at least one first-line drug.[86,87] An estimated 20–25 per cent of these prisoners, mostly men, have MDR-TB, but even more harrowing is the fact that TB is the leading cause of death among these young men; it may soon also be the leading cause of death of their jailors, doctors and nurses.

In one prison in Western Siberia, DST performed at initiation of therapy demonstrated that only 25 per cent of patients have pan-susceptible disease. The rest of these patient-prisoners were found to have drug-resistant disease, many of them MDR-TB (Figure 18.6). In another prison in the region, at least 23 per cent of patients had MDR-TB at the beginning of therapy. Despite access to

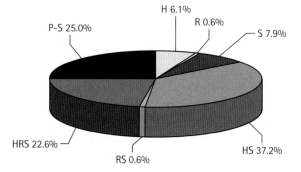

Figure 18.6   Drug-susceptibility results at treatment initiation, Mariinsk prison, Kemerovo, Russia (*n* = 164). H, isoniazid; P-S, pan-susceptibility; R, rifampicin; S, streptomycin. (Reproduced with permission from Kimerling ME, Kluge H, Vazhnina N *et al*. Inadequacy of the current WHO retreatment regimen in a central Siberian prison: treatment failure and MDR TB. *Int J Tuberc Lung Dis* 1999; **3**: 451–3.)

these data, clinicians – many of them non-Russians – insisted that all patients receive standardized short-course chemotherapy with one drug added to 'reinforce' the regimen. That additional drug, SM, was the very one to which most of the patients were already resistant. Not surprisingly, only 46 per cent of these patients were cured (as defined by smear microscopy).[88]

As these statistics surfaced, more transnational collaborations were forged. In 2000, Partners In Health was invited to implement a DOTS-Plus programme in the Tomsk Oblast of Western Siberia. A retrospective analysis of the 244 patients (both civilians and prisoners) who initiated individualized directly observed therapy between September 2000 and September 2002 revealed that 77 per cent were cured. Among the 230 patients who had positive baseline cultures, 218 (94.8 per cent) achieved culture conversion after a median of 2 months of therapy.[89]

Second, the recent outbreak of XDR-TB in KwaZulu Natal, South Africa, sounded an alarm within the international TB community. The convergence of nearly pan-resistant TB with endemic HIV was truly the perfect storm.[90] In autumn 2006, several months after the KwaZulu Natal findings were announced at the

International AIDS Society conference in Toronto, experts established a case definition for XDR-TB: those strains with resistance to the quinolones and at least one second-line injectable agent, in addition to INH and RIF. Although the term was new, XDR-TB had long been in existence, as we had observed in the mid-1990s in Peru. To date, XDR-TB has been reported in 35 countries.[91] Estimates based on reports of the global incidence of MDR-TB suggest that almost 30 000 cases of XDR-TB existed in 2004, representing 0.4 per cent of the global TB burden.[92] The most sobering aspect of this outbreak is the recognition that MDR-TB and XDR-TB are firmly entrenched in HIV-endemic areas. Before this outbreak, efforts to implement the MDR-TB treatment programme had focused on countries with strong DOTS programmes; these recent events clearly illustrate the urgent need for access to MDR-TB treatment in regions with minimal infrastructure. Strong laboratory capacity, coordinated case management between TB and HIV programme, aggressive case finding and vigilant infection control are all sorely needed. In order to meet these challenges, additional resources and technical assistance are critical. The international response to the outbreak in Peru may provide important lessons in transnational collaboration.

CONCLUSION: BEYOND DOTS AND DOTS-PLUS

The three chief objections to the treatment of MDR-TB – regarding relative transmissibility, cost and efficacy – have all been mitigated or even dismissed entirely. Furthermore, the spectre of amplified resistance and the convergence of the TB and HIV epidemics in the poorest regions of the world has further spurred the international public health community to action.

The decline of TB in much of the industrialized world and, more recently, the full characterization of the *M. tuberculosis* genome, reminds us that much has already been accomplished. However, the future of the global TB pandemic will be determined by the success of control measures in high-prevalence, resource-poor areas. It is shocking that TB remains one of the world's leading infectious causes of adult deaths fully 50 years after the development of effective chemotherapy. The convergence of HIV and XDR-TB remind us of the need for new and more effective tools for the treatment and control of these persistent plagues. Applying these tools where the burden of disease is greatest will remain the central task of twenty-first century TB control.

LEARNING POINTS

- MDR-TB is increasing morbidity and mortality due to TB.
- MDR-TB is decreasing cure rates of short-course chemotherapy.

- Experience from Peru has shown populations of patients with MDR disease resistant to at least four drugs after failure of the standard short-course directly observed therapy regimen.
- While DOTS may prevent the development of drug resistance, its efficacy is diminished where significant drug resistance is already present.
- Drug-resistant strains may be passed between family members, causing high mortality.
- Where some drug resistance is present, the DOTS regimen can amplify the number of drugs to which bacteria are resistant: the so-called amplifier effect.
- Not treating MDR-TB may eventually prove more costly than treating appropriately with second-line drugs.
- From the Lima experience, adverse events from second-line drug therapy were fewer than expected.
- Pressure on pharmaceutical companies to reduce the costs of the second-line drugs is proving successful.
- The New York experience has shown that MDR-TB can be eliminated from a community by appropriate treatment, which includes improved DOT and early detection and effective treatment of drug-resistant cases.
- Evidence for diminished or normal 'infectiousness' of MDR-TB is mixed.
- Once drug resistance is established, DOTS alone will not provide success, though 'DOTS-Plus' – the treatment of MDR-TB patients with second-line drugs based on sensitivity testing – has been shown to provide good cure rates where an effective DOTS infrastructure is present.

ACKNOWLEDGEMENTS

We would like to thank Thomas White, the Bill and Melinda Gates Foundation, and our many partners who seek to promote the rational use of antituberculosis drugs for those who need them most. We are particularly grateful to the Partners In Health, Zanmi Lasante and Socios En Salud staff who first implemented 'DOTS-Plus' in Haiti and Peru.

REFERENCES

1. World Health Organization. *WHO report on the tuberculosis epidemic*. Geneva: World Health Organization, 1997.
2. Vailway S, Greifinger R, Papania M *et al*. Multidrug-resistant tuberculosis in the New York state prison system, 1990–1991. *J Infect Dis* 1994; **170**: 151–6.
3. Nardell E, McInnis B, Thomas B, Widhass S. Exogenous reinfection with tuberculosis in a shelter for the homeless. *N Engl J Med* 1986; **315**: 1570–3.

4. Beck-Sague C, Dooley S, Hotton M et al. Hospital outbreak of multidrug-resistant *Mycobacterium tuberculosis* infections: Factors in transmission to staff and HIV-infected patients. *J Am Med Assoc* 1992; **268**: 1280–6.

5. Barnes P, El-Hajj H, Preston-Martin S et al. Transmission of tuberculosis among the urban homeless. *J Am Med Assoc* 1996; **275**: 305–307.

6. Pablos-Mendez A, Raviglione M, Battan R et al. Drug resistant tuberculosis among the homeless in New York City. *N Y State J Med* 1990; **90**: 351–5.

7. Kritski A, Marques MJ, Rabahi MF et al. Transmission of tuberculosis to close contacts of patients with multidrug-resistant tuberculosis. *Am J Respir Crit Care Med* 1996; **153**: 331–5.

8. Rullán J, Herrera D, Cano R et al. Nosocomial transmission of multidrug-resistant tuberculosis in Spain. *Emerg Infect Dis* 1996; **2**: 125–9.

9. Gandhi NR, Moll A, Sturm AW et al. Extensively drug-resistant tuberculosis as a cause of death in patients co-infected with tuberculosis and HIV in a rural area of South Africa. *Lancet* 2006; **368**: 1575–80.

10. Case definition for extensively drug-resistant tuberculosis. *Wkly Epidemiol Rec* 2006; **81**: 408.

11. World Health Organization. *Anti-tuberculosis drug resistance in the world. Report No. 2: The WHO/IUATLD global project on anti-tuberculosis drug resistance surveillance 2000.* Geneva: World Health Organization, 2000.

12. Li X, Zhang Y, Shen X et al. Transmission of drug-resistant tuberculosis among treated patients in Shanghai, China. *J Infect Dis* 2007; **195**: 864–9.

13. Zignol M, Hosseini MS, Wright A et al. Global incidence of multidrug-resistant tuberculosis. *J Infect Dis* 2006; **194**: 479–85.

14. Farmer PE, Bayona J, Becerra M et al. Poverty, inequality, and drug resistance: Meeting community needs. Proceedings of the International Union Tuberculosis and Lung Disease, North American Regional Conference, 27 February–2 March, 1997: 88–102.

15. Johnson JL, Okwera A, Nsubuga P et al. Efficacy of an unsupervised 8-month rifampicin-containing regimen for the treatment of pulmonary tuberculosis in HIV-infected adults. *Int J Tuberc Lung Dis* 2000; **4**: 1032–40.

16. Kassim S, Sassan-Morokro M, Ackah A et al. Two-year follow-up of persons with HIV-1- and HIV-2-associated pulmonary tuberculosis treated with short-course chemotherapy in West Africa. *AIDS* 1995; **9**: 1185–91.

17. Perriëns JH, St. Louis ME, Mukadi YB et al. Pulmonary tuberculosis in HIV-infected patients in Zaire: A controlled trial of treatment for either 6 or 12 months. *N Engl J Med* 1995; **332**: 779–84.

18. Centers for Disease Control and Prevention. *Reported tuberculosis in the United States, 2005.* Atlanta: US Department of Health and Human Services, CDC, 2006.

19. Talbot EA, Moore M, McCray E et al. Tuberculosis among foreign-born persons in the United States, 1993–1998. *J Am Med Assoc* 2000; **284**: 2894–900.

20. Becerra MC, Bayona J, Farmer PE et al. Defusing a time-bomb: The challenge of antituberculosis drug resistance in Peru. In: *The global impact of drug-resistant tuberculosis.* Program in Infectious Disease and Social Change. Boston, MA: Harvard Medical School and the Open Society Institute, 1999; 107–26.

21. Becerra MC, Freeman J, Bayona J et al. Using treatment failure under effective directly observed short-course chemotherapy programs to identify patients with multidrug-resistant tuberculosis. *Int J Tuberc Lung Dis* 2000; **4**: 108–14.

22. Farmer PE, Palacios E, Shin SS et al. Innovative community-based treatment for multidrug resistant TB in a resource-poor setting (oral presentation). American Public Health Association Annual Meeting, Boston, MA, 15 November 2000.

23. World Health Organization. *TB treatment observer.* Geneva: World Health Organization, 24 March 1997: 2.

24. Farmer P. *Infections and inequalities: the modern plagues.* Berkeley: University of California Press, 2001.

25. Furin JJ, Becerra MC, Shin SS et al. Amplifying resistance? Effect of administering short-course standardized resistance regimens in individuals infected with drug-resistant *Mycobacterium tuberculosis* strains. *Eur J Clin Microbiol Infect Dis* 2000; **19**: 132–6.

26. Becerra MC. Epidemiology of tuberculosis in the northern shantytowns of Lima, Peru (ScD thesis). Boston, MA: Harvard University, 1999..

27. World Health Organization. *TB/HIV: A clinical care manual.* Geneva: World Health Organization, 1996.

28. Farmer PE, Bayona J, Becerra M et al. The dilemma of MDRTB in the global era. *Int J Tuberc Lung Dis* 1998; **2**: 869–76.

29. Farmer PE, Furin JJ, Shin SS. Managing multidrug-resistant tuberculosis. *J Respir Dis* 2000; **21**: 53–6.

30. Partners In Health. *The PIH guide to the medical management of multidrug-resistant tuberculosis.* Boston: Partners In Health, 2003.

31. World Health Organization. WHO Fact Sheet No. 104: Tuberculosis. Geneva: World Health Organization, 1998.

32. Furin J, Mitnick C, Shin S et al. Occurrence of serious adverse effects in patients receiving community-based therapy for multidrug-resistant tuberculosis. *Int J Tuberc Lung Dis* 2001; **5**: 648–54.

33. Mitnick CD, Bayona J, Palacios E et al. Community-based therapy for multidrug-resistant tuberculosis in Lima, Peru. *N Engl J Med* 2003; **348**: 119–28.

34. Farmer PE, Kim JY. Community-based approaches to the control of multidrug-resistant tuberculosis: introducing 'DOTS-Plus'. *Br Med J* 1998; **317**: 671–4.

35. Garner P, Alejandria M, Lansang MA. Is DOTS-plus a feasible and cost-effective strategy? *PLoS Med* 2006; **3**: e350.

36. Bottger EC, Pletschette M, Andersson D. Drug resistance and fitness in *Mycobacterium tuberculosis* infection. *J Infect Dis* 2005; **191**: 823–4.

37. Espinal MA, Dye C, Raviglione M et al. Rational 'DOTS Plus' for the control of MDR-TB. *Int J Tuberc Lung Dis* 1999; **3**: 561–3.

38. Crofton J, Chaulet P, Maher D et al. *Guidelines for the management of drug-resistant tuberculosis.* WHO/GTB/96.210. Geneva: World Health Organization, 1997.

39. Pablos-Mendez A, Raviglione MC, Laszlo A et al. Global surveillance for antituberculosis-drug resistance, 1994–1997. *N Engl J Med* 1998; **338**: 1641–9.

40. Wolinsky E, Smith M, Steenken W. Isoniazid susceptibility, catalase activity, and guinea pig virulence of recently isolated cultures of tubercle bacilli. *Am Rev Tuberc* 1956; **73**: 768–72.

41. Pym A, Domenech P, Honore N et al. Regulation of catalase-peroxidase (*KatG*) expression, isoniazid sensitivity and virulence by *furA* of *Mycobacterium tuberculosis*. *Mol Microbiol* 2001; **40**: 879–89.

42. Wilson T, de Lisle G, Collins D. Effect of *inhA* and *katG* on isoniazid resistance and virulence of *Mycobacterium bovis*. *Mol Microbiol* 1995; **15**: 1009–15.

43. Billington O, McHugh T, Gillespie S. Physiological cost of rifampin resistance induced *in vitro* in *Mycobacterium tuberculosis*. *Antimicrob Agents Chemother* 1999; **43**: 1866–9.

44. Gagneux S, Burgos MV, DeRiemer K et al. Impact of bacterial genetics on the transmission of isoniazid-resistant *Mycobacterium tuberculosis*. *PLoS Pathog* 2006; **2**: e61.

45. Bjorkman J, Nagaev I, Berg OG et al. Effects of environment on compensatory mutations to ameliorate costs of antibiotic resistance. *Science* 2000; **287**: 1479–82.

46. Mariam DH, Mengistu Y, Hoffner SE et al. Effect of rpoB mutations conferring rifampin resistance on fitness of *Mycobacterium tuberculosis*. *Antimicrob Agents Chemother* 2004; **48**: 1289–94.

47. Gillespie SH, Billington OJ, Breathnach A et al. Multiple drug-resistant *Mycobacterium tuberculosis*: Evidence for changing

fitness following passage through human hosts. *Microb Drug Resist* 2002; **8**: 273–9.

48. Gagneux S, Long CD, Small PM *et al*. The competitive cost of antibiotic resistance in *Mycobacterium tuberculosis*. *Science* 2006; **312**: 1944–6.

49. Cohen T, Sommers B, Murray M. The effect of drug resistance on the fitness of *Mycobacterium tuberculosis*. *Lancet Infect Dis* 2003; **3**: 13–21.

50. van Soolingen D, Borgdorff M, de Haas P *et al*. Molecular epidemiology of tuberculosis in the Netherlands: A nationwide study from 1993–1997. *J Infect Dis* 1999; **180**: 726–36.

51. van Soolingen D, de Haas PE, van Doorn HR *et al*. Mutations at amino acid position 315 of the *katG* gene are associated with high-level resistance to isoniazid, other drug resistance, and successful transmission of *Mycobacterium tuberculosis* in the Netherlands. *J Infect Dis* 2000; **182**: 1788–90.

52. van Doorn HR, de Haas PE, Kremer K *et al*. Public health impact of isoniazid-resistant *Mycobacterium tuberculosis* strains with a mutation at amino-acid position 315 of *katG*: A decade of experience in the Netherlands. *Clin Microbiol Infect* 2006; **12**: 769–75.

53. Cohen T, Becerra MC, Murray MB. Isoniazid resistance and the future of drug-resistant tuberculosis. *Microb Drug Resist* 2004; **10**: 280–5.

54. Toungoussova OS, Caugant DA, Sandven P *et al*. Impact of drug resistance on fitness of *Mycobacterium tuberculosis* strains of the W-Beijing genotype. *FEMS Immunol Med Microbiol* 2004; **42**: 281–90.

55. Narvskaya O, Otten T, Limeschenko E *et al*. Nosocomial outbreak of multidrug-resistant tuberculosis caused by a strain of *Mycobacterium tuberculosis* W-Beijing family in St Petersburg, Russia. *Eur J Clin Microbiol Infect Dis* 2002; **21**: 596–602.

56. Marais BJ, Victor TC, Hesseling AC *et al*. Beijing and Haarlem genotypes are overrepresented among children with drug-resistant tuberculosis in the Western Cape Province of South Africa. *J Clin Microbiol* 2006; **44**: 3539–43.

57. Nikolayevskyy VV, Brown TJ, Bazhora YI *et al*. Molecular epidemiology and prevalence of mutations conferring rifampicin and isoniazid resistance in *Mycobacterium tuberculosis* strains from the southern Ukraine. *Clin Microbiol Infect* 2007; **13**: 129–38.

58. Johnson R, Warren R, Strauss OJ *et al*. An outbreak of drug-resistant tuberculosis caused by a Beijing strain in the western Cape, South Africa. *Int J Tuberc Lung Dis* 2006; **10**: 1412–14.

59. Drobniewski F, Balabanova Y, Nikolayevsky V *et al*. Drug-resistant tuberculosis, clinical virulence, and the dominance of the Beijing strain family in Russia. *J Am Med Assoc* 2005; **293**: 2726–31.

60. Snider DE, Kelly GD, Cauthen GM *et al*. Infection and disease among contacts of tuberculosis cases with drug-resistant and drug-susceptible bacilli. *Am Rev Respir Dis* 1985; **132**: 125–32.

61. Teixeira L, Perkins MD, Johnson JL *et al*. Infection and disease among household contacts of patients with multidrug-resistant tuberculosis. *Int J Tuberc Lung Dis* 2001; **5**: 321–8.

62. Palmero D, Cusmano L, Bucci Z *et al*. Infectiousness and virulence of multidrug-resistant and drug susceptible tuberculosis in adult contacts. *Medicina* 2002; **62**: 221–5.

63. Blower SM, Gerberding JL. Understanding, predicting and controlling the emergency of drug-resistant tuberculosis: A theoretical framework. *J Mol Med* 1999; **76**: 624–36.

64. Cohen T, Murray M. Modeling epidemics of multidrug-resistant *M. tuberculosis* of heterogeneous fitness. *Nat Med* 2004; **10**: 1117–21.

65. Blower S, Koelle K, Lietman T. Antibiotic resistance – to treat or not to treat? *Nat Med* 1999; **5**: 358.

66. Kim JY, Shakow A, Castro A *et al*. Tuberculosis control. In: Smith R, Beaglehole R, Woodward D, Drager N (eds). *Global public goods for health: Health economic and public health perspectives*. New York: Oxford University Press for the World Health Organization, 2003: 54–72.

67. World Health Organization. The concept of essential medicines. *Report of the WHO expert committee on the selection and use of essential medicines*. Geneva: World Health Organization, 19–23 March 2007 (unedited prepublication).

68. Gupta R, Kim JY, Espinal MA *et al*. Responding to market failures in tuberculosis control. *Science* 2001; **293**: 1049–51.

69. Sterling TR, Lehmann HP, Frieden TR. Impact of DOTS compared with DOTS-plus on multidrug resistant tuberculosis and tuberculosis deaths: Decision analysis. *Br Med J* 2003; **326**: 574.

70. Coker R. Should tuberculosis programs invest in second-line treatments for multidrug-resistant tuberculosis (MDR-TB)? *Int J Tuberc Lung Dis* 2002; **6**: 649–50.

71. Garner P, Alejandria M, Lansang MA. Is DOTS-plus a feasible and cost-effective strategy? *PLoS Med* 2006; **3**: e350.

72. Suarez PG, Floyd K, Portocarrero J *et al*. Feasibility and cost-effectiveness of standardized second-line drug treatment for chronic tuberculosis patients: A national cohort study in Peru. *Lancet* 2002; **359**: 1980–9.

73. World Health Organization. The feasibility and efficiency of controlling MDR-TB using the DOTS-Plus strategy in the Russian Federation. Geneva: World Health Organization, 2005.

74. Wilton P, Smith RD, Coast J *et al*. Directly observed treatment for multidrug-resistant tuberculosis: An economic evaluation in the United States of America and South Africa. *Int J Tuberc Lung Dis* 2001; **5**: 1137–42.

75. Baltussen R, Floyd K, Dye C. Cost effectiveness analysis of strategies for tuberculosis control in developing countries. *Br Med J* 2005; **331**: 1364.

76. Resch SC, Salomon JA, Murray M *et al*. Cost-effectiveness of treating multidrug-resistant tuberculosis. *PLoS Med* 2006; **3**: e241.

77. Stop TB Partnership. *The global plan to stop TB: 2006–2015*. Geneva: World Health Organization, 2006.

78. World Health Organization. *TB/HIV: A clinical care manual*. Geneva: World Health Organization, 1996.

79. World Health Organization. *WHO report on the tuberculosis epidemic*. Geneva: World Health Organization, 1996.

80. Sterling TR, Lehmann HP, Frieden TR. Impact of DOTS compared with DOTS-plus on multidrug resistant tuberculosis and tuberculosis deaths: Decision analysis. *Br Med J* 2003; 326: 574.

81. Garrett L. *The coming plague*. New York: Farrar, Straus and Giroux, 1994.

82. Leimane V, Leimans J. Tuberculosis control in Latvia: Integrated DOTS and DOTS-plus programs. *Euro Surveill* 2006; **11**: 29–33.

83. Keshavjee S, Gelmanova I, Peremitin I *et al*. Using DOTS-Plus to improve DOTS and expand access to effective tuberculosis treatment in Tomsk Oblast, Russia. Presented at the 35th World Conference on Lung Health and 5th DOTS Expansion Working Group Meeting, 28 October–1 November 2004, Paris, France.

84. Farmer PE, Furin JJ, Bayona J *et al*. Management of MDR-TB in resource-poor countries. *Int J Tuberc Lung Dis* 1999; **3**: 643–5.

85. Farmer PE, Bayona J, Becerra M *et al*. DOTS plus strategy in resource-poor countries. *Int J Tuberc Lung Dis* 1999; **3**: 844.

86. Farmer PE, Kononets AS, Borisov SE *et al*. Recrudescent tuberculosis in the Russian Federation. In: *The global impact of drug-resistant tuberculosis*. Program in Infectious Disease and Social Change. Boston, MA: Harvard Medical School and the Open Society Institute, 1999: 39–84.

87. Farmer PE. Cruel and unusual: Drug-resistant tuberculosis as punishment. In: Stern V (ed.). *Sentenced to die? The problem of TB in prisons in East and Central Europe and Central Asia*. London: International Centre for Prison Studies, 1999: 70–88.

88. Kimerling ME, Kluge H, Vezhnina N *et al*. Inadequacy of the current WHO re-treatment regimen in a central Siberian prison: Treatment failure and MDR-TB. *Int J Tuberc Lung Dis* 1999; **3**: 451–3. See also comment in: Farmer PE. Managerial successes, clinical failures. *Int J Tuberc Lung Dis* 1999; **3**: 365–7.

89. Shin SS, Pasechnikov AD, Gelmanova IY *et al.* Treatment outcomes in an integrated civilian and prison MDR-TB treatment program in Russia. *Int J Tuberc Lung Dis* 2006; **10**: 402–408.

90. Fierer J. MDR-TB and HIV: The perfect storm? *Am J Trop Med Hyg* 2006; **75**: 1025–6.

91. Glusker A. Global tuberculosis levels plateau while extensively drug resistant strains increase. *Br Med J* 2007; **334**: 659.

92. Van Rie A, Enarson D. XDR tuberculosis: An indicator of public-health negligence. *Lancet* 2007; **369**: 272–3.

PART 5

TUBERCULOSIS IN SPECIAL SITUATIONS

19

The association between HIV and tuberculosis in the developing world, with a special focus on sub-Saharan Africa

ANTHONY D HARRIES AND RONY ZACHARIAH

INTRODUCTION

Tuberculosis has for many years caused considerable morbidity and mortality in the developing countries of the world. Between the 1930s and 1940s in sub-Saharan Africa, a virus, which we now know as the human immunodeficiency virus (HIV), made the species jump from chimpanzees (to cause HIV-1) and macaques and sooty mangabeys (to cause HIV-2) to man. The first known case of the acquired immunodeficiency syndrome (AIDS) was traced to a blood sample of a man who died in the Democratic Republic of the Congo in 1959, but the official start of the epidemic was in June 1981 when *Pneumocystis carinii* (now called *jeroveci*) pneumonia (PCP) and Kaposi's sarcoma were diagnosed in homosexual men in New York and California. The subsequent devastating spread of the virus, particularly in sub-Saharan Africa, during the last 25 years has had, and continues to have, a profound effect on the epidemiology, clinical features and management of tuberculosis. This chapter addresses the important interactions which arise from dual infection with HIV and *Mycobacterium tuberculosis* and discusses the strategies and interventions which may help to mitigate the serious consequences of this dual epidemic in the developing world. Most attention is paid to sub-Saharan Africa, which is the region most severely affected by this global pandemic.

Table 19.1 Adults and children living with HIV and adult HIV-prevalence by region: December 2005.[1]

Region	Adults and children living with HIV	Adult HIV prevalence (%)
Sub-Saharan Africa	25.8 million	7.2
North Africa and Middle East	510 000	0.2
South and South-East Asia	7.4 million	0.7
East Asia	870 000	0.1
Oceania	74 000	0.5
Latin America	1.8 million	0.6
Caribbean	300 000	1.6
Eastern Europe and Central Asia	1.6 million	0.9
Western and Central Europe	720 000	0.3
North America	1.2 million	0.7
Total	40.3 million	1.1

THE HIV AND AIDS PANDEMIC

Epidemiological perspective

HIV/AIDS is the modern world's greatest pandemic. Twenty-five years after first being recognized, it has claimed 25 million lives and the number of people infected with HIV worldwide has reached 40.3 million, the majority of whom live in the developing world (Table 19.1).[1] In 2005 alone, there were 4.9 million new HIV infections and 3.1 million AIDS deaths.

Sub-Saharan Africa bears the brunt of this global catastrophe.[1] With less than 10 per cent of the world's population, the region is home to nearly 65 per cent of people living with HIV/AIDS (25.8 million in 2005). In 2005, there were 3.2 million new HIV infections in this region and 2.4 million people with HIV/AIDS died, representing 77 per cent of global AIDS deaths for that year. In the last 10 years, an increasing proportion of HIV infections has occurred in women, which has additional implications for mother-to-child transmission. Among young people aged 15–24 years, an estimated 4.6 per cent of women and 1.7 per cent of men were living with HIV in 2005. These higher rates in women are because HIV is transmitted more easily from men to women than vice versa, sexual activity starts earlier for women, and young women have sex with older partners. Within the region, Southern Africa is the epicentre of the epidemic, where HIV-prevalence rates of 30 per cent or more are being recorded in pregnant women in the countries of South Africa, Botswana, Lesotho, Namibia and Swaziland.

The majority of HIV infections in sub-Saharan Africa are a result of HIV-1. HIV-2, which is much less common, is primarily found in West Africa, although HIV-2 infections have also been confirmed in other African countries, including Angola and Mozambique. HIV-2 is the more slowly growing of the two viruses, is less easily transmitted, has a slower progression to AIDS and is associated with reduced mortality.[2]

Modes of transmission

In sub-Saharan Africa, virus transmission is principally by heterosexual intercourse, although mother-to-child transmission, infected blood transfusions,[3] and injections and scarification play their role. Specific sexual transmission risk factors include sexual behaviour patterns, sexual intercourse between older men and younger women, lack of circumcision and the presence of sexually transmitted infections – both ulcerative and non-ulcerative.[4] Cervical ectopy and the frequent presence of genital ulcers due to herpes simplex type 2 put young women particularly at risk of HIV infection. Recent observations in Southern Africa in particular have pointed out that men and women often have more than one – typically two or even three – concurrent sexual partnerships that can overlap for months or years.[5] This pattern differs from that of the serial monogamy, which is more common in western society, or the one-off casual or commercial sexual encounters that occur everywhere. Mathematical modelling suggests that HIV transmission is much more rapid (and the resulting epidemic 10 times greater) with long-term concurrent sexual relationships than with serial monogamous relationships. This can be explained biologically by the fact that infectivity is much higher during the initial weeks or months after infection, and thus as soon as one person in a network of concurrent relationships contracts HIV, everyone else in the network is placed at high risk. By contrast, serial monogamy traps the virus within a single relationship for months or years.

These observations provide some explanation as to why the HIV epidemic is still rampant in sub-Saharan Africa. In Asia, 8.3 million people are infected with HIV,[1] with the epidemic largely concentrated in injecting drug users, men who have sex with men, sex workers, clients of sex workers and their immediate sexual partners. However, Asia, and particularly the large countries of India and China, is at a crossroads, where there is the potential for a massive increase in HIV infection rates unless comprehensive prevention packages are implemented. In Latin America and the Caribbean, 2.1 million people are infected with HIV,[1] with transmission in Latin America being principally through injecting drug use and men who have sex with men, while in the Caribbean mechanisms of transmission are similar to those seen in sub-Saharan Africa.

Impact of HIV in sub-Saharan Africa

The impact of HIV in sub-Saharan Africa is immense. Over the last 25 years, HIV-related disease and AIDS have become increasingly responsible for hospital admissions. In a large central hospital in Malawi, 70 per cent of all adult medical admissions were HIV-positive and 45 per cent had AIDS, while 36 per cent of all surgical admissions were HIV-positive and 8 per cent had AIDS.[6] In the same hospital in Malawi, nearly 20 per cent of admissions to a paediatric ward were HIV-positive with HIV infection being most common in children aged less than 6 months.[7]

Over 15 years ago, AIDS was the leading cause of adult death in Abidjan, Côte d'Ivoire,[8] and autopsy studies since then in other countries, such as Botswana,[9] have continued to confirm these findings. High mortality rates are being recorded in rural communities where the HIV epidemic is well established, particularly among young and better-educated adults.[10] A study from seven randomized mother-to-child transmission intervention trials in the region highlighted the very high mortality experienced in African children born to HIV-infected mothers.[11] By 1 year of age, 35 per cent of HIV-infected children had died and by 2 years of age, this had increased to 52 per cent; the corresponding death rates for uninfected children were 5 and 8 per cent, respectively.

This considerable adult-, and to a certain extent child-, related mortality has resulted in substantial reductions in life expectancy in African urban and rural settings. In Botswana, Zimbabwe and South Africa, life expectancy is estimated to plummet from 60 years in 1990 to about 30 years in 2010.[12] By killing adults in their most productive years, AIDS is depriving the region of the skills and knowledge base that are so essential for economic development. The living standards of poor people are being increasingly threatened by HIV/AIDS, where AIDS care-related expenses may absorb one-third of a household's monthly income. Education is being undermined since teachers die at almost the same rate as they can be trained. Already weak health-care systems have to try and cope with a workforce that suffers the ravages of the epidemic just as much as the rest of the community. The orphan problem is huge and large numbers of children have to be brought up by their grandparents. Many orphans cannot attend school, suffer from poverty and malnutrition, and are drawn into a spiral of crime, violence and commercial sex. AIDS retards development and creates conditions ripe for political instability.

ASSOCIATION OF TB AND HIV INFECTION

Infection with *M. tuberculosis* and HIV

About one-third of the world's population is infected with *M. tuberculosis*.[13] In general, 5–10 per cent of individuals infected with *M. tuberculosis* will develop symptomatic tuberculosis (TB) at some time during their lives, the greatest risk being within the first 5 years of infection. Factors that enhance the risk of developing TB following infection are age, malnutrition, alcohol, immunosuppressive drugs and diseases, such as silicosis and diabetes mellitus. However, all pale into insignificance compared with HIV infection. HIV, by targeting CD4 T-lymphocytes and reducing cellular immune function, is by far the strongest risk factor for development of TB. Not only does HIV increase the risk that latent *M. tuberculosis* will be reactivated, but it also increases the risk of rapid development of TB soon after infection or reinfection with the tubercle bacillus.

In individuals co-infected with HIV and *M. tuberculosis*, the annual risk of active TB is 5–15 per cent. The risk starts within the first year of HIV infection,[14] increases as the immune system becomes more compromised and over the course of an infected person's life is approximately 50 per cent. HIV appears to be shifting the balance of TB between men and women. Women aged 15–24 years are making up a relatively high proportion of reported TB cases in the African countries with a high-prevalence of HIV infection, this being consistent with the observation that HIV infection tends to be more common in women in this age group compared with men. As the prevalence of HIV infection in adults increases so does the female proportion of all adult TB cases. In 2000, it was estimated that

11.4 million adults aged 15–49 years were co-infected with HIV and *M. tuberculosis*, the majority of these adults living in sub-Saharan Africa.[15]

Extent of HIV–TB interaction in sub-Saharan Africa

Initial reports of HIV-associated TB in sub-Saharan Africa were in immigrants receiving treatment overseas. For example, HIV infection was reported in 17 per cent of African immigrants with TB who were being treated in Brussels in the early 1980s.[16] However, during the 1980s, reports started to come from Ethiopia,[17] Zimbabwe,[18] Malawi[19] and Zambia,[20] indicating that TB was being found at presentation in approximately one-third of patients infected with HIV, and the strong association between the two infections became recognized. Autopsy studies around the continent confirmed these findings, with TB being found at autopsy in 41 per cent of selected AIDS patients in Zaire,[21] 40 per cent of HIV-positive patients in Côte d'Ivoire[22] and 40 per cent of HIV-positive patients in Botswana.[9] In Abidjan, Côte d'Ivoire, TB was the prime cause of death in 32 per cent of HIV-positive cadavers and in 54 per cent of HIV-positive patients who died with an AIDS defining illness.[23] Similarly in Botswana, TB was the cause of death in 38 per cent of HIV-positive patients.[9]

The extent of the interaction between HIV and TB in sub-Saharan Africa can also be seen in HIV-seroprevalence studies conducted in patients with TB from various countries between 1986 and 2003 (Table 19.2).[24–46] For countries in East and Central Africa, HIV-seropositivity refers to infection with HIV-1. However, in some West African countries, HIV-seropositivity indicates infection with HIV-1, HIV-2 or both. The studies summarized in Table 19.2 are heterogeneous and include patients (1) with different ages and therefore different degrees of risk for HIV infection, (2) with bacteriologically proven disease or with suspected disease, (3) with newly diagnosed or with previously treated disease and (4) from urban and rural areas. This heterogeneity explains in part some of the variation in HIV-seropositivity rates. However, it is clear from these studies and national reports that there are countries in Southern Africa where HIV seroprevalence in TB patients has climbed to 50 per cent or higher, while other countries particularly in West Africa have lower HIV seroprevalence rates. The first large countrywide survey of HIV-seroprevalence in TB patients was conducted in Tanzania between 1991 and 1993.[47] In 6928 TB cases, there was an overall HIV-seroprevalence rate of 32 per cent, with regional differences that varied from 10 to 59 per cent. Overall, prevalence of HIV infection was higher in women (35 versus 30 per cent), those aged 25–34 years (45 per cent) and residents in urban areas (37 versus 28 per cent). Patients with new pulmonary smear-negative and extra-pulmonary disease had a higher prevalence of HIV infection (40 per cent) than those with new smear-positive pul-

Table 19.2   HIV-seroprevalence in patients with TB in sub-Saharan Africa: 1986–2003.

Year of study	Country	No. with TB	% HIV–positive	Ref.
1986	Malawi	125	26	24
1987	Zambia	131	58[a]	25
1987	Zaire (now DRC)	287	36	26
1987	Central African Republic	220	28[a]	27
1987	Côte d'Ivoire	193	51	28
1988–89	Malawi	152	52[a]	29
1988–89	Zambia	346	60	30
1988–89	Zimbabwe	1434	45	31
1989–90	Côte d'Ivoire	2043	40	32
1989–91	Zaire	1666	22[a]	33
1989–90	Cote d'Ivoire	4504	44[a]	34
1989	Zambia	249	73[a]	35
1989–90	Kenya	281	38	36
1989–91	Zaire	561	64	37
1990–91	Uganda	330	66	38
1990	Burkina Faso	Not given	25	39
1992	Guinea-Bissau	168	24[a]	40
1992–93	Côte d'Ivoire	559	44[a]	41
1993–94	Malawi	665	75	42
1995	Malawi	793	77	43
1995–96	Botswana	188	51[a]	44
1997	South Africa	Not given	66	45
2003	Malawi	1404	68	46

[a]Studies in which only new patients with tuberculosis were included.

monary (28 per cent) or relapse smear-positive (30 per cent) disease. Similar findings were reported in two other countrywide surveys, one conducted in Kenya between 1993 and 1994 showing an overall HIV-seroprevalence rate of 41 per cent,[48] and one in Malawi in 2000 showing an overall HIV-seroprevalence rate of 77 per cent.[49]

In contrast to autopsy data in HIV-infected African adults, tuberculosis had been reported as a relatively uncommon cause of death in HIV-infected African children.[50] However, sampling in these studies may cause potential bias, as an autopsy study reported from Botswana identified TB in 12 per cent of HIV-seropositive children,[51] and a post-mortem study from Zambia found TB in a fifth of children dying of respiratory illness, with almost 60 per cent being HIV-positive.[52] A number of cross-sectional studies which have taken children with tuberculosis as their starting population have shown high rates of association with HIV. HIV-1 seroprevalence in children with TB in Zambia aged 1 month to 14 years was 37 per cent compared with an HIV-seroprevalence rate of 10.7 per cent amongst controls.[53] In Zambia, the highest overall age-specific HIV-seroprevalence was 53 per cent in the 12–18 month age group. In Côte d'Ivoire,[54] 11.8 per cent of children with TB were HIV-seropositive (10 per cent with HIV-1, 0.7 per cent with HIV-2 and 1 per cent with both viruses). The highest overall age-specific HIV-seroprevalence was in children aged 1–4 years (23.4 per

cent). In South Africa[55] and Malawi,[56] HIV-seroprevalence in children hospitalized with tuberculosis was 42 and 64 per cent, respectively.

The increase in tuberculosis in Africa

TB case notifications mirror increases in HIV prevalence, and in sub-Saharan Africa, this strong association between the two infections has led to an upsurge of TB in most countries in the region. In countries with high HIV infection rates, estimated TB incidence rates have risen from 140 per 100 000 in 1991 to 400 per 100 000 in 2003.[57] This is in marked contrast to the situation in established market economies, which have seen a gradual decline in case notification rates in the last 20 years, and other regions in the world where, apart from Eastern Europe, rates have also declined or stabilized. Programmes in Tanzania and Malawi have allowed accurate surveillance of the situation.[57] The increase in case notifications for all forms of TB are shown for Tanzania (Figure 19.1) and for Malawi (Figure 19.2). In Tanzania, the case notification rate per 100 000 people has increased from 62 in 1985 to 167 in 2003, and in Malawi has increased from 74 in 1985 to 213 in 2003. Programme surveillance in these two countries showed that TB cases rose dramatically in the 1980s and 1990s, but in the last few years TB case notifications have

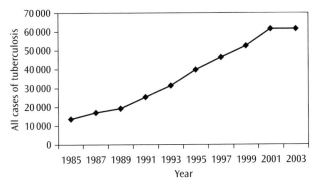

Figure 19.1 Tuberculosis in Tanzania: 1985–2003.[57]

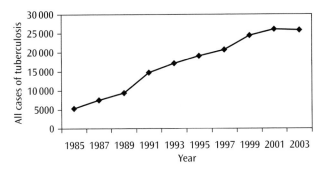

Figure 19.2 Tuberculosis in Malawi: 1985–2003.[57]

begun to plateau. Of note, HIV-prevalence rates in the two countries began to plateau 5 or more years previously. Data from Kenya has shown that increases in TB cases follow rises in HIV prevalence by approximately 7 years, and similarly plateaus in TB cases occur approximately 7 years after HIV rates have plateaued.[58] This delay is explained by the fact that healthy people have approximately 1000 CD4 T-lymphocytes per microlitre of blood, which decline at the rate of about 100 cells per microlitre per year after HIV infection, and the median level CD4-lymphocyte count at which people develop TB is 190 per microlitre.[58]

HIV–TB interactions in other developing countries

HIV–TB interactions in other developing countries mirror HIV-prevalence rates and rates of infection with *M. tuberculosis*. India has the second highest number of HIV-TB co-infected adults in the world after South Africa.[15] With an estimated 3 per cent of its tuberculosis patients being HIV-seropositive, there are genuine fears that the HIV epidemic may undermine TB control efforts in that vast country.[59] In Chiang Rai, northern Thailand, HIV seroprevalence in TB patients increased from 1.5 per cent in 1990, to 19 per cent in 1992 to 45.5 per cent in 1994.[60] However, in other large Asian countries, such as China, Indonesia and Bangladesh, HIV infection rates have

remained below 1 per cent in TB patients.[61] In Haiti in the Caribbean, high HIV seroprevalence rates are found in patients with TB[62] – similar findings to those reported in sub-Saharan Africa. In Latin America, Brazil records the highest HIV-seropositivity rates in TB patients in the region, estimated countrywide to be about 5 per cent.[13]

CLINICAL FEATURES

Tuberculosis in Africa before the advent of HIV/AIDS

Large surveys carried out in Kenya and Tanzania between 1964 and 1984 by the British Medical Research Council (MRC) and East African Research Centres[63–66] provide excellent data on the pattern of TB in Africa prior to the AIDS epidemic (Table 19.3). Almost 90 per cent of all patients had pulmonary disease. Of those with extrapulmonary TB (EPTB), lymphadenopathy (mainly cervical in distribution) (Figure 19.3), bone/joint disease (Figure 19.4) and pleural effusion were responsible for 85 per cent of the total. In Kenya, pericardial and/or peritoneal disease (Figure 19.5) was seen in 5 per cent of patients with EPTB. Amongst adults and children older than 15 years with pulmonary tuberculosis (PTB), almost 80 per cent had positive sputum smears for acid fast bacilli on Ziehl–Neelsen stain and 66 per cent had cavitation on chest x-ray (Figure 19.6). There were highly significant associations in the different

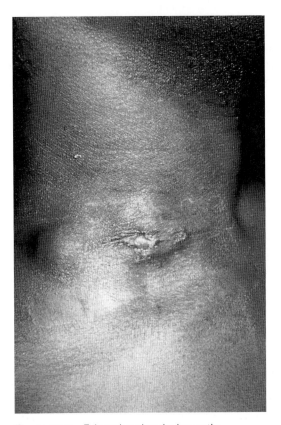

Figure 19.3 Tuberculous lymphadenopathy.

Table 19.3 Tuberculosis in East Africa before the advent of AIDS (East African/MRC Co-operative studies).[63–66]

Country	Year	No. of patients	Pattern of disease %		
			PTB	PTB + EPTB	EPTB
Kenya	1964	1164	89.8	2.5	7.7
	1974	1490	88.5	3.0	8.5
	1984	1961	85.4	2.5	12.1
Tanzania	1970	1884	87.4	2.5	10.1
	1980	2242	91.5	0.6	7.9
Total		8741	88.5	2.1	9.4

Country	Year	No. of patients	Extrapulmonary tuberculosis		
			Lymphadenopathy	Bone/joint	Pleura
Kenya	1964	132	48	21	15
	1974	172	51	25	9
	1984	286	52	22	8
Tanzania	1970	237	54	28	7
	1980	191	40	26	19
Total		1018	49.5	24.5	10.9

PTB, pulmonary tuberculosis; EPTB, extrapulmonary tuberculosis.

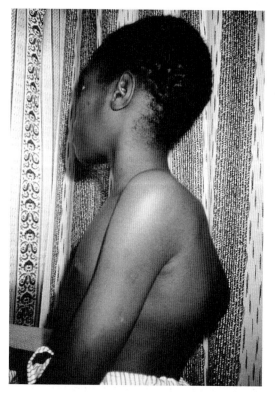

Figure 19.4   Tuberculous spondylitis.

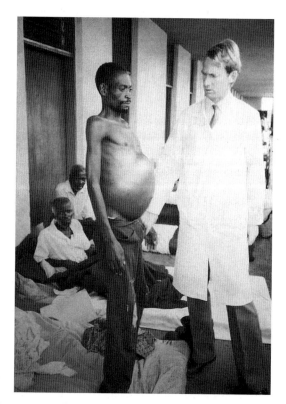

Figure 19.5   Tuberculous ascites in a patient on a general medical ward.

surveys between extent of radiological cavitation and sputum smear-positivity; these findings are in accord with the clinical observation that in cavitatory tuberculosis, the majority of patients have positive sputum smears for acid-fast bacilli (AFB). Extensive disease involving more than three radiographic zones was found in 30 per cent of patients. Miliary disease was uncommon, and in Kenyan adults it was present in only 1.7 per cent of TB patients.

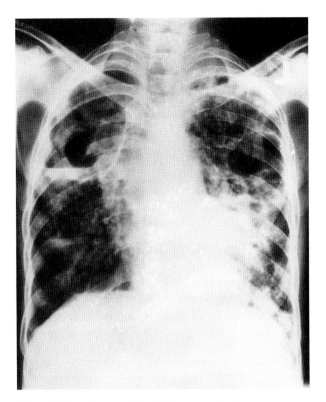

Figure 19.6 Characteristic chest x-ray of pulmonary tuberculosis in Africa. HIV-negative, smear-positive patient.

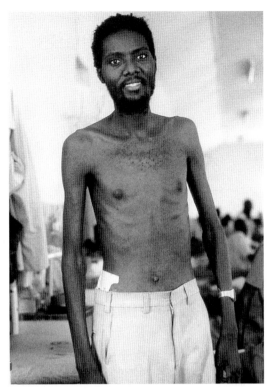

Figure 19.7 Malnourished patient with pulmonary tuberculosis.

Tuberculosis in association with HIV infection in Africa

In the HIV-positive patient, TB is said to be an early manifestation of illness (owing to the relative virulence of *M. tuberculosis*). However, studies in sub-Saharan Africa which have measured CD4-lymphocyte counts at diagnosis in HIV-infected smear-positive PTB patients have found that patients may present across a wide spectrum of immunodeficiency. In Zaire, approximately one-third of patients had less than 200 CD4-lymphocytes/µL, one-third between 200–499 and one-third 500 or more.[33] In Côte d'Ivoire, 43 per cent of patients had CD4-lymphocyte counts below 200/µL while 18 per cent had CD4-lymphocyte counts of 500/µL.[41]

The clinical pattern of TB correlates with the host immune status and this is reflected in the microbiological and histological characteristics of the tuberculous lesions. If TB occurs in the early stages of HIV infection when the patient's immunity is only partially compromised, the features are characteristic of post-primary TB and resemble those seen in the pre-AIDS era. Usually, the patient has typical symptoms; chest radiography shows extensive lung destruction, cavitation and upper lobe involvement; sputum smears are positive for AFB. The histological appearances are usually those of the classic tuberculous lesion with caseating, giant cell and epithelioid granulomas. As CD4-lymphocyte counts decline (indicating more advanced immunodeficiency), HIV-positive patients present with atypical pulmonary disease resembling primary pulmonary TB (i.e. pulmonary infiltrates with no cavities, lower lobe involvement, intrathoracic adenopathy, negative sputum smears) or extrapulmonary, disseminated disease.[67]

GENERAL FEATURES

Formal studies have shown that certain social variables and clinical features are significantly more common in HIV-positive TB patients compared with HIV-negative TB patients.[30,34,36,48,49] Social features associated with HIV infection include a good education, living in good housing and being divorced or widowed. Past medical history suggesting HIV infection includes the presence of sexually transmitted infections, herpes zoster (shingles), recurrent pneumonia and bacteraemia (especially *Salmonella typhimurium*). Symptoms and signs strongly associated with HIV infection are: diarrhoea for longer than 1 month, pain on swallowing (suggesting oesophageal candidiasis), burning sensation of the feet (suggesting peripheral neuropathy), a scar of herpes zoster, pruritic papular rash, Kaposi's sarcoma, symmetrical generalized lymphadenopathy and oral candidiasis. Irrespective of HIV status, many patients with TB have weight loss.[30,36] However, severe weight loss – more than 20 per cent or more than 10 kg – is more often associated with HIV-seropositivity.[26,34] Significant malnutrition in HIV-positive

Table 19.4 Pattern of tuberculosis in association with HIV infection.

Country	No. of HIV-positive patients	No. with PTB (%)	No. with EPTB (%)	Ref.
Zambia	239	116 (49)	123 (51)	20
Zaire	176	154 (87)	22 (13)	26
Malawi	80	34 (42)	46 (58)	29
Zambia	229	133 (58)	96 (42)	30
Côte d'Ivoire	821	662 (81)	159 (19)	32
Côte d'Ivoire	4504	3718 (82)	786 (18)	34
Kenya	70	50 (71)	20 (29)	36
Malawi	612	432 (71)	180 (29)	43

PTB, pulmonary tuberculosis; EPTB, extrapulmonary tuberculosis.

Table 19.5 Proportion of pulmonary TB patients with negative sputum smears – relation with HIV-serostatus.

Country	PTB patients with negative sputum smears (%)		Ref.
	HIV-positive	HIV-negative	
Zaire	39	27	26
Zambia	45	35	30
Côte d'Ivoire	8	6	32
Kenya	28	17	36
Malawi	37	32	43
Senegal	35	17	71

TB patients as judged by weight, anthropometry and low body mass index is also a common observation (Figure 19.7).[68,69] Although these demonstrable differences allow differentiation between groups, their value in distinguishing the HIV-positive from the HIV-negative TB patient is less apparent. Furthermore, up to half of HIV-positive patients with TB will have no clinical features specifically suggestive of HIV infection.[36]

PATTERN OF TUBERCULOSIS

There have been a number of studies in different African countries examining the pattern of TB in relation to HIV infection in consecutive patients attending hospital (Table 19.4). The findings show that EPTB is more common in HIV-positive patients. The ratio of pulmonary to extrapulmonary disease in HIV-negative patients is in general similar to that observed in the MRC studies carried out in East Africa in the pre-AIDS era.

The pattern of HIV-associated EPTB reported from studies in East and Central Africa is pleural disease (60 per cent), lymphadenopathy (14 per cent), pericardial disease (11 per cent) and miliary disease (10 per cent).[19,20,29,30,36,43] This pattern may vary in different geographical regions. In the USA, lymphadenopathy, pleural effusions and miliary disease are the most common types of extrapulmonary disease, with involvement of the central nervous system, genitourinary tract and bone marrow being additional significant problems.[70] These may be genuine differences, or merely reflect patient selection and differences in the availability of diagnostic capacity.

PTB IN ADULTS

Initial impressions were that HIV infection in Africa was associated with a large and predominant increase in smear-negative PTB. However, it is apparent from cross-sectional studies that the majority of HIV-positive PTB patients are sputum smear-positive, although the proportion of patients with smear-negative PTB is greater in those with HIV infection compared with those who are HIV-negative (Table 19.5).[26,30,32,36,43,71] A study in Zambia[72] which examined over 100 patients with culture positive PTB found that 24 per cent of those who were HIV-negative had a negative

---

Case history 1

A 21-year-old African female presented to hospital with a 6-month history of gradual increasing shortness of breath on exertion, cough and haemoptysis. There had been no response to several courses of antibiotics. Three sputum specimens were negative for AFB and the chest radiograph showed a normal sized heart with patchy infiltrates in the lower zones.

The patient was diagnosed with smear-negative pulmonary TB and started on antituberculosis treatment. One month after starting treatment, there was no improvement and the patient continued to have haemoptysis.

On review, the patient was found to have a tapping apex beat, a loud first heart sound and a low pitched rumbling diastolic murmur at the apex. There was clinical evidence of pulmonary congestion.

The patient was diagnosed with mitral stenosis and pulmonary congestion. Antituberculosis treatment was discontinued and the patient was treated with digoxin and diuretics. The patient became less breathless and haemoptysis stopped.

Practice point: patients with valvular heart disease and heart failure can be misdiagnosed as having smear-negative pulmonary tuberculosis unless a thorough clinical assessment is carried out.

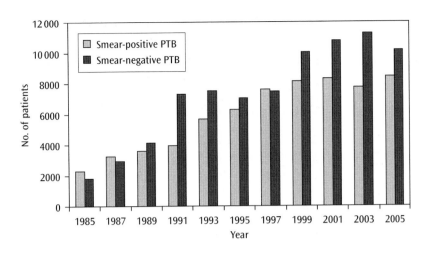

Figure 19.8 Smear-negative and smear-positive pulmonary tuberculosis (PTB) in Malawi: 1985–2005. *Source*, Malawi NTP.

sputum smear compared with 43 per cent of those who were HIV-positive, low sputum bacillary load being related to the absence of radiographic cavitation. In Tanzania, another study in 433 HIV-positive TB patients found that sputum bacillary density was inversely related to CD4-lymphocyte counts, the lower the CD4 count the more likely the sputum would be smear-negative.[73]

Countries with good reporting systems, such as Tanzania and Malawi, have found that under routine conditions there has been a larger increase in new cases with smear-negative PTB compared with smear-positive PTB in the last 10–15 years (Figure 19.8). It is not clear whether these figures reflect the true pattern of PTB or whether there is an over-diagnosis or an under-diagnosis of smear-negative TB cases. Reports from national TB programmes of the pattern of PTB are influenced by various factors, such as (1) the criteria used to diagnose smear-negative PTB, (2) the extent to which these criteria are actually followed in clinical practice, (3) the proportion of positive sputum smears falsely read as negative, (4) the correct interpretation of chest radiographs and (5) the number of other respiratory diseases which can resemble and be misdiagnosed as PTB. An operational research study in Malawi on patients registered as smear-negative PTB concluded that 78 per cent were diagnosed correctly according to TB programme guidelines, 8 per cent were considered to have EPTB and had therefore been misclassified and 14 per cent had another non-TB diagnosis (see Case history 1).[74]

The diagnostic process

The diagnosis of adult PTB in most African countries is based on simple techniques such as clinical assessment, sputum smear microscopy and chest radiography. Tuberculin skin testing is not useful for individual diagnosis. Cutaneous anergy increases as the CD4-lymphocyte count declines: in Zaire over 50 per cent of HIV-positive PTB patients with a CD4-lymphocyte count <200/µL were found to have a negative tuberculin test.[33] Techniques which are widely available in industrialized countries for obtaining pulmonary specimens (e.g. fibreoptic bron-

choscopy with bronchoalveolar lavage) and for analysing such specimens (culture, polymerase chain reaction) are beyond the resources of most hospitals in sub-Saharan Africa.

Patients are considered to be PTB suspects if there is a cough for 3 weeks or longer (particularly if associated with weight loss and no response to a course of antibiotics), haemoptysis or acute diffuse pneumonia which has not responded to penicillin or broad-spectrum antibiotics. Among adults presenting with a chronic cough for more than 3 weeks to primary health-care clinics in Harare, the prevalence of HIV infection was 83 per cent and TB was diagnosed in 43 per cent with over 70 per cent having smear-positive disease.[75] Studies in Burundi and Tanzania suggest that TB suspects whose initial sputum smears are negative for AFB have a high chance of having TB if two out of four clinical features are found – cough more than 3 weeks, chest pain longer than 2 weeks, absence of expectoration and absence of shortness of breath.[76]

Sputum smear microscopy

The most cost-effective method of screening TB suspects in low-income countries is first by sputum smear microscopy, and, if the sputum smears are negative, to proceed to a chest radiograph. It has always been standard practice to examine three early-morning sputum specimens for tubercle bacilli. However, the effectiveness of the third smear has been called into question,[77] and studies conducted in both Malawi[78] and Zambia[79] have clearly shown that a policy of screening TB suspects using two sputum smears is as effective as using three sputum smears, and also less costly and labour intensive.

Most hospital laboratories in Africa screen sputum smears for AFB using light microscopy and the Ziehl–Neelsen stain. However, to pronounce a sputum smear as negative 100 high-power fields must be examined. The maximum number of Ziehl–Neelsen-stained smears that a microscopist can properly examine in 1 day is about 30–40. Laboratories handling large numbers of specimens each day usually invest in a fluorescent microscope. Fluorescent microscopy using phenolic auramine

Table 19.6 Causes of false-negative sputum smears in sub-Saharan Africa.

Sputum collection	Inadequate sputum sample
	Inappropriate sputum container
	Sputum stored too long before microscopy
	Incorrect labelling of sample
Sputum processing	Faulty sampling of sputum specimen for smear
	Faulty sputum smear preparation and staining
Sputum smear examination	Inadequate time spent examining smears
	Inadequate attention to smear examination
Laboratory	Shortage of trained laboratory personnel
	Poorly functioning microscopes
	Shortage of laboratory supplies
	Lack of quality control

stains enables smears to be examined quickly under low magnification, and a microscopist can examine 200 or more smears per day with this technique. The data from sub-Saharan Africa about the sensitivity or specificity of sputum smear examination is sparse. In Kenya and Malawi, a re-examination with two repeat sputum smears in patients registered as smear-negative PTB found that 26 and 22 per cent, respectively, of patients were smear-positive.[80,81] The reasons for the false-negative smear results were not investigated, but Table 19.6 summarizes some of the important causes.

Chest radiography

Although the classical radiographic hallmarks of PTB are cavitation, apical distribution, bilateral distribution, pulmonary fibrosis, shrinkage and calcification, no pattern is absolutely diagnostic of TB. Patients with HIV infection may have atypical radiographic findings of TB such as infiltrates without cavitation, involving particularly the lower lobes (Figure 19.9), and hilar and/or paratracheal lymphadenopathy (Figure 19.10). The radiographic presentation is related to the CD4-lymphocyte count. A study in Canada found that the mean CD4-lymphocyte count in HIV-positive PTB patients was 323 cells/μL when the chest radiograph was 'typical' and 69 cells/μL when the chest radiograph was 'atypical'.[82] Similar findings have been reported from South Africa[83] and from the Côte d'Ivoire.[84] The lack of trained radiologists in Africa coupled with the non-specific findings of pulmonary infiltrates in HIV-positive patients makes for difficulties in correct radiographic diagnosis.

It is also well recognized in industrialized countries[85] and in countries in sub-Saharan Africa[81,83] that the chest radiograph can be normal in HIV-positive PTB patients

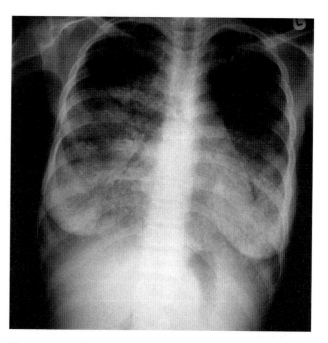

Figure 19.9 Chest x-ray in HIV-positive, smear-negative pulmonary tuberculosis (culture-positive for *M. tuberculosis*) showing bilateral lower lobe infiltrates.

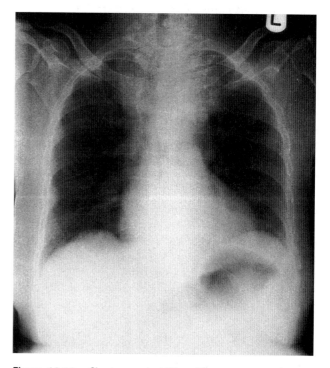

Figure 19.10 Chest x-ray in HIV-positive, smear-negative pulmonary tuberculosis (culture-positive for *M. tuberculosis*) showing paratracheal lymphadenopathy.

(Figure 19.11). In health facilities where mycobacterial cultures are not available, such patients will probably not be recognized as having PTB and will not therefore receive antituberculosis treatment.

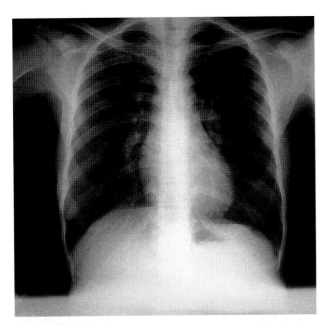

Figure 19.11 Chest x-ray in HIV-positive, smear-negative pulmonary tuberculosis (culture-positive for *M. tuberculosis*) showing normal appearance.

Differential diagnosis of smear-negative PTB

Over the last 20 years there have been a number of research studies, using either induced sputum or fibreoptic bronchoscopy with bronchoalveolar lavage and transbronchial biopsy, in sub-Saharan Africa to determine the range of pulmonary diseases found in patients with respiratory illness and negative AFB sputum smears.[86,87] In these studies, about one-quarter to one-third of patients were found to have microbiologically proven TB. Other pathogens or diseases identified have included PCP, bacterial pneumonia due to a wide range of pathogens, Kaposi's sarcoma, nocardiosis and fungal infections with *Cryptococcus neoformans* and *Aspergillus fumigatus*.

A study in Malawi investigated 353 patients about to be registered for smear-negative PTB, diagnosed according to routine programme conditions.[81] Eighty-nine per cent of the patients assessed were HIV-positive. Microbiologically confirmed TB was found in 39 per cent. Diagnoses other than PTB were made in 22 per cent and no diagnosis in 39 per cent. Among the other diagnoses were PCP, bacterial pneumonia, Kaposi's sarcoma, asthma, oesophageal conditions and cardiac failure. A further study in Botswana in people with suspected TB and an abnormal chest radiograph, of whom 86 per cent were HIV-positive, found TB in 52 per cent, *Mycoplasma pneumoniae* in 17 per cent, and PCP in 3 per cent: many of these patients had dual infections.[88]

EPTB IN ADULTS

The pattern of EPTB and the degree of diagnostic certainty depend on available diagnostic tools, such as specialized radiographs, laboratory investigations and histology services. In most district hospitals in Africa, definitive diagnosis is difficult: in one study in Tanzania in the early 1990s only 18 per cent of patients with EPTB had laboratory confirmation of the diagnosis.[89] Radiographic and laboratory capacity in most of sub-Saharan Africa has stagnated or deteriorated in the last 15 years, and the situation with respect to a definitive diagnosis remains largely the same.[90]

TB lymphadenopathy

Peripheral lymphadenopathy is a frequent form of EPTB and in patients being investigated for peripheral lymphadenopathy, TB can be found in 60–70 per cent of cases.[91–93] Regardless of HIV-serostatus, cervical lymph node involvement (scrofula) is the most common presentation. In the immunosuppressed patient, the lymphadenitis may be acute and resemble an acute pyogenic infection.

Symmetrical generalized lymphadenopathy (PGL) is common in HIV-infected patients, usually due to follicular hyperplasia. A clinical study in Zambia[92] found that while HIV-negative TB patients had focal, asymmetrical cervical lymphadenopathy (clearly distinguishable from PGL), in HIV-positive patients there was much overlap in the presentation of TB-lymphadenopathy and PGL. For example, in HIV-positive TB lymphadenopathy lymph node enlargement was symmetrical in 29 per cent; cervical lymph nodes were enlarged in 99 per cent, axillary nodes in 82 per cent, epitrochlear nodes in 36 per cent and inguinal nodes in 54 per cent; the largest nodes were less than 3 cm in 30 per cent. These findings suggest that greater use of lymph node aspiration or biopsy is indicated if the diagnosis of TB is not to be missed.

Wide-needle aspiration of lymph nodes for AFB or macroscopic caseation is recommended as the first-line investigation. AFB and/or caseous material have been found in nearly 75 per cent of lymph nodes which have subsequently been proven to be tuberculous in aetiology.[94] However, much lower diagnostic yields have been found elsewhere,[93] probably reflecting investigator experience and technique. If diagnostic aspiration is not rewarding, lymph node biopsy is indicated. The presence of macroscopic caseation in excised lymph nodes has a diagnostic yield of 60–80 per cent,[91,93] and simple inspection of cut-lymph nodes may expedite a diagnosis of TB pending results of histological or culture examination.

TB pleural effusion

Studies in Zambia,[35] Rwanda,[95] Tanzania,[96] Uganda[97] and the Côte d'Ivoire[84] have shown a strong association between HIV infection and TB pleural effusion, which probably accounts for the increased incidence of pleural disease in many African countries. It has been widely believed that TB pleurisy may be a manifestation of primary infection in HIV-infected patients, but this is controversial and difficult to prove. TB is the main cause of unilateral pleural effusion in Africa. In a prospective study of 118 patients with pleural effusion in Tanzania,[96] TB was diagnosed in 112: in 84 patients the diagnosis was confirmed microbiologically or histologically, and in 28 patients on the basis of a good response to antituberculosis chemotherapy. In district hospitals with poor facilities, a pleural fluid protein >50 g/L has been shown to have a high predictive value for tuberculosis.[96] Clinical and diagnostic findings of TB pleurisy are largely similar between HIV-positive and HIV-negative patients, although the former group tend to have a more severe illness.[97]

TB pericardial effusion

A pericardial effusion most commonly develops as a result of rupture of a mediastinal lymph node into the pericardial space. Like the development of a pleural effusion, in HIV infection it is probably the result of a primary infection,[98] but may also be seen in association with miliary spread.[99] A large increase in the number of patients with pericardial effusion has been seen since the HIV era (Figure 19.12) and the disease appears to be strongly associated with HIV.[98–100] Between 65 and 90 per cent of patients with TB pericardial effusion are HIV-seropositive. The presentation and diagnosis of pericardial effusion is similar in HIV-positive and HIV-negative patients (Figure 19.13), although HIV-positive patients with pericardial disease more often have TB in another clinically obvious site.[99]

Miliary or disseminated TB

Classical miliary TB is reported more frequently in HIV-positive patients.[19,20] The clinical illness is non-specific, and in most African hospitals, the diagnosis will be made on the basis of the chest x-ray. However, miliary infiltrates on chest x-ray can be atypical and some patients can present with a normal chest x-ray (see Case history 2).[101] Definitive diagnosis can be difficult requiring the use of fibreoptic bronchoscopy, liver biopsy, bone marrow examination and special blood cultures.

Cryptic miliary TB is an insidious illness with fever and weight loss. Physical examination and chest x-ray are usually normal. This disease is likely to be more prevalent in HIV-positive African patients with advanced immunosuppression than is currently thought and is likely to be an important cause of the 'HIV wasting syndrome'. In the Côte d'Ivoire, disseminated tuberculosis was found in 44 per cent of patients diagnosed with the HIV wasting syndrome who came to autopsy, the diagnosis not having been made ante mortem.[102] In Malawi, *M. tuberculosis* bacteraemia was found in 10 per cent of adults admitted to hospital with a febrile illness[103] and in over half these patients the diagnosis would not have been made if it had not been for mycobacterial blood cultures, a laboratory tool which is unavailable outside the research setting. Severe anaemia in adults admitted to medical wards in Blantyre, Malawi, was associated with TB in one-third of cases, and in almost 10 per cent of these patients the diagnosis of TB was only made on mycobacterial bone marrow culture.[104] How to diagnose TB in patients with such

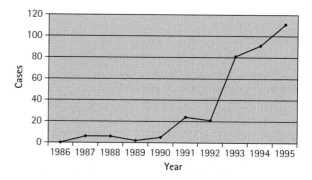

Figure 19.12   Tuberculous pericardial effusion diagnosed in Queen Elizabeth Central Hospital, Blantyre, Malawi: 1986–1995.

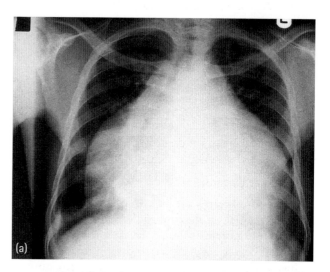

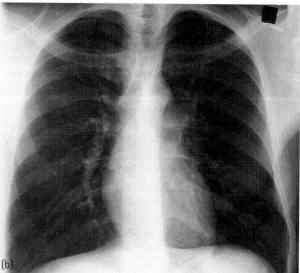

Figure 19.13   Tuberculous pericardial effusion in an HIV-positive African patient. Chest x-rays (a) before and (b) after antituberculosis treatment.

advanced immunodeficiency is of crucial importance, particularly with the advent of antiretroviral therapy (see below), and whether antituberculosis treatment at this stage of the illness will reduce the otherwise high mortality,

Case history 2

A 35-year-old African man was admitted to hospital with a 3-month history of weight loss, a 2-month history of fever and night sweats and a 4-week history of cough. Past medical history revealed that he had been treated several times for genital ulceration and 1 year previously had developed ophthalmic herpes zoster. He had been counselled and tested for antibodies against HIV-1 and HIV-2, and had been found to be HIV-seropositive.

On examination he was thin, with a facial scar of herpes zoster and oral candidiasis. He had a sinus tachycardia, but otherwise no other abnormalities were found.

A full blood count, blood film for malaria parasites, three sputa for AFB and a chest x-ray were all normal. There were no facilities for blood cultures.

He was treated with sulfadoxine-pyrimethamine for presumptive malaria, followed by a 10-day course of chloramphenicol and gentamicin for presumptive bacteraemia. He remained unwell with a high intermittent fever. Two weeks after admission an empirical diagnosis of disseminated tuberculosis was made. He was treated with antituberculosis short-course chemotherapy.

Three weeks later he was much improved, the fever had subsided and a repeat x-ray showed miliary shadowing. A firm diagnosis of miliary TB was made. He completed treatment.

Practice point: Miliary TB, especially in immunosuppressed patients, may present with a normal chest radiograph. With effective treatment, immunity may improve and the chest radiograph may then show miliary shadowing.

---

are important clinical and research questions which need to be answered.

Other forms of EPTB

Other forms of HIV-related EPTB appear not to be common in Africa. For example, in industrialized countries, HIV-infected patients with TB are said to be at increased risk for TB meningitis, but there are few cases of TB meningitis reported from high HIV-TB prevalence areas in Africa.[20,56,90,105] The reason for this is not entirely clear, but may relate to the difficulties in searching for or establishing a diagnosis. The same argument may apply to the low frequency of reported cases of TB ascites given the large number of causes of ascites in African patients. Interestingly, there is no evidence from sub-Saharan Africa that bone/joint TB is strongly associated with HIV infection.[20,105] Indeed, the proportion of extrapulmonary cases with spinal TB has decreased,[56] possibly because of the large numbers of patients now presenting with lymphadenopathy and serous effusions.

CHILDHOOD TB

In a high HIV-prevalent area, childhood TB accounts for 10–15 per cent of national TB notifications,[106] and therefore contributes to a significant proportion of disease burden. In HIV-positive children, PTB is the most common manifestation of disease, although there is a propensity for extrapulmonary disease.[53,54,107,108] The patterns of EPTB in children and the diagnostic problems encountered are similar to those described for adults.

The diagnosis of childhood PTB has always been difficult, but the diagnostic challenge is compounded by the advent of HIV infection leading to a high probability of missed diagnoses unless a high index of clinical suspicion is maintained.[109] An autopsy study on children dying with HIV-related lung disease in South Africa found that 77 per cent of children with post-mortem-diagnosed TB had not been diagnosed or treated for TB while alive.[110] The highest rates of HIV infection are observed in children aged 1–4 years. Because of the high incidence of cutaneous anergy to tuberculin testing,[55] the majority of cases in this age group are diagnosed according to clinical and radiographic criteria, which are often non-specific, along with a positive family history of contact with a case of TB. Chest radiographic abnormalities do not differ significantly between HIV-positive and HIV-negative children with PTB. With the recognized importance of PCP as an important cause of acute severe lung illness and death in HIV-infected infants and the emergence of HIV-related conditions, such as lymphoid interstitial pneumonitis (LIP) in older children, the chest x-ray is even less specific for TB than it was before the HIV epidemic.[111]

There have been a number of approaches to this conundrum. Gastric aspiration, induced sputum, nasopharyngeal aspiration all show some promise as alternative diagnostic techniques in the clinical research setting,[111] and there has been huge effort in developing and testing point scoring systems, diagnostic classifications and diagnostic algorithms.[112] However, in the routine clinical arena, these potentially useful diagnostic interventions are rarely used, and the developing world awaits the development of a simple, affordable dipstick test that can be used for children and also adults with smear-negative TB.[113]

Tuberculosis and HIV infection in other developing countries

Disease patterns and presentation of clinical disease are very similar to those described in sub-Saharan Africa, and again depend on resources available for diagnosis. As an example, in Thailand, the proportion with pulmonary smear-negative TB is higher in HIV-positive than HIV-negative patients, and EPTB is also more frequent in HIV-infected patients.[60]

TREATMENT OF TB USING THE DOTS STRATEGY ONLY

Tuberculosis control: the DOTS strategy

In 1993, the World Health Organization (WHO) took the unprecedented step of declaring TB to be a global emergency, and along with its various partners advocated for rapid and widespread expansion of the DOTS strategy for global TB control.

The overall objective of this TB control strategy is to reduce mortality, morbidity and transmission of the disease until it no longer poses a threat to public health. The strategy is straightforward. Standardized combination chemotherapy is provided to, at least, all sputum smear-positive TB patients (Table 19.7).[114] This treatment should cure the disease and prevent future transmission of infection within the community. Targets have been set for TB control, which focus on new cases of smear-positive PTB with the aim to (1) cure 85 per cent of detected new cases and (2) detect 70 per cent of existing cases.

Achieving the targets for TB control should lead to a substantial decrease in infected TB contacts and, as a result, to a decline in TB incidence by 5–10 per cent per year. The targets have thus been embraced by the Millennium Development Goals (MDG) of the United Nations, and a new Stop TB Strategy (Table 19.8)[115] has been designed to achieve the targets set for the period 2006–2015. Partly based on the expectation of a decline in TB incidence, the MDG also embrace the objectives of halving TB prevalence and mortality by 2015.[116] In countries with little or no HIV infection, it is apparent that

good progress is being made, both in terms of case detection, TB incidence and treatment success.[57] However, and largely due to HIV infection, the situation in sub-Saharan Africa is quite different. The large case burdens, which stress the TB control programmes, have already been described, but HIV also compromises the chances of successful outcomes of antituberculosis treatment.

Treatment of the HIV-infected TB patient using antituberculosis drugs only

Before the advent of HIV infection, treatment with antituberculosis drugs was straightforward and was generally associated with good cure and treatment completion rates. However, HIV has forced a change in the way antituberculosis treatment is provided and has rendered antituberculosis treatment on its own less effective than before.

DECENTRALIZATION OF THE INITIAL PHASE OF TREATMENT AND CHANGING TO FULL ORAL REGIMENS

In the pre-AIDS era, many TB programmes in Africa kept the patient in hospital for the initial phase of treatment for

Table 19.8 Revised STOP TB Strategy: components of strategy and implementation approaches.[115]

1. Pursue high-quality DOTS expansion and enhancement:
    Political commitment with enhanced and sustained funding
    Case detection through quality-assured bacteriology
    Standardized treatment, with supervision and patient support
    An effective system of drug supply and management
    Monitoring and evaluation system, and impact measurement
2. Address TB/HIV, MDR-TB and other challenges:
    Implement collaborative TB/HIV activities
    Prevent and control MDR-TB
    Address prisoners, refugees and other high-risk groups
3. Contribute to health system strengthening:
    Actively participate in the whole process of health system strengthening
    Share innovations that strengthen systems
    Adapt innovations from other fields
4. Engage all care providers:
    Public–public and public–private mix approaches
    International standards for TB care
5. Empower people with TB, and communities
    Advocacy, communication and social mobilization
    Community participation in TB care
    Patient's charter for TB care
6. Enable and promote research:
    Programme-based operational research
    Research to develop new diagnostics, drugs and vaccines

Table 19.7 WHO-recommended standardized treatment regimens for new cases of smear-positive pulmonary tuberculosis.

Initial phase of treatment (daily or three times a week)	Continuation phase of treatment
2 EHRZ (SHRZ)	6 HE
2 EHRZ (SHRZ)	4 HR
2 EHRZ (SHRZ)	4 H_3R_3

S, streptomycin; H, isoniazid; R, rifampicin; Z, pyrazinamide; E, ethambutol.
The number before the first letter of each phase of the regimen is the duration in months of that phase.
The number in subscript after the letters is the number of doses per week.

up to 2 months. This was for a number of reasons that included the need to administer daily intramuscular streptomycin and to ensure regular supervised drug intake in areas where a patient might have to walk 20 km to get health care. The growing case load, the concomitant intense overcrowding in TB wards and concerns about the safety of intramuscular injections in the presence of HIV infection resulted in a radical rethinking of this policy.

Thus, in the last 10 years, most TB programmes in Africa have decentralized treatment to peripheral health centres and the community.[117] This has been helped by the fact that in many programmes oral ethambutol has replaced intramuscular streptomycin for the initial phase of treatment of new patients. A decentralized approach using oral medication is undoubtedly patient-friendly. However, the logistics of observed drug administration, drug security (especially of rifampicin), supervision, monitoring and recording in the community are difficult. In a country like Malawi that has embraced the concept on a national scale, decentralization has been well accepted, has resulted in a marked decrease in TB bed occupancy rates, but on the other hand has been associated with an increase in rates of treatment default.[118] Time will tell as to whether this approach is associated with an increase in drug-resistant TB.

REACTIONS TO ANTITUBERCULOSIS CHEMOTHERAPY

Short-course chemotherapy regimens using rifampicin, isoniazid, pyrazinamide and ethambutol

In industrialized countries, there is a higher incidence of adverse drug reactions in HIV-positive compared with HIV-negative patients, with 90 per cent of reactions occurring in the first 2 months of treatment.[119] Reactions are most common with rifampicin (12 per cent) followed by pyrazinamide (6 per cent), isoniazid (4 per cent) and ethambutol (2 per cent). In sub-Saharan Africa, the frequency of adverse reactions seems to be lower. Using clinical monitoring in Uganda, the incidence of adverse drug reactions in HIV-positive patients receiving rifampicin, isoniazid and pyrazinamide (RHZ) was 1.6 per cent per year.[38] Severe reactions to RHZ were reported to be rare in Zimbabwe.[120] However, HIV-infected children may be at greater risk of adverse effects. In 65 HIV-positive Zambian children who were treated with streptomycin and RHZ, seven patients (11 per cent) developed cutaneous reactions within 8 weeks of commencing therapy, two of whom developed a fatal Stevens–Johnson syndrome.[107]

'Standard' treatment regimens using streptomycin, thiacetazone and isoniazid

In the pre-HIV era, cutaneous reactions with standard chemotherapy regimens (streptomycin, isoniazid and thiacetazone) occurred in less than 5 per cent of patients, and severe reactions such as toxic epidermal necrolysis and Stevens–Johnson syndrome (with involvement of the mucous membranes) were very rare. If cutaneous reac-

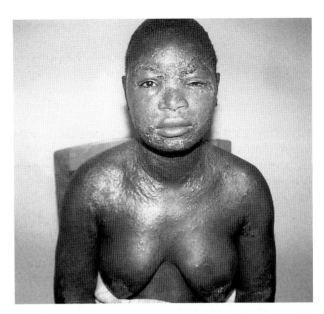

Figure 19.14 Cutaneous drug reaction. This HIV-positive patient developed a severe cutaneous reaction 3 weeks after starting therapy with streptomycin, isoniazid and thiacetazone for a tuberculous pleural effusion.

tions did occur, thiacetazone was the drug most often implicated.

With the advent of HIV in Africa, a large increase was observed in the incidence of cutaneous reactions in patients receiving standard chemotherapy. Several clinical studies documented a high frequency of cutaneous hypersensitivity reactions of the order of 15–20 per cent in HIV-positive adults treated with 'standard' chemotherapy; up 6 per cent of these reactions were severe with Stevens–Johnson syndrome or toxic epidermal necrolysis, and there was a significant mortality (Figure 19.14).[20,26,30,36,120–123] Cutaneous hypersensitivity reactions were also found frequently in HIV-positive children. In Zambia, 19 (21 per cent) of 88 HIV-positive children had a cutaneous skin reaction compared with 2 per cent of HIV-negative children.[124] Twelve (63 per cent) of the HIV-positive children with skin reactions had a Stevens–Johnson syndrome, 11 of whom died.

Drug reactions, including those due to thiacetazone, are more common in HIV-infected patients with more advanced degrees of immunosuppression[38,122] and are thought to be due to the parent compound itself, the reactive derivatives, impairment of detoxification processes which deteriorate with advancing immunosuppression or a combination of these mechanisms. Whatever the mechanisms, in the 1990s thiacetazone (such a useful and cheap bacteriostatic antituberculosis drug in the pre-AIDS era) was correctly perceived to be dangerous, and in 1992 the WHO issued guidelines emphasizing that thiacetazone should not be given to patients known to be infected with HIV or at increased risk of HIV infection, i.e. young adults from countries with a high-prevalence of HIV infection.[125]

This marked a turning point in the use of thiacetazone in sub-Saharan Africa, and almost all TB programmes in the region have now abandoned thiacetazone, replacing the drug with ethambutol.

INCREASED MORBIDITY AND MORTALITY

HIV-positive TB patients often run a stormy course while on antituberculosis treatment with fever, chest infections, oral/oesophageal candidiasis, diarrhoea and bacteraemia. The pattern and type of infections causing illness in HIV-infected patients with TB may vary from country to country. A cross-sectional study in Kenya showed that bacteraemia (usually with *Salmonella typhimurium* or *Streptococcus pneumoniae*) occurred in 18 per cent of HIV-positive patients compared with 6 per cent of HIV-negative patients.[126] In Côte d'Ivoire, enteritis (with isosporiasis and non-typhoidal salmonellosis) and bacteraemia (with non-typhoidal salmonellae) were the principal causes of morbidity, followed by bacterial chest infections, urinary tract infections and anaemia.[127]

Given the high morbidity, it is not surprising that HIV-positive patients have a much higher mortality during and after antituberculosis treatment compared with HIV-negative patients. In sub-Saharan Africa, approximately 20–30 per cent of HIV-positive smear-positive TB patients die by 12 months of treatment.[37,43,128–131] In Kenya, more profound clinical immunosuppression was, not surprisingly, associated with increased risk of death,[128] and in both Zaire[37] and Côte d'Ivoire,[41] a low CD4-lymphocyte count at diagnosis in HIV-positive, smear-positive patients was associated with a higher mortality (Table 19.9).

In the pre-HIV era, smear-negative PTB was a disease with a good treatment outcome. However, studies from sub-Saharan Africa show that HIV-positive patients who present with smear-negative TB or atypical radiographic appearances have even higher case fatality rates (25–60 per cent) than patients who present with smear-positive disease or typical radiographic appearances.[43,130,132,133] This higher attrition persists well after antituberculosis treatment has been completed.[134] This is probably because such patients are more immunosuppressed than those with smear-positive disease. The higher mortality rates may also relate to misdiagnosis,[74,81] and the fact that patients with smear-negative TB were previously often treated with inferior 'standard treatment' regimens. HIV-positive patients treated with standard regimens consisting of streptomycin, isoniazid and thiacetazone had higher death rates than those given rifampicin-containing regimens.[38,128,129] Rifampicin-containing regimens might offer survival advantages because they have stronger activity against *M. tuberculosis* and, through the broad-spectrum antibiotic activity of rifampicin, may prevent and treat other bacterial infections.

The precise cause of death in patients with HIV-related TB in Africa has been difficult to determine because of the lack of substantial autopsy studies. One autopsy study on 14 adult HIV-infected patients treated for TB in Côte

Table 19.9 Mortality rates in HIV-positive, smear-positive pulmonary tuberculosis patients in relation to CD4-lymphocyte counts at the start of antituberculosis treatment.

Country	CD4-lymphocyte counts/µL			Ref.
	<200	200–499	500 or more	
Zaire: 24-month mortality	67%	22%	8%	37
Côte d'Ivoire: 6-month mortality	10%	4%	3%	41

d'Ivoire found the causes of death to be TB in four, bacterial infections in three, cerebral toxoplasmosis in two, nocardiosis in two, PCP in one, atypical mycobacteriosis in one and wasting syndrome in one patient.[135] In a clinical/autopsy study in HIV-positive South African miners with TB, the causes of death were TB (22 per cent), pneumonia (16 per cent) and other opportunistic infections (56 per cent), of which cryptococcal disease was the most frequent.[136] A further post-mortem study in South Africa showed that deaths occurring within the first month of treatment were mainly caused by TB, whereas late deaths were most commonly due to other infections, such as cryptococcal meningitis.[137]

There is an urgent need for more research to determine the causes of death in HIV-positive TB patients and to investigate strategies and interventions which might reduce death rates. Such interventions include reducing diagnostic delays, improving antituberculosis treatment, provision of adjunctive treatments and antiretroviral therapy and improving quality of care.[131]

RECURRENCE OF TUBERCULOSIS AFTER COMPLETING TREATMENT

Several studies in sub-Saharan Africa have shown that recurrence rates are increased in HIV-positive compared with HIV-negative TB patients (Table 19.10).[121,138–143] Various risk factors for recurrence have been identified. In Kenya,[138] there was a strong association between recurrence and a cutaneous hypersensitivity reaction due to thiacetazone during initial treatment, although the reasons for this association were not clear. In one of the South African gold miners' studies,[141] initial treatment with RHZ was associated with higher recurrence rates than treatment with rifampicin, isoniazid, pyrazinamide and ethambutol (RHZE), although these results need to be interpreted with caution as the allocation to treatment regimens was not randomized. In Uganda, older age, poor treatment compliance and thiacetazone-containing regimens were associated with increased recurrence rates in HIV-positive patients.[144] Finally, in a large multicentre study in Africa and Asia, which included small numbers of HIV-infected patients, a rifampicin-throughout antituberculosis treat-

Table 19.10 Recurrence of tuberculosis (TB) after completing antituberculosis treatment.

Country	Rates of recurrent TB per 100 person-years		Ref.
	HIV-positive	HIV-negative	
Zaire	18.1	6	121
Kenya	16.7	0.5	138
Zambia	22	6	139
Malawi	18.2	1.7	140
South Africa	8.2	2.2	141
South Africa	16.0	6.4	142
Malawi	18.2	1.7	143

ment regimen had a significantly lower recurrent rate of TB compared with a regimen using isoniazid and ethambutol in the continuation phase.[145] These results suggest that factors such as the initial treatment regimen, drugs used in the continuation phase and poor adherence/compliance are associated with increased recurrence, maybe due to reactivation of inadequately treated disease.

Recurrence may be due to reactivation of disease or reinfection. DNA fingerprinting is the only available method to distinguish between these two mechanisms. Unfortunately, the data on which of these two mechanisms is the most important are rather limited. A study in South Africa on mainly HIV-seronegative patients found that exogenous reinfection was the major cause of recurrent TB after previous cure.[146] Another study from the same country found that 62 per cent of recurrences in HIV-positive patients were due to reinfection, in contrast to HIV-negative patients in whom 94 per cent of recurrences were due to reactivation.[142] The majority of recurrences in the first 6 months after treatment completion were due to reactivation of disease, while those occurring later were more often due to reinfection.

In a TB programme which properly documents its cases as new or previously treated, there is growing evidence that HIV leads to an increase in recurrent TB.[147] These cases add to the case burden and to the complexity of management, particularly if the recurrent case needs a retreatment antituberculosis treatment regimen.

HIV AND DRUG-RESISTANT TUBERCULOSIS

Several outbreaks of multidrug-resistant tuberculosis (MDR-TB) have been reported from industrialized countries amongst patients with HIV infection. HIV does not itself cause MDR-TB, but it fuels the spread of this dangerous condition by increasing susceptibility to infection and accelerating the progression from infection to disease. Global surveys carried out by the WHO and the International Union against TB and Lung Disease (IUATLD) have in general shown low levels of drug resis-

tance in new patients with TB in sub-Saharan Africa.[148] However, there are a few countries where the situation is of concern: for example, Côte d'Ivoire, Zimbabwe and Sierra Leone are recognized to be 'hot spots' for MDR-TB.[149] The situation is also dynamic and data from Botswana suggest that primary MDR-TB may be a growing problem.[150]

Towards the end of 2006, a new chapter to the story of drug-resistant TB was added by a report of extensively drug resistant (XDR) TB in a rural area of KwaZulu Natal, South Africa.[151] XDR-TB is defined as *M. tuberculosis* resistant to isoniazid and rifampicin plus resistant to any fluoroquinolone and at least one of three injectable second-line drugs (i.e. amikacin, kanamycin or capreomycin). Six per cent of 475 patients with active culture-positive TB were found to have XDR-TB. All the patients with XDR-TB who were tested for HIV were co-infected. All but one of the patients with XDR-TB died, with a median survival of 16 days from time of diagnosis. Fifty-five per cent of patients had never previously received treatment for TB and 67 per cent had been admitted to hospital for any cause in the 2 years preceding their presentation with XDR-TB. This study provides disturbing and new evidence of the presence and serious consequences of drug-resistant TB in a resource-poor setting. It is likely that XDR-TB is transmitted within hospital settings and is a serious threat to HIV-infected patients.

MDR and XDR-TB have the same root causes: namely, negligent case management and poorly functioning public health services.[152] The emergence of XDR-TB should act as a stimulus for more comprehensive surveillance, better access to drug sensitivity testing and above all a strengthening of basic control measures.

DECREASING THE DUAL BURDEN OF TB AND HIV

The new strategy to control TB in high HIV-prevalent areas

It is clear that the DOTS strategy alone will not be sufficient to control tuberculosis in areas with epidemic HIV infection, and in sub-Saharan Africa the MDG will not be met unless an additional set of tactics is introduced and implemented. Under the leadership of WHO and the Stop-TB partnership, TB-HIV guidelines,[153] a TB-HIV strategic framework[154] and an interim policy on TB-HIV coordination[155] have all been developed to try and reduce the burden of HIV-TB disease in those countries most hard hit by the epidemic. The policy goal is to decrease the burden of TB and HIV by joint collaborative activities outlined in Table 19.11. Mechanisms of collaboration are needed at all levels and include planning, monitoring and evaluation. The specific interventions that need to be implemented to reduce the dual burden of disease are discussed briefly below.

Table 19.11 Recommended collaborative TB/HIV activities to reduce the burden of tuberculosis (TB) and HIV in affected communities.

Mechanisms for collaboration
  Set up coordinating bodies for TB/HIV at all levels
  Conduct surveillance of HIV prevalence in TB patients
  Carry out joint TB/HIV planning
  Conduct monitoring and evaluation
Decrease the burden of TB in people with HIV infection
  Establish intensified TB case finding
  Introduce isoniazid preventive therapy
  Ensure TB infection control in health care or congregate settings
  Scale up antiretroviral therapy
Decrease the burden of HIV in patients with TB
  Provide HIV testing and counselling
  Introduce methods of HIV prevention, care and support
  Introduce cotrimoxazole preventive therapy
  Introduce antiretroviral therapy

Decreasing the burden of TB in people living with HIV/AIDS

INTENSIFIED TB CASE FINDING

This intervention comprises screening for symptoms and signs of TB in settings where HIV-infected people are concentrated. Early identification of TB, followed by diagnosis and prompt treatment in people living with HIV/AIDS, their household contacts, groups at high risk of HIV and those in congregate settings (for example, prisons, workers' hostels, police and military barracks, and hospitals and clinics) increases the chances of survival, improves the quality of life and reduces transmission of TB in the community. It has been shown that intensified case finding is feasible, not time-consuming and can be done at little additional cost in existing health service settings.[156] In all HIV testing and counselling settings, trained counsellors and other lay workers can be trained to administer a simple set of questions to identify suspected TB cases as soon as possible.

ISONIAZID PREVENTIVE THERAPY

Isoniazid preventive therapy (IPT) linked particularly to counselling and HIV testing, is used to prevent the progression of latent *M. tuberculosis* to active disease. Several randomized trials have shown that IPT is efficacious in reducing the incidence of TB and death from tuberculosis in HIV-infected patients with a positive tuberculin skin test.[157] Isoniazid is as effective and safer than rifampicin- and pyrazinamide-containing regimens, and is the preferred drug. However, IPT requires several steps to be taken, including identification of HIV-positive subjects, screening to exclude active TB and provision of information to promote adherence.[158] While IPT can be success-

fully set up and implemented with good results in the setting of the workplace, as shown in South African gold mines,[159] the structures for providing IPT within the general health sector of most resource-poor countries are sorely lacking, rendering the feasibility of this intervention on a large scale not clear.

Studies in Haiti[62] and South Africa[160] found that post-treatment isoniazid for 6–12 months significantly reduced the rate of recurrent TB in HIV-positive patients who successfully completed antituberculosis treatment. However, this intervention has yet to find a place in the routine management of TB. If the main mechanism of recurrence is reinfection, which appears to be the case in many HIV-infected individuals who develop recurrent TB several months after completing treatment, then isoniazid may need to be given for life. Again, the structures for delivering and monitoring such an intervention do not exist.

TB INFECTION CONTROL IN HEALTH-CARE AND CONGREGATE SETTINGS (E.G. PRISONS)

Infection control measures can reduce the increased risk of TB which occurs when people with TB and HIV are crowded together, such as in prisons and health-care institutions. Measures to reduce TB transmission in a health-care setting include administrative, environmental and personal protection measures (Table 19.12).

ANTIRETROVIRAL THERAPY FOR HIV-INFECTED NON-TB PATIENTS

In industrialized countries, antiretroviral therapy (ART) significantly reduces the risk of TB in HIV-infected persons.[161] In the high HIV-TB burden arena of sub-Saharan Africa, cohort studies have found similar results. In South Africa, ART reduced the risk of TB from 9.7 to 2.4 cases per 100 person-years, although the risk was not reduced to levels seen in HIV-uninfected persons.[162] In a follow-up study in the same cohort of patients, the risk of TB decreased from 3.4 per 100 person-years in the first year of ART to 1.0 per 100 person-years by the fifth year of treatment, the best results being found in those with the most impressive immunological responses to therapy.[163] Whether ART will reduce the incidence of TB at a national level will depend on the degree of scale up and coverage of ART.

Decreasing the burden of HIV in patients with TB

THE PROVISION OF HIV COUNSELLING AND TESTING

The use of rapid HIV tests has revolutionized the practice of HIV counselling and testing (CT), and has greatly improved the type of service that can be offered to patients compared with the days when ELISA testing was the norm.

Table 19.12 Measures for control of tuberculosis (TB) in health-care settings.

Administrative measures	Prompt diagnosis and treatment of infectious pulmonary tuberculous (PTB) patients
	    Investigating PTB suspects as out-patients
	    Decreasing delays between submission of sputum and sputum results
	    Keeping PTB suspects away from other patients
	Separation of PTB cases from others (e.g. in TB wards)

Environmental protection	Maximizing natural cross-ventilation Using ultraviolet radiation (if applicable) Isolation of known drug-resistant TB cases

Personal protection	Simple measures to avoid inhalation of droplet nuclei (e.g. patient cough hygiene, examining patients
	    with their faces turned away from the health-care worker
	HIV-testing of health care workers and minimising exposure of HIV-positive health-care workers to
	    medical and tuberculosis wards
	Isoniazid preventive therapy and antiretroviral therapy for HIV-positive health-care workers

A positive HIV test provides the all important entry point for a continuum of prevention, care, support and treatment for HIV/AIDS, as well as for TB. Unfortunately, less than 10 per cent of African patients with TB are tested for HIV,[57] although operational studies have shown that HIV testing is acceptable to most people when offered in a convenient and confidential way. UNAIDS and WHO have recommended that CT should be offered routinely to all TB patients.[155,164]

Routine and diagnostic HIV testing has been found acceptable in TB patients living in countries like Malawi[165] and Kenya[166] and it is hoped that with this new found momentum the service will be expanded to many more patients in Africa.

HIV PREVENTION, CARE AND SUPPORT SERVICES

These services must accompany the process of CT. Reduction of sexual, parenteral and vertical transmission of HIV builds on broad-based programmes of education about HIV/AIDS. In principle, all clients attending TB clinics should be screened for sexually transmitted infections (STI) using a simple questionnaire or other recommended approaches. Those with symptoms of STI should be treated or referred to the relevant treatment providers, as effective STI treatment reduces the risk of both the acquisition and transmission of HIV. TB control programmes should implement harm-reduction measures for TB patients when injecting drug use is a problem or should establish a referral linkage with HIV/AIDS programmes to do so. TB programmes can also ensure a marked reduction in mother-to-child vertical transmission of HIV by getting HIV-infected pregnant women with TB on to ART (see below). Access to HIV care and support includes good clinical management of opportunistic infections and malignancies, nursing care, nutritional support, home care and palliative care. Unfortunately, these services at health facility or community level are in general not particularly good[167] and there needs to be better collaboration between

programmes if these are ever to be effectively implemented.

COTRIMOXAZOLE PREVENTIVE THERAPY

Cotrimoxazole is a cheap, broad-spectrum antibiotic that has important activity against a range of HIV- and non HIV-related pathogens. It is used in HIV-infected persons in industrialized countries as primary and secondary prophylaxis against PCP and *Toxoplasma gondii* encephalitis. Its use in sub-Saharan Africa was almost non-existent, until a randomized placebo-controlled study in Côte d'Ivoire in 1998 showed that cotrimoxazole in HIV-positive patients with TB was associated with a 48 per cent reduction in deaths.[127] There were significantly fewer hospital admissions due to septicaemia and enteritis in the cotrimoxazole group compared to placebo, and the drug was also well tolerated with only 1 per cent of patients reporting skin reactions. The results of this study were an important factor in persuading WHO and UNAIDS in 2000 to issue provisional recommendations that cotrimoxazole preventive therapy (CPT) be given to all patients in Africa living with AIDS including HIV-positive patients with TB.[168]

Despite this recommendation, its routine use in most African countries remained minimal because of concerns about efficacy in areas with high rates of bacterial resistance to the antibiotic and a fear that widespread use of cotrimoxazole would cause malaria parasites to become cross-resistant to sulfadoxine-pyrimethamine ((SP) Fansidar®), a drug that is still first-line therapy for malaria in several endemic countries. However, the last 5 years have seen a number of published studies from countries such as Malawi,[169] Uganda[170] and Zambia[171] on the efficacy, effectiveness, safety and feasibility of CPT. These and other studies have been well summarized in a recent review paper[172] and have all shown significant benefits in terms of a reduction in morbidity and mortality in HIV-infected patients, including those with TB. Furthermore, the

Table 19.13 Cotrimoxazole preventive therapy (CPT) recommendations.

Adults	CPT to all symptomatic HIV-positive adults
	CPT to HIV-positive adults with CD4-count of 500 cells/μL or less
Children	CPT to all children born to HIV-positive mothers
	CPT to all HIV-positive children <5 years, regardless of symptoms
	CPT to all symptomatic HIV-positive children 5 years or above

concerns about CPT selecting for sulfadoxine-pyrimethamine-resistant malaria parasites have so far been unfounded. In 2004, an expert WHO consultation on CPT firmly recommended the use of cotrimoxazole in HIV-infected adults and children (Table 19.13).[173] Once started it is recommended that CPT should be given indefinitely if a CD4 count is not available for patient monitoring. If a CD4 count is available then CPT can be discontinued if the CD4 count rises above the threshold for starting the intervention.

If the health sector is serious about providing CPT to HIV-infected patients, it must set in motion the logistics of long-term provision of the drug as an essential part of HIV care, as with ART, and not just for the duration of antituberculosis treatment. Other issues, such as easy dispensing of tablets and methods of monitoring, need to be worked out if CPT is ever going to reach the thousands of patients who would benefit from it.

The provision of highly active antiretroviral therapy (HAART) to HIV-positive TB patients is the intervention which is likely to have the greatest impact in improving the quality of life and reducing death rates in HIV-positive TB patients (Case history 3) (see below Provision of antiretroviral therapy to HIV-infected TB patients).

Provision of antiretroviral therapy to HIV-infected TB patients

ART may improve antituberculosis treatment outcomes by reducing HIV-related morbidity and mortality and decreasing the risk of recurrent TB. HIV-positive PTB is classified in WHO clinical stage 3 and extrapulmonary TB in WHO clinical stage 4, and HIV-infected patients in stage 3 and 4 are all potentially eligible for ART.[174] Many countries in Africa are scaling up ART using a first-line regimen consisting of two nucleoside reverse transciptase inhibitors (NRTI) and one non-nucleoside reverse transcriptase inhibitor (NNRTI): by December 2005, 810 000 African patients had been started on this life-saving medication.[175] The preferred first-line regimen in nearly two-thirds of African countries is a triple combination of stavudine/ lamivudine/nevirapine, which is manufactured generically and relatively cheaply as a fixed-dose tablet, taken twice a day. Other first-line regimens substitute zidovudine for stavudine and efavirenz for nevirapine.

The problem with treating TB patients and using the preferred ART option is that a proportion of HIV-infected TB patients have CD4-lymphocyte counts that are greater than

---

Case history 3

A 32-year-old African man is diagnosed with smear-positive pulmonary tuberculosis and is admitted for the first 2 weeks of initial phase antituberculosis treatment to a TB ward of a district hospital. He is referred for HIV testing and counselling 3 days after starting treatment and is found to be HIV-positive. He is started on long-term cotrimoxazole preventive therapy, 480 mg twice a day which he takes with his anti-TB drugs.

He is discharged home and completes the initial phase of anti-TB treatment as an outpatient. On the day that he starts the continuation phase of anti-TB treatment with isoniazid and ethambutol, he is referred to the antiretroviral treatment clinic where he is assessed to be in WHO clinical stage 3. There are no facilities for performing a CD4-lymphocyte count. He is referred for a group counselling education session and 2 weeks later starts ART. He is commenced on one tablet of stavudine/lamivudine/nevirapine in the morning and one tablet of stavudine/lamivudine in the evening for the first 2 weeks: this starter phase with half-dose nevirapine is to reduce the risk of nevirapine-induced skin rash. He completes the 2 weeks with no problems and when he returns to collect his monthly supply of isoniazid and ethambutol he also starts and collects his monthly supply of stavudine/lamivudine/nevirapine, one tablet twice a day.

The following month he complains of burning sensation in his feet and pyridoxine 25 mg daily is added, with symptomatic improvement over the next few weeks.

The rest of his treatment for TB continues without problems, except that he has to collect antituberculosis drugs from the TB office and ART drugs from the ART clinic. When the TB treatment is finished, he continues on ART drugs and cotrimoxazole. When last seen, 12 months later he is well.

Practice point: HIV-positive TB patients must all be considered for ART and cotrimoxazole preventive therapy to take alongside their anti-TB treatment. Ways to integrate this treatment need to be found so that patients do not have to go to separate clinics to receive drugs.

Table 19.14 Additive adverse drug reactions in HIV-positive tuberculosis patients taking antiretroviral therapy (ART) and antituberculosis treatment.[176,177]

Adverse reaction	Main ART drug involved	Main anti-TB drug involved
Peripheral neuropathy	Stavudine	Isoniazid
Skin rash	Nevirapine	Rifampicin, isoniazid, pyrazinamide
Gastrointestinal dysfunction	All drugs	All drugs
Hepatitis	Nevirapine	Rifampicin, isoniazid, pyrazinamide
Central nervous system dysfunction	Efavirenz	Isoniazid
Anaemia	Zidovudine	Rifampicin

350 cells/mm^3 and in these patients ART may be unnecessary and potentially dangerous if nevirapine-based treatment is used.[176,177] Nevirapine-induced toxicity (including skin reactions and hepatic dysfunction) occurs at higher rates in women with CD4 counts greater than 250 cells/mm^3 and men with CD4 counts greater than 400 cells/mm^3. The lack of access to CD4 count testing in most African hospitals means that many TB patients will start ART without CD4 count results, and therefore in some patients there is a potential risk of drug-induced toxicity. There is limited information to date from sub-Saharan Africa about the effectiveness and safety of ART in HIV-positive TB patients.

Concomitant use of ART during antituberculosis treatment is also not easy and there are a number of issues which need to be considered in every patient receiving dual treatment.

ADDITIVE ADVERSE DRUG REACTIONS

ART and antituberculosis drugs may result in overlapping toxicity (see Table 19.14). Particularly important is the peripheral neuropathy caused by both isoniazid and stavudine. This can be partly prevented by ensuring that the patient also takes pyridoxine at a dose of 12.5 mg daily.

Drug–drug interactions

The NNRTIs (and also protease inhibitors, which are being used in second-line regimens in resource-poor countries) are metabolized mainly through cytochrome P450 (CYP450) enzymes. Rifampicin induces CYP450, leading to a reduction in the plasma concentration of nevirapine by 30–40 per cent and efavirenz by 20–25 per cent.[176,177] There is concern that reduced nevirapine concentrations will lead to emerging drug resistance and treatment failure. Increasing the dose of nevirapine to compensate for this interaction may increase the risk of toxicity and it also makes administration of therapy more complicated. Efavirenz could be substituted for nevirapine. Efavirenz is generally well tolerated, but the drug is teratogenic (and at least half of treated patients are women). There is still debate about whether the dose should be 600 or 800 mg daily.[176] There is currently no fixed-dose generic combination with stavudine and lamivudine and the drug regimen is more expensive than the fixed-dose combination of stavudine/lamivudine/nevirapine. Data from Thailand[178] and Brazil[179] suggest that the standard 600 mg dose of efavirenz is sufficient in patients whose mean body weight is below 60 kg and the general consensus is that 600 mg of efavirenz should be used until further data are accumulated to support alternative dosing. Other options such as substituting rifabutin for rifampicin (rifabutin is a less potent inducer of CYP450) or using triple NRTIs (e.g. zidovudine/lamivudine/abacavir) are not currently feasible in Africa because of cost.

Although nevirapine levels are reduced by rifampicin, they may still be in the effective range. Given the simplicity of being able to continue with the fixed dose combination of stavudine/lamivudine/nevirapine, further studies on safety, pharmacokinetics and efficacy of concomitant nevirapine and rifampicin are urgently needed to provide answers to these problems.

IMMUNE RECONSTITUTION DISEASE

The initiation of ART during antituberculosis treatment can lead to immune reconstitution disease (IRD), manifested as worsening of symptoms and signs or the appearance of new TB lesions. This problem occurs more frequently if ART is started early in the course of antituberculosis treatment and if the patient has an initial low CD4-lymphocyte count.[180,181] The majority of cases have been reported to occur within the first 2 months of ART, with a median duration of ART of 4 weeks. The illness is generally managed with anti-inflammatory drugs, including corticosteroids in severe cases.

WHEN TO START ART

The optimal time to start ART in HIV-positive TB patients is not known, and there are arguments for early as well as delayed antiretroviral therapy (Table 19.15). Current WHO guidelines recommend that patients with a CD4 count <200 cells/mm^3 should initiate ART as soon as antituberculosis treatment is tolerated, i.e. within 2–4 weeks.[182] For patients with CD4 counts >200 cells/mm^3, ART should be started after the initial 2 months of antituberculosis treatment has been completed. In patients for whom CD4 counts are not available, ART should be initiated after the first 2 months of antituberculosis treatment.

Table 19.15 Arguments for early or delayed start of antiretroviral therapy (ART) in HIV-positive patients with tuberculosis.

	Start ART early 2–4 weeks after start of antituberculosis treatment during the initial phase	Start ART later: 8 weeks after start of antituberculosis treatment during the continuation phase
Advantages	May reduce early TB-HIV mortality	Patient more stable Pill burden less Continuation phase may not have rifampicin Less risk of immune reconstitution disease
Disadvantages	High pill burden Additive toxicities due to more anti-TB drugs Rifampicin-nevirapine interaction Increased risk of immune reconstitution disease	May have limited impact on case fatality

WHERE TO PROVIDE ART

In most of sub-Saharan Africa, ART is delivered in hospital clinics while antituberculosis treatment is delivered in the continuation phase from health centres as a result of decentralized management over the last 5–10 years. TB patients find it difficult to collect their antituberculosis drugs from health centres and then make a separate journey to collect ART drugs from the hospital, and this is one of the reasons why few HIV-positive TB patients are currently accessing ART in Africa. Innovative solutions to these problems must be found if HIV-positive TB patients are to be properly served.[183,184]

THE NEED FOR ADJUNCTIVE TREATMENT WITH ART

Is there a need to provide CPT and/or IPT with ART? Certainly, the addition of CPT to ART in HIV-infected adults in Uganda reduced the incidence of malaria compared with ART alone,[185] and a modelling exercise in Côte d'Ivoire showed that CPT and ART together was a cost-effective strategy and one associated with major survival benefits.[186] Whether IPT confers additional benefit in preventing a recurrent episode of TB in patients on ART who have completed antituberculosis treatment is not known.

CONCLUSIONS

HIV and AIDS continue to pose enormous challenges for TB control in sub-Saharan Africa. The already large case burden continues to grow in marked contrast to the other regions of the world where TB incidence is stable or falling.[57] High recurrent rates of TB in high HIV-prevalent areas add to the increasing number of new cases being registered for treatment. The difficulties of diagnosing smear-negative PTB and EPTB contribute to this problem. HIV-related morbidity increases the complexity of care needed during antituberculosis treatment, and high mortality

rates mean that cure rate targets cannot be reached, threatening the credibility of TB programmes in the eyes of health workers, patients and the wider community.

However, in the same way that HIV has fundamentally changed the epidemiology and management of TB in Africa, so now the arrival of ART must start to change the way in which TB control should be approached.[187] Previously, little in the way of HIV diagnosis or care has been offered to TB patients in the region, as TB control efforts have continued to focus solely on implementing DOTS. It is high time for a paradigm shift, hopefully spurred on by the scaling up of ART throughout the continent. The task ahead will not be easy. There are many barriers, from drug interactions to the historic differences in the way TB and HIV are perceived and managed, and the working arena in the African health sector is the most challenging in the world. However, failure to grasp the opportunities offered by ART and other HIV-related interventions will be to deny dually infected patients a much better standard of care and a longer and better quality life.

STATEMENT

The views expressed in this book are those of the authors alone and do not necessarily reflect the stated policy of the institutions with which they are affiliated.

LEARNING POINTS

- The HIV became established in humans in sub-Saharan Africa between the 1930s and 1940s, although the first written report of patients with AIDS was in 1981 from the USA.
- The subsequent devastating spread of HIV globally has had, and continues to have, a profound effect on the epidemiology, clinical features and management of TB, particularly in sub-Saharan Africa.

- By the end of 2005, there were an estimated 40.3 million adults and children living with HIV, of whom 25.8 million (64 per cent) lived in sub-Saharan Africa. Within the African region, Southern Africa is the epicentre of the epidemic with HIV-prevalence rates of 30 per cent or higher being recorded in pregnant women in countries such as South Africa, Botswana, Lesotho, and Swaziland.

- In sub-Saharan Africa, HIV is principally transmitted by heterosexual intercourse, although mother-to-child transmission, infected blood transfusions, injections and scarifications play their role.

- The considerable adult- and, to a lesser extent, child-related mortality as a result of HIV-related disease and AIDS has resulted in substantial reductions in life expectancy, that in Botswana, Zimbabwe and South Africa is expected to plummet from 60 years in 1990 to about 30–40 years in 2010.

- About one-third of the world's population is infected with *M. tuberculosis*. Over 11 million people were thought to be co-infected with HIV and *M. tuberculosis* in 2000, the majority of whom lived in sub-Saharan Africa.

- In people co-infected with HIV and *M. tuberculosis*, the annual risk of developing active TB is 5–15 per cent, this risk becoming apparent within the first year of HIV infection and increasing as the immune system becomes more immunocompromised. This compares with a life-time risk of developing active TB of 5–10 per cent in people with *M. tuberculosis* who are not infected with HIV.

- HIV-seroprevalence rates are high in TB patients in sub-Saharan Africa, and in countries of Southern Africa may be 50 per cent or higher. Patients with smear-negative pulmonary tuberculosis and extrapulmonary tuberculosis have higher HIV-seroprevalence rates compared with patients who have smear-positive pulmonary tuberculosis.

- In countries with high HIV prevalence rates in the general population, TB incidence rates have climbed on average from 140 per 100 000 in 1991 to 400 per 100 000 in 2003.

- In the HIV-infected individual, the clinical pattern of TB correlates with the host immune status. If TB occurs early, the pattern is similar to that seen in HIV-negative disease. If TB occurs later in the course of HIV infection, atypical pulmonary disease and disseminated extrapulmonary disease tend to develop.

- The immunosuppressed patient with pulmonary TB often has negative sputum smears for AFB and chest x-rays that show lower lobe infiltrates, intrathoracic lymphadenopathy or even a normal appearance.

- The most common extrapulmonary manifestations of TB in HIV-seropositive people are pleural effusion, lymphadenopathy, pericardial disease and miliary disease.

- HIV-positive patients diagnosed with the HIV-wasting syndrome may have disseminated TB, which is difficult to diagnose because of an atypical presentation.

- Patterns of TB in HIV-seropositive children are similar to those seen in HIV-seropositive adults. Because HIV infection causes similar symptoms in children with TB – failure to thrive, fever and cough not responsive to antibiotics – it may be difficult to distinguish the two conditions.

- Treatment of the HIV-infected TB patient using antituberculosis drugs only in sub-Saharan Africa is not associated with outcomes as good as those seen in non-HIV infected patients. In particular, the HIV-infected TB patient has more morbidity, an increased frequency of drug reactions, a higher case fatality and a higher recurrence rate of disease after treatment has been completed.

- The finding of XDR-TB in rural South Africa that is associated with an alarmingly high mortality rate in HIV-infected patients and appears to be rapidly spread within hospital settings is a serious cause for concern and poses additional challenges for TB control in high HIV-TB burden areas.

- With 'DOTS' alone, TB control efforts in sub-Saharan Africa will fail to achieve agreed targets, and the Millennium Development Goals of reducing the prevalence and death rate of TB by 50 per cent in 2015 will not be met. Other interventions are therefore needed.

- There is a need to decrease the burden of TB in people living with HIV and AIDS through (1) intensified TB case finding, (2) isoniazid preventive therapy and (3) TB infection control measures in health-care and congregate settings.

- There is a need to decrease the burden of HIV in patients with TB by (1) the provision of diagnostic HIV testing and counselling, (2) HIV prevention, care and support activities, (3) cotrimoxazole preventive therapy and (4) ART.

- ART may improve TB treatment outcomes by reducing HIV-related mortality and by reducing the risk of recurrent TB after antituberculosis treatment has been completed. The extent of this improvement will depend on coverage and on when in the course of antituberculosis treatment ART is commenced.

- Concomitant use of ART and antituberculosis treatment is not easy because of (1) additive adverse drug reactions, (2) drug–drug interactions particularly between rifampicin and nevirapine, (3) immune reconstitution disease, (4) the optimal timing for initiation of ART, (5) the issue of whether ART and antituberculosis treatment can be delivered from the same clinic and (6) the uncertainty of the need for adjunctive treatment, such as cotrimoxazole and isoniazid preventive therapies.

REFERENCES

1. UNAIDS and WHO. AIDS epidemic update. December 2005. (available from www.unaids.org).

2. Bock PJ, Markovitz DM. Infection with HIV-2. AIDS 2001; 15 (Suppl. 5): S35–45.

3. Moore A, Herrera G, Nyamongo J et al. Estimated risk of HIV transmission by blood transfusion in Kenya. Lancet 2001; 358: 657–60.

4. Buve A, Carael M, Hayes RJ et al. Multicentre study on factors determining differences in rate and spread of HIV in sub-Saharan Africa: summary and conclusions. AIDS 2001; 15 (Suppl. 4): S127–31.

5. Halperin DT, Epstein H. Concurrent sexual partnerships help to explain Africa's high HIV prevalence: implications for prevention. Lancet 2004; 364: 4–6.

6. Lewis DK, Callaghan M, Phiri K et al. Prevalence and indicators of HIV and AIDS among adults admitted to medical and surgical wards in Blantyre, Malawi. Trans Roy Soc Trop Med Hyg 2003; 97: 91–6.

7. Rogerson S, Gladstone M, Callaghan M et al. HIV infection among paediatric in-patients in Blantyre, Malawi. Trans Roy Soc Trop Med Hyg 2004; 98: 544–52.

8. De Cock KM, Barrere B, Diaby L et al. AIDS – the leading cause of adult death in the West African city of Abidjan, Ivory Coast. Science 1990; 249: 793–6.

9. Ansari NA, Kombe AH, Kenyon TA et al. Pathology and causes of death in a group of 128 predominately HIV-positive patients in Botswana, 1997–1998. Int J Tuberc Lung Dis 2002; 6: 55–63.

10. Sewankambo NK, Gray RH, Ahmad S et al. Mortality associated with HIV infection in rural Rakai district, Uganda. AIDS 2000; 14: 2391–400.

11. Newell M-L, Coovadia H, Cortina-Borja M et al. Mortality of infected and uninfected infants born to HIV-infected mothers in Africa: a pooled analysis. Lancet 2004; 364: 1236–43.

12. Buve A, Bishikwabo-Nsarhaza K, Mutangadura G. The spread and effect of HIV-1 infection in sub-Saharan Africa. Lancet 2002; 359: 2011–17.

13. Dye C, Scheele S, Dolin P et al. Global burden of tuberculosis: estimated incidence, prevalence and mortality by country. J Am Med Assoc 1999; 282: 677–86.

14. Sonnenberg P, Glynn JR, Fielding K et al. How soon after infection with HIV does the risk of tuberculosis start to increase? A retrospective cohort study in South African Gold Miners. J Infect Dis 2005; 191: 150–8.

15. Corbett EL, Watt CJ, Walker N et al. The growing burden of tuberculosis: global trends and interactions with the HIV epidemic. Arch Intern Med 2003; 163: 1009–21.

16. Clumeck N, Sonnet J, Taelman H et al. Acquired immunodeficiency syndrome in African patients. N Eng J Med 1984; 310: 492–7.

17. Lester FT, Ayehunie S, Debrework Z. Acquired immunodeficiency syndrome: seven cases in Addis Ababa (Ethiopia) hospital. Ethiop Med J 1988; 26: 139–47.

18. McLeod DT, Latif A, Neill P, Lucas S. Pulmonary diseases in AIDS patients in Central Africa. Am Rev Respir Dis 1988; 137: 119.

19. Reeve PA. HIV infection in patients admitted to a general hospital in Malawi. Br Med J 1989; 298: 1567–8.

20. Wadhawan D, Hira SK. Tuberculosis and HIV-1 in medical wards. Med J Zambia 1989; 24: 16–18.

21. Nelson AM, Perriens JH, Kapita B et al. A clinical and pathological comparison of the WHO and CDC case definitions for AIDS in Kinshasa, Zaire: is passive surveillance valid? AIDS 1993; 7: 1241–5.

22. Abouya YL, Blaumel A, Lucas S et al. Pneumocystis carinii pneumonia. An uncommon cause of death in African patients with acquired immunodeficiency syndrome. Am Rev Respir Dis 1992; 145: 617–20.

23. Lucas SB, Hounnou A, Peacock C et al. The mortality and pathology of HIV infection in a West African city. AIDS 1993; 7: 1569–79.

24. Kool HE, Bloemkolk D, Reeve PA, Danner SA. HIV seropositivity and tuberculosis in a large general hospital in Malawi. Trop Geogr Med 1990; 42: 128–32.

25. Simooya OO, Maboshe MN, Kaoma RB, Chimfwembe EC, Thurairajah A, Mukunyandela M. HIV infection in newly diagnosed tuberculosis patients in Ndola, Zambia. Cent Afr J Med 1991; 37: 4–7.

26. Colebunders RL, Ryder RW, Nzilambi N et al. HIV infection in patients with tuberculosis in Kinshasa, Zaire. Am Rev Respir Dis 1989; 139: 1082–5.

27. Cathebras P, Vohito JA, Yete ML et al. Tuberculose et infection par le virus de l'immunodeficience humaine en Republique Centrafricaine. Med Trop (Mars) 1988; 48: 401–407.

28. Ouattara SA, Diallo D, Meite M et al. Epidemiologie des infections par le virus de l'immunodeficience humaine VIH-I et VIH-2 en Cote d'Ivoire. Med Trop (Mars) 1988; 48: 375–9.

29. Kelly P, Burnham G, Radford C. HIV seropositivity and tuberculosis in a rural Malawi hospital. Trans Roy Soc Trop Med Hyg 1990; 84: 725–7.

30. Elliott AM, Luo N, Tembo G et al. Impact of HIV on tuberculosis in Zambia: a cross-sectional study. Br Med J 1990; 301: 412–15.

31. Houston S, Roy S, Mahari M et al. The association of tuberculosis and HIV infection in Harare, Zimbabwe. Tuberc Lung Dis 1994; 75: 220–6.

32. De Cock KM, Gnaore E, Adjorlolo G et al. Risk of tuberculosis in patients with HIV-I and HIV-II infections in Abidjan, Ivory Coast. Br Med J 1991; 301: 496–9.

33. Mukadi Y, Perriens JH, St Louis ME et al. Spectrum of immunodeficiency in HIV-1 infected patients with pulmonary tuberculosis in Zaire. Lancet 1993; 342: 143–6.

34. Gnaore E, Sassan-Morokro M, Kassim S et al. A comparison of clinical features in tuberculosis associated with infection with human immunodeficiency viruses 1 and 2. Trans Roy Soc Trop Med Hyg 1993; 87: 57–9.

35. Elliott AM, Halwiindi B, Hayes RJ et al. The impact of human immunodeficiency virus on presentation and diagnosis of tuberculosis in a cohort study in Zambia. J Trop Med Hyg 1993; 96: 1–11.

36. Nunn P, Gicheha C, Hayes R et al. Cross-sectional survey of HIV infection among patients with tuberculosis in Nairobi, Kenya. Tuberc Lung Dis 1992; 73: 45–51.

37. Perriens JH, St Louis ME, Mukadi YB et al. Pulmonary tuberculosis in HIV-infected patients in Zaire. A controlled trial of treatment for either 6 or 12 months. N Engl J Med 1995; 332: 779–84.

38. Okwera A, Whalen C, Byekwaso F et al. Randomised trial of thiacetazone and rifampicin-containing regimens for pulmonary tuberculosis in HIV-infected Ugandans. Lancet 1994; 344: 1323–8.

39. Malkin JE, Prazuck T, Simmonet F et al. Tuberculosis and human immunodeficiency virus infection in West Burkina Faso: clinical presentation and clinical evolution. Int J Tuberc Lung Dis 1997; 1: 68–74

40. Winqvist N, Naucler A, Gomes V et al. Three-year follow up of patients with pulmonary tuberculosis in Guinea-Bissau, West Africa. Int J Tuberc Lung Dis 2000; 4: 845–52.

41. Ackah AN, Coulibaly D, Digbeu H et al. Response to treatment, mortality, and CD4 lymphocyte counts in HIV-infected persons with tuberculosis in Abidjan, Cote d'Ivoire. Lancet 1995; 345: 607–10.

42. Harries AD, Maher D, Mvula B, Nyangulu DS. An audit of HIV testing and HIV serostatus in tuberculosis patients, Blantyre, Malawi. Tuberc Lung Dis 1995; 76: 413–17.

43. Harries AD, Nyangulu DS, Kang'ombe C et al. Treatment outcome of an unselected cohort of tuberculosis patients in relation to human immunodeficiency virus serostatus in Zomba hospital, Malawi. Trans Roy Soc Trop Med Hyg 1998; 92: 343–7.

44. Kenyon TA, Mwasekaga MJ, Huebner R et al. Low levels of drug resistance amindst rapidly increasing tuberculosis and human immunodeficiency virus co-epidemics in Botswana. Int J Tuberc Lung Dis 1999; 3: 4–11.

45. Connolly C, Davies GR, Wilkinson D. Impact of human immunodeficiency virus epidemic on mortality among adults with tuberculosis in rural South Africa, 1991–1995. Int J Tuberc Lung Dis 1998; 2: 919–25.

46. Chimzizi RB, Harries AD, Manda E et al. Counselling, HIV testing and adjunctive cotrimoxazole for TB patients in Malawi: from research to routine implementation. Int J Tuberc Lung Dis 2004; 8: 938–44.

47. Chum HJ, O'Brien RJ, Chonde TM et al. An epidemiological study of tuberculosis and HIV infection in Tanzania, 1991–1993. AIDS 1996; 10: 299–309.

48. van Gorkom J, Kibuga DK. HIV infection among patients with tuberculosis in Kenya. Int J Tuberc Lung Dis 1999; 3: 741–2.

49. Kwanjana JK, Harries AD, Gausi F, Nyangulu DS, Salaniponi FM. TB-HIV seroprevalence in patients with tuberculosis in Malawi. Malawi Med J 2001; 13: 7–10.

50. Lucas SB, Peacock CS, Hounnou A et al. Disease in children infected with HIV in Abidjan, Cote d'Ivoire. Br Med J 1996; 312: 335–8.

51. Ansari NA, Kombe AH, Kenyon TA et al. Mortality and pulmonary pathology of children with HIV infection in Francistown, Botswana. Int J Tuberc Lung Dis 1999; 3 (Suppl. 1): S201.

52. Chintu C, Mudenda V, Lucas S et al. Lung diseases at necropsy in African children dying from respiratory illnesses: a descriptive necropsy study. Lancet 2002; 360: 985–90.

53. Chintu C, Bhat G, Luo C et al. Seroprevalence of human immunodeficiency virus type 1 infection in Zambian children with tuberculosis. Paediatr Infect Dis J 1993; 12: 499–504.

54. Sassan-Morokro M, De Cock KM, Ackah A et al. Tuberculosis and HIV infection in children in Abidjan, Cote d'Ivoire. Trans Roy Soc Trop Med Hyg 1994; 88: 178–81.

55. Madhi SA, Huebner RE, Doedens L et al. HIV-1 co-infection in children hospitalised with tuberculosis in South Africa. Int J Tuberc Lung Dis 2000; 4: 448–54.

56. Harries AD, Parry C, Nyong'onya Mbewe L et al. The pattern of tuberculosis in Queen Elizabeth Central Hospital, Blantyre, Malawi: 1986–1995. Int J Tuberc Lung Dis 1997; 1: 346–51.

57. World Health Organization. WHO Report 2005. Global tuberculosis control. Surveillance, planning, financing. WHO/HTM/TB/2005.349. Geneva: WHO.

58. Nunn P, Williams B, Floyd K et al. Tuberculosis control in the era of HIV. Nat Rev 2005; 5: 819–26.

59. Khatri GR, Frieden TR. Controlling tuberculosis in India. N Eng J Med 2002; 347: 1420–5.

60. Yanai H, Uthaivoravit W, Panich V et al. Rapid increase in HIV-related tuberculosis, Chiang Rai, Thailand, 1990–1994. AIDS 1996; 10: 527–31.

61. Frieden TR, Sterling TR, Munsiff SS et al. Tuberculosis. Lancet 2003; 362: 887–99.

62. Fitzgerald DW, Desvarieux M, Severe P et al. Effect of post-treatment isoniazid on prevention of recurrent tuberculosis in HIV-1-infected individuals: a randomised trial. Lancet 2000; 356: 1470–4.

63. East African and British Medical Research Council co-operative investigation. Tuberculosis in Kenya. A second national sampling survey of drug resistance and other factors, and a comparison with the prevalence data from the first national sampling survey. Tubercle 1978; 59: 155–77.

64. Kenya/British Medical Research Council co-operative investigation. Tuberculosis in Kenya 1984: a third national survey and a comparison with earlier surveys in 1964 and 1974. Tubercle 1989; 70: 5–20.

65. East African and British Medical Research Council co-operative investigation. Tuberculosis in Tanzania: a national sampling survey of drug resistance and other factors. Tubercle 1975; 56: 269–94.

66. Tanzanian/British Medical Research Council collaborative study. Tuberculosis in Tanzania: a national survey of newly notified cases. Tubercle 1985; 66: 161–78.

67. De Cock KM, Soro B, Coulibaly IM, Lucas SB. Tuberculosis and HIV infection in sub-Saharan Africa. J Am Med Assoc 1992; 268: 1581–7.

68. Kennedy N, Ramsay A, Uiso L et al. Nutritional status and weight gain in patients with pulmonary tuberculosis in Tanzania. Trans Roy Soc Trop Med Hyg 1996; 90: 162–6.

69. Zachariah R, Spielmann MP, Harries AD, Salaniponi FML. Moderate to severe malnutrition in patients with tuberculosis is a risk factor associated with early death. Trans Roy Soc Trop Med Hyg 2002; 96: 291–4.

70. Barnes PF, Bloch AB, Davidson PT, Snider DE. Tuberculosis in patients with human immunodeficiency virus infection. N Eng J Med 1991; 324: 1644–50.

71. Samb B, Sow PS, Kony S et al. Risk factors for negative sputum acid-fast bacilli smears in pulmonary tuberculosis: results from Dakar, Senegal, a city with low HIV seroprevalence. Int J Tuberc Lung Dis 1999; 3: 330–6.

72. Elliott AM, Namaambo K, Allen BW et al. Negative sputum smear results in HIV-positive patients with pulmonary tuberculosis in Lusaka, Zambia. Tuberc Lung Dis 1993; 74: 191–4.

73. Mugusi F, Villamor E, Urassa W et al. HIV co-infection, CD4 cell counts and clinical correlates of bacillary density in pulmonary tuberculosis. Int J Tuberc Lung Dis 2006; 10: 663–9.

74. Harries AD, Hargreaves NJ, Kwanjana JH, Salaniponi FM. Clinical diagnosis of smear-negative pulmonary tuberculosis: an audit of diagnostic practice in hospitals in Malawi. Int J Tuberc Lung Dis 2001; 5: 1143–7.

75. Munyati SS, Dhoba T, Makanza ED et al. Chronic cough in primary health care attendees, Harare, Zimbabwe: diagnosis and impact of HIV infection. Clin Infect Dis 2005; 40: 1818–27.

76. Samb B, Henzel D, Daley CL et al. Methods for diagnosing tuberculosis among patients in Eastern Africa whose sputum smears are negative. Int J Tuberc Lung Dis 1997; 1: 25–30.

77. Mabaera B, Naranbat N, Dhliwayo P, Rieder HL. Efficiency of serial smear examinations in excluding sputum smear-positive tuberculosis. Int J Tuberc Lung Dis 2006; 9: 1030–35.

78. Harries AD, Mphasa NB, Mundy C et al. Screening tuberculosis suspects using two sputum smears. Int J Tuberc Lung Dis 2000; 4: 36–40.

79. Walker D, McNerney R, Mwembo MK et al. An incremental cost-effectiveness analysis of the first, second and third sputum examination in the diagnosis of pulmonary tuberculosis. Int J Tuberc Lung Dis 2000; 4: 246–51.

80. Hawken MP, Muhindi DW, Chakaya JM et al. Under- diagnosis of smear-positive pulmonary tuberculosis in Nairobi, Kenya. Int J Tuberc Lung Dis 2001; 5: 360–3.

81. Hargreaves NJ, Kadzakumanja O, Phiri S et al. What causes smear-negative pulmonary tuberculosis in Malawi, an area of high HIV seroprevalence? Int J Tuberc Lung Dis 2001; 5: 1–10.

82. Kelper MD, Beumont M, Elshami A et al. CD4 T lymphocyte count and the radiographic presentation of pulmonary tuberculosis. Chest 1995; 107: 74–80.

83. Post FA, Wood R, Pillay GP. Pulmonary tuberculosis in HIV infection: radiographic appearance is related to CD4+ T-lymphocyte count. Tuberc Lung Dis 1995; 76: 518–21.

84. Abouya L, Coulibaly IM, Coulibaly D et al. Radiologic manifestations of pulmonary tuberculosis in HIV-1- and HIV-2-infected patients in Abidjan, Cote d'Ivoire. Tuberc Lung Dis 1995; 76: 436–40.

85. Pedro-Botet J, Gutierrez J, Miralles R et al. Pulmonary tuberculosis in HIV-infected patients with normal chest radiographs. AIDS 1992; 6: 91–3.

86. Harries AD, Maher D, Nunn P. An approach to the problems of diagnosing and treating adult smear-negative pulmonary tuberculosis in high-HIV-prevalence settings in sub-Saharan Africa. Bull World Health Organ 1998; 76: 651–62.

87. Colebunders R, Bastian I. A review of the diagnosis and treatment of smear-negative pulmonary tuberculosis. *Int J Tuberc Lung Dis* 2000; **4**: 97–107.

88. Lockman S, Hone N, Kenyon TA *et al.* Etiology of pulmonary infections in predominately HIV-infected adults with suspected tuberculosis, Botswana. *Int J Tuberc Lung Dis* 2003; **7**: 714–23.

89. Richter C, Ndosi B, Mwammy AS, Mbwambo RK. Extrapulmonary tuberculosis – a simple diagnosis? *Trop Geogr Med* 1991; **43**: 375–8.

90. Harries AD, Hargreaves NJ, Kwanjana JH, Salaniponi FM. The diagnosis of extrapulmonary tuberculosis in Malawi. *Trop Doctor* 2003; **33**: 7–11.

91. Perenboom RM, Richter C, Swai ABU *et al.* Diagnosis of tuberculous lymphadenitis in an area of HIV infection and limited diagnostic facilities. *Trop Geogr Med* 1994; **46**: 288–92.

92. Bem C. Human immunodeficiency virus-positive tuberculous lymphadenitis in Central Africa: clinical presentation of 157 cases. *Int J Tuberc Lung Dis* 1997; **1**: 215–19.

93. Bekedam HJ, Boeree M, Kamenya A *et al.* Tuberculous lymphadenitis, a diagnostic problem in areas of high prevalence of HIV and tuberculosis. *Trans Roy Soc Trop Med Hyg* 1997; **91**: 294–7.

94. Bem C, Patil PS, Elliott AM *et al.* The value of wide-needle aspiration in the diagnosis of tuberculosis lymphadenitis in Africa. *AIDS* 1993; **7**: 1221–5.

95. Batungwanayo J, Taelman H, Allen S *et al.* Pleural effusion, tuberculosis and HIV-1 infection in Kigali, Rwanda. *AIDS* 1993; **7**: 73–9.

96. Richter C, Perenboom R, Swai ABM *et al.* Diagnosis of tuberculosis in patients with pleural effusion in an area of HIV infection and limited diagnostic facilities. *Trop Geogr Med* 1994; **46**: 293–7.

97. Luzze H, Elliott AM, Joloba ML *et al.* Evaluation of suspected tuberculous pleurisy: clinical and diagnostic findings in HIV-1-positive and HIV-negative adults in Uganda. *Int J Tuberc Lung Dis* 2001; **5**: 746–53.

98. Cegielski JP, Lwakatare J, Dukes CS *et al.* Tuberculous pericarditis in Tanzanian patients with and without HIV infection. *Tuberc Lung Dis* 1994; **75**: 429–34.

99. Pozniak AL, Weinberg J, Mahari M *et al.* Tuberculous pericardial effusion associated with HIV infection: a sign of disseminated disease. *Tuberc Lung Dis* 1994; **75**: 297–300.

100. Maher D, Harries. Tuberculous pericardial effusion: a prospective clinical study in a low-resource setting–Blantyre, Malawi. *Int J Tuberc Lung Dis* 1997; **1**: 358–64.

101. Maartens G, Willcox PA, Benatar SR. Miliary tuberculosis: rapid diagnosis, haematologic abnormalities, and outcome in 109 treated adults. *Am J Med* 1990; **89**: 291–6.

102. Lucas SB, De Cock KM, Hounnou A *et al.* Contribution of tuberculosis to slim disease in Africa. *Br Med J* 1994; **308**: 1531–3.

103. McDonald LC, Archibald LK, Rheanpumikankit S *et al.* Unrecognised *Mycobacterium tuberculosis* bacteraemia among hospital inpatients in less developed countries. *Lancet* 1999; **354**: 1159–63.

104. Lewis DK, Whitty CJM, Walsh AL *et al.* Treatable factors associated with severe anaemia in adults admitted to medical wards in Blantyre, Malawi, an area of high HIV seroprevalence. *Trans Roy Soc Trop Med Hyg* 2005; **99**: 561–7.

105. Harries AD, Nyangulu DS, Kangombe C *et al.* The scourge of HIV-related tuberculosis: a cohort study in a district general hospital in Malawi. *Ann Trop Med Hyg* 1997; **91**: 771–6.

106. Harries AD, Hargreaves NJ, Graham SM *et al.* Childhood tuberculosis in Malawi: nationwide case finding and treatment outcomes. *Int J Tuberc Lung Dis* 2002; **6**: 424–31.

107. Luo C, Chintu C, Bhat G *et al.* Human immunodeficiency virus type-I infection in Zambian children with tuberculosis: changing seroprevalence and evaluation of a thiacetazone-free regimen. *Tuberc Lung Dis* 1994; **75**: 110–15.

108. Mukadi YD, Wiktor SZ, Coulibaly I-M *et al.* Impact of HIV infection on the development, clinical presentation, and outcome of tuberculosis among children in Abidjan, Cote d'Ivoire. *AIDS* 1997; **11**: 1151–8.

109. Jeena PM, Pillay P, Pillay T, Coovadia HM. Impact of HIV-1 coinfection on presentation and hospital-related mortality in children with culture proven pulmonary tuberculosis in Durban, South Africa. *Int J Tuberc Lung Dis* 2002; **6**: 672–8.

110. Rennert WP, Kilner D, Hale M *et al.* Tuberculosis in children dying with HIV-related lung disease: clinical-pathological correlations. *Int J Tuberc Lung Dis* 2002; **6**: 806–13.

111. Graham SM, Coulter JBS, Gilks CF. Pulmonary disease in HIV-infected African children. *Int J Tuberc Lung Dis* 2001; **5**: 12–23.

112. Hesseling AC, Schaaf HS, Gie RP *et al.* A critical review of diagnostic approaches used in the diagnosis of childhood tuberculosis. *Int J Tuberc Lung Dis* 2002; **6**: 1038–45.

113. Mwinga A. Challenges and hope for the diagnosis of tuberculosis in infants and young children. *Lancet* 2005; **365**: 97–8.

114. World Health Organization. *Treatment of tuberculosis. Guidelines for national programmes*, 3rd edn. WHO/CDS/TB/ 2003.313. Geneva: World Health Organization, 2003.

115. World Health Organization and Stop TB Partnership. *The stop TB strategy.* WHO/HTM/TB/2006.368. Geneva: WHO, 2006.

116. Dye C, Watt CJ, Bleed DM *et al.* Evolution of tuberculosis control and prospects for reducing tuberculosis incidence, prevalence and deaths globally. *J Am Med Assoc* 2005; **293**: 2767–75.

117. Maher D, van Gorkom JLC, Gondrie PCFM, Raviglione M. Community contribution to tuberculosis care in countries with high tuberculosis prevalence: past, present and future. *Int J Tuberc Lung Dis* 1999; **3**: 762–8.

118. Nyirenda TE, Harries AD, Gausi F *et al.* Auditing the new decentralised oral treatment regimens in Malawi. *Int J Tuberc Lung Dis* 2004; **8**: 1089–94.

119. Grosset JH. Treatment of tuberculosis in HIV infection. *Tuberc Lung Dis* 1992; **73**: 378–83.

120. Pozniak AL, MacLeod GA, Mahari M *et al.* The influence of HIV status on single and multiple drug reactions to antituberculosis therapy in Africa. *AIDS* 1992; **6**: 809–14.

121. Perriens JH, Colebunders RL, Karahunga C *et al.* Increased mortality and tuberculosis treatment failure rate among human immunodeficiency virus (HIV) seropositive compared with HIV seronegative patients with pulmonary tuberculosis treated with 'standard' chemotherapy in Kinshasa, Zaire. *Am Rev Respir Dis* 1991; **144**: 750–5.

122. Nunn P, Kibuga D, Gathua S *et al.* Cutaneous hypersensitivity reactions due to thiacetazone in HIV-1 seropositive patients treated for tuberculosis. *Lancet* 1991; **337**: 627–30.

123. Kelly P, Buve A, Foster SD *et al.* Cutaneous reactions to thiacetazone in Zambia – implications for tuberculosis treatment strategies. *Trans Roy Soc Trop Med Hyg* 1994; **88**: 113–15.

124. Chintu C, Luo C, Bhat G *et al.* Cutaneous hypersensitivity reactions due to thiacetazone in the treatment of tuberculosis in Zambian children infected with HIV-1. *Arch Dis Child* 1993; **68**: 665–8.

125. World Health Organization. Severe hypersensitivity reactions among HIV-seropositive patients with tuberculosis treated with thioacetazone. *Wkly Epidemiol Rec* 1992; **67**: 1–3.

126. Brindle RJ, Nunn PP, Batchelor BIF *et al.* Infection and morbidity in patients with tuberculosis in Nairobi, Kenya. *AIDS* 1993; **7**: 1469–74.

127. Wiktor SZ, Sassan-Morokro M, Grant AD *et al.* Efficacy of trimethoprim-sulphmethoxazole prophylaxis to decrease morbidity and mortality in HIV-1-infected patients with tuberculosis in Abidjan, Cote d'Ivoire: a randomised controlled trial. *Lancet* 1999; **353**: 1469–75.

128. Nunn P, Brindle R, Carpenter L *et al.* Cohort study of human immunodeficiency virus infection in patients with tuberculosis in Nairobi, Kenya. *Am Rev Respir Dis* 1992; **146**: 849–54.

129. Elliott AM, Halwiindi B, Hayes RJ *et al.* The impact of human

immunodeficiency virus on mortality of patients treated for tuberculosis in a cohort study in Zambia. *Trans Roy Soc Trop Med Hyg* 1995; **89**: 78–82.

130. Mukadi YD, Maher D, Harries AD. Tuberculosis case fatality rates in high HIV prevalence populations in sub-Saharan Africa. *AIDS* 2001; **15**: 143–52.

131. Harries AD, Hargreaves NJ, Kemp J *et al.* Deaths from tuberculosis in sub-Saharan African countries with a high prevalence of HIV-1. *Lancet* 2001; **357**: 1519–23.

132. Connolly C, Davies GR, Wilkinson D. Impact of human immunodeficiency virus epidemic on mortality among adults with tuberculosis in rural South Africa, 1991–1995. *Int J Tuberc Lung Dis* 1998; **2**: 919–25.

133. Hargreaves NJ, Kadzakumanja O, Whitty CJM *et al.* 'Smear-negative' pulmonary tuberculosis in a DOTS programme: poor outcomes in an area of high HIV seroprevalence. *Int J Tuberc Lung Dis* 2001; **5**: 847–54.

134. Kang'ombe CT, Harries AD, Ito K *et al.* Long-term outcomes in patients registered with tuberculosis in Zomba, Malawi: mortality at 7 years according to initial HIV status and type of TB. *Int J Tuberc Lung Dis* 2004; **8**: 829–36.

135. Greenberg AE, Lucas S, Tossou O *et al.* Autopsy-proven causes of death in HIV-infected patients treated for tuberculosis in Abidjan, Cote d'Ivoire. *AIDS* 1995; **9**: 1251–4.

136. Churchyard GJ, Kleinschmidt I, Corbett EL *et al.* Factors associated with an increased case-fatality rate in HIV-infected and non-infected South African gold miners with pulmonary tuberculosis. *Int J Tuberc Lung Dis* 2000; **4**: 705–12.

137. Murray J, Sonnenberg P, Shearer SC, Godfrey-Faussett P. Human immunodeficiency virus and the outcome of treatment for new and recurrent pulmonary tuberculosis in African patients. *Am J Respir Crit Care Med* 1999; **159**: 733–40.

138. Hawken M, Nunn P, Gathua S *et al.* Increased recurrence of tuberculosis in HIV-1-infected patients in Kenya. *Lancet* 1993; **342**: 332–7.

139. Elliott AM, Halwiindi B, Hayes RJ *et al.* The impact of human immunodeficiency virus on response to treatment and recurrence rate in patients treated for tuberculosis: two-year follow-up of a cohort in Lusaka, Zambia. *J Trop Med Hyg* 1995; **98**: 9–21.

140. Kelly PM, Cumming RG, Kaldor JM. HIV and tuberculosis in rural sub-Saharan Africa: a cohort study with two year follow-up. *Trans Roy Soc Trop Med Hyg* 1999; **93**: 287–93.

141. Mallory KF, Churchyard GJ, Kleinschmidt I *et al.* The impact of HIV infection on recurrence of tuberculosis in South African gold miners. *Int J Tuberc Lung Dis* 2000; **4**: 455–62.

142. Sonnenberg P, Murray J, Glynn JR *et al.* HIV-1 and recurrence, relapse, and reinfection of tuberculosis after cure: a cohort study in South African mineworkers. *Lancet* 2001; **358**: 1687–93.

143. Banda H, Kang'ombe C, Harries AD *et al.* Mortality rates and recurrent rates of tuberculosis in patients with smear-negative pulmonary tuberculosis and tuberculosis pleural effusion who have completed treatment. *Int J Tuberc Lung Dis* 2000; **4**: 968–74.

144. Johnson JL, Okwera A, Vjecha MJ *et al.* Risk factors for relapse in human immunodeficiency virus type 1 infected adults with pulmonary tuberculosis. *Int J Tuberc Lung Dis* 1997; **1**: 446–53.

145. Jindani A, Nunn AJ, Enarson DA. Two 8-month regimens of chemotherapy for treatment of newly diagnosed pulmonary tuberculosis: international multicentre randomised trial. *Lancet* 2004; **364**: 1244–51.

146. van Rie A, Warren R, Richardson M *et al.* Exogenous reinfection as a cause of recurrent tuberculosis after curative treatment. *N Eng J Med* 1999; **341**: 1174–9.

147. Harries AD, Chimzizi RB, Nyirenda TE *et al.* Preventing recurrent tuberculosis in high HIV-prevalent areas in sub-Saharan Africa: what are the options for tuberculosis control programmes. *Int J Tuberc Lung Dis* 2003; **7**: 616–22.

148. Espinal MA, Laszlo A, Simonsen L *et al.* Global trends in resistance to antituberculosis drugs. *N Engl J Med* 2001; **344**: 1294–303.

149. Becerra MC, Bayona J, Freeman J *et al.* Redefining MDR-TB transmission 'hot spots'. *Int J Tuberc Lung Dis* 2000; **4**: 387–94.

150. Nelson LJ, Talbot EA, Mwasekaga MJ *et al.* Antituberculosis drug resistance and anonymous HIV surveillance in tuberculosis patients in Botswana, 2002. *Lancet* 2005; **366**: 488–90.

151. Gandhi NR, Moll A, Sturm AW *et al.* Extensively drug-resistant tuberculosis as a cause of death in patients co-infected with tuberculosis and HIV in a rural area of South Africa. *Lancet* 2006; **368**: 1575–80.

152. van Rie A, Enarson D. XDR tuberculosis: an indicator of public-health negligence. *Lancet* 2006; **368**: 1554–5.

153. World Health Organization. *Guidelines for implementing collaborative TB and HIV programme activities.* WHO/CDS/TB/2003.319; WHO/HIV/2003.01.2003. Geneva: WHO, 2003.

154. World Health Organization. *Strategic framework to decrease the burden of TB/HIV.* WHO/CDS/TB/2002.296; WHO/HIV_AIDS/2002.2. 2002, Geneva: WHO, 2002.

155. World Health Organization. *Interim policy on collaborative TB/HIV activities.* WHO/HTM/TB/2004.330.2004. Geneva: WHO, 2004.

156. World Health Organization. *Guidelines for HIV surveillance among tuberculosis patients*, 2nd edn. WHO/HTM/TB/2004.339; WHO/HIV/2004.06; UNAIDS/04.30E. Geneva: WHO, 2004.

157. Woldehanna S, Volmink J. Treatment of latent tuberculosis infection in HIV-infected persons. *Cochrane Database Syst Rev* 2004 (1); CD000171.

158. Ayles H, Muyoyeta M. Isoniazid to prevent first and recurrent episodes of TB. *Trop Doctor* 2006; **36**: 83–6.

159. Grant AD, Charalambous S, Fielding KL *et al.* Effect of routine isoniazid preventive therapy on tuberculosis incidence among HIV-infected men in South Africa. A novel randomized incremental recruitment study. *J Am Med Assoc* 2005; **293**: 2719–25.

160. Churchyard GJ, Fielding K, Charalambous S *et al.* Efficacy of secondary isoniazid preventive therapy among HIV-infected Southern Africans: time to change policy? *AIDS* 2003; **17**: 1–8.

161. Girardi E, Antonucci G, Vanacore P *et al.* Impact of combination antiretroviral therapy on the risk of tuberculosis among persons with HIV infection. *AIDS* 2000; **14**: 1985–91.

162. Badri M, Wilson D, Wood R. Effect of highly active antiretroviral therapy on incidence of tuberculosis in South Africa: a cohort study. *Lancet* 2002; **359**: 2059–64.

163. Lawn SD, Badri M, Wood R. Tuberculosis among HIV-infected patients receiving HAART: long term incidence and risk factors in a South African cohort. *AIDS* 2005; **19**: 2109–16.

164. WHO/UNAIDS. *UNAIDS/WHO policy statement on HIV testing.* Geneva: World Health Organization. www.unaids.org/html/pub/una-docs/hivtestingpolicy_en_pdf.htm, 2004.

165. Chimzizi R, Harries AD, Gausi F *et al.* Scaling up HIV/AIDS and joint HIV-TB services in Malawi. *Int J Tuberc Lung Dis* 2005; **9**: 582–4.

166. De Cock KM, Odhiambo J. HIV testing in patients with TB. *Trop Doctor* 2006; **36**: 71–3.

167. Chimzizi RB, Harries AD, Hargreaves NJ *et al.* Care of HIV complications in patients receiving anti-tuberculosis treatment in hospitals in Malawi. *Int J Tuberc Lung Dis* 2001; **5**: 979–81.

168. World Health Organization and UNAIDS. *Provisional WHO/UNAIDS Secretariat recommendations on the use of cotrimoxazole prophylaxis in adults and children living with HIV/AIDS in Africa.* Geneva: WHO/UNAIDS, 2000.

169. Zachariah R, Spielmann M-P, Chinji C *et al.* Voluntary counseling, HIV testing and adjunctive cotrimoxazole reduces mortality in tuberculosis patients in Thyolo, Malawi. *AIDS* 2003; **17**: 1053–61.

170. Mermin J, Lule J, Ekwaru P *et al.* Effect of cotrimoxazole prophylaxis on morbidity, mortality, CD4-cell count, and viral load in HIV infection in rural Uganda. *Lancet* 2004; **364**: 1428–34.

171. Chintu C, Bhat GJ, Walker AS *et al.* Co-trimoxazole as prophylaxis against opportunistic infections in HIV-infected Zambian children

(CHAP): a double-blind randomized placebo-controlled trial. *Lancet* 2004; **364**: 1865–71.

172. Zacharian R, Massaquoi M. Cotrimoxazole prophylaxis for HIV-positive TB patients in developing countries. *Trop Doctor* 2006; **36**: 79–82.

173. World Health Organization. *Report of a WHO expert consultation on cotrimoxazole prophylaxis in HIV infection.* Geneva: WHO, May 2005.

174. Swaminathan S, Luetkemeyer A, Srikantiah P *et al.* Antiretroviral therapy and TB. *Trop Doctor* 2006; **36**: 73–9.

175. World Health Organization and UNAIDS. *Progress on global access to HIV antiretroviral therapy. A report on '3 by 5' and beyond.* Geneva: World Health Organization, March 2006.

176. Kwara A, Flanigan TP, Carter EJ. Highly active antiretroviral therapy (HAART) in adults with tuberculosis: current status. *Int J Tuberc Lung Dis* 2005; **9**: 248–57.

177. Harries AD, Chimzizi R, Zachariah R. Safety, effectiveness, and outcomes of concomitant use of highly active antiretroviral therapy with drugs for tuberculosis in resource-poor settings. *Lancet* 2006; **367**: 944–5.

178. Manosuthi W, Sungkanuparph S, Thakkinstian A *et al.* Efavirenz levels and 24-week efficacy in HIV-infected patients with tuberculosis receiving highly active antiretroviral therapy and rifampicin. *AIDS* 2005; **19**: 1481–6.

179. Pedral-Sampaio DB, Alves C, Netto EM *et al.* Efficacy and safety of efavirenz in HIV patients on rifampin for tuberculosis. *Braz J Infect Dis* 2004; **8**: 211–16.

180. Lawn SD, Gail-Bekker L, Miller R. Immune reconstitution disease associated with mycobacterial infections in HIV-infected individuals receiving antiretrovirals. *Lancet Infect Dis* 2005; **5**: 361–73.

181. Colebunders R, John L, Huyst V *et al.* Tuberculosis immune reconstitution inflammatory syndrome in countries with limited resources. *Int J Tuberc Lung Dis* 2006; **10**: 946–53.

182. World Health Organization. *Antiretroviral therapy for HIV infection in adults and adolescents in resource-limited settings: towards universal access. Recommendations for a public health approach* (2006 version). Geneva: World Health Organization.

183. Zachariah R, Teck R, Ascurra O *et al.* Can we get more HIV-positive tuberculosis patients on antiretroviral treatment in a rural district of Malawi? *Int J Tuberc Lung Dis* 2005; **9**: 238–47.

184. Friedland G, Abdool Karim S, Abdool Karim Q *et al.* Utility of tuberculosis directly observed therapy programs as sites for access to and provision of antiretroviral therapy in resource-limited countries. *Clin Infect Dis* 2004; **38**: S421–8.

185. Mermin J, Ekwaru JP, Liechty CA *et al.* Effect of co-trimoxazole prophylaxis, antiretroviral therapy, and insecticide-treated bed nets on the frequency of malaria in HIV-1-infected adults in Uganda: a prospective cohort study. *Lancet* 2006; **367**: 1256–61.

186. Goldie SJ, Yazdanpanah Y, Losina E *et al.* Cost-effectiveness of HIV treatment in resource-poor settings – the case of Cote d'Ivoire. *N Engl J Med* 2006; **355**: 1141–53.

187. Corbett E, Marston B, Churchyard GJ, De Cock KM. Tuberculosis in sub-Saharan Africa: opportunities, challenges, and change in the era of antiretroviral treatment. *Lancet* 2006; **367**: 926–37.

20

HIV and TB in industrialized countries

ANTON POZNIAK

INTRODUCTION

Tuberculosis (TB) is one of the leading causes of illness in HIV-infected patients living in industrialized countries. Its management in co-infected patients is complicated by the underlying immunosuppression, complex drug–drug interactions and side effects. Some major social and political issues are raised by this 'duet of diseases' and include stigma, health policy, immigration and funding.

EPIDEMIOLOGY

Worldwide, it is estimated that approximately 9 per cent of all new TB cases in adults (aged 15–49 years) are attributable to human immunodeficiency virus (HIV) infection. This proportion is much greater in Africa and some industrialized countries where it has been estimated at around 31 per cent and TB-HIV killed nearly 200 000 people in 2005.[1] Surveillance of HIV incidence among TB patients is vital in understanding the trends of these dual epidemics and critical in informing and monitoring control strategies. There are major problems when it comes to reliable epidemiological monitoring of TB in HIV-positive people as less than 0.5 per cent of people living with HIV were screened for TB and there is a need to expand HIV testing in TB patients whether the TB is confirmed or diagnosed clinically (www.who.int/gtb/tbestimates/index).

While TB and HIV co-infection remains a major public health problem in many parts of the world, there are still no accurate figures for the TB-HIV co-infection rates in any industrialized country, including the USA. In 1998, it was estimated that 20 per cent of all patients with TB in the USA were HIV co-infected.[2] Data from the Bureau of HIV/AIDS Prevention and Control indicate that in 2000, TB was second only to *Pneumocystis pneumoniae* (PCP) as the most common opportunistic infection in HIV/AIDS patients in New York City. The Centers for Disease Control and Prevention (CDC) reported that in the USA from 2005 to 2006, among TB cases with HIV status reported, the percentage of TB cases with HIV infection decreased from 13 to 12.4 per cent, but the percentage of TB cases with unknown HIV status increased from 28.7 to 31.7 per cent. The decline in the percentage of TB cases with HIV infection might reflect incomplete reporting of HIV test results because of a lack of HIV testing or HIV reporting.[3]

There are other data from the same report which help as a pointer to why more focused epidemiological data are needed. In 2006, a total of 13 767 TB cases were reported which was down from 14 085 cases in 2005. The TB rate among foreign-born people was 21.9 compared with 2.3 cases per 100 000 people for those born in the USA, which is almost 10 times the rate. However, no breakdown of these communities by HIV status was published and it is hard not to speculate that there was a substantial number who were HIV-infected.[3] In New York City from 1992 to 2005, the percentage of TB cases who were also HIV-infected has decreased and is now around 15–18 per cent of all cases.[4] The percentage of US-born TB cases infected with HIV has only dropped 13 per cent, from 43 per cent in 1994 to 30 per cent in 2005. Most of this recent decrease reflects the extensive transmission that occurred in the late 1980s and early 1990s in New York.

The percentage of patients with an unknown HIV status in New York has also decreased from 51 per cent in 1992, but still remains high at 28 per cent in 2005. There are concerns in the USA about the large number of people with undiagnosed HIV infection who may only present when they are severely immunodeficient and may unknowingly transmit HIV to others. A new policy has been recommended in the USA where HIV screening is recommended for patients aged 13–64 years in all health-care settings unless the patient declines so-called 'opt-out screening'. People at high risk of HIV will be offered testing annually. This should enable better data on TB-HIV co-infection rates to be collected and ensure that those patients who are found to be positive can access appropriate care and treatment.

In spite of much investment in public health measures, ongoing TB transmission among HIV-infected people continues in large cities, such as New York. There have been several outbreaks of TB in residential facilities for HIV-infected people where extensive transmission occurred. In 2004 and 2005, 19 investigations were conducted using molecular epidemiology. Data from New York have shown that 60 per cent of HIV-infected TB cases from 2001 to 2005 were genotypically clustered, compared to 40 per cent of HIV-negative cases. While some clustered TB strains do not indicate recent transmission because they are endemic in New York City and may have been acquired several years earlier, the data are consistent with evidence of ongoing TB transmission in this population.[5]

In Europe, a postal survey of 20 cities using contacts identified through the EURO-TB surveillance network showed that the rates of TB overall ranged from less than 10 per 100 000 in Reykjavik and Belfast to over 70 per 100 000 in Lisbon and that the proportion of TB patients estimated to be HIV-positive ranged from less than 5 per cent in many countries to over 20 per cent in Milan. TB appeared to be concentrated in these big cities and there were major variations in control policy.[6]

Although the prevalence of HIV among TB patients in Holland remained stable between 1993 and 2001 at around 4 per cent, the distribution of risk groups changed over this period with increasing prevalence amongst immigrant patients from African countries. The highest prevalence was observed among drug users (29.2 per cent), homeless patients (20.1 per cent) and patients residing illegally in the country (9.1 per cent).[7]

TB is now a leading cause of HIV-related morbidity in the UK and was the most common AIDS-defining illness

in 2002. A study of 30 670 tuberculosis patients aged 15 years and over in England and Wales between 1999 and 2003 described trends in the proportion of individuals with HIV infection. There were an estimated 1743 (5.7 per cent) co-infected with HIV and a year-on-year increase in the proportion from 3.1 per cent (169/5388) in 1999 reaching 8.3 per cent (548/6584) in 2003. TB-HIV patients were predominantly those born abroad regardless of ethnic origin and contributed to almost a third of the increase in the number of total TB cases during the 5-year period.[8]

UK CHIC is an observational cohort of HIV-positive patients from major UK clinics in the UK. In this cohort from 1996 to 2005, 9 per cent of black Africans and 1.3 per cent of white patients had at least one episode of TB. Multivariate analysis showed that, compared to white patients, black Africans had an adjusted risk ratio of tuberculosis of 2.49. The median time from HIV diagnosis to TB diagnosis was only 0.7 months for black Africans, but 38 months for white patients. This difference can be explained by the fact that most TB episodes in Africans were diagnosed at the time of, or close to, their diagnosis of HIV infection. The study also showed that black African ethnicity and low CD4 were the main risk factors for TB incidence.[9]

Co-infection with TB and HIV is an increasing problem in London. In 1998, 5.4 per cent of patients with TB were co-infected with HIV and this had increased to 6.5 per cent by 2001. Reports from hospitals in London revealed rates of co-infection as high as 17–25 per cent.[10]

THE IMPACT OF HAART ON THE INCIDENCE OF TB

Since the introduction of highly active antiviral therapy (HAART), AIDS-related mortality and morbidity has decreased by 60–90 per cent in Europe among HIV-infected patients taking highly active antiretroviral therapy.[11]

Although the incidence of all HIV-related opportunistic infections has declined significantly in the HAART era, *Mycobacterium tuberculosis* may cause disease at any stage of HIV infection, and the beneficial influence of HAART on its incidence seems to be smaller than for other opportunistic infections.

The risk of TB was up to 80 per cent lower among people prescribed HAART and 40 per cent lower among people prescribed other non-HAART antiretroviral therapy than the risk in people not prescribed antiretroviral therapy (Table 20.1).[12,14] The protective effect of HAART was greatest in symptomatic patients and those with advanced immune suppression, but was not apparent in those with CD4 counts of more than 350 cells/µL.[15]

In Spain, the use of antiviral therapy and improved TB control has seen a marked decrease in reported HIV-TB cases.[16–18]

Table 20.1 Effect of highly active antiviral therapy (HAART) on tuberculosis (TB) incidence.

Country (Ref.)	Population (patient years)	TB incidence without HAART (per 100 patient years)	Adjusted % reduction (95% CI)
USA[12]	16 032	0.19	80 (50–90)
Italy[13]	2272 62% asymptomatic 7% TST+	0.79 overall	92 (12–99)
Brazil[14]	255 CD4 <15%	8.4	80 (–13–96)
South Africa[15]	375	9.7	81 (62–91)

The incidence of TB during the first 3 years after initiation of HAART among 17 142 treatment-naive patients and AIDS-free people starting HAART enrolled in 12 cohorts from Europe and North America was studied. During the first 3 years (36 906 person-years), 173 patients developed TB (incidence, 4.69 cases per 1000 person-years)., the incidence rate was lower for men who have sex with men, compared with injection drug users (relative rate, 2.46; 95 per cent confidence interval [CI], 1.51–4.01), heterosexuals (relative rate, 2.42; 95 per cent CI, 1.64–3.59). It was important to note that the level of immunodeficiency at which HAART is initiated and the response to HAART were important determinants of the risk of TB. During 28 846 person-years of follow up after the first 6 months of HAART, 88 patients developed TB (incidence, 3.1 cases per 1000 person-years of follow up). Rates were higher in those who were more immunodeficient with a lower $CD4^+$ count at the time of HAART initiation and in those whose $CD4^+$ count remained low at 6 months. However, even in those with good responses to HAART, the risk of TB remains appreciable and HAART is only one of the interventions needed to control the TB epidemic in the HIV-infected population.[19]

Similar effects of HAART have been seen in South Africa, which has a large TB-HIV epidemic and limited resources. Where HAART was available, the incidence of TB decreased during the first 5 years of therapy. This does suggest that as a control strategy HAART is an important component, as it may contribute more to TB control in low-income countries than was previously estimated from short-term follow up.[20]

HAART's effect is almost certainly by increasing the CD4 count above which the risk of new or reinfection is greatly diminished. One untested but pragmatic approach to those HIV patients who are of increased risk of tuberculosis, e.g. immigrants, is to give isoniazid prophylaxis until the CD4 count has risen to above a reasonable threshold of 200–300 CD4 cells/mm³ on HAART. Data are needed on what the threshold might be as patients may require being on isoniazid for more than 1 year and the effects of this are unknown.

Whether the widespread availability of antiviral medication plus strategies to detect and treat HIV-infected people will have a substantial impact on the incidence of TB in HIV patients is still unknown. Problems such as health-care access, poverty, overcrowding, homelessness, poor nutrition and inadequate immigrant screening are all factors that may keep TB incidence high in this population. HAART should be seen as one of the strategies used to control TB and close working between HIV and TB control programmes is essential.

RESPONSE TO HAART

Do patients with TB have a similar response to HAART as those without TB? In spite of all the potential problems of treating both TB and HIV together, successful virological outcomes on antiretroviral therapy in patients on TB treatment have been reported.

In a study from Taiwan, virological, immunological and clinical responses to HAART and prognosis of 46 HIV-1-infected TB patients who were concurrently treated with antituberculous therapy and HAART were similar to those of 230 non-TB patients started on HAART.[21]

Despite starting with a lower baseline CD4 cell count, patients with HIV-related TB on HAART showed similar CD4 and antiviral responses to antiretroviral therapy as patients without TB. Two-thirds of both groups achieved viral suppression, less than 500 copies/mL HIV-RNA.[17,22]

INFECTIOUSNESS OF HIV-TB-CO-INFECTED PATIENTS

Whether HIV increases the infectiousness of pulmonary tuberculosis (PTB) is controversial. In Brazil, 104 close contacts of patients with PTB who were also HIV-seropositive and 256 close contacts of patients with PTB who were HIV-seronegative were enrolled into a study to examine this question.[23] Infection with TB was equivalent among contacts of patients who were HIV-seropositive and HIV-seronegative: 27 versus 35 per cent. On follow up after at least 1 year, 8 per cent of the contacts of the HIV-seropositive index cases had converted their tuberculin skin test as compared with 26 per cent of the contacts of the HIV-seronegative index cases – a significant difference. Active TB was diagnosed in nine of these, eight in contact with HIV seronegative index cases. Another prospective study from the Dominican Republic, using tuberculin induration of 5 mm or greater as evidence of transmission, showed a positive skin test in 153 (61 per cent) of 252 household contacts of HIV-1-positive index cases and in 418 (76 per cent) of 551 household contacts of HIV-1-negative index cases.

The authors concluded that HIV-1-positive individuals with TB are less likely than HIV-1-negative individuals with TB to transmit *M. tuberculosis* to their close contacts.[24]

In two large meta-analyses of health-care workers and household contacts, skin test data suggested that TB-HIV patients are not intrinsically more infectious to their contacts than are HIV-1-negative TB patients.[25]

A small pilot study based on tuberculin tests supports this theory as it showed that HIV-infected PTB patients are less infectious to their contacts than HIV-negative patients.[26]

One conclusion from these studies is that patients with PTB who are also HIV-seropositive are less likely to infect their close contacts compared with patients with TB who are HIV-seronegative. This would fit in with the data that HIV-positive patients are less likely to have both cavitatory disease and be sputum-positive than HIV-negative patients. However, if family members of seropositive individuals are also seropositive then they may die of other causes before the TB is obvious. Furthermore, the tuberculin test as a diagnostic tool would be less useful in those contacts who are themselves seropositive. Finally, the decreased infectivity could be related to the duration of infection in sputum-positive patients. This was addressed in a study from Cape Town which identified a huge unrecognized burden of TB in the community, predominantly among HIV-infected people. However for those with sputum smear-positive TB, the mean time spent in the community before accessing TB treatment, the duration of infectivity, was estimated to be no longer for HIV-positive than for HIV-negative individuals, even after accounting for increased HIV mortality.[27]

TREATMENT

HAART has transformed the management of HIV disease in developed countries from an invariably fatal illness to a long-term chronic disease. Unfortunately, the use of antiretroviral therapy is not without problems especially those of long-term adherence and toxicity. HAART has the potential to substantially improve the outcome for co-infected patients, as well as reducing the risk of developing TB in those who are significantly immunosuppressed. The use of concurrent antiretroviral and tuberculosis treatment is complicated by overlapping toxicity profiles and drug–drug interactions of some antituberculosis and antiretroviral drugs.[28–30]

There are also concerns about drug malabsorption, the timing of commencement of HAART in relation to the start of TB treatment because of the risk of further HIV-related morbidity and the occurrence of paradoxical reactions. The use of HAART in patients who have tuberculosis and require antituberculosis therapy is complex and in managing such patients detailed knowledge and skills in the use of both antiretroviral and TB therapies are essential as is a multidisciplinary approach to care.

Table 20.2   Currently licensed HIV drugs.

Nucleos(t)ides
Abacavir (ABC)
Didanosine (ddI)
Emtricitabine (FTC)
Lamivudine (3TC)
Stavudine (d4T)
Tenofovir (TDF)
Zidovudine (ZDV)
3TC/ABC combination
FTC/TDF

Non-nucleoside reverse transcriptase inhibitors
Efavirenz (EFV)
Nevirapine (NVP)
EFV/FTC/TDF combination

Protease inhibitors[a]
Amprenavir (APV)
Atazanavir (ATV)
Darunavir (DRV)
Fosamprenavir (FPV)
Indinavir (IDV)
Lopinavir/ritonavir (LPV/RTV)
Nelfinavir (NFV)
Ritonavir (RTV)
Saquinavir (SQV)
Tipranavir (TPV)

Entry inhibitors
Enfuvirtide (ENF)
Maraviroc (MVC)

Integrase inhibitors
Raltegravir (RAL)

[a]Almost always used in conjunction with low-dose ritonavir.

DRUG–DRUG INTERACTION

Most drug–drug interactions between HIV and TB therapy are through induction or inhibition of metabolic enzymes in the liver and intestine. The most important family of enzymes is cytochrome P450 (CYP). CYP3A4 is the isoform involved in the metabolism of many drugs including the protease inhibitors and non-nucleoside reverse transcriptase inhibitors (NNRTIs), which makes up the core of most HAART regimens.

HAART usually consists of three or more drugs in combination. There are five different classes of drugs currently licensed, nucleoside/nucleotide analogues, non-nucleoside reverse-transcriptase inhibitors, the protease inhibitors, entry inhibitors and integrase inhibitors. The non-nucleoside reverse-transcriptase inhibitors and protease inhibitors have clinically important drug interactions with the rifamycins,[31,32] as do Maraviroc and potentially Raltegravir but few data are available.

Rifamycins are potent inducers of CYP3A4 and the drug transporter P-glycoprotein in the liver and intestinal wall. Of all the drugs used in clinical medicine, rifampicin is probably the most potent inducer of this isoform and several important pharmacokinetic interactions must be considered when starting antiretroviral (ARV) therapy in HIV patients with TB treated with a regimen including rifampicin. Its use leads to decrease in the serum concentrations of drugs metabolized by the CYP3A4 enzyme system.[33] Rifampacin brings broad changes in the pattern of gene expression and induces CYP1A2, CYP2C8, CYP2C9, CYP2E1, 2C19, P-glycoprotein activity, phase II metabolism (transferase enzymes).[34]

Another important issue to consider is that the inducing effect of rifampicin not only takes up to 2 weeks to become maximal, but will also persist for about 2 weeks after rifampicin has been stopped. If antivirals are being started or changed at the end of TB treatment, this time effect on enzyme induction should be taken into consideration.

Rifabutin is a less potent inducer of CYP3A4, but unlike rifampicin is also a substrate of it. Therefore, any 3A4 inhibitors will increase the concentration of rifabutin, but will have no effect on rifampicin metabolism. Thus, when rifabutin is given with the protease inhibitors, which are inhibitors of 3A4, its concentration and that of its metabolites can increase to cause toxicity.[35]

Rifapentine has a long serum half-life allowing once-weekly directly observed therapy during the continuation phase of treatment. There are few data regarding its interaction with HAART. Rifapentine is a CYP3A inducer, but is not a substrate for this enzyme. It may decrease levels of anitvirals but its own concentration would remain unaffected. A problem with increased rates of rifapentine resistance has been seen when used in the initial phase of therapy and more data are needed before rifapentine can be recommended for use in HIV patients.[36]

The individual drug–drug interactions between rifamycins and antiretroviral agents are shown in Tables 20.3, 20.4 and 20.5. The complexity of the drug–drug interaction requires much in the way of expertise in managing the dosing of both antiretroviral agents and TB drugs (Table 20.5).

Those diagnosed with TB often have a low CD4 T-cell count and guidelines for these patients recommend starting HIV therapy at or around the same time as therapy for TB. Combining treatment for TB and HIV is often difficult, particularly as both infections involve treatment with multiple medications. Drug interactions between medications used to treat HIV and TB mean that interactions can occur resulting in subtherapeutic drug concentrations. This may not only lead to persistent or relapsing illness, but also to the emergence of HIV drug resistance.

Patients with HIV and TB co-infection often present with advanced immunodeficiency and require antiviral therapy. Although the optimal timing of this is still unclear, most such patients will commence HAART whilst on rifampicin. The most common antiviral combination used in this situation is based on non-nucleoside reverse-

Table 20.3 Drug–drug interactions with currently licensed antiretroviral drugs.

Drug	Rifampicin	Rifabutin
Nevirapine	37% NVP	No change
Efavirenz	26% QFV	No change[a]
Nucleos(t)ide reverse transcriptase inhibitors	No effect	No effect

[a]Dose of RBT can be increased to 450 mg a day if >60 kg but this is not universal policy.

transcriptase inhibitors either nevirapine or efavirenz. The NNRTI nevaripine is both partially metabolized by CYP3A4 and an inducer of this enzyme system. The other commonly used NNRTI efavirenz behaves in a similar way. Because of this inducing effect, the clinical use of these drugs together with the rifamycins is complex.

Efavirenz and rifampicin

The pharmacokinetics and the safety of coadministration of the NNRTI efavirenz (EFV) and rifampicin (RIF) have not been well characterized. Rifamycins are an essential component of short-course TB therapy. RIF is a potent inducer of the CYP3A4 enzyme, thus has significant interactions with many anti-HIV drugs and is often substituted with rifabutin for HIV-infected individuals with TB, as rifabutin is a less potent enzyme inducer. EFV-containing antiretroviral regimens are recommended and proven effective first-line regimens for treatment of HIV.

Current guidelines vary, but some recommend increasing the EFV dose from 600 to 800 mg once daily when coadministering with RIF.[37] This recommendation was initially made on the basis of a Spanish study which found evidence of a significant drug interaction between EFV and RIF, with daily RIF, isoniazid and pyrazinamide reducing efavirenz concentrations by 20 per cent in a group of 97 HIV-infected patients from full 24-hour pharmacokinetic (PK) sampling.[38] The same researchers subsequently found that dosing EFV at 800 mg a day in people receiving TB treatment, including RIF, is effective and safe.[39]

These results are supported by an intensive prospective, controlled PK study from Spain of 24 patients showing that EFV oral clearance was 30 per cent faster when RIF was present, supporting a 30 per cent increase in EFV dosage from 600 to 800 mg in HIV-infected patients requiring RIF treatment for TB.[40]

A prospective, comparative study of EFV pharmacokinetics in HIV and TB co-infected adults taking 600 or 800 mg once daily (16 cases) or on EFV at a standard 600 mg dose without RIF (13 controls) showed that cases had a significantly higher oral clearance of EFV but otherwise, dose-dependent pharmacokinetic parameters of EFV were similar between cases and controls. No increased EFV

Table 20.4   Protease inhibitors.

PI	Rifampicin	Rifabutin	Comment
ATV	↓ ATV C_{min} by 93% (300/100), 80% (300/200), 60% (400/200)	↑ rifabutin AUC (205%)	(1) Avoid coadministration with rifampicin (2) Reduce rifabutin dose[b]
FPV	↓ APV AUC by 82%	↑ rifabutin AUC (193%)	(1) Avoid coadministration with rifampicin (2) ↓ rifabutin dose[c] or if boosted[b]
IDV	↓ IDV AUC by 89% (unboosted)/87% (boosted)	↓ IDV AUC by 32%, compensated by low-dose R; ↑ rifabutin AUC (204%)	(1) Avoid coadministration with rifampicin (2) ↓ rifabutin dose[c]
LPV/r	↓ LPV AUC by 75%; increased doses to 400/400 or 800/200 b.i.d. compensate ↓	↑ rifabutin AUC (303%)	(1) ↑ toxicity during co-administration of rifampicin and increased dose of LPV/R (2) ↓ rifabutin dose[b]
NFV	↓ NFV AUC by 82%	↓ NFV AUC by 32%; ↑ rifabutin AUC (207%)	(1) Avoid coadministration with rifampicin (2) TDM of NFV; ↓ rifabutin dose[b]
SQV	↓ SQV AUC by 84%; induction partly compensate by SQV/R 400/400 mg b.i.d.	↓ SQV AUC by 43%; compensated by R	(1) Hepatotoxicity during co-administration of rifampicin and SQV/R (2) ↓ rifabutin dose in presence of R[b]
TPV/r	↓ TPV by 80%	↔ TPV; ↑ rifabutin AUC (190%), C_{max} (70%), and C_{min} (114%)	(1) Avoid coadministration with rifampicin (2) ↓ rifabutin dose[b]

[a]25-O-desacetyl-rifabutin.
[b]150 mg every other day or 150 mg 3 times per week.
[c]150 mg every other day or 300 mg 3 times per week.
ATV, atazanavir; AUC, area under the curve; C_{max} and C_{min}, maximum and minimum concentrations; FPV, fosamprenavir; IDV, indinavir; LPV, lopinavir; NFV, nelfinavir; R, ritonavir; SQV, saquinavir; TDM, therapeutic drug monitoring; TPV, tipranavir.

Table 20.5   Drug–drug interactions with new antiretroviral drugs.

Drug	Rifampicin	Rifabutin	Comment
TMC 125	Not done	Little change	Use normal doses with rifabutin; don't use with rifampicin
TMC 278	↓1 AUC, C_{max} and C_{min} decreased by 80/69/89%	↓C_{min} by 49%	Avoid coadmistration with rifampicin; ?double dose 278 with rbt
Raltegravir	reduced the C_{min} AUC and C_{max} of MK-0518 by 61, 40 and 38%, respectively	Not done	?Avoid coadministration with rifampicin
GS 9137	Not done	Not done	
Maraviroc	6.6-fold increase in CYP3A4 induction		Double dose of maraviroc will compensate
Darunavir with ritonavir	Not done	Not done	Use rifabutin as with other ritonavir boosted PIs
Enfurvitide	No change	No change	Can use

AUC, area under the curve; C_{max} and C_{min}, maximum and minimum concentrations; TDM, therapeutic drug monitoring.

toxicity was observed. The mean weight of cases was 64 kg and the results suggest that a dose of 800 mg of EFV in association with RIF may be appropriate for patients of weight >60 kg in Europe. Again this study concluded that therapeutic drug monitoring may be beneficial for patients on EFV with RIF.[41]

However, data from a Thai study of 84 HIV-infected individuals also showed that the standard dose of 600 mg EFV did not cause lower drug exposure or efficacy than 800 mg once daily, but was in patients with a low body weight (mean 50–53 kg).[42] Other studies from Brazil and India have found no detrimental effect of coadministering EFV at the standard dose of 600 mg once daily and RIF on the clinical efficacy of either drug.[43,44]

The mean body weight of the Brazilian subjects was 51 kg, but was not reported in the India cohort. A retrospective analysis of EFV concentrations in patients taking RIF in a therapeutic drug monitoring (TDM) database from Canada also found no difference in EFV concentrations between patients taking 600 or 800 mg.[45] A very similar database analysis from the UK also found EFV concentrations were comparable in patients taking RIF with either 800 or 600 mg EFV, although there was a trend towards a higher proportion of patients with body weight <60 kg having high EFV concentrations compared to those ≥60 kg.[46]

Finally, a small prospective study assessing clinical toxicity and EFV concentrations in HIV-TB co-infected patients found that seven of nine patients receiving RIF and EFV developed significant clinical toxicity and that in all seven patients EFV trough concentrations were elevated significantly beyond the therapeutic range.[47] All but one of the patients in this group was black.

It has been suggested that the different results from these studies are due not only to the numbers and study design but also to variability in pharmacokinetics, therapeutic response and side effects in HIV-infected patients from distinct ethnic origins. One potential mechanism that may contribute to increased toxicity is single nucleotide polymorphisms in the cytochrome P450 2B6 genes, which appear to modulate EFV central nervous system (CNS) toxicity. Patients with a TT genotype (20 per cent of the black population compared with 3 per cent of white individuals) have an extended clearance of EFV.[48,49]

Nevirapine and rifampicin

Based on PK and limited clinical data, most physicians prefer the combination of EFV with RIF rather than nevirapine. There are limited data available about whether or not nevirapine and RIF can be safely coadministered without the plasma concentration of nevirapine falling below therapeutic levels. Early PK data suggested that daily RIF should not be used with nevirapine.[50] There are data on a few patients who received RIF twice a week with nevirapine-based regimens, but this type of TB regimen is not optimal for HIV-positive patients.[51]

In countries with high numbers of HIV-TB co-infection, nevirapine and RIF are used extensively. In a study from Thailand, blood plasma concentrations were collected from samples of patients using nevirapine 200 mg twice daily with or without concomitant RIF. The use of RIF was significantly associated with lower nevirapine plasma concentrations. In the RIF group, the mean nevirapine concentration was 5.47 ± 2.66 mg/L, whereas in the control group the mean nevirapine concentration was 8.72 ± 3.98 mg/L. In the RIF group, seven nevirapine trough concentrations were low (<3.1 mg/L), while in the control group two patients had low nevirapine trough concentrations. However, the majority of Thai co-infected patients have low body mass indices (BMI) and may maintain nevirapine plasma concentrations that are adequate for treatment of HIV. The problem is that to ensure patients of all BMIs have adequate trough levels, nevirapine plasma concentration monitoring should be performed.[52]

To overcome the problem of potentially low nevirapine (NVP) trough levels with concomitant RIF, the effect of administering higher doses of nevirapine has been studied.[53] There was a lower C_{min} at week 2 for the 400-mg group, but no differences at weeks 4 and 12 compared with the the 600-mg group. The higher dose was associated with a high frequency of NVP hypersensitivity in the early dose escalation period. A dose of 400 mg daily might well be sufficient in Asian patients (whose body weight was 46 to 55 kg), but higher dose lead-in dosing must be avoided. Recent data from South Africa shows that patients on rifampicin and nevirapine have a 3-fold risk of HAART failure compared with patients on rifampicin and efavirenz.

Interaction between rifamycin and nucleoside analogues

Most nucleosides have either unknown or little change in pharmacokinetics when given together with RIF-based regimens. RIF reduces the area under the curve (AUC) and increases the clearance of zidovudine via the mechanism of RIF-induced, increased glucuronidation of zidovudine. This is not clinically significant and dose alteration is not required. In contrast, rifabutin does not appear to affect the clearance of zidovudine.[54]

Rifamycins and protease inhibitors

Protease inhibitors (PIs) are mainly metabolized by CYP3A4 and they are also P-glycoprotein substrates. RIF decreases levels of saquinavir (Invirase®), indinavir (Crixivan®), nelfinavir (Viracept®) and amprenavir (Agenerase®) by >75 per cent, leading to subtherapeutic concentrations of all these agents. Such reductions would lead to loss of antiviral activity of the protease-containing regimen and consequently result in the emergence of resistance to one or more of the other drugs in the HAART regimen.

Today, protease inhibitors are rarely used without boosting with low-dose ritonavir (100–200 mg total daily dose) which markedly improves their pharmacokinetics by inhibiting CYP3A4 and P-glycoprotein.

Ritonavir is an exception because it is a potent inhibitor of cytochrome P450 and when used in full dose, 600 mg twice daily can be given with RIF by balancing out the inducing effect.[55] However, the problem with this therapeutic approach is that full-dose ritonavir is very poorly tolerated and rarely if ever used in clinical practice.[56]

Ritonavir-boosted saquinavir and rifampicin

A dose of 400-mg ritonavir with 400-mg saquinavir has been given with full-dose RIF in a few patients only and appeared not to affect the PK of either protease inhibitor adversely.[57]

The use of saquinavir as a soft gel capsule once daily (1600 mg) with ritonavir (200 mg) in HIV-infected patients who are taking concomitant HIV treatment has been examined in a pilot study from Spain in 32 adult antiretroviral naive subjects who were on daily RIF and isonaizid. The medium saquinavir C trough level was 44 per cent lower with RIF and interestingly two patients had hepatotoxicity leading to discontinuation.[58] Although this might have been a possible treatment option, events overtook any thought of using saquinavir with RIF when a PK study performed in healthy volunteers had to be stopped because of severe hepatitic reaction. Roche performed a phase 1 randomized open-label multidose clinical pharmacological study in healthy volunteers. Eleven of 28 (39.3 per cent of subjects) exposed to RIF 600 mg once a day taken with ritonavir 100 mg and saquinavir 1000 mg given twice daily developed significant hepatotoxicity during the 28-day study period. There were transaminase elevations up to >20 times the upper limit of normal and one subject was admitted to hospital. Following drug discontinuation, liver function tests in all affected subjects returned to normal. There were no deaths (www.inverase.com).[59]

Ritonavir-boosted lopinavir and rifampicin

The data from the drug–drug interaction of RIF with lopinavir and ritonavir would suggest that ritonavir at this low dose is not able to compensate for the induction effect of RIF on lopinavir metabolism.[60]

However, if the dose of ritonavir is increased to 400 mg twice a day, the trough levels of lopinavir were adequate in 9/10 subjects, but there were high rates of elevated transaminases. Gastrointestinal toxicity and lipid perturbations were also noted.[61]

A recent PK study in normal healthy volunteers was reminiscent of the saquinavir study with high rates of severe transaminitis occurring leading to termination of the study.[62]

Atazanavir with and without boosting by ritonavir and rifampicin

Recent data were consistent with that from the other protease inhibitors and showed that atazanavir with or without ritonavir boosting had unfavourable pharmacokinetics when given with concomitant RIF to 15 healthy volunteers. The atazanavir C_{min} was reduced to greater than 80 per cent whether low-dose ritonavir was given or not.[63,64]

In a three-patient PK study of boosted atazanavir given with RIF, the atazanavir level was below the minimum recommended trough plasma level (150 ng/mL) for more than 50 per cent of the time.[65]

Rifabutin and HAART

As far as TB is concerned, rifabutin appeared to be as effective as RIF in a small study in HIV-infected patients.[66]

There is little long-term outcome data from other studies where rifabutin has been used in HIV patients, but it appears to be effective in these patients.

Rifabutin is expensive. The cost of 4 days of treatment with rifabutin is the equivalent cost of an entire 6-month RIF regimen. Rifabutin toxicites include marrow suppression, arthralgias and uveitis. It has a complex drug–drug interaction profile as it is both an inhibitor and substrate of cytochrome P450 enzymes.

If rifabutin is used with efavirenz, the rifabutin dose should be increased to 450 mg a day because of the induction effect of EFZ.

Rifabutin can be used with single (unboosted) protease inhibitors, except saquinavir.[32,67]

However, because of the balance between rifabutin induction and protease inhibition of CYP3A4, when single unboosted protease inhibitors are used with rifabutin a modification in the dose of the protease inhibitor may be required (see Table 20.4) and the dose of rifabutin should be decreased by half to 150 mg.[68] If protease inhibitors are used with 100-mg ritonavir boosting, then the dose of rifabutin should be reduced to 150 mg and should only be given two or three times a week.[69]

There is still debate as to whether this dose of rifabutin is adequate. Data from a small PK study in London showed that the 4-hour levels of rifabutin were below predicted. One conclusion from this would be that the dose should be increased to 300 mg. No good data exist to settle this issue.[70]

Other interactions

Complex interactions may occur when a rifamycin is given with two protease inhibitors plus boosted ritonavir, or with a protease inhibitor boosted or not and a nonnucleoside reverse-transcriptase inhibitor. These combinations are used in patients who have had virological failure or intolerance to simpler regimens. These multiple interactions have yet to be fully studied and there are no clear guidelines regarding dosing of rifabutin when used with such regimens.[32] Rifabutin and nevirapine have been given together with no adjustment in either of their dosages.[71]

Newer PIs

DARUNAVIR (TMC 114)

To date, these interactions have not been investigated. Concomitant use of rifabutin with darunavir and ritonavir is expected to increase rifabutin plasma concentrations. It is recommended to administer rifabutin at a dosage of 150-mg rifabutin once every other day when coadministered with darunavir, and ritonavir administration with RIF is contraindicated.[72]

TIPRANAVIR

Administration with RIF is contraindicated as concentrations of tipranavir were decreased by tipranavir by 80 per cent. Rifabutin had no significant effect on tipranavir levels, but the rifabutin AUC was increased by 190 per cent, C_{max} by 70 per cent and C_{min} by 114 per cent, suggesting three times weekly dosing at 150 mg may be adequate.[73]

Non-rifamycin regimens

Finally, HIV-related TB can be treated with non-rifamycin-containing regimens. The use of non-rifamycin-containing regimens should be only contemplated in patients with serious toxicity to rifamycins where desensitization has failed or in those with rifamycin-resistant isolates. Drug–drug interactions might be fewer but a non-rifamycin regimen is inferior to a rifampicin-based regimen for treatment of HIV-related TB. If non-rifamycin treatment regimens of 1 year's duration are used, then streptomycin should be given. In addition, high relapse rates of greater than 15 per cent have been seen even when after the initial 2 months with a RIF-containing regimen and then is switched in the continuation phase to isoniazid and ethambutol.

Nucleoside/nucleotide only regimens

Because of inadequate potency triple nucleoside regimens are not recommended for the treatment of HIV. In some patients a quadruple nucleoside/nucleotide regimen, commonly abacavir, lamivudine, zidovudine and tenofovir has been given to patients on antituberculous therapy with rifampicin to avoid drug interactions. This has had some anecdotal success.

New drugs

NNRTIS TMC 125 (ETRAVIRINE)

This is a diarylpyrimidine derivative whose metabolism of etravirine involves both cytochrome P450 3A4 and glucuronidation. Etravirine is an inducer of CYP3A4. Etravirine is a substrate and inducer of CYP3A4 and a substrate and inhibitor of CYP2C, and has a different drug interaction profile compared with nevirapine and efavirenz. The metabolism of etravirine is moderately reduced by pure CYP3A4 inhibitors (i.e. indinavir (IDV)) and increased by CYP3A4 inducers (i.e. nevirapine).

There are no substantial changes required with rifabutin, but there are, as yet, no data on RIF and no study is planned.

TMC 278

TMC 278 is the newest NNRTI. The drug–drug interaction potential is limited in that it has not been found to induce or inhibit CYP isoforms. The drug has an oral tablet formulation.

When given with RIF, the AUC, C_{max} and C_{min} of TMC 278 decreased by 80, 69 and 89 per cent, respectively, so the drugs should not be used together. Rifabutin decreases the C_{min} by 49 per cent, so a double dose of 278 mg may be adequate.[74]

Integrase inhibitors

Raltegravir is metabolized by UGT 1A1 glucuronidation and has to be administered twice daily for optimal efficacy. RIF modestly reduces plasma levels of raltegravir. The effect of RIF at 600 mg once daily for 14 days on the PK of a single dose of the integrase inhibitor at 400 mg was studied in 10 HIV-negative subjects.

RIF reduced the C_{min}, AUC and C_{max} of MK-0518 by 61, 40 and 38 per cent, respectively. Coadministration should probably be avoided.

Elvitegravir is another integrase inhibitor which is a modified quinolone antibiotic with potent activity against HIV-1, is metabolized by CYP3A4 and is an inducer of that CYP isoform. To date, no interactions have been performed with rifamycins.

CCR5 antagonists

MARAVORIC (UK-427,857)

The drug is metabolized by CYP3A4. RIF lowers levels of maravoric and doubling the dose of maravoric may compensate for this inducing effect.[75]

Non-rifamycin regimens and interaction with HAART

There is a theoretical interaction between abacavir and isoniazid. Both drugs may be metabolized by cytosolic enzymes. Isoniazid may act both as a substrate for alcohol dehydrogenase (ADH) and induce uridine diphosphate glucorosyltransferase (UDPGT). Abacavir is metabolized by both ADH and UDPGT. An increase in plasma concentration of isoniazid and a decrease in abacavir concentration may occur if they are coadministered. However, because abacavir can be glucoronidated, this interaction is probably of little significance. Another theoretical interaction is with the coadministration of protease inhibitors with isoniazid which may result in greater potential for isoniazid-induced side effects as a result of inhibition of isoniazid metabolism by the protease inhibitors.

Overlapping toxicity profiles of antiretroviral drugs with antituberculous therapy

Adverse reactions to drugs are common among patients with HIV-related TB, especially if taking HAART concomitantly.

The nucleoside analogues ddI and D4T may all cause peripheral neuropathy and an additive toxicity of isoniazid when used with D4T has been demonstrated.[76] It is probably best to avoid these therapies if possible when treating patients for HIV who are on antituberculosis treatment. Rash, fever and hepatitis are common side effects of antituberculosis drugs especially RIF, isoniazid and pyrazinamide. The NNRTIs can also cause similar side effects. The coadministration of these drugs can lead to difficult clinical management decisions if these side effects occur, especially when HAART and TB drugs are started together. To compound the problem, cotrimoxazole is usually given to patients with low CD4 counts to prevent pneumoysitis and can also cause rash and fever. Hepatotoxicity due to isoniazid in the general population increases with age, occurring in less than 0.3 per cent of those under 35 years versus about 2.3 per cent in those older than 50 years. It is also more likely in those with a heavy alcohol intake, with hepatitis C co-infection and in those who are receiving cotherapy with RIF. High rates of adverse reaction requiring changes in therapy have been reported in HIV-infected patients who are likely to have some or all of the other risk factors noted above. The rates of adverse reaction were 26 per cent in one HIV cohort compared with 3 per cent in the uninfected group and other studies have shown similar results.

A total of 167 adverse events were recorded in 99 (54 per cent) of the 183 patients for whom data on therapy were available in a study from the south east of England.[77]

Adverse events led to cessation or interruption of either their TB or HIV therapy in 63 (34 per cent) of the 183 patients. The most common side effects usually occurred in the first 2 months of treatment and were peripheral neuropathy (21 per cent), rash in 31 patients (17 per cent), gastrointestinal in 18 patients (10 per cent), hepatitis in 11 patients (6 per cent) and neurological events in 12 patients (7 per cent).

The majority of adverse reactions have occurred within the first 2 months of starting concurrent therapies and RIF was frequently implicated accounting for almost two-thirds of adverse events.

When HIV-negative TB patients have been compared with HIV-positive patients, a greater rate of serious (grade III/IV) adverse events among HIV-infected individuals. However, discontinuation of antituberculosis treatment occurred with a similar frequency in both groups of individuals. The reasons for discontinuation were different and the groups are difficult to compare as they have obvious different characteristics, such as degree of immunosuppression and co-medications.[78]

DRUG ABSORPTION

Malabsorption of antimycobacterial drugs, including all first-line therapies as well as ethionamide and cycloserine, has been reported in people with AIDS and *M. tuberculosis*.

Absorption of drugs may be less in those patients with a low CD4 count, whether it be due to HIV enteropathy or other specific HIV-related gut diseases, resulting in subtherapeutic serum and drug levels and consequently associated with treatment failure and drug resistance.[79,80]

Although some studies show lower peak concentrations of RIF and ethambutol, as well as lower AUCs compared with controls,[81–85] there are other data suggesting that RIF is absorbed well in HIV patients even those with AIDS or with diarrhoea.[86]

Based on the limited amount of available data, TB drug therapeutic monitoring might be useful in patients who are at high risk of malabsorption of their TB drugs, in those who are having an inadequate response to directly observed therapy with first-line drugs and in patients being treated for multidrug-resistant TB.[79,87,88]

One of the problems with monitoring antimycobacterial drugs in HIV-positive patient is that the kinetics of absorption are not predictable. It is therefore difficult to know at what time-point to measure a peak serum dose and it is probably best to measure levels at more than one time-point post dose.

Some patients find it difficult to take the antituberculosis therapy on an empty stomach (which aids the absorption of isoniazid and RIF) because of severe problems of nausea and vomiting. The antituberculosis therapy can be taken with food in these circumstances but it is also possible to modify the first-line treatment to rifabutin, ethambutol, pyrazinamide and a fluoroquinolone as all of these can be taken with food.

WHEN TO START HAART

In HIV patients without TB, HAART is usually started when the CD4 count is between 200 and 350 cells/μL as the risk of AIDS and death starts to significantly increase below the 200-cell threshold (Table 20.8). The optimal time to start HAART in TB-HIV patients is not known and physicians try and balance the risk of progression against the risk of having to discontinue therapies because of toxicities, side effects or unforeseen drug–drug interactions. Similar routes of metabolism and elimination and extensive drug interactions may result in subtherapeutic plasma levels of antituberculous or antiviral agents and furthermore, overlapping toxicity profiles may result in the interruption or alteration of TB and HIV regimens with potential subsequent microbiological or virological failure. In co-infected patients, delaying the start of HAART can simplify patient management, limit the development of side effects and drug interactions and the risk of immune restoration reactions.

Patients with HIV disease and a CD4 cell count of greater than 200/μL cells have a low risk of HIV disease progression or death during the subsequent 6 months of TB treatment and they should have their CD4 cell count,

Table 20.6 TB treatment regimens: HAART/rifampicin.

HAART	Dose	TB therapy	Dose
4NRTI	No change	RIF	No change
Nevirapine	200 mg b.d.	RIF	600 mg o.d.
Nevirapine	?300 mg b.d.	RIF	600 mg o.d.
Efavirenz[a]	600–800 mg o.d.	RIF	600 mg o.d.

[a]Dose adjusted.

Table 20.7 TB treatment regimens: HAART/rifabutin.

HAART	Dose	TB therapy	Dose
4NRTI	No change	RBT	No change
Ritonavir-boosted PI	No change	RBT	150 mg 2–3× a week
Nevirapine	200 mg b.d.	RBT	300 mg o.d.
Efavirenz	600 mg o.d.	RBT	450 mg o.d.

Table 20.8 TB and HIV: immediate versus delayed HAART – proposed algorithm.

CD4 count	When to treat with HAART
CD4 cells/mm^3 <100	As soon as possible
100–200	After 2 months of TB treatment
200–350	After completing 6 months TB treatment
>350	None

Note: Regular CD4 monitoring should be performed.

monitored regularly and antiretroviral therapy withheld if possible during the short-course TB treatment.

Most co-infected patients, however, present with a low CD4 count often below 100 cells/mL. In such patients, HAART improves survival, but can be complicated by immune reconstitution inflammatory syndrome (IRD) and drug toxicity. Some recommend that antiretroviral therapy be delayed until the first 2 months of TB therapy has been completed,[17,89,90] but others would only recommend this strategy for those with a CD4 >100 and <200 cells/mL because of the short-term risk of developing further AIDS and death. Starting HAART early in severely immunosuppressed HIV-positive patients presenting with TB is associated with decreased mortality and a lowering of the rates of progression.[51]

In one study modelling early versus deferred HAART in patients with TB and CD4 counts <200 lymphocytes/mm, early HAART was favoured. Deferred HAART was only favoured over early HAART if the IRD-related mortality rate in the early group exceeded 4.6 per cent.[91] Most data from cohorts reveal an IRD-related mortality of <2 per cent.

There are currently several studies organized by the USA, the French National Agency for AIDS Research

(ANRS) and others looking at the question of when to start HAART. These are mainly based in the developing world and data should be available in the next year.

TYPE AND LENGTH OF TREATMENT

Type of treatment

The data on the efficacy of a 6-month regimen of RIF are well researched in HIV-uninfected individuals.[92]

The recommended drug regimen of RIF, isoniazid and pyrazinamide together with ethambutol (where the population isoniazid-resistant rate is significant) is used for the first 2 months followed by RIF and isoniazid for 4 months. This drug combination should be recommended to all HIV-positive patients with TB wherever possible. For those on complex antiretroviral regimens, where there is a risk of drug–drug interactions with RIF, rifabutin may sometimes be substituted although there are limited data for its use in HIV-positive patients. An uncontrolled study of 50 HIV-positive cases in Uganda showed similar efficacy to historical data on RIF.[66]

Although rifabutin seemed to perform as well as RIF, there was no long-term follow-up data to make more detailed comparisons as not all patients in the trial had reached 24 months of evaluation after completion of TB treatment.

In spite of the uncertainty regarding the utility of rifabutin in HIV patients, the Centers for Disease Control and Prevention (CDC) has taken a pragmatic approach and recommended the use of rifabutin in place of RIF in multidrug regimens for the treatment of active TB in HIV-TB because rifabutin can be administered with antiretroviral treatment regimens that include protease inhibitors. Non-protease regimens are now available and some have little or no major interaction with RIF which for most TB physicians would remain the drug of choice whenever practicable.[32,93]

Directly observed therapy

The use of directly observed therapy (DOT) should be the gold standard for treatment of HIV-related TB especially with the use of intermittent dosing.[94,95]

There are few data to support intermittent dosing of rifabutin-based regimens for HIV-related TB, but they have been used with success in patients without HIV.[96] However, in a study of patients with culture-confirmed TB treated under direct supervision with 2 months of rifabutin, isoniazid, pyrazinamide and ethambutol (given daily, three times weekly or twice weekly), followed by 4 months of twice-weekly rifabutin plus isoniazid, showed that although it was well tolerated, it was associated with a high risk of treatment failure or relapse with acquired rifamycin resistance especially among patients with a CD4 lymphocyte count below 100 cells/mm^3. In a pharmacokinetic substudy, lower plasma concentrations of rifabutin were associated with treatment failure or relapse in association with acquired rifamycin resistance.[97]

Most physicians do not use use twice-weekly regimens in HIV-positive patients and should avoid this strategy in those with low CD4 counts.

Length of treatment

The optimal length of TB treatment in patients co-infected with HIV is unknown and guidelines therefore vary. There are few data to suggest that the duration of treatment for fully drug-sensitive TB should be prolonged in HIV-positive patients.[95,98,99]

One study[100] supported a 12-month total treatment period, which appears to be the basis of some other recommendations. The apparently better results with 12-month regimens may be related to overall adherence and that in the short follow-up period, reinfection is less likely as they were, in effect, on secondary prevention for the last 6 months of therapy.

The US Centers for Disease Control and Prevention suggest 6 months for most patients and 9 months for those with continued clinical signs or a positive culture after 2 months of therapy.[32]

The British Thoracic Society recommend standard short-course TB treatment regimens.[101]

To try and clarify better how long to give treatment, there has been a review of six studies of patients with HIV infection and three studies of patients without HIV infection given 6 months of treatment or longer.[102] The analysis showed that the studies differed in terms of design, eligibility criteria, site of disease, frequency of dosing, dose administration methods and outcome definitions. HIV-infected patients had cure rates of 59–97 per cent; treatment success, 34–100 per cent and relapse, 0–10 per cent. In those without HIV infection, cure was 62.3–88.0 per cent, treatment success 91.2–98.8 per cent and relapse 0–3.4 per cent. Although the rate of relapse appeared to be higher in some studies of co-infected patients, other outcomes were comparable using only 6-month regimens.

The data from these studies are difficult to interpret as there are an excess of early deaths in patients treated for TB in HIV patients related to severe immune deficiency. There is also an increased risk of adverse events leading to interruptions or discontinuation in treatment suppression which may make 6-month regimens appear less efficacious than HIV-negative controls. Importantly, there is a higher rate of reinfection post treatment from other index cases especially in situations where antiretroviral therapy is not routinely available. This then makes the use of 2-year microbiological relapse rates difficult to interpret without molecular typing to distinguish true relapse from reinfection.

Some or all of these factors have a role in explaining the present data. A multicentre study from the USA found no difference between TB relapses with 6- and 9-month regimens.[103] However, the numbers who relapsed were only two and one patient, respectively. In light of the potency of the isoniazid- and RIF-based regimens, long-term randomized trials are needed to answer this question of therapy duration but the use of HAART, the risks of increased drug toxicity and the problems of reinfection versus relapse have to be addressed in any trial design.

More recent data cast doubt on the use of 6-month short-course therapy. A retrospective review of data from 1990 to 2001 from the USA evaluated treatment outcomes for HIV-infected patients with TB stratified by duration of rifamycin-based TB therapy. It showed that HIV-infected individuals who received a standard 6-month rifamycin-based regimen were four times more likely to relapse than those treated longer. HIV-infected individuals who received intermittent therapy were also more likely to relapse than those treated on a daily basis. Interestingly, the use of highly active antiretroviral therapy was associated with more rapid conversion of smears and cultures, as well as improved survival. The conclusion drawn from this was that the standard 6-month TB therapy may be insufficient to prevent relapse in patients with HIV. However, the data were generated from a relatively small subset of patients as only 17 per cent of the HIV-infected and 37 per cent of the HIV-uninfected/unknown patients received 6 months of rifamycin-based therapy. DOT for all doses was given to 56.9 per cent of the cases. There were no formal adherence analyses, but HIV-infected patients were significantly more likely to experience adverse reactions to anti-tuberculosis medications and to acquire drug resistance as compared with the HIV-uninfected/unknown subjects.[104]

In Spain, a study of HIV-infected patients receiving a 9-month TB regimen and concomitant HAART demonstrated that achieving both an undetectable viral load and increasing CD4 cell counts with HAART were associated with prevention of TB relapses.[105]

The optimal duration of treatment for HIV-related TB with a rifamycin-containing regimen remains controversial. In the absence of a definitive comparative trial, it is not known if a longer duration of therapy should be used to treat TB in HIV-infected patients.

INTERMITTENT THERAPY

There appears to be a relationship between the frequency of dosing and the risk for acquired TB resistance. In a study of once-weekly rifapentine plus isoniazid in the treatment of HIV-TB, acquired rifamycin resistance was common.[36]

Acquired rifamycin resistance also occurred in another study of HIV-TB treated with twice-weekly RIF plus isoniazid.[102]

It is not known whether the risk for acquired rifamycin resistance is greater with rifabutin than with RIF. The occurrence of five cases of acquired rifamycin resistance among patients enrolled in the TBTC Study 23, a single-arm trial of twice-weekly rifabutin-based therapy for treatment of HIV-TB study has been of concern.[106] Further data on 169 patients with culture-confirmed TB were treated under direct supervision with 2 months of rifabutin, isoniazid, pyrazinamide and ethambutol given daily, three times weekly or twice weekly followed by 4 months of twice-weekly rifabutin plus isoniazid. Most had advanced HIV disease with a median CD4 cell count of 90 cells/mm^3 (interquartile range, 35–175). Three had culture-positive treatment failure and six relapse. Eight of these nine cases had isolates with acquired rifamycin resistance. Treatment failure or relapse was associated with a baseline CD4 lymphocyte count of <100 and intermittent rifabutin-based treatment.[97]

In these studies, patients with acquired rifamycin resistance had very low CD4 cell counts at the time of TB diagnosis. These data have led to the CDC in the USA to recommend that people with HIV-TB and CD4 cell counts <100/mm^3 should not be treated with highly intermittent (i.e. once- or twice-weekly) regimens. These patients should receive DOT with daily therapy during the intensive phase, and daily or three doses a week during the continuation phase. Patients already on highly intermittent regimens should switch over to daily or three times a week.[106]

Clinicians should treat suspected relapse in such patients with regimens active against rifamycin-resistant TB until results of susceptibility testing are available.

Diagnostic tests

Despite the effectiveness of HAART, HIV-infected individuals with latent TB infection are much more likely to progress to active TB than HIV-uninfected people.[107] Detection and treatment of latent TB infection is important in this population.

In the pre-HIV era, patients newly diagnosed with PTB reacted to 5 units intermediate-strength purified protein derivative (PPD) testing in about 75–85 per cent of cases.[108]

In HIV and TB co-infection, there is a reduction in the proportion of those reacting to PPD as the CD4 count falls, from 50–90 per cent who have a CD4 count of 500 cells or over, down to 0–20 per cent in those patients who have AIDS or advanced HIV infection with a CD4 count of less than 200 cells/µL.[109–112]

An American national survey of HIV-infected people showed that tuberculin reactivity was four times lower overall compared with controls (2.7 versus 10 per cent).[113] To clarify whether non-reactivity to PPD was part of the general poor immune responsiveness seen in HIV patients, anergy testing using a panel of antigens has been used to distinguish true anergy from non-reactivity to tuberculin.[114–117]

However, because of inconsistent and ambiguous results in several studies, this is not a recommended strategy.

HAART can improve immunological respones to TB, but in one study only 7 per cent of patients[17] treated with antiretroviral therapy had reversion of their negative tuberculin tests to positive. It was interesting to note that the patients most likely to revert to a positive PPD were those with a rise in CD4 count of >200 cells/mL from baseline.

Who should have tuberculin testing?

The US Public Health Service and Infection Disease site of America guidelines[106] recommended that all newly diagnosed HIV patients should have a tuberculin skin test so that those with a positive test (>5 mm induration) can be given isoniazid or other chemopreventative therapy. Whether this policy has any long-term public health impact on TB control in countries where TB has a relatively low prevalence is not known. The reason for a tuberculin test it is to identify those patients who may have latent infection and prevent reactivation. However, there are many different factors which may affect the usefulness of such a strategy, such as the lower PPD-positive rates in HIV-positive patients, the effect of bacillus Calmette–Guèrin (BCG) immunization on PPD reactivity, the relative short-term impact of any chemopreventative therapy because of the high rates of exogenous infection in some populations and the effect of HAART in preventing TB reactivation and progression to infection by improving immune function. Recently, new diagnostic tests have been developed which may be more helpful than tuberculin testing in HIV-positive patients.

Interferon-γ tests

There is a specific region of difference in the DNA sequence (RD1) existing between MTB and *Mycobacterium bovis* type of BCG. This results in production of antigens, such as early secreted antigen target-6 (ESAT-6) and culture filtrate protein-10 (CFP-10), by MTB, but not by *M. bovis* and forms the basis of a number of commercially available immunodiagnostic tests for both latent and active TB by measuring interferon-γ (IFN-γ) released from T cells after stimulation with these specific antigens. Because these antigens are absent from BCG, the test is performed with greater specificity than the tuberculin skin test and differentiates exposure to BCG alone from exposure to MTB.[118]

Tuberculin testing is complex and requires specific skills and training and the patient has to come back for the tuberculin test to be read. The advantage of these tests is that only a single blood test is needed and the result is available the next day. Although IFN-γ release assays are approved for the diagnosis of latent tuberculosis infection (LTBI), limited data exist regarding their performance in HIV infection.

Studies which have investigated IFN-γ release tests in HIV patients suggest that they are more sensitive than the tuberculin tests and that they may well be more reliable to detect MTB exposure in patients with relatively low CD4 counts, although the lower threshold for this has not yet been set.[119,120]

Other data suggest combining both tuberculin and IFN tests would give better specificity. There is a problem with some of the assays as in this study 5 per cent had indeterminant IFN results, and this rose to 16.1 per cent in individuals with a CD4+ cell count <100 cells/mm³.[121]

CHEMOPREVENTATIVE THERAPY

The historical data on the use of 6–12 months of isoniazid in non-HIV patients in preventing latent TB from becoming active showed an effect that lasted at least 19 years. Eleven trials involving 73 375 patients were included in a Cochrane review to show that in the HIV-negative population there was no significant difference between 6- and 12-month courses in preventing TB with a reduction of about 60 per cent for both time periods.[122] Preventive therapy reduced deaths from TB, but this effect was not seen for all causes of mortality and INH was associated with hepatotoxicity in 0.36 per cent of people on 6 months treatment and in 0.52 per cent of people treated for 12 months.[123]

There have been several short-term controlled trials in HIV-positive people showing the protective effect of chemoprevention and the data are interesting in many ways.[124,125]

The protective effect of isoniazid is apparent only in those who are tuberculin skin test positive and this protective affect appears to only last 2.5–4 years. The reason isoniazid may only have such a short-term effect in HIV-positive patients may be related to the fact that the majority of infections in the populations studied are not from reactivation of latent TB but are new. In the developing world, the feasibility of undertaking such widespread prophylaxis faces great problems with only 30–40 per cent completing 6 months of isoniazid treatment in studies in Uganda and Kenya.

Chemopreventative therapy seemed to have no effect on HIV progression or mortality in the long term[126] and its implementation on a large scale poses major operational difficulties.[127,128]

Another difficulty is in screening patients for active TB prior to chemopreventive therpay. This requires x-ray and sputum examination facilities.

In the UK, a study trying to investigate whether chemopreventative therapy would be useful in patients at high risk of developing TB ran into difficulties as isoniazid supplies became short.

However, in certain populations that are well defined and are part of a comprehensive health-care system, many of the logistic problems can be overcome and larger proportions of eligible patients can be recruited into these programmes. In South African gold mines, a 34 per cent reduction in the rates of TB was seen after the introduction of a chemopreventative programme.[129]

To help overcome adherence problems, shorter courses of chemopreventative therapy using other drugs have been recommended. Unfortunately, RIF and pyrazinamide given three times a week for 2 months have been associated with severe and fatal hepatic reactions in five non-HIV patients with a total of 21 cases of liver injury reported to CDC.[130] This complication has not been seen in the studies of HIV-positive patients using this regimen.[131–133]

It is known from RFLP studies that many TB infections in HIV-positive patients appear to be new infections rather than reactivation of the original TB.[134,135]

Isoniazid may prevent such exogenous infection, but would then have to be given long term, at least until there was a substantial CD4 rise on HAART. There are no current data to support such a strategy.

Even though isoniazid preventive therapy for HIV-TB-co-infected individuals may reduce the reactivation of latent *M. tuberculosis* infections, a mathematical model predicted that community-wide isoniazid preventive therapy might reduce the incidence of TB in the short term, but may also speed the emergence of drug-resistant TB. This may particularly apply to developing countries unless diagnostic and treatment policies designed to accurately identify and treat patients with drug-resistant TB are employed.[136]

POST-TREATMENT PROPHYLAXIS

Studies have shown that by using isoniazid prophylaxis post treatment, short-term reductions in rates of recurrence of TB can be achieved. Such a strategy may prevent reinfection rather than true reactivation in settings of high TB transmission. Arguments for this approach are that eligible patients are easier to identify as an HIV test could be undertaken at TB diagnosis. Sputum smears are undertaken routinely at treatment completion, so there would be no need to rescreen for active TB. However, the issues regarding logistics, drug resistance, durability and sustainability are the same as for primary prevention. An unblinded randomized controlled trial in Haiti showed that prophylaxis with isoniazid after treatment for TB decreased the risk of recurrent TB in HIV-infected individuals, but did not prolong survival. However, the recurrences were mainly diagnosed on clinical grounds and there was no culture confirmation and no molecular studies that they were not reinfections.[137,138]

Antiviral therapy might be preferable in the developed world for this situation.[139]

IMMUNE RECONSTITUTION DISEASE OR IRIS

It was noticed that some patients experienced a clinical decline soon after starting HAART, even though these individuals had decreasing HIV RNA levels and rising CD4 T-cell counts. In these individuals, being on HAART was associated with a pathological inflammatory response to either previously treated infections or subclinical infections. The inflammation, which can result in adverse clinical outcomes, has been labelled 'immune reconstitution disease (IRD)' or 'immune reconstitution inflammatory syndrome (IRIS)'.

These syndromes do not have a widely accepted definition, although an international attempt is being made to standardize one.[140] They are characterized by worsening or appearance of new signs, symptoms or radiographic manifestations of TB that occur after initiation of HAART and are not the direct result of TB treatment failure or another disease process.[141–146]

They are often defined as transient, but can last many months. They are usually seen when the TB is microbiologically controlled, but cases can rarely occur with viable organisms isolated on culture. These reactions are thought to represent an abnormal immune response to tubercle antigens released by dead or dying bacilli. Such paradoxical reactions have been reported in immunocompetent patients before HIV became prevalent. Worsening of nodal disease occurred in around 10 per cent of some populations and central nervous system disease with enlarging tuberculoma was sometimes seen.[147–151]

In the HAART era, IRD has been reported widely and occurred in 36 per cent (12/33)[152] and 32 per cent (6/19)[153] of patients in two studies, but in another study paradoxical worsening was not significantly more common in patients receiving HAART (3 of 28 cases or 11 per cent) compared with 3 of 44 cases (7 per cent) in patients not receiving antiretroviral treatment.[154]

The majority of cases of IRD occur within the first 60 days of initiating HAART, with a median of 15 days.[142] IRD can continue for up to 2 years following the initiation of HAART.

IRD does not appear to be associated with any particular antiretroviral regimen or drug class.[155] Most patients with IRD have advanced HIV infection; and a median baseline CD4 cell count of 35 cells/mm^3 and a median HIV-RNA level of 581 694 copies/mL. Its relationship to the initiation of antiretroviral therapy[142] suggests that as the immune system recovers from profound immunosuppression, abnormal responses toward mycobacterial antigens occur.[156]

These reactions may be caused by the restored proliferation of T cells and elaboration of proinflammatory cytokines in response to TB antigens. In one small study, the immune response to *M. tuberculosis* antigens was restored in HIV-infected patients following HAART, but the restoration was delayed compared with virological and CD4 count response, and was frequently incomplete. Proliferative responses to stimulation with a strain of *M. tuberculosis* after 6 months of treatment were not as pronounced compared with controls. IFN-γ release peaked at near normal levels only after 8 months of anti-HIV therapy. Production of interleukin (IL)-12 was more delayed

and of a smaller increase compared with that of IFN-γ and the IL-2 response was even more muted.[157]

Data support the theory that there is an acute exacerbation of mycobacteria-specific T_H1 responses after HIV is controlled by HAART and this causes immune restoration syndrome in HIV-TB co-infected patients.[158]

Other preliminary data suggest that in patients who develop IRD after HAART expansions of an anergic abnormal T-cell clone may lead to inadequate, abnormal antigen responses and cell signalling, which can be improved with IL-2 and granulocyte–macrophage colony-stimulating factor (GM-CSF).[159]

In another study, evidence of TB recovering host immunity was seen after initiation of HAART with increased proliferation of peripheral blood mononuclear cells and IFN-γ production in response to *M. tuberculosis* antigens.[160]

French *et al.* have shown that distinct cytokine-mediated mechanisms contribute to IRD. Patients with mycobacterial disease and IRD never carried the polymorphism in the cytokine gene *TNFA-308*2*. Increased levels of IL-6 have also been found.[161] These studies suggest that the cause for IRD is complex, involving CD4 cells, cytokine regulation and expression, abnormal antigen responses and cell signalling.[162,163]

IRD most often presents with fever and increased or new lymphadenopathy. The skin over the nodes is often inflamed and the nodes can spontaneously rupture. Pleural and pericardial effusions, ascites, psoas abcess, cutaneous lesions and new or expanding central nervous system tuberculomata have also been described[141] as have worsening pulmonary lesions.[164]

With such small datasets in the literature, it is difficult to know who is at risk of IRD, but a low baseline CD4 cell count, a rapid recovery in CD4 numbers and having extrapulmonary or disseminated TB appear to be relevant,[155–166] as does a rapid decline in HIV-1 RNA level.[167] Cases with dissemination outside the lung may also be of increased risk.[154] HAART started within the first 2 months of TB treatment was associated with an increased risk of a IRD. This may be due to the high burden of bacilli inducing immunologic changes associated with the rapid rise in CD4 cells.

The diagnosis of IRD must be one of exclusion, as it can be confused with recrudescence of TB due to treatment failure and with drug hypersensitivity. Other infections common among immunocompromised patients should be excluded. The management of patients with IRD is usually with high-dose corticosteroids to control symptoms. Non-steroidal anti-inflammatory agents tend not to be helpful. Leucotriene overactivity has been implicated in IRD and montelukast can be considered as a treatment as an alternative to steroids and/or where these are not effective, but may need to be continued for a prolonged period.[78] Temporary discontinuation of antiretroviral therapy[168] has also been advocated but can cause precipitous falls in CD4 counts. Recurrent needle aspiration of nodes or abscesses, especially if they become tense and/or inflamed, can prevent spontaneous rupture which if it occurs can lead to long-term sinus formation and scarring. Cytokine treatment with IL-2 and GM-CSF has had benefit in some patients.[159]

There has been a concerted effort to come up with a unifying definition of IRD and this may help with its associations and pathogenesis. Trials of early or deferred HAART may also give useful insights, but studies into its optimum management are lacking.

DRUG-RESISTANT TB

The proportion of cases of TB that were multidrug-resistant (MDR) – defined as TB that is resistant to at least two first-line therapies (isoniazid and RIF) – remained stable in the USA from 2004 to 2005 and accounts for 1.2 per cent of all TB cases for which drug-susceptibility data were available.

Extensively-drug resistant TB (XDR-TB) is defined as TB that is resistant to at least isoniazid and RIF among the first-line antituberculosis drugs (MDR-TB) and, among second-line drugs, is resistant to any fluoroquinolone and at least one of three injectable drugs.

Between 1993 and 2006, there were a total of 49 XDR-TB reported cases in the USA, representing 2.9 per cent of MDR-TB cases for which sufficient resistance data were available. Because drug-susceptibility results are often incomplete, this figure is probably an underestimate.

XDR-TB is widely distributed geographically. The bulk of the problem of XDR-TB resides in those countries with high numbers of MDR-TB and two-thirds of MDR is in just three countries – China, India and the Russian Federation.

The most well-known XDR-TB data are from South Africa. It is extremely disturbing and has major implications for TB control. In 1539 patients from January 2005 to March 2006, MDR-TB was found in 221 patients, of whom 53 had XDR-TB. Prevalence among 475 patients with culture-confirmed TB was 39 per cent (185 patients) for MDR and 6 per cent (30 patients) for XDR-TB. Of concern only 55 per cent of patients with XDR-TB had never been previously treated for tuberculosis; all 44 patients with XDR-TB who were tested for HIV were co-infected. The disease was almost universally fatal with 52 of 53 XDR-TB patients dying. The median survival was only 16 days from time of diagnosis among the 42 HIV-positive patients with confirmed dates of death. Genotyping of isolates showed that 39 of 46 (85 per cent) patients with XDR-TB had similar strains.[169]

HIV is strongly associated with MDR-TB through outbreaks. One factor for these to occur is that HIV-positive patients have an increased risk of developing active tuberculous disease once infected with *M. tuberculosis*. The annual risk from infection to clinical disease for HIV-infected people is about the same as the lifetime risk for HIV-uninfected individuals at about 10 per cent.

Outbreaks of multidrug resistance tuberculosis among HIV-positive patients in the early 1990s in the USA and Europe highlighted the problems in public health and hospital control of infection policies. The factors which led to the outbreaks included (1) putting all the immune-suppressed patients in one location without contol of infection facilities, such as a clinic, prison block or open hospital ward, (2) having a low index suspicion for TB and (3) little investment in laboratory and clinical management, research, development and education in TB. The outbreaks have led to an increase in health-care spending and investment in TB and consequently most developed countries have a comprehensive TB control strategy for immunocompromised people so that the risk of such incidents occurring in health-care settings or institutions are minimized.

Outbreaks have occurred in hospitals in Europe,[170–173] American clinics[173–175] and in hostels for HIV-positive patients and for substance abusers[176] in prisons[177] and homeless shelters. From 1990 to 1992, nine large outbreaks of MDR-TB were reported from the USA. The HIV infection rate amongst these patients was from 20 to 100 per cent and the mortality was from 60 to 89 per cent. The interval from TB diagnosis to death was between 4 and 16 weeks.

By definition, all organisms isolated were resistant to RIF and isoniazid and most also had streptomycin and ethambutol resistance. Various genotypic strains of MDR-TB were circulating during this period of time, especially the notorious 'W' strain, which infected 199 patients in New York from 1991 to 1994 and involved 30 hospitals.[178] Other types, 'N2', 'W1' and 'AB', infected a large number of patients in 10–16 hospitals. These outbreaks were mainly controlled using public health and administrative measures, including infection control policies for patients with HIV who have a cough, segregation of potential infectious patients, the use of negative-pressure rooms and submicron masks.[179–182]

Procedures, such as nebulization of pentamidine for PCP prophylaxis, saline for induced sputums or even salbutamol for those with obstructive airway disease was confined to negative-pressure rooms.

In Europe, there have been about six outbreaks involving around 225 patients and these have had major implications for resource utilization and public health. They occupied a large number of staff in contact tracing and case finding. It was interesting to note that in the second outbreak in the UK, very few people took up TB prophylaxis and, of those who did, almost all of them stopped by 2 weeks because of drug toxicity.

One of the largest outbreaks of MDR-TB occurred in Argentina over a 15-month period[183] and 101 patients had resistance to five drugs and survival was around 10 per cent. Most of these patients were in contact with one intravenous drug user who was poorly adherent to treatment and had developed sequential TB drug resistance.

There have also been cases of immunosuppressed patients with fully drug-sensitive TB and, whilst on effective treatment, are then exposed to and acquire a drug-resistant strain.[184]

Outbreaks of multidrug-resistant *M. bovis* in HIV patients have been reported in Spain involving 19 cases over 15 months of resistance to 11 drugs. All the patients died with a median survival of 44 days. The major risk factor was severe immune suppression.[185]

Treatment

The drug treatment regimens used for outbreak patients have been based on drug-sensitivity patterns. Most of them included an 8-quinolone, such as ofloxacin, together with amikacin and, if sensitive, pyrazinamide. Other drugs, such as ethionamide, have been used. The long-term efficacy of many of these combinations is unknown.

The optimum duration of treatment for MDR-TB in HIV has not been determined, but many cases are treated for at least 2 years after cultures convert to negative.

Surgery and interferon

As most HIV patients have multisite disease, surgery, which is usually reserved for those patients with localized disease and a low bacterial burden, is not an option. Nebulized interferon has been used in rendering sputum smears negative in some patients before surgery. It has also been used as a method to prevent spread of infection when all other drug treatments have failed in non-HIV-infected MDR-TB cases.

Prognosis and predictors

The major risk factors for MDR-TB in HIV patients are the same as in the general population. These include previous TB treatment, birth, travel or work in an area endemic for MDR-TB, history of poor adherence, sputum positivity, continuing at 2 months or culture positive at 3 months.

Other factors relevant to the HIV population have also been recognized as predictors of MDR-TB. Severely immune-suppressed HIV-positive patients seem more likely to develop MDR-TB probably related to the high risk of progression to disease once infected.

A failure to become apyrexial by 2 weeks of treatment and development of hilar lymph nodes are clinical clues pointing towards possible MDR-TB in HIV patients.[186,187]

One of the best predictors of survival is starting on at least two drugs to which the organism is susceptible within 2 weeks of diagnosis. This often means a patient is given multiple drugs prior to the drug sensitivity patterns being available.[188,189] However, the prognosis in HIV patients with MDR-TB overall has been very poor and only 25–30 per cent of people survive 6 months if they are severely immune suppressed.[190]

Chemopreventative therapy for MDR-TB

If given at all, this should be based on the drug sensitivity pattern of the case isolate. If MDR-TB is suspected and not yet confirmed, some suggest the use of fluoroquinolone and pyrazinamide.

CONCLUSIONS

MDR-TB in HIV is an outbreak phenomenon and it is important that public health procedures are enforced to safeguard the health of HIV patients, their carers and health-care staff from transmission of TB. The spectre of XDR-TB may lead to worsening TB control as it is difficult to treat and in much of the world is difficult to diagnose, as there is no drug resistance service available. Urgent interventions are needed, as XDR-TB threatens the success of treatment programmes for TB and HIV.

LEARNING POINTS

- HIV infection has been a contributory factor to increases in TB in a number of industrialized countries.
- Since the introduction of HAART, AIDS-related mortality and mobidity has decreased by 60–90 per cent in Europe among HIV-infected patients taking therapy.
- Whether or not infection with HIV increases the infectiousness of pulmonary TB is controversial.
- Overlapping toxicity profiles and drug–drug interactions of some antituberculosis and antiretroviral drugs complicates the use of concurrent antiretroviral and TB treatment.
- Most drug–drug interactions between HIV and TB therapy are through induction or inhibition of metabolic enzymes in the liver and intestine.
- Rifabutin appears to be as effective as rifampicin in the treatment of TB in HIV-infected patients, but data are limited.
- Rates of adverse reactions to TB/HAART treatment are high. The rate of adverse reaction was 26 per cent in one HIV cohort compared with 3 per cent HIV in the uninfected group and other studies have showed similar results.
- In the HIV-positive patients, HAART should be started as soon as possible if the CD4 count is less than 100 cells/mm^3.
- The standard four-drug regimen should be used for TB in the presence of HIV wherever possible.
- There are few data to suggest that the duration of treatment for fully drug-sensitive TB should be prolonged in HIV-positive patients. In

uncomplicated non-CNS TB, 6 months appears satisfactory.

- Widespread use of HAART has reduced the risk of developing clinical TB among people infected with HIV.
- In HIV and TB co-infection, there is a reduction in the proportion of those reacting to PPD.
- From RFLP studies, it seems that many TB infections in HIV-positive patients appear to be new infections rather than reactivation of the original TB.
- The use of directly observed therapy should be the gold standard for treatment of HIV-related TB, especially with the use of intermittent dosing.
- Paradoxical reactions (apparent worsening) may occur as HAART is given to TB patients on treatment due to a reconstitution of the immune process: IRIS.
- HIV is strongly associated with MDR-TB through outbreaks.
- The optimum duration of treatment for MDR-TB in HIV has not been determined, but many cases are treated for at least 2 years after cultures convert to negative.

REFERENCES

1. World Health Organization. *Global tuberculosis control, surveillance, planning, financing.* Geneva: World Health Organization, 2007.
2. Kaplan JE, Hanson D, Dworkin MS *et al.* Epidemiology of human immunodeficiency virus-associated opportunistic infections in the United States in the era of highly active antiretroviral therapy. *Clin Infect Dis* 2000; 30: S5–14.
3. Centers for Disease Control and Prevention (CDC). Trends in tuberculosis incidence – United States, 2006. *MMWR Morb Mortal Wkly Rep* 2007; 56: 245–50
4. New York City Department of Health and Mental Hygiene. TB annual summary. http://www.NYC.gov/html/doh/downloads/pdf/tb/tb2005.pdf
5. Driver CR, Kreiswirth B, Macaraig MM *et al.* Molecular epidemiology of tuberculosis after declining incidence, New York City, 2001–2003. *Epidemiol Infect* 2007; 135: 634–43.
6. Hayward AC, Darton T, Van-Tam JN *et al.* Epidemiology and control of tuberculosis in Western European cities, 1. *Int J Tuberc Lung Dis* 2003; 7: 751–7.
7. Haar CH, Cobelens FG, Kalisvaart NA *et al.* HIV prevalence among tuberculosis patients in The Netherlands, 1993–2001: trends and risk factors. *Int J Tuberc Lung Dis* 2006; 10: 768–74
8. Ahmed AB, Abubakar I, Delpech V *et al.* The growing impact of HIV infection on the epidemiology of tuberculosis in England and Wales. *Thorax* 2007; 62: 672–6.
9. Grant A, Bansi L, Sabin C. TB incidence among HIV-infected Africans in the United Kingdom. Fourteenth Conference on Retroviruses and Opportunistic Infections, Los Angeles, 2007 (Abstr. 846).
10. Anderson SA, Maguire H, Carless J. Tuberculosis in London: a decade and a half of no decline. *Thorax* 2007; 62: 162–7.
11. Mocroft A, Ledergerber B, Katlama C *et al.* EuroSIDA study group. Decline in the AIDS and death rates in the Eurosida study an observational cohort. *Lancet* 2003; 362: 22–9.
12. Jones JL, Hanson DL, Dworkin MS, DeCock KM, the Adult/Adolescent Spectrum of HIV Disease Group. HIV-associated tuberculosis in the era of highly active antiretroviral therapy. *Int J Tuberc Lung Dis* 2000; 11: 1026–31.
13. Girardi E, Antonucci G, Vanacore P *et al.* Gruppo Italiano di Studio Tubercolosi e AIDS (GISTA). Impact of combination antiretroviral therapy on the risk of tuberculosis among persons with HIV infection. *AIDS* 2000; 14: 1985–91.
14. Santoro-Lopes G, de Pinho AM, Harrison LH, Schechter M. Reduced risk of tuberculosis among Brazilian patients with advanced human immunodeficiency virus infection treated with highly active antiretroviral therapy. *Clin Infect Dis* 2002; 34: 543–6.
15. Badri M, Wilson D, Wood R. Effect of highly active antiretroviral therapy on incidence of tuberculosis in South Africa: a cohort study. *Lancet* 2002; 35: 2059–64.
16. Calpe JL, Chiner E, Marin-Pardo J, Calpe A, Armero V. Impact of the human immunodeficiency virus on the epidemiology of tuberculosis in area 15 of the Valencian community in Spain. *Int J Tuberc Lung Dis* 2004; 8: 1204–12.
17. Moreno S. Management of TB in HIV persons. World AIDS Conference, Barcelona, Spain, 2002 (Abstr. TUOR 171).
18. Calpe J, Chiner E, Marin J, Armero V, Calpe A. Tuberculosis epidemiology in area 15 of the Spanish autonomous community of Valencia: evolution from 1987 through 2001. *Arch Bronconeumol* 2005; 41: 118–24
19. Girardi E, Sabin CA, d'Arminio Monforte A *et al.* Antiretroviral Therapy Cohort Collaboration. Incidence of tuberculosis among HIV-infected patients receiving highly active antiretroviral therapy in Europe and North America. *Clin Infect Dis* 2005; 41: 1772–82.
20. Lawn SD, Badri M, Wood R. Tuberculosis among HIV-infected patients receiving HAART: long-term incidence and risk factors in a South African cohort. *AIDS* 2005; 19: 2109–16.
21. Hung CC, Chen MY, Hsiao CF *et al.* Improved outcomes of HIV-1-infected adults with tuberculosis in the era of highly active antiretroviral therapy. *AIDS* 2003; 17: 2615–22.
22. Edwards S, Dean G, Matthews G *et al.* Does tuberculosis treatment alter immunological and virological responses to HAART? 7th Conference on Retroviruses and Opportunistic Infections, San Francisco, 2000 (Abstr. 256).
23. Carvalho AC, De Riemer K, Nunes ZB *et al.* Transmission of *Mycobacterium tuberculosis* patients. *Am J Respir Crit Care Med* 2001; 164: 2166–71.
24. Espinal MA, Perez EN, Baez J *et al.* Infectiousness of *Mycobacterium tuberculosis* in HIV-1-infected patients with tuberculosis: a prospective study. *Lancet* 2000; 355: 275–80.
25. Cruciani M, Malena M, Bosco O *et al.* The impact of human immunodeficiency virus type 1 on infectiousness of tuberculosis: a meta-analysis. *Clin Infect Dis* 2001; 33: 1922–30.
26. Mohammad Z, Naing NN, Salleh R *et al.* A preliminary study of the influence of HIV infection in the transmission of tuberculosis. *Southeast Asian J Trop Med Public Health* 2002; 33: 92–8.
27. Wood R, Middelkoop K, Myer L *et al.* Undiagnosed tuberculosis in a community with high HIV prevalence: implications for tuberculosis control *Am J Respir Crit Care Med* 2007; 175: 87–93.
28. Pozniak AL, Miller R, Ormerod LP. The treatment of tuberculosis in HIV-infected persons. *AIDS* 1999; 13: 435–45.
29. Moreno S, Hernandez B, Dronda F. Antiretroviral therapy in AIDS patients with tuberculosis. *AIDS Rev* 2006; 8: 115–24.
30. Kwara A, Flanigan TP, Carter EJ. Highly active antiretroviral therapy (HAART) in adults with tuberculosis: current status. *Int J Tuberc Lung Dis* 2005; 9: 248–57
31. Burman WJ, Gallicano K, Peloquin C. Therapeutic implications of drug interactions in the treatment of HIV-related tuberculosis. *Clin Infect Dis* 1999; 28: 419–30.
32. Centers for Disease Control and Prevention (CDC). Updated guidelines for the use of rifabutin or rifampin for the treatment and prevention of tuberculosis among HIV-infected patients taking

protease inhibitors or nonnucleoside reverse transcriptase inhibitors. *MMWR Morb Mortal Wkly Rep* 2000; **49**: 185–9.

33. Li AP, Reith MK, Rasmussen A *et al.* Primary human hepatocytes as a tool for the evaluation of structure-activity relationship in cytochrome P450 induction potential of xenobiotics: evaluation of rifampicin, rifapentine, rifabutin. *Chemico-Biol Interact* 1997; **107**: 17–30.

34. Rae JM, Johnson MD, Lippman ME, Flockhart DA. Rifampin is a selective, pleiotropic inducer of drug metabolism genes in human hepatocytes: studies with cDNA and oligonucleotide expression arrays. *J Pharmacol Exp Ther* 2001; **299**: 849–57.

35. Sun E, Heath-Chiozzi M, Cameron DW *et al.* Concurrent ritonavir and rifabutin increases risk of rifabutin-associated adverse events. XI International Conference on AIDS, Vancouver, Canada, 1996 (Abstr. MoB171).

36. Vernon A, Burman W, Benator D *et al.* Relapse with rifamycin mono-resistant tuberculosis in HIV-infected patients treated with supervised once-weekly rifapentine and isoniazid. *Lancet* 1999; **353**: 1843–7.

37. Pozniak AL, Miller RF, Lipman MCI *et al.* on behalf of the BHIVA Guidelines Writing Committee. BHIVA treatment guidelines for TB/HIV infection. London: British HIV Association, 2005 (www.bhiva.org/guidelines/2005).

38. Lopez-Cortes LF, Ruiz R, Viciana P *et al.* Pharmacokinetic interactions between rifampin and efavirenz in patients with tuberculosis and HIV infection. Eighth Conference on Retroviruses and Opportunistic Infections, Chicago, 2001 (Abstr. 32).

39. Lopez-Cortes LF, Ruiz-Valderas R, Viciana P *et al.* Pharmacokinetic interactions between efavirenz and rifampicin in HIV-infected patients with tuberculosis. *Clin Pharmacokinet* 2002; **41**: 681–90.

40. Soy D, Lopez E, Sarasa M *et al.* Population pharmacokinetic modeling in HIV patients with tuberculosis treated with efavirenz and rifampicin. Program and Abstracts of the 6th International Workshop on Clinical Pharmacology of HIV Therapy, Quebec City, Canada, 28–30 April, 2005 (Abstr. 15).

41. Matteelli A, Regazzi M, Villani P *et al.* Multiple-dose pharmacokinetics of efavirenz with and without the use of rifampicin in HIV-positive patients. *Curr HIV Res* 2007; **5**: 349–53.

42. Manosuthi W, Kiertiburanakul S, Sungkanuparph S *et al.* Efavirenz 600 mg/day versus efavirenz 800 mg/day in HIV-infected patients with tuberculosis receiving rifampicin: 48 weeks results. *AIDS* 2006; **20**: 131–2.

43. Pedral-Samapio D, Alves C, Netto E *et al.* Efficacy of efavirenz 600 mg dose in ARV therapy regimen for HIV patients receiving rifampicin in the treatment of tuberculosis. Tenth Conference on Retroviruses and Opportunistic Infections, Boston, 2003 (Abstr. 784).

44. Patel A, Patel K, Patel J *et al.* Safety and antiretroviral effectiveness of concomitant use of rifampicin and efavirenz for antiretroviral-naive patients in India who are coinfected with tuberculosis and HIV-1. *J Acquir Immune Defic Syndr* 2004; **37**: 1166–9.

45. Sheehan NL, Richter C, Koopmans P, Burger DM. Efavirenz (EFV) in not associated with subtherapeutic EFV concentrations when given concomitantly with rifampin (RFP). Program and Abstracts of the 6th International Workshop on Clinical Pharmacology of HIV Therapy, Quebec City, Canada, 28–30 April, 2005 (Abstr. 28).

46. Almond L, Gibbons S, Davies G *et al.* A retrospective survey of Liverpool TDM service: Factors influencing efavirenz concentrations in patients taking rifampicin. Program and Abstracts of the 6th International Workshop on Clinical Pharmacology of HIV Therapy, Quebec City, Canada, 28–30 April, 2005 (Abstr. 19).

47. Brennan-Benson P, Lys R, Harrison T *et al.* Pharmacokinetic interactions between efavirenz and rifampicin in the treatment of HIV and tuberculosis: one size does not fit all. *AIDS* 2005; **19**: 1541.

48. Ribaudo H, Clifford D, Gulick R *et al.* Relationship between efavirenz pharmacokinetics, side effects, drug discontinuation, virologic response and race: results from ACTG A5095/A5097s. 11th Conference on Retroviruses and Opportunistic Infections, San Francisco, 8–11 February 2004 [Abstr. 132].

49. Haas D, Ribaudo H, Kim R *et al.* A common CYP2B variant is associated with efavirenz pharmacokinetics and central nervous system side effects: AACTG Study NWCS214. 11th Conference on Retroviruses and Opportunistic Infections, San Francisco, 8–11 February 2004 (Abstr. 133).

50. Robinson P, Lamson M, Gigliotti M *et al.* Pharmacokinetic interaction between nevirapine and rifampicin. Program and abstracts of the 12th World AIDS Conference, Geneva, Switzerland, 1998 (Abstr.).

51. Dean GL, Back DJ, de Ruiter A. Effect of tuberculosis therapy on nevirapine trough plasma concentrations. *AIDS* 1999; **13**: 2489–90.

52. Wit FW, Sankote J, Mahanontharit A *et al.* Nevirapine plasma concentrations and concomitant use of rifampin in patients coinfected with HIV-1 and tuberculosis. *AIDS* 2005; **19**: 1541–3.

53. Avihingsanon A, Manosuthi W, Kantipong P *et al.* PK and 12 weeks efficacy of NVP 400 vs. 600 mg daily in HIV+ patients with active TB receiving rifampin. 14th Conference on Retroviruses and Opportunistic Infections, Los Angeles, 2007 (Abstr. 576).

54. Burger DM, Meenhorst PL, Koks CHW, Beijnen JH. Pharmacokinetic interaction between rifampicin and zidovudine. *Antimicrob Agents Chemother* 1993; **37**: 1426–31.

55. Moreno S, Podzamczer D, Blazquez R *et al.* Treatment of tuberculosis in HIV-infected patients: safety and antiretroviral efficacy of the concomitant use of ritonavir and rifampin. *AIDS* 2001; **15**: 1185–7.

56. Bonfanti P, Valsecchi L, Parazzini F *et al.* Incidence of adverse reactions in HIV patients treated with protease inhibitors: a cohort study. Coordinamento Italiano Studio Allergia e Infezione da HIV (CISAI) Group. *J Acquir Immun Defic Syndr* 2000; **23**: 236–45.

57. Veldkcamp AI, Hoetelmans RM, Beijnen JH *et al.* Ritonavir enables combined therapy with rifampicin and saquinavir. *Clin Infect Dis* 1999; **29**: 1586.

58. Ribera E, Azuaje C, Lopez RM *et al.* Once-daily regimen of saquinavir, ritonavir, didanosine, and lamivudine in HIV-infected patients with standard tuberculosis therapy (TBQD study). *J Acquir Immun Defic Syndr* 2005; **40**: 317–23.

59. Gray A, Abdool Karim SS, Gengiah TN. Ritonavir/saquinavir safety concerns curtail antiretroviral therapy options for tuberculosis-HIV-co-infected patients in resource-constrained settings. *AIDS* 2006; **20**: 302–3.

60. Bertz R, Hsu A, Lam W *et al.* Pharmacokinetic interactions between lopinavir/ritonavir (ABT-378r) and other non-HIV drugs. *AIDS* 2000; **14** (Suppl. 4): S100 (Abstr.).

61. La Porte CJ, Colbers EP, Bertz R *et al.* Pharmacokinetics of adjusted-dose lopinavir-ritonavir combined with rifampin in healthy volunteers. *Antimicrob Agents Chemother* 2004; **48**: 1553–60.

62. Nijland H, L'homme R, Rongen G *et al.* Unexpected high incidence of nausea, vomiting and asymptomatic elevations of AST/ALT enzymes in healthy volunteers receiving rifampin and adjusted doses of lopinavir/ritonavir tablets. International Workshop on Clinical Pharmacology of HIV Therapy, Budapest, 2007 (Abstr. 51).

63. Acosta E, Kendall M, Gerber J *et al.* and the A5213 Study Team. Effect of rifampin on pharmacokinetics and safety of twice-daily atazanavir: ACTG Protocol A5213. 14th Conference on Retroviruses and Opportunistic Infections, Los Angeles, 2007 (Abstr. 575).

64. Burger DM, Agarwala S, Child M *et al.* Effect of rifampin on steady-state pharmacokinetics of atazanavir with ritonavir in healthy volunteers. *Antimicrob Agents Chemother* 2006; **50**: 3336–42.

65. Mallolas J, Sarasa M, Nomdedeu M *et al.* Pharmacokinetic interaction between rifampicin and ritonavir-boosted atazanavir in HIV-infected patients. *HIV Med* 2007; **8**: 131–4.

66. Schwander S, Rusch-Gerdes S, Mateega A et al. A pilot study of antituberculosis combinations comparing rifabutin with rifampicin in the treatment of HIV-1-associated tuberculosis: a single-blind randomized evaluation in Ugandan patients with HIV-1 infection and pulmonary tuberculosis. Tuberc Lung Dis 1995; 76: 210–18.

67. Narita M, Stambaugh JJ, Hollender ES et al. Use of rifabutin with protease inhibitors for human immunodeficiency virus-infected patients with tuberculosis. Clin Infect Dis 2000; 30: 779–83.

68. Kerr BM, Daniels R, Clendeninn N. Pharmacokinetic interaction of nelfinavir with half-dose rifabutin. Can J Infect Dis 1999; 10 (Suppl. B): 21B (Abstr.).

69. Gallicano K, Khaliq Y, Carignan G et al. A pharmacokinetic study of intermittent rifabutin dosing with a combination of ritonavir and saquinavir in patients infected with human immunodeficiency virus. Clin Pharmacol Ther 2001; 70: 149–58.

70. Khachi H, Ladenheim D, Orkin C et al. Pharmacokinetic interactions between rifabutin and lopinavir/ritonavir in HIV-infected patients with mycobacterial co-infection. HIV Med 2006; 7 (Suppl. 1): 3 (Oral abstr. O12).

71. Sanz J, Oliva J, Perez-Molina J et al. Treatment of tuberculosis in HIV-1-infected patients. Safety and antiretroviral efficacy of concomitant use of navirapine and rifampin. XIV International AIDS Conference, Barcelona, 2002 (Abstr. TuPeB4543).

72. Tibotec I. Prezista™ package insert. Raritan, NJ: Ortho Biotech Products, 2006.

73. Boehringer Ingelheim Pharmaceuticals Inc. Aptivus® package insert. Ridgefield, CT: Boehringer Ingelheim International, 2005.

74. van Heeswijk R. The effects of CYP3A4 modulation on the pharmacokinetics of TMC278, an investigational non-nucleoside reverse transcriptase inhibitor (NNRTI). Programme and Abstracts of the 7th International Workshop on Clinical Pharmacology of HIV Therapy, Lisbon, 20–22 April 2006 (Abstr. 74).

75. Abel S, Russell D, Ridgway C, Muirhead G. Overview of the drug–drug interaction data for maraviroc (UK-427,857). 6th International Workshop on Clinical Pharmacology of HIV Therapy, Quebec, 28–30 April 2005 (Abstr. 76).

76. Breen RAM, Lipman MCI, Johnson MA. Increased incidence of peripheral neuropathy with co-administration of stavudine and isoniazid in HIV infected individuals. AIDS 2000; 14: 615.

77. Dean GL, Edwards SG, Ives NJ et al. Treatment of tuberculosis in HIV-1 infected persons in the era of highly active antiretroviral therapy. AIDS 2002; 16: 75–83.

78. Breen RA, Miller RF, Gorsuch T et al. Adverse events and treatment interruption in tuberculosis patients with and without HIV co-infection. Thorax 2006; 61: 791.

79. Peloquin CA, MacPhee AA, Berning SE. Malabsorption of antimycobacterial medications. N Engl J Med 1993; 329: 1122–3 (letter).

80. Patel KB, Belmonte R, Grove HM. Drug malabsorption and resistant tuberculosis in HIV-infected patients. N Engl J Med 1995; 332: 336–7.

81. Berning SE, Huitt GA, Iseman MD, Peloquin CA. Malabsorption of antituberculosis medications by a patient with AIDS. N Engl J Med 1992; 327: 1817–18.

82. Peloquin CA, Nitta AT, Burman WJ et al. Low antituberculosis drug concentrations in patients with AIDS. Ann Pharmacother 1996; 30: 919–25.

83. Sahai J, Gallicano K, Swick L et al. Reduced plasma concentrations of antituberculous drugs in patients with HIV infection. Ann Intern Med 1997; 127: 289–93.

84. Perlman DC, Segal Y, Rosenkranz S et al. AIDS Clinical Trials Group 309 Team. The clinical pharmacokinetics of rifampin and ethambutol in HIV-infected persons with tuberculosis. Clin Infect Dis 2005; 41: 1638–47.

85. Tappero JW, Bradford WZ, Agerton TB et al. Serum concentrations of antimycobacterial drugs in patients with pulmonary tuberculosis in Botswana. Clin Infect Dis 2005; 41: 461–9.

86. Taylor J, Smith PJ. Does AIDS impair the absorption of antituberculosis agents? Int J Tuberc Lung Dis 1998; 2: 670–5.

87. Peloquin CA. Using therapeutic drug monitoring to dose the antimycobacterial drugs. Clin Chest Med 1997; 18: 79–87.

88. Peloquin CA. Therapeutic drug monitoring in the treatment of tuberculosis. Drugs 2002; 62: 2169–83.

89. Burman WJ, Jones BE. Treatment of HIV-related tuberculosis in the era of effective antiretroviral therapy. Am J Respir Crit Care Med 2001; 164: 7–12.

90. Navas E, Oliva J, Miralles P et al. Antiretroviral therapy in AIDS patient. XIV International AIDS Conference, Barcelona, 2002 (Abstr. THPeB7271).

91. Schiffer JT, Sterling TR. Timing of antiretroviral therapy initiation in tuberculosis patients with AIDS: a decision analysis. J Acquir Immun Defic Syndr 2007; 44: 229–34.

92. Fox W, Ellard GA, Mitchison DA. Studies on the treatment of tuberculosis undertaken by the British Medical Research Council Tuberculosis Units, 1946–1986, with relevant subsequent publications. Int J Tuberc Lung Dis 1999; 3: S231–79.

93. Centers for Disease Control. Prevention and treatment of tuberculosis among patients infected with human immunodeficiency virus: principles of therapy and revised recommendations. MMWR Morb Mortal Wkly Rep 1998; 47: RR-20.

94. Jones B, Otaya M, Rayos E et al. Directly observed therapy of highly active antiretroviral therapy in patients with HIV and tuberculosis. 12th World AIDS Conference, Geneva, 1998 (Abstr. 60582).

95. Chaisson RE, Clermont HC, Holt EA et al. Six-month supervised intermittent tuberculosis therapy in Haitian patients with and without HIV infection. Am J Respir Crit Care Med 1996; 154: 1034–8.

96. McGregor MM, Olliaro P, Wolmarans L et al. Efficacy and safety of rifabutin in the treatment of patients with newly diagnosed pulmonary tuberculosis. Am J Respir Crit Care Med 1996; 154: 1462–7.

97. Burman W, Benator D, Vernon A et al. Tuberculosis Trials Consortium. Acquired rifamycin resistance with twice-weekly treatment of HIV-related tuberculosis. Am J Respir Crit Care Med 2006; 173: 350.

98. Sterling TR, Alwood K, Gachuhi R et al. Relapse rates after short-course (6-month) treatment of tuberculosis in HIV-infected and uninfected persons. AIDS 1999; 13: 1899–904.

99. Kassim S, Sassan-Morokro M, Ackah A et al. Two-year follow-up of persons with HIV-1- and HIV-2-associated pulmonary tuberculosis treated with short-course chemotherapy in West Africa. AIDS 1995; 9: 1185–91.

100. Perriens JH, St Louis ME, Mukadi YB et al. Pulmonary tuberculosis in HIV infected patients in Zaire: a controlled trial of treatment for either 6 or 12 months. N Engl J Med 1995; 332: 779–84.

101. Joint Tuberculosis Committee of the British Thoracic Society. Chemotherapy and management of tuberculosis in the United Kingdom: recommendations 1998. Thorax 1998; 53: 536–48.

102. El-Sadr WM, Perlman DC, Denning E et al. A review of efficacy studies of 6-month short-course therapy for tuberculosis among patients infected with human immunodeficiency virus: differences in study outcomes. Clin Infect Dis 2001; 32: 623–32.

103. El-Sadr WM, Perlman DC, Matts JP et al. Evaluation of an intensive intermittent-induction regimen and duration of short course treatment for human immunodeficiency virus-related pulmonary tuberculosis. Clin Infect Dis 1998; 26: 148–58.

104. Nahid P, Gonzalez LC, Rudoy I et al. Treatment outcomes of patients with HIV and tuberculosis. Am J Respir Crit Care Med 2007; 175: 1199–206.

105. Lopez-Cortes LF, Marin-Niebla A, Lopez-Cortes LE et al. Influence of treatment and immunological recovery on tuberculosis relapses in HIV-infected patients. Int J Tuberc Lung Dis 2005; 9: 1385–90.

106. Anonymous. Acquired rifamycin resistance in persons with

advanced hiv disease being treated for active tuberculosis with intermittent rifamycin-based regimens. *MMWR Morb Mortal Wkly Rep* 2002; **51**: 214–15.

107. Collins KR, Quinones-Mateu ME, Toossi Z, Arts EJ. Impact of tuberculosis on HIV-1 replication, diversity, and disease progression. *AIDS Rev* 2002; **4**: 165–76.

108. Holden M, Dubin MR, Diamond PH. Frequency of negative intermediate-strength tuberculin sensitivity in patients with active tuberculosis. *N Engl J Med* 1971; **285**: 1506–509.

109. Graham NMH, Nelson KE, Solomon L *et al.* Prevalence of tuberculin positivity and skin test anergy in HIV-1-seropositive and seronegative intravenous drug users. *J Am Med Assoc* 1992; **267**: 369–73.

110. Markowitz N, Hansen NI, Wilcosky TC *et al.* Tuberculin and anergy testing in HIV-seropositive and HIV-seronegative persons. *Ann Intern Med* 1993; **119**: 185–93.

111. Huebner RE, Schein MF, Hall CA, Barnes SA. Delayed-type hypersensitivity anergy in human immunodeficiency virus-infected persons screened for infection with *Mycobacterium tuberculosis*. *Clin Infect Dis* 1994; **19**: 26–32.

112. Johnson MP, Coberly JS, Clermont HC *et al.* Tuberculin skin test reactivity among adults infected with human immunodeficiency virus. *J Infect Dis* 1992; **166**: 194–8.

113. Markowitz N, Hansen NI, Wilcosky TC *et al.* Tuberculin and anergy testing in HIV seropositive and HIV seronegative persons. Pulmonary complications of HIV infection study group. *Ann Intern Med* 1993; **119**: 241–3.

114. Chin DP, Osmond D, Page-Shafer K *et al.* Reliability of anergy skin testing in persons with HIV infection. *Am J Respir Crit Care Med* 1996; **153**: 1982–4.

115. Yanai H, Uthaivoravit W, Mastro TD *et al.* Utility of tuberculin and anergy skin testing in predicting tuberculosis infection inhuman immunodeficiency virus-infected persons in Thailand. *Int J Tuberc Lung Dis* 1997; **1**: 427–34.

116. Caiaffa WT, Graham NMH, Galai N, Rizzo RT, Nelson KE, Vlahov D. Instability of delayed-type hypersensitivity skin test anergy in human immunodeficiency virus infection. *Arch Intern Med* 1995; **155**: 2111–17.

117. Moreno S, Bavaia-Etxabury J, Bouza E *et al.* Risk for developing tuberculosis among anergic patients infected with HIV. *Ann Intern Med* 1993; **119**: 194–8.

118. Tsiouris SJ, Coetzee D, Toro PL, Austin J, Stein Z, El-Sadr W. Sensitivity analysis and potential uses of a novel gamma interferon release assay for diagnosis of tuberculosis. *J Clin Microbiol* 2006; **44**: 2844–50.

119. Rangaka MX, Diwakar L, Seldon R *et al.* Clinical, immunological, and epidemiological importance of antituberculosis T cell responses in HIV-infected Africans. *Clin Infect Dis* 2007; **44**: 1639–46.

120. Brock I, Ruhwald M, Lundgren B *et al.* Latent tuberculosis in HIV positive, diagnosed by the *M. tuberculosis* specific interferon-gamma test. *Respir Res* 2006; **7**: 56.

121. Luetkemeyer AF, Charlebois ED, Flores LL *et al.* Comparison of an interferon-gamma release assay with tuberculin skin testing in HIV-infected individuals. *Am J Respir Crit Care Med* 2007; **175**: 737–42.

122. Chaisson RE, Schecter GF, Theuer CP *et al.* Tuberculosis in patients with acquired immunodeficiency syndrome: clinical features, response to therapy, and survival. *Am Rev Respir Dis* 1987; **136**: 570–74.

123. Smieja MJ, Marchetti CA, Cook DJ, Smaill FM. Isoniazid for preventing tuberculosis in non-HIV infected persons. *Cochrane Database Syst Rev* 2000; (2): CD001363.

124. Gordin FM, Matts JP, Miller C *et al.* A controlled trial of isoniazid in persons with anergy and human immunodeficiency virus infection who are at high risk for tuberculosis. *N Engl J Med* 1997; **37**: 315–20.

125. Jordon TJ, Levit EM, Montgomery EL, Reichman LB. Isoniazid as

126. Quigley MA, Mwinga A, Hosp M *et al.* Long-term effect of preventive therapy for tuberculosis in a cohort of HIV-infected Zambian adults. *AIDS* 2001; **15**: 215–22.

127. Aisu T, Raviglione MC, van Praag E *et al.* Preventive chemotherapy for HIV-associated tuberculosis in Uganda: an operational assessment at a voluntary counselling and testing centre. *AIDS* 1995; **9**: 267–73.

128. Ayles H, Mukumbo D, Godfrey-Fausset P. Is it feasible to administer TB preventive therapy in Lusaka? XIII International AIDS Conference, Durban, 2000 (Abstr. ThPeB5212).

129. Charalambou SS, Fielding K, Day JH *et al.* Effectiveness of primary prophylaxis regimes among HIV infected employees in South Africa. XIV International Conference on AIDS, Barcelona, 2002 (Abstr. MoOrB1006).

130. Update: fatal and severe liver injuries associated with rifampicin and pyrazinamide for latent tuberculosis infection, and revisions in American Thoracic Society/CDC recommendations, United States, 2001. *Am J Respir Crit Care Med* 2001; **164**: 1319–20.

131. Gordin F, Chaisson RE, Matts JP *et al.* Rifampicin and pyrazinamide versus isoniazid for prevention of tuberculosis in HIV infected persons: an international randomized trial. *J Am Med Assoc* 2000; **283**: 1445–50.

132. Mwinga A, Hosp M, Godfrey-Faussett P *et al.* Twice weekly tuberculosis preventive therapy in HIV infection in Zambia. *AIDS* 1998; **12**: 2447–57.

133. Halsey NA, Coberly JS, Desormeaux J *et al.* Randomized trial of isoniazid versus rifampicin and pyrazinamide for the prevention of tuberculosis in HIV-1 infection. *Lancet* 1998; **351**: 786–92.

134. Sonnerbery P, Murray J, Glynn JR *et al.* HIV-1 and recurrence, relapse and reinfection of tuberculosis after cure: a cohort study in South African Mineworkers. *Lancet* 2001; **358**: 1687–93.

135. Warren RM, Van Helden PD. HIV-1 and tuberculosis infection. *Lancet* 2002; **359**: 1619–20.

136. Cohen T, Lipsitch M, Walensky RP, Murray M. Beneficial and perverse effects of isoniazid preventive therapy for latent tuberculosis infection in HIV-tuberculosis coinfected populations. *Proc Natl Acad Sci U S A* 2006; **103**: 7042–7.

137. Fitzgerald D, Desvarieux M, Severe P *et al.* Effect of post-treatment isoniazid on prevention of recurrent tuberculosis in HIV-1-infected individuals: a randomized trial. *Lancet* 2000; **356**: 1470–4.

138. Fielding KL, Hayes RJ, Charalambou SS *et al.* Efficacy of secondary isoniazid preventative therapy among HIV infected South Africans. XIV International AIDS Conference, Barcelona, 2002 (Abstr. ThPeB7275).

139. Haller L, Sossouhounto R, Coulibaly IM *et al.* Isoniazid plus sulphodoxine-pyrimethamine can reduce morbidity of HIV-positive patients treated for tuberculosis in Africa. A controlled clinical trial. *Chemotherapy* 1999; **45**: 452–65.

140. Lawn SD, Bekker LG, Miller RF. Immune reconstitution disease associated with mycobacterial infections in HIV-infected individuals receiving antiretrovirals. *Lancet Infect Dis* 2005; **5**: 361–73.

141. Crump JA, Tyrer MJ, Lloyd-Owen SJ *et al.* Miliary tuberculosis with paradoxical expansion of intracranial tuberculomas complicating human immunodeficiency virus infection in a patient receiving highly active antiretroviral therapy. *Clin Infect Dis* 1998; **26**: 1008–1009.

142. Furrer H, Malinverni R. Systemic inflammatory reaction after starting highly active antiretroviral therapy in AIDS patients treated for extrapulmonary tuberculosis. *Am J Med* 1999; **106**: 371–2.

143. John M, French MA. Exacerbation of the inflammatory response to *Mycobacterium tuberculosis* after antiretroviral therapy. *Med J Aust* 1998; **169**: 473–4.

144. Kunimoto DY, Chui L, Nobert E *et al.* Immune mediated 'HAART'

attack during treatment for tuberculosis: highly active antiretroviral therapy. *Int J Tuberc Lung Dis* 1999; **3**: 944–7.

145. Mofredj A, Guerin JM, Leibinger F *et al.* Paradoxical worsening in tuberculosis during therapy in an HIV-infected patient. *Infection* 1996; **24**: 390–91 (letter).

146. Ramdas K, Minamoto GY. Paradoxical presentation of intracranial tuberculomas after chemotherapy in a patient with AIDS. *Clin Infect Dis* 1994; **19**: 793–4 (letter).

147. Campbell IA, Dyson AJ. Lymph node tuberculosis: a comparison of various methods of treatment. *Tubercle* 1977; **58**: 171–9.

148. Choremis CB, Padiatellis C, Zoumboulakis D, Yannakos D. Transitory exacerbation of fever and roentgenographic findings during treatment of tuberculosis in children. *Am Rev Tuberc* 1955; **72**: 527–36.

149. Chambers ST, Record C, Hendricks WA *et al.* Paradoxical expansion of intracranial tuberculomas during chemotherapy. *Lancet* 1984; **2**: 181–4.

150. Afghani B, Lieberman JM. Paradoxical enlargement or development of intracranial tuberculomas during therapy: case report and review. *Clin Infect Dis* 1994; **19**: 1092–9.

151. Minguez C, Roca B, Gonzalez-Mino C *et al.* Superior vena cava syndrome during the treatment of pulmonary tuberculosis in an HIV-1 infected patient. *J Infect* 2000; **40**: 187–9.

152. Narita M, Ashkin D, Hollender ES *et al.* Paradoxical worsening of tuberculosis following antiretroviral therapy in patients with AIDS. *Am J Respir Crit Care Med* 1998; **158**: 157–61.

153. Navos S, Moreno L, Martin-Davila V *et al.* TB reactivation in AIDS patients treated with HAART. 39th Interscience Conference on Antimicrobial Agents and Chemotherapy, San Francisco, 1999.

154. Wendel KA, Alwood KS, Gachuhi R *et al.* Paradoxical worsening of tuberculosis in HIV-infected persons. *Chest* 2001; **120**: 193–7.

155. Michailidis C, Pozniak AL, Mandalia S *et al.* Clinical characteristics of IRD syndrome in patients with HIV and tuberculosis. *Antivir Ther* 2005; **10**: 417–22.

156. Foudraine NA, Hovenkamp E, Notermans DW *et al.* Immunopathology as a result of highly active antiretroviral therapy in HIV-1-infected patients. *AIDS* 1999; **13**: 177–84.

157. Judson MA. Highly active antiretroviral therapy for HIV with tuberculosis: pardon the granuloma. *Chest* 2002; **122**: 399–400, 597–602.

158. Bourgarit A, Carcelain G, Martinez V *et al.* Explosion of tuberculin-specific Th1-responses induces immune restoration syndrome in tuberculosis and HIV co-infected patients. *AIDS* 2006; **20**: F1–7.

159. Pires A, Nelson M, Pozniak AL *et al.* Mycobacterial immune reconstitution inflammatory syndrome in HIV-1 infection after antiretroviral therapy is associated with deregulated specific T-cell responses: beneficial effect of IL-2 and GM-CSF immunotherapy. *J Immune Based Ther Vaccines* 2005; **3**: 7.

160. Perez D, Liu Y, Jung T *et al.* Reconstitution of host immunity to *M. tuberculosis* in HIV-infected individuals. *Am J Respir Crit Care Med* 2000; **161**: A224 (Abstr.).

161. Price P, Mathiot N, Krueger R *et al.* Immune restoration disease in HIV patients given highly active antiretroviral therapy. *J Clin Virol* 2001; **22**: 279–87.

162. Price P, Morahan G, Huang D *et al.* Polymorphisms in cytokine genes define subpopulations of HIV-1 patients who experienced immune restoration diseases. *AIDS* 2002; **16**: 2043–7.

163. French MA, Price P, Stone SF. Immune restoration disease after antiretroviral therapy. *AIDS* 2004; **18**: 1615–27.

164. Fishman JE, Saraf-Lavi E, Narita M *et al.* Transient chest radiographic worsening after initiation of antiretroviral therapy. *AJR Am J Roentgenol* 2000; **174**: 43–9.

165. Manosuthi W, Kiertiburanakul S, Phoorisri T, Sungkanuparph S. Immune reconstitution inflammatory syndrome of tuberculosis among HIV-infected patients receiving antituberculous and antiretroviral therapy. *J Infect* 2006; **53**: 357–63.

166. Lawn SD, Myer L, Bekker LG, Wood R. Tuberculosis-associated immune reconstitution disease: incidence, risk factors and impact in an antiretroviral treatment service in South Africa. *AIDS* 2007; **21**: 335–41.

167. Shelburne SA, Visnegarwala F, Darcourt J *et al.* Incidence and risk factors for immune reconstitution inflammatory syndrome during highly active antiretroviral therapy. *AIDS* 2005; **19**: 399–406.

168. Hollender E, Narita M, Ashkin D *et al.* CNS manifestations of paradoxical reactions in HIV+ TB patients on HAART. 7th Conference on Retroviruses and Opportunistic Infections, San Francisco, 2000 (Abstr. 258).

169. Gandhi NR, Moll A, Sturm AW *et al.* Extensively drug-resistant tuberculosis as a cause of death in patients co-infected with tuberculosis and HIV in a rural area of South Africa. *Lancet* 2006; **368**: 1575–80.

170. Hannan MM, Peres H, Maltez F *et al.* Investigation and control of a large outbreak of multi-drug resistant tuberculosis at a central Lisbon hospital. *J Hosp Infect* 2001; **72**: 91–7.

171. Moro ML, Errante I, Infuso A *et al.* Effectiveness of infection control measures in controlling a nosocomial outbreak of multidrug-resistant tuberculosis among HIV patients in Italy. *Int J Tuberc Lung Dis* 2000; **41**: 61–8.

172. Breathnach AS, de Ruiter A, Holdsworth GM *et al.* An outbreak of multi-drug-resistant tuberculosis in a London teaching hospital. *J Hosp Infect* 1998; **92**: 111–7.

173. Coronado VG, Beck-Sague CM, Hutton MD *et al.* Transmission of multidrug-resistant *Mycobacterium tuberculosis* among persons with human immunodeficiency virus infection in an urban hospital: epidemiologic and restriction fragment length polymorphism analysis. *J Infect Dis* 1993; **1684**: 1052–5.

174. Centers for Disease Control. Outbreak of multidrug-resistant tuberculosis at a hospital – New York City, 1991. *MMWR Morb Mortal Wkly Rep* 1993; **427**: 433–4.

175. Pitchenik AE, Burr J, Laufer M *et al.* Outbreaks of drug-resistant tuberculosis at AIDS centre. *Lancet* 1990; **336**: 440–1.

176. Conover C, Ridzon R, Valway S *et al.* Outbreak of multidrug-resistant tuberculosis at a methadone treatment program. *Int J Tuberc Lung Dis* 2001; **1**: 59–64.

177. Centers for Disease Control. Transmission of multidrug-resistant tuberculosis among immunocompromised persons in a correctional system – New York, 1991. *MMWR Morb Mortal Wkly Rep* 1992; **4128**: 507–9.

178. Shafer RW, Small PM, Larkin C *et al.* Temporal trends and transmission patterns during the emergence of multidrug-resistant tuberculosis in New York City: a molecular epidemiologic assessment. *J Infect Dis* 1995; **171**: 170–6.

179. Moro ML, Gori A, Errante I *et al.* An outbreak of multidrug-resistant tuberculosis involving HIV-infected patients of two hospitals in Milan, Italy. Italian Multidrug-Resistant Tuberculosis Outbreak Study Group. *AIDS* 1998; **129**: 1095–102.

180. Maloney SA, Pearson ML, Gordon MT *et al.* Efficacy of control measures in preventing nosocomial transmission of multidrug-resistant tuberculosis to patients and health care workers. *Ann Intern Med* 1995; **122**: 90–95.

181. Stroud LA, Tokars JI, Grieco MH *et al.* Evaluation of infection control measures in preventing the nosocomial transmission of multidrug-resistant *Mycobacterium tuberculosis* in a New York City hospital. *Infect Control Hosp Epidemiol* 1995; **16**: 141–7.

182. Passannante MR, Gallagher CT, Reichman LB. Preventive therapy for contacts of multidrug-resistant tuberculosis. A Delphi survey. *Chest* 1994; **1062**: 431–4.

183. Ritacco V, Di Lonardo M, Reniero A *et al.* Nosocomial spread of human munodeficiency virus-related multidrug-resistant tuberculosis in Buenos Aires. *J Infect Dis* 1997; **176**: 637–42.

184. Small PM, Shafer RW, Hopewell PC *et al.* Exogenous reinfection with multidrug-resistant *Mycobacterium tuberculosis* in patients with advanced HIV infection. *N Engl J Med* 1993; **328**: 1137–44.

185. Cobo J, Asensio A, Moreno S *et al.* Risk factors for nosocomial transmission of multidrug-resistant tuberculosis due to

Mycobacterium bovis among HIV-infected patients. *Int J Tuberc Lung Dis* 2001; **5**: 413–8.

186. Telzak EE, Chirgwin KD, Nelson ET *et al.* Predictors for multidrug-resistant tuberculosis among HIV-infected patients and response to specific drug regimens. Terry Beirn Community Programs for Clinical Research on AIDS. CPCRA and the AIDS Clinical Trials Group. ACTG, National Institutes for Health. *Int J Tuberc Lung Dis* 1999; **4**: 337–43.

187. Salomon N, Perlman DC, Friedmann P *et al.* Predictors and outcome of multidrug-resistant tuberculosis. *Clin Infect Dis* 1995; **215**: 1245–52.

188. Park MM, Davis AL, Schluger NW *et al.* Outcome of MDR-TB patients, 1983–1993. Prolonged survival with appropriate therapy. *Am J Respir Crit Care Med* 1996; **153**: 317–24.

189. Turett GS, Telzak EE, Torian LV *et al.* Improved outcomes for patients with multidrug-resistant tuberculosis. *Clin Infect Dis* 1995; **215**: 1238–44.

190. Fischl MA, Daikos GL, Uttamchandani RB *et al.* Clinical presentation and outcome of patients with HIV infection and tuberculosis caused by multiple-drug-resistant bacilli. *Ann Intern Med* 1992; **117**: 184–90.

21

Tuberculosis and migration

PAUL ALBERT AND PETER DO DAVIES

INTRODUCTION

Tuberculosis (TB) has been infecting humans for many centuries. Evidence for this includes the finding of a TB complex in 1990 in a 1000-year-old mummified Peruvian,[1] centuries before Columbus discovered the New World, and DNA analysis confirming the presence of *Mycobacterium tuberculosis* in Egyptian mummies up to 4500 years old.[2] In the early seventeenth century, the incidence of TB in Western Europe began to increase, probably reflecting overcrowding as populations became more urbanized. From the 1700s, as Western Europeans explored, traded and colonized, they carried their diseases with them, including TB. The British took the disease to the Australian Aborigines[3] and New Zealand Maoris.[4] European traders took the disease to Africa,[5] India[6] and to the native Indians of North America. As recently as the 1950s, non-natives were still introducing TB to the Inuit Eskimos of Canada[7] and natives of the highlands of Papua New Guinea.[4] This led to considerable morbidity and mortality from TB and devastating epidemics amongst populations which had previously had very little exposure to the disease.[8]

In Western Europe, rates of the disease peaked in the early 1800s, when approximately one death in four was caused by TB. However, a combination of advances in medical science, public health and socioeconomic development resulted in better disease contol. By 1850, TB accounted for 12 per cent of deaths, and this had fallen to 9 per cent by the beginning of the twentieth century. In the UK, TB incidence continued to fall through the twentieth century: the TB notification system for England and Wales (implemented in 1913) recorded 300 new cases per 100 000 people per year in the early twentieth century. By 1987, this had fallen to 10 new cases per 100 000 people. A similar declining incidence was observed in the native-born population of most developed nations, with only small pockets of high incidence, mostly among disadvantaged groups, such as the homeless[9] and indigenous populations.[10]

This led many to believe that TB could soon be entirely eradicated, in the developed world at least. However, in the past two decades, this downward trend has reversed in many developed countries. The major reasons for this are HIV/AIDS, large-scale immigration and drug resistance.

EXPERIENCE OF IMMIGRATION AND TB IN THE UK

Immigration in the 1950s onwards

Since the end of the Second World War, there have been high rates of migration to the UK from its former colonies. Generally, this has meant a population flow from areas of high TB incidence to a low-incidence area.

The first group to come under scrutiny were the Irish.[11] In a study of TB hospital patients in London, a higher proportion of Irish immigrants were found to be tuberculin negative than the English. The immigrant Irish had higher rates of TB than those born to Irish parents in the UK. There was also a higher incidence of pleural infection and primary disease in the Irish than in English patients of similar age. The authors suggested that TB had passed through the UK in a 'wave-like epidemic' affecting the English population first, which at that time resulted in a more resistant

English and a more susceptible Irish population. A mass miniature radiography (MMR) study in 1958 confirmed the high TB rates in the Irish and also identified higher rates in immigrants from the West Indies.[12] In a paper looking at epidemiological trends in TB and sarcoidosis in London from 1958 to 1963, Brett observed a decline in rates among the Irish, but an increase among West Indian immigrants.[13] A paper looking at immigrant workers (mostly Chinese) in Soho in 1961 found rates of TB to be twice as high in immigrant workers compared with the indigenous population and more than 10 times as high in workers from Hong Kong.[14]

TB in immigrants from the Indian subcontinent

In a review of TB notifications in Birmingham in 1958, Springett et al.[15] showed a steady rise in the proportion of notifications among immigrants born in India and Pakistan, with rates four to six times higher than the white population. The authors suggested that immigrants brought their disease with them and higher rates reflected rates in the countries of origin. Nicol Roe[16] made similar observations in 1959, but found that the majority of immigrants did not develop disease until a year or more after entry to the UK, and that a large proportion of contacts were tuberculin negative, leading him to conclude that the disease was acquired mainly in the UK. Further studies by Springett et al. in Birmingham,[17] Stevenson in Bradford[18] and Aspin in Wolverhampton[19] confirmed increasing incidence in immigrants from the Indian subcontinent. The British Tuberculosis Association survey[20] of all new cases of TB in England and Wales in 1965 found that 16.5 per cent of the 3806 TB cases were in immigrants (who made up 4 per cent of the population). Of the notifications, 9.6 per cent were among those born in India and Pakistan (who made up less than 1 per cent of the population). A similar survey in 1971 looked at 3521 notifications in a 4-month period. At that point, 5 per cent of the population were born outside the UK, but they made up 32 per cent of notifications.

Springett[21] continued to monitor TB rates in Birmingham. He found a fall in the annual rates for UK-born males from 0.68 to 0.28 per 1000 per year between 1961 and 1971, and a fall in UK-born females from 0.39 to 0.18. However, the rate among Indian-born males in that time period increased from 4.5 to 5.1 and for Indian-born females from 4.2 to 8.3 per 1000 per year. Overall, the rates in the immigrant population were highest in young adults. Springett believed that the increased incidence rates would cease when the immigration of dependents was completed. He also showed that non-respiratory TB accounted for 11 per cent of cases among the UK born, but 40 per cent of those born in the Indian subcontinent. McNicol et al.[22] in Brent demonstrated a rising trend in notification rates in the Asian population from 1964 to 1970, but also showed that immigrants had less extensive disease than the white

population and were more likely to be sputum smear negative.

A 1971 survey[23] found that notification rates for immigrant groups tended to be highest for recent arrivals, reducing progressively for immigrants who had been in the UK for longer. Pakistani and Bangladeshi females showed the highest incidence (1109 per 100 000 per annum), of whom 80 per cent had entered the country during the previous 2 years. In comparison, the rate for Indian males was 414 per 100 000 per annum, of whom 65 per cent had entered the country in the previous 2 years.

Non-respiratory disease

In 1961, Silver and Steel[24] noted the high incidence of mediastinal involvement in Asians. A survey of the 4172 TB notifications in a 6-month period in 1978–79 found that the incidence of bone or joint TB was 29 per 100 000 per year for those of Indian subcontinent ethnic origin, and 0.34 per 100 000 in the white group.[25] Among patients in Bradford with gastrointestinal TB (1967–77), 45 of 52 affected patients were Asian.[26] However, a more recent survey of the Bangladeshi community of East London found a significant fall in the incidence of abdominal TB from 7.4 per 100 000 per year for the period 1985–89 to 2.5 per 100 000 per year for 1997–2001.[27]

The phenomenon of increased extrathoracic disease in immigrants has been seen elsewhere. Among 3982 cases of TB in New York City in 1995–96, patients born in the Middle East (odds ratio 3.9, $p = 0.0001$), India (odds ratio 2.5, $p = 0.0007$), sub-Saharan Africa (odds ratio 2.6, $p = 0.0001$) and the Caribbean (odds ratio 2.0, $p = 0.0001$) were more likely to have extrapulmonary disease than patients born in the USA.[28]

Trends in the 1970s and 1980s

Although the initial studies in the 1950s and 1960s were based on where patients were born, by the 1970s, as their offspring were born in the UK, it became important to assess the ethnic origin when carrying out epidemiological studies. The Medical Research Council Tuberculosis and Chest Diseases Unit surveyed all TB notifications in England and Wales from October 1978 to March 1979[29] and, using estimates of ethnic origin from a housing survey for England,[30] concluded the following:

1 Of patients with 'new' disease, 57 per cent were white and 35 per cent of Indian subcontinent (ISC) origin (who made up 2 per cent of the population).
2 Rates of disease were 30 times higher for respiratory disease and 80 times higher for non-respiratory disease among those of ISC origin than the white population.
3 Rates for respiratory disease were higher in white men than white women, whereas the sex incidence for respiratory disease was equal in the ISC population. Rates

Table 21.1   Annual notification rates for newly notified previously untreated patients for England.

Ethnic origin	1978/9 Population estimate (000)	1978/9 Rate per 100 000	1983 Population estimate (000)	1983 Rate per 100 000	1988 Population estimate (000)	1988 Rate per 100 000
White	43 320	9.4	42 994	6.9	43 938	4.7
Indian	525	354.0	773	178.0	800	134.6
Pakistani/ Bangladeshi	248	353.0	422	169.0	541	100.5
West Indian	514	30.0	494	30.0	464	29.2
Other	425	97.0	634	47.0	792	25.9
Total[a]	45 779	16.4	46 164	12.2	46 829	8.6

[a]Includes patients whose ethnic origin was unclassified.

for non-respiratory disease were much higher in ISC females than males, but similar in white males and females.

4 Fifty-six per cent of the ISC group with non-respiratory disease had lymph node disease. Genitourinary disease was more common in the white group, affecting 30 per cent of those with non-respiratory TB.

5 The extent of disease on chest x-ray was on average less in the ISC group compared with the white group and cavitation was less frequent.

6 Patients with pulmonary disease were more likely to be sputum smear and culture positive in the white group compared with the ISC group.

7 Children born to ISC parents in the UK had rates three times those of white children. ISC children born abroad had rates that were 10 times greater.

8 Drug resistance in the white group was 1.6 per cent of isolates, compared with 7.5 per cent in the ISC group.

Subsequent studies in the 1980s painted an optimistic picture of the trends. This showed a halving of the rates in the white population between 1978 and 1988. Rates among the ISC group decreased three-fold (Table 21.1).

Declining figures were seen elsewhere in the Western world, leading many to believe that TB in these parts could soon be eradicated. There were still small pockets of disease, such as among the homeless.

Further immigration and increasing TB notifications in the UK

The term 'immigrant' encompasses many different groups. The majority of immigration to the UK in the 1950s–1970s comprised mostly of regulated migration patterns, mainly people moving to the former colonial motherland for economic or family reasons. However, particularly in the past two decades, there have been large flows of irregular migration movements, in the form of refugee claimants and asylum seekers, people who have been trafficked and smuggled, along with migrant workers and foreign students.[31] Many of these people originate from countries with high TB incidence (Figure 21.1). Since the early 1990s, there have been large increases in migrants from several sub-Saharan African countries.[32] Many of these countries have experienced large increases in TB incidence (fuelled to a large extent by the HIV epidemic) in recent years.[33] The majority of immigrants to the UK in recent years have settled in London.

A total of 8113 TB cases were reported in England, Wales and Northern Ireland in 2005 (14.7 per 100 000 population), an 11 per cent increase compared with 2004. The rate among UK-born cases is stable at 4.2 per 100 000; the increase is predominantly among individuals born outside the UK (Figures 21.2 and 21.3).

Of the UK TB cases in 2001–2003, 67 per cent were foreign born. Additionally, rates of TB among UK-born

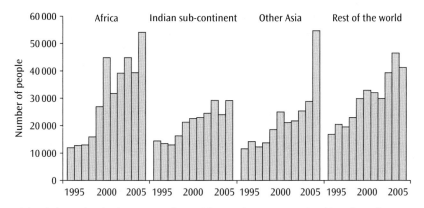

Figure 21.1   Grants of settlement in the UK 1995–2005, excluding European Economic Area Nationals and Switzerland. *Source*: Home Office Control of Immigration Statistics 2005.

(1) Includes nationals of Cyprus, Czech Republic, Estoria, Hugary, Latvia, Lithuania, Malta, Poland, Slovakia and Slovenia before 1 May 2004, but excludes them from this date.

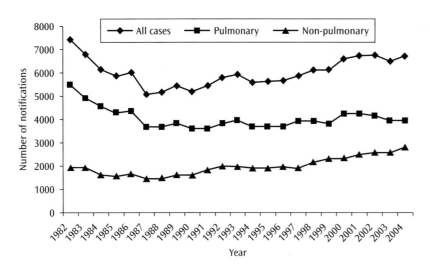

Figure 21.2 Pulmonary and non-pulmonary tuberculosis notifications, England and Wales, 1982–2004. *Source*: Statutory Notifications of Infectious Diseases (NOIDs). Prepared by Communicable Disease Surveillance Centre (CDSC), Health Protection Agency Centre for Infections.

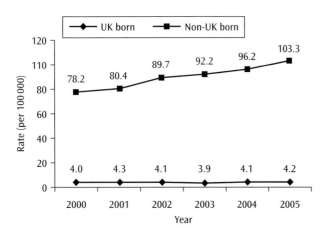

Figure 21.3 Tuberculosis rates by place of birth (UK born versus non-UK born), England, Wales and Northern Ireland, 2000–2005. *Sources*: Enhanced Tuberculosis Surveillance, Labour Force Survey population estimates. Prepared by Health Protection Agency Centre for Infections.

ethnic minority groups remain higher than rates in the white population.[34] This may be due to close contact with infectious cases within the UK or travel to high incidence areas (for example, to visit family).

The highest number of TB cases is seen in the ISC group (Figure 21.4). However, the rate per 100 000 population is twice as high in the black African group compared with the ISC group (Figure 21.5). Many of these people originated from conflict areas of sub-Saharan Africa, where years of civil war have led to poverty and breakdown of the social and health structures, leading to a surge in disease including TB. The fall of the Iron Curtain in 1989 followed by expansion of the European Union and relaxation of immigration controls within Europe has resulted in large-volume migration from former Eastern Bloc countries to Western Europe, including the UK. The UK has also taken migrants fleeing the troubles in the Balkans in the 1990s. Many of these migrants have come from areas of higher TB incidence than the UK. However, their impact in terms of new TB cases is far smaller than the numbers contributed by the black African, Indian, Pakistani and Bangladeshi groups (Figure 21.4).

The UK data reflect the two different populations of UK-born and non-UK-born cases being affected in different ways. Figure 21.6 demonstrates the peak incidence in

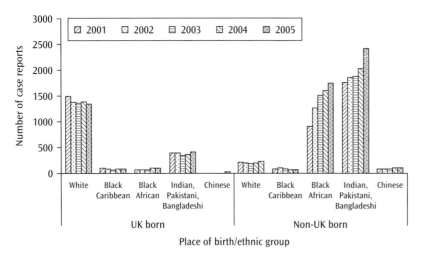

Figure 21.4 Tuberculosis case reports by place of birth and ethnic group, England, Wales and Northern Ireland, 2001–2005. 'Other' ethnic groups not shown. *Source*: Enhanced Tuberculosis Surveillance. Prepared by Health Protection Agency Centre for Infections.

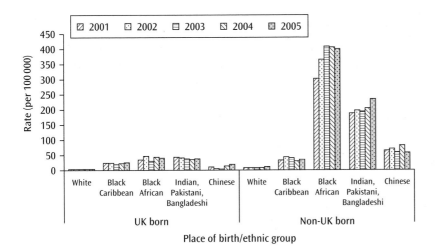

Figure 21.5 Tuberculosis rates by place of birth and ethnic group, England, Wales and Northern Ireland, 2001–2005. 'Other' ethnic groups not shown. *Sources*: Enhanced Tuberculosis Surveillance, Labour Force Survey population estimates. Prepared by Health Protection Agency Centre for Infections.

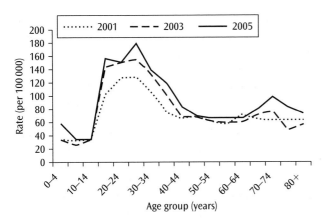

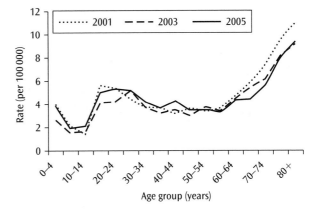

Figure 21.6 Tuberculosis rates in non-UK born people by age group, England, Wales and Northern Ireland, 2001–2005. *Sources*: Enhanced Tuberculosis Surveillance, Labour Force Survey population estimates. Prepared by Health Protection Agency Centre for Infections.

Figure 21.7 Tuberculosis rates in people born in the UK by age group, England, Wales and Northern Ireland, 2001–2005. *Sources*: Enhanced Tuberculosis Surveillance, Labour Force Survey population estimates. Prepared by Health Protection Agency Centre for Infections, Drug Resistance and Immigration.

the younger age group (20–30 years) for non-UK born. This pattern would have been similar for UK-born cases in the eighteenth, nineteenth and early twentieth centuries.

For the UK-born population, peak incidence is now occurring in the later decades (Figure 21.7), largely reflecting reactivation of the disease in a group of people who grew up when TB was more widespread.

The 2005 surveillance figures show that the proportion of TB cases with isoniazid resistance in patients who had previously had TB was three times greater in the non-UK born group than those born in the UK. More than 4 per cent of non-UK-born cases who had previously had TB had multidrug resistance (MDR): there were no cases of MDR in the UK-born group who had previously had TB (Figure 21.8).

EXPERIENCE OF IMMIGRATION AND TB IN THE USA

Most migrants to the USA originate from Mexico, the Philippines, Vietnam, India and China (Table 21.2) and

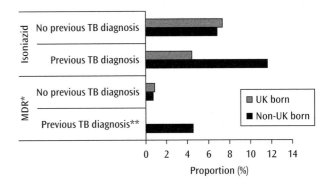

Figure 21.8 Proportion of antituberculosis drug resistance at start of treatment, by place of birth and previous tuberculosis (TB) diagnosis status, England, Wales and Northern Ireland, 2005. *Multidrug resistant (resistance to at least isoniazid and rifampicin); **no UK-born MDR cases with a previous TB diagnosis. *Sources*: Enhanced Tuberculosis Surveillance, MycobNet. Prepared by Health Protection Agency Centre for Infections.

Table 21.2 Tuberculosis in foreign-born people in 2004 by country of origin and time in the USA.

Country	Time in the USA (years)	Cases in 2004[a] No. (%)	Population	Case rate (per 100 000)	Estimated case rate in country of origin (per 100 000)
Mexico	Total	1976	10 404 919	19.0	33
	1	362 (22)	482 926	75.0	
	>1 to ≤5	435 (26)	1 974 036	22.0	
	>5	876 (52)	7 947 958	11.0	
Philippines	Total	829	1 594 083	52.0	296
	≤1	216 (27)	39 804	542.7	
	>1 to ≤5	124 (15)	187 778	66.0	
	>5	414 (51)	1 366 500	30.3	
Vietnam	Total	619	1 067	58.0	178
	≤1	113 (21)	21 711	520.5	
	>1 to ≤5	71 (13)	81 606	87.0	
	>5	352 (66)	964 328	36.5	
India	Total	557	1 386 321	40.2	168
	≤1	104 (22)	69 398	149.9	
	>1 to ≤5	165 (35)	326 999	50.5	
	>5	205 (43)	989 924	20.7	
China	Total	352	1 239 346	28.4	102
	≤1	63 (21)	48 850	129.0	
	>1 to ≤5	58 (19)	218 521	26.5	
	>5	186 (61)	971 975	19.1	
Haiti	Total	248	450 366	55.1	323
	≤1	42 (19)	9809	428.2	
	>1 to ≤5	74 (34)	75 278	98.3	
	>5	103 (47)	365 279	28.2	
South Korea	Total	219	430 491	50.9	87
	≤1	28 (15)	17 692	158.3	
	>1 to ≤5	41 (22)	61 298	66.9	
	>5	114 (62)	351 501	32.4	
Guatemala	Total	190	593 271	32.0	74
	≤1	49 (28)	28 360	172.8	
	>1 to ≤5	69 (40)	118 275	58.3	
	>5	55 (32)	446 636	12.3	
Ethiopia	Total	169	106 310	159.0	356
	≤1	68 (43)	4488	1515.2	
	>1 to ≤5	42 (27)	22 239	188.9	
	>5	47 (30)	79 583	59.1	
Peru	Total	159	338 041	47.0	188
	≤1	27 (18)	11 572	233.3	
	>1 to ≤5	63 (43)	69 778	90.3	
	>5	58 (39)	256 691	22.6	

[a]Total cases includes people with unknown year of entry into the United States. These people are excluded from further analysis.
Source: Ref. 46.

the increased TB rates in these groups compared with the USA-born population have been well documented since the 1970s.[35–37] Particularly high rates of disease and drug resistance have been described in refugees.[38,39] As in the UK, extrapulmonary TB was seen more frequently in ethnic minorities and the foreign born, the most common site being the lymph system.[40] Of foreign-born people

entering the USA, 51.5 per cent present with TB within 5 years.[41]

Particularly high rates of disease and multidrug resistance have been noted in Haitian immigrants, attributed in part to the high rates of HIV in this group.[42,43]

Since the 1950s, a steady decline in TB rates in the USA was observed. However, a resurgence occurred between

Table 21.3 Case rate for foreign-born people by world region of origin in 2004.

Region		Time in the United States		
	Overall rate	≤1 year	>1 to ≤5 years	>5 years
Sub-Saharan Africa	79.0	1186.9	91.5	28.0
South Asia	35.5	178.5	51.6	21.6
East Asia and the Pacific	37.0	286.6	48.7	26.3
Latin America, South America and the Caribbean	16.1	81.8	26.2	10.2
Eastern Europe and Central Asia	16.8	65.4	19.2	12.6
Middle East and North Africa	7.5	46.8	14.6	5.2
Low-incidence countries (Canada, Japan, New Zealand, Australia, Western Europe)	1.7	3.0	2.0	1.6

Source: Ref. 46.

1985 and 1992. This increase was attributed to the HIV epidemic, deficient infrastructure, immigration and widespread occurrence of multidrug-resistant TB strains. As a result, a national action plan to combat multidrug resistance was devised and increased resources channelled into TB control. This has led to a fall in TB rates since 1992.[44]

In 2005, there were 14 093 reported cases of TB (4.8 cases per 100 000 population). This was the lowest recorded rate since 1953, when national reporting began. The incidence rate was 8.7 times greater in foreign-born people than US born. Hispanics, black people and Asians had TB rates 7.3, 8.3 and 19.6 times higher than white people, respectively. The number of multidrug-resistant TB cases increased 13.3 per cent compared with 2004.[45]

Guidelines from the Centers for Disease Control and Prevention (CDC) and the American Thoracic Society recommend testing for (and treating) latent TB infection only among foreign-born people from high-incidence countries who have been in the USA for 5 years or less. However, data from 2004 showed that almost 25 per cent of all TB cases in the USA occurred in foreign-born people who had resided in the USA for longer than 5 years,[46] which would mean that a number of TB cases that are yet to activate would be missed by following this recommendation. Table 21.3 demonstrates that certain 'high-risk' populations who had lived in the USA for more than 5 years (such as individuals born in the Philippines, Vietnam, South Korea and Ethiopia) had a higher TB incidence than other 'high-risk' foreign-born populations who had lived in the USA for less than 5 years (such as individuals born in Mexico and China). As such, there would be a case for offering latent TB screening to all foreign-born populations from these 'very-high-risk' groups even if they have been resident for more than 5 years.

Since 1993, the total foreign-born population in the USA has increased by 61.6 per cent and this population accounted for 54.3 per cent of TB notifications for 2005. However, despite this increase, the total number of TB cases reported in this population has not changed substantially, resulting in a decline of 36 per cent in the TB rate among foreign-born people (from 34 per 100 000 in 1993

to 21.8 in 2005). Tables 21.2 and 21.3 may help explain why the USA has experienced improvement in TB incidence compared with the UK: the two countries receive their immigrants from very different populations. In 2004, the largest immigrant group to the USA came from Mexico (approximately 10.5 million individuals) with a TB incidence rate of 19 per 100 000. In contrast, the majority of the UK's immigrants in 2005 originated in Africa, the ISC and Asia (with TB incidence rates of up to 400 per 100 000 in some groups, Figure 21.1). However, there is some concern in the USA about the increased MDR rates and a slowing in the annual incidence decline. There are also calls for more to be done to address the disproportionately high rates in the US-born Hispanic, black and Asian populations.

EXPERIENCE OF IMMIGRATION AND TB IN CANADA

The indigenous population of Canada (Indians and Inuit) were exposed to TB by European arrivals in the sixteenth and seventeenth centuries, causing significant morbidity and mortality. High rates in this population persist.[47] A wave of immigration came in the mid-1960s with easing of immigration restrictions. High TB rates up to 6800 per 100 000 were described in Chinese immigrants between 1964 and 1968.[48]

Canada also received a number of Ugandan Asians in the early 1970s. TB prevalence was high in this group,[49] as well as increased drug resistance and lymphadenitis.[50] In the 1970s, Enarson and colleagues found that TB rates in Scandinavian immigrants to Canada, even after a long duration of residence in their country of adoption, were very similar to rates in the country of birth. They found that the majority of cases became infected before the age of 20 years and concluded that the early experience of TB predetermines future susceptibility of the disease throughout the lifespan of the immigrant group. The question 'where did you live in your childhood?' is therefore very important.[51,52]

Currently, Canada receives more than 200 000 immigrants per year and these account for 92 per cent of TB

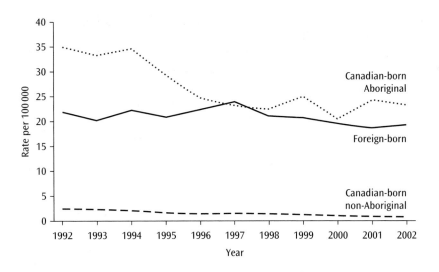

Figure 21.9 Tuberculosis incidence by origin (Canada): 1992–2002. *Source:* Tuberculosis in Canada 2002: Public Agency of Canada.

cases in Toronto. A retrospective study of immigrants to Ontario between 1990 and 1997 showed that TB rates in recent immigrants was 23 times higher than in Canadian-born, non-aboriginal people.[53] The highest rates were seen in the 16–30 years and >65 years age groups, and in immigrants from sub-Saharan Africa (followed by India and Asia). The risk decreased significantly in the first 1–2 years after arrival.

Overall, Canada has seen small falls in the incidence rate of TB in recent years in overall, foreign-born and Canadian-born (both aboriginal and non-aboriginal) groups (Figure 21.9).

EXPERIENCE OF IMMIGRATION AND TB IN EUROPE

Generally, a similar picture to that seen in the UK is seen elsewhere in Western Europe and Scandinavia where there has been significant immigration from high-incidence countries. In Norway, the proportion of immigrants in the total population increased from 2.4 per cent in the mid-1970s to 6.9 per cent in 2002.[54] The majority of immigrants came from Africa (mostly from Somalia) and Asia (mostly from Pakistan and Vietnam). In 2002, the TB incidence was 1.4 per 100 000 among those born in Norway (one of the lowest figures in the world) and 61.9 per 100 000 among immigrants.[55] Most cases presented within the first 2 years after migration, although the risk for developing TB remained much higher than the native population for many years after immigration. DNA probing of the strains of *M. tuberculosis* isolated between 1994 and 1998 suggested that most immigrants were infected before arrival in Norway, with low transmission after arrival.[56]

Denmark has seen a small fall in native-born incidence rates between 1985 and 2000, but a large increase among immigrant groups, particularly Somalis, leading to increases in the overall TB incidence rates. Overall, 9.5 per cent of all Somalis who arrived in Denmark were diagnosed with TB during their first 7 years of residence.[57] The

rate within the Somali immigrant population was comparable with, or even higher than, the estimated incidence within Somalia. Only a gradual reduction in incidence was seen after migration. Using DNA probing on isolates (1996–98), Lillebaek and colleagues[58] concluded that, among the Somalis with TB, 74.9 per cent appeared to have been infected outside Denmark, 23.3 per cent could have been infected in Denmark by other Somalis, and 1.8 per cent could have been infected by Danes. Likewise, they calculated that only 0.9 per cent of all Danish TB patients appeared to be infected by Somalis.

A retrospective study in the Netherlands reported 2661 legal immigrants identified with pulmonary TB between 1996 and 2000 (in 2000 there were just under 2 million immigrants residing in the Netherlands, of a total population of nearly 16 million). Average incidence rates after immigration were 379 per 100 000 per year in Somalis in comparison with approximately 3 per 100 000 in the indigenous Dutch population.[59] As a whole, there was a gradual reduction in incidence rates with years after migration, although the decline was not as steep as might be expected, bearing in mind that recent infection (more likely in the high-prevalence country of origin) is a known risk factor for developing active TB.[60] The authors postulate three reasons for this: (1) The proportion of immigrants who were recently infected or reinfected may already have been low at the time of immigration. (2) The risk of reactivation of latent TB infection in immigrant populations may be higher than the risk in white non-immigrant populations. (3) Immigrants residing in the Netherlands may have acquired new infections or reinfections, either through transmission from TB contacts within the Netherlands or through frequent visits to their country of origin.

There is mounting concern about the relationship between immigration and the development of multidrug-resistant TB. Surveillance of TB in France between 1992 and 1999 reported that the prevalence of multidrug-resistant TB was low (<1 per cent), but 55.7 per cent of cases were foreign born. However, the authors reflect that a number of such cases had come to France specifically to be treated for the multidrug-resistant TB.[61] In 2006, a systematic review of multidrug-resistant TB in Europe found that multidrug-resistant TB patients were more likely to be foreign born, but this may be confounded by previous treatment.[62] A UK study found that cases treated abroad were at higher risk of multidrug-resistant TB than those treated in the UK, regardless of birthplace.[63]

EXPERIENCE OF IMMIGRATION AND TB IN AUSTRALIA AND NEW ZEALAND

As in Canada, the indigenous people of Australia and New Zealand suffered large-scale morbidity and mortality from TB brought over by European colonizers.

The countries which neighbour Australia account for one-quarter of the world's TB notifications.[64] The majority of Australia's migrant population (and majority of TB cases) originate from Asia. Among immigrants from Vietnam and the Philippines, there is a high incidence of drug resistance.[65,66]

Australia has one of the most stringent immigration systems in the world. Surveillance for TB among candidate immigrants is governed by the migration regulations of the Migration Act 1958 and consists of premigration screening and post-arrival assessment of high-risk individuals identified in the original screening.

In Australia, the National Notifiable Disease Surveillance System received 1076 TB notifications in 2004. Of these, 1043 were new cases and 33 were relapses. The overall incidence rate was 5.4 cases per 100 000 population. The rate was 1.0 cases per 100 000 among the non-indigenous Australian-born population, 21.7 per 100 000 among people born overseas and 8.1 per 100 000 among indigenous Australians.[67] Among 71 cases with a drug-resistant strain (in 2004) 8 were Australian, 60 were overseas born and 3 were of unknown origin.[68]

Australia sometimes attracts criticism for a 'heavy-handed' approach towards migrants, particularly the mandatory detention of unauthorized arrivals. However, it has managed to maintain low TB incidence rates and has not experienced the increases seen elsewhere in the world.

In New Zealand, TB notifications have fallen from 2600 cases in 1943 to a low of 295 in 1988. However, numbers have been increasing since then, with 300–500 new cases being reported each year.[69] Immigration to New Zealand from overseas has increased since the early 1990s and 69 per cent of all cases of TB in New Zealand are born overseas.[70] In a review of paediatric TB cases between 1992 and 2001, average annual TB rates per 100 000 by ethnicity were as follows: African 575.2, Pacific Island 15.2, Maori 6.4, Asian 5.6 and European 0.6.[71]

In response to this, the New Zealand Government strengthened TB screening for people from countries with a high TB rate. Since 2004 all those intending to stay in New Zealand for 6 months or more need screening. Before this, only those intending to stay 2 years or more were screened.

EXPERIENCE OF IMMIGRATION AND TB IN ISRAEL

Since Israel's formation in 1948, the population has grown seven-fold, from 872 000 in 1948 to more than 6.3 million in 2000. The first waves of immigration in 1948 consisted of Jewish migrants from Eastern Europe and neighbouring Arab countries. This led to an increase in the TB incidence rate from 50 per 100 000 in 1948 to 210 per 100 000 in 1950.[72] With effective treatment strategies and improved socioeconomic status, the incidence rate had fallen to 5 per 100 000 in 1990.

Since the mid-1980s, more than 1 million immigrants have settled in Israel. Many of these migrants have come from high-prevalence areas. There was a peak in TB notifications in 1985, coinciding with a wave of immigration from Ethiopia, and a further peak in the early 1990s when a large number of immigrants came over from the former Soviet Union.[73] In 1999, 86 per cent of TB patients in Israel were of foreign origin (30 per cent of Israeli citizens were foreign born).[74] DNA probing suggested that most cases of active TB in immigrants were reactivation of strains native to the country of origin, with little evidence of spread to the native population.[75]

The number of cases of TB notified to WHO in 2003 is indicated in Table 21.4.

NON-DOCUMENTED IMMIGRANTS

Most of the data provided relate to immigrants who are registered with the authorities. However, a significant number of migrants are not registered. In the Netherlands, at least 5 per cent of TB cases are estimated to be in the country illegally.[76] A figure of 20 per cent undocumented patients has been reported in California.[77] This group of

Table 21.4 Number of cases of tuberculosis notified to the World Health Organization in 2003 and estimated percentage of toral cases by foreign birth.

Country	Reported cases of tuberculosis in 2003	Total cases in foreign born (%)
Australia	1013	80
Canada	1451	66
France	5740	41
Germany	6526	38
Israel	505	85
Netherlands	1282	61
Norway	320	76
Switzerland	554	51
UK	6400	64
USA	14 861	51

Adapted from the World Health Organization.

people will tend to live in poverty, with restricted access to treatment and contact-tracing programmes, and are less likely to complete a course of TB chemotherapy than documented immigrants.

TRANSMISSION OF DISEASE

The World Health Organization estimates that 2 billion people carry TB bacteria and that more than 8 million people develop active TB each year. One-third of new cases occur in South East Asia, but the estimated incidence is highest in sub-Saharan Africa.

There is often a misconception among the media and the public in countries experiencing increased TB rates that the disease is being spread from immigrants to the native population. There is, however, very little evidence for transmission between ethnic groups. TB is not as contagious as many other transmissible diseases and it only tends to be household contacts or close associates of a sputum smear-positive case who are at appreciable risk of contracting the disease. A study from the UK suggested that the infection rate of white people by a white index case may be higher than that of Asian contacts from an Asian case.[78] Perhaps this is because pulmonary disease in Asians in the UK tends to be less extensive and less often smear positive than in white people.[22]

Three processes may be behind the high incidence of TB among immigrants after settling in low-incidence countries:[79]

1 reactivation of pre-existing TB infection (related to the country of origin, age at migration, sociodemographic characteristics and time since arrival);
2 recent TB infection or reinfection due to periodic travel to the home country;
3 recent TB infection within the new country from close contacts.

With the development of DNA probing of *M. tuberculosis* isolates in recent years, it is now possible to distinguish cases due to recent infection (these cases are likely to have clustered isolates suggesting a transmission chain) from cases of reactivated disease (who would tend to have unique non-clustered isolates).

Epidemiologic studies using these molecular techniques have shown that foreign-born people are more likely to have unique isolates than clustered ones and that there is little evidence that TB has spread from foreign-born people to those born in the host country.[80-82] DNA probing from 2490 TB cases in London (1995–97) broke down the isolates into 12 large 'superfamilies'. The data suggested that there had been relatively little transmission of TB in London from immigrant communities into the indigenous population. The data also showed that certain isolate 'superfamilies' were significantly associated with pulmonary rather than extrapulmonary disease, or with

sputum smear negativity, independently of country of birth or ethnicity, suggesting that the properties of the infecting organism play a role in the nature of the disease process.[83]

However, some studies have shown that significant new infections after migration also occur. In Lillebaek *et al.*'s[57] study of TB transmission among Somali immigrants, 55 per cent of the TB cases were clustered. Although some of these clustered cases may have been acquired in Somalia, the likelihood is that TB is also being transmitted within immigrant communities in the host country. This may be especially likely among very recent immigrants, possibly because the socioeconomic conditions in which they find themselves led to transmission of airborne infectious diseases. It has been suggested that the very stress of migration may predispose to infections such as TB.[54,84]

ENVIRONMENTAL FACTORS INFLUENCING TRANSMISSION

SOCIOECONOMIC FACTORS

In addition to the very stress of migration, socioeconomic factors do influence the transmission of TB. TB is still strongly associated with poverty.[85] Immigrant families will also tend to live together often in cramped conditions, particularly in the early stages of arrival in the new country: these are optimal conditions for transmission of airborne diseases. Among Senegalise immigrants living in Italy, poor living conditions were related to increased TB incidence.[86] Studies in the UK have found that socioeconomic factors, such as overcrowding and unemployment, are associated with increased TB rates.[87,88]

THE HIV EPIDEMIC AND OTHER IMMUNE-COMPROMISING CONDITIONS

The World Health Organization attributes the increased rates of TB in South East Asia and sub-Saharan Africa largely to the HIV epidemic. Not only is increased HIV associated with increased TB incidence, but TB itself has a significant adverse affect on HIV progression.[89] Managing patients with both HIV and TB brings its own challenges, particularly due to interactions of chemotherapy. Studies demonstrating the impact on immigrants are limited and appear to show a mixed picture. Anonymous testing of stored serum from 39 immigrant TB cases (1991–94) in London found no cases of HIV.[90] However, the UK's Health Protection Agency reported in 2004 that 10 per cent of London's TB cases were likely to be co-infected with HIV, although a proportion will have been UK born. A survey of three USA counties in 1995 found that half of the TB patients were foreign born and of these 52 per cent were co-infected with HIV.[91]

Other immune-compromising conditions can also increase the risk of active TB. A study looking at the incidence of TB in renal dialysis patients in London 1994–99 found that all the TB cases had been born overseas. The incidence of TB was calculated at 1187 cases per 100 000 renal patients per year.[92] The authors noted that there was a high incidence of diabetes in this group, which was itself a likely contributor to impaired immunity. They also raise concern about the frequent hospital visits for these patients, with close contact with other renal patients, giving high potential for nosocomial spread. The authors advocate early screening for latent TB in renal failure patients from endemic TB areas. This recommendation is in line with those of the American Thoracic Society, CDC and the Council of the Infectious Diseases Society of America.[93]

NUTRITIONAL FACTORS

In some immigrant groups in the newly adopted country, the incidence of TB is far higher than the WHO reported rates for their country of origin.[94] It has also been noted that Hindus (many of whom eat a vegetarian diet) appear to have a higher incidence of TB than Muslims.[95] A likely contributor is vitamin D_3 deficiency. *In vitro* work has shown that vitamin D_3 has a role in activating macrophages to destroy mycobacteria.[96,97] Additionally, a peptide called lipocalin 2 has been identified which appears to contribute to neutrophil-mediated antituberculosis activity; this peptide is vitamin D inducible.[98]

Vitamin D3 deficiency can arise from poor dietary intake (the main sources are fish, meat and dairy products), decreased intestinal absorption of cholecalciferol or a lack of sunlight exposure.

It may be the case that vitamin D deficiency contributes towards an 'acquired immunodeficiency of immigration'.[99] In many overseas groups with latent TB, plentiful sunlight maintains adequate vitamin D levels and hence maintains immunity against TB infection. However, after migrating to a country with a more temperate climate and less sunlight, vitamin D levels fall, compromising antituberculosis immunity and leading to latent TB flaring into overt disease. This could also explain why non-respiratory disease is more prevalent in the immigrant group: a small number of mycobacteria may disperse from the lung to distant sites via the bloodstream, the blood-borne macrophages and neutrophils being too immunodeficient to kill the organism. Several investigators have found increased rates of vitamin D3 deficiency among patients with TB compared to matched controls.[100,101] A review of TB patients in London by Ustionawski et al.[102] found that, of 210 patients diagnosed with TB, 76 per cent were vitamin D3 deficient and 56 per cent had undetectable levels: 70/82 Indian, 24/28 East African Asian, 29/34 Somali, 14/19 Pakistani and Afghani, 16/22 Sri Lankan and 2/6 other African patients were vitamin D3 deficient. Compared with darker-skinned individuals, lighter-skinned people produce more $25(OH)D_3$ for a similar degree of sunlight exposure[103–105] and the authors suggest that this might explain the relatively normal levels found in the pale-skinned European and Chinese/South East Asian patients.

TB control in immigrants

The high TB rate in many immigrant groups has led to revision of screening programmes in many countries in recent years. Although there is a strong argument for trying to control TB on a global scale – that is, programmes to detect, treat and eradicate the disease in the high-incidence counties of origin, most immigrant-receiving countries focus on detecting the disease in individuals who are about to, or already have migrated to the receiving country. Government policy-makers need to balance the benefits of greater investment in domestic elimination with support for international strategies to reduce the total global burden of the disease.[106]

An ideal screening process should achieve three aims:[107]

1 to identify individuals with active TB disease (pulmonary and extrapulmonary) who are in need of treatment;
2 to identify those with latent TB infection (these individuals may benefit from chemoprophylaxis to reduce the risk of later progression to active TB disease);
3 to identify those with neither evidence of disease nor infection (some of these individuals will benefit from BCG vaccination).

For the past century, many immigrant-receiving countries included a medical examination of the migrant as part of the initial immigration process. This often took place in quarantine and medical stations at the port of origin, such as Ellis Island in the USA.[108]

PRE–ENTRY SCREENING

Some countries (including the USA, Canada, Australia and New Zealand) now employ pre-entry screening usually involving a chest x-ray. If the x-ray suggests active TB, sputum samples are obtained (usually for smear, but some screening programmes culture the samples too). If a diagnosis of TB is made, then treatment must be taken and repeated smears shown to be negative before the individual is allowed entry to the country. If the x-ray shows evidence of previous TB, the individual is required to contact the local health department shortly after arrival for further evaluation.

Pre-entry screening allows prompt identification and treatment of an infectious TB case and enables contact tracing in the country of origin. However, supervising treatment is more difficult than doing so in the receiving country and there is a possibility of individuals developing active TB between the initial screening and arrival in the country of destination.

Table 21.5 Assessment and management of tuberculosis for new UK entrants.

Chest x-ray if the person has not had one recently – unless younger than 11 years or possibly pregnant

Clinical assessment for anyone with an abnormal chest x-ray

Risk assessment for HIV – take into account for Mantoux testing and BCG vaccination

Mantoux test if recent chest x-ray is normal and person is:

    younger than 16 years, or

    aged 16–35 years and from sub-Saharan Africa or a country with a TB incidence greater than 500 per 100 000

Mantoux test for children younger than 11 years and pregnant women

Interferon-γ test (if available) if Mantoux test is positive (unvaccinated person) or strongly positive (vaccinated person)

Assessment for active tuberculosis if interferon-γ test is positive; interpret chest x-ray first if it is not contraindicated

Treatment for latent tuberculosis infection in people aged 35 or younger after excluding active tuberculosis, if person has positive Mantoux test inconsistent with their BCG history, and positive interferon-γ test and is:

    younger than 16 years, or

    aged 16–35 years, from sub-Saharan Africa or a country with a tuberculosis incidence greater than 500 per 100 000

Consideration of BCG if unvacinnated and Mountex negative

'Inform and advise' if not being offered treatment or vaccination

Source: Tuberculosis: Clinical diagnosis and management of tuberculosis and measures for its prevention and control. National Institute for Health and Clinical Excellence, March 2006.

POST-ARRIVAL SCREENING

Most European countries have a post-arrival screening programme, although there is wide variation between countries regarding the clinical approach, which individuals to screen and the screening site.[109] Some countries screen immediately at the port of entry, others refer individuals to be screened elsewhere some time after arrival. All programmes use a chest x-ray to find active disease, although a number of countries do not have organized screening programmes. Some countries will also screen for latent TB infection with the Mantoux test. In the Netherlands, migrants continue to have 6-monthly chest x-rays (even if the initial x-ray is normal) for the first 2 years. A review of the Netherlands screening programme found that it detected TB cases earlier, resulting in fewer hospital admissions, shorter duration of symptoms and probably reduced TB transmission compared with cases detected passively.[110]

Screening programmes do have limitations. They will miss temporary visitors and non-legal immigrants. Some countries enforce TB screening more rigidly than others, or may not allow access to benefits, health care or employment without screening. Nonetheless, a number of migrants do 'slip the net' either through poor compliance with the screening programme or due to getting lost in the system as a result of moving address.

Screening for TB will find only a small proportion of individuals to have active disease. Of 46 424 asylum seekers entering the Netherlands between 1994 and 1997, 103 pulmonary TB cases were identified by screening (0.2 per cent).[111] Screening by chest x-ray will not identify extrapulmonary TB or latent infection. A large proportion of migrants will have latent TB infection at the time of arrival and may not develop active disease until many years after arrival. Marks *et al*.[112] found that, on reviewing South East Asian refugees in Sydney between 1984 and 1994, short-term screening for active cases of TB identified fewer than one-third of the cases destined to occur within a decade of arrival. In the UK, only one-fifth of the 5300 immigrant TB cases in 2005 occurred within 2 years of the first arrival.[107]

SCREENING PROGRAMMES IN THE UK

Screening and management of potential or actual migrants to the UK is a complex issue and is often the subject of significant media and political attention. There has been a policy of offering screening to new arrivals from high-incidence countries since 1983.[113] In the UK, around half of immigrants are screened at the port of entry (a number of entry ports do not have operative chest x-ray machines). The remainder (and those with an abnormal chest x-ray) are invited to attend the local chest clinic for a clinical evaluation. The UK now has national guidelines[114] on the management of TB within which there is guidance on screening new entrants from high-risk areas (TB incidence 40 per 100 000 per year or greater) (Table 21.5).

The Home Office, which is the government department responsible for immigration policy in the UK, has been running a trial of pre-entry screening in Tanzania, Sudan, Thailand, Cambodia and Bangladesh, with a planned extension of the scheme to 12 other countries. Potential immigrants undergo a chest x-ray, followed by sputum testing if abnormal. Individuals who are sputum smear positive must undergo a 6-month period of treatment in their nation of origin before reapplying. The effectiveness and cost-effectiveness has been called into question, bearing in mind the small numbers of active disease that are being detected, and the fact that latent TB and extrapulmonary disease will not be identified.[107]

CONCLUSIONS

Much of the developed world, having seen falling TB rates in the late twentieth century, with the real hope of complete eradication, is now seeing a resurgence of the disease. This is mainly attributable to increased immigration from high-incidence countries. This has led to enhanced immigration screening in many nations, but there is much variation from one country to another. Meanwhile, as individual countries focus introspectively to tackle their own problem, the wider picture – how to address the high TB rates and the HIV epidemic in the source countries, along with their underlying health and social deficiencies – is often forgotten.

LEARNING POINTS

- For many centuries, migrants have brought their diseases with them, including TB.
- Many developed countries, having seen declining TB rates in the latter half of the twentieth century, are experiencing increased incidence rates, mainly due to immigrants arriving from high-incidence areas.
- Not all migrant-receiving countries are experiencing increased TB incidence. This is probably because different populations migrate to different countries and some migrant populations have a much higher TB incidence than others.
- In the UK, migrants from sub-Saharan Africa carry the highest TB incidence rate (100 times the indigenous white population).
- Increased rates of TB in South East Asia and sub-Saharan Africa are largely attributable to the HIV epidemic.
- DNA probing suggests that most TB cases in immigrants represent reactivation of latent TB rather than recent infection in the host country.
- The highest TB rates occur in recent entrants (within the first 2 years of entry), although the risk of developing the disease remains high for many years after arrival in the receiving country.
- Multidrug resistance is more common in immigrant groups.
- Nutritional factors, in particular Vitamin D deficiency, appear to contribute towards latent TB flaring into active disease.
- Rates of TB being spread from immigrants to the indigenous population of the host nation are minimal.
- Many countries have developed stricter immigration policies and enhanced TB screening programmes with the aim of controlling the disease.

REFERENCES

1. Choraton F. Peruvian mummy shows TB preceded Columbus. *Br Med J* 1994; **308**: 808.
2. Zink AR, Sola C, Reischl U *et al.* Characterization of *Mycobacterium tuberculosis* complex DNAs from Egyptian mummies by spoligotyping. *J Clin Microbiol* 2003; **41**: 5350–51.
3. O'Brien EM. *The foundation of Australia.* Sidney: Angus and Robertson, 1950.
4. Proust AJ. History of tuberculosis in Australia, New Zealand and Papua New Guinea. Canberra: Brolga Press, 1991.
5. Metcalf C. *A century of tuberculosis. South African perspectives.* Cape Town: Oxford University Press, 1991.
6. Cummins SL. Tuberculosis in primitive tribes and its bearing on tuberculosis of the civilised communities. *Int J Publ Health* 1920; **1**: 10–171.
7. Grzybowski S, Styblo K, Dorken E. Tuberculosis in eskimos. *Tubercle* 1976; **57** (Suppl. 4).
8. Bates JH, Stead WW. The history of tuberculosis as a global epidemic. *Med Clin North Am* 1993; **77**: 1205–17.
9. Diel R, Meywald-Walter K, Gottschalk R *et al.* Ongoing outbreak of tuberculosis in a low-incidence community: a molecular-epidemiological evaluation. *Int J Tuberc Lung Dis* 2004; **8**: 855–61.
10. Nguyen D, Proulx JF, Westley J *et al.* Tuberculosis in the Inuit Community of Quebec, Canada. *Am J Respir Crit Care Med* 2003; **168**: 1353–7.
11. Hess EV, MacDonald N. Pulmonary tuberculosis in Irish Immigrants in Londoners; comparison of hospital patients. *Lancet* 1954; **267**: 132–7.
12. Brett GZ. Pulmonary tuberculosis in immigrants: a mass radiography study survey in 1956. *Tubercle* 1956; **39**: 24–8.
13. Brett GZ. Epidemiology trends in tuberculosis and sarcoidosis in a district of London between 1958 and 1963. *Tubercle* 1965; **46**: 412–16.
14. Emerson PA, Beath G, Tomkins JG. Tuberculosis in Soho. *Br Med J* 1961; **2**: 148–52.
15. Springett VH, Adams JCS, D'Costa TB, Hemming M. Tuberculosis in immigrants in Birmingham. *Br J Prev Soc Med* 1958; **12**: 135–40.
16. Roe N. Tuberculosis in Indian immigrants. *Tubercle* 1959; **40**: 387–8.
17. Springett VH. Tuberculosis in immigrants. *Lancet* 1964; **1**: 1091–5.
18. Stevenson DK. Tuberculosis in Pakistanis in Bradford. *Br Med J* 1962; **1**: 1382–6.
19. Aspin J. Tuberculosis among Indian immigrants to Midland industrial areas. *Br Med J* 1962; **1**: 1386–8.
20. British Tuberculous Association. Tuberculosis among immigrants to England and Wales: a national survey in 1965. *Tubercle* 1966; **47**: 145–6.
21. Springett VH. Tuberculosis in immigrants in Birmingham 1970–72. *Br J Prev Soc Med* 1973; **27**: 242–6.
22. McNicol MW, Mikhail JR, Sutherland I. Tuberculosis in Brent. *Postgrad Med J* 1971; **47**: 591–3.
23. British Thoracic and Tuberculosis Association. Tuberculosis among immigrants related to length of residence in England and Wales. A report from the Research Committee of the British Thoracic and Tuberculosis Association. *Br Med J* 1975; **ii**: 698–9.
24. Silver CP, Steel SJ. Mediastinal lymphatic gland tuberculosis in Asian and coloured immigrants. *Lancet* 1961; **i**: 1254–6.
25. Davies PD, Humphries MJ, Byfield SP *et al.* Bone and joint tuberculosis. A survey of notifications in England and Wales. *J Bone Joint Surg* 1984; **66**: 326–30.
26. Findlay JM, Stevenson DK, Addison NV, Mirza ZA. Tuberculosis of the gastrointestinal tract in Bradford 1967–77. *J Roy Soc Med* 1979; **72**: 587–91.
27. Tsironi E, Feakins RM, Probert CSJ, Rampton D. Incidence of inflammatory bowel disease is rising and abdominal tuberculosis is falling in Bangladeshis in East London, United Kingdom. *Am J Gastroenterol* 2004; **99**: 1749–55.
28. Wilberschied LA, Kaye K, Fujiwara PI, Frieden TR. Extrapulmonary

tuberculosis among foreign-born patients, New York City, 1995-1996. *J Immigr Health* 1999; **1**: 65-75.

29. Medical Research Council Tuberculosis and Chest Diseases Unit. National survey of tuberculosis notifications in England and Wales 1978-9. *Br Med J* 1980; **281**: 895-8.

30. Department of the Environment. *National dwelling and housing survey*. London: HMSO, 1979.

31. MacPherson DW, Gushulak BD. Balancing prevention and screening among international migrants with tuberculosis: Population mobility as the major epidemiological influence in low-incidence nations. Public Health 2006; **120**: 712-23.

32. Rose AMC, Watson JM, Graham C et al. Tuberculosis at the end of the 20th century in England and Wales: results of a national survey in 1998. *Thorax* 2001; **56**: 173-9.

33. World Health Organization. *Global tuberculosis control: surveillance, planning, financing*. Geneva: World Health Organization, 2005.

34. French CE, Antoine D, Gelb D et al. Tuberculosis in foreign-born persons, England and Wales, 2001-2003. *Int J Tuberc Lung Dis* 2007; **11**: 577-84.

35. Massachusetts Department of Public Health. Tuberculosis and the new citizen. *N Engl J Med* 1971; **285**: 919-20.

36. Reichman LB, Felton CP, Hammarsten JF et al. Tuberculosis in the foreign born. *Am Rev Respir Dis* 1977; **116**: 561-4.

37. Powell KE, Brown ED, Farer LS. Tuberculosis among Indo-Chinese refugees in the United States. *J Am Med Assoc* 1983; **249**: 1455-60.

38. Byrd RB, Fisk DE, Roethe RA et al. Tuberculosis in oriental immigrants. *Chest* 1979; **72**: 136-9.

39. Snider DE, Farer LS. Tuberculosis in oriental immigrants. *Chest* 1980; **77**: 812 (Correspondence).

40. Rieder HL, Snider DE, Cauthen GM. Extrapulmonary tuberculosis in the United States. *Am Rev Respir Dis* 1990; **141**: 347-51.

41. Talbot EA, Moore M, McCray E, Binkin NJ. Tuberculosis among foreign-born persons in the United States, 1993-1998. *J Am Med Assoc* 2000; **284**: 2894-900.

42. Pitchenick AE, Russell BW, Cleary T et al. The prevalence of tuberculosis and drug resistance among Hiatians. *N Engl J Med* 1987; **307**: 162-5.

43. Pitchenick AE, Cole C, Russell BW et al. Tuberculosis, atypical mycobacteriosis, and the acquired immunodeficiency syndrome among Hiatian and non-Hiatian patients in South Florida. *Ann Intern Med* 1984; **101**: 641-5.

44. Iademarco MF, Castro KG. Epidemiology of tuberculosis. *Semin Respir Infect* 2003; **18**: 225-40.

45. Centers for Disease Control and Prevention. Trends in tuberculosis – United States 2005. *MMWR Morb Mortal Wkly Rep* 2006; **55**: 305-308.

46. Cain KP, Haley CA, Armstrong LR et al. Tuberculosis among foreign-born persons in the United States: achieving tuberculosis elimination. *Am J Respir Crit Care Med* 2007; **175**: 75-9.

47. Enarson DA, Wang JS, Grzybowski S. Case finding in the elimination phase of tuberculosis: tuberculosis in displaced people. *IUATLD* 1990; **65**: 71-2.

48. Willis JS, Duncan RA. Medical status of Chinese immigrants 1964-1968. *Can J Publ Hlth* 1972; **63**: 237-47.

49. Barr JWB. Arrival of Uganda Asians. *Can Med Assoc J* 1972; **107**: 1062 (editorial).

50. Hershfield ES, Eidus L, Helbecque DM. Canadian survey to determine the rate of drug resistance to isoniazid, PAS, streptomycin in newly detected untreated tuberculosis patients and retreatment cases. *Int J Clin Pharmacol* 1979; **17**: 387-93.

51. Enarson D, Ashley MJ, Grzybowski S. Tuberculosis in immigrants to Canada. *Am Rev Respir Dis* 1979; **119**: 11-18.

52. Enarson D, Sjogren I, Grzybowski S. Incidence of tuberculosis among Scandinavian immigrants in Canada. *Eur J Respir Dis* 1980; **61**: 139-42.

53. Creatore MI, Lam M, Wobeser WL. Patterns of tuberculosis risk over time among recent immigrants to Ontario, Canada. *Int J Tuberc Lung Dis* 2005; **9**: 667-72.

54. Farah MG, Meyer HE, Selmer R et al. Long-term risk of tuberculosis among immigrants in Norway. *Int J Epidemiol* 2005; **34**: 1005-1011.

55. Winje BA, Heldal E. *Tuberculosis disease in Norway 2002*. MSIS-rapport No. 23. Oslo: Norwegian Institute of Public Health, 2003 (in Norwegian).

56. Dahle UR, Sandven P, Heldal E, Caugant DA. Molecular epidemiology of *Mycobacterium tuberculosis* in Norway. *J Clin Microbiol* 2001; **39**: 1802-807.

57. Lillebaek T, Anderson AB, Dirksen A et al. Persistent high incidence of tuberculosis in immigrants in a low-incidence country. *Emerg Infect Dis* 2002; **8**: 679-84.

58. Lillebaek T, Andersen AB, Bauer J et al. Risk of *Mycobacterium tuberculosis* transmission in a low-incidence country due to immigration from high-incidence areas. *J Clin Microbiol* 2001; **39**: 855-61.

59. Vos AM, Meima A, Verver S et al. High incidence of pulmonary tuberculosis persists a decade after immigration, the Netherlands. *Emerg Infect Dis* 2004; **10**: 736-9.

60. Sutherland I. The ten-year incidence of clinical tuberculosis following 'conversion' in 2550 individuals aged 14 to 19 at the time of conversion. TSRU progress report. The Hague: KNCV, 1968.

61. Robert J, Trystram D, Truffot-Pernot C, Jarlier V. Multidrug-resistant tuberculosis: eight years of surveillance in France. *Eur Respir J* 2003; **22**: 833-7.

62. Faustini A, Hall AJ, Perucci CA. Risk factors for multidrug resistant tuberculosis in Europe: a systematic review. *Thorax* 2006; **61**: 158-63.

63. Hayward AC, Herbert J, Watson JM. Tuberculosis drug resistance in England and Wales. How much is 'home-grown'? *Epidemiol Infect* 2000; **125**: 463-4.

64. O'Connor B, Christensen A, McAnulty J. Epireview: Tuberculosis in New South Wales, 1991-2002. *NSW Public Health Bull* 2004; **15**: 138-43.

65. Plant AJ, Rushworth RL, Wan Q, Thomas M. Tuberculosis in New South Wales. *Med J Austr* 1991; **154**: 86-9.

66. Chest Service of the Government Medical and Health Department (Australia). Annual report, 1987.

67. Roche PW, Antic R, Bastian I et al. Tuberculosis notifications in Australia, 2004. *Commun Dis Intell* 2006; **30**: 93-101.

68. Lumb R, Bastian I, Crighton T et al. Tuberculosis in Australia: bacteriologically confirmed cases and drug resistance, 2004: a report of the Australian Mycobacterium Reference Laboratory Network. *Commun Dis Intell* 2006; **30**: 102-108.

69. Turnbull F. The epidemiology and surveillance of tuberculosis in New Zealand. In: Harrison A, Calder L (eds). *Guidelines for tuberculosis control in New Zealand 2003*. Wellington: Ministry of Health, 2002: 4.

70. Carr H. Tuberculosis control in people from countries with a high incidence of tuberculosis. In: Harrison A, Calder L (eds). *Guidelines for tuberculosis control in New Zealand 2003*. Wellington: Ministry of Health, 2002: 12.

71. Howie S, Voss L, Baker M, Calder L. Tuberculosis in New Zealand, 1992-2001: a resurgence. *Arch Dis Child* 2005; **90**: 1157-61.

72. Wartski SA. Epidemiology and control of tuberculosis in Israel. *Publ Health Rev* 1995; **23**: 297-341.

73. Chemtob D, Leventhal A, Berlowitz Y et al. The new National Tuberculosis Programme in Israel, a country of high immigration. *Int J Tuberc Lung Dis* 2003; **7**: 828-36.

74. Surveillance of tuberculosis in Europe. Report on tuberculosis cases notified in 1999. Saint Maurice: EuroTB, 2002.

75. Ravins M, Bercovier H, Chemtob D et al. Molecular epidemiology of *Mycobacterium tuberculosis* infection in Israel. *J Clin Microbiol* 2001; **39**: 1175-1177.

76. Borgdorff MW, Lambregts-van Weezenbeek CSB, Broekmans JF.

Number of illegal TB patients in the Netherlands at the time of diagnosis. *Tegen de Tuberculose* 2000; **96**: 9–11 (in Dutch).

77. Asch S, Leake B, Gelberg L. Does fear of immigration authorites deter tuberculosis patients from seeking care? *West J Med* 1994; **161**: 373–6.

78. BTS Research Committee. A study of standardised contact procedure in tuberculosis. *Tubercle* 1978; **59**: 245–59.

79. Verver S, Veen J. Tuberculosis control and migration. In: Reichman LB, Hershfield ES (eds). *Reichman and Hershfield's tuberculosis – a comprehensive international approach*. Informa Healthcare USA 2006.

80. Hopewell PC. Using conventional and molecular epidemiological analyses to target tuberculosis control interventions in a low incidence area. *Novartis Found Symp* 1998; **217**: 42–54.

81. Alland D, Kalkut GE, Moss AR *et al*. Transmission of tuberculosis in New York City. An analysis by DNA fingerprinting and conventional epidemiologic methods. *N Engl J Med* 1994; **330**: 1710–6.

82. Borgdorff MW, Behr MA, Nagelkerke NJ *et al*. Transmission of tuberculosis in San Francisco and its association with immigration and ethnicity. *Int J Tuberc Lung Dis* 2000; **4**: 287–94.

83. Dale JW, Bothamley GH, Drobniewski F *et al*. Origins and properties of *Mycobacterium tuberculosis* isolates in London. *J Med Microbiol* 2005; **54**: 575–82.

84. Hertz DG. Bio-psycho-social consequences of migration stress: a multidimensional approach. *Isr J Psychiatry Relat Sci* 1993; **30**: 204–12.

85. Spence DS, Williams CSD, Hotchkis J, Davies PDO. Tuberculosis and poverty. *Br Med J* 1993; **307**: 759–61.

86. Scolari C, El-Hamad I, Matteelli A *et al*. Incidence of tuberculosis in a community of Senegalise immigrants in northen Italy. *Int J Tuberc Lung Dis* 1999; **3**: 18–22.

87. Mangtani P, Jolley DJ, Watson JM, Rodrigues LC. Socioeconomic deprivation and notification rates for tuberculosis in London during 1982–1991. *Br Med J* 1995; **310**: 963–6.

88. Bhatti N, Law MR, Halliday R, Moore-Gillon J. Increasing incidence of tuberculosis in England and Wales: a study of the likely causes. *Br Med J* 1995; **310**: 967–9.

89. Harries AD, Maher D, Graham S. *TB/HIV, a clinical manual*, 2nd edn. Geneva: World Health Organization, 2004.

90. Bonington A, Harden S, Anderson S *et al*. HIV-testing study of immigrants with pulmonary tuberculosis. *Scand J Infect Dis* 1997; **29**: 461–3.

91. Granich RM, Zuber PL, McMillan M *et al*. Tuberculosis among foreign-born residents of southern Florida, 1995. *Public Health Rep* 1998; **113**: 552–6.

92. Moore DA, Lightstone L, Javid B, Friedland JS. High rates of tuberculosis in end-stage renal failure: the impact of international migration. *Emerg Infect Dis* 2002; **8**: 77–8.

93. Centers for Disease Control and Prevention. Targeted tuberculin testing and treatment of latent tuberculosis infection. *MMWR Morb Mortal Wkly Rep* 2000; **49**: 1–51.

94. Rose AM, Watson JM, Graham C *et al*. Tuberculosis at the end of the 20th century in England and Wales: results of a national survey in 1998. *Thorax* 2001; **56**: 173–9.

95. Finch PJ, Millard FJ, Maxwell JD. Risk of tuberculosis in immigrant Asians: culturally acquired immunodeficiency? *Thorax* 1991; **46**: 1–5.

96. Rook GA, Taverne J, Leveton C, Steele J. The role of gamma-interferon, vitamin D_3 metabolites and tumour necrosis factor in the pathogenesis of tuberculosis. *Immunology* 1987; **62**: 229–34.

97. Crowle AJ, Ross EJ, May MH. Inhibition by 1,25(OH)$_2$-vitamin D_3 of the multiplication of virulent tubercle bacilli in cultured human macrophages. *Infect Immun* 1987; **55**: 2945–50.

98. Martineua MR, Wilkinson KA, Kampmann B *et al*. Neutrophil-mediated immunity to *Mycobacterium tuberculosis* infection: role of lipocalin 2. *Thorax* 2006; **61**: ii, 25–6.

99. Davies PDO. A possible link between vitamin D deficiency and impaired host defence to *Mycobacterium tuberculosis*. *Tubercle* 1985; **66**: 301–6.

100. Wilkinson RJ, Llewelyn M, Toossi Z *et al*. Influence of vitamin D deficiency and vitamin D receptor polymorphisms on tuberculosis among Gujarati Asians in west London: a case–control study. *Lancet* 2000; **355**: 618–21.

101. Sasidharan PK, Rajeev E, Vijayakumari V. Tuberculosis and vitamin D deficiency. *J Assoc Phys India* 2002; **50**: 554–8.

102. Ustianowski A, Shaffer R, Collin S *et al*. Prevalence and associations of vitamin D deficiency in foreign-born persons with tuberculosis in London. *J Infect* 2005; **50**: 432–7.

103. Meulmeester JF, van den Berg H, Wedel M *et al*. Vitamin D status, parathyroid hormone and sunlight in Turkish, Moroccan and Caucasian children in The Netherlands. *Eur J Clin Nutr* 1990; **44**: 461–70.

104. Jablonski NG, Chaplin G. The evolution of human skin coloration. *J Hum Evol* 2000; **39**: 57–106.

105. Holick MF, MacLaughlin JA, Clark MB *et al*. Photosynthesis of previtamin D_3 in human skin and the physiologic consequences. *Science* 1980; **210**: 203–205.

106. Schwartzman K, Oxlade O, Barr RG *et al*. Domestic returns from investment in the control of tuberculosis in other countrie. *N Engl J Med* 2005; **353**: 1008–20.

107. Moore-Gillon J, Davies PDO, Ormerod P. Screening for tuberculosis in new arrivals to the UK: practicalities, politics and the newspapers. *Br Med J* 2007 (in press).

108. Moreno B. *Encyclopaedia of Ellis Island*. Westpoint, CT: Greenwood Press, 2004.

109. Coker R, Bell A, Pitman R *et al*. Tuberculosis screening in migrants in selected European countries shows wide disparities. *Eur Respir J* 2006; **27**: 801–807.

110. Verver S, Bwire R, Borgdorff MW. Screening for pulmonary tuberculosis among immigrants: estimated effect on severity of disease and duration of infectiousness. *Int J Tuberc Lung Dis* 2001; **5**: 419–25.

111. van Burg J L, Verver S, Borgdorff MW. The epidemiology of tuberculosis among asylum seekers in the Netherlands: implications for screening. *Int J Tuberc Lung Dis* 2003; **7**: 139–144.

112. Marks GB, Bai J, Stewart GJ *et al*. Effectiveness of postmigration screening in controlling tuberculosis among refugees: a historical cohort study, 1984–1998. *Am J Public Health* 2001; **91**: 1797–9.

113. Joint Tuberculosis Committee of the British Thoracic Society. Control and prevention of tuberculosis: a code of practice. *Br Med J* 1983; **287**: 1118–21.

114. National Institute for Health and Clinical Excellence. *Tuberculosis: clinical diagnosis and management of tuberculosis, and measures for its prevention and control*. London: National Institute for Health and Clinical Excellence, 2006.

PART 6

PREVENTION

22

Preventive therapy

JEAN-PIERRE ZELLWEGER

INTRODUCTION

The idea of preventing the occurrence of tuberculosis (TB) by treating infected subjects before clinical expression of the disease has long been discussed, based on the fact that infected subjects (historically defined as subjects with a positive tuberculin skin test or a significant exposure to tuberculosis or fibrotic lesions on chest x-ray) have an increased risk of tuberculosis (Figure 22.1).[1–6] The risk, estimated at 10 per cent over lifetime, is increased in children,[2] in the presence of fibrotic lesions on chest x-ray[7]

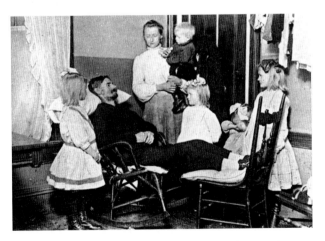

Figure 22.1 In the days when this photograph was taken, there was no treatment, no prevention of transmission, no screening, no preventive therapy – and many deaths among the young relatives of a TB patient. The only useful measure was sending the children away from their homes, sometimes for years, until the sick parents died! From Dubos R, Dubos J. *The white plague*, New Brunswick, J: Rutgers University Press, 2nd reprint, 1992 .

and in immunocompromised individuals.[8] It is maximal during the first 2 years after infection and decreases over time.[1,3,4] Soon after the introduction of antibiotics active against TB (as early as 1959), trials have been conducted which demonstrate that, if properly prescribed and taken, preventive treatment decreases the risk of future disease.[9,10] In theory at least, if applied rigorously to infected individuals or to whole populations with a high rate of latent infection, this policy could result in a decrease in TB incidence in the future.[11]

The obstacles which need to be overcome to reach this target are numerous. Some of them will be discussed here. These are:

1 the definition of latent TB infection;
2 the estimation of the risk of reactivation;
3 the evaluation of the efficacy and cost-effectiveness of preventive treatment (and the number of patients to be treated to avoid one case of TB);
4 the choice of the appropriate treatment;
5 the potential side effects of the treatment;
6 the adherence to treatment;
7 the possible impact of preventive treatment on the sensitivity of mycobacteria.

Definition of latent TB infection and estimation of the risk are discussed in Chapter 5, The diagnosis of tuberculosis.

EFFICACY OF PREVENTIVE TREATMENT

The efficacy of preventive treatment (this term is to be preferred to chemoprevention or chemoprophylaxis, which refers to the administration of a protective drug to an uninfected individual), has been established in large population groups in the USA,[10] in Alaska,[11] in Asia,[12,13] in

Africa[14] and in Europe.[9] Some studies were conducted in individuals with positive tuberculin skin tests and normal chest x-ray[10] or a history of exposure to TB, or in subjects with fibrotic lesions compatible with untreated, spontaneously healed previous TB[9] or in whole population groups with high risk of exposure, irrespective of tuberculin status.[11,15] Some studies selected individuals with a special risk factor for TB progression, such as silicosis,[16] renal dialysis,[17] renal transplant,[18,19] haematopoietic stem cell transplant,[20] drug abuse[21] or human immunodeficiency virus (HIV).[22,23]

The review of the main controlled trials with isoniazid in non-HIV-infected people revealed an average risk ratio of TB within the next 2 or more years of 0.40 in the active group compared with the placebo group.[24] In patients receiving anti-tumour necrosis factor (TNF) therapy, known for increasing the risk of TB reactivation,[25,26] the preventive treatment only partially reduced the risk of future disease.[27]

In HIV-infected people, some studies demonstrated a decrease in the risk of progression to TB,[22,28–30] but the rate of disease remained high[31] and the mortality or rate of HIV progression were not significantly modified.[32–34] In a randomized prospective study, preventive treatment with isoniazid in HIV-positive patients with anergy did not modify the rate of development of active TB.[23]

CHOICE OF APPROPRIATE TREATMENT

Isoniazid

Most studies on preventive treatment have used isoniazid in a dose of 5 mg/kg. Historical studies, all performed before the emergence of HIV, used a duration of treatment of 12 months, and demonstrated a reduction of the risk of active TB during the follow-up period of 25–70 per cent, depending on the duration of the observation period and the adherence to treatment.[35] The highest reduction was observed in a study among young members of the Dutch navy with recent tuberculin conversion, where the reduction reached 96 per cent.[36] One large study in Europe compared the effect of 3 versus 6 versus 12 months of treatment among subjects with positive tuberculin skin tests and fibrotic lesions. The reduction was 21 per cent after 3 months, but reached 65 per cent after 6 months and 75 per cent after 12 months.[9] Based on the first trials, a duration of treatment of 6 months was initially recommended as the best balance between risk and efficacy.[37] This regimen is recommended by the British guidelines.[38] In US guidelines, the recommended duration was increased to 9 months, although no controlled study compared this duration of treatment with 6 or 12 months.[39]

For HIV-positive subjects, the reduction in risk of TB during the follow-up period varied between 36 and 78 per cent in tuberculin-positive individuals, but could not be demonstrated among tuberculin-negative individuals.[30,35]

The recommended duration of treatment is the same as for HIV-negative individuals. Treatment of HIV-positive individuals with negative tuberculin skin test is currently not recommended.

Soon after the completion of the first trials, reports were issued about the hepatotoxicity of isoniazid, drug-induced hepatitis and deaths.[40] Analysis of the reports has demonstrated that severe adverse events and deaths were associated with irregular clinical follow up[41,42] and with several risk factors such as age, postpartum period, ethnicity, hepatitis B and alcohol abuse.[43–46] The incidence of severe adverse events seemed to decrease over time, probably due to better monitoring of the patients. Patients prescribed isoniazid preventive therapy should therefore be regularly monitored.[42]

Addition of vitamin B_6 is recommended for the prevention of neurotoxicity of isoniazid in patients predisposed to neuropathy such as pregnant women, elderly, diabetics and alcoholics.[47,48]

Rifampicin

Rifampicin has been proposed as an alternative to isoniazid in individuals unable to tolerate this drug, in contacts of TB patients with isoniazid-resistant strains and in the aim of improving the adherence to preventive treatment by offering a shorter duration of treatment (4 months versus 9 months). There is only limited evidence of the efficacy of rifampicin as a preventive treatment. A study conducted in Hong Kong among subjects with positive tuberculin skin test and silicosis demonstrated a reduction of 50 per cent of the risk of TB over 5 years in the group receiving rifampicin for 3 months compared to placebo.[49] Two studies demonstrated a reduction of the risk of TB among contacts of cases of smear-positive, isoniazid-resistant TB, but both used a duration of treatment of 6 months.[50,51] No study has assessed the efficacy of a treatment duration of 4 months, as currently recommended by the American Thoracic Society (ATS) guidelines[39] and there is no study among HIV-positive individuals. Therefore, rifampicin is not recommended in these individuals.

Toxicity of rifampicin is lower than toxicity of isoniazid.

Rifampicin and isoniazid

The efficacy of the combination of isoniazid and rifampicin for 3 months has been demonstrated among children in contact with smear-positive cases of TB[52] and in HIV-negative adults.[49] In HIV-positive adults, a regimen of isoniazid and rifampicin for 3 months was equally effective as a regimen of isoniazid for 12 months, with a lower rate of hepatotoxicity.[53] The regimen is currently recommended and used mainly in the UK.[38,54]

Rifampicin and pyrazinamide

The combination of rifampicin and pyrazinamide for 2 months has been studied among HIV-positive subjects, who have the greatest risk of TB reactivation and where a regimen of short duration offers a chance of better adherence. Further trials were conducted among patients with latent infection and silicosis.[55] The trials demonstrated an efficacy similar to 12 months of isoniazid.[56–59] The regimen was therefore recommended for use in HIV-positive subjects;[39] however, due to a high rate of severe adverse reactions with fatal hepatic insufficiency, it is no longer recommended.[60]

INDICATIONS FOR PREVENTIVE TREATMENT

The preventive chemotherapy or treatment of latent tuberculosis infection is recommended for individuals who (1) are infected with *Mycobacterium tuberculosis* and (2) have a demonstrated risk of reactivation. Considering the statistical risk of reactivation, the indications for preventive therapy are, by decreasing order of magnitude:

- HIV-positive patients with positive tuberculin skin test (or positive interferon-γ test);
- recent contacts of smear-positive cases of TB with tuberculin conversion (or positive interferon-γ test);
- children with positive tuberculin skin test (or positive interferon-γ test);
- subjects with fibrotic lesions compatible with untreated pulmonary TB;
- subjects with natural, viral or drug-induced immune depression and with a positive tuberculin skin test (or positive interferon-γ test).

In other groups of population (individuals with a positive tuberculin skin test without a clear history of exposure, such as immigrants who have recently arrived from countries with a high incidence of TB), the indication for preventive treatment is a matter of individual appreciation. It may be indicated if the subject has an additional risk factor for TB reactivation (diabetes, severe malnutrition, cancer, gastrectomy, smoking).

Special situations

- *Pregnancy*: isoniazid is safe in pregnant women, the only problem in practice being the possible increase of nausea if the treatment is prescribed during the first trimester.
- *Children*: isoniazid is effective and usually well tolerated in children and is considered the drug of choice.[61]
- *Contacts of index cases with isoniazid-resistant cases*: a study among immigrants demonstrated that about half of the cases of TB occurring during or after the prescription of isoniazid preventive treatment were due to isoniazid-resistant strains.[62] Therefore, prior knowledge of isoniazid resistance in the index case or evaluation of the risk of isoniazid resistance in a population group is useful in the selection of the proper treatment regimen.
- *Contacts of cases with multidrug-resistant tuberculosis (MDR-TB)*: no clinical trial has been performed to assess the efficacy of any regimen in preventing the development of TB among contacts of index cases with strains resistant to isoniazid and rifampicine.[63] A prospective cohort study in children contacts of MDR-TB demonstrated a decrease of TB among subjects who received a preventive treatment tailored according to the susceptibility of the index case.[64] A regimen of 6–12 months with a combination of pyrazinamide and a fluoroquinolone or pyrazinamide with ethambutol has been recommended.[65] Other guidelines recommend close observation of contacts without preventive treatment.[38]

ADHERENCE TO TREATMENT

The main problem associated in practice with preventive treatment of latent TB infection is the low level of compliance of both health-care professionals and patients with the recommended treatment.[66] Only a proportion of the patients who could benefit from preventive treatment receive it[67,68] and only a proportion of those who receive it take it long enough to benefit from it, even among the groups with the highest risk, such as small children[69] or HIV-positive patients.[28] The consequence is that only a proportion of the expected cases of TB are really prevented.[66] Failure to prescribe preventive treatment among population groups with a high risk of reactivation means that cases will occur which could have been avoided.[70]

Several strategies have been proposed for increasing the adherence to treatment of subjects with latent TB infection. Several studies have demonstrated that the rate of adherence can be increased by shortening the duration of treatment and replacing isoniazid by one of the shorter regimens (rifampicin 4 months, rifampicin and isoniazid 3 months, rifampicin and pyrazinamide 2 months, weekly isoniazid with rifapentine).[20,56,71–74] Concerns have been expressed regarding the potential induction of rifampicin resistance in HIV-positive patients with atypical forms of TB mistakenly considered as latently infected and treated by a single drug.[75] Therefore, excluding active TB by careful clinical, radiogical and bacteriological (if appropriate) examination is an important prerequisite before institution of preventive treatment.[76,77]

Other studies have tried to identify the factors associated with non-completion of treatment. Some of the factors, like the perception of the risk of progression to active disease, can be detected before initiating the treatment.[78] Employing cultural mediators able to understand the needs of the patients originating from foreign countries with different cultural backgrounds,[79] intervention by specially

Case history

A foreign-born man of 48 years, known for alcohol abuse, was treated for smear-positive pulmonary TB. Under directly observed therapy, he had a slow recovery, with a prolonged period of smear positivity but final cure.

The contact-tracing investigations performed in the family revealed a positive tuberculin skin test in his wife, aged 45 years, his daughter, aged 11 years and his son, aged 14 years.

The wife and both children received preventive therapy with isoniazid. One month later, the daughter experienced a seizure and isoniazid treatment was stopped. The neurologist in charge of further antiepileptic treatment is not informed of the TB contact and does not consider an alternative preventive treatment. No follow up is organized.

Three years later, the girl developed progressive cough, weight loss and dyspnoea. Viral bronchitis, then asthma, were considered and symptomatic treatment prescribed, without success. After 3 months, a chest x-ray revealed extensive infiltrate with cavities in the right upper lobe (Figure 22.2). Direct smear was positive for *M. tuberculosis*. The patient was treated with standard anti-tuberculous chemotherapy. The treatment was well tolerated, without recurrence of seizures.

A contact investigation among students and staff at school discovered 23 cases of latent infection and one secondary case of TB.

Lessons from this case:

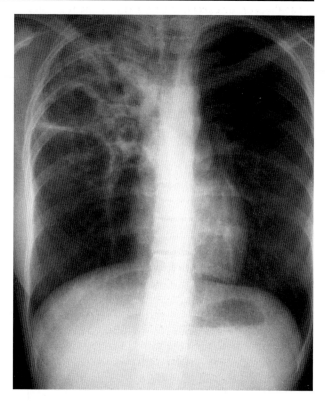

Figure 22.2 Chest x-ray of a 14-year-old girl with prolonged cough, treated for bronchitis for 3 months.

1 TB is transmissible.
2 Contact tracing among the family members and preventive treatment of infected contacts is useful.
3 If the preventive treatment is not tolerated (which may happen), the infected contacts should be offered an alternative treatment or close supervision (which was not performed in this case).
4 The development of TB in this 14-year-old girl could have been avoided, as well as the infection of a further 23 schoolfriends and one more case of TB.
5 Prolonged cough may be the expression of TB in an adolescent. Previous history of exposure to TB with untreated infection, should have alerted the family and the physician!

trained nurses,[80] monetary incentives,[81,82] and direct supervision of intake[21] can increase the adherence rate, particularly in groups of patients who are difficult to control, such as injecting drug users.

External control of the drug intake, by checking the presence of isoniazid in urine[83] or the use of electronic devices[84] have also been proposed.

COST-EFFECTIVENESS OF PREVENTIVE TREATMENT

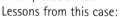

Ideally, detecting and treating all individuals in a population who have been infected with *M. tuberculosis* could contribute to the eradication of the disease by decreasing the number of future cases.[85] As screening of large populations is not feasible in practice, unless we have cheap, reliable and highly specific tests, detecting recently infected people who were in contact with a case of infectious TB is considered currently as a cost-effective intervention, if good case-finding and treatment of TB exists and if resources permit.[86] In the USA, it has been estimated that the current use of preventive treatment of latent TB infection, assuming a life risk of reactivation of 5 per cent and an effectiveness of 20–60 per cent, can prevent the future emergence of 4000–11 000 cases of TB each year.[87] The benefit of preventive treatment is particularly high for young individuals with a high risk of reactivation, and may even be associated with monetary savings, whereas the benefit for older individuals or people with a low risk of reactivation is smaller or is associated with expense.[88,89] A recent analysis of the effect of preventive treatment among TB contacts concluded that the intervention is highly cost-effective.[90] Increasing the efficacy of the contact-tracing procedure by using more specific detection methods such as interferon-γ assays to confirm the positive tuberculin skin test increases the cost-effectiveness of the intervention and decreases the number of cases needed to treat to prevent one future case.[91,92]

LEARNING POINTS

- Preventive chemotherapy is an efficient intervention for reducing the reservoir of future cases of TB.
- It is particularly indicated in patients or population groups with the highest risk of progression to TB after infection, such as HIV-positive patients, immunosuppressed patients, small children, recent contacts of smear-positive cases and patients with fibrotic lesions from previous untreated TB.
- The effectiveness of preventive treatment seems to decrease with age.
- Because adverse effects of isoniazid may be severe, close monitoring of the patients during treatment is essential.
- The efficacy is dependent on the adherence to the prescribed treatment. If necessary, incentives or other methods for improving the adherence should be used.
- Although isoniazid for 6 or 9 months is the recommended treatment, regimens of shorter duration (rifampin for 4 months or rifampicin and isoniazid for 3 months) may be equally effective and improve the adherence to treatment making them more efficient.
- A better selection of the cases with suspected latent infection, by integration of the interferon-γ release assays, may improve the cost-efficacy.

REFERENCES

1. Horwitz O, Wilbek E, Erickson PA. Epidemiological basis of tuberculosis eradication. Bull World Health Organ 1969; 41: 95–113.
2. Comstock GW, Livesay VT, Woolpert SF. The prognosis of a positive tuberculin reaction in childhood and adolescence. Am J Epidemiol 1974; 99: 131–8.
3. Sutherland I, Svandova E, Radhakrishna S. The development of clinical tuberculosis following infection with tubercle bacilli. Tubercle 1982; 63: 255–68.
4. Morán-Mendoza O, Marion SA, Elwood K et al. Tuberculin skin test and risk of tuberculosis development: a large population-based study in contacts. Int J Tuberc Lung Dis 2007; 11: 1014–20.

5. Horsburgh CR Jr. Priorities for the treatment of latent tuberculosis infection in the United States. N Engl J Med 2004; 350: 2060–2067.
6. Radhakrishna S, Frieden TR, Subramani R. Association of initial tuberculin sensitivity, age and sex with the incidence of tuberculosis in south India: a 15-year follow-up. Int J Tuberc Lung Dis 2003; 7: 1083–91.
7. Norregaard J, Heckscher T, Viskum K. Abacillary pulmonary tuberculosis. Tubercle 1990; 71: 35–8.
8. Del Amo J, Petruckevitch A, Phillips AN et al. Risk factors for tuberculosis in patients with AIDS in London: a case- control study. Int J Tuberc Lung Dis 1999; 3: 12–17.
9. International Union Against Tuberculosis Committee on Prophylaxis. Efficacy of various durations of isoniazid preventive therapy for tuberculosis: five years of follow-up in the IUAT trial. Bull World Health Organ 1982; 60: 555–64.
10. Ferebee SH. Controlled chemoprophylaxis trials in tuberculosis A general review. Adv Tuberc Res 1970; 17: 28–106.
11. Comstock GW, Baum C, Snider DE Jr. Isoniazid prophylaxis among Alaskan Eskimos: a final report of the Bethel Isoniazid studies. Am Rev Respir Dis 1979; 119: 827–30.
12. del Castillo H, Bautista LD, Jacinto CP. Chemoprophylaxis in the Philippines. A controlled pilot study among household contacts of tuberculosis cases. Bull Quezon Inst 1965; 7: 277–90.
13. Chiba Y, Takahara T, Kondo K. Chemoprophylaxis of tuberculosis for adults in Japan. Bull Int Union Tuberc 1963; 69: 91–3.
14. Egsmose T, Ang'awa JOW, Poti SJ. The use of isoniazid among household contacts of open cases of pulmonary tuberculosis. Bull World Health Organ 1965; 33: 419–33.
15. Comstock GW, Ferebee SH, Hammes LM. A controlled trial of community-wide isoniazid prophylaxis in Alaska. Am Rev Respir Dis 1967; 95: 935–43.
16. Girling DJ. Double-blind controlled trial of chemoprophylaxis against tuberculosis in patients with silicosis in Hong Kong. Am Rev Respir Dis 1990; 141: A438.
17. Dervisoglu E, Yilmaz A, Sengul E. The spectrum of tuberculosis in dialysis patients. Scand J Infect Dis 2006; 38: 1040–44.
18. Naqvi R, Akhtar S, Noor H et al. Efficacy of isoniazid prophylaxis in renal allograft recipients. Transplant Proc 2006; 38: 2057–8.
19. Vikrant S, Agarwal SK, Gupta S et al. Prospective randomized control trial of isoniazid chemoprophylaxis during renal replacement therapy. Transpl Infect Dis 2005; 7: 99–108.
20. Cook PP, Maldonado RA, Yarnell CT, Holbert D. Safety and completion rate of short-course therapy for treatment of latent tuberculosis infection. Clin Infect Dis 2006; 43: 271–5.
21. Chaisson RE, Barnes GL, Hackman J et al. A randomized, controlled trial of interventions to improve adherence to isoniazid therapy to prevent tuberculosis in injection drug users. Am J Med 2001; 110: 610–15.
22. Pape JW, Jean SS, Ho JL et al. Effect of isoniazid prophylaxis on incidence of active tuberculosis and progression of HIV infection. Lancet 1993; 342: 268–72.
23. Gordin FM, Matts JP, Miller C et al. A controlled trial of isoniazid in persons with anergy and human immunodeficiency virus infection who are at high risk for tuberculosis. Terry Beirn Community Programs for Clinical Research on AIDS. N Engl J Med 1997; 337: 315–20.
24. Smieja MJ, Marchetti CA, Cook DJ, Smaill FM. Isoniazid for preventing tuberculosis in non-HIV infected persons. Cochrane Database Syst Rev 1999; CD001363.
25. Keane J, Gershon S, Wise RP et al. Tuberculosis associated with infliximab, a tumor necrosis factor alpha-neutralizing agent. N Engl J Med 2001; 345: 1098–104.
26. Gomez-Reino JJ, Carmona L, Valverde VR et al. Treatment of rheumatoid arthritis with tumor necrosis factor inhibitors may predispose to significant increase in tuberculosis risk: a multicenter active-surveillance report. Arthritis Rheum 2003; 48: 2122–7.

27. Sichletidis L, Settas L, Chloros D, Patakas D. Tuberculosis in patients receiving anti-TNF agents despite chemoprophylaxis. *Int J Tuberc Lung Dis* 2006; **10**: 1127–32.

28. Elzi L, Schlegel M, Weber R *et al.* Reducing tuberculosis incidence by tuberculin skin testing, preventive treatment, and antiretroviral therapy in an area of low tuberculosis transmission. *Clin Infect Dis* 2007; **44**: 94–102.

29. Whalen CC, Johnson JL, Okwera A *et al.* A trial of three regimens to prevent tuberculosis in Ugandan adults infected with the human immunodeficiency virus. Uganda–Case Western Reserve University Research Collaboration. *N Engl J Med* 1997; **337**: 801–808.

30. Bucher HC, Griffith LE, Guyatt GH *et al.* Isoniazid prophylaxis for tuberculosis in HIV infection: a meta-analysis of randomized controlled trials. *AIDS* 1999; **13**: 501–507.

31. Grant AD, Charalambous S, Fielding KL *et al.* Effect of routine isoniazid preventive therapy on tuberculosis incidence among HIV-infected men in South Africa: a novel randomized incremental recruitment study. *J Am Med Assoc* 2005; **293**: 2719–25.

32. Quigley MA, Mwinga A, Hosp M *et al.* Long-term effect of preventive therapy for tuberculosis in a cohort of HIV-infected Zambian adults. *AIDS* 2001; **15**: 215–22.

33. Lim HJ, Okwera A, Mayanja-Kizza H *et al.* Effect of tuberculosis preventive therapy on HIV disease progression and survival in HIV-infected adults. *HIV Clin Trials* 2006; **7**: 172–83.

34. Woldehanna S, Volmink J. Treatment of latent tuberculosis infection in HIV infected persons. *Cochrane Database Syst Rev* 2004; CD000171.

35. Dooley KE, Sterling TR. Treatment of latent tuberculosis infection: challenges and prospects. *Clin Chest Med* 2005; **26**: 313–26, vii.

36. Veening GJJ. Long term isoniazid prophylaxis. Controlled trial of INH prophylaxis after recent tuberculin conversion in young adults. *Bull Int Union Tuberc* 1968; **41**: 169–71.

37. Comstock GW. How much isoniazid is needed for prevention of tuberculosis among immunocompetent adults? *Int J Tuberc Lung Dis* 1999; **3**: 847–50.

38. National Collaborating Centre for Chronic Conditions. *Tuberculosis: clinical diagnosis and management of tuberculosis, and measures for its prevention and control.* London: Royal College of Physicians, 2006.

39. American Thoracic Society, Centers for Disease Control and Prevention. Targeted tuberculin testing and treatment of latent tuberculosis infection. *Am J Respir Crit Care Med* 2000; **161**: S221–47.

40. Kopanoff DE, Snider DE, Caras GJ. Isoniazid-related hepatitis. *Am Rev Respir Dis* 1978; **117**: 991–1001.

41. Moulding TS, Redeker AG, Kanel GC. Twenty isoniazid associated death in one state. *Am Rev Respir Dis* 1989; **140**: 700–705.

42. Snider DE Jr, Caras GJ. Isoniazid-associated hepatitis deaths: a review of available information. *Am Rev Respir Dis* 1992; **145**: 494–7.

43. Fountain FF, Tolley E, Chrisman CR, Self TH. Isoniazid hepatotoxicity associated with treatment of latent tuberculosis infection: a 7-year evaluation from a public health tuberculosis clinic. *Chest* 2005; **128**: 116–23.

44. Dossing M, Wilcke JTR, Askgaard DS, Nybo B. Liver injury during antituberculosis treatment: an 11-year study. *Tubercle Lung Dis* 1996; **77**: 335–40.

45. Fernandez-Villar A, Sopena B, Fernandez-Villar J *et al.* The influence of risk factors on the severity of anti-tuberculosis drug-induced hepatotoxicity. *Int J Tuberc Lung Dis* 2004; **8**: 1499–505.

46. Saukkonen JJ, Cohn DL, Jasmer RM *et al.* An official ATS statement: hepatotoxicity of antituberculosis therapy. *Am J Respir Crit Care Med* 2006; **174**: 935–52.

47. Snider DE Jr. Pyridoxine supplementation during isoniazid therapy. *Tubercle* 1980; **61**: 191.

48. Leuenberger P, Zellweger JP. Drugs used in tuberculosis and leprosy. In: Dukes MNG, Aronson JK (eds). *Meyler's side effects of drugs*, 14th edn. Oxford: Elsevier Science, 2001: 1005–1029.

49. Hong Kong Chest Service TRCM. A double-blind placebo-controlled clinical trial of three antituberculosis chemoprophylaxis regimens in patients with silicosis in Hong Kong. *Am Rev Respir Dis* 1992; **145**: 36–41.

50. Polesky A, Farber HW, Gottlieb DJ *et al.* Rifampin preventive therapy for tuberculosis in Boston's homeless. *Am J Respir Crit Care Med* 1996; **154**: 1473–7.

51. Villarino ME, Ridszon R, Weismuller PC *et al.* Rifampin preventive therapy for tuverculosis infection. Experience with 157 adolescents. *Am J Respir Crit Care Med* 1997; **155**: 1735–8.

52. Ormerod LP. Rifampicin and isoniazid prophylactic chemotherapy for tuberculosis. *Arch Dis Child* 1998; **78**: 169–71.

53. Martinez Alfaro EM, Cuadra F, Solera J *et al.* [Evaluation of 2 tuberculosis chemoprophylaxis regimens in patients infected with human immunodeficiency virus. The GECMEI Group]. *Med Clin (Barc)* 2000; **115**: 161–5.

54. Ormerod LP. Chemotherapy and management of tuberculosis in the United Kingdom: recommendations of the Joint Tuberculosis Committee of the British Thoracic Society. *Thorax* 1990; **45**: 403–408.

55. Leung CC, Law WS, Chang KC *et al.* Initial experience on rifampin and pyrazinamide vs isoniazid in the treatment of latent tuberculosis infection among patients with silicosis in Hong Kong. *Chest* 2003; **124**: 2112–18.

56. Gordin F, Chaisson RE, Matts JP *et al.* Rifampin and pyrazinamide vs isoniazid for prevention of tuberculosis in HIV-infected persons: an international randomized trial. Terry Beirn Community Programs for Clinical Research on AIDS, the Adult AIDS Clinical Trials Group, the Pan American Health Organization, and the Centers for Disease Control and Prevention Study Group. *J Am Med Assoc* 2000; **283**: 1445–50.

57. Mwinga A, Hosp M, Godfrey-Faussett P *et al.* Twice weekly tuberculosis preventive therapy in HIV infection in Zambia. *AIDS* 1998; **12**: 2447–57.

58. Halsey NA, Coberly JS, Desormeaux J *et al.* Randomised trial of isoniazid versus rifampicin and pyrazinamide for prevention of tuberculosis in HIV-1 infection. *Lancet* 1998; **351**: 786–92.

59. Gao XF, Wang L, Liu GJ *et al.* Rifampicin plus pyrazinamide versus isoniazid for treating latent tuberculosis infection: a meta-analysis. *Int J Tuberc Lung Dis* 2006; **10**: 1080–90.

60. American Thoracic Society, Centers for Disease Control and Prevention. Update: fatal and severe liver injuries associated with rifampin and pyrazinamide for latent tuberculosis infection, and revisions in American Thoracic Society/CDC recommendations – United States 2001. *Am J Respir Crit Care Med* 2001; **164**: 1319–20.

61. Mount FW, Ferebee SH. Preventive effects of isoniazid in the treatment of primary tuberculosis in children. *N Engl J Med* 1961; **265**: 713–21.

62. Nolan CM, Aitken ML, Elarth AM *et al.* Active tuberculosis after isoniazid chemoprophylaxis of southeast asian refugees. *Am Rev Respir Dis* 1986; **133**: 431–6.

63. Fraser A, Paul M, Attamna A, Leibovici L. Treatment of latent tuberculosis in persons at risk for multidrug-resistant tuberculosis: systematic review. *Int J Tuberc Lung Dis* 2006; **10**: 19–23.

64. Schaaf HS, Gie RP, Kennedy M *et al.* Evaluation of young children in contact with adult multidrug-resistant pulmonary tuberculosis: a 30-month follow-up. *Pediatrics* 2002; **109**: 765–71.

65. Centers for Disease Control. Management of persons exposed to multidrug-resistant tuberculosis. *MMWR Morbid Mortal Wkly Rep* 1992; **41**: 61–70.

66. Rieder HL. Preventing latent tuberculosis among HIV-infected patients: efficacious and effective, yet inefficient? *Clin Infect Dis* 2007; **44**: 103–104.

67. Breuss E, Helbling P, Altpeter E, Zellweger JP. Screening and treatment for latent tuberculosis infection among asylum seekers entering Switzerland. *Swiss Med Wkly* 2002; **132**: 197–200.

68. MacIntyre CR, Plant AJ, Yung A, Streeton JA. Missed opportunities

for prevention of tuberculosis in Victoria, Australia. *Int J Tuberc Lung Dis* 1997; **1**: 135–41.

69. Marais BJ, van ZS, Schaaf HS *et al*. Adherence to isoniazid preventive chemotherapy: a prospective community based study. *Arch Dis Child* 2006; **91**: 762–5.

70. Marks GB, Bai J, Simpson SE, Sullivan EA, Stewart GJ. Incidence of tuberculosis among a cohort of tuberculin-positive refugees in Australia. Reappraising the estimates of risk. *Am J Respir Crit Care Med* 2000; **162**: 1851–4.

71. Jasmer RM, Snyder DC, Chin DP *et al*. Twelve months of isoniazid compared with four months of isoniazid and rifampin for persons with radiographic evidence of previous tuberculosis. An outcome and cost-effectiveness analysis. *Am J Respir Crit Care Med* 2000; **162**: 1648–52.

72. Lardizabal A, Passannante M, Kojakali F *et al*. Enhancement of treatment completion for latent tuberculosis infection with 4 months of rifampin. *Chest* 2006; **130**: 1712–17.

73. Menzies D, Dion MJ, Rabinovitch B *et al*. Treatment completion and costs of a randomized trial of rifampin for 4 months versus isoniazid for 9 months. *Am J Respir Crit Care Med* 2004; **170**: 445–9.

74. Schechter M, Zajdenverg R, Falco G *et al*. Weekly rifapentine/isoniazid or daily rifampin/pyrazinamide for latent tuberculosis in household contacts. *Am J Respir Crit Care Med* 2006; **173**: 922–6.

75. Davies P, Ormerod P. The role of four months of rifampicin in the treatment of latent tuberculosis infection. *Am J Respir Crit Care Med* 2005; **172**: 509–10.

76. Reichman LB, Lardizabal A, Hayden CH. Considering the role of four months of rifampin in the treatment of latent tuberculosis infection. *Am J Respir Crit Care Med* 2004; **170**: 832–35.

77. Ashkin D, Julien J, Lauzardo M, Hollender E. Consider rifampin BUT be cautious. *Chest* 2006; **130**: 1638–40.

78. Shieh FK, Snyder G, Horsburgh CR *et al*. Predicting non-completion of treatment for latent tuberculous infection: a prospective survey. *Am J Respir Crit Care Med* 2006; **174**: 717–21.

79. Goldberg SV, Wallace J, Jackson JC *et al*. Cultural case management of latent tuberculosis infection. *Int J Tuberc Lung Dis* 2004; **8**: 76–82.

80. Nyamathi AM, Christiani A, Nahid P *et al*. A randomized controlled trial of two treatment programs for homeless adults with latent tuberculosis infection. *Int J Tuberc Lung Dis* 2006; **10**: 775–82.

81. Malotte CK, Hollingshead JR, Larro M. Incentives vs outreach workers for latent tuberculosis treatment in drug users. *Am J Prev Med* 2001; **20**: 103–107.

82. Tulsky JP, Pilote L, Hahn JA *et al*. Adherence to isoniazid prophylaxis in the homeless: a randomized controlled trial. *Arch Intern Med* 2000; **160**: 697–702.

83. Eidlitz-Markus T, Zeharia A, Baum G *et al*. Use of the urine color test to monitor compliance with isoniazid treatment of latent tuberculosis infection. *Chest* 2003; **123**: 736–9.

84. Fallab-Stubi CL, Zellweger JP, Sauty A *et al*. Electronic monitoring of adherence to treatment in the preventive chemotherapy of tuberculosis. *Int J Tuberc Lung Dis* 1998; **2**: 525–30.

85. Ziv E, Daley CL, Blower SM. Early therapy for latent tuberculosis infection. *Am J Epidemiol* 2001; **153**: 381–5.

86. Chee CB, Teleman MD, Boudville IC *et al*. Treatment of latent TB infection for close contacts as a complementary TB control strategy in Singapore. *Int J Tuberc Lung Dis* 2004; **8**: 226–31.

87. Sterling TR, Bethel J, Goldberg S *et al*. The scope and impact of treatment of latent tuberculosis infection in the United States and Canada. *Am J Respir Crit Care Med* 2006; **173**: 927–31.

88. Rose DN, Schechter CB, Silver A, Fahs MC. Cost effectiveness of isoniazid chemoprophylaxis. In: Goldbloom RB, Lawrence RS (eds). *Preventing disease – beyond the rethoric*. New York: Springer Verlag, 1990: 446–54.

89. Salpeter SR, Sanders GD, Salpeter EE, Owens DK. Monitored isoniazid prophylaxis for low-risk tuberculin reactors older than 35 years of age: a risk–benefit and cost-effectiveness analysis. *Ann Intern Med* 1997; **127**: 1051–61.

90. Diel R, Nienhaus A, Schaberg T. Cost-effectiveness of isoniazid chemoprevention in close contacts. *Eur Respir J* 2005; **26**: 465–73.

91. Wrighton-Smith P, Zellweger JP. Direct costs of three models for the screening of latent tuberculosis infection. *Eur Respir J* 2006; **28**: 45–50.

92. Diel R, Wrighton-Smith P, Zellweger JP. Cost-effectiveness of interferon-gamma release assay testing for the treatment of latent tuberculosis. *Eur Res J* 2007; **30**: 321–32.

23

Clinical interpretation of tests for latent tuberculosis infection

VICTORIA J COOK, J MARK FITZGERALD AND DICK MENZIES

INTRODUCTION

The accurate diagnosis of people with latent tuberculosis infection (LTBI), and subsequent initiation of treatment, is essential to prevent new active tuberculosis (TB) cases arising from endogenous reactivation. Historically, the diagnosis of LTBI has relied on the tuberculin skin test (TST), the default 'gold standard'. Limitations of the TST are well described and have fuelled interest in the development and implementation of alternative means by which to diagnose people infected with *Mycobacterium tuberculosis* (MTB). *In vitro* diagnostic aids for detecting LTBI, based on T cell-mediated immunity to MTB, are now commercially available as adjunctive diagnostic tools. Available blood tests are referred to as interferon-γ release assays (IGRAs). This chapter will review TST and IGRA interpretation in the diagnosis of LTBI.

TUBERCULIN SKIN TESTING

Sir Robert Koch developed an extract from heat-killed *M. tuberculosis*, which he hoped might prove useful as therapy for TB disease.[1] In fact this substance, termed 'old tuberculin' (OT), proved ineffective for treatment. However, as first described by von Pirquet in 1907, this substance could be used as a skin test to detect TB infection.[2] Since then, there have been considerable refinements in tuberculin test materials and techniques, but uncertainty and controversy persist regarding the utility and interpretation of the TST in different populations and clinical situations.

The principle purpose for the TST is to diagnose tuberculous infection. The skin test has only a secondary role in the diagnosis of active disease, especially in subjects from high-prevalence countries where there is a high-prevalence of tuberculous infection in the at-risk population. The primary role of the TST is therefore to identify subjects who have been recently infected. Most commonly, this is in the context of a contact investigation where the source case has pulmonary TB. A second major group of subjects where the TST is used is in the screening of groups at high risk of tuberculous exposure and infection (i.e. human immunodeficiency virus (HIV)-infected people). Skin testing may also be used to establish whether people are uninfected before potential exposure to TB, such as health-care workers or travellers to endemic areas. The size of tuberculin reaction is not helpful in distinguishing latent infection from disease, but can predict the risk of progression to active disease.[3] Finally, TST is used as a surveillance tool among at-risk populations to define the current prevalence of infection and with serial TST surveys to estimate the annual risk of infection.

An undocumented history of a positive tuberculin test is not a contraindication to skin testing, as this history is often unreliable.[4] In most subjects, TST can be safely carried out, but there are certain groups for which a repeat skin test should not be considered. These people include those in whom active TB has been diagnosed or in whom treatment of active disease or infection has occurred in the past. Because of difficulties in interpretation, a skin test should not be planted on patients with significant skin conditions, such as eczema or extensive burns. In the presence of a previous history of a blistering reaction, the

Table 23.1   Tuberculin skin test technique.

(a) *Materials*

OT	Old Tuberculin. First prepared by Robert Koch.[1] Not purified, nor standardized. Had poor specificity.
PPD	Purified protein derivative. From culture of mycobacterial species, filtered, and purified by precipitation with ammonium sulphate or trichloroacetic acid.
PPD-S	Standard lot of PPD produced from *M. tuberculosis* by Dr Florence Seibert in 1941.[7] Stored by FDA (in USA) and used as worldwide standard lot. A Tuberculin Unit (1 TU) is defined as 0.02 µg of PPD-S (so 5 TU 5 0.1 µg). All commercial lots of PPD must be tested for bioequivalence against PPD-S.
PPD-T	Commercial PPD produced from *M. tuberculosis*, and used mainly in North America. There are two major manufacturers: Pasteur-Merieux-Connaught (Tubersol); Parke-Davis (Aplisol)
RT-23	Commercial PPD produced from *M. tuberculosis*, validated against PPD-S, and standardized by WHO.[14] This tuberculin test material is the most commonly used outside North America. Manufacturer: Statens Serum Institute (Copenhagen, Denmark).
PPD-B	Also known as PPD-Battey, because it was first produced at the Battey Institute from a non-tuberculous mycobacteria – *Mycobacterium intracellulare* (part of the *Mycobacterium avium-intracellulare* complex (MAC). This antigen is of little or no clinical use, and is used primarily for epidemiological surveys to determine prevalence of non-tuberculous mycobacteria and potential for false-positive tuberculin tests.
PPD-G	Also known as PPD-Gause, produced from *Mycobacterium scrofulaceum*. This antigen is of little clinical utility, and is used primarily for epidemiological surveys, although less commonly than PPD-B.

(b) *Techniques*

Mantoux	Intradermal injection of tuberculin material and reading of transverse diameter of induration after 48–72 hours. First described by Mantoux in 1912.[21]
Tine	Multi-puncture test in which four prongs or tines are coated with tuberculin material and dried. The prongs are pressed into the skin for about 2 seconds.
Heaf	Multi-puncture test – first introduced by Heaf in 1951.[25] The prongs are dipped in tuberculin solution and then the applicator is pressed into the skin.

TST should also not be repeated. Recent (within 1 month) viral infection or immunization with a live virus vaccination precludes TST. Clinicians often express uncertainty regarding skin testing in certain situations, but a previous history of bacillus Calmette–Guérin, current pregnancy or recent immunization with a non-live virus vaccination are not contraindications to a current TST being planted.

TUBERCULIN TEST MATERIALS

As summarized in Table 23.1, many different materials have been used for TST. Old tuberculin, originally developed by Dr Koch, has now been abandoned because this was a very impure product containing carbohydrates and nucleic acids, as well as tuberculin proteins. These impurities resulted in many non-specific reactions and considerable difficulty in standardizing the product. Purified protein derivative (PPD) is now the accepted standard. This material is prepared from a culture of a reference strain of *M. tuberculosis* that is killed with steam and then filtered. The filtrate is precipitated with trichloroacetic acid or ammonium sulphate, centrifuged, then dissolved in buffer containing stabilizer and preservative. This is then washed with buffer by ultrafiltration and finally lyophilized. The most important step in purification of the tuberculin proteins is the precipitation.[5] Early tuberculin testing materials were not well standardized,[5,6] but in 1941 Dr Florence

Seibert prepared a large batch of tuberculin which became the international standard (PPD-S). One tuberculin unit (1 TU) is defined as 0.02 µg of PPD-S.[7] Therefore, 5 TU is equivalent to 0.1 µg of PPD-S.[7] All commercial tuberculin test materials are compared with this reference batch of tuberculin to ensure bio-equivalence.

In North America, there are two major manufacturers of tuberculin materials. Of the two materials, Tubersol® and Aplisol® have equivalent sensitivity,[8,9] but Tubersol has 99 per cent specificity, while the specificity of Aplisol is 98 per cent.[9] This difference is too small to be clinically significant in most situations. The only exception appears to be when serial testing (e.g. for a cohort of workers with occupational TB exposure) has been performed with Tubersol, and then Aplisol is used. This has been associated with apparent 'outbreaks' of conversions, when several individuals who had never responded to Tubersol reacted to Aplisol.[10–13] This problem might be avoided by consistently using the same product. Outside North America, the most commonly used tuberculin material is RT-23 manufactured by Statens Serum Institute, Copenhagen. This material has been standardized against PPD-S by the World Health Organization[14] and in one comparative study had similar sensitivity but lower specificity than PPD-S.[15] Tuberculins, such as PPD-B and PPD-G, are prepared from non-tuberculous mycobacteria. These materials have little or no clinical utility, but are useful for epidemiologic surveys to ascertain the prevalence of sensitivity to environmental non-tuberculous mycobacteria (NTM) (i.e. *Mycobacterium xenopi* or *Mycobacterium kansasii*) and the potential effect this may have, through cross-reactivity, on TST reactions. This is especially important when interpreting TST reactions in a region with a low-prevalence of MTB, but high-prevalence of NTM, such as in the southern United States.

DOSE

The standard recommended dose is 5 TU of PPD-S or equivalent.[16] This means 5 TU (0.1 µg) of North American manufactured PPD, or 2 TU of RT-23 (0.04 µg). Use of 1 TU had been suggested to minimize adverse reactions, such as severe blistering. However, this preparation is much less sensitive[17,18] and there is no evidence that it will, in fact, reduce adverse events.[19] Testing with 100 TU or 250 TU has been associated with a large number of non-specific reactions, unrelated to TB exposure.[20] Therefore, the only recommended dose is that which is bio-equivalent to 5 TU of PPDS.[16]

METHOD OF ADMINISTRATION

The Mantoux method, first described by Mantoux in 1912,[21] consists of the intradermal injection of tuberculin material. Injection is usually on the volar (inside) aspect of the forearm, and should produce a small bleb with *peau d'orange*, which is absorbed within 15 minutes. The size of the bleb is not a reliable indicator of the amount injected. Errors in administration include injection of an inadequate amount, which has a surprisingly small effect on the resultant reaction (more dependent on the concentration of the tuberculin material) or subcutaneous injection. Subcutaneous injections, which are too deep, result in more diffuse reactions that are difficult to measure[22] and can be smaller, but are often larger.[23] Although smaller needles may be less painful and result in less bleeding or bruising, errors in administration and resultant variability in tuberculin reactions are greater with needles smaller than 27 gauge (the standard size for a tuberculin syringe).[24] The major limitation of the Mantoux technique is that it requires a slow injection, meaning the subject must be cooperative making it less practical for paediatric populations.

Table 23.2 Comparison of Heaf and Mantoux tests.

	Mantoux – PPD 5 TU		Accuracy of Heaf[a]	
	Positive (51mm)	Negative (0–4mm)	Sensitivity (%)	Specificity (%)
Older adults and adolescent boys in New York, USA[b]				
Heaf				
Grade 0	36	245		
Grades 1–4	323	248	90	50
Grades 0–1	90	413		
Grades 2–4	269	80	75	84
Grades 0–2	123	431		
Grades 3–4	236	62	66	87
Grades 0–3	306	484		
Grade 4	53	9	15	98

	Mantoux – PPD 5 TU		Accuracy of Heaf	
	Positive (91mm)	Negative (0–8mm)	Sensitivity (%)	Specificity (%)
School children in Australia[c]				
Heaf (OT or PPD)				
Grade 0	36	6886		
Grades 1–4	477	406	93	94
Grades 0–1	147	7158		
Grades 2–4	366	134	71	98
Grades 0–2	337	7274		
Grades 3–4	176	18	34	99.7
Grades 0–3	476	7290		
Grade 4	37	2	7	99.9

[a]In these comparisons the Mantoux is taken as the gold or reference standard.
[b]From Katz et al.[27]
[c]From Carruthers 1969.[26]
PPD, purified protein derivative.

Table 23.3 Comparison of Tine testing with Mantoux.

Author (year)	No. tested	Mantoux – 5 TU		Tine			
		Criteria for positive (mm)	% Positive	Material	Criteria (mm)	Sensitivity[a] (%)	Specificity[a] (%)
Badger et al. (1962)[99]	1001	10	43	OT	2	97	66
					6	78	86
Furcolow et al. (1966)[36]	770	10	46	OT	2	97	90
Fine et al. (1972)[100]	589	10	64	OT	2	98	66
					5	90	86
Donaldson and Elliot (1976)[101]	135	10	100	OT	2	84	–
				PPD	2	90	–
Ackerman (1981)[b,102]	6239	10	41	PPD		76	–
Hansen et al. (1982)[103]	829	10	5	OT	2	69	98
Rudd et al. (1982)[†39]	100	5	70	OT	2	96	83

[a]In these comparisons, the Mantoux is taken as the gold or reference standard.
[b]In these studies Mantoux performed with 10 TU of PPD instead of 5 TU as in all others.

Table 23.4 Variability of tuberculin readings between readers.

Author	No. tested	Technique	No. readers	Misclassified positive/negative (%)	Comments
Loudon et al. (1963)[30]	53	Mantoux 5 TU	7	9	–
Fine et al. (1972)[100]	189	Mantoux 5 TU	4	12	–
Erdtmann et al. (1974)[32]	121	Mantoux 5 TU	4	(standard deviation) 2.5 mm	–
Perez-Stable and Slutkin (1985)[33]	537	Mantoux 5 TU	6	4	–
Howard and Solomon (1988)[34]	806	Mantoux 5 TU	2	11	–
Carruthers (1970)[104]	69	Heaf	3	25–35	1 Grade
	46	Mantoux 5 TU	3	20	3 mm
	46	Mantoux 5 TU	3	10	4 mm
Griffith (1963)[105]		Heaf	2	21	(inter-observer)
		Heaf	1	7	(intra-observer)

Multiple puncture tests were believed to have the advantages of simpler administration and easier, more reliable, reading of reactions. The most commonly used in North America is the Tine test, while the Heaf test[25] is commonly used in Britain. Both are small single-use devices with multiple prongs or tines which are coated with tuberculin material. These are pressed into the skin for 1–2 seconds, making this technique easier to administer and more practical for paediatric populations. However, there are a number of limitations. Relative to the Mantoux test, sensitivity and specificity of the Heaf test are suboptimal (Table 23.2).[26,27] Sensitivity is improved if lower grades are considered positive, but this reduces specificity. Compared to the Mantoux, sensitivity of the Tine test has ranged from 75 to 95 per cent, depending on the size of reaction considered positive, while specificity has shown a considerable range as well, largely determined by the criterion for a positive test (Table 23.3). There is further variability because of variable coating of tuberculin

material on the tines[28] and difficulties in standardizing the depth and time of injection.[29] Although it was assumed that reading of these multiple puncture tests would be easier and therefore more reliable than with the Mantoux technique, this has not been the case (Table 23.4). Inter-reader[30–35] and intrareader[36,37] variability of readings are low with the Mantoux technique. In two studies, agreement between readers of the Tine test was 93 per cent[38] and 98 per cent.[39] However, in studies comparing variability of readings of the Mantoux and multipuncture tests, variability has been higher with the multipuncture techniques.[26,27,36,38]

One of the most important advantages of the Mantoux test is the wealth of information derived from large-scale epidemiologic surveys. As shown in Figure 23.1, the risk of TB is associated with the size of tuberculin reaction in a nearly linear relationship, although modified by the clinical situation.[40] There are no similar prospective data of TB incidence associated with size of reaction to Tine tests (or

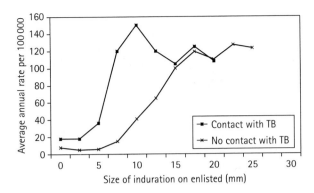

Figure 23.1 Average annual incidence of tuberculosis among navy recruits by size of tuberculin reaction and history of household contact. (Reproduced with permission from Comstock GW, Edwards LB, Livesay VT. Tuberculosis morbidity in the US Navy: its distribution and decline. *Am Rev Respir Dis* 1974; **110**: 572–80.)

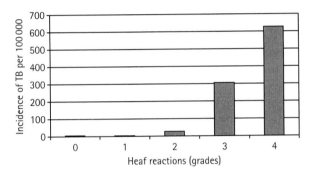

Figure 23.2 Incidence of tuberculosis (TB) by Heaf reactions (5308 positive and 65692 negative who were BCG vaccinated all tested/vaccinated in Britain at 13 years of age). Data from reference 41.

with the IGRAs as described later in this chapter and in Chapter 6, Immunodiagnostic tests). As shown in Figure 23.2, a gradient in risk has also been demonstrated for different Heaf grades,[41] although the differences in risk were by orders of magnitude for each increase by one grade. This means that a single Heaf grade difference in reading would have major implications in terms of prognosis. Given the inter-reader differences (21 per cent) in reading the Heaf, this could lead to a substantial misclassification of risk. In summary, given its greater reliability and prognostic information for different size reactions, the Mantoux technique has been the recommended diagnostic tool of choice to diagnose LTBI.[16]

READING OF MANTOUX TEST

The transverse diameter of induration should be measured after 48–72 hours.[16] Three techniques have been proposed:

the palpation, ballpoint and inspection methods. The palpation method is the oldest technique, while the ballpoint method was first proposed by Sokal in 1975.[42] Comstock *et al.*[40] proposed simple inspection from the side of the arm in order to visually delimit the edges of induration. When the palpation and ballpoint methods were directly compared by experienced readers, there were remarkably small differences in readings.[43,44] With less experienced readers, use of the ballpoint technique is associated with less interreader variability.[34,35,45] If tuberculin reactions are read 12–24 hours after administration, sensitivity is considerably reduced.[18,34,46] After 4 days or more, reactions begin to wane,[18,27] reducing sensitivity. Blistered reactions, read after 48–72 hours, should be considered significant. Interestingly, Heaf test reactions appear to persist longer, remaining constant for up to 1 week.[27] Self-reading of tuberculin reactions is strongly discouraged, as patients substantially under-read positive reactions.[34,47]

ADVERSE REACTIONS

Following Mantoux testing, local allergic reactions occurred in 2.3 per cent of patients seen in an allergy clinic.[48] These allergic reactions were most often associated with history of atopy, occurred within the first 24 hours and were not related to true tuberculin reactions measured at 42–78 hours. Generalized rash may occur in less than 0.1 per cent of all patients tuberculin tested.

Severe local reactions with blistering occur in less than 5 per cent of those with a positive tuberculin test. More severe blistering can lead to ulceration, though lymphangitis is extremely rare.[49] The presence of blistering generally indicates true infection, but otherwise has no particular prognostic significance (i.e. these individuals are not necessarily at increased risk of disease). Steroid cream is often used, but in the only available randomized controlled trial, was of no benefit.[50] Cold compresses can provide symptomatic relief. Any blistering should be covered with a dry dressing to avoid scratching and abrasion, as this could result in secondary infection.

Anaphylaxis is extremely rare. Two cases of anaphylaxis, one of them fatal, have been reported following Tine testing.[51,52] The survivor did not have serum IgE or other evidence of allergy to tuberculin, and the authors attributed the anaphylaxis to the gum or resin used to fix the tuberculin material to the Tines.[51] There has been one report of non-fatal anaphylaxis following Mantoux testing – with a 1-TU dose.[19] Tuberculin skin testing is felt to be very safe and is a well-studied diagnostic tool. Recent reports of allergic reactions in Canada prompted an advisory statement issued by Health Canada regarding potential serious reactions to Tubersol. This advisory statement suggests that any person administering Tubersol should be prepared to immediately treat systemic allergic reactions. All clients should be monitored for a period of 15 minutes following administration of Tubersol to observe for the possible onset of allergy, including anaphylaxis, angioedema, urticaria and dyspnoea. The risk of allergic reaction should be discussed with each client as part of the informed consent for skin testing.

The tuberculin test can be administered to pregnant women. There is no evidence that the test is in any way harmful – to the mother or fetus[53] and pregnancy has no effect on tuberculin reactions.[54]

INTERPRETATION OF SINGLE- AND MULTIPUNCTURE TINE TEST RESULTS

In most reports, a reaction of 2 mm or more has been considered positive. With this criterion, sensitivity has been 96–98 per cent in several series, but values of only 69–84 per cent have also been reported. A criterion of 5 or 6 mm has had higher specificity, but reduced sensitivity (Table 23.3). There is no prospective cohort study looking at the incidence of active TB by size of reaction to the Tine test.

HEAF TEST

- grade 0: 0–3 papules;
- grade 1: 4 or more papules;
- grade 2: papules coalesce to form a ring of induration;
- grade 3: papules coalesce to form a plaque of induration;
- grade 4: papules coalesce to form a plaque of induration, 15 mm or greater.

Compared to the Mantoux test, if grade 1 reactions are considered positive, sensitivity will be 90–93 per cent, but will be only 71–75 per cent if grade 2 reactions are considered the threshold, and 34–66 per cent if grade 3 or more are considered positive.[26,27] Higher-grade reactions have higher specificity, but reduced sensitivity (Table 23.2). Incidence of active TB was strongly associated with size of reaction among non-vaccinated British adolescents,[41] with the largest increment in incidence occurring between grades 2 and 3 (Figure 23.2).

INTERPRETATION OF TUBERCULIN TESTING

In general, the TST should be interpreted in the context of why it is being done and the risk profile of the person in whom the TST has been planted. The accuracy of a true positive TST result depends on *M. tuberculosis* prevalence in a community: a low-prevalence community has a low probability of accuracy; conversely, a high-prevalence community has a high probability of accuracy. The significance of different reactions is shown in Table 23.5.[55] Different cut-points are used depending on the patient's risk for having LTBI and the size of induration in millimetres.

The skin test should be read at 48–72 hours by an experienced health-care professional. Although reactions may

Table 23.5 Interpretation of different size tuberculin skin test reactions with the size of reactions that are considered significant.

Skin test reaction size in mm of induration	Factors associated with the population at risk
0–4	In general, not considered significant but in the presence of HIV infection and a history of contact with an active infectious case of tuberculosis
5–9	HIV infection, contact of an active tuberculosis case, abnormal chest x-ray with apical fibronodular changes
>10	In all other settings

Adapted from Ref. 55.

persist for longer, a significant minority negative at 1 week will have been positive at the recommended reading time. It is not recommended that people interpret their own skin test, rather this should be done by a health professional experienced in reading skin tests. The primary measurement is one of induration and not the presence of redness or bruising. Blistering rarely occurs, but when it does its presence should be noted and the person cautioned against any future skin tests.

False-negative tests

As summarized in Table 23.6, technical causes of false-negative TSTs can be corrected with careful attention to technique. Problems in production, contamination or inadequate concentration of tuberculin materials can be avoided by use of well-standardized materials from recognized manufacturers. Even the best-quality material will degrade if stored for prolonged periods, particularly if exposed to sunlight.[16] Refrigeration is less important than avoidance of light exposure.[16] The technique of administration is rarely the cause of false-negative tests, because the errors must be quite major, although drawing tuberculin material up in syringes more than 20 minutes before administration is a common mistake. Errors in reading are more common, as this requires more training. Rounding errors are a particularly common problem; these can be avoided by use of simple calipers, with which readers demarcate the diameter of the induration while unable to read the scale. Only after the calipers are set, can the reader look at the scale and determine the size in millimetres.

Biologic problems are much more common and generally not correctable. Immune suppression leading to anergy, an inability to react to injected antigens, is of great concern with interpreting the TST. Of these, the most

Table 23.6 Causes of false–negative tests.

Technical (can be corrected)

Material	Poor quality production, or contamination.
	Inadequate concentration (e.g. 1 TU)
	Improper storage (exposure to light or heat), non-stabilized (no Tween), or use after expiry date
Administration	Material not injected properly, e.g. too deep (usually this causes larger reactions)
	Interval between drawing up in syringe and administration too long (>20 min)
Reading	Inexperienced or biased reading, rounding error
	Reading too soon (<40 hours) or too late (>80 hours)
	Error in recording result

Biological (cannot be corrected)

Viral infections	HIV infection most important. Also measles, mumps, chicken pox
	Live virus vaccination
Tuberculosis	Active TB disease – particularly if more advanced pulmonary, or miliary
Other illnesses	Malignancies especially lymphomas, renal failure, malnutrition, major surgery
Therapy	Immune suppression – corticosteroid, cancer therapy, transplant therapy, infliximab
Age	Very young (infants), or elderly

Table 23.7 Risk factors for the development of active tuberculosis based on the presence of additional risk factors.

Risk factor	Estimate of risk of infection compared to a person with no risk factor
AIDS	170
HIV infection	113
Organ transplant	20–74
Silicosis	30
Chronic renal failure or dialysis	10–25.3
Carcinoma of head and neck	16
Recent infection (within 2 years)	15
Apical fibronodular changes on chest x-ray	9–19
Diabetes mellitus	2–3.6
Underweight (<90% of ideal body weight)	2.0–3.0
Infected in childhood	2.2–5.0
Presence of granuloma on chest x-ray	2.0
No documented risk factor	1.0

important clinical scenario is HIV infection. Patients with HIV infection are at greater risk of acquiring infection in the face of TB exposure, as well as developing active disease once infected. Accurate TST interpretation in this group is vital. The likelihood of a false-negative tuberculin test is greater with lower CD4 counts; when the CD4 count is less than 200 almost all individuals with TB infection will have a false-negative tuberculin test.[56–59] Another important cause of false-negative tests is the presence of active TB itself. With minimal, smear-negative pulmonary disease, 10 per cent will have false-negative TST,[60] compared to 23–47 per cent[61–63] of individuals with more extensive disease. False-negative results are also associated with age extremes or recent viral infections or vaccinations with live virus in the past month (e.g. mumps or measles). Recent TB infection can lead to a 'false-negative' response as the immune system has not had time to respond appropriately. In this situation, a repeat TST in 8–12 weeks from the date of last exposure is recommended.

Once a significant reaction is documented, active TB should be excluded and there should be consideration for the initiation of treatment of latent TB infection (see Chapter 17, Directly observed therapy and other aspects of management of tuberculosis care). A key factor in making such a recommendation is the presence of a coexisting risk factor for the development of active TB (Table 23.7).

False-positive results

Previous immunization with BCG is an important consideration when interpreting a TST. Although not used widely in North America, many other countries still use BCG as part of their TB control programme. Foreign-born subjects presenting in North America for immigration screening or with suspected TB will often have a history of BCG vaccination. Published meta-analyses[64,65] have provided guidance with interpretating a TST in the presence of BCG. People who had received BCG were more likely to have a positive TST, regardless of the antigen used. Immunization in infancy was much less likely to be associated with a positive TST, especially 10–15 years later. BCG received after infancy leads to more frequent, persistent and larger TST responses. In people given BCG after infancy or in adulthood, or in the event of repeated vaccinations, IGRAs will be of great diagnostic importance in accurately identifying patients with true latent TB infection. TST interpretation should also integrate the background prevalence of infection, contact history and whether the person being evaluated is from a high-prevalence group. In the presence of a high-risk population, a positive TST is more likely to be on the basis of true infection and not BCG.

In some locations (i.e. southern United States), infection with NTM is prevalent and can give rise to false-positive TST results. In most situations, these reactions will be less than 10 mm and will not interfere with the interpretation of the skin test results. A recent meta-analysis including more than 1 million subjects confirmed that NTM are not a clinically important cause of false-positive TST in populations

Table 23.8 Occurrence of positive tuberculin tests on two-step testing ('boosting')

Population	Countries	No. subjects	Initial (PPD1)[a] 10+ mm %	Two-step (PPD2)[b] 10+ mm %	References
Health-care workers	USA, Canada	4357	6	2.1	73, 74, 106–109
Nursing home residents	USA, Holland	2870	29	14	75, 76, 110–112
Foreign born	USA, Canada, Holland	3537	37	30	69, 77, 113, 114
HIV infected	USA	95	13	8	115, 116
	Uganda	345	71	29	

[a]Denominator is all persons tested.
[b]Denominator is all persons undergoing PPD2 who were negative on PPD1.

Table 23.9 Effect of BCG vaccination and non-tuberculous mycobacteria on two-step tuberculin testing.

Population	No. subjects	Initial (PPD1) 10+ mm %	Two-step (PPD2) 10+ mm %	References
BCG vaccination				
Never vaccinated[a]	3699	5.9	4.0	74, 106, 117–127
BCG in infancy	1469	6.3	9.9	
BCG after age 5 years	3159	43	18	
Non-tuberculous mycobacterial (NTM) sensitivity				
Not sensitive to NTM	362	2.2	1.4	74, 109
Reacts to NTM antigens	128	1.6	12.7	

[a]Data for never vaccinated from two studies in Canadian-born populations in Montreal, Canada: schoolchildren and young adults[72] and health-care workers.[104]

with a low-prevalence of NTM sensitization and in the absence of a very low-prevalence of TB infection.[65]

REPEATED OR SERIAL TUBERCULIN SKIN TESTS

Indications

The major reason to repeat the tuberculin test is to detect new TB infections in situations of potential exposure. This includes contact investigations (recent exposure), when close or high-risk contacts are tested soon after diagnosis of the index case. At the time of this first test, some of the tuberculin-negative contacts may have been infected just before the end of exposure, and so would not yet manifest a tuberculin reaction. These contacts should be retested 8 weeks after the end of exposure, by which time all newly infected contacts with intact immune systems should manifest tuberculin conversion.[66] Repeated TSTs are also performed in individuals at risk for future TB exposure, such as health-care or prison workers, or travellers to TB-endemic countries.

Non-specific variation

Two tuberculin tests administered simultaneously in different sites in the same individuals, will result in small test-to-test differences because of differences in administration, and reading, as well as biologic variation. These factors result in variation with a standard deviation of less than 3 mm. Given these sources of variability, 95 per cent of repeated tests should fall within 6 mm of each other, representing two standard deviations. Therefore, it is conventional to consider that reactions that increase by 6 mm or more represent a true biologic phenomenon – either boosting or conversion.[67]

Boosting

Boosting is defined as an increase of 6 mm or more on repeated tests, due to anamnestic recall of waned cellular immunity in the absence of new infection. This phenomenon is common in many populations and roughly correlates with the prevalence of positive initial tuberculin reactions (PPD1) as shown in Table 23.8. Boosting is common in the elderly and foreign born, most probably because of remote TB infection, but is also associated with BCG vaccination[64] and non-tuberculous mycobacteria as shown in Table 23.9. Because the phenomenon is less specific and associated with remote, rather than recent TB infection, the likelihood of developing TB disease is substantially lower in people manifesting the boosting phenomenon, than in people whose initial TST is positive.[68]

For optimum detection of the boosting phenomenon, a second TST should be performed between 1 and 4 weeks after an initially negative first TST.[66,68,69] The same technique and same dose (i.e. 5 TU should be used), although the site of injection should be different. Use of the same site can result in spurious increased reactions.[70] The booster phenomenon will be substantially less frequent if the second test is administered only 2 days,[71] or 2 months[69] or more after the first TST. However, the phenomenon can occur after intervals of 1 year[71-73] and possibly longer.[74] In addition, boosting has been reported with a third and even a fourth tuberculin test in the very elderly[75,76] and malnourished South East Asian refugees.[77] This has not been reported in younger healthy adults (e.g. workers or travellers).

Conversion

Tuberculin conversion is defined as a biologic increase in tuberculin reactions as a result of a new mycobacterial infection. This can be the result of BCG vaccination, non-tuberculous mycobacteria or true TB infection. If the TST response is due to new TB infection, tuberculin conversion is associated with substantially increased risk of disease.[68,78,79] Furthermore, the absolute size of the TST response in millimetres is directly correlated to the risk of developing active TB. Conversion most often occurs within 3–7 weeks following new TB infection[80-84] or BCG vaccination.[85] All available evidence suggests that tuberculin conversion is completed within 8 weeks after the moment of primary infection.[67]

Distinguishing conversion from boosting

One of the most difficult aspects of repeated tuberculin tests is the interpretation of increased reactions – specifically to distinguish boosting from conversion. The importance of the distinction is considerable – given the very different risks of developing active TB. Boosting is associated with a lower risk of active TB, so therapy for LTBI may not be recommended. Conversion is associated with a very high risk of disease and so therapy for LTBI would be strongly recommended, regardless of age. There are three approaches to distinguishing boosting from conversion:

1 *Initial two-step testing*: If initial two-step testing has been carried out and both tests were negative, then a substantial increase in size (≥5 mm) on a third or subsequent TST is highly likely to represent true conversion.[73] This reinforces the importance of two-step testing of people who are at risk for future TB exposure. This will enhance the accuracy of diagnosing conversion and thereby reduce the likelihood of unnecessary and potentially harmful LTBI therapy for the individual involved. In an occupational health programme, this will also reduce the chances of needlessly investigating apparent nosocomial transmission.

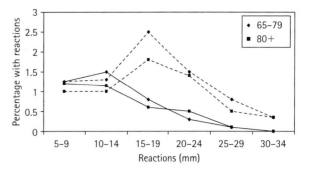

Figure 23.3   Conversion and two-step tuberculin skin test (TST) reactions. Arkansas nursing home residents, by age. Solid line, 38262 two-step TST; dashed line, 38182 repeat skin tests for conversion. Data from W Stead, Little Rock, Arkansas.

2 *Size*: As shown in Figure 23.3, among elderly nursing home residents, reactions to the second TST in two-step testing have a very different frequency distribution compared to conversion reactions. Most two-step reactions are small (6–9 mm increase) and larger reactions are progressively less frequent. This is also true of two-step reactions in health professional students and workers.[74] On the other hand, conversion reactions are most frequently 10–15 mm or 16–20 mm in size, in the elderly or younger populations.[86] Therefore, at progressively larger reaction sizes, conversion is increasingly likely. This means that using larger reaction sizes to define tuberculin conversion will result in greater specificity, but reduced sensitivity. For example, if tuberculin conversion is defined as an increase in reaction size of 6 mm, this will detect almost all individuals with true tuberculin conversion, but will also include the majority of those with boosting reactions. Using a definition of 10 mm will eliminate a small number of individuals with true tuberculin conversion, and a large number of people with boosting. Setting a criteria of 15 mm will eliminate virtually all those with boosting, but will correctly identify only 50 per cent of those with conversion. Selection of an appropriate cut-point therefore depends upon the population and clinical situation.

3 *Clinical situation*: The occurrence of tuberculin conversions has varied considerably in different studies, as summarized in Table 23.10. Contacts of an active case in the same household[87-90] or in an outbreak situation[91-94] have very high rates of tuberculin conversion. On the other hand, health-care workers, even in 'high risk' hospitals have a much lower risk of tuberculin conversion.[86,95-97] It is possible to make a very rough and ready estimate of the relative likelihood of conversion versus boosting in different situations, by comparing the expected occurrence of conversion (Table 23.10) with boosting (Table 23.8) for the same population. Using this crude method, one can estimate that an increased reaction on annual testing among hospital workers may be much more likely to represent boosting

Table 23.10 Occurrence of tuberculin conversion.

Populations	Author	No. subjects	Conversion	
			Cumulative (%)	Per unit time
Household contacts[a]				
	Shaw and Wynn-Williams (1954)[88]	161 (0–4 years)	54	Not given
	Zaki *et al.* (1976)[90]	727 (all ages)	22	Not given
	Van Geuns *et al.* (1975)[89]	46 (0–14 years)	50	Not given
	Grzybowski *et al.* (1970)[87]	309 (0–4 years)	28	Not given
Health-care workers				
High-risk hospitals	Blumberg *et al.* (1998)[95]	2144	2.4	0.7% annually
	Boudreau *et al.* (1997)[96]	209	14.5	3.2% annually
	Menzies *et al.* (2000)[86]	1216	18.8	1.7% annually
Low-risk hospitals	Aitkin *et al.* (1987)[98]	124 869[b]	0.3	0.1% annually
Working in endemic country	de Silva *et al.* (2000)[97]	455	12	2.9% annually
Travelling to endemic countries	Cobelens *et al.* (2000)[128]	65	6.2	9.5% annually
Outbreak investigations				
Airplanes – work contacts	Driver *et al.* (1994)[94]	274	25	2.1%/hour
Airplanes – passengers	Miller *et al.* (1996)[91]	121	2	0.2%/hour
	Driver *et al.* (1994)[94]	59	7	0.3%/hour
	Kenyon *et al.* (1996)[93]	358	2	0.2%/hour
University classmates	Braden (1995)[92]	302	21	0.4–1.8%/hour

[a] In only one study of household contacts (Zaki *et al.*[90]) was documented conversion measured, in contacts whose first tuberculin skin test (TST) was negative. For the other three studies, results of all positive TSTs are shown together, but only for youngest contacts, and prevalence of positive TSTs in a control group of the same age without contact was subtracted.
[b] This represents the number of TSTs placed and read over a 3-year period. Many workers were tested annually, although not all, so the number of workers was not less than 42 000.

than conversion. This is particularly true if these workers had previous BCG vaccination and/or were foreign born, and/or lived in regions endemic for non-tuberculous sensitivity, and/or did not undergo initial two-step testing at hiring. For workers in lower-risk hospitals with even lower risk of conversion,[97] the likelihood that an increased reaction represented boosting would be even higher. Therefore, in these groups use of a higher, more specific cut-point to define conversion would be appropriate, whereas in household contacts or an outbreak situation the lowest cut-point would be most appropriate. The same logic might be applied to casual contacts or recently returned travellers.

In summary, serial tuberculin testing should be performed only when clearly indicated. Boosting is common in almost all populations, particularly when the prevalence of positive initial tuberculin tests is high. The likelihood that an increased reaction represents conversion depends upon the amount of increase in the tuberculin reaction (in millimetres) and the pretest likelihood of conversion; the latter is dependent on the clinical situation. In populations with a relatively low risk of tuberculin conversion, such as health-care workers and travellers, baseline two-step testing is strongly recommended and more stringent criteria for definition of conversion used (≥10 mm). Among household contacts, the relative importance of boosting is low, so two-step testing should be avoided, and a lower cut-point used to define conversion (≥5 mm). Decisions regarding therapy for latent TB infection should be based not only on the amount of increase in size of tuberculin reaction, but also on the clinical situation which determines the relative likelihood that this represents new TB infection or boosting from remote mycobacterial exposure of any type. In addition, the likelihood of development of TB disease must be balanced against the risks of therapy on a case-by-case basis.

IGRAs: NOVEL TESTS FOR THE DIAGNOSIS OF LATENT TB INFECTION

In vitro diagnostic aides for detecting LTBI, based on T-cell mediated immunity to MTB, have been rapidly refined and are now commercially available as adjunctive diagnostic tools. As a group, these blood tests are referred to as interferon-γ release assays or IGRAs and can be used to diagnose both latent infection and active disease. In late 2005, the US Centers for Disease Control and Prevention released a statement that the TST can now be replaced by a blood test (QuantiFERON-TB Gold Test or QFT-G) for diagnosing latent TB infection.[129] And in the UK, a National Institute for Clinical Excellence statement recommended that the IGRAs should be used as an adjunct test to confirm a positive TST.[130]

Commercially Available Tests (Table 23.11)

QUANTIFERON®-TB GOLD TEST (CELLESTIS LTD, AUSTRALIA)

In 2001, the US Food and Drug Administration first approved an *in vitro* diagnostic aid for detecting latent infection with MTB. This first generation test, known as the QuantiFERON®-TB Test (Cellestis Ltd, Australia), was based on the quantification of interferon-γ (IFN-γ) released from sensitized lymphocytes when whole-blood containing peripheral blood monocytes was incubated overnight with tuberculin (purified protein derivative from MTB), an avian antigen, and controls using an enzyme-linked immunosorbent assay (ELISA). The results measured the amount of IFN-γ released in response to tuberculin compared with the other antigens. This test has been refined since its introduction and the QuantiFERON®-TB Test is no longer commercially available.

The QuantiFERON®-TB Gold Test (Cellestis Ltd, Australia) was developed as a second generation IGRA with synthetic peptides mimicking two MTB specific proteins: the early secretory antigenic target 6 (ESAT-6) and culture filtrate protein 10 (CFP-10), both present in MTB, as well positive (phytohemaglutinin mitogen) and negative (saline) controls. These peptides are encoded by genes located within the region of difference 1 (RD1) segment of the genome of MTB complex. These genes are absent in the *Mycobacterium bovis* strain used in the preparation of BCG vaccine, and several common non-tuberculous mycobacteria such as *M avium*, but are present in several other NTM including *M. kansasii*, *M. szulgai*, *M. marinarum* and *M. leprae*. These modifications have improved test specificity as test results are unaffected by BCG status. A positive QFT-G test is recorded when the IFN-γ level in whole blood incubated with ESAT-6 or CFP-10 minus the IFN-γ concentration in blood mixed with saline is ≥0.35 IU/ml (and 50 per cent above nil).

QUANTIFERON IN-TUBE (CELLESTIS LTD, AUSTRALIA)

A third generation test, the QuantiFERON In-Tube (Cellestis Ltd, Australia), is now available. The test incorporates ESAT-6, and CFP-10 and a third MTB specific antigen TB7.7 (Rv2654). The test kit enables blood to be collected directly into tubes containing these MTB-specific antigens, as well as positive and negative controls. This minimizes handling and lends itself to large-scale automation. Also available are portable blood stimulation and test-specific incubators which may improve processing in remote communities.

T-SPOT.TB ASSAY (OXFORD IMMUNOTEC, UK)

The T-SPOT.TB assay, which also relies on the ESAT-6 and CFP-10 antigens, is also widely available now. Earlier versions were based on the ESAT-6 antigen alone. The present assay involves incubating peripheral blood mononuclear cells with ESAT-6 and CFP-10 antigens and measuring the number of IFN-γ-producing cells using an enzyme-linked immunospot (Elispot) assay. A positive test result is recorded when > 6 IFN-γ spot forming cells are counted. The manufacturer's suggested use of this test includes screening of immune-compromised persons (e.g. HIV/AIDS, transplant, anti-TNF-α treatment and chronic renal failure), as a 'rule-out' test for TB infection in active TB suspects and as a means to monitor treatment response in active TB disease.

Sensitivity and specificity

Pooled sensitivity and specificity results for IGRAs were reviewed in a recently published meta-analysis (Tables 23.12 and 23.13). Sensitivity was estimated from studies of patients with active TB, as a proxy of LTBI, since they must have infection. Using newly-diagnosed active TB as a surrogate marker for latent infection, the pooled estimates of sensitivity were lowest for the TST, slightly higher for QFT and highest for Elispot. The sensitivity of the TST exceeded that of IGRAs in 3 studies of previously treated patients.[65] However, IGRAs, like the TST, are not recommended to diagnose active disease but rather to diagnose latent TB infection.[131] The biggest weakness of all studies evaluating the sensitivity of IGRAs is their cross-sectional design, because there is no gold standard for latent TB infection. Using a gradient of exposure among contacts of patients with active TB as a clinical gold standard, TST and IGRA sensitivity was similar in subjects with the highest exposure – the prevalence of positive results were highest in the most exposed. In less exposed groups, the prevalence of positive TSTs was higher than IGRAs – but only in BCG vaccinated populations.[132,133]

Among immune-compromised populations, the T-SPOT. TB assay was more sensitive than TST, particularly in subjects with greater levels of immune-suppression.[134-138] Indeterminate results were frequently noted with use of the QFT-G in HIV infected persons whose CD4 counts were <100. Insufficient information is available to evaluate IGRA use in children. A key point is that no test (IGRA or TST) is able to distinguish active TB disease from latent TB infection.

Specificity was estimated from studies of healthy subjects with a very low likelihood of exposure (i.e. no contact history, originating from low-prevalence country). In these populations at very low risk for LTBI, IGRA using RD1 antigens had very high specificity. The pooled average specificity of QFT was 97.7 per cent (95 per cent confidence interval: 96–99 per cent) and Elispot was 92.5 per cent (86–99 per cent), and was unaffected by BCG vaccination. Both were far more specific than TST in BCG vaccinated populations, especially if the vaccine was given after infancy,[131] given the greater effect of BCG at a later age on subsequent TST reactions.[65] The effect of non-

Table 23.11 *Characteristics of the three tests for latent TB infection*[a]

	TST	QFT-Gold QFT-Gold In-Tube	Elispot T-SPOT.TB
Administration	*In vivo* (intradermal)	*Ex vivo*; ELISA based	*Ex vivo*; Elispot based
Antigens	PPDS or RT-23	ESAT-6 + CFT-10 ± TB 7.7	ESAT-6 + CFP-10
Standardized	Mostly	Yes	Yes
Units of measurement	Millimetres of induration	International Units of IFN-γ	IFN-γ Spot forming cells (SFC)
Definition of positive test	5, 10, 15 mm	Patient's IFN-γ ≥ 0.35 IU /ml (after subtracting IFN-γ response in nil control)	≥6 SFC in the antigen wells, with 250 000 cells/well, and at least double negative well
Indeterminate	If anergy (rarely tested)	Poor response to mitogen: (<0.5 IU/mL in positive control) or high background response (>8.0 IU/mL in nil well)	Poor response to mitogen (<20 SFC in positive control well) or high background (>10 SFC in negative well)
Time to result	48–72 hours	16–24 hours (but longer if run in batches)	16–24 hours (but longer if run in batches)
Cost per test[b]			
– Materials		$19 (3)	$63 (3)
– Labour/other		$22 (1;3)	$22 (1)
– Total cost	$12.73 (1;2)	$41	$85

[a]Adapted from Reference 131 with permission.
[b]All costs in Canadian dollars (1$ Canadian = 0.91 US). For the IGRA tests, the materials cost is based on quotes from the manufacturers for shipment to a Canadian centre in September 2006. The cost for IGRA labour, shipping, and handling is taken from published field experience with Quantiferon testing, as reported by San Francisco TB program.[157] Costs may vary widely in different countries.

tuberculous mycobacteria on IGRA response remains poorly studied.

SERIAL TESTING

Several studies have reported conversions and reversions with repeated IGRA testing. In two studies, reversion occurred in untreated persons over 18 months to 4 years in 20 per cent of those with initially positive IGRA; this was associated with weaker initial IGRA response, and initially negative TST.[139,140] In one small study, 9 per cent of patients with positive T-SPOT. TB assay reverted within a week.[141] Other studies have reported IGRA reversion in patients treated for active TB, but not in those treated for latent TB infection.[141–144] However, the effect of treatment cannot be ascertained until the biologic and random variability of IGRA response has been better characterized.

Concordance of IGRA and TST

In studies with cross-sectional designs, there is no gold standard for the diagnosis of latent tuberculosis infection. IGRAs and the TST are composed of different combinations of antigens measuring different components of the T-cell immune response. As such, discordant results are expected.[132,133,139–151] If the IGRA is more specific then some

TST positive/IGRA negative discordance is expected. If IGRAs are more sensitive then the reverse would also be seen (i.e. IGRA positive and TST negative). As reported in a recent meta-analysis,[131] when the tests are performed concurrently, substantial discordance has been found both in high- and low-risk populations. These discordant TST and IGRA reactions were largely unexplained, although some may be related to variation around the definitions of positive tests, and some positive TST with negative IGRA results can be explained by prior BCG vaccination or exposure to environmental mycobacteria. Thus, although some discordance may be explained by superior specificity of IGRA it would be overly simplistic to assume that the IGRA tests were always correct and the TST incorrect.

Economic evaluations

Published analyses have concluded that the additional use of QFT-G is cost-effective in the context of contact investigations,[152,153] especially if its use is confined to TST positive persons or those with previous BCG vaccination.[154] A reduction in the number of patients treated for LTBI with false positive TST accounts for the cost savings. Screening for LTBI with the TST followed by T-SPOT.TB assay for confirmation was also less costly for similar reasons.[155] The use of IGRAs for screening lower risk populations, such as

Table 23.12 *Summary of sensitivity and specificity from pooled estimates from all studies – Patients with active TB used as surrogate for Latent TB Infection[a]*

	Studies (n)	Sensitivity	95% Conference interval[b]
Tuberculin Skin Testing			
All studies	14	0.71	0.65–0.74
Size of TST			
5 mm	9	0.74	0.66–0.82
10 mm	4	0.72	0.50–0.95
15 mm	1	0.40	0.25–0.56
Age			
Paediatric	4	0.55	0.43–0.67
Adult	10	0.73	0.68–0.78
Quantiferon			
All studies	13	0.76	0.7–0.83
Antigens			
ESAT-6 only	1	0.58	0.34–0.80
ESAT-6/CFP10	9	0.80	0.73–0.87
ESAT-6/CFP10 + 7.7	3	0.67	0.56–0.78
Age			
Paediatric	4	0.66	0.5–0.83
Adult	10	0.76	0.7–0.83
Elispot or T-SPOT.TB			
All studies	12	0.88	0.81–0.95
Antigens			
ESAT-6	3	0.93	0.91–0.96
ESAT-6 / CFP10	9	0.87	0.78–0.95
Age			
Paediatric	2	0.62	0.43–0.81
Adult	10	0.92	0.88–0.95

[a]Adapted from Reference 131 with permission.
[b]All 95% conference intervals are corrected for over-dispersion.

Table 23.13 *Summary of specificity from pooled estimates from all studies[a]*

Grouping	Studies (n)	Specificity	95% Conference interval
Tuberculin Skin Testing			
All studies	8	0.66	0.46–0.86
BCG:			
Not vaccinated	3	0.98	0.96–1.0
Vaccinated	5	0.56	0.34–0.78
TST criteria:			
Positive ≥ 10 mm	6[b]	0.58	0.37–0.79
Positive ≥ 15 mm	3[b]	0.87	0.7–1.0
Quantiferon			
All studies	9[c]	0.97	0.95–0.99
ESAT-6	2	1.0	0.94–1.0
ESAT-6 + CFP10	7	0.96	0.94–0.99
BCG:			
Not vaccinated	3	1.0	0.94–1.0
Vaccinated	6	0.96	0.93–0.99
Elispot or T-SPOT.TB			
All studies	4	0.92	0.88–0.95

[a]Adapted from Reference 131 with permission.
[b]In one study[132] data for 2 TST cut points are given.
[c]In each of two studies (Brock *et al*,[147] and Johnson *et al*[158]) 2 different very low risk populations were tested. These were counted as separate studies.

immigrants from high- to low-incidence, will not be cost-effective[154] – similar to the use of TST. The cost-effectiveness of the use of IGRA in periodic screening (e.g. healthcare workers) is unknown, but data on the utility of IGRA for this indication are needed first.

Operational advantages and disadvantages of IGRA compared to TST

In addition to improved specificity, the IGRAs have a number of operational advantages compared to TB skin testing.[156] Only a single patient visit is required to draw the blood sample, the results can be available within 24 hours, and should be less subject to observer bias (i.e. reader variability). Because antigens are not given to patients they eliminate any risk of adverse events such as allergy or anaphylaxis. As well, if they are to be used in serial testing to detect new TB infection in exposed populations, there is no 'boosting phenomenon', because the antigens are not administered in vivo to the subjects. This reduces problems in interpretation, and eliminates the need for baseline two-step skin testing. The response to multiple antigens can be assessed simultaneously.

However several important disadvantages do exist.[156] Blood draws can be unacceptable or unsuccessful with some patients, especially children. Whole blood must be transported to the lab, and processed within 8 to 12 hours after collection while the circulating mononuclear cells remain viable. This means that IGRAs may not be practical for use in remote communities, where incidence of active TB may be higher. Initial capital expenses for equipment are high, the unit costs of the assays are much more than the TST, and performance of the assays requires well trained technical staff. Patients may refuse to give a blood sample, or it can not be obtained, while other errors in specimen collection and transportation, as well as assay performance and interpretation are inevitable. As well, indeterminate results (neither negative nor positive) can occur due to low mitogen response (failure of the positive control) or high background response in the saline control.

Areas for Future Research

There are limited data evaluating the use of IGRAs in: young children (i.e. especially those under the age of 5 years); patients with impaired immunity (such as those with HIV infection or AIDS) or taking immune-modulating medications (i.e. TNF-α antagonists); persons recently exposed to M. tuberculosis; and persons with haematological disorders, malignancies, diabetes, silicosis, and chronic renal failure. Since these conditions place patients at greatest risk for reactivation of active TB, this knowledge gap is critical. The incidence of active TB after a positive or negative IGRA is unknown; of particular interest is the long-term risk in persons with discordant IGRA-TST results.

The length of time between the acquisition of latent TB infection, and emergence of a positive IGRA has not been determined. This is relevant in the context of a contact evaluation, if the initial IGRA is negative – how long to wait before repeating the test to determine if infection occurred just before the exposure ended? The performance and practicality of periodic screening, targeted testing (i.e. recent immigrants from high-incidence countries), and contact investigations are areas for investigation. The variability of IGRA over days, months and years is unknown. This must be known before the changes in IFN-γ release during treatment for active or latent TB can be estimated. This will also help in the evaluation of serial IGRA, which will require substantial validation before these tests can be used for periodic screening, such as for health care workers.

Conclusions

Commercially available IGRAs have evolved rapidly over the last decade. The latest versions use more specific M. tuberculosis antigens not present in BCG or in certain non-tuberculous mycobacteria. The commercial IGRAs are relatively simple to perform and have been successfully used under field conditions by independent investigators in many settings. Additional studies are needed to better define their performance in high-risk populations and in serial testing. Longitudinal studies are needed to define the value of IGRAs in predicting risk of TB disease.

LEARNING POINTS

- The principle role of the TST is to identify subjects infected with M. tuberculosis. The TST has only a secondary role in the diagnosis of active disease, especially in subjects from high-prevalence countries.
- The accepted standard TST uses 5 tuberculin units (5 TU) of purified protein derivative (PPD-S) via the Mantoux method of administration.
- The Heaf test, commonly used in the UK is considered unreliable by some authorities.
- False negatives may be due to technical reasons, such as injecting into the wrong site, or biological reasons, such as HIV infection. The presence of active TB can be a reason for a false negative.
- Previous BCG is likely to result in a positive skin test, particularly if the vaccine is given after infancy or with repeated doses. By choosing an appropriate cut-off point, in terms of the size of the reaction to the skin test, the presence of infection can usually be distinguished from the effect of BCG alone. A TST measured ≥10 mm in an individual vaccinated in infancy should be considered a true positive. Exposure to environmental mycobacteria can also lead to false-positive TST responses.

- Tuberculin conversion is an increase in the tuberculin reaction as a result of a new mycobacterial infection. It is completed within eight weeks of a primary infection.
- In North America, a two-step Mantoux test to detect boosting where previous TB infection has taken place, is recommended. The reading at the second test is measured to detect the presence of infection. Care is needed to distinguish a booster phenomenon (caused by remote infection) from infection occuring between tests. The two-step tuberculin test is a practice not considered necessary by other authorities.
- Due to well-described limitations in sensitivity and specificity of the TST, there has been considerable interest for many decades in developing a blood test to detect tuberculous infection.
- IGRAs are now commercially available and can be used to diagnose both latent infection and active disease.
- IGRAs appear to have the greatest use in determining true latent infection from previous BCG vaccination or exposure to environmental mycobacteria.
- Additional studies are needed to better define IGRA performance in high-risk populations and in serial testing. Longitudinal studies are needed to define the predictive value of IGRAs.
- None of the available tests for diagnosing latent TB infection (neither TST nor IGRA) can distinguish active TB disease from latent TB infection.

REFERENCES

1. Koch R. An address on bacteriological research. *Br Med J* 1890; **2**: 380–3.
2. von Pirquet C. Frequency of tuberculosis in childhood. *J Am Med Assoc* 1907; **52**: 675–8.
3. Al-Zahrani K, Al Jahdali H, Menzies D. Does size matter? Utility of size of tuberculin reactions for the diagnosis of mycobacterial disease. *Am J Respir Crit Care Med* 2000; **162**: 1419–22.
4. Reichman LB, O'Day R. The influence of a history of a previous test on the prevalence and size of reactions to tuberculin. *Am Rev Respir Dis* 1977; **115**: 737–41.
5. Landi S, Gupta KC, Held HR. Production and standardization of tuberculin (a brief history). The multi-facets of tuberculin standardization. International WHO IABS Symposium on Standardization and Control of Allergens Administered to Man, Geneva, 1974.
6. Grzybowski S, Dorken E, Bates C. Disparities of tuberculins. *Am Rev Respir Dis* 1969; **100**: 86–7.
7. Seibert SB, Glenn JT. Tuberculin puncture protein derivative: preparation and analysis of a large quantity for standard. *Am Rev Tuberc* 1941; 44: 9–25.
8. Duchin JS, Jereb JA, Nolan CM *et al.* Comparison of sensitivities to two commercially available tuberculin skin test reagents in persons with recent tuberculosis. *Clin Infect Dis* 1997; **25**: 661–3.
9. Villarino ME, Burman W, Wang YC *et al.* Comparable specificity of 2 commercial tuberculin reagents in persons at low risk for tuberculosis infection. *J Am Med Assoc* 1999; **281**: 169–71.
10. Grabau J, Burrows D, Kern M. A pseudo-outbreak of purified protein derivative skin-test conversions caused by inappropriate testing materials. *Infect Control Hosp Epidemiol* 1997; **18**: 571.
11. Lifson AR, Watters JK, Thompson S, Crane CM, Wise F. Discrepancies in tuberculin skin test results with two commercial products in a population of intravenous drug users. *J Infect Dis* 1993; **168**: 1048–51.
12. Lanphear BP, Linnemann CC, Cannon CG. A high false-positive rate of tuberculosis associated with Aplisol: an investigation among health care workers. *J Infect Dis* 1994; **169**: 703–704.
13. Rupp ME, Schultz AW, Davis JC. Discordance between tuberculin skin test results with two commercial puriried protein derivative preparations. *J Infect Dis* 1994; **169**: 1174–5.
14. Guld J, Bentzon MW, Bleiker MA *et al.* Standardization of a new batch of purified tuberculin (PPD) intended for international use. *Bull World Health Organ* 1958; **19**: 845–951.
15. Comstock GW, Edwards LB, Philip RN, Winn WA. A comparison in the United States of America of two tuberculins, PPD-S and PPD-RT 23. *Bull World Health Organ* 1964; **31**: 161–70.
16. World Health Organization. *The WHO standard tuberculin test.* Geneva: World Health Organization, 1963.
17. Murtagh K. Unreliability of the Mantoux test using 1 TU PPD in excluding childhood tuberculosis in Papua New Guinea. *Arch Dis Child* 1980; **55**: 795–9.
18. Duboczy BO, Brown BT. Multiple readings and determination of maximal intensity of tuberculin reaction. *Am Rev Respir Dis* 1960; **82**: 60–67.
19. Spiteri MA, Bowman A, Assefi AR, Clarke SW. Life threatening reaction to tuberculin testing. *Br Med J* 1986; **293**: 243–4.
20. Palmer CE. Tuberculin sensitivity and contact with tuberculosis. *Am Rev Tuberc* 1953; **68**: 678–94.
21. Mantoux MC. La voie intradermique en tubercalinothérapie. *Presse Med* 1912; **20**: 146–8.
22. Guld J. Quantitative aspects of the intradermal tuberculin test in humans. *Acta Tuberc Scand* 1954; **30**: 26–36.
23. Rhoades EV, Bryant RE. The influence of local factors on the reaction to tuberculin. 1. The effect of injection. *Chest* 1980; **77**: 190–3.
24. Flynn P, Shenep J, Mao L *et al.* Influence of needle gauge in Mantoux skin testing. *Chest* 1994; **106**: 1463–5.
25. Heaf F. The multiple puncture tuberculin test. *Lancet* 1951; **21**: 151–3.
26. Carruthers KJM. Comparison of the Heaf (multiple puncture) and Mantoux tests using several tuberculins. *Tubercle* 1969; **50**: 22–41.
27. Katz J, Krasnitz A, Kunofsky S. Comparative study of the Heaf and Mantoux tests. *Am Rev Respir Dis* 1967; **96**: 1033–8.
28. Herzog C. Reason for variable response to tuberculin tine test. *Lancet* 1981; **2**: 417–18.
29. Chaparas SD. Multiple puncture tuberculin tests. *Pediatr Infect Dis J* 1987; **6**: 496–7.
30. Loudon RG, Lawson JR, Brown J. Variation in tuberculin test reading. *Am Rev Respir Dis* 1963; **87**: 852–61.
31. Fine MH, Furcolow ML, Chick EW *et al.* Tuberculin skin test reactions. *Am Rev Respir Dis* 1972; **106**: 752–8.
32. Erdtmann FJ, Dixon KE, Liewellyn CH. Skin testing for tuberculosis. Antigen and observer variability. *J Am Med Assoc* 1974; **228**: 479–81.
33. Perez-Stable EJ, Slutkin G. A demonstration of lack of variability among six tuberculin skin test readers. *Am J Public Health* 1985; **75**: 1341–3.
34. Howard TP, Solomon DA. Reading the tuberculin skin test: who, when, and how? *Arch Intern Med* 1988; **148**: 2457–9.
35. Pouchot J, Grasland A, Collet C *et al.* Reliability of tuberculin skin test measurement. *Ann Intern Med* 1997; **126**: 210–14.
36. Furcolow ML, Watson KA, Charron T, Lowe J. A comparison of the tine and mono-vacc tests with the intradermal tuberculin test. *Am Rev Respir Dis* 1967; **96**: 1009–27.
37. Bearman JE, Kleinman H, Glyer VV, LaCroix OM. A study of

variability in tuberculin test reading. *Am Rev Respir Dis* 1964; **90**: 913–18.

38. Research Committee of the British Thoracic Association. Reproducibility of the Tine tuberculin test. *Br J Dis Chest* 1982; **76**: 75–8.

39. Rudd RB, Gellert AR, Venning M. Comparison of Mantoux, Tine, and 'Imotest' tuberculin tests. *Lancet* 1982; **2**: 515–18.

40. Comstock GW, Edwards LB, Livesay VT. Tuberculosis morbidity in the US navy: its distribution and decline. *Am Rev Respir Dis* 1974; **110**: 572–80.

41. Capewell S, France A, Uzel N, Leitch AG. The current value of tuberculin testing and BCG vaccination in school children. *Br J Dis Chest* 1986; **80**: 254–64.

42. Sokal JE. Measurement of delayed skin-test responses. *New Engl J Med* 1975; **293**: 501–502.

43. Bouros D, Zeros G, Panaretos C *et al*. Palpation vs pen method for the measurement of skin tuberculin reaction (Mantoux test). *Chest* 1991; **99**: 416–19.

44. Bouros D, Maltezakis G, Tzanakis N *et al*. The role of inexperience in measuring tuberculin skin reaction (Mantoux test) by the pen or palpation technique. *Respir Med* 1992; **86**: 219–23.

45. Jordan TJ, Sunderam G, Thomas L, Reichman LB. Tuberculin reaction size measurement by the pen method compared to traditional palpation. *Chest* 1987; **92**: 234–6.

46. Kardjito T, Grange JM. A clinical evaluation of the diagnostic usefulness of an early dermal reaction to tuberculin: a failure to distinguish between tuberculosis and other respiratory disease. *Tubercle* 1985; **66**: 129–32.

47. Colp C, Goldfarb A, Wei I, Graney J. Patient's self-interpretation of tuberculin skin tests. *Chest* 1996; **110**: 1275–7.

48. Tarlo SM, Day JH, Mann P, Day MP. Immediate hypersensitivity to tuberculin in vivo and in vitro studies. *Chest* 1977; **71**: 33–7.

49. Morrison JB. Lymphangitis after tuberculin tests. *Br Med J* 1984; **289**: 413.

50. Hanson ML, Comstock GW. Efficacy of hydrocortisone ointment in the treatment of local reactions to tuberculin skin tests. *Am Rev Respir Dis* 1968; **97**: 472–3.

51. Wright DN, Ledford DK, Lockey RF. Systemic and local allergic reactions to the tine test purified protein derivative. *J Am Med Assoc* 1989; **262**: 2999–3000.

52. DiMaio VJM, Froede CRC. Allergic reactions to the tine test. *J Am Med Assoc* 1975; **233**: 769.

53. Snider DE. The tuberculin skin test. *Am Rev Respir Dis* 1982; **125**: 108–12.

54. Present PA, Comstock GW. Tuberculin sensitivity in pregnancy. *Am Rev Respir Dis* 1975; **112**: 413–16.

55. Long R (ed.). *Canadian tuberculosis standards*, 5th edn. Ottawa: Canadian Lung Association, 2000.

56. Graham NMH, Nelson KE, Solomon L *et al*. Prevalence of tuberculin positivity and skin test anergy in HIV-1-seropositive and -seronegative intravenous drug users. *J Am Med Assoc* 1992; **267**: 369–73.

57. Huebner RE, Schein MF, Hall CA, Barnes SA. Delayed-type hypersensitivity anergy in human immunodeficiency virus-infected persons screened for infection with Mycobacterium tuberculosis. *Clin Infect Dis* 1994; **19**: 26–32.

58. Markowitz N, Hansen NI, Wilcosky TC *et al*. Tuberculin and anergy testing in HIV-seropositive and HIV-seronegative persons. *Ann Intern Med* 1993; **119**: 185–93.

59. Caiaffa WT, Graham NMH, Galai N *et al*. Instability of delayed-type hypesensitivity skin test anergy in human immunodeficiency virus infection. *Arch Intern Med* 1995; **155**: 2111–17.

60. Zahrani KA, Jahdali HA, Poirier L *et al*. Accuracy and utility of commercially available amplification and serologic tests for the diagnosis of minimal pulmonary tuberculosis. *Am J Resp Crit Care Med* 2000; **162**: 1323–9.

61. Holden M, Dubin MR, Diamond PH. Frequency of negative intermediate-strength tuberculin sensitivity in patients with active tuberculosis. *New Engl J Med* 1971; **285**: 1506–509.

62. Stead WW, To T. The significance of the tuberculin skin test in elderly persons. *Ann Int Med* 1987; **107**: 837–42.

63. Kardjito T, Donosepoetro M. The Mantoux test in tuberculosis: correlations between the diameters of the dermal responses and the serum protein levels. *Tubercle* 1981; **62**: 31–5.

64. Wang L, Turner MO, Elwood RK *et al*. A meta-analysis of the effect of bacille Calmette Guerin vaccination on tuberculin skin test measurements. *Thorax* 2002; **57**: 804–809.

65. Farhat M, Greenaway C, Pai M, Menzies D. False positive tuberculin skin tests – what is the absolute effect of BCG and non-tuberculous mycobacteria? *Int J Tuber Lung Dis* 2006; **10**: 1–13.

66. Narain RO. Interpretation of the repeat tuberculin test. *Tubercle* 1968; **49**: 92.

67. Menzies D. Interpretation of repeated tuberculin tests. *Am J Respir Crit Care Med* 1999; **159**: 15–21.

68. Ferebee SH. Controlled chemoprophylaxis trials in tuberculosis. *Adv Tuberc Res* 1969; **17**: 28–106.

69. Cauthen GM, Snider DE, Onorato IM. Boosting of tuberculin sensitivity among Southeast Asian refugees. *Am J Respir Crit Care Med* 1994; **149**: 1597–600.

70. Duboczy BO. Repeated tuberculin tests at the same site in tuberculin-positive patients. *Am Rev Respir Dis* 1964; **90**: 77–86.

71. Thompson NJ, Glassroth JL, Snider DE, Farer LS. The booster phenomenon in serial tuberculin testing. *Am Rev Respir Dis* 1979; **119**: 587–97.

72. Magnus K, Edwards LB. The effect of repeated tuberculin testing on post-vaccination allergy. *Lancet* 1955; **ii**: 643–4.

73. Bass JB, Serio RA. The use of repeated skin tests to eliminate the booster phenomenon in serial tuberculin testing. *Am Rev Respir Dis* 1981; **123**: 394–6.

74. Menzies RI, Vissandjee B, Rocher I, St Germain Y. The booster effect in two-step tuberculin testing among young adults in Montreal. *Ann Intern Med* 1994; **120**: 190–8.

75. Gordin FM, Perez-Stable EJ, Flaherty D *et al*. Evaluation of a third sequential tuberculin skin test in a chronic care population. *Am Rev Respir Dis* 1988; **137**: 153–7.

76. Van den Brande P, Demedts M. Four-stage tuberculin testing in elderly subjects induces age-dependent progressive boosting. *Chest* 1992; **101**: 447–50.

77. Veen J. Aspects of temporary specific anergy to tuberculin in Vietnamese refugees. Amsterdam: Royal Netherlands Tuberculosis Association (KNCV), 1992: 1–119.

78. MacIntyre CR, Plant AJ. Preventability of incident cases of tuberculosis in recently exposed contacts. *Int J Tuberc Lung Dis* 1998; **21**: 56–61.

79. Sutherland I. The evolution of clinical tuberculosis in adolescents. *Tubercle* 1966; **47**: 308.

80. Youmans GP. *Tuberculosis*. Philadelphia, PA: WB Saunders, 1979.

81. Triep WA. *De tuberculinereactie*. The Hague: Royal Netherlands Tuberculosis Association (KNCV), 1957 (in Dutch).

82. Wasz-Hockert O. On the period of incubation in tuberculosis. *Ann Med Fenn* 1947; **96**: 764–72.

83. Wallgren A. The time-table of tuberculosis. *Tubercle* 1948; **29**: 245–51.

84. Poulsen A. Some clinical features of tuberculosis. I. Incubation period. *Acta Tuberc Scand* 1954; **24**: 311–46.

85. Guld J. Response to BCG vaccination. In: Palmer CE, Magnus K, Edwards LB (eds). *Studies by the WHO Tuberculosis Research Office*. Geneva: World Health Organization, 1953: 51–6.

86. Menzies RI, Fanning A, Yuan L, FitzGerald JM. Hospital ventilation and risk of tuberculous infection in Canadian health care workers. *Ann Intern Med* 2000; **133**: 779–89.

87. Grzybowski S, Barnett GD, Styblo K. Contacts of cases of active pulmonary tuberculosis. *Bull Int Union Tuberc* 1975; **50**: 90–106.

88. Shaw JB, Wynn-Williams N. Infectivity of pulmonary tuberculosis in relation to sputum status. *Am Rev Tuberc* 1954; **69**: 724–32.

89. Van Geuns HA, Meijer J, Styblo K. Results of contact examination in Rotterdam, 1967–1969. *Bull Int Union Tuberc* 1975; **50**: 107–21.

90. Zaki MH, Lyons HA, Robins AB, Brown EP. *Tuberculin sensitivity. N Y State J Med* 1976; **76**: 2138–43.

91. Miller MA, Valway S, Onorato IM. Tuberculosis risk after exposure on airplanes. *Tuber Lung Dis* 1996; **77**: 414–19.

92. Braden CR. Infectiousness of a university student with laryngeal and cavitary tuberculosis. *Clin Infect Dis* 1995; **21**: 565–70.

93. Kenyon TA, Valway SE, Ihle WW *et al.* Transmission of multidrug-resistant *Mycobacterium tuberculosis* during a long airplane flight. *New Engl J Med* 1996; **334**: 933–38.

94. Driver CR, Valway SE, Morgan WM *et al.* Transmission of *Mycobacterium tuberculosis* associated with air travel. *J Am Med Assoc* 1994; **272**: 1031–5.

95. Blumberg HM, Sotir M, Erwin M, Bachman R, Shulman JA. Risk of house staff tuberculin skin test conversion in an area with a high incidence of tuberculosis. *Clin Infect Dis* 1998; **27**: 826–33.

96. Bourdreau AY, Baron SL, Steenland NK *et al.* Occupational risk of *Mycobacterium tuberculosis* infection in hospital workers. *Am J Ind Med* 1997; **32**: 528–34.

97. Silva VMC, Cunha AJLA, Oliveira JR *et al.* Medical students at risk of nosocomial transmission of *Mycobacterium tuberculosis*. *Int J Tuberc Lung Dis* 2000; **4**: 420–6.

98. Aitken ML, Anderson KM, Albert RK. Is the tuberculosis screening program of hospital employees still required? *Am Rev Respir Dis* 1987; **136**: 805–807.

99. Badger TL, Breitwieser ER, Muench H. Tuberculin Tine test: multiple-puncture intradermal technique compared with PPD-S, intermediate strength. *Am Rev Respir Dis* 1963; **87**: 338–51.

100. Fine MH, Furcolow ML, Chick EW *et al.* Tuberculin skin test reactions. *Am Rev Respir Dis* 1972; **106**: 752–8.

101. Donaldson JC, Elliot RC. A study of co-positivity of three multipuncture techniques with intradermal PPD tuberculin. *Am Rev Respir Dis* 1978; **118**: 843–6.

102. Ackerman-Liebrich U. Tuberculin skin testing. *Lancet* 1982; ii: 934.

103. Hansen JP, Falconer JA, Gallis HA, Hamilton JD. Inadequate sensitivity of tuberculin tine test for screening employee populations. *J Occup Med* 1982; **24**: 602–604.

104. Carruthers KJM. Observer and experimental variation in tuberculin testing. *Tubercle* 1970; **51**: 48–67.

105. Griffith AH. Heaf test studies. *Med Off* 1963; **110**: 161.

106. Menzies D, Fanning A, Yuan L, FitzGerald JM and the Canadian Collaborative Group in Nosocomial Transmission of Tuberculosis. Tuberculosis in health care workers: a multicentre Canadian prevalence survey: preliminary results. *Int J Tuberc Lung Dis* 1998; **2**: S98–S102.

107. Valenti WM, Andrews BA, Presley BA, Reifler CB. Absence of the booster phenomenon in serial tuberculin skin testing. *Am Rev Respir Dis* 1982; **125**: 323–5.

108. Gross TP, Israel E, Powers P *et al.* Low prevalence of the booster phenomenon in nursing-home employees in Maryland. *Maryland Med J* 1984; **35**: 107–109.

109. Richards NM, Nelson KE, Batt MD *et al.* Tuberculin test conversion during repeated skin testing, associated with sensitivity to non-tuberculous mycobacteria. *Am Rev Respir Dis* 1979; **120**: 59–65.

110. Slutkin G, Perez-Stable EJ, Hopewell PC. Time course and boosting of tuberculin reactions in nursing home residents. *Am Rev Respir Dis* 1986; **134**: 1048–51.

111. Barry MA, Regan AM, Kunches LM *et al.* Two-stage tuberculin testing with control antigens in patients residing in two chronic disease hospitals. *J Am Geriatr Soc* 1987; **35**: 147–53.

112. Alvarez S, Karprzyk DR, Freundl M. Two-stage skin testing for tuberculosis in a domiciliary population. *Am Rev Respir Dis* 1987; **136**: 1193–6.

113. Menzies RI, Vissandjee B, Amyot D. Factors associated with tuberculin reactivity among the foreign-born in Montreal. *Am Rev Respir Dis* 1992; **146**: 752–6.

114. Morse DL, Hansen RE, Swalbach G *et al.* High rate of tuberculin conversion in Indochinese refugees. *J Am Med Assoc* 1982; **248**: 2983–6.

115. Lifson AR, Grant SM, Lorvick J *et al.* Two-step tuberculin skin testing of injection drug users recruited from community-based settings. *Int J Tuberc Lung Dis* 1997; **1**: 128–34.

116. Hecker MT, Johnson JL, Whalen CC *et al.* Two-step tuberculin skin testing in HIV-infected persons in Uganda. *Am J Respir Crit Care Med* 1997; **155**: 81–6.

117. Lifschitz M. The value of the tuberculin skin test as a screening test for tuberculosis among BCG-vaccinated children. *Pediatrics* 1965; **36**: 624–7.

118. Margus JH, Khassis Y. The tuberculin sensitivity in BCG-vaccinated infants and children in Israel. *Acta Tuberc Pneumonol Scand* 1965; **46**: 113–22.

119. Joncas JH, Robitaille R, Gauthier T. Interpretation of the PPD skin test in BCG-vaccinated children. *Can Med Assoc J* 1975; **113**: 127–8.

120. Karalliede S, Katugha LP, Uragoda CG. The tuberculin response of Sri Lankan children after BCG vaccination at birth. *Tubercle* 1987; **68**: 33–8.

121. Comstock GW, Edwards LB, Nabangwang H. Tuberculin sensitivity eight to fifteen years after BCG vaccination. *Am Rev Respir Dis* 1971; **103**: 572–5.

122. Bahr GM, Chugh TD, Behbehani K *et al.* Unexpected findings amongst the skin test responses to mycobacteria of BCG vaccinated Kuwaiti school children. *Tubercle* 1968; **68**: 105–12.

123. Horwitz O, Bunch-Christensen K. Correlation between tuberculin sensitivity after 2 months and 5 years among BCG vaccinated subjects. *Bull World Health Organ* 1972; **47**: 49–58.

124. Menzies RI, Vissandjee B. Effect of bacille Calmette–Guerin vaccination on tuberculin reactivity. *Am Rev Respir Dis* 1992; **145**: 621–5.

125. Sepulveda RL, Burr C, Ferrer X, Sorensen RU. Booster effect of tuberculin testing in health 6-year-old school children vaccinated with bacillus Calmette–Guerin at birth in Santiago, Chile. *Pediatr Infect Dis J* 1988; **7**: 581.

126. Sepulveda R, Ferrer X, Latrach C, Sorensen R. The influence of Calmette–Guerin bacillus immunization on the booster effect of tuberculin testing in healthy young adults. *Am Rev Respir Dis* 1990; **142**: 24–8.

127. Friedland IR. The booster effect with repeat tuberculin testing in children and its relationship to BCG vaccination. *S Afr Med J* 1990; **77**: 387–9.

128. Cobelens FGJ, van Deutekom H, Draayer-Jansen IWE *et al.* Risk of infection with *Mycobacterium tuberculosis* in travellers to areas of high tuberculosis endemicity. *Lancet* 2000; **356**: 461–5.

129. Mazurek G, Jereb J, LoBue P *et al.* Guidelines for the investigation of contacts of persons with infectious tuberculosis; Recommendations from the National Tuberculosis Controllers Association and CDC; Guidelines for using the QuantiFERON-TB Gold Test for detecting *Mycobacterium Tuberculosis* infection, United States. *Morb Mortal Wkly Rep* 2005; **54**: 49–55.

130. Royal College of Physicians. Tuberculosis: National clinical guidelines for diagnosis, management, prevention, and control. London: http://www.nice.org.uk, 2006 (published September 2005).

131. Menzies D, Pai M, Comstock G. Meta-analysis: new tests for the diagnosis of latent tuberculosis infection: areas of uncertainty and recommendations for research. *Annals Intern Med* 2007; **146**: 340–54.

132. Kang YA, Lee HW, Yoon HI *et al.* Discrepancy between the tuberculin skin test and the whole-blood interferon gamma assay for the diagnosis of latent tuberculosis infection in an intermediate tuberculosis-burden country. *J Am Med Assoc* 2005; **293**: 2756–61.

133. Lalvani A, Pathan AA, Durkan H *et al.* Enhanced contact tracing and spatial tracking of *Mycobacterium tuberculosis* infection by enumeration of antigen-specific T cells. *Lancet* 2001; **357**: 2017–21.

134. Liebeschuetz S, Bamber S, Ewer K *et al.* Diagnosis of tuberculosis in South African children with a T-cell-based assay: a prospective cohort study. *Lancet* 2004; **364**: 2196–203.

135. Chapman AL, Munkanta M, Wilkinson KA *et al.* Rapid detection of active and latent tuberculosis infection in HIV-positive individuals

by enumeration of *Mycobacterium tuberculosis*-specific T cells. *AIDS* 2002; **16**: 2285–93.

136. Piana F, Codecasa LR, Cavallerio P *et al.* Use of a T-cell-based test for detection of tuberculosis infection among immunocompromised patients. *Eur Respir J* 2006; **28**: 31–4.

137. Passalent L, Khan K, Richardson R *et al.* Detecting latent tuberculosis infection in hemodialysis patients: a head-to-head comparison of the T-SPOT.TB test, tuberculin skin test, and expert physician panel. *Clin J Am Soc Nephrol* 2007; **2**: 68–73.

138. Brock I, Ruhwald M, Lundgren B *et al.* Latent tuberculosis in HIV positive, diagnosed by the *M. Tuberculosis* specific interferon gamma test. *Respir Res* 2006; **7**: 56.

139. Pai M, Joshi R, Dogra S *et al.* Serial testing of health care workers for tuberculosis using interferon-gamma assay. *Am J Respir Crit Care Med* 2006; **174**: 349–55.

140. Ewer K, Millington KA, Deeks JJ *et al.* Dynamic antigen-specific T-cell responses after point-source exposure to *Mycobacterium tuberculosis*. *Am J Respir Crit Care Med* 2006; **174**: 831–9.

141. Aiken AM, Hill PC, Fox A *et al.* Reversion of the ELISPOT test after treatment in Gambian tuberculosis cases. *BMC Infect Dis* 2006; **6**: 66.

142. Pathan AA, Wilkinson KA, Klenerman P *et al.* Direct *ex vivo* analysis of antigen-specific IFN-γ-secreting CD4 T cells in *Mycobacterium tuberculosis*-infected individuals: associations with clinical disease state and effect of treatment. *The Journal of Immunology* 2001; **167**: 5217–25.

143. Ewer K, Deeks J, Alvarez L *et al.* Comparison of T-cell-based assay with tuberculin skin test for diagnosis of *Mycobacterium tuberculosis* infection in a school tuberculosis outbreak. *Lancet* 2003; **361**: 1168–73.

144. Pai M, Joshi R, Dogra S *et al.* Persistently elevated T cell interferon-gamma responses after treatment for latent tuberculosis infection among health care workers in India: a preliminary report. *J Occup Med Toxicol* 2006; **1**: 7.

145. Harada N, Nakajima Y, Higuchi K *et al.* Screening for tuberculosis infection using whole-blood interferon-gamma and Mantoux testing among Japanese healthcare workers. *Infect Control Hosp Epidemiol* 2006; **27**: 442–8.

146. Diel R, Nienhaus A, Lange C *et al.* Tuberculosis contact investigation with a new, specific blood test in a low-incidence population containing a high proportion of BCG-vaccinated persons. *Respir Res* 2006; **7**: 77.

147. Brock I, Weldingh K, Lillebaek T *et al.* Comparison of tuberculin skin test and new specific blood test in tuberculosis contacts. *Am J Respir Crit Care Med* 2004; **170**: 65–9.

148. Porsa E, Cheng L, Seale MM *et al.* Comparison of a new ESAT-6/CFP-10 peptide-based gamma interferon assay and a tuberculin skin test for tuberculosis screening in a moderate-risk population. *Clin Vaccine Immunol* 2006; **13**: 53–8.

149. Hill PC, Brookes RH, Adetifa IM *et al.* Comparison of enzyme-linked immunospot assay and tuberculin skin test in healthy children exposed to *Mycobacterium tuberculosis*. *Pediatrics* 2006; **117**: 1542–8.

150. Cellestis. QuantiFERON Precision and reproducibility report. http://www.cellestis.com/IRM/content/gold/Precisionproductivity.pdf Date Accessed: February 27, 2006.

151. Nicol MP, Pienaar D, Wood K *et al.* Enzyme-linked immunospot assay responses to early secretory antigenic target 6, culture filtrate protein 10, and purified protein derivative among children with tuberculosis: implications for diagnosis and monitoring of therapy. *Clin Infect Dis* 2005; **40**: 1301–8.

152. Mori T, Harada N. Cost-effectiveness analysis of Quantiferon-TB 2nd generation used for detection of tuberculosis infection in contact investigations. *Kekkaku* 2005; **80**: 675–86.

153. Diel R, Neinhaus A, Lange C, Schaberg T. Cost-optimization of screening for latent tuberculosis in close contacts. *Eur Respir J* 2006; **28**: 35–44.

154. Oxlade O, Schwartzman K, Menzies D. Interferon gamma release assays and TB screening in high-income countries: a cost-effectiveness analysis. *Int J Tuberc Lung Dis* 2007; **11**: 16–26.

155. Wrighton-Smith P, Zellweger JP. Direct costs of three models for the screening of latent tuberculosis infection. *Eur Respir J* 2006; **28**: 45–50.

156. Pai M, Kalantri S, Dheda D. New tools and emerging technologies for the diagnosis of tuberculosis: Part 1. Latent Tuberculosis. *Expert Rev Mol Diagn* 2006; **6**: 413–22.

157. Dewan PK, Grinsdale J, Liska S *et al.* Feasibility, acceptability and cost of TB testing by whole blood interferon gamma assay. *BMC Infect Dis* 2006; **6**: 47.

158. Johnson PDR, Stuart RL, Grayson ML *et al.* Tuberculin-PPD, MPT-64, and ESAT-6 stimulated gamma interferon responses in medical students before and after BCG vaccination and in TB patients. *Clin Diag Lab Immunol* 1999; **6(6)**: 934–7.

24

BCG vaccination

HANS L RIEDER

EARLY VACCINE DEVELOPMENT

Vaccination with *Mycobacterium tuberculosis*

Early in the twentieth century, von Behring attempted vaccination (or as he called it, 'Jennerization') of cattle by utilizing increasing doses of living *Mycobacterium tuberculosis*.[1,2] Similar to these attempts, Webb in the United States tried to make experimental animals resistant to rechallenge with increasing doses of virulent *M. tuberculosis*. A few children were also 'vaccinated' with this approach, apparently with no adverse outcome.[3] While this approach seemed indeed to provide some protection against a subsequent challenge in cattle and other experimental animals compared to controls, protection was incomplete in the case of von Behring's 'bovo-vaccination' and in the guinea pig. Furthermore, with 'Jennerization' in cattle, there was the potential that the microorganism would appear in milk.[4] Theobald Smith also pointed out that the unknown duration of the incubation period carried great dangers, even if the immediate effect seemed to be innocuous.[4] This approach was therefore only short-lived.

Vaccination with BCG

VACCINE DEVELOPMENT

A virulent strain of *Mycobacterium bovis*, isolated by Nocard in 1902, from milk obtained from a cow with tuberculous mastitis[5] was inoculated for the first time on 8

January 1908 by Albert Calmette (1863–1933) and Camille Guérin (1872–1961)[6] at the Pasteur Institute in Lille, France,[7] on to a medium consisting of cooked potato and glycerinated bile.

The strain, to become known as bacille Calmette–Guérin (BCG), was subcultured in 230 passages on bile potato medium until 1921, when it no longer changed its characteristics.

After 30 passages, the strain ceased to kill guinea pigs, after 60 it was still slightly virulent for rabbits and horses, but avirulent for guinea pigs, monkeys and calves.[5] From 1912 onwards, experiments were conducted among calves, demonstrating their resistance to subsequent infection with virulent bacilli.[5] It may be noted that the main objective in the development of this vaccine was to obtain an effective vaccine against tuberculosis (TB) in goats[8] and cattle.[8,9] It is now clear that it was not the glycerinated bile medium that was the reason for the loss of virulence.[10,11] By subculturing four bovine strains on Calmette's bile–potato medium over 6 years, Griffith[12] failed to reproduce Calmette's finding and to induce stable attenuation. The reasons for the loss of virulence of *M. bovis* BCG remained unclear until today.

On 1 July 1921, Weill-Hallé, a paediatrician, requested the vaccine for use in an infant born to a mother who had died of TB shortly after delivery. The child was to be brought up by a grandmother who was herself suffering from TB.[13] The child was given 6 mg of BCG orally and developed normally over the next 6 months without any sign of illness, either from the vaccine or from TB.[5,13] Over the next 3 years, 317 infants (67 of whom were born into and brought up by families with TB patients) were vaccinated with 30 mg of oral BCG vaccine, given in three portions at 48-hour intervals.

Following these early experiments in humans, BCG was distributed to a large number of laboratories, largely in Europe, and given to hundreds of thousands of children within a decade after its introduction.[14–17] Trials to evaluate its impact began in Europe[18–20] and North America.[21,22]

Controlled assessment of the vaccine's efficacy was conspicuously absent and one of its most critical opponents was Petroff in the USA, who doubted both the vaccine's innocuousness and efficacy.[23,24] Despite the justified concerns about the quality of the data on efficacy given all the methodological problems (such as selection bias), it seemed apparent that BCG reduced case fatality from TB among exposed children in a variety of settings.[16] It also seemed to protect adult student nurses heavily exposed to TB from both death and disease.[18–20,25]

The assumption of the safety of BCG vaccination was severely challenged when 72 of 251 children who were presumably vaccinated with BCG between 10 December 1929 and 30 April 1930 died from tuberculosis in Lübeck, Germany.[26–28] While not all circumstances surrounding this disaster have ever become public,[29] it soon became apparent that BCG was not the cause, and two physicians intimately involved were later sentenced to prison.[30] The preliminary epidemiologic analysis in July 1930 already showed large differences in case fatality by week of vaccination, indicating that strains with different virulence had been mixed.[31] This was bacteriologically confirmed by demonstrating that virulent tubercle bacilli, but not BCG, were consistently isolated on autopsy.[26] The epidemiologic and bacteriologic investigations demonstrated conclusively that batches containing both BCG and *M. tuberculosis* in varying proportions had been fed to the infants during the epidemic.[26,28,32,33] Among the 53 fatal cases ascertained by mid-July 1930, the interval between vaccination and death ranged from 34 to 129 days with a median of 79 days.

Petroff's concerns about a reversion to virulence of BCG have never been confirmed, and his observation of different colony morphology with virulent and avirulent colonies[23] have not been confirmed elsewhere.[26]

THE BCG STRAIN FAMILY

Until the introduction of freeze-drying in Japan in 1943,[34] the only means of maintaining a viable strain was through subculturing. With the distribution of the vaccine strain to multiple laboratories in the world, each using slightly different techniques for strain maintenance, it is not surprising that the BCG family shows large diversity.[10] The first freeze-dried French strain (1949) from the Pasteur Institute in Paris was strain 1173-P$_2$, from which the Glaxo and Danish strains descended.[35]

Recent work based on molecular characterization of the various substrains points to various mutations that have

occurred at different points in time[36–38] and indicates that the various BCG substrains are morphologically and genetically different from each other.

SAFETY RECORD OF BCG VACCINATION

A large review has shown BCG to be one of the safest vaccines.[39,40] The demarcation between a normal reaction and an adverse reaction is not always clear.[41] The normal reaction is a red indurated area measuring 5–15 mm. A crust is formed around this induration, which is soft at the centre for 3–4 weeks. At 6–10 weeks, the crust falls off, leaving a flat scar measuring 3–7 mm.[41] Regional lymphadenopathy in the absence of erythema or vesicle formation should also be considered a normal reaction to the vaccine.[42] Complications include cutaneous lesions and regional suppurative lymphadenitis, more severe localized or multiple lesions (such as musculoskeletal lesions),[43–45] and non-fatal and fatal complications resulting from hypersensitivity reactions or mycobacterial dissemination.[39,40,46–53] The risk of complications varies with the type of vaccine and with the age at vaccination. The risk of osteomyelitis ranged from 0.01 to 50 per 1 million vaccinations, that of multiple or generalized lesions from 0.01 to 2 and that of fatal cases from 0.01 to 1 per million vaccinated individuals.[39,40] The lowest complication rates were reported with the Tokyo strain, and the highest with the Gothenburg strain produced in Denmark.[43,54]

In a prospective study in South Africa among 10 000 neonates receiving the Copenhagen strain intradermally at birth, the vaccination scar had healed in more than 95 per cent of children at 6 weeks after vaccination, 1.5 per cent had no vaccination scar, and in 3 per cent adverse events were noted.[55] All adverse events were local (oozing, abscesses, rarely combined with lymphadenopathy).

Because BCG is a live vaccine, concerns were raised early on about the safety of its use in people infected with HIV,[56–58] and several case reports about disseminated mycobacteriosis[59–65] and mycobacterial meningitis due to BCG[59,61,66] have been published. A study among mother–child pairs with and without HIV infection has shown that children of mothers with HIV infection who also had HIV infection themselves had a slightly increased risk of suppurative lymphadenitis, but the manifestations were mild and easily manageable.[67] Apparently, living BCG can persist for decades and cause localized[68] or disseminated[69] complications after acquisition of immunosuppression. Nevertheless, most of these case reports appear to be isolated events, although it has been argued that disseminated disease attributable to BCG vaccination in HIV-infected children might be exceedingly difficult to diagnose.[70] However, a study in Zambia among HIV-symptomatic children with a median age of 15 months, showed that mycobacteraemia due to BCG must be exceedingly rare.[71]

In 2007, the Global Advisory on Vaccine Safety revised its previous guidelines. As populations with a high-prevalence of HIV infection in general also have the greatest burden of tuberculosis, HIV-uninfected children in such populations will particularly benefit from BCG vaccination. Within these populations, three groups of children might be distinguished:[72]

- Infants in whom the benefits outweigh the risk of BCG vaccination should be vaccinated. These are children born to mothers with unknown HIV status.
- Infants in whom the benefits usually outweigh the risks. These are infants whose HIV infection status is unknown and who demonstrate no signs or reported symptoms suggestive of HIV infection but who are born to known HIV-infected women. These infants should be immunized after consideration of locally determined factors.
- Infants in whom the risks outweigh the benefit of BCG vaccination. These are infants who are known to be HIV infected with or without signs or reported symptoms of HIV infection. These infants should not be immunized.

MANAGEMENT OF ADVERSE REACTIONS DUE TO BCG VACCINATION

Children with lymphadenitis due to BCG were randomly allocated to receive either isoniazid or no treatment.[73] There was no difference in the duration of lymphadenitis between the two groups, nor did isoniazid prevent the occurrence of suppuration. Similarly, children with abscess formation were randomly assigned to receive either isoniazid or erythromycin (serving as placebo).[74] The response in each treatment group was the same. In another study, comparing excision, excision plus isoniazid, and isoniazid alone compared to a control group without intervention, no significant differences were observed between the various interventions, and in particular, isoniazid offered no advantage.[75] Non-suppurative lymphadenitis is a normal reaction, and is best left without antibiotic treatment.[41,76]

Patients with suppurative lymphadenitis following BCG vaccination were randomly assigned to treatment with simple needle aspiration, introducing the needle subcutaneously 2–3 cm distant from the node, versus no treatment.[77] Regression was significantly faster in the treated than in the non-treated group and spontaneous drainage was less frequent.

For osteoarticular mycobacteriosis due to BCG, combination therapy is indicated, but results were not always favourable (both in terms of sequelae and relapses) in a case series from Sweden.[78]

A standard course of treatment (as for clinically manifest TB) is also indicated in disseminated mycobacteriosis due to BCG. As this is a rare complication, however, treatment regimens have not been amenable to formal study. In

treatment, it should be kept in mind that BCG is, like its parent organism, *M. bovis*, naturally resistant to pyrazinamide.

EFFICACY AND EFFECTIVENESS OF BCG VACCINATION

Efficacy is the extent to which an intervention produces a beneficial result under ideal conditions. The best setting to address efficacy is thus prospectively, in a controlled clinical trial. In contrast, effectiveness takes the various constraints that are found in the field into account in the actual routine delivery of the intervention.[79] Effectiveness is often ascertained retrospectively, such as in case–control studies. Efficacy (in clinical trials) and effectiveness (in case–control studies) have been ascertained in various settings. These trials were supplemented by community trials and contact studies. The variation in estimates of protection ranged widely, from harm (more cases among the vaccinated than among controls) to a high level of protection.

Briefly, clinical trials are a prospective ascertainment of cases occurring among the exposed. Clinical trials thus start with looking at the exposure (BCG vaccination given or not) and then ascertain the outcome (TB) in a group of individuals, preferably randomly assigned to exposure.[80] These are population-based studies and the denominator is the number of person-years of observation. The measures are incidence rates among the exposed and unexposed and the summary measure is the relative risk (the risk among the exposed divided by the risk among the unexposed). Vaccine efficacy (as a percentage) is calculated as $(1 - \text{relative risk}) \times 100$.[81] The 95 per cent confidence intervals were calculated (or recalculated, where appropriate) using the formula proposed by Orenstein *et al.*[81] in their review on assessment of vaccine efficacy, unless adjusted or stratified summary estimates were provided by the authors.

To defray the costs incurred in clinical trials and to obtain results more quickly, it was proposed to ascertain the effectiveness of BCG vaccination by means of (retrospective) case–control studies.[82] Briefly, case–control studies start with looking at the outcome (TB) and then ascertain exposure (BCG vaccination given or not) in a group of patients with the outcome, compared to an appropriately selected control group of people without the outcome.[83] A relative risk cannot be calculated as this measurement is confined to population-based studies with person-time of observation. The measurement of risk in a case–control study is the odds ratio (or relative odds). For rare diseases, the odds ratio approximates the relative risk in a clinical trial.

The advantages and disadvantages in the use of the case–control approach are linked to its being observational, having subjects selected on the basis of disease status, and using controls from the population from which the cases emanated.[84] The advantages of case–control studies include avoidance of ethical problems arising in situations where there is already evidence that the vaccine is better than placebo, allowing much faster conduct than randomized trials, and requiring a much smaller number of subjects. They are thus substantially cheaper to conduct than randomized clinical trials.[84]

The most challenging difficulty in the design of case–control studies is the selection of appropriate controls in that they have to be selected in such a way that they are comparable to cases in every respect except for the outcome. Selection bias resulting from a failure to ensure this comparability may thus invalidate any findings.

The results of some of these case–control studies are summarized below. Vaccine effectiveness (as a percentage) from a case–control study is estimated as (1 – odds ratio) × 100.[81] For unmatched case–control studies, the 95 per cent confidence intervals were calculated (or recalculated where appropriate) using Woolf's method.[83] For matched and adjusted analyses, the confidence interval published by the authors of the study was chosen. If not stated for matched studies, the confidence interval around the crude odds ratio was calculated as above.

PROSPECTIVE AND RETROSPECTIVE STUDIES ON BCG VACCINATION

In one of the first clinical trials with a methodologically fairly acceptable design (systematic alternate allocation), BCG was given to children exposed to a parent with TB and compared with a similar group who did not receive the vaccine.[85] The impact on fatality was dramatic, with an 82 per cent reduction in the risk. Nevertheless, suspicion about the efficacy of BCG vaccination persisted, particularly in the United States,[86] but also in the United Kingdom,[29] largely because the design of many studies was dubious at best.

One of the most conspicuous differences observed in the protection afforded by BCG reveals that age at vaccination is important. Of further crucial importance is the type of TB that is targeted for protection by vaccination.

In the following summary of the best-known studies in the English literature, the studies are identified as being prospective or retrospective. For each of these two study types, five classes were examined:

1   protection against disseminated and meningeal TB, and against death from TB;
2   protection afforded to children by vaccination of newborns or infants;
3   protection afforded by vaccinating children beyond the age of 1 year;
4   protection afforded by vaccinating adolescents or adults;
5   protection afforded by vaccinating people of various ages.

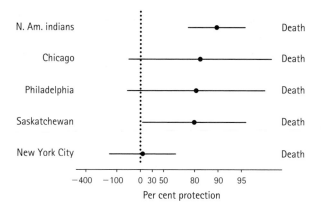

Figure 24.1   Results from five controlled clinical trials to evaluate the efficacy of bacillus Calmette–Guérin vaccination against death from tuberculosis, meningeal or disseminated tuberculosis.[85,90–93]

Protection conferred by BCG vaccination against disseminated and meningeal TB, and against death from TB

Five major prospective studies have examined the protection afforded by BCG vaccination against death from TB (Figure 24.1).[85,87–93] All of these studies were conducted before the advent of curative chemotherapy. Four of the studies showed a point estimate of the protective efficacy of 80 per cent and above, and one afforded no protection. The confidence interval was wide in all studies, because the number of events was small.

Several retrospective studies (including two using two different control groups) examined the protection against disseminated and meningeal TB (Figure 24.2).[94–102] The protective effectiveness was usually in excess of 80 per cent and in no case did the 95 per cent confidence interval include zero.

It may be concluded from these studies that BCG affords very good protection against death from TB, and against disseminated and meningeal TB.

Protection conferred by BCG vaccination of newborns and infants

Three prospective studies looked into the protective efficacy of BCG given to newborns or infants against all forms of TB or morbidity (Figure 24.3).[91,92,103] The point estimate of the efficacy was between 50 and 80 per cent.

Several retrospective studies examined the effectiveness of newborn or infant vaccination (Figure 24.4).[96,97,102,104–111] The level of protection in these studies varies widely, but is frequently above 50 per cent. Noteworthy is the study from Zambia, which stratified effectiveness estimates by HIV status,[109] showing that HIV-infected children had no protection as compared to 60 per cent protection among HIV-negative children.

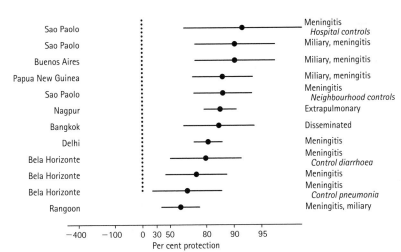

Figure 24.2   Results from retrospective studies on the effectiveness of bacillus Calmette–Guérin vaccination against death from tuberculosis, meningeal or disseminated tuberculosis.[94–102]

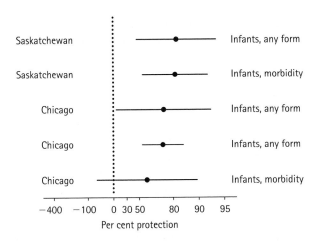

Figure 24.3   Results from prospective studies on the efficacy of bacillus Calmette–Guérin vaccination against tuberculosis in the newborn and infants.[91,92,103]

Protection conferred by BCG vaccination of children over 1 year of age

Only three prospective studies of BCG vaccination of older children are available (Figure 24.5).[112–117] All three showed a very low level of protection, of less than 30 per cent. In Chingleput, south India, where BCG gave little or no protection, there was a tendency to provide some protection in children below the age of 15 years, but a similar tendency towards harm (more cases in the vaccinated than the non-vaccinated) in older people (Figure 24.6).[114]

Three retrospective studies among children also showed very variable levels of protection, from 16 to 74 per cent (Figure 24.7).[99,118,119]

These studies seem to show that vaccination of older children does not offer protection against TB that is as reliable as vaccination at an earlier age.

Protection conferred by BCG vaccination among adolescents and adults

Six prospective studies have examined the protection of BCG vaccination against TB among adolescents or adults

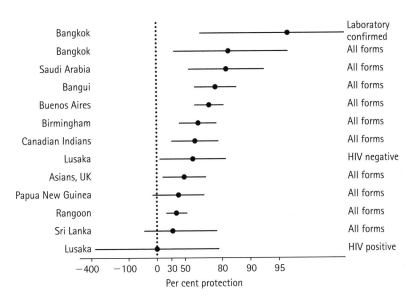

Figure 24.4   Results from retrospective studies on the effectiveness of bacillus Calmette–Guérin vaccination against tuberculosis in the newborn and infants.[96,97,102,104–111]

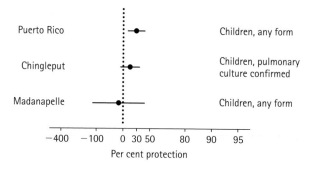

Figure 24.5 Results from prospective studies on the efficacy of bacillus Calmette–Guérin vaccination against tuberculosis in children other than infants.[112–117]

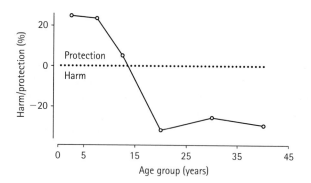

Figure 24.6 Protection from bacillus Calmette–Guérin vaccination by age, Chingleput, India.[114]

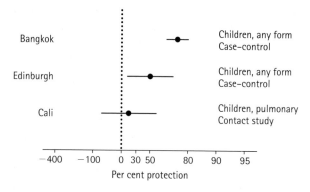

Figure 24.7 Results from retrospective studies on the effectiveness of bacillus Calmette–Guérin vaccination against tuberculosis in children other than infants.[99,118,119]

(Figure 24.8).[18,20,112–114,116,117,120–127] The study in Ulleval, Norway, was the first ever conducted prospective study.[18,20] It does, however, not live up to current requirements for a controlled trial, as student nurses with a negative tuberculin skin test at entry could choose whether to be vaccinated or not. In this context, the study conducted in England (where, in addition to BCG, *Mycobacterium microti* was given to a subset of participants) remains the only study of high standard that has shown a very high level of protection, of close to 80 per cent, in this age group.[120–125] The other studies

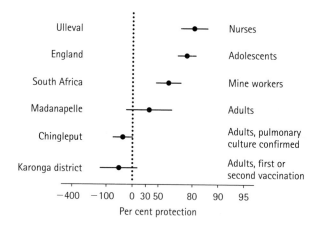

Figure 24.8 Results from prospective studies on the efficacy of bacillus Calmette–Guérin vaccination against tuberculosis in adults.[18,20,112–114,116,117,120–127]

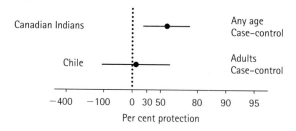

Figure 24.9 Results from retrospective studies on the efficacy of bacillus Calmette–Guérin vaccination against tuberculosis in adults.[128,129]

show little or no protection, with a tendency to reveal a potentially harmful effect in India.[112–114,126] In England, protection appeared to last for about 10 years before dropping rapidly.[125] In contrast, in Chingleput, where there was no overall protection, vaccination appeared to confer harm (more cases than in the control group) in the first 5 years and minimal protection subsequently.[114]

The two retrospective studies show a protective effectiveness of 10 per cent[128] and close to 60 per cent,[129] respectively (Figure 24.9).

These studies seem to indicate that vaccination of adolescents or adults is rarely a useful intervention.

Protection conferred by BCG vaccination across various age groups

Of the seven clinical trials studying protective efficacy across a wide range of age groups, with a preponderance of people other than infants, two showed a high level of protection, of around 80 per cent, while all of the others showed little or no protection (Figure 24.10).[89,112–114,116,117,130–136]

These observations reconfirm that utilization of BCG vaccination in age groups other than infants is rarely an effective intervention.

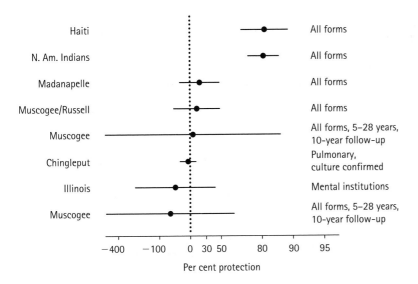

Figure 24.10   Results from prospective studies on the efficacy of bacillus Calmette–Guérin vaccination against tuberculosis in all ages.[89,112–114,116,117,130–136]

One retrospective study from the Gambia reported that 35 patients among 200 without a BCG scar died during chemotherapy, while none of 85 with a BCG scar did so.[137] While considerable attention was paid to adjustment for potential confounding factors (yet the effect remained), the authors were still cautious in concluding that BCG vaccination reduces case fatality from pulmonary TB.

HYPOTHESES ABOUT THE VARIATION IN THE EFFICACY OF BCG VACCINATION

While the overall evidence is quite clearly in favour of a protective effect of BCG vaccination, the observed variations are large in both prospective and retrospective studies. A number of hypotheses have been formulated to address these discrepancies. Smith[138] and Smith and Fine[139] have comprehensively reviewed the evidence and the following outline is guided by, and draws heavily on, their assessment.

The principal hypotheses to explain the variations observed in the protection offered by BCG include:

- differences in methodological stringency;
- differences in vaccine strains;
- differences in vaccine dose;
- differences in virulence of *M. tuberculosis* strains;
- differences in risk attributable to exogenous reinfection tuberculosis;
- differences in genetic make up of vaccinees;
- differences in nutritional status of vaccinees;
- differences in prevalence of infection with environmental mycobacteria;
- other factors.

Differences in methodological stringency

Quite obviously, not every study can be methodologically as rigorously conducted as ideal standards of study design and conduct call for.[80,83] Among the clinical trials, several

have been excluded from major reviews and meta-analyses, such as those conducted by Colditz and collaborators.[140,141] These authors found that study validity score explained 66 per cent of the variation in prospective clinical trials and 36 per cent in retrospective case–control studies[140] and only 15 per cent in case–control studies on BCG protection against infant TB.[141] Nevertheless, perhaps the most relevant trial showing no protection against bacteriologically confirmed TB, conducted in Chingleput, India, was judged to be of high scientific quality by a World Health Organization (WHO) expert committee specifically charged to ascertain the trial's validity.[142]

It must be kept in mind that the range of protection cannot be taken at face value, but must also be seen in the context of what the study in question sought to address. BCG trials (be they prospective or retrospective) ascertained protection against various outcomes such as morbid state (TB or death from TB) and site of disease, e.g. pulmonary, extrapulmonary single site and disseminated TB, taking into account such aspects as bacteriologic certainty of the case, age of the patients and time elapsed since vaccination. What seems apparent from the studies is the tendency of BCG to provide its greatest protection within the few years following vaccination, against death from TB, disseminated disease manifestations and bacteriologically unconfirmed TB. In summarizing these effects, BCG is generally most effective against serious forms of TB occurring shortly after infection acquired at an early age. Thus, any evaluation of the protective efficacy of BCG vaccination should be stratified according to these variables.

Differences in vaccine strains

The available BCG vaccine strains differ widely in phenotype and genotype.[10,11,36,37] It has been proposed[143] that differences in vaccine strains may account for observed variations in vaccine efficacy. In the rabbit model, not all BCG (and *M. microti*) strains provided the same level of protection.[144] However, the most powerful argument against this hypothesis arises from the Chingleput study, where two vaccine strains were used[112–114] that had documented high efficacy in other settings, but were not shown to be efficacious in Chingleput. Furthermore, one of the studies (a case–control study from Indonesia) cited for evidence of differential effectiveness of strains, examined successive vaccination policies, and was thus by necessity a non-concurrent study which additionally failed to adjust for time elapsed since vaccination.[145]

Differences in vaccine dose

BCG has been administered through various routes, initially orally, then parenterally. The latter administration may have been given intradermally or transdermally via multipuncture devices. The dosage reaching the target thus may well have varied. Nevertheless, the following observations seem to contradict the argument of an influence of differential dosage effect. Three controlled clinical trials with low efficacy used multipuncture administration,[117,134,135] and one with high efficacy did so too.[91] Furthermore, the trial in Chingleput specifically considered in its design the possibility of deterioration of vaccine potency in the field, and allocated vaccinees also to two arms receiving a 10-fold difference in dose, with no difference in effect.[112–114]

Differences in virulence of *M. tuberculosis* strains

That not all tubercle bacilli are equally virulent has been demonstrated repeatedly for both *M. bovis* BCG[146] and *M. tuberculosis* in general[147,148] and for isoniazid-resistant strains in particular.[149–152]

The hypothesis that the relative frequency of more or less virulent tubercle bacilli affects the observed protective efficacy of BCG vaccination is based on the assumption that tubercle bacilli of lower virulence might also cause tuberculin skin test reactions of smaller size. Such people then might be classified as 'non-reactors', i.e. people not infected with tubercle bacilli, thus becoming eligible for vaccination. Vaccination of actually infected people may thus mask any protective effect of BCG vaccination, as vaccination is not expected to provide protection against those who are already infected.[153]

The argument fails to account for the fact that BCG provided no protection at all in some trials. Depending on the proportion of individuals who had escaped infection with environmental mycobacteria at the point of BCG vaccination, masking of protection by BCG vaccination would be expected to be incomplete.

Differences in risk attributable to exogenous reinfection TB

BCG vaccination is expected to provide protection against TB resulting from infection acquired subsequent to vaccination. It is not expected to provide greater protection than a naturally acquired primary infection. Protection conferred by a primary infection against disease from reinfection is incomplete.[154–161] Thus, the protective efficacy of BCG might be increasingly masked as the contributory fraction of cases attributable to reinfection increases.[162,163] Thus, following this argument, the protection afforded by BCG is expected to be lower where the risk of infection with *M. tuberculosis* (and thus reinfection) is high.

This is not borne out by observations. The annual risk of infection in the UK decreased considerably over time,[164] yet the level of protection afforded by BCG remained high and virtually unchanged.[110]

Differences in genetic make up of vaccinees

Because differences in protection from BCG among males and females were observed in at least one study,[115] other genetic factors may also play a role in the differential protection conferred by BCG. Nevertheless, the finding that BCG gave virtually no protection to children in Chingleput,[114] but high protection in children from the Indian subcontinent living in the UK[107,110] would tend to disfavour this hypothesis.

Differences in nutritional status of vaccinees

As nutritional status affects the functioning of the cellular immune system, it might be expected that poor nutritional status would adversely affect the protective efficacy of BCG vaccination. However, BCG provided very high protection against TB death among poorly nourished Native American children, even somewhat higher than among well-nourished British adolescents,[125] a finding that would tend to contradict this hypothesis.

Differences in prevalence of infection with environmental mycobacteria

BCG vaccination has been used not only for protection against TB, but also against leprosy,[165–171] often with more success than in the prevention of TB.[126,172,173] It is thus apparent that different mycobacterial species (in this case *M. tuberculosis*, *M. bovis* BCG, *M. microti* and *M. leprae*) exert a modification of the immunologic response to infection with another mycobacterial species.[174] It is thus postulated that infection with one species of mycobacterium triggers a cellular immune response prepared to act more swiftly in the killing of mycobacteria of another species acquired during a subsequent infection. This is most apparent from the (albeit limited) protection provided by infection with *M. tuberculosis* against superinfection with tubercle bacilli[160] and the apparently similar effect of *M. bovis* BCG under certain circumstances. That BCG can also afford protection against leprosy would indicate that cross-protection is not limited to closely related mycobacterial species.

It has been postulated that different mycobacterial species induce different immunologic responses, some beneficially increasing protection against superinfection with another mycobacterial infection, while others may increase susceptibility to progression to clinically overt disease.[175] In experimental models, protection afforded by vaccination with *M. bovis* BCG, *M. fortuitum*, *M. avium*, *M. kansasii* and *M. scrofulaceum* against *M. tuberculosis* was examined in the guinea pig.[176] All environmental mycobacteria used in this study provided some protection, but with a wide variation, yet none provided as high a level of protection as BCG vaccination. It has therefore been postulated that the low protection afforded by BCG in Georgia as compared to the high protection observed in Britain may be attributable to a differential prevalence of infection with environmental mycobacteria.[176] Edwards *et al.*[177] demonstrated similar protection by vaccinating with *M. avium* complex against *M. tuberculosis* isolated in Chingleput as with the Danish BCG strain. Orme and Collins[178] demonstrated that airborne infection with *M. avium* in mice was as effective as intravenous BCG in protection against a challenge with virulent tubercle bacilli. Brown *et al.*[179] administered *M. vaccae* in drinking water to mice, subsequently challenged them with BCG and measured the proliferative response of spleen cells.[179] The results showed that, depending on the timing of the exposure of the mice to *M. vaccae* before BCG vaccination, *M. vaccae* could enhance, mask or interfere with the expression of sensitization by BCG.

If environmental mycobacteria do indeed provide some protection against *M. tuberculosis* and infection with them occurs before the administration of BCG, then the effect of the latter will be at least partially masked.[163] This may explain the larger protection conferred by BCG given earlier in life than if given later, as demonstrated in Chingleput.[114]

Furthermore, the risk of TB would be expected to be greater in initially tuberculin-negative people than in individuals with small tuberculin skin test reaction sizes (more likely attributable to infection with environmental than tubercle bacilli).

In Puerto Rico, protection from BCG was lower in rural areas, where non-specific sensitivity was higher than in urban areas, where protection from BCG was higher.[180] However, in Chingleput, the rate of TB among people with a reaction size of more than 9 mm to a sensitin produced from *M. avium* complex (PPD-B) was identical to that among those with zero to 9 mm reaction sizes.[114]

In the UK, the risk of TB was higher among initially tuberculin skin test-negative adolescents than among those reacting to 100 tuberculin units only, but the risk decreased over time.[125] The protection afforded against TB by a tuberculin skin test reaction that can be elicited only by this large dose of tuberculin is remarkably similar (but smaller) to that imparted by BCG vaccination (Figure 24.11).

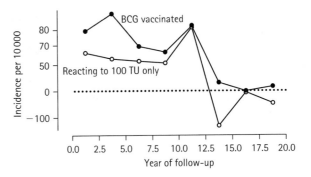

Figure 24.11 Comparative protection from bacillus Calmette–Guérin vaccination and presumed infection with environmental mycobacteria among British school children during follow up.[125]

In the Karonga, Malawi, trial the risk of TB during follow up was lowest among those with an initial tuberculin skin test reaction size of 6–10 mm.[181] After adjustment for age and sex, the risk was also lower among those with reactions of 1–5 mm than among non-reactors.[182]

That different species of mycobacteria seem to act on the immune system has also been demonstrated by observations from Sweden. After the cessation of mass BCG vaccination, there was a large increase in peripheral lymphadenitis due to environmental mycobacteria (Figure 24.12)[54,183,184] (also V Romanus, personal written communication, 18 February 2000). Similarly, in the Czech Republic, the incidence of lymphadenitis among children due to *M. avium* following cessation of BCG vaccination was 3.6, compared to 0.2 per 100 000 person-years among children vaccinated on the insistence of their parents,[185] suggesting a protection of 95 per cent (95 per cent confidence interval, 88–98 per cent) from BCG against lymphadenits due to *M. avium*.

While not all findings are consistent with the hypothesis that environmental mycobacteria may mask the protection that BCG can confer in their absence,[182] it may explain to a considerable extent certain variations in observed efficacy.

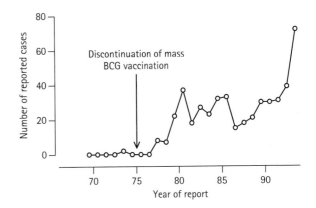

Figure 24.12 Reported cases of mycobacteriosis due to *M. avium* complex, Sweden, 1969–93. Data courtesy of Victoria Romanus, Swedish Institute for Infectious Diseases.

This hypothesis has aptly been called the 'masking hypothesis'. Alternatively, to explain the role of environmental mycobacteria in the variation of protection, Andersen and Doherty[186] have proposed the 'blocking hypothesis'. BCG must replicate to induce the desired immunological response. Previous sensitization with environmental mycobacteria might be sufficient to block successful replication and dissemination of BCG, thereby reducing its full potential for protective immunity. Conversely, sensitization with environmental mycobacteria might have only minimal influence on the replication of virulent *M. tuberculosis*. Thus, the heterologous immunity induced by environmental mycobacteria suffices to block the immune-inducing replication of BCG but will not suffice to do so successfully if an individual becomes infected with *M. tuberculosis*.

Other factors

It has been suggested that infestation with parasites, in particular with helminths, may affect the human T-cell immune responses to mycobacterial antigens.[187] Treatment of helminths resulted in significant improvement of T-cell proliferation and interferon-γ production. To some extent, this could explain the reduced efficacy of BCG in countries in the world where helminthic infestation is common.[187]

BCG REVACCINATION

It is or has been the policy in many countries to revaccinate with BCG at school entry or later in life. There is no evidence that this increases protection against TB,[188–190] but in northern Malawi it has been shown to considerably increase protection against leprosy.[126] A large study of revaccination in school children who had first been vaccinated as infants has been conducted in Brazil.[191] There was no benefit from revaccination.

Revaccination schemes have frequently been used for children in the lowest TB risk period in life (at 5–14 years of age). Furthermore, with this age group they target a population where primary protection from BCG vaccination has been dubious or variable at best.

EFFECTS OF BCG OTHER THAN THOSE DIRECTED AGAINST TB

BCG has been shown to be protective against leprosy in some situations[165–168,192] but not in others.[169] It has also shown to be effective against *M. ulcerans*, albeit with an apparently very short-lived protection.[193]

The best known indications for BCG against other than mycobacterial diseases are its use as an immunotherapeutic agent in the treatment of superficial bladder cancer[194–203]

and, to a lesser extent, malignant melanoma.[204] It has also been suggested that BCG reduces the risk of atopy and asthma,[205–207] and reductions in the risk of intestinal nematodes in children[208] and HIV-infected patients have been reported.[209,210]

INDICATIONS AND RECOMMENDATIONS FOR THE USE OF BCG VACCINATION

Approximately 100 million children now receive BCG every year.[188] The number of doses produced in the year 2000, in descending order, were the Copenhagen 1331 strain, D2PB302, Tokyo 172, Sofia SL 222, Pasteur 1173, Glaxo 1077 and the Russian strain.[188]

While there have been wide variations in the protection afforded by BCG vaccination in different trials, the evidence is overwhelming that BCG provides protection against TB, especially against tuberculous meningitis and death from disseminated TB in children. Where it worked, its protective effect waned over time, to disappear after 15–20 years. The evidence for protection against bacteriologically confirmed TB in adults has been less consistent.

Because BCG vaccination is given early in life, the protection afforded is limited in time, and its effect on bacteriologically confirmed TB in adults is inconsistent, it cannot be expected to have a great impact on the epidemiology of TB.[211,212]

It seems inappropriate to conclude from meta-analyses that BCG provides some average protection.[140,141] The observed range in protection is real and remains largely unexplained.

In light of the evidence, WHO recommends its use in newborn children or as early in life as possible.[142,213] This is still sound policy for those countries in the world where TB is highly prevalent and tuberculous meningitis is a frequent, disabling or fatal occurrence. It fails to address the role of BCG where TB in children has become a rare occurrence.

The International Union Against Tuberculosis and Lung Disease has developed recommendations on criteria for the discontinuation of mass BCG vaccination.[214] Three key issues enter into the decision-making process on the discontinuation of BCG vaccination.

The first is the extent of protection BCG actually imparts in a given location. In the USA, the low efficacy of BCG vaccination in Georgia, Georgia-Alabama and Puerto Rico had an important impact on the decision not to routinely utilize BCG vaccination. As such prospective studies are usually beyond the realm of resource availability, effectiveness might alternatively be studied utilizing the case–control or contact study approach.

The second is the frequency of serious forms of TB in children (meningitis, disseminated forms) weighted against the frequency of adverse reactions from the vaccine itself. This has been best studied in Sweden where the frequency of serious adverse reactions from BCG vaccination (osteoarticular and disseminated mycobacteriosis due to BCG) outweighed the incidence of cases that the vaccine was intended to prevent.[54] Similarly, BCG vaccination may become non-cost-effective as the frequency of childhood TB decreases, so that an increasing number of children need to be vaccinated to prevent one case.

The third consideration is the value attached to the preservation of the utility of the interpretation of tuberculin skin test results. BCG vaccination induces tuberculin sensitivity and complicates the interpretation of tuberculin skin testing results. In industrialized countries with an elimination strategy in mind, the tuberculin skin test is an important means of identifying people with tuberculous infection at a high risk of progression to TB who would benefit from preventive chemotherapy. This argument will nevertheless become irrelevant with the development of interferon-γ release assays that contain antigens which are not found in the BCG strain.[215]

The WHO discourages revaccination because there is no evidence of its usefulness.[216] Lack of evidence is, however, not synonymous with lack of efficacy. Revaccination at school entry is likely to be inefficient (even if it were efficacious), because it falls into the period in life when the risk of TB is lowest.

Finally, concerning HIV infection, the WHO has concluded after careful review of available data, that BCG vaccination schemes do not need to be altered, unless HIV infection is symptomatic (AIDS).[72] Where the mother is known to be HIV infected, but the infant's HIV status is unknown but is free of signs or symptoms of HIV infection, vaccination is usually indicated. If the infant is known to be HIV infected, with or without signs or symptoms, the infant should not be vaccinated with BCG. This, too, seems to be a reasonable recommendation given the lack of evidence of an increased frequency of serious adverse events in BCG-vaccinated children who also have acquired HIV infection from their mother. However, it appears that HIV infection lowers or indeed annihilates the protective effect against extrapulmonary TB.[217] In industrialized countries, where the need for BCG vaccination is generally lower, it is usually recommended not to give BCG vaccination to individuals known to have HIV infection.[218]

The freeze-dried vaccine should be kept refrigerated and protected from light, and diluted only immediately before vaccination. In most countries, BCG vaccine is given by the intradermal route, generally by injection with a 25- or 26-gauge needle, in the deltoid insertion region of the upper arm.[219] Most manufacturers (including all those who provide vaccine for UNICEF, the largest purchaser in the world) recommend a 0.05-mL dose for infants, and double the dose for children.

Difficulties have arisen for decision-makers about the value of vaccinating health-care workers at increased risk of infection with *M. tuberculosis*, particularly in settings where multidrug-resistant TB is common. The uncertainty stems from the scarcity of data on protection against TB among adults, and the generally low level of protection (or none at all) among adults in clinical trials. While decision analyses appear to favour the use of BCG vaccination in such settings,[220] such a conclusion has been disputed, largely based on the argument that it deprives those vaccinated from ever learning whether they have acquired tuberculous infection or not (loss of specificity of the tuberculin test).[221] Nevertheless, in areas where BCG has been demonstrated to provide appreciable protection against TB among adults, where there is a high risk for health-care workers of becoming infected, and where multidrug-resistant TB is common, a BCG vaccination policy for health-care workers might deserve consideration. Where these conditions are not met, non-vaccination of health-care workers might be more appropriate.

In summary, barring a better alternative, BCG vaccination remains a useful adjunct for the individual protection against disabling and lethal forms of childhood TB in most parts of the world where TB remains highly prevalent. It cannot be expected, however, to have great impact on the epidemiologic situation of TB.[211,212]

NOTE

This chapter has been modified from a chapter in a monograph originally published in *Interventions for tuberculosis control and elimination*, published by the International Union Against Tuberculosis and Lung Disease, Paris, France, 2002, and reproduced with permission.

LEARNING POINTS

- BCG was created by the passage of a virulent strain of *M. bovis* after 230 passages from 1908 until 1921 when it no longer changed its characteristics.
- An oral form of BCG was first used which gave satisfactory results in terms of preventing TB deaths in infants.
- Its safety was wrongly challenged when 72 of 251 children died in Lübeck, Germany after being given an oral BCG contaminated with a virulent strain of *M. tuberculosis* in error.
- Successive subculturing has meant that strains across the world differ considerably in their genetic make up.
- BCG is a live vaccine, so there is a potential danger in vaccinating immunocompromised hosts, such as those who are HIV infected. WHO recommends that BCG be given at birth or as early in life unless children are known to be HIV infected.
- No intervention has been shown to speed up the resolution of minor adverse effects of BCG, such as local abscess formation of lymphadenopathy.

- When given to infants, BCG affords good protection against death from TB and against disseminated and meningeal TB.
- Vaccination of older children is not as reliable as vaccination of infants.
- In randomized clinical trials with BCG among adolescents and young adults, only the study carried out in the UK in the 1950s has shown good protection.
- Hypotheses as to why there is such variation in BCG efficacy are many and varied. None provides a sufficient explanation, although some, such as the role of heterologous immunity resulting from infection with environmental mycobacteria deserve further study.
- The efficacy of BCG should not be 'averaged' across different trials. The fact is that some trials have shown protective efficacy of 80 per cent and some none.
- No trial has shown BCG to have important harmful effects.
- BCG is recommended for infants in developing countries where TB is common. It continues to be given in some countries where the prevalence is low, but the majority of low-incidence countries in Western Europe have relinquished its use and in others this policy is under some review.
- Some countries, such as the USA and The Netherlands, have never routinely used BCG.

REFERENCES

1. von Behring E. Tuberkulose. Einleitung. *Beitr Exp Ther* 1902; **5**: V–XVIII.
2. von Behring E, Römer P, Ruppel WG. Tuberkulose. *Beitr Exp Ther* 1902; **5**: 1–90.
3. Webb GB, Williams WW. Immunity in tuberculosis. Its production in monkeys and children. *J Am Med Assoc* 1911; **57**: 1431–5.
4. Smith T. Certain aspects of natural and acquired resistance to tuberculosis and their bearing on preventive measures. *J Am Med Assoc* 1917; **68**: 669–74/764–9.
5. Calmette A. Preventive vaccination against tuberculosis with BCG. *Proc Roy Soc Med* 1931; **24**: 85–94.
6. Sakula A. BCG: who were Calmette and Guérin? *Thorax* 1983; **38**: 806–12.
7. Calmette A, Guérin C. Vaccination des bovidés contre la tuberculose et méthode nouvelle de prophylaxie de la tuberculose bovine. *Ann Inst Pasteur* 1924; **38**: 371–98.
8. Calmette A, Guérin C, Breton M. Contribution à l'étude de la tuberculose expérimentale du cobaye. (Infection et essais de vaccination par la voie digestive). *Ann Inst Pasteur* 1907; **21**: 401–16.
9. Calmette A, Guérin C. Nouvelles recherches expérimentales sur la vaccination des bovidés contre la tuberculose. *Ann Inst Pasteur* 1920; **34**: 553–60.
10. Osborn TW. Changes in BCG strains. *Tubercle* 1983; **64**: 1–13.
11. Grange JM, Gibson J, Osborn TW *et al*. What is BCG? *Tubercle* 1983; **64**: 129–39.
12. Griffith AS. A study of the BCG strain of tubercle bacillus. With an account of two immunity experiments and a preliminary report on the cultivation of tubercle bacilli on bile media. *Lancet* 1932; **1**: 361–3.
13. Weill-Hallé B, Turpin R. Premiers essais de vaccination antituberculeuse de l'enfant par le bacille Calmette-Guérin (BCG). *Bull Soc Méd Hôpitaux (France)* 1925; **49**: 1589–601.
14. Calmette A, Guérin C, Nègre L, Boquet A. Prémunition des nouveau-nés contre la tuberculose par le vaccin BCG (1921 à 1926). *Ann Inst Pasteur* 1926; **40**: 89–134.
15. Calmette A. La vaccination préventive de la tuberculose par le BCG dans les familles de médecins 1924–1932. *Ann Inst Pasteur* 1932; **49** (Suppl.): 1–62.
16. Institut Pasteur. *Vaccination préventive de la tuberculose de l'homme et des animaux par le BCG. Rapports et documents provenant des divers pays (France exceptée) transmis à l'Institut Pateur en 1932*. Paris: Masson et Cie, 1932.
17. Calmette A. *L'infection bacillaire et la tuberculose chez l'homme et chez les animaux. Processus d'infection et de défense, étude biologique et expérimentale, vaccination préventive*. Paris: Masson et Cie, 1928.
18. Heimbeck J. Sur la vaccination préventive de la tuberculose par injection sous-cutanée de BCG chez les élèves-infirmières de l'hôpital Ulleval, à Oslo (Norvège). *Ann Inst Pasteur* 1929; **43**: 1229–32.
19. Heimbeck J. Tuberculosis in hospital nurses. *Tubercle* 1936; **18**: 97–9.
20. Heimbeck J. BCG vaccination in nurses. *Tubercle* 1948; **29**: 84–8.
21. Kereszturi C, Park WH, Levine M *et al*. Clinical study of BCG vaccination. *N Y State J Med* 1933; **33**: 375–81.
22. Baudouin JA. Vaccination against tuberculosis with the BCG vaccine. *Can J Public Health* 1936; **27**: 20–6.
23. Petroff SA. A new analysis of the value and safety of protective immunization with BCG (Bacillus Calmette-Guérin). *Am Rev Tuberc* 1929; **20**: 275–96.
24. Petroff SA, Branch A, Steenken W Jr. A study of bacillus Calmette-Guérin (BCG). I. Biological characteristics, cultural 'dissociation' and animal experimentation. *Am Rev Tuberc* 1929; **19**: 9–46.
25. Heimbeck J. Immunity to tuberculosis. *Arch Intern Med* 1928; **41**: 336–42.
26. Lange B. Untersuchungen zur Klärung der Ursachen der im Anschluss an die Calmette-Impfung aufgetretenen Säuglingserkrankungen in Lübeck. *Zeitschr Tuberkulose* 1930; **59**: 1–18.
27. Calmette A. Epilogue de la catastrophe de Lubeck. *Presse Méd* 1931; **2**: 17–18.
28. Moegling A. Die 'Epidemiologie' der Lübecker Säuglingstuberkulose. *Arb Reichsges-Amt* 1935; **69**: 1–24.
29. Dormandy T. *The white death*. London and Rio Grande: The Hambledon Press, 1999.
30. Edelhoff J. *Der Calmette-Prozess. Der Wagen. Ein Lübeckisches Jahrbuch*. Lübeck: Hansisches Verlagskontor, 1984: 62–8.
31. Lange L. Zu den Tuberkuloseschutzimpfungen in Lübeck. *Zeitschr Tuberkulose* 1930; **57**: 305–10.
32. Schürmann P, Kleinschmidt H. Pathologie und Klinik der Lübecker Säuglingstuberkuloseerkrankungen. *Arb Reichsges-Amt* 1935; **69**: 25–204.
33. Lange L, Pescatore H. Bakteriologische Untersuchungen zur Lübecker Säuglingstuberkulose. *Arb Reichsges-Amt* 1935; **69**: 205–305.
34. Hashimoto T. *The vaccination, theory and practice. BCG*. Tokyo: International Medical Foundation, 1975.
35. Gheorghiu M, Augier J, Lagrange PH. Maintenance and control of the French BCG strain 1173-P$_2$ (primary and secondary seed-lots). *Bull Inst Pasteur* 1983; **81**: 281–8.
36. Behr MA, Small PM. A historical and molecular phylogeny of BCG strains. *Vaccine* 1999; **17**: 915–22.
37. Oettinger T, Jørgensen M, Ladefoged A *et al*. Development of the *Mycobacterium bovis* BCG vaccine: review of the historical and

biochemical evidence for a genealogical tree. *Tuber Lung Dis* 1999; **79**: 243–50.

38. Behr MA, Schroeder BG, Brinkman JB *et al.* A point mutation in the *mma3* gene is responsible for impaired methoxymycolic acid production in *Mycobacterium bovis* BCG strains obtained after 1927. *J Bacteriol* 2000; **182**: 3394–9.

39. Lotte A, Wasz-Höckert O, Poisson N *et al.* BCG complications. Estimates of the risks among vaccinated subjects and statistical analysis of their main characteristics. *Adv Tuberc Res* 1984; **21**: 107–93.

40. Lotte A, Wasz-Höckert O, Poisson N *et al.* A bibliography of the complications of BCG vaccination. A comprehensive list of the World Literature since the introduction of BCG up to July 1982, supplemented by over 100 personal communications. *Adv Tuberc Res* 1984; **21**: 194–245.

41. FitzGerald JM. Management of adverse reactions to bacille Calmette–Guérin vaccine. *Clin Infect Dis* 2000; **31** (Suppl.): S75–6.

42. Lotte A, Wasz-Höckert O, Poisson N *et al.* Second IUATLD study on complications induced by intradermal BCG-vaccination. *Bull Int Union Tuberc Lung Dis* 1988; **63**: 47–59.

43. Böttiger M, Romanus V, De Verdier C, Boman G. Osteitis and other complications caused by generalized BCG-itis. Experiences in Sweden. *Acta Paediatr Scand* 1982; **71**: 471–8.

44. Schopfer K, Matter L, Brunner C *et al.* BCG osteomyelitis. Case report and review. *Helv Paediatr Acta* 1982; **37**: 73–81.

45. Kröger L, Korppi M, Brander E *et al.* Osteitis caused by bacille Calmette–Guérin vaccination: a retrospective analysis of 222 cases. *J Infect Dis* 1995; **172**: 574–6.

46. Horwitz O, Meyer J. The safety record of BCG vaccination and untoward reactions observed after vaccination. *Adv Tuberc Res* 1957; **8**: 245–71.

47. Tardieu M, Truffot-Pernot C, Carrière JP *et al.* Tuberculous meningitis due to BCG in two previously healthy children. *Lancet* 1988; **1**: 440–41.

48. Abramowsky C, Gonzalez B, Sorensen RU. Disseminated bacillus Calmette–Guérin infections in patients with primary immunodeficiencies. *Am J Clin Pathol* 1993; **100**: 52–6.

49. Stone MM, Vannier AM, Storch SK *et al.* Brief report: meningitis due to iatrogenic BCG infection in two immunocompromised children. *N Engl J Med* 1995; **333**: 561–3.

50. Gonzalez B, Moreno S, Budach R *et al.* Clinical presentation of bacillus Calmette–Guérin infections in patients with immunodeficiency syndromes. *Pediatr Infect Dis J* 1989; **8**: 201–206.

51. Jouanguy E, Altare F, Lamhamedi S *et al.* Interferon-gamma-receptor deficiency in an infant with fatal bacille Calmette–Guérin infection. *N Engl J Med* 1996; **335**: 1956–61.

52. Casanova JL, Blanche S, Emile JF *et al.* Idiopathic disseminated bacillus Calmette–Guérin infection: a French national retrospective study. *Pediatrics* 1996; **98**: 774–8.

53. Talbot EA, Perkins MD, Fagundes M *et al.* Disseminated bacille Calmette–Guérin disease after vaccination: case report and review. *Clin Infect Dis* 1997; **24**: 1139–46.

54. Romanus V. *The impact of BCG vaccination on mycobacterial disease among children born in Sweden between 1969 and 1993*. Stockholm: Smittskyddsinstitutet, 1995.

55. Jeena PM, Chhagan MK, Topley J, Coovadia HM. Safety of the intradermal Copenhagen 1331 BCG vaccine in neonates in Durban, South Africa. *Bull World Health Organ* 2001; **79**: 337–43.

56. Nousbaum JB, Garre M, Boles JM *et al.* Deux manifestations inhabituelles d'une infection par le virus LAV-HTLV III: BCGite et varicelle pulmonaire. *Rev Pneumol Clin* 1986; **42**: 310–311.

57. von Reyn CF, Mann JM, Clements CJ. Human immunodeficiency virus infection and routine childhood immunisation. *Lancet* 1987; **2**: 669–71.

58. Weltman AC, Rose DN. The safety of bacille Calmette–Guérin vaccination in HIV infection and AIDS. *AIDS* 1993; **7**: 149–57.

59. Houde C, Dery P. *Mycobacterium bovis* sepsis in an infant with

human immunodeficiency virus infection. *Pediatr Infect Dis J* 1988; **7**: 810–811.

60. Boudes P, Sobel A, Deforges L, Leblic E. Disseminated *Mycobacterium bovis* infection from BCG vaccination and HIV infection. *J Am Med Assoc* 1989; **262**: 2386 (correspondence).

61. Ninane J, Grymonprez A, Burtonboy G *et al.* Disseminated BCG in HIV infection. *Arch Dis Child* 1988; **63**: 1268–9.

62. Lallemant-Le Coeur S, Lallemant M, Cheynier D *et al.* Bacillus Calmette–Guérin immunization in infants born to HIV-1-seropositive mothers. *AIDS* 1991; **5**: 195–9.

63. Besnard M, Sauvion S, Offredo C *et al.* Bacillus Calmette–Guérin infection after vaccination of human immunodeficiency virus-infected children. *Pediatr Infect Dis J* 1993; **12**: 993–7.

64. Rosenfeldt V, Pærregaard A, Valerius NH. Disseminated infection with bacillus Calmette–Guérin in a child with advanced HIV disease. *Scand J Infect Dis* 1997; **29**: 526–7.

65. Romanus V, Fasth A, Tordai P, Wiholm BE. Adverse reactions in healthy and immunocompromised children under six years of age vaccinated with the Danish BCG vaccine, strain Copenhagen 1331: implications for the vaccination policy in Sweden. *Acta Paediatr* 1993; **82**: 1043–52.

66. van Deutekom H, Smulders YM, Roozendaal KJ, van Soolingen D. Bacille Calmette–Guérin (BCG) meningitis in an AIDS patient 12 years after vaccination with BCG. *Clin Infect Dis* 1996; **22**: 870–1 (correspondence).

67. O'Brien KL, Ruff AJ, Louis MA *et al.* Bacillus Calmette–Guérin complications in children born to HIV-1-infected women with a review of the literature. *Pediatrics* 1995; **95**: 414–8.

68. Reynes J, Perez C, Lamaury I, Janbon F, Bertrand A. Bacille Calmette–Guérin adenitis 30 years after immunization in a patient with AIDS. *J Infect Dis* 1989; **160**: 727 (correspondence).

69. Armbruster C, Junker W, Vetter N, Jaksch G. Disseminated bacille Calmette–Guérin infection in an AIDS patient 30 years after BCG vaccination. *J Infect Dis* 1990; **162**: 1216 (correspondence).

70. Reichman LB. Why hasn't BCG proved dangerous in HIV-infected patients? *J Am Med Assoc* 1989; **261**: 3246 (correspondence).

71. Waddell RD, Lishimpi K, von Reyn CF *et al.* Bacteremia due to *Mycobacterium tuberculosis* or *M. bovis*, bacille Calmette–Guérin (BCG) among HIV-positive children and adults in Zambia. *AIDS* 2001; **15**: 55–60.

72. World Health Organization. Revised BCG vaccination guidelines for infants at risk for HIV infection. *Wkly Epidem Rec* 2007; **82**: 193–6.

73. Close GC, Nasiiro R. Management of BCG adenitis in infancy. *J Trop Pediatr* 1985; **31**: 286 (correspondence).

74. Hanley SP, Gumb J, Macfarlane JT. Comparison of erythromycin and isoniazid in treatment of adverse reactions to BCG vaccination. *Br Med J* 1985; **290**: 970.

75. Oguz F, Müjgan S, Alper G *et al.* Treatment of bacille Calmette–Guérin-associated lymphadenitis. *Pediatr Infect Dis J* 1992; **11**: 887–8.

76. Victoria MS, Shah BR. Bacillus Calmette–Guérin lymphadenitis: a case report and review of the literature. *Pediatr Infect Dis J* 1985; **4**: 295–6.

77. Banani SA, Alborzi A. Needle aspiration for suppurative post-BCG adenitis. *Arch Dis Child* 1994; **71**: 446–7.

78. Boman G, Sjögren I, Dahlström G. A follow-up study of BCG-induced osteo-articular lesions in children. *Bull Int Union Tuberc Lung Dis* 1984; **59**: 198–200.

79. Last JM. *A dictionary of epidemiology*. New York: Oxford University Press, 1995.

80. Rothman KJ, Greenland S. *Modern epidemiology*. Philadelphia: Lippincott-Raven, 1998.

81. Orenstein WA, Bernier RH, Dondero TJ *et al.* Field evaluation of vaccine efficacy. *Bull World Health Organ* 1985; **63**: 1055–68.

82. Smith PG. Retrospective assessment of the effectiveness of BCG vaccination against tuberculosis using the case-control method. *Tubercle* 1982; **63**: 23–35.

83. Schlesselman JJ. *Case–control studies. Design, conduct, analysis.* New York: Oxford University Press, 1982.

84. Rodrigues LC, Smith PG. Use of the case–control approach in vaccine evaluation: efficacy and adverse effects. *Epidemiol Rev* 1999; 21: 56–72.

85. Aronson JD, Dannenberg AM. Effect of vaccination with BCG on tuberculosis in infancy and in childhood. Correlation of reactions to tuberculin tests, roentgenologic diagnosis and mortality. *Am J Dis Child* 1935; 50: 1117–30.

86. Feldberg GD. *Disease and class. Tuberculosis and the shaping of modern North American society.* New Jersey: Rutgers University Press, 1995.

87. Aronson JD, Palmer CE. Experience with BCG vaccine in the control of tuberculosis among North American Indians. *Public Health Rep* 1946; 61: 802–20.

88. Townsend JG, Aronson JD, Saylor R, Parr I. Tuberculosis control among the North American Indians. *Am Rev Tuberc* 1942; 45: 41–52.

89. Aronson JD, Aronson CF, Taylor HC. A twenty-year appraisal of BCG vaccination in the control of tuberculosis. *Arch Intern Med* 1958; 101: 881–93.

90. Aronson JD. Protective vaccination against tuberculosis with special reference to BCG vaccination. *Am Rev Tuberc* 1948; 58: 255–81.

91. Rosenthal SR, Loewinsohn E, Graham ML *et al.* BCG vaccination against tuberculosis in Chicago. A twenty-year study statistically analyzed. *Pediatrics* 1961; 28: 624–41.

92. Ferguson RG, Simes AB. BCG vaccination of Indian infants in Saskatchewan. *Tubercle* 1949; 30: 5–11.

93. Levine MI, Sackett MF. Results of BCG immunization in New York City. *Am Rev Tuberc* 1946; 53: 517–32.

94. Wünsch Filho V, de Castilho EA, Rodrigues LC, Huttly SRA. Effectiveness of BCG vaccination against tuberculous meningitis: a case–control study in São Paulo, Brazil. *Bull World Health Organ* 1990; 68: 69–74.

95. Wünsch-Filho V, Moncau JEC, Nakao N. Methodological considerations in case–control studies to evaluate BCG vaccine effectiveness. *Int J Epidemiol* 1993; 22: 149–55.

96. Miceli I, De Kantor IN, Colaiácovo D *et al.* Evaluation of the effectiveness of BCG vaccination using the case–control method in Buenos Aires, Argentina. *Int J Epidemiol* 1988; 17: 629–34.

97. Murtagh K. Efficacy of BCG. *Lancet* 1980; 1: 423 (correspondence).

98. Zodpey SP, Maldhure BR, Dehankar AG, Shrikhande SN. Effectiveness of bacillus Calmette Guerin (BCG) vaccination against extra-pulmonary tuberculosis: a case–control study. *J Commun Dis* 1996; 28: 77–84.

99. Chavalittamrong B, Chearskul S, Tuchinda M. Protective value of BCG vaccination in children in Bangkok, Thailand. *Pediatr Pulmonol* 1986; 2: 202–205.

100. Sharma RS, Srivastava DK, Asunkanta Singh A *et al.* Epidemiological evaluation of BCG vaccine efficacy in Delhi – 1989. *J Commun Dis* 1989; 21: 200–206.

101. Camargos PAM, Guimaraes MDC, Antunes CMF. Risk assessment for acquiring meningitis tuberculosis among children not vaccinated with BCG: a case–control study. *Int J Epidemiol* 1988; 17: 193–7.

102. Myint TT, Win H, Aye HH, Kyaw-Mint TO. Case–control study on evaluation of BCG vaccination of newborn in Rangoon, Burma. *Ann Trop Paediatr* 1987; 7: 159–66.

103. Rosenthal SR, Loewinsohn E, Graham ML *et al.* BCG vaccination in tuberculous households. *Am Rev Respir Dis* 1961; 84: 690–704.

104. Sirinavin S, Chotpitayasunondh T, Suwanjutha S *et al.* Protective efficacy of neonatal bacillus Calmette-Guérin vaccination against tuberculosis. *Pediatr Infect Dis J* 1991; 10: 359–65.

105. Al-Kassimi FA, Al-Hajjaj MS, Al-Orainey IO, Bamgboye EA. Does the protective effect of neonatal BCG correlate with vaccine-induced tuberculin reaction? *Am J Respir Crit Care Med* 1995; 152: 1575–8.

106. Lanckriet C, Lévy-Bruhl D, Bingono E, Siopathis RM, Guérin N. Efficacy of BCG vaccination of the newborn: evaluation by a follow-up study of contacts in Bangui. Int J Epidemiol 1995; 24: 1042–9.

107. Packe GE, Innes JA. Protective effect of BCG vaccination in infant Asians: a case–control study. *Arch Dis Child* 1988; 63: 277–81.

108. Young TK, Hershfield ES. A case–control study to evaluate the effectiveness of mass neonatal BCG vaccination among Canadian Indians. *Am J Public Health* 1986; 76: 783–6.

109. Bhat GJ, Diwan VK, Chintu C, Kabika M, Masona J. HIV, BCG and TB in children: a case control study in Lusaka, Zambia. *J Trop Pediatr* 1993; 39: 219–23.

110. Rodrigues LC, Gill ON, Smith PG. BCG vaccination in the first year of life protects children of Indian subcontinent ethnic origin against tuberculosis in England. *J Epidemiol Comm Health* 1991; 45: 78–80.

111. Smith PG. Evaluating interventions against tropical diseases. *Int J Epidemiol* 1987; 16: 159–66.

112. Tuberculosis Prevention Trial. Trial of BCG vaccines in south India for tuberculosis prevention: first report. *Bull World Health Organ* 1979; 57: 819–27.

113. Tuberculosis Prevention Trial Madras. Trial of BCG vaccines in south India for tuberculosis prevention. *Indian J Med Res* 1980; 72 (Suppl.): 1–74.

114. Tuberculosis Research Centre (ICMR) Chennai. Fifteen year follow up of trial of BCG vaccines in south India for tuberculosis prevention. *Indian J Med Res* 1999; 110: 56–69.

115. Comstock GW, Livesay VT, Woolpert SF. Evaluation of BCG vaccination among Puerto Rican children. *Am J Public Health* 1974; 64: 283–91.

116. Frimodt-Møller J, Thomas J, Parthasarathy R. Observations on the protective effect of BCG vaccination in a South Indian rural population. *Bull World Health Organ* 1964; 30: 545–74.

117. Frimodt-Møller J, Acharyulu GS, Pillai KK. Observations on the protective effect of BCG vaccination in a South Indian rural population: fourth report. *Bull Int Union Tuberc* 1973; 48: 40–49.

118. Shapiro C, Cook N, Evans D *et al.* A case–control study of BCG and childhood tuberculosis in Cali, Colombia. *Int J Epidemiol* 1985; 14: 441–6.

119. Capewell S, Leitch AG. The value of contact procedures for tuberculosis in Edinburgh. *Br J Dis Chest* 1984; 78: 317–29.

120. Hart PD, Pollock TM, Sutherland IC. Assessment of the first results of the Medical Research Council's trial of tuberculosis vaccines in adolescents in Great Britain. *Adv Tuberc Res* 1957; 8: 171–89.

121. British Medical Association. BCG. and vole bacillus vaccines in the prevention of tuberculosis in adolescents. First (progress) report to the Medical Research Council by their Tuberculosis Vaccines Clinical Trials Committee. *Br Med J* 1956; 1: 413–27.

122. British Medical Association. BCG and vole bacillus vaccines in the prevention of tuberculosis in adolescents. Second report to the Medical Research Council by their Tuberculosis Vaccines Clinical Trials Committee. *Br Med J* 1959; 2: 379–96.

123. British Medical Association. BCG and vole bacillus vaccines in the prevention of tuberculosis in adolescence and early adult life. Third report to the Medical Research Council by their Tuberculosis Vaccines Clinical Trials Committee. *Br Med J* 1963; 1: 973–8.

124. Medical Research Council Tuberculosis Vaccines Clinical Trials Committee. BCG and vole bacillus vaccines in the prevention of tuberculosis in adolescence and early adult life. Fourth report to the Medical Research Council by its Tuberculosis Vaccines Clinical Trials Committee. *Bull World Health Organ* 1972; 46: 371–85.

125. Hart PD, Sutherland I. BCG and vole bacillus vaccines in the prevention of tuberculosis in adolescence and early adult life. Final report to the Medical Research Council. *Br Med J* 1977; 2: 293–5.

126. Karonga Prevention Trial Group. Randomised controlled trial of single BCG, repeated BCG, or combined BCG and killed *Mycobacterium leprae* vaccine for prevention of leprosy and tuberculosis in Malawi. *Lancet* 1996; 348: 17–24.

127. Coetzee AM, Berjak J. BCG in the prevention of tuberculosis in an adult population. *Proc Mine Med Off Assoc* 1968; **48**: 41–53.

128. Sepulveda RL, Parcha C, Sorensen RU. Case-control study of the efficacy of BCG immunization against pulmonary tuberculosis in young adults in Santiago, Chile. *Tuberc Lung Dis* 1992; **73**: 372–7.

129. Houston S, Fanning A, Soskolne CL, Fraser N. The effectiveness of bacillus Calmette–Guérin (BCG) vaccination against tuberculosis. A case-control study in treaty Indians, Alberta, Canada. *Am J Epidemiol* 1990; **131**: 340–8.

130. Palmer CE, Shaw LW, Comstock GW. Community trials of BCG vaccination. *Am Rev Tuberc Pulm Dis* 1958; **77**: 877–907.

131. Comstock GW, Palmer CE. Long-term results of BCG vaccination in the southern United States. *Am Rev Respir Dis* 1966; **93**: 171–83.

132. Comstock GW, Shaw LW. Controlled trial of BCG vaccination in a school population. *Public Health Rep* 1960; **75**: 583–94.

133. Comstock GW, Woolpert SF, Livesay VT. Tuberculosis studies in Muscogee County, Georgia. Twenty-year evaluation of a community trial of BCG vaccination. *Public Health Rep* 1976; **91**: 276–80.

134. Comstock GW, Webster RG. Tuberculosis studies in Muscogee County, Georgia. VII. A twenty-year evaluation of BCG vaccination in a school population. *Am Rev Respir Dis* 1969; **100**: 839–45.

135. Bettag OL, Kaluzny AA, Morse D, Radner DB. BCG study at a state school for mentally retarded. *Dis Chest* 1964; **45**: 503–507.

136. Vandiviere HM, Dworski M, Melvin IG et al. Efficacy of bacille Calmette–Guérin and isoniazid-resistant bacille Calmette–Guérin with and without isoniazid chemoprophylaxis from day of vaccination. II. Field trial in man. *Am Rev Respir Dis* 1973; **108**: 301–13.

137. Corrah T, Byass P, Jaffar S et al. Prior BCG vaccination improves survival of Gambian patients treated for pulmonary tuberculosis. *Trop Med Intern Health* 2000; **5**: 413–17.

138. Smith PG. BCG vaccination. In: Davies PDO (ed.). *Clinical tuberculosis*. London: Chapman & Hall Medical, 1994: 297–310.

139. Smith PG, Fine PEM. BCG vaccination. In: Davies PDO (ed.). *Clinical tuberculosis*. London: Chapman & Hall Medical, 1998: 417–31.

140. Colditz GA, Brewer TF, Berkey CS et al. Efficacy of BCG vaccine in the prevention of tuberculosis. Meta-analysis of the published literature. *J Am Med Assoc* 1994; **271**: 698–702.

141. Colditz GA, Berkey CS, Mosteller F et al. The efficacy of bacillus Calmette–Guérin vaccination of newborns and infants in the prevention of tuberculosis: meta-analyses of the published literature. *Pediatrics* 1995; **96**: 29–35.

142. World Health Organization. Vaccination against tuberculosis. Report of an ICMR/WHO Scientific Group. *Tech Rep Ser* 1980; **651**: 1–21.

143. Comstock GW. Identification of an effective vaccine against tuberculosis. *Am Rev Respir Dis* 1988; **138**: 479–80.

144. Dannenberg AM Jr, Bishai WR, Parrish WR et al. Efficacies of BCG and vole bacillus (*Mycobacterium microti*) vaccines in preventing clinically apparent pulmonary tuberculosis in rabbits: a preliminary report. *Vaccine* 2001; **19**: 796–800.

145. Sutrisna B, Utomo P, Komalarini S, Swatrinai S. Penelitan efectifitas vaksin BCG can beberapa faktor lainnya pada anak yang menderita TBC berat di 3 rumah sakit di Jakarta 1981–1982. *Medika* 1983; **9**: 143–50.

146. Bøe J. Variations in the virulence of BCG. *Acta Tuberc Scand* 1947; **21**: 123–33.

147. Mitchison DA, Wallace JG, Bhatia AL et al. A comparison of the virulence in guinea-pigs of South Indian and British tubercle bacilli. *Tubercle* 1960; **41**: 1–22.

148. Dickinson JM, Lefford MJ, Lloyd J, Mitchison DA. The virulence in the guinea-pig of tubercle bacilli from patients with pulmonary tuberculosis in Hong Kong. *Tubercle* 1963; **44**: 446–51.

149. Middlebrook G, Cohn ML. Some observations on the pathogenicity of isoniazid-resistant variants of tubercle bacilli. *Science* 1953; **118**: 297–9.

150. Middlebrook G. Isoniazid-resistance and catalase activity of tubercle bacilli. A preliminary report. *Am Rev Tuberc* 1954; **69**: 471–2.

151. Ordway DJ, Sonnenberg MG, Donahue SA et al. Drug-resistant strains of *Mycobacterium tuberculosis* exhibit a range of virulence for mice. *Infect Immun* 1995; **63**: 741–3.

152. Cohn ML, Davis CL. Infectivity and pathogenicity of drug-resistant strains of tubercle bacilli studied by aerogenic infection of guinea pigs. *Am Rev Respir Dis* 1970; **102**: 97–100.

153. Sutherland I, Lindgren I. The protective effect of BCG vaccination as indicated by autopsy studies. *Tubercle* 1979; **60**: 225–31.

154. Raleigh JW, Wichelhausen R. Exogenous reinfection with *Mycobacterium tuberculosis* confirmed by phage typing. *Am Rev Respir Dis* 1973; **108**: 639–42.

155. Romeyn JA. Exogenous reinfection in tuberculosis. *Am Rev Respir Dis* 1970; **101**: 923–7.

156. Small PM, Shafer RW, Hopewell PC et al. Exogenous reinfection with multidrug-resistant *Mycobacterium tuberculosis* in patients with advanced HIV infection. *N Engl J Med* 1993; **328**: 1137–44.

157. Nardell E, McInnis B, Thomas B, Weidhaas S. Exogenous reinfection with tuberculosis in a shelter for the homeless. *N Engl J Med* 1986; **315**: 1570–75.

158. Godfrey-Faussett P, Githui W, Batchelor B et al. Recurrence of HIV-related tuberculosis in an endemic area may be due to relapse or reinfection. *Tuber Lung Dis* 1994; **75**: 199–202.

159. Nolan CM. Reinfection with multidrug-resistant tuberculosis. *N Engl J Med* 1993; **329**: 811 (correspondence).

160. Vynnycky E, Fine PEM. The natural history of tuberculosis: the implications of age-dependent risks of disease and the role of reinfection. *Epidemiol Infect* 1997; **119**: 183–201.

161. Sutherland I, Švandová E, Radhakrishna S. The development of clinical tuberculosis following infection with tubercle bacilli. 1. A theoretical model of clinical tuberculosis following infection, linking data on the risk of tuberculous infection and the incidence of clinical tuberculosis in the Netherlands. *Tubercle* 1982; **63**: 255–68.

162. ten Dam HG, Pio A. Pathogenesis of tuberculosis and effectiveness of BCG vaccination. *Tubercle* 1982; **63**: 225–33.

163. Smith D, Wiegeshaus E, Balasubramanian V. An analysis of some hypotheses to the Chingleput bacille Calmette–Guérin trial. *Clin Infect Dis* 2000; **31** (Suppl. 3): S77–S80.

164. Vynnycky E, Fine PEM. The annual risk of infection with *Mycobacterium tuberculosis* in England and Wales since 1901. *Int J Tuberc Lung Dis* 1997; **1**: 389–96.

165. Abel L, Cua VV, Oberti J et al. Leprosy and BCG in southern Vietnam. *Lancet* 1990; **335**: 1536 (correspondence).

166. Brown JAK, Stone MM, Sutherland I. BCG vaccination of children against leprosy in Uganda: results at end of second follow-up. *Br Med J* 1968; **1**: 24–7.

167. Fine PEM, Maine N, Ponnighaus JM et al. Protective efficacy of BCG against leprosy in northern Malawi. *Lancet* 1986; **2**: 499–502.

168. Lwin K, Sundaresan T, Mg Gyi MG et al. BCG vaccination of children against leprosy: fourteen-year findings of the trial in Burma. *Bull World Health Organ* 1985; **63**: 1069–78.

169. Orege PA, Fine PEM, Lucas SB, Obura M, Okelo C, Okuku P. Case-control study of BCG vaccination as a risk factor for leprosy and tuberculosis in Western Kenya. *Int J Leprosy* 1993; **61**: 542–9.

170. Sutherland I. Research into the control of tuberculosis and leprosy in the community. *Br Med Bull* 1988; **44**: 665–78.

171. Zodpey SP, Bansod BS, Shrikhande SN et al. Protective effect of bacillus Calmette Guerin (BCG) against leprosy: a population-based case–control study in Nagpur, India. *Lepr Rev* 1999; **70**: 287–94.

172. Pönnighaus JM, Fine PEM, Bliss L et al. The Karonga prevention trial: a leprosy and tuberculosis vaccine trial in Northern Malawi. I. Methods of the vaccination phase. *Lepr Rev* 1993; **64**: 338–56.

173. Pönnighaus JM, Fine PEM, Sterne JAC et al. Efficacy of BCG vaccine against leprosy and tuberculosis in northern Malawi. Lancet 1992; 339: 636–9.

174. Black GF, Dockrell HM, Crampin AC et al. Patterns and implications of naturally acquired immune responses to environmental and tuberculous mycobacterial antigens in Northern Malawi. J Infect Dis 2001; 184: 322–9.

175. Stanford JL, Shield MJ, Rook GAW. How environmental mycobacteria may predetermine the protective efficacy of BCG. Tubercle 1981; 62: 55–67.

176. Palmer CE, Long MW. Effects of infection with atypical mycobacteria on BCG vaccination and tuberculosis. Am Rev Respir Dis 1966; 94: 553–68.

177. Edwards ML, Goodrich JM, Muller D et al. Infection with Mycobacterium avium-intracellulare and the protective effects of bacille Calmette–Guérin. J Infect Dis 1982; 145: 733–41.

178. Orme I, Collins FM. Efficacy of Mycobacterium bovis BCG vaccination in mice undergoing prior pulmonary infection with atypical mycobacteria. Infect Immun 1984; 44: 28–32.

179. Brown CA, Brown IN, Swinburne S. The effect of oral Mycobacterium vaccae on subsequent responses of mice to BCG sensitization. Tubercle 1985; 66: 251–60.

180. Comstock GW, Edwards PQ. An American view of BCG vaccination, illustrated by results of a controlled trial in Puerto Rico. Scand J Respir Dis 1972; 53: 207–17.

181. Fine PEM, Sterne JAC, Ponnighaus JM, Rees RJW. Delayed-type hypersensitivity, mycobacterial vaccines and protective immunity. Lancet 1994; 344: 1245–9.

182. Fine PEM. Variation in protection by BCG: implications of and for heterologous immunity. Lancet 1995; 346: 1339–45 (published erratum appears in Lancet 1996; 347: 340).

183. Romanus V, Hallander HO, Wåhlén P et al. Atypical mycobacteria in extrapulmonary disease among children. Incidence in Sweden from 1969 to 1990, related to changing BCG vaccination coverage. Tuber Lung Dis 1995; 76: 300–10.

184. Tala E, Romanus V, Tala-Heikkilä M. Bacille Calmette–Guérin vaccination in the 21st century. Eur Respir Mon 1997; 4: 327–53.

185. Trnka L, Dankova D, Svandová E. Six years' experience with the discontinuation of BCG vaccination. 4. Protective effect of BCG vaccination against the Mycobacterium avium intracellulare complex. Tuber Lung Dis 1994; 75: 348–52.

186. Andersen P, Doherty TM. The success and failure of BCG – implications for a novel tuberculosis vaccine. Nature Rev 2005; 3: 656–62.

187. Elias D, Wolday D, Akuffo H et al. Effect of deworming on human T cell responses to mycobacterial antigens in helminth-exposed individuals before and after bacille Calmette–Guérin (BCG) vaccination. Clin Exp Immunol 2001; 123: 219–25.

188. World Health Organization. BCG in immunization programmes. Wkly Epidem Rec 2001; 76: 33–9.

189. Tala-Heikkilä M. Evaluation of the Finnish BCG-revaccination programme in schoolchildren. Ann Univ Turkuensis 1993; 119: 5–65.

190. Tala-Heikkilä M, Tuominen JE, Tala EOJ. Bacillus Calmette–Guérin revaccination questionable with low tuberculosis incidence. Am J Respir Crit Care Med 1998; 157: 1324–7.

191. Rodrigues LC, Pereira SM, Cunha SS et al. Effect of BCG revaccination on incidence of tuberculosis in school-aged children in Brazil: the BCG-REVA cluster-randomised trial. Lancet 2005; 366: 1290–95.

192. Fine PEM. BCG vaccination against tuberculosis and leprosy. Br Med Bull 1988; 44: 691–703.

193. Smith PG, Revill WDL, Lukwago E, Rykushin YP. The protective effect of BCG against Mycobacterium ulcerans disease: a controlled trial in an endemic area of Uganda. Trans R Soc Trop Med Hyg 1976; 70: 449–57.

194. Anonymous. Topical BCG for recurrent superficial bladder cancer. Lancet 1991; 337: 821–2 (editorial).

195. Melekos MD, Chionis H, Pantazakos A et al. Intravesical bacillus Calmette–Guérin immunoprophylaxis of superficial bladder cancer: results of a controlled prospective trial with modified treatment schedule. J Urology 1993; 149: 744–8.

196. Talic RF, Hargreve TB, Bishop MC et al. Intravesical Evans bacille Calmette–Guérin for carcinoma in situ of the urinary bladder. Br J Urology 1994; 73: 645–8.

197. Wishahi MM, Ismail IMH, El-Sherbini M. Immunotherapy with bacille Calmette–Guérin in patients with superficial transitional cell carcinoma of the bladder associated with bilharziasis. Br J Urology 1994; 73: 649–54.

198. Fellows GJ, Parmar MKB, Grigor KM et al. Marker tumour response to Evans and Pasteur bacille Calmette–Guérin in multiple recurrent pTa/pTI bladder tumours: report from the Medical Research Council Subgroup on Superficial Bladder Cancer (Urological Cancer Working Party). Br J Urology 1994; 73: 639–44.

199. Rogerson JW. Intravesical bacille Calmette–Guérin in the treatment of superficial transitional cell carcinoma of the bladder. Br J Urology 1994; 73: 655–8.

200. Mack D, Frick J. Five-year results of a phase II study with low-dose bacille Calmette–Guérin therapy in high-risk superficial bladder cancer. Urology 1995; 45: 958–61.

201. Witjes JA, van den Meijden APM, Collette L et al. Long-term follow-up of an EORTC randomized prospective trial comparing intravesical bacille Calmette–Guérin-RIVM and mitomycin C in superficial bladder cancer. Urology 1998; 52: 403–10.

202. Alexandroff AB, Jackson AM, O'Donnell MA, James K. BCG immunotherapy of bladder cancer: 20 years on. Lancet 1999; 353: 1689–94.

203. Malström PU, Wijkström H, Lundholm C et al. 5-year follow-up of a randomized prospective study comparing mitomycin C and bacillus Calmette–Guérin in patients with superficial bladder carcinoma. J Urol 1999; 161: 1124–7.

204. Czarnetzki BM, Macher E, Suciu S et al. Long-term adjuvant immunotherapy in stage I high risk malignant melanoma, comparing two BCG preparations versus non-treatment in a randomised multicentre study. (EORTC Protocol 18781). Eur J Cancer 1993; 29A: 1237–42.

205. Shirakawa T, Enomoto T, Shimazu S, Hopkin JM. The inverse association between tuberculin responses and atopic disorders. Science 1997; 275: 77–9.

206. Alm JS, Lilja G, Scheynus A. Early BCG vaccination and development of atopy. Lancet 1997; 350: 400–403.

207. Aaby P, Shaheen SO, Heyes CB et al. Early BCG vaccination and reduction in atopy in Guinea-Bissau. Clin Exp Allergy 2000; 30: 644–50.

208. Barreto ML, Rodrigues LC, Silva PCR et al. Lower hookworm incidence, prevalence, and intensitiy of infection in children with a bacillus Calmette–Guérin vaccination scar. J Infect Dis 2000; 182: 1800–1803.

209. Elliott AM, Nakiyingi J, Quigley MA et al. Inverse association between BCG immunisation and intestinal nematode infestation among HIV-1-positive individuals in Uganda. Lancet 1999; 354: 1000–1001.

210. Odent M. Future of BCG. Lancet 1999; 354: 2170 (correspondence).

211. Styblo K, Meijer J. Impact of BCG vaccination programmes in children and young adults on the tuberculosis problem. Tubercle 1976; 57: 17–43.

212. Rouillon A, Waaler H. BCG vaccination and epidemiological situation. Adv Tuberc Res 1976; 19: 64–126.

213. World Health Organization. BCG vaccination policies. Report of a WHO Study Group. Tech Rep Ser 1980; 652: 1–17.

214. International Union Against Tuberculosis and Lung Disease. Criteria for discontinuation of vaccination programmes using bacille Calmette–Guerin (BCG) in countries with a low prevalence of tuberculosis. A statement of the International Union Against Tuberculosis and Lung Disease. Tuber Lung Dis 1994; 75: 179–80.

215. Pai M, Kalantri S, Dheda K. New tools and emerging technologies for the diagnosis of tuberculosis: Part I. Latent tuberculosis. *Exp Rev Mol Diagn* 2006; **6**: 413–22.

216. World Health Organization. Global Tuberculosis Programme and Global Programme on Vaccines. Statement on BCG revaccination for the prevention of tuberculosis. *WHO Wkly Epidem Rec* 1995; **70**: 229–31.

217. Arbeláez MP, Nelson KE, Muñoz A. BCG vaccine effectiveness on preventing tuberculosis and its interaction with human immunodeficiency virus infection. *Int J Epidemiol* 2000; **29**: 1085–91.

218. Centers for Disease Control and Prevention. The role of BCG vaccine in the prevention and control of tuberculosis in the United States: a joint statement by the Advisory Council for the Elimination of Tuberculosis and the Advisory Committee on Immunization Practices. *MMWR Morb Mortal Wkly Rep* 1996; **45** (RR-4): 1–18.

219. Fine PEM, Carneiro IAM, Milstien JB, Clements CJ. *Issues relating to the use of BCG in immunization programmes. A discussion document.* World Health Organization Document, WHO/V&B/99.23, 1999: 1–42.

220. Greenberg PD, Lax KG, Schechter CB. Tuberculosis in house staff. A decision analysis comparing the tuberculin screening strategy with the BCG vaccination. *Am Rev Respir Dis* 1991; **143**: 490–5.

221. Reichman LB, Jordan TJ, Greenberg PD. Decision analysis comparing the tuberculin screening strategy with BCG vaccine. *Am Rev Respir Dis* 1992; **145**: 732–3 (correspondence).

PART 7

CONTROL

25

Control of tuberculosis in low-prevalence countries

DANIEL SAGEBIEL

INTRODUCTION

The objective of tuberculosis (TB) control is the elimination of TB by preventing the transmission of tubercle bacilli and the emergence of drug resistance.[1–4] The lowest TB incidences in the world in 2004 are reported from the European Union (EU) and Western Europe (12.6), the USA (5), Canada (5), Australia (5) and New Zealand (9).[5,6] In these regions there has been a steady decline in TB cases for many years and today the situation is characterized by a low prevalence associated with little public awareness of TB and decreasing knowledge about the disease. Recently, this steady decrease has stopped in some countries and the resurgence of TB in several industrialized countries[6–10] has shown that the disease today occurs most frequently in specific groups, such as foreign-born persons from countries with a high TB prevalence, socially marginalized people and intravenous drug users.[7] The rise of new TB cases is mainly observed in the foreign-born population.[6]

Early diagnosis, adequate treatment and documented cure of infectious patients with pulmonary TB are necessary to reduce transmission of *Mycobacterium tuberculosis* and ultimately to eliminate TB.[7,11,12] The World Health Organization (WHO) defines an effective national TB programme as having a high cure rate, a low level of acquired drug resistance and a high case-detection rate.[7,13] In order to prevent the emergence of drug-resistant TB, each new case of sputum-positive pulmonary TB must be given an effective chemotherapy regimen for a sufficient period of time.

As the possibility of drug resistance is high in chronic or relapsing patients, special precautions need to be taken for this group.[14] As various studies have shown, the use of standardized drugs and dosages, as well as strict patient adherence through directly observed treatment (DOT), constitute an efficient approach, even in the industrialized countries, where its role is less clear.[1,7,15] In addition, the necessary infrastructure needs to be available and to be supported by adequate training and organizational facilities to ensure programme success.[14]

DEFINITIONS

TB control and elimination strategies aim to diminish the incidence and prevalence of active TB and latent infection to reduce the pool of those with TB infection from which future cases of TB will emanate.

Tuberculosis control strategies

These aim to reduce the incidence of new infection with *M. tuberculosis* complex by rapid identification of sources of infection (e.g. risk-group management and prevention of transmission in institutional settings), and by rendering them non-infectious through curative treatment.[11]

Tuberculosis elimination strategies

These include additional elements to reduce the prevalence of latent TB infection, such as preventive therapy for specified groups and individuals with an increased risk of progression from latent infection to overt clinical TB, and outbreak management.[11]

Low tuberculosis incidence countries

While low TB incidence countries (low-prevalence countries) have been defined as those with a crude case notification rate below 10 (all cases) per 100 000 inhabitants and declining,[2,11] the definition has been extended to include all countries in Europe with a crude notification rate below 20 per 100 000 population in the 'European framework'.[1,2,7,11] As the vast majority of patients in low-prevalence countries are cured, the prevalence is estimated to be comparable with the case notification rate.

Tuberculosis elimination

TB elimination will be reached when less than one infectious (sputum smear-positive) case per 1 000 000 inhabitants emerges annually in the general population.[2]

REASONS FOR DECLINE OF TB

During the last century, a decline in TB was described in many parts of the world, especially in Western Europe and the USA. In most European low-incidence countries, TB morbidity among the native population declined dramatically in the twentieth century.[11,16] The main reasons for this decline are improved social and economic structures – in particular, better housing and sanitary conditions, a better nourished population and more information about TB and its transmission. The declining mortality curves over the last centuries may also be explained by genetic selection towards a less susceptible population ('survival of the fittest').[17–20]

Furthermore, the confinement of TB patients to closed spaces in the sixteenth to eighteenth century,[18] the establishment of the sanatorium as a curative institution in the nineteenth century (since 1859), as well as the establishment of TB dispensaries and finally the era of chemotherapy for TB, contributed to the decline of TB.[21,22] Thus, a significant role in the second half of the twentieth century can be attributed to the use of combined chemotherapy and to TB control programmes incorporating elements of passive and active case finding to treat disease at early stages and thereby prevent spreading. Increasing use of effective anti-tuberculosis drugs led to a further fall in new cases and mortality rates until the end of the 1980s. For example, the mortality from TB in Germany fell from 3.2/100 000 (1980) to 0.3/100 000 inhabitants (2004).[23,24] In Germany, a transient increase of TB morbidity and mortality occurred during the First and Second World Wars.[21]

EPIDEMIOLOGY

TB in the world

Despite falling mortality rates in industrialized countries, TB is increasing worldwide and remains one of the most common fatal infectious diseases along with human immunodeficiency virus (HIV) and malaria. TB causes a quarter of all avoidable deaths. The WHO estimates that one-third of the world's population is infected with TB. Approximately 5–10 per cent of the 100 million people newly infected with TB each year develop active TB in the course of their lives. In 2004, 8.9 million people developed TB, of whom more than 80 per cent lived in the developing countries of Africa or Asia. Approximately 1.7 million people died of TB in 2004, among them 100 000 children.[5,25,26] The TB case notification rates are unevenly distributed worldwide, with under 15/100 000 cases in the industrialized countries and over 400/100 000 cases in some sub-Saharan African countries.[5]

TB in Europe

Out of all TB cases notified to the WHO in 2004, 7 per cent (354 954) were from Europe ('Europe region' by WHO definition, including Central and Eastern Europe), with an average incidence of 40/100 000. This represents a slight decrease since the year 2000 (373 081; 43/100 000), but a considerable increase compared with 1991 (231 608; 27/100 000). The incidence in Western European countries ranged from 0 (San Marino) to 34/100 000 (Portugal) – including the new member states to 68/100 000 (Latvia).[5] According to EuroTB, the notification rate in 2004 amounted to 12.6/100 000 in Western Europe (the 25 countries of the EU, Andorra, Iceland, Israel, Malta, Norway, San Marino and Switzerland; no data from Monaco).[6] On average overall, TB rates decreased by 4.8 per cent annually between 2000 and 2004, but less in young adults (–3 per cent between 1998 and 2004) than in the older age groups (–31 per cent between 1998 and 2004). TB rates were stable in Belgium and Ireland and increased in Greece, Norway and the United Kingdom due to rising numbers of foreign-born cases.[6] Stable or decreasing case notification rates and rather low levels of drug resistance in most low-prevalence countries indicate that TB control remains effective overall. Rates were highest in those over 64 years of age, reflecting reactivation of old *M. tuberculosis* infection, and in the male population. Twenty-nine per cent of TB cases were of foreign origin. Pulmonary cases represented 77 per cent of TB cases in the West and out of these 42 per cent were sputum smear-positive.[6] In comparison, the Russian Federation, the largest country of the Europe region, had an incidence of 106/100 000. The highest incidence within this WHO region was reported by Kazakhstan (217/100 000).[6] TB crosses borders and its increase in the countries of the former Soviet Union remains to be of particular epidemiological importance to some Western European countries.[5,21,27-29]

Low-prevalence countries

In 2004, the definition of a low-incidence country with a crude case notification rate below 10/100 000[2] was fulfilled by Australia (5), Canada (5), Cyprus (4), Denmark (7), Finland (6), France (8), Germany (8), Greece (6), Iceland (4), Ireland (9), Israel (8), Italy (7), Luxembourg (7), Malta (5), the Netherlands (8), New Zealand (9), Norway (6), San Marino (0), Sweden (5), Switzerland (7) and the USA (5).[5] The extended definition of a crude case notification rate below 20 per 100 000[1,11] included all 25 EU and Western European countries (with the exception of Estonia (40), Hungary (22), Latvia (68), Lithuania (59), Poland (23) and Portugal (34)), as well as Albania (18). Higher rates were also notified from the new EU member states of 2007, Bulgaria (39) and Romania (131).[5]

The TB situation in Germany

In Germany, the TB incidence and mortality rates have decreased continuously during the past decades and reached the lowest point so far with 8/100 000 inhabitants in the year 2004 (6583 cases). One-third of the TB patients were of foreign nationality (35 per cent), and the case-notification rate in this group amounted to 30.6/100 000, 5.5 times higher than in German nationals (5.5/100 000).[24] During the early 1990s, a slight rise of TB was observed in Germany due to increased migration after the fall of the Iron Curtain (resettlers and asylum seekers).[21]

Comparison with WHO predictions

In the 1960s, international organizations and experts declared that TB was to be eradicated as a public health problem by the year 2000.[30] In 1994, the WHO predicted the number of new TB cases worldwide to rise from 7.5 million in 1990 to 10.2 million by the year 2000. In industrialized countries (Western Europe, USA, Canada, Japan, Australia and New Zealand), they expected a rise from 196 000 new TB cases in 1990 to 204 000 in 1995 and to 211 000 in the year 2000.[31] However, the amount of new TB cases reported in the same industrialized countries decreased and amounted to 194 722 in 1980, 137 848 in 1990, 103 079 in 2000 and 85 186 in 2004 (including new EU member states 102 257) (Table 25.1).[5] Worldwide, the estimated new cases increased to 8.9 million in the year 2004,[5] and are projected to rise to over 10 million by 2015.[32,33]

TARGET: ELIMINATION OF TB

The target of TB control is the elimination of TB. The age-specific case notification rate indicates how far a specific country or population segment is away from this target. At present in European and other low-prevalence countries, TB in the indigenous population is mainly a problem of the older generations with the highest prevalence of latent TB infection acquired during their youth.[11,34] They were born during the war and post-war periods, when the risk of TB infection was high, and have had a long cumulative probability of acquiring infection.[11] Disease in children and teenagers, the youngest generations, occurs far less frequently, as the prevalence and risk of newly acquired TB infection is now assumed to be very low in those born in low-prevalence countries. The situation is different in the foreign-born population from countries with a high TB prevalence, where young generations have a high risk of TB infection and may spread TB in the case of progression to active disease.[35]

As long as the risk of infection in the general population continues to decline, each generation will be replaced by one with a lower prevalence of infection. To ensure the continuation of this decline, it is essential to minimize, through early identification, the risk of new generations becoming infected and to cure newly emerging infectious cases. Newly acquired TB infection must be prevented from progressing to overt disease, to accelerate the progress towards elimination of TB in low-prevalence countries.[11] It has been estimated that, without additional efforts, it may still take another 50–60 years until TB elimination in low-prevalence countries is reached.[2,11]

FACTORS COUNTERACTING DECLINE OF TB

The causes for the worldwide increase of TB include demographic factors such as population growth, the surge in HIV infection, and deteriorating socioeconomic conditions with the resulting impoverishment of large areas of the world. Medical care in the affected countries is usually inappropriate, with inadequate therapeutic facilities and unsuccessful TB control.[13,21,36] There are, by contrast, positive examples showing successes of improved TB control programmes (e.g. Peru and India).[37-44]

The spread of TB is also facilitated by global migration and civil conflicts. The situation is worsened considerably by the increase in resistant TB strains as a consequence of inadequate treatment regimens. Furthermore, approximately one-third of the increase in TB cases can be attributed to the HIV epidemic, and TB is the most common cause of death for HIV patients: 30 per cent of deaths from the acquired immunodeficiency syndrome (AIDS) worldwide are thought to result from TB.[5,21,33,45]

Today, low-prevalence countries face specific challenges resulting from declining TB rates in the native population, the gradually increasing role of imported TB and

Table 25.1   TB cases reported in industrialized countries from 1980 to 2004.[5]

Country	1980		1990		2000		2004	
	No. cases	Rate[a]	No. cases	Rate[a]	No. cases	Rate[a]	No. cases	Rate[a]
Western Europe								
Andorra	–	–	23	44	12	18	7	10
Austria	2191	29	1521	20	1185	15	895	11
Belgium	2687	27	1577	16	1278	12	1128	11
Denmark	430	8	350	7	587	11	356	7
Finland	2247	47	772	15	527	10	319	6
France	17 199	32	9030	16	6122	10	5004	8
Germany	29 991	38	14 653	18	9064	11	6583[b]	8
Greece	5412	56	877	9	703	6	668	6
Iceland	25	11	18	7	13	5	11	4
Ireland	1152	34	624	18	386	10	380	9
Italy	3311	6	4246	7	3501	6	3968	7
Luxembourg	71	20	48	13	44	10	31	7
Malta	24	7	13	4	16	4	18	5
Monaco	1	4	1	3	0	0	–	–
Netherlands	1701	12	1369	9	1244	8	1316	8
Norway	499	12	285	7	221	5	278	6
Portugal	6873	70	6214	62	4227	41	3600	34
San Marino	–	–	1	4	1	4	0	0
Spain	4853	13	7600	19	7993	20	6015	14
Sweden	926	11	557	7	417	5	416	5
Switzerland	1160	18	1278	19	544	8	528	7
United Kingdom	10 488	19	5908	10	6220	11	7039	12
New EU member states								
Cyprus	69	11	29	4	33	4	30	4
Czech Republic	4962	48	1937	19	1414	14	1027	10
Estonia	614	42	423	27	791	58	537	40
Hungary	5412	51	3588	35	3073	30	2251	22
Latvia	1194	48	906	33	1982	84	1579	68
Lithuania	1636	48	1471	40	2657	76	2036	59
Poland	25 807	73	16 136	42	10 931	28	8698	23
Slovakia	2465	50	1448	31	1010	19	664	12
Slovenia	1085	59	722	30	368	19	249	13
Outside Europe								
USA	27 749	12	25 701	10	16 309	6	14 517	5
Canada	2885	12	1997	7	1694	6	1517	5
Australia	1457	10	1016	6	1043	5	1059	5
New Zeland	474	15	348	10	344	9	373	9
Japan	70 916	61	51 821	42	39 384	31	29 736	23
Total: Western Europe	91 241		56 965		44 305		38 560	
Total: New EU member states	43 244		26 660		22 259		17 071	
Total: Outside Europe	103 481		80 883		58 774		47 202	
Total: Industrialized countries	237 966		164 508		125 338		102 833	

[a]Rate per 100 000 population.
[b]From Ref. 24.
–, data not available.

latent TB infection (LTBI),[6,11,46] and the importation of (multi)drug-resistant (MDR)-TB mainly from Eastern European countries. In addition, the increasing visibility of high-risk groups for TB (e.g. HIV-infected patients, homeless people, prisoners, etc.) needs to be taken into account.[11,47–49]

Reasons for the increase of TB

Recent notification data indicate that the previously observed regular decline slowed down or stopped in several low-incidence countries of Europe in the 1990s.[5,8,11] After an average annual decrease of 5.4 per cent of new TB cases between 1974 and 1991,[8] some Western European countries were faced with increasing numbers of new TB cases in the 1990s (Austria, Denmark, Germany, Ireland, Italy, the Netherlands, Norway, Switzerland).[5,6] This was mainly due to increasing numbers of cases of foreign origin; for example, in Germany, refugees and asylum seekers originating from high-burden countries.[21] In addition, several other reasons may be responsible which are summarized in Table 25.2 and described in detail below.

Table 25.2 Reasons for the increase of tuberculosis (TB) in low-prevalence countries.

HIV in the population at risk

Increase of poverty (e.g. homelessness, drug abuse), especially in large cities

Migration

Low priority given to TB control

Dismantling of TB control services

Neglect of control measures (e.g. prisons, (illegal) migrants (see Screening of migrants)

Increase of resistant strains

Increase of more virulent strains

Decrease of host immunity

The influence of HIV was of importance in some low-prevalence countries, especially in the USA. However, this remained mainly a localized problem and its importance was shown to be related to the prevalence of *M. tuberculosis* infection in the at-risk population.[14] In Western Europe, where HIV prevalence has reached 0.3 per cent in adults, HIV co-infection only plays a marginal role except for a few densely populated areas with a widespread addiction to intravenous drugs, e.g. Spain, Portugal.[8,21,45,50]

Large cities are confronted with a high number of TB cases, not only because of higher rates of HIV-infected people and migrants from high-prevalence regions, but also due to a higher level of poverty, intravenous drug users and homelessness.[14,51]

The dangers of giving low priority to TB control and of dismantling TB control services have been demonstrated in the USA, where after an average yearly decrease in TB notifications of 5.7 per cent between 1975 and 1984, a sharp increase of TB cases was noticed after 1985. Between 1985 and 1992, the total increase reached 20 per cent (1985: 22 201 cases; 1992: 26 673 cases).[5] Here the effects of reduced public health efforts – severe underfinancing and consequent understaffing of the TB control services – socioeconomic developments, an increase of poverty and

homelessness combined with an escalating rate of HIV infections and migration played a part. A weakened and disseminated service without appropriate resources was unable to respond to a changing situation, eventually leading to the MDR-TB epidemic in New York City in the late 1980s and early 1990s.[14,18,29,52–55] The USA as the first country to realize that TB control had slipped had to put a large effort into correcting the apparent failures (the U-shaped curve of concern).[14,56] Authorities estimate that New York City alone spent about US$1 billion (1 000 000 000) in the early 1990s to regain control of TB.[18,57] Post-outbreak cases seem to have represented a reasonable amount of MDR-TB cases (28 per cent) in the years 1993 to 1999.[58] From 26 673 cases in 1992 (case notification rate 10/100 000), the number of new TB cases decreased to 14 517 cases in the year 2004 (case notification rate 5/100 000).[5] This reduction is largely attributable to a comprehensive strengthening of control activities resulting in a decrease of transmission and the distribution of cases has been limited to identifiable populations, primarily in urban and immigrant communities.[58–61] Nowadays, the USA are trying very hard to eliminate TB in their country and have formulated a strategy for the treatment of latent TB infection (LTBI).[61–63]

Western Europe, together with the WHO and the International Union Against Tuberculosis and Lung Disease (the Union), has formulated a joint strategy to deal with an unexpected resurgence of TB, and its elimination.[2,8,11,12,29]

The development of drug resistance is usually man-made and the result of medical or public health malpractice. Because drug resistance develops fast, inadequate treatment or non-adherence to treatment commonly leads to the development of drug-resistant disease with subsequent transmission of drug-resistant strains in the community. This may result from several overlapping programmatic factors, including poor medical management of treatment, non-establishment of recommended regimens, lack of supervised treatment, limited or interrupted drug supply, use of substandard quality drugs with inferior bioavailability, widespread availability of antituberculosis drugs without prescription and inadequate patient monitoring and case management in poorly managed and supported national TB control programmes.[33,48,55,64–66]

The treatment of drug-resistant patients may be the most expensive component of any TB service.[15,67] The knowledge of drug resistance patterns is of utmost importance for effective treatment regimens. A special effort should be made to prevent drug resistance by following simple strategies. Appropriate drugs in the correct doses should be delivered to the patients for the required duration. Directly observed treatment can play an important role, although without accompanying measures its role in low-prevalence countries may be limited.[68–71]

The greatest threat in this connection is combined resistance to at least the two main antituberculosis drugs isoniazid and rifampicin, the so-called multidrug resistant

(MDR) and especially the extensively drug-resistant TB (XDR-TB).[66] XDR-TB is defined as MDR-TB plus additional resistance to any fluoroquinolone and at least one of the three injectable second-line drugs capreomycin, kanamycin and amikacin. The treatment of MDR-TB and XDR-TB is difficult, prolonged and very expensive due to the need for second-line drugs.[43,44,49,66,72-75] Up to 50 million people worldwide are already infected with MDR-TB bacteria. WHO estimates the annual burden of MDR-TB at 300 000 to 600 000 cases and the prevalence to be three-fold higher.[66,76] For 2004, it has been estimated that 424 000 cases (95 per cent CI 376 000–620 000) of MDR-TB have emerged worldwide, 4.3 per cent (95 per cent CI 3.8–6.1) of all new and previously treated TB cases globally.[66] In a survey conducted by the WHO and the Centers for Disease Control (CDC) between 2000 and 2004, XDR-TB has been shown to occur worldwide and rates for XDR-TB among MDR-TB cases have been found to be between 1 and 15 per cent.[74] Risk factors for MDR and XDR-TB are previous treatment or relapse, origin from 'hot spot' areas, history of imprisonment, homelessness and possibly immunosuppressive diseases, like HIV[72,73,77,78] and diabetes mellitus,[79] all directly related to problems in TB control.[55]

As TB does not respect borders, the increase in drug resistance in the former Soviet Union (Newly Independent States, NIS) influences other industrialized countries and, for geographic reasons, in particular Western Europe. Here, resistance is more frequent not only among previously treated cases but in particular among cases of foreign origin. In 2004, cases of foreign origin accounted for the vast majority of MDR-TB cases, e.g. in Austria (100 per cent), Belgium (92 per cent), Germany (91 per cent), Israel (100 per cent), Sweden (100 per cent) and the UK (77 per cent).[6] In Austria, for example, MDR-TB among all cases (combined resistance) rose from 0.5 per cent in 2000 to 3.1 per cent in 2004.[6,76]

In Germany, a slight increase in overall resistance rates has been observed and the rate of any resistance (HRZES) in 2004 amounted to 13.9 per cent (2003, 13.2 per cent; 2002, 12.1 per cent). MDR-TB was found in 2.5 per cent (2003, 2.1 per cent; 2002, 2.0 per cent). Significantly higher ($p < 0.001$) resistance rates were found in the foreign-born population with 20.4 per cent resistance to first-line drugs (HRZES) compared to 8.2 per cent in the German-born population and MDR-TB rates of 4.7 per cent (foreign borns) compared to 0.4 per cent (German borns).[24] Rates were highest in those born in the NIS with 14.3 per cent MDR-TB and 38.3 per cent 'any resistance' in 2004.[80] These results demonstrate how the worldwide incidence of drug resistance affects low-prevalence countries today and may continue to do so in the future. Due to the dramatic development in the NIS, we have seen an increase of drug resistance in Germany since 1996 and can expect a future increase, even though no increase has been found in German-born patients and substantial transmission between these population subgroups has not been detected

so far.[55] A similar experience has been made in Israel with its many migrants from the former Soviet Union.[6,81]

Given the recent trend of transnational migration and the potential spread of MDR and XDR-TB across continents, industrialized countries have started to review their national policies of TB control in foreign-born populations.[58,61,82] A similar trend was observed for MDR-TB, where the combined rate of MDR-TB in 2004 varied between countries from 0 to 3.8 per cent (Spain).[6] Higher MDR-TB rates in the EU countries were observed in the Baltic States of Lithuania (20 per cent), Estonia (19.9 per cent), Latvia (17.7 per cent) and in the new member states of 2007, Bulgaria (5.7 per cent) and Romania (5.3 per cent).[6] For example, Germany, in 2004, reported 0.4 per cent MDR-TB prevalence among indigenous cases and 4.7 per cent among foreign-born cases; Norway reported 0 and 2.1 per cent, respectively.[6] In the USA, MDR-TB was reported at 1.2 per cent in 2004, a 13.3 per cent increase from 2003. It was 0.6 per cent in US-born and 1.6 per cent in foreign-born persons, respectively.[83] In Israel, a higher MDR-TB prevalence among recent immigrants, mainly from the NIS, was reported and in 2004 amounted to 0 per cent among the indigenous population and 5.3 per cent among foreign borns.[6] The prevalence of drug-resistant TB in industrialized countries is generally higher among the foreign-born than in the indigenous population, reaffirming that TB control is a global issue.[6,66,76,84] This is also shown for the USA, were 76 per cent of MDR-TB cases ($n = 128$) in 2004 were foreign born.[83] In a study from Los Angeles, MDR-TB cases ($n = 102$) were significantly more likely to be foreign born (80 per cent), non-white, and of Hispanic or Asian ethnicity. This may indicate poor public health infrastructure in the countries of origin.[85]

In recent years, there are indications of the emergence of *M. tuberculosis* strains with increased virulence for humans, spreading through the community faster than strains of standard virulence.[86] Results of molecular epidemiological studies also suggest that certain *M. tuberculosis* strains have an enhanced capacity to spread within a community. One of these strains, the Beijing genotype, has been associated with outbreaks in several communities throughout the world. On a Canary Island (Gran Canaria) between 1993 and 1996, the rapid dissemination of this Beijing genotype has been described. This strain became the most common isolate of the island, even though it was not known there before 1993. The authors suspect a higher level of virulence of the Beijing strain, but a correlation with drug resistance could not be confirmed.[87] In a different setting, Pfyffer *et al.*[88] found a high rate of infection with Beijing strains (70.8 per cent) associated with high rates of MDR-TB (60.9 per cent) in Azerbaijan prisons ($n = 65$). Due to the limitations of the study in this special setting, these results have to be interpreted with care. It is not known whether the Beijing strain turns out to be more virulent and resistant due to its greater fitness, or is spreading because primary TB control has failed and patients have been subjected to years of poor treatment.[89] The most likely explanation is a combination of both.[55]

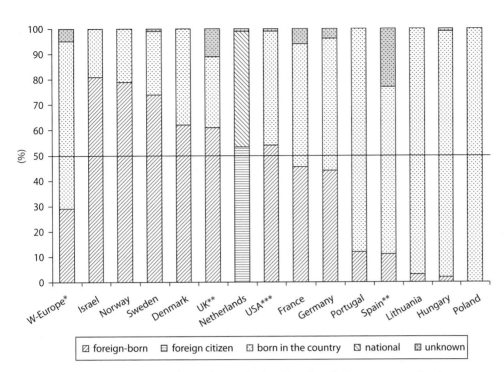

Figure 25.1 Tuberculosis cases by geographic origin 2004.[6,83]

*EU and West (32 countries), foreign-born or foreign citizen/born in the country or national;
**provisional data;
***83

Several factors may decrease host immunity. Due to a weakened immune defence, people infected with both *M. tuberculosis* and HIV are at higher risk of developing TB. HIV infection is the strongest factor for developing active TB and advanced immunosuppression may also lead to higher numbers of reinfection. Up to now there is no clear evidence that HIV infection is a risk factor of developing MDR or XDR-TB in proper treatment settings,[48,78] but some factors may contribute to an increased risk of drug-resistant TB in HIV-infected people. Less virulent *M. tuberculosis* strains may appear only in immunosuppressed individuals and TB due to recent infection with a higher fraction of resistant strains is more likely to develop in immunocompromised people.[89] Additionally, there might be shared risk factors between HIV infection and resistant TB (e.g. intravenous drug injection, homelessness, hospitalization).[55,89] Malnutrition, economic crises, civil conflicts, genetic factors and the use of corticosteroids or TNF-α blockers may also contribute to a decrease of host immunity and thus be cofactors for developing active TB.

TB IN THE POPULATION OF FOREIGN ORIGIN

The influence of migrants from high-prevalence regions has become obvious as the proportion of new TB cases continues to shift from the indigenous to the migrant population in most low-prevalence countries.[14] While the incidence of TB continues to decline in the indigenous population, a relative increase in the foreign-born population can be noticed in many countries.[6]

Most low-incidence countries report substantial numbers of TB cases among their foreign-born populations, particularly highlighted by increased international migration from high- to low-incidence countries.[11,29] The proportion of immigrants among TB cases notified in 2004 exceeded 50 per cent in Andorra, Cyprus, Denmark, Iceland, Israel, Luxembourg, Norway, Sweden, Switzerland and the UK (notified as foreign born), as well as in Belgium, Malta and the Netherlands (notified as foreign citizens) (Figure 25.1).[6] In Germany, 33.9 per cent of TB cases in the year 2004 were among foreign nationals (1991, 21.5 per cent) and 43.7 per cent were foreign born.[24] Substantial numbers are also reported from Australia and New Zealand. In Australia, high-incidence groups were identified to be foreign born and indigenous Australians[90] and in New South Wales the proportion of all TB notifications occurring in residents born overseas increased from 30 to 79 per cent between 1975 and 1995.[91] Between 1995 and 2004 in New Zealand, 64.6 per cent of people with TB were foreign born and migration has been identified as the main reason for non-decreasing TB incidence rates.[92,93] Notification rates in 31 countries of Western Europe (EU 25 and Andorra, Iceland, Israel, Norway, San Marino and Switzerland) providing population statistics in 2004 were overall 12 times higher in foreigners (57.0/100 000) than in nationals (4.8/100 000).[6] In the USA, nearly the entire decline in the number of TB cases since 1993 is accounted for by a decline in cases among US-born people (decrease of 63.4 per cent), while the absolute number of cases in people born outside the USA has not changed substantially.[83,94] The proportion of foreign-born cases has increased each year to 54.3 per cent and the notification rate of foreign-born people was 8.7 times that of USA-born people in 2005.[83]

PRINCIPLES OF CONTROL STRATEGIES

TB control strategies are aimed at the reduction of transmission of *M. tuberculosis* complex in the community through rapid identification of infectious patients and fast, adequate diagnostic measures, followed by immediate treatment with effective drugs according to resistance and documented cure, as long as sufficient protection by vaccination is not available.[4,7,11,12,55] This will also reduce the risk of drug resistance.[11,95]

A national programme for the control and elimination of TB including the organization of services is important in achieving TB control even in countries with a low TB prevalence.[11,14] The previous 'vertical' approach towards TB control has mainly been replaced by new integrated approaches since the 1970s.[11] A nationally agreed programme integrated into existing infrastructures and planned, coordinated, supervised and evaluated by a core group of experienced professionals (national TB committee)[11] is essential. Bacteriological services and epidemiological surveillance as well as clinical services need to be included, supported by advice from those with expertise in high-risk groups, such as immigrants and hostel dwellers.[15,96] The strategic approach also includes a focus on settings such as metropolitan areas.[96,97] Good, reliable information is a key element, implying that a nationwide, computer-based information and collection system must be in place.[12,14] Funding and political support of a central or national TB programme unit remains important and the organization of TB services needs strengthening rather than dismantling in order to meet the challenges of future TB control.[56,96,97] Figure 25.2 shows the organization of TB control in Germany.

In the twenty-first century, the global dynamics of the TB epidemic show a considerable need to accelerate the

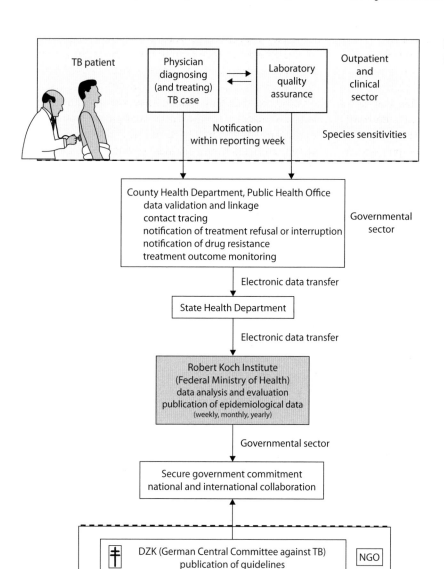

Figure 25.2 Tuberculosis (TB) control in Germany.

approach of TB elimination in low-incidence countries with a common, preferably international, approach to control policies and activities.[2,11] Important steps of close international cooperation are compulsory notification of TB cases,[11,12] free access to medical care and medication,[1,11,29] strict control of rifampicin supplies[11] and country-specific strategies on how to deal with patients with poor treatment adherence, who pose a public health threat.[15]

In October 2005, the WHO introduced a new DOTS-based STOP TB strategy, which addresses TB-HIV infection, MDR-TB and other challenges. It aims to engage all care providers and thus strengthen the health system and promote research.[75,98]

Surveillance

Surveillance must ensure that a minimum data set is collected without delay on all TB patients on an individual basis (Table 25.3). Physicians' compulsory notifications should be supplemented by laboratory notifications and the two systems should be linked.[11,12] Diagnosis and treatment outcome monitoring should be based on bacteriological confirmation wherever possible, and therefore the case definition of TB in Europe is based on culture.[11,12] A reliable, standardized surveillance system of TB cases and drug resistance patterns, including treatment outcome monitoring, together with adequate reporting by medical and laboratory staff, is available in most low-prevalence countries.

Prevalence of drug resistance to first-line drugs and of MDR-TB among incident cases should be routinely evaluated within surveillance activities.[11,49,66,96,99–101] As MDR-TB and XDR-TB represent a threat for TB control, the prevalence of MDR-TB, and if available XDR-TB, at country level is a useful indicator of the performance of the treatment programme and for planning proper public health action.[11,74,99]

Surveillance should result in public health action. The WHO's global target is the detection of 70 per cent of new sputum smear-positive cases and a cure rate of 85 per cent for infectious cases. In the absence of HIV infection, this should lead to a substantial decrease of TB prevalence and incidence.[33,102] If a 5 per cent death rate is accepted as

unavoidable, the maximum rate of unsatisfactory outcome is 10 per cent. This implies that an unsatisfactory outcome rate >10 per cent should lead to investigation of the reasons and development of interventions for improvement by the National TB Programme.[7]

Outcome data

Treatment outcome monitoring is based on six mutually exclusive categories evaluated by cohort analysis.[7,11,103] Treatment outcome is expressed as a percentage of the total number of notified cases. A separate analysis should be available for new and retreatment cases. In order to evaluate the effectiveness of the intervention, it is essential to monitor the treatment outcome, and the evaluation of treatment results should be a component of national monitoring of the programme performance.[7] Data collection, analysis and interpretation of treatment outcome allow more focused interventions and contribute to improved quality of care. Monitoring should be standardized to allow international comparison.[7] Table 25.4 shows the recommended categories of treatment outcome monitoring.

Treatment outcome data, in the same way as case notification data, have to be collected at the local level and passed on to regional and national authorities continuously.[7] Treatment with short-course chemotherapy usually lasts 6 months (up to 9 months) and patients are allowed to interrupt treatment for up to 2 months before classification as interruption. Because of the long duration of treatment, outcome analysis can only take place 1 year after closure of the calendar year of notification. Thus, it is recommended that analysis is carried out in the first quarter of the calendar year following a full year after the last patient was enrolled. Treatment outcome results should become an inseparable part of the annual report on TB, even though they will always refer to cases reported 1 year earlier.[7]

There has been substantial improvement since 1995, when standardized treatment outcome data in Western Europe were available from five countries (Italy, Malta, the Netherlands, Norway and Portugal) and, in addition, non-standardized treatment outcome results from Iceland and Luxembourg.[1] By 2006, standardized treatment outcome monitoring data were provided by 24 EU and Western European countries for the year 2003 (UK, 2002) and Italy reported data from selected centres.[6]

Table 25.3 Minimum data collection set.[11]

Date of starting treatment
Place of residence
Date of birth
Sex
Country of origin
Site of disease
Bacteriological status
History of previous antituberculosis treatment

Table 25.4 Categories of treatment outcome monitoring.

Cure[a]
Treatment completion[a]
Treatment interruption
Failure
Death
Transfer out

[a]Cure and treatment completion combined represent treatment success.

Due to the higher socioeconomic status in low-prevalence countries, these countries should use their potential to reduce the proportion of patients with an unfavourable outcome (failure, default, death (particularly from TB)), to less than 10 per cent. This may be achieved by putting a special focus on high-risk groups, where the proposed target is to screen 95 per cent of cases belonging to these groups and to treat 95 per cent.[11]

However, these recommendations may not be transferable to low-prevalence countries as unsatisfactory outcomes in the elderly are high because of 'death due to other causes than TB' and therefore may not indicate poorly functioning TB control programmes. For the year 2002, a treatment success rate of 76.5 per cent has been reported in 'established markets' countries, with a death rate of 9.7 per cent – the highest of all regions.[33] In Germany, for example, the treatment success rate in 2003 was only 77.4 per cent overall and 59 per cent in the elderly (>69 years of age). The largest proportion of unfavourable treatment outcomes was attributed to 'death due to other causes than TB' with 8.3 per cent (death due to TB 4.3 per cent) overall and increasing with age.[24]

Case finding

Screening measures aim to interrupt the spread of infection through proper treatment of infectious cases.[14] As the incidence of TB is declining in low-prevalence countries, case detection should take place through case finding among symptomatic individuals presenting at health services and active case finding in special high-risk groups. Therefore, prompt diagnosis of TB cases requires good-quality laboratory and radiology services, as well as well-qualified staff in the health service.[11]

There are basically two approaches to case finding: active and passive.

1 *Passive case finding.* Case finding limited to individuals presenting at health services with symptoms suggestive of TB remains the basis of the case-detection policy and is commonly considered the most cost-effective approach[11] and the most common method of TB detection. The cornerstones of diagnosis are chest radiography, sputum microscopy and, if available, culture of *M. tuberculosis* for full identification and drug susceptibility testing. The role of tuberculin skin testing, as well as that of interferon-γ release assays, in the diagnosis of active TB is rather limited and it is mainly used for surveillance and screening purposes.[14,104,105]

2 *Active case finding.* In low-prevalence countries, active case finding should not be used for the general population. However, it is justified for contact tracing and in special high-prevalence groups (TB incidence higher than that of the general population), identified by a national team of experts.[2,11] Where available, this selection should be based on cost-effectiveness evaluation.[11]

Risk group management

In low-prevalence countries, it is desirable to identify groups at special risk. Active case finding should only take place in these groups and not as general mass screening.[2,106] As TB declines in a community, groups at particularly high risk become more visible, providing an opportunity for targeted intervention.[11] Risk group management involves active rather than solely passive case finding aimed at detecting both those with active disease and those with latent infection.[11] This depends to a large degree on reliable methods of surveillance.[2]

Although there are significant differences between countries, a large fraction of cases in low-prevalence countries arises from groups with a high-prevalence of latent TB infection and of active disease:[11,61] migrants from high-prevalence countries,[6,11,29,107,108] ethnic minorities,[11,109,110] displaced people,[14,111] residents of jails and prisons,[11,108,112–115] hospital staff,[11] residents of nursing homes and homeless shelters,[11,110] as well as the elderly[11,14,116] and immunocompromised (e.g. HIV-infected) people.[55,108] In addition, transmission of TB infection in institutional settings, such as jails and prisons, hospitals, lodging houses, hostels and shelters for the homeless as well as for new immigrants (both within the institutionalized population and to the staff), occurs more frequently than in the general population, because people staying in these places are at special risk of having active TB and have frequent and close contacts with people at special risk for having active TB.[11,14] An increased risk of transmission in nursing homes/residential homes for the elderly remains controversial.[117–119] The probability of developing TB also depends on socio-economic factors, such as nutrition, housing, access to health-care facilities, as well as immunological factors.[14,111]

A special focus should be put on TB-HIV co-infection, as TB is fuelled by the HIV epidemic and interactions have to be fully understood to develop effective control programmes not only in low-prevalence countries, but worldwide.[14,98,120,121] For political reasons, general screening measures and case reporting may not be feasible in this group.

SCREENING OF MIGRANTS

People born in high-prevalence countries have by far the highest risk of developing TB, even though the relative risk varies considerably according to the country of origin and duration of stay in the host country.[15,29] As the detection of active pulmonary TB is the primary goal, chest radiography combined with a consultation and clinical examination is usually carried out (e.g. the USA, Canada, the UK, Switzerland).[61,122] Tuberculin skin testing or, where recommended, interferon-γ release assays should be used in children and pregnant women. Screening of immigrants is best carried out at the point of entry to a country. Because there are usually multiple entry points, this can be difficult to organize. The screening results should not be used as a criterion for entry or exclusion of access to a country,[14,29] but active disease must lead to immediate treatment of the patient. However, the US Government, for example, requires that people planning to emigrate to the USA must be screened for active TB before departure (see Chapter 21, Tuberculosis and migration).[61,94]

ILLEGAL MIGRANTS

Another important and not easily accessible risk group is illegal or undocumented migrants, who do not have access to medical services and are under the permanent threat of being discovered and expelled from their country of choice. They therefore tend to seek medical advice too late or not at all and in case of having active TB may infect others.[51] As for all risk groups, barriers of access to treatment should be reduced.

PRISONS

In prisons, the problem is multifactorial and notification rates are generally far higher than in the civilian population – up to 84 times as estimated by a recent European survey.[114] In particular, the increase in incidence of HIV and the high resistance rates pose a major threat in the prison setting.[55] Many inmates in low-prevalence countries are sentenced for drug-related offences with a higher probability of dual TB-HIV infection. As HIV is the greatest risk factor for TB-infected people to develop active disease, the potential for spread is very serious. In addition, high rates of drug resistance and MDR-TB have been reported from prison settings. In comparison, an MDR-TB rate of 5.9 per cent was reported in a Spanish prison in 1994,[113] and during the 1991 outbreak in New York City, 32 per cent of prisoners were reported to suffer from MDR-TB.[123]

Many sentences are relatively short, posing a great challenge to public health services to implement proper treatment and patient follow up. This is further aggravated because prisons are often controlled by ministries of justice and not ministries of health in low-prevalence countries, and a comprehensive national policy usually does not exist.[14] All these factors make infection prevention in institutional settings a public health priority. Administrative measures, such as active screening by chest radiography, tuberculin skin testing or interferon-γ release assays and questionnaires for residents and staff followed by preventive interventions may be considered.[11,14,47,124]

SOURCE CONTROL

Transmission is greatly influenced by characteristics of the source case (e.g. number of bacteria excreted) and the nature of the encounter (e.g. duration and closeness of exposure).[59] By nature of their activities, certain groups of people are more prone to transmitting the disease than others.[108,110,125] These groups include health-care workers, teachers, people working with children and immunocompromised people.

Most studies concerning the risk of infection in hospitals and high-risk settings (e.g. laboratories, pathology) show a slightly increased risk of TB for health-care workers.[126–129] Between 1984 and 1992, an increased yearly risk of tuberculin skin test conversion was described in the USA for health-care workers compared with the general population.[130] In 1994, the CDC recommended infection control measures, which were implemented widely in health-care facilities. Since then, a reduction of health-care worker associated transmission of TB has been observed, resulting in guidelines stressing the need to maintain expertise in order to avert another TB resurgence.[131] In Canada, as well as in England and Wales, an increased relative risk for manifest TB disease of health-care workers[132,133] and in Germany a highly significant association between health-care work and clustering was found.[134] A recent study from Italy found small room size and infectiousness of the index case to be the strongest predictors for tuberculin skin test conversion among health-care workers.[135] In contradiction, a study from Finland showed a reduced risk of TB in health-care personnel,[136] possibly attributable to the 'healthy worker' effect.

Nurses, doctors and dentists generally have close contacts with immunocompromised patients who are more susceptible to infection. Therefore, when first employed, health-care workers should be screened on a regular basis with a tuberculin skin test, an interferon-γ release assay or, in case of a positive test, by chest x-ray.[14,131] Additionally, protection measures, e.g. masks, should be mandatory if health-care workers are likely to deal with TB patients. On the occurrence of conversion of a skin test or interferon-γ release assays, preventive therapy is usually recommended in low-prevalence countries.[14,62,131]

Treatment

Prompt and accurate diagnosis and effective treatment are the key elements of the public health response to TB and therefore the cornerstone of TB control.[108] Successful treatment of TB should be provided within a clinical and social framework based on the patient's circumstances, as it depends on more than the science of chemotherapy alone. The responsibility for ensuring treatment completion is mainly assigned to the public health programme and the treatment provider, not to the patient.[137] After diagnosing a case of active, sputum-positive pulmonary TB, the most important control measure – besides isolation – is the immediate employment of an appropriate antituberculosis treatment to render the patient non-contagious. Comprehensive treatment is based on a complex interaction between clinical care and public health. In all low-incidence countries, cases of TB should be reported to public health authorities as soon as possible, leading to a range of activities designed not only for treatment but also for protection of the health of other people in the community. Care provided by the private medical sector should also be monitored by public health officials to ensure adherence, provide patient education, coordinate contact evaluation, identify possible outbreaks, prevent the emergence and monitor patterns of drug resistance in the community.[59,61]

Before treatment is initiated, every effort should be made to obtain adequate specimens for culture and susceptibility testing.[59] Translation and support during the case management should be provided for migrants by professional translators to ensure rapid diagnosis and to strengthen treatment adherence in foreign-born patients from the first contact to the final cure.[11]

Modern antituberculosis treatment is based on proper administration of selected standardized drug combinations at correct dosages and frequency for a sufficient duration.[1,11] The rates of drug resistance, the nature of the most important risk groups in a country and the schedule of administration most likely to ensure adherence should be considered by the physician and will influence the national recommendations for the treatment regimen.[11,59,138]

A 6- (up to 9-) month regimen has been determined to be the most efficacious in fully susceptible patients, and is appropriate in most countries in the elimination phase.[1,11,13] Here treatment should consist of isoniazid, rifampicin, pyrazinamide and either ethambutol or streptomycin for the initial 2 months followed by isoniazid and rifampicin for another 4 (to 7) months in the continuation phase.[13,137] Adequate short-course chemotherapy regimens, in some cases standardized, are used in the USA, Canada, Australia and most of the 25 EU member states, as well as other Western European countries (e.g. Andorra, Denmark, Finland, Germany, Ireland, Israel, Italy, Malta, Norway, Portugal, Sweden, Switzerland, the Netherlands and the UK) for both new and retreatment cases.[1] Treatment should be closely monitored and preferably the drug intake should be directly observed.[13,137]

As recommended by the WHO and the Union, fixed-dose combinations of proven bioavailability containing at least isoniazid and rifampicin can be prescribed to ensure that these drugs are given together, in order to prevent the development of drug resistance.[1,13] The treatment of (multi)drug-resistant TB and especially XDR-TB cases should be based on drug susceptibility test results.[11,49,66,96,139,140] Preferably polyresistant, MDR-TB and XDR-TB patients should only be treated by specially qualified experts in centres of expertise.[11,49,55] In any case, every TB patient should have free access to diagnostic and treatment services[11] during the whole treatment course. With the development of the International Standards for Tuberculosis Care (ISTC), an important step has been taken to effectively engage all care providers in delivering high-quality care for all patients.[141]

DIRECTLY OBSERVED TREATMENT

Even though DOT is widely promoted by the WHO throughout the world, its role in low-prevalence countries is less clear.[15,54] The WHO recommends exclusively DOT during the whole treatment course, while the 'European Framework' recommends DOT at least for patients with doubtful treatment adherence during both the intensive and the continuation phase of treatment, and close supervision of all patients during the intensive phase of treatment.[11,95]

The USA considers DOT by a trained health-care worker for all patients part of a comprehensive patient-centred programme.[59,61,137] This includes features encouraging patients to complete therapy (e.g. incentives), as well as staff members who can communicate in the patient's native language and who are sensitive to cultural issues, as well as a mechanism ensuring immediate follow up of patients not adhering to the treatment regimen.[59] In Germany, for example, DOT is recommended for patients with dubious treatment adherence and/or poly-, multi- or extensively drug-resistant TB.[139]

However, its place is undisputed in difficult therapeutic settings in rich and urban areas of the developed world to ensure treatment, early detection and management of adverse reactions and to evaluate the treatment response, as well as the programme performance.[1,7,13,14,44,76]

Contact tracing

While active case finding is ineffective, impracticable and expensive in the general population, it is highly effective when used as part of a contact-tracing procedure. For the initiation of contact tracing, it is important that all cases of active TB are immediately notified. Most countries with a low TB prevalence have notification systems requiring the diagnosing physician to notify the case.[12,14] In many countries, laboratories also have to notify cases, e.g. Germany. After notification to the appropriate authorities, effective contact-tracing procedures need to be designed and initiated, taking into account the local epidemiology. Therefore, variations of contact-tracing measures in different regions and population segments (e.g. homeless, immunocompromised, HIV-positive persons) are common.[14,142] Contact tracing will also be influenced by the type of TB notified. Usually only pulmonary TB has a significant potential of being infectious and the greatest risk occurs in patients with sputum smear-positive pulmonary TB, especially with extensive cavitary disease.[137,143] Contacts may also be described as close or casual. This is not only determined by the proximity, but also by the duration of exposure.[142,144,145] Family and others sharing the household are generally viewed as close contacts and included in contact-tracing procedures. However, a detailed case history is necessary to assess who else should be categorized as a close contact. Other contacts are viewed as casual and contact tracing in this group should only take place if the prevalence of infection is higher in the close contacts than in the general population.[14,144,145]

Clear guidelines describing when and how to perform contact tracing, as well as adequate responses to the varying screening outcomes are of substantial help and

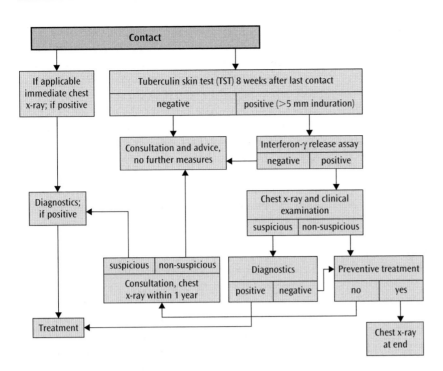

Figure 25.3 Tuberculin diagnostics in 15-to 49-year-olds after exposure to infectious tuberculosis (TB) (modified from Refs 144, 145 and 146).

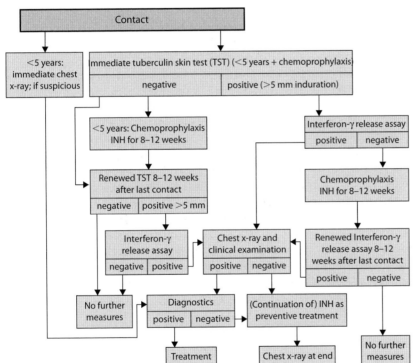

Figure 25.4 Tuberculin diagnostics in children <15 years after exposure to infectious tuberculosis (TB) (modified from Refs 144 and 145). INH, isoniazid.

thus extremely important. Figures 25.3 and 25.4 show, as an example, the recommended screening procedures for contacts of TB patients in Germany.[144–146] Medical, nursing and administrative personnel are involved and sufficient resources need to be available. In addition, proper documentation is essential to allow decision-making. Emerging new TB cases during the screening need to be treated, but the appropriate response to contacts only found to be infected (latent TB) is often less clear.[14] However, in recent years more low-prevalence countries recommend the treatment of people with latent TB infection.[61,62,137,147]

Methods commonly used for contact tracing are the tuberculin skin test and chest radiography,[14,144] possibly combined with interferon-γ release assays, as recommended more frequently in recent years.[61,104,145,148]

Tuberculin skin test

So far the tuberculin skin test (TST) has been the principal method to identify TB infection, despite the limitations of sensitivity and specificity (due to its cross-reactivity with

Table 25.5 Targeted tuberculin testing in high-risk groups for tuberculosis (TB).[59,61,137,147,151]

Close contacts/recent exposures of patients with active TB (especially children)
Persons living or working in long-term care facilities
Immunosuppressed persons
Health-care professionals
HIV-infected persons
Homeless persons
Migrants from high-prevalence regions

BCG and environmental mycobacteria). In most low-prevalence countries, the intradermal Mantoux test is used. While in most European countries, as recommended by the WHO, two tuberculin units (TU) of purified protein derivative (PPD) RT-23 are used, in France and in the USA five TU PPD-S are used. Therefore cut-offs are not necessarily comparable.[149]

Because of the limited specificity of screening procedures, their widespread application to low-risk populations is likely to generate false-positive results in low-prevalence countries, in most cases due to contact with *Mycobacteria* other than tuberculosis (MOTT). Therefore, testing for TB infection should be performed only in people who are at high risk of infection and who would benefit from treatment.[150] A decision to test a person should reflect a commitment to treat the patient if the test is positive.[59] Due to its limitation in HIV-infected patients and the elderly, the test should be interpreted with caution in these groups. A positive test should possibly be followed by an interferon-γ release assay and a chest radiograph to exclude active disease (Figures 25.3 and 25.4).[61,144,145]

Each national programme should define which groups are particularly at risk and the appropriate cut-off values taking into account the likely compliance to preventive therapy.[1] Groups that are at high risk of TB infection, and which should be targeted for tuberculin testing, are shown in Table 25.5.

The cut-off for defining a 'positive' TST, and thus whether an individual should be given preventive chemotherapy, is related to the probability that the reaction represents true infection and to the likelihood that the individual, if truly infected, will develop TB.[1] In low-prevalence countries, the prevalence of infection in children and juveniles is estimated to be very low, while people born in high-prevalence settings have often acquired an infection with *M. tuberculosis* in their country of origin.[35]

Interferon-γ release assays

Up to a few years ago, the diagnosis of LTBI was based solely on the TST. In recent years, whole blood antigen-specific T cell-based interferon-γ release assays (QuantiFERON®-TB Gold In-Tube, T SPOT-TB test) have been shown to be as sensitive and more specific than the TST for the detection of LTBI.[104,148,152–159] Interferon-γ release assays have been shown to correlate closer with exposition to *M. tuberculosis*,[160] to show no cross-reaction with BCG, and to be less influenced by infection with MOTT.[148,161,162]

Despite ongoing research, interferon-γ release assays have not yet been evaluated sufficiently in selected populations of interest and prospective research is needed to determine whether interferon-γ responses are predictors for progression to active disease, to determine the usefulness in specialized subgroups of patients (e.g. HIV-infected people,[163] children), and whether treating LTBI based on interferon-γ results will reduce the TB burden in low-incidence countries.[104,137,148,155] As with the TST, negative results should be interpreted with specific caution and may not be sufficient to exclude *M. tuberculosis* infection in certain clinical situations (e.g. immunocompromised people, people being treated with tumour necrosis factor alpha (TNF-α) antagonists).[104,158]

In the USA, the use of QuantiFERON-TB Gold has been approved and is recommended by the CDC in all circumstances in which the TST has been used so far, including contact investigations and screening of migrants, correctional facility inmates and health-care workers.[148] In Europe, both the T SPOT-TB test and the QuantiFERON-TB Gold In-Tube test have been approved. In Germany, interferon-γ release assays have been recommended as a useful additional diagnostic method.[147,164]

Concerning the detection of TB disease, interferon-γ release assays and the TST have suboptimal sensitivity.[104,105] They are both based on cellular immune response and are thus incapable of distinguishing between LTBI and active disease.[104] Therefore, a negative test result cannot be used alone to exclude the diagnosis of active TB and additional diagnostic tests should be performed without delay.[104,105,148] However, interferon-γ release assays have shown a great potential to act as an additional diagnostic tool, and may be able to replace the TST in the near future.

Chest x-ray

Abnormal chest x-rays detected by screening need careful attention by specialists, followed by a detailed patient assessment by an experienced respiratory clinician to differentiate between TB, carcinoma or various other respiratory diseases.[14]

Role of molecular epidemiology (DNA fingerprinting)

Reliable molecular methods (DNA fingerprinting) can distinguish between different strains of *M. tuberculosis*. DNA fingerprinting can also be used in culture-positive cases to distinguish newly acquired infections and exogenous reinfections from reactivations and to discover chains of transmission and clusters not detected by traditional epidemiology and contact tracing. Thus, targeted DNA fingerprinting can be used to confirm or disprove suspected relationships among cases. Universal typing of isolates can be used to identify unsuspected transmission and broaden the scope of contact investigations.[165] In addition, false-positive culture results, perhaps due to cross-contamination in the laboratory, can be assessed.[166,167] Identifying related cases using DNA-fingerprint technology opens the way to identify transmitters and to improve control by identifying so-called 'cluster epidemics'.[11,168] Furthermore, this technique shows which TB cases are more likely to be due to reactivation of remotely acquired infection and which to recent transmission.[11,107,116,169,170]

For example, in different low-prevalence countries, it has been shown that predictors of non-cluster status included birth outside the country of residence. Among foreign-born people, TB was largely caused by reactivation of latent infection, whereas among those born in the country of residence, many cases resulted from recent transmission.[94,171–175] In an area with a high-prevalence of TB, it was shown by bacterial genotyping that exogenous reinfection is a cause of recurrent TB after curative therapy.[59,170,176]

Outbreak management

An important group of people with recent infection are people associated with a common, infectious source case in a recognized outbreak of TB. Outbreak management requires the identification of people with probable recent infection (starting with close household contacts or equivalent) and extending the circle, if necessary, according to the 'stone in the pond' principle.[177] This should be followed by adequate treatment if disease is present and preventive chemotherapy for those found to be infected.[11,107,116,169]

DNA fingerprinting of isolated *M. tuberculosis* strains with molecular methods and their comparison with each other can be used as an additional tool of outbreak management. Therefore, all isolates of an outbreak should be collected in a laboratory where DNA fingerprinting can be carried out. The results should be notified to the responsible public health office. Joint surveillance to detect outbreaks at an international level using DNA-based typing results stored in data banks is an additional component of international and European collaboration.[11]

Maintenance of a good control system

The maintenance of effective TB control in low-incidence countries and the possible achievement of TB elimination will partially depend on the implementation of a TB policy package. This should basically be comparable to that for high-prevalence settings. DOTS is acknowledged as one of the most cost-effective public health approaches by the World Bank, and includes:

- government and private sector commitment towards TB control and elimination;
- case detection through case finding among symptomatic individuals presenting at health services and active case finding in special groups;
- access to TB diagnostic and treatment services;
- standard approach to treatment of disease and infection;
- surveillance and treatment outcome monitoring.[11]

Efficient TB control and elimination will not be possible without government commitment. To allow TB care and control, the necessary basic infrastructure (funding, human resources and facilities) should be provided. An effective national TB network with international collaboration, an adequate legal framework, as well as research and health education should be maintained.[11] Additionally, if not in place, a coherent, consensus-based national TB control and elimination policy should be developed in collaboration with the private sector. A special focus should be put on the maintenance of high and timely case-finding rates, high treatment success rates (and low unsuccessful outcome rates), risk group management, outbreak management, enhanced infection prevention in institutional settings, and provision of preventive therapy, if feasible.[11] The new Stop TB strategy of the WHO contains the following elements in order to reduce the global burden of TB by 2015: (1) pursuing of high-quality DOTS expansion and enhancement; (2) addressing TB-HIV and MDR-TB and other special challenges; (3) contributing to health system strengthening; (4) engagement of all care providers; (5) empowerment of people with TB, and communities; (6) enabling and promoting research.[96,97]

Treatment of latent TB infection

LTBI (see also Chapter 23, Clinical interpretation of tests for latent tuberculosis infection) is defined as a subclinical infection with *M. tuberculosis* complex without clinical, bacteriological or radiological signs of active disease.[2,62] It has been recognized for over 30 years that cases of subclinical, latent infection with *M. tuberculosis* are at the centre of the TB dynamics.[11,178] The incidence of TB infection in the community is most effectively reduced by identification of potential sources of infection in the community at the earliest possible time and interruption of the chain of transmission. The development of active disease in people with LTBI poses a continuous threat of transmission and its control is particularly difficult in regions where low case rates have resulted in decreased expertise in the identification and control of TB outbreaks.[59] Therefore, TB elimination strategies in low-incidence countries aim at reducing the prevalence of LTBI, particularly among those at high risk of progression to manifest disease.

Because preventive chemotherapy has proven very effective in preventing progression to manifest TB or reactivation of disease,[1,62] the treatment of LTBI is both a basic component of preventive health care for individual patients and an increasingly important public health intervention. An emphasis on the diagnosis and treatment of LTBI represents a substantial shift in the approach to TB control,[59] and a policy of preventive chemotherapy in selected patients is essential in countries approaching the elimination phase.[11] Recommendations should be based on evidence from clinical trials and the regimen as well as the management strategy should be elaborated at national level.[11]

As preventive therapy in all infected people without active disease is rational, but impractical in many situations, special efforts are made to identify groups considered to be at an increased risk of developing active TB. The decision whether or not to treat latent TB is usually based on several factors: has the contact been infected by the source case or was she/he already infected? The chest radiograph, the age, the immune status, the risk of developing TB and the risks associated with treatment should also be taken into account. Preventive treatment should be offered to recently infected contacts of cases,[2,62,137] HIV-infected individuals,[11,62,147,169] and people with pulmonary fibrotic lesions from previously untreated, but spontaneously healed TB.[11,147] Other groups include patients with silicosis, chronic renal failure, diabetes mellitus, individuals treated with corticosteroids or other immunosuppressive drugs and intravenous drug users.[14,62,147] Another major group may be recent migrants from high-prevalence regions.[62,137,151] In the USA the guidelines by the CDC, the ATS and the Infectious Disease Society of America encourage testing for and treatment of latent infection in people from countries with a high TB prevalence who have been in the USA for less than 5 years.[62,94,137] As almost one-quarter of all TB cases in the USA have been found to occur among foreign-born people who have resided in the USA for longer than 5 years, the question of addressing the burden of LTBI in this group has been raised.[179]

For preventive therapy in those infected, but not having active disease, a regimen with isoniazid 300 mg for 1 year has been shown in several prospective clinical trials to be effective in reducing the risk of TB and is recommended by the 'European Framework for TB Control and Elimination in Countries with a Low Incidence'.[11] In the USA and in Germany, 9 months are recommended.[62,94,137,147] However, prevention of TB with a regimen lasting twice as long as the proper treatment of disease does not seem practical[15] and some experts recommend shorter regimens for the treatment of LTBI, such as a 3-month regimen of isoniazid and rifampicin, even though these are less well researched.[15,180] Due to high rates of hospitalization and deaths from liver injury associated with the treatment of LTBI with a combination of rifampicin and pyrazinamide,

in 2003 the CDC recommended not to use this regimen for people with LTBI.[63] It must be ensured that patients under treatment for LTBI complete the whole treatment, implying the availability of necessary resources and TB control services.[14] However, in certain high-risk groups, supervised treatment may even lower treatment adherence. Because of the long duration of treatment, adherence is often lacking and additional strategies such as monetary incentives are needed.[151] In countries aiming for the eradication of TB, this intervention is assumed to speed up the process substantially.[2,14]

INDICATION FOR PROPHYLACTIC TREATMENT

Prophylactic treatment is defined as treatment to prevent acquisition of infection with *M. tuberculosis* in a person exposed to tubercle bacilli, thus minimizing the risk of acquiring LTBI. There is little evidence for the efficacy of prophylactic treatment and therefore it is rarely indicated. However, the Union recommends prophylactic treatment for newborns and children under the age of 5 years in case of contact to a potentially infectious parent or household member for up to 3 months after relevant exposure has ended.[181–183]

Immunization/BCG vaccination

Bacille Calmette–Guérin (BCG) is an attenuated strain of *Mycobacterium bovis* which underwent one or more critical mutations during its subcultivations up to the year 1921, when it lost its virulence. BCG is the most widely used vaccine in the world[59] and its use has been recommended by the WHO. BCG vaccination generally provides protection of 80 per cent and more against meningeal and miliary TB if given before acquisition of infection with *M. tuberculosis*. The main use of BCG is in the prevention of severe forms of TB in children.[184] Thus BCG is preventing deaths. The protective value against other forms of TB is much smaller and it decreases with increasing age. It rarely protects against pulmonary TB in the adult as shown in several BCG trials.[185] The role of BCG vaccination in low-prevalence countries is of limited value and remains debatable.[11,14,186,187] In addition, it causes confusion in diagnosing latent TB infection when using the TST.[59]

In 1995, mass-scale BCG vaccination was not applied in most low-prevalence European countries, nor was revaccination used. Today BCG revaccination is no longer recommended because the protective value could not be demonstrated.[185] In 2005, a survey among all 25 EU member states and Andorra, Norway, Romania and Switzerland showed that BCG vaccination was still recommended in 12 countries for all children under the age of 12 months. In five countries, it was recommended for older children and in 10 countries for children at increased risk (country of origin, TB contacts, travel). In some countries, several of the above recommendations are used. In seven

European countries, it is not regarded as a reasonable protective strategy (Andorra, Belgium, Denmark, Germany, Luxembourg, Austria and Spain). Eleven countries are discussing changes in their vaccination policy.[188] In the USA, it has never been recommended for TB control.[59]

In those low-incidence countries continuing the use of BCG vaccination programmes, the cost-effectiveness should be evaluated and the frequency of adverse effects assessed.[11,186] While there is progress in the development of alternative vaccines against TB, the actual implementation of a superior product has still a long way to go.[185]

Isolation of infectious patients

Patients with infectious TB must be prevented from infecting others. Depending on the setting in which the patient is being treated, the need for isolation varies. Patients in hospitals must be isolated due to the high possibility of contact with susceptible, immunocompromised people. They should usually be admitted to hospital not only for isolation, but might also need to be hospitalized for the severity of disease, diagnostic services, care, toxicity of antituberculosis drugs, MDR and XDR-TB, concomitant diseases or directly observed treatment.[14,139,189] When treated at home, further spread to contacts after initiation of treatment will be rather unlikely. Outpatients living in lodging houses or hostels, or homeless people, are at special risk of transmitting TB unless suitable accommodation is provided.[14,125]

Technical interventions

TB control measures are largely aimed at preventing the development of infectious droplet nuclei. The number of nuclei can be reduced by cough discipline of the patient.[14] FFP2 or 3 masks should be worn by the staff whenever exposure to cough of infectious patients cannot be avoided (e.g. endoscopy, transport, non-cooperative patients). Staff and patients should wear FFP2 or 3 masks during transportation of infectious patients[14] and/or in case of polydrug resistance and MDR or XDR-TB. Patient adherence should be particularly emphasized because the use of masks can be stigmatizing.[61,131,140,190]

Patients should be isolated in a single room. Risk areas within hospitals are endoscopy, respiratory therapy wards, operating theatres and respiratory function laboratories. Instruments used in these facilities must be sterilized with particular care.[14]

According to the 'European Framework', adequate methods to prevent transmission of resistant strains to patients and health staff, such as proper ventilation and negative pressure rooms, are desirable.[11,140] For effective negative-pressure ventilation, at least six changes of room air per hour, with two consisting of outside air, are recommended for isolation. However, even in low-incidence countries only very few hospitals have these facilities.[14]

Germicidal ultraviolet radiation (254-nm wavelength) rapidly inactivates airborne microorganisms, including virulent *M. tuberculosis* and BCG.[191–196] It may well be ineffective and even dangerous, causing skin and eye irritations, if not appropriately installed and used.[2,195,196] However, air disinfection can only be effective if installed at the principal site of transmission.[195] Appropriate settings include prisons, shelters for the homeless and certain hospital units like TB laboratories, operating theatres, bronchoscopy rooms and ICUs.[2]

Combined approach in HIV and TB

The activities of TB and HIV services should be coordinated at all levels and close collaboration between the civilian, military and prison health services is necessary to ensure the same quality of health care for all patients.[11] In the 'European Framework to Decrease the Burden of TB-HIV', three specific preventive interventions are recommended for collaborative action: isoniazide preventive therapy, environmental measures and post-exposure prophylaxis.[50] However, despite large improvements in recent years, the main problem in the management of TB-HIV co-infection may still be the need for better cooperation and communication between both programmes.[15]

Cost-effectiveness

Free access to health services (diagnostic procedures, treatment and follow up) for all TB patients has been strongly recommended[1,11] and economic evaluation should guide the physician in selecting the most cost-effective option during clinical activity.[1] In the last few years, a great deal of progress has been made concerning treatment outcome monitoring in low-prevalence countries, and for most European countries individual data are available.[6] Further operative research on the cost-effectiveness of screening procedures is still needed[15] as new challenges for treatment and management of patients with drug resistance are emerging and pose constraints on infrastructure, policy and resources.[11,44,48,49,66,197,198] The most expensive component of any TB service may be the treatment of drug-resistant patients.[15,67]

TB EDUCATION AND TRAINING

Despite the availability of diagnostic tools and effective treatment, some patients in low-prevalence countries remain undiagnosed until their death from or with TB. This shows how the decline in TB can adversely affect the clinical index of suspicion, pointing to the need for continuing professional education.[11]

The steady decline of TB in many low-prevalence countries may lead to complacency and neglect of TB control, resulting in loss of expertise.[11] In many low-prevalence countries, health professionals have neglected teaching clinical and epidemiological facts about TB, leading to a lack of basic skills needed in diagnosis and management in doctors, nurses and medical workers.[15] Today, relevant expertise in TB management and control in low-prevalence countries can be found in governmental, as well as in non-governmental agencies, professional and scientific societies. Carefully planned TB education and centres of expertise with international support and advice need to be further established.[11] These 'centres of expertise' should act as a resource to improve surveillance and to monitor and evaluate national TB programmes. In addition, they should provide service guidance, training and support for all health-care workers dealing with TB, as well as for patients.[14] A close link between the public health level and the medical and research communities is required. At university and hospital level, better education about TB, drug resistance and the risks of nosocomial transmission is necessary.[55,72]

Health education

Failures of basic treatment principles may be due to errors by the health-care providers as well as the patient. Strategies to avoid these mistakes include appropriate education and training beyond medical professionals and include patients as well as the public. Not only should the medical and public health sectors be included in the work, but also non-governmental organizations (NGOs) and charity organizations. Patients should be able to recognize the main symptoms of TB and thus present at an early stage of disease for diagnosis and treatment.[14,15]

Modern health education material (brochures, videos, etc.) should be well known and widely available to facilitate TB control and elimination activities. This should also be available in the original languages of foreign-born communities. The design, print and distribution of educational material for patients and medical staff should be coordinated by a team of experts, in order to ensure the fulfilment of local and national needs.[11]

Specific training should be planned for both medical and non-medical staff (e.g. charity organizations, religious groups, retired people, volunteers) who can be involved in the provision of directly observed therapy on a voluntary basis.[11,50]

Professional/university teaching

The importance of TB in the education of medical students and nurses has greatly diminished in low-prevalence countries, aggravated by fewer opportunities to learn from experience. Decreased teaching combined with reduced learning opportunities reduces the capability of public health services to deal with TB effectively.[14] In Germany, a study among medical students showed that the occurrence of TB was greatly underestimated, especially towards the end of medical school.[199] Therefore, adequate teaching at medical and nursing schools should include

- the essential knowledge, skills and attitudes needed in provision of care, decision-making, communication, community leadership and management;
- development of practical guidelines;
- continuing education opportunities after formal training.[11,200]

Adequate graduate and postgraduate education for staff directly (e.g. control officers, public health nurses, chest physicians and bacteriologists) and for those indirectly involved (e.g. students, physicians and nurses caring for asylum seekers, prisoners, etc.) in TB control and elimination should be developed in collaboration with universities, training institutes, professional societies and other non-governmental agencies.[11,200]

Research

Research is essential in all public health programmes. Worldwide research activities on TB have been on the rise in recent years with increased funding by governmental bodies and NGOs. Key areas requiring additional research include: (1) diagnosis and case finding; (2) treatment, monitoring and support; (3) public health and operational research.[141] Epidemiological research and surveillance should form the priorities set among interventions and monitor their impact, whereas clinical research may improve diagnosis and treatment.[50]

OPERATIONAL RESEARCH AND PUBLIC HEALTH

Operational and epidemiological research should address key constraints in the implementation of control and elimination policies and evaluate the impact of specific interventions and the introduction of new technologies and tools.[11]

Priorities include research projects focusing on public health and operational aspects of TB control, e.g. setting up of notification systems (including cross-notification with laboratories and surveillance of drug resistance), setting up of systems to monitor treatment results on a national scale, how to ensure adherence to treatment in certain parts of the TB population, how to ensure preventive and treatment services for immigrants, how to improve TB management practices in private practitioners, how to find optimal models to integrate TB-HIV care and how to document the outcome of screening activities.[11,141] In addition, cost-effectiveness research should be further addressed.

GENOME SEQUENCING

The combination of a fully sequenced genome, efficient methods for genetic manipulation, and a variety of *in vitro* and *in vivo* models will provide further insight into fundamental issues, such as virulence and latency of TB.[59,72] Increasing knowledge on various mycobacterial virulence genes will promote the progression in the identification of genes that code for new drug targets.

IMMUNOMODULATORS

Preliminary clinical trials of adjunctive therapy with immunomodulators (e.g. cytokine therapy) have shown highly debatable results and further clinical trials are needed before some of these advances may be incorporated into clinical practice.[55,59,201–203] However, some promising results have been shown for adjunctive therapy, including IFN-γ, interleukin (IL)-2 and IL-12 in the treatment of pulmonary TB.[204–207]

NEW DRUGS AND VACCINES

The development of new, more effective drugs, which can shorten the treatment, and may therefore have a positive impact on treatment adherence, is urgently needed.[208] After many years of neglect, there is now some ongoing research on new drugs. The use of the new fluoroquinolones (moxifloxacin and gatifloxacin) may lead to a substantial shortening of treatment duration. Another new candidate could be a diarylquinolone (207910), which considerably reduces the treatment duration of TB in mice.[209] However, further studies are needed to find out if this potential will be met in humans.[137] Today, the effort for drug development is mainly being coordinated by the 'Global Alliance for TB Drug Development'. Building on public–private partnership, its main objective is the creation of new TB drugs. The current drug pipeline contains 27 new candidates, compared with none 5 years ago.[210] However, due to a lack of clinical trials capacity, the first new antituberculosis drug is not expected to be on the market before 2010.[96] Active research for a more effective vaccine is a key element in the struggle against TB in times of increasing drug resistance and probably the key issue towards elimination, but, despite a great deal of ongoing research, it will still be many years before a new vaccine will be widely available.[185]

LABORATORY METHODS

The development and application of effective new diagnostic tools and laboratory techniques for TB is important. However, their use and cost-effectiveness should be clearly demonstrated before reallocation of scarce resources.[14,211] For example, the microscopic-observation drug susceptibility (MODS) assay for the detection of *M. tuberculosis* directly from sputum has been shown to offer fast and sensitive detection of TB and MDR-TB.[212] Insight into the molecular mechanisms of drug resistance has led to the development of rapid, nucleic acid-based methods of susceptibility testing.[59,213]

International and European collaboration

TB is and remains a global problem. High-prevalence countries are facing enormous problems in controlling TB, and may therefore negatively influence the TB epidemiology in low-prevalence areas. Expertise in TB management and control can be maintained and increased in low-prevalence countries by collaborating with TB control programmes in high-prevalence countries. Cooperation can also lead to improved programme monitoring and raised awareness. TB elimination will not be reached without a coordinated global approach by low-prevalence countries towards TB control in high-prevalence countries.[11,96]

CONCLUSIONS

Major challenges of current TB control in some low-prevalence countries are shown in Table 25.6. To ensure continued progress towards TB elimination, the public health infrastructure must be maintained or even extended. Local health services must be able to provide all the components of a comprehensive TB control programme, including education and training of health-care providers, case finding, surveillance, laboratory monitoring, as well as measures to improve treatment adherence. The development of new, fast diagnostic tests, effective antituberculosis drugs which are easy to use, and the development of an efficient vaccine with few side effects would constitute an additional important step in the management and control of TB. Moreover, the collaboration between TB and HIV programmes must be further strengthened.

Table 25.6 Major challenges of current tuberculosis (TB) control.[51,61]

Maintaining clinical and public health expertise in an era of declining TB incidence
Prevalence of TB among foreign-born persons
Difficulties in follow up of special patient groups ((illegal) migrants, prisoners, homeless)
Delay in detecting, treating and reporting TB cases
Deficiencies in TB management practices (e.g. often non-standardized treatment regimens used, patient support/supervision)
Deficiencies in preventing and responding to TB outbreaks
Population with latent tuberculosis infection who are at risk for progression to TB disease
Uncertain cause of death (from or with TB)
Little information on HIV co-infection rate, integration of TB/HIV care
Poor information on TB in health-care workers

Country-specific guidelines (e.g. treatment, risk group management, TB-HIV, outbreak management, infection prevention in institutional settings, occupational protection and provision of preventive therapy) based on the national epidemiology and cost-effectiveness evaluation should be developed and the need for better education among politicians and the public should be further emphasized.

TB preferably strikes the poorest segments of the population, and therefore comprehensive health-care services should be provided free of charge or covered by comprehensive insurance schemes. Through poverty reduction, risk factors such as malnutrition and poor sanitation can be influenced and access to health-care services can be improved. However, TB control programmes alone will never have the possibility to influence the socioeconomic status of whole populations.

The overall goal of public health programmes must be not merely the provision of health care for marginalized persons, but a systematic commitment to protect the health of the general public in a time of increasing globalization.[59]

Because TB among foreign-born people from high-prevalence countries is causing a large proportion of new TB cases in low-prevalence countries (the returning home of a western pandemic, created during the industrial revolution), culturally sensitive services are essential and a coordinated global approach by low-prevalence countries to control TB in high-prevalence countries is needed.

LEARNING POINTS

- TB control strategies aim to reduce the incidence of new infection by identifying the source cases and curing them.
- Elimination strategies include additional elements such as the use of preventive therapy for individuals with latent TB infection at risk of developing disease.
- The decline of TB in developed countries before the advent of chemotherapy has been attributed to improved socioeconomic conditions and genetic selection.
- The most important cause of the decline of TB in the second half of the twentieth century was the introduction of specific chemotherapy.
- Stable or decreasing notification rates and low levels of MDR-TB indicates that TB control in most developed countries is effective.
- Within Europe, rates are highest in countries of the former Soviet Union and in Romania.
- If the definition of a low incidence of 20/100 000 cases a year is accepted, only Australia, Albania, Canada, Cyprus, Israel, New Zealand, the USA

and the countries of Western Europe (EU 27), except for Bulgaria, Estonia, Hungary, Latvia, Lithuania, Poland, Portugal and Romania, qualify.

- Among the indigenous population of these countries, the highest incidence is in the elderly due to reactivation of infection acquired in earlier years.
- The decline of TB has slowed down or stopped in some developed countries as a result of immigration from developing countries where population increase, HIV infection, poverty and a decline in the medical infrastructure is causing TB to increase.
- The USA during the 1970s and 1980s showed how a decline in the infrastructure of TB control can lead to an increase in cases.
- The emergence of MDR and XDR-TB is due to poor medical management. The rise in countries of the former Soviet Union is having an impact on Western Europe, especially Germany.
- In most developed countries, rates among the indigenous population decline, while rates among immigrant groups are stable or increase. Whether overall numbers increase or decline depends on the balance between these two factors.
- Important factors in the control of disease are compulsory notification, free access to care and medication, strict control of supplies of rifampicin and specific strategies to help patients with poor adherence.
- The prevalence of drug resistance in a country should be routinely evaluated.
- In treated patients, if rates of interruption (default) and failure exceed 10 per cent, investigation of the causes and appropriate interventions should be made.
- Monitoring of outcomes should be standardized to enable international comparisons to be made.
- Case finding takes place in symptomatic patients presenting to the health services (passive case finding), while active case finding is the screening of specific groups with an increased risk of TB.
- High-risk groups which should be screened include migrants from high-incidence countries, ethnic minorities, prisoners and residents of shelters for the homeless.
- Screening of high-risk groups should comprise an interview and chest x-ray for adults. Children and pregnant women should have a skin test, or where recommended an interferon-γ release assay, and only be x-rayed if the skin test or the interferon-γ release assay suggests the presence of infection.
- Most patients can be treated in the community. Hospital admission may be necessary to make the

diagnosis, to monitor and alleviate adverse effects of treatment, if the patient is seriously ill or if compliance is in doubt.

- Before treatment is begun, full social support should be provided for the patient, for example translation services if needed.
- MDR and XDR-TB should only be treated at specific specialized centres.
- Directly observed therapy should be considered for all patients.
- Compulsory notification of cases allows contact tracing and screening to take place.
- Sufficient medical and nursing personnel must be provided to ensure that an efficient contact tracing service is in place.
- The skin test or, where recommended, the interferon-γ release assay, is the basis of screening for infection. The Mantoux test is universal.
- DNA fingerprinting which distinguishes between different strains of *M. tuberculosis* is useful in tracing transmission of disease.
- The identification and where appropriate the giving of preventive therapy to individuals with LTBI is an important component of disease elimination in well-resourced countries.
- The best preventive regimen for LTBI is disputed. Most countries prefer 9–12 months of isoniazid alone, while some use 3 months of isoniazid and rifampicin together.
- BCG is still used to prevent disease in many developed countries, sometimes for all children, but in others for high-risk groups only.
- Unless drug resistance is suspected, isolation of patients while in hospital is only required for 2–4 weeks.
- Negative-pressure rooms are recommended for isolating cases of MDR and XDR-TB.
- TB and HIV services should be coordinated.
- Lack of experience and knowledge of TB is leading to frequently missed diagnosis in developed countries.
- Medical schools should ensure that medical students have adequate training in TB.

REFERENCES

1. Migliori GB, Raviglione MC, Schaberg T et al. Recommendations of a task force of the ERS, WHO and IUATLD (Europe region): TB management in Europe. Eur Respir J 1999; 14: 978–92.
2. Clancy L, Rieder HL, Enarson DA, Spinaci S. Tuberculosis elimination in the countries of Europe and other industrialized countries. Eur Respir J 1991; 4: 1288–95.
3. Enarson DA. The International Union against Tuberculosis and Lung Disease model: National Tuberculosis Programmes. Tuberc Lung Dis 1995; 76: 95–99.
4. World Health Organization. WHO framework for effective tuberculosis control. Geneva: World Health Organization, WHO/TB/94.179, 1994: 1–13.
5. World Health Organization. Global tuberculosis control: surveillance, planning, financing. WHO Report 2006. Geneva: World Health Organization, WHO/HTM/TB2006.362, 2006.
6. EuroTB and the national coordinators for tuberculosis surveillance in the WHO European Region. Surveillance of tuberculosis in Europe. Report on tuberculosis cases notified in 2004. Saint-Maurice, France: Institut de Veille Sanitaire, February 2006.
7. Veen J, Raviglione MC, Rieder HL et al. Standardised outcome monitoring in Europe. Recommendations of a working group of the WHO and the IUATLD (Europe Region). Eur Resp J 1998; 12: 505–10.
8. Raviglione MC, Sudre P, Rieder HL et al. Secular trends of tuberculosis in Western Europe. Bull World Health Organ 1993; 71: 297–306.
9. Bhatti N, Law MR, Morris JK et al. Increasing incidence of tuberculosis in England and Wales: a study of the likely causes. Br Med J 1995; 310: 967–9.
10. Anderson S, Maguire H, Carless J. Tuberculosis in London: a decade and a half of no decline – TB epidemiology and control. Thorax 2006; 62: 162–7.
11. Broekmans JF, Migliori GB, Rieder HL et al. European framework for tuberculosis control and elimination in countries with a low-incidence. Eur Respir J 2002; 19: 765–75.
12. Rieder HL, Watson JM, Raviglione MC et al. Surveillance of tuberculosis in Europe. Recommendations of a working group of the WHO and the European Region of the IUATLD for uniform reporting on tuberculosis cases. Eur Respir J 1996; 9: 1097–104 .
13. World Health Organization. Treatment of tuberculosis. Guidelines for national programmes. Geneva: World Health Organization, WHO/CDS/TB/2003.313, 2003.
14. Clancy L. Control of tuberculosis in low-prevalence countries. In: Davies PDO (ed.). Clinical tuberculosis, 2nd edn. London: Chapman & Hall, 1998: 435–50.
15. Davies PDO. A European framework for effective tuberculosis control. Eur Respir J 2002; 19: 590–92 (editorial).
16. Rieder HL. Epidemiologic basis of tuberculosis control. Paris: International Union Against Tuberculosis and Lung Disease, 1999: 1–162.
17. Davies RPO, Tocque K, Bellis MA, Rimmington T, Davies PDO. Historical declines in tuberculosis in England and Wales: improving social conditions or natural selection? Int J Tuberc Lung Dis 1999; 3: 1051–4.
18. Iseman MD. A clinician's guide to tuberculosis. Philadelphia, PA: Lippincott, Williams & Wilkins 2000.
19. Grigg ERN. The arcana of tuberculosis with a brief epidemiologic history of the disease in the USA. Am Rev Tuberc Pulm Dis 1958; 78:151–72; 426–53; 583–603.
20. Dubos R, Dubos J. The white plague. Tuberculosis, man and society. New Brunswick, NJ: Rutgers University Press, 1987.
21. Loddenkemper R, Hauer B, Sagebiel D, Forßbohm M. Tuberkuloseepidemiologie in Deutschland und der Welt mit Schwerpunkt Osteuropa. Bundesgesundheitsbl Gesundheitsforsch Gesundheitsschutz 1999; 42: 683–93.
22. Ferlinz R. Die Tuberkulose in Deutschland und das Deutsche Zentralkomitee zur Bekämpfung der Tuberkulose. Pneumologie 1995; 49: 617–32.
23. Deutsches Zentralkomitee zur Bekämpfung der Tuberkulose. 27. Informationsbericht. Frankfurt/Main: pmi Verlagsgruppe, 2002.
24. Robert Koch Institute. Bericht zur Epidemiologie der Tuberkulose in Deutschland für 2004. Berlin: Robert Koch Institute, 2006: 1–80.
25. Drobniewski F, Pablos-Méndez A, Raviglione MC. Epidemiology of tuberculosis in the world. Sem Resp Crit Care Med 1997; 18: 419–29.
26. Raviglione MC, Snider DE, Kochi A. Global epidemiology of tuberculosis. Morbidity and mortality of a worldwide epidemic. J Am Med Assoc 1995; 273: 220–26.
27. Migliori GB, Raviglione MC. Specific problems in developing areas

of the world. Central and Eastern Europe. In: Davies PDO (ed.). *Clinical tuberculosis*, 2nd edn. London: Chapman & Hall Medical, 1998: 643–60.

28. Raviglione MC, Rieder HL, Styblo K et al. Tuberculosis trends in eastern Europe and the former USSR. *Tuberc Lung Dis* 1994; **75**: 400–16.

29. Rieder HL, Zellweger JP, Raviglione MC et al. Tuberculosis control in Europe and international migration. *Eur Respir J* 1994; **7**: 1545–53.

30. Waaler HT. Tuberculosis and poverty. *Int J Tuberc Lung Dis* 2002; **6**: 745–6.

31. Dolin PJ, Raviglione MC, Kochi A. Global tuberculosis incidence and mortality during 1990–2000. *Bull World Health Organ* 1994; **72**: 213–20.

32. Dye C. Tuberculosis 2000–2010: control, but not elimination. *Int J Tuberc Lung Dis* 2000; **4**: S146–52.

33. Dye C, Watt C, Bleed D, Hosseini S, Raviglione M. Evolution of tuberculosis control and prospects for reducing tuberculosis incidence, prevalence, and deaths globally. *J Am Med Assoc* 2005; **293**: 2767–75.

34. Sudre P, ten Dam G, Kochi A. Tuberculosis: a global overview of the situation today. *Bull World Health Organ* 1992; **70**: 149–59.

35. Sagebiel D, Hauer B, Forßbohm M, Loddenkemper R. Grundzüge der Epidemiologie der Tuberkulose und aktuelle Tuberkulose-Situation in der Welt und in Deutschland. In: Forßbohm M, Loytved G, Königstein B (eds). *Praxisleitfaden Tuberkulose.* Düsseldorf: Akademie für öffentliches Gesundheitswesen, 2001: 135–56.

36. Maher D, Kochi A. Combating tuberculosis. A global view of tuberculosis and ways to fight this threatening disease. *RT International* 1997; **80–81**, 110.

37. Suárez PG, Floyd K, Portocarrero J et al. Feasibility and cost effectiveness of standardised second-line drug treatment for chronic tuberculosis patients: a national cohort study in Peru. *Lancet* 2002; **359**: 1980–89.

38. Santha T, Garg R, Frieden TR et al. Risk factors associated with default, failure and death among tuberculosis patients treated in a DOTS programme in Tiruvallur District, South India, 2000. *Int J Tuberc Lung Dis* 2002; **6**: 780–88.

39. Khatri GR, Frieden TR. Controlling tuberculosis in India. *N Engl J Med* 2002; **347**: 1420–25.

40. Floyd K, Arora V, Murthy K et al. Cost and cost-effectiveness of PPM-DOTS for tuberculosis control: evidence from India. *Bull World Health Organ* 2006; **84**: 427.

41. Sisodia R, Wares D, Sahu S et al. Source of retreatment cases under the revised national TB control programme in Rajasthan, India, 2003. *Int J Tuberc Lung Dis* 2006; **10**: 1373–9.

42. Balasubramanian R, Rajeswari R, Vijayabaskara R et al. A rural public–private partnership model in tuberculosis control in south India. *Int J Tuberc Lung Dis* 2006; **10**: 1380–5.

43. Nathanson E, Lambregts-van Weezenbeek C, Rich M et al. Multidrug resistant tuberculosis management in resource-limited settings. *Emerg Infect Dis* 2006; **12**: 1389–97.

44. Resch S, Salomon J, Murray M, Weinstein M. Cost-effectiveness of treating multidrug-resistant tuberculosis. *PLoS Med* 2006; **3**: e241.

45. EuroHIV. *HIV/AIDS surveillance in Europe. End-year report 2004.* Saint-Maurice, France: Institut de Veille Sanitaire, 2005: No. 71.

46. Lillebaek T, Andersen AB, Bauer J et al. Risk of *Mycobacterium tuberculosis* transmission in a low-incidence country due to immigration from high-incidence areas. *J Clin Microbiol* 2001; **39**: 855–61.

47. World Health Organization. *Tuberculosis control in prisons.* Geneva: World Health Organization, WHO/CDS/TB/2001.281, 2001.

48. Espinal M, Laszlo A, Simonsen L et al. Global trends in resistance to antituberculosis drugs. *N Engl J Med* 2001; **344**: 1294–303.

49. World Health Organization. *Guidelines for the programmatic management of drug-resistant tuberculosis.* Geneva: World Health Organization, WHO/HTM/TB/2006.361, 2006.

50. de Colombani P, Banatvala N, Zaleskis R, Maher D. European framework to decrease the burden of TB/HIV. *Eur Respir J* 2004; **24**: 493–501.

51. Loddenkemper R, Sagebiel D. Control in low-prevalence countries. In: Davies PDO (ed.). *Clinical tuberculosis*, 3rd edn. London: Arnold, 2003: 357–80.

52. Centers for Disease Control and Prevention. Division of TB elimination: Tuberculosis morbidity, United States, 1997. *MMWR Morb Mortal Wkly Rep* 1998; **47**: 253–7.

53. Frieden TR, Sterling T, Pablos-Méndez A et al. The emergence of drug-resistant tuberculosis in New York City. *N Engl J Med* 1993; **328**: 521–6.

54. Frieden TR, Fujiwara PI, Washko RM, Hamburg MA. Tuberculosis in New York City – turning the tide. *N Engl J Med* 1995; **333**: 229–33.

55. Loddenkemper R, Sagebiel D, Brendel A. Strategies against multidrug-resistant tuberculosis. *Eur Respir J* 2002; **20** (Suppl. 36), 66s–77s.

56. Reichman LB. The U-shaped curve of concern. *Am Rev Respir Dis* 1991; **144**: 141–2.

57. Garret L. *The coming plague. Newly emerging diseases in a world out of balance.* New York: Penguin Books, 1994.

58. Munsiff S, Nivin B, Sacajiu G et al. Persistence of a highly resistant strain of tuberculosis in New York City during 1990–1999. *J Infect Dis* 2003; **188**: 356–63.

59. Small PM, Fujiwara PI. Management of tuberculosis in the United States. *N Engl J Med* 2001; **345**: 189–200.

60. Zuber PL, McKenna MT, Binkin NJ et al. Longterm risk of tuberculosis among foreign-born persons in the United States. *J Am Med Assoc* 1997; **278**: 304–307.

61. Centers for Disease Control and Prevention, American Thoracic Society, Infectious Diseases Society of America. Controlling tuberculosis in the United States: Recommendations from the American Thoracic Society, CDC, and the Infectious Diseases Society of America. *MMWR Morb Mortal Wkly Rep* 2005; **54**: 1–81.

62. American Thoracic Society, Centers for Disease Control and Prevention. Targeted tuberculin testing and treatment of latent tuberculosis infection. *Am J Crit Care Med* 2000; **161**: S221–47.

63. Centers for Disease Control and Prevention. Update: adverse event data and revised American Thoracic Society/CDC recommendations against the use of rifampin and pyrazinamide for treatment of latent tuberculosis infection – United States, 2003. *MMWR Morb Mortal Wkly Rep* 2003; **52**: 735–9.

64. O'Brian RJ, Nunn PP. The need for new drugs against tuberculosis. Obstacles, opportunities, and next steps. *Am J Respir Crit Care Med* 2001; **163**: 1055–8.

65. Lambregts-van weezenbeek CSB, Veen J. Control of drug-resistant tuberculosis. *Tuberc Lung Dis* 1995; **76**: 455–9.

66. Aziz M, Wright A, Laszlo A et al. Epidemiology of antituberculosis drug resistance (the global project on anti-tuberculosis drug resistance surveillance): an updated analysis. *Lancet* 2006; **368**: 2142–54.

67. White VLC, Moore-Gillon J. Resource implications of patients with multidrug resistant tuberculosis. *Thorax* 2000; **55**: 962–3.

68. Iseman MD, Cohn DL, Sbarbaro JA. Directly observed treatment of tuberculosis. We can't afford not to try it. *N Engl J Med* 1993; **328**: 576–8.

69. Mangura B, Napolitano E, Passannante M et al. Directly observed treatment (DOT) is not the entire answer: an operational cohort analysis. *Int J Tuberc Lung Dis* 2002; **6**: 662–5.

70. Ormerod LP, Horsfield N, Green RM. Tuberculosis treatment outcome monitoring: Blackburn 1988–2000. *Int J Tuberc Lung Dis* 2002; –: 662–5.

71. Dèruaz J, Zellweger J. Directly observed therapy for tuberculosis in a low prevalence region: first experience at the Tuberculosis Dispensary in Lausanne. *Swiss Med Wkly* 2004; **134**: 552–8.

72. Cole ST, Telenti A. Drug resistance in *Mycobacterium tuberculosis.* *Eur Respir J* 1995; **8** (Suppl. 20): 701s–13s.

73. Schaberg T, Gloger G, Reichert B et al. Drug-resistant tuberculosis in Berlin, Germany, 1987–1993. Eur Respir J 1995; 8: 278–84.

74. Centers for Disease Control and Prevention. Emergence of Mycobacterium tuberculosis with extensive resistance to second-line drugs – worldwide, 2000–2004. MMWR Morb Mortal Wkly Rep 2006; 55: 301–305.

75. Raviglione M, Uplekar M. WHO's new STOP TB strategy. Lancet 2006; 367: 952–5.

76. WHO/IUATLD. Antituberculosis drug resistance in the world: Report No 3. Prevalence and trends. Geneva: World Health Organization, WHO/HTM/TB/2004.343, 2004.

77. Albino JA, Reichman LB. The treatment of tuberculosis. Respiration 1998; 65: 237–55.

78. Faustini A, Hall A, Perucci C. Risk factors for multidrug resistant tuberculosis in Europe: a systematic review. Thorax 2006; 61: 158–63.

79. Bashar M, Alcabes P, Rom WN, Condos R. Increased incidence of multidrug-resistant tuberculosis in diabetic patients on the Bellevue Chest Service, 1987 to 1997. Chest 2001; 120: 1514–19.

80. Brodhun B, Kunitz F, Altmann D et al. Epidemiologie der Tuberkulose in Deutschland und weltweit. Pneumologe 2006; 3: 257–65.

81. Gilad J, Borer A, Riesenberg K et al. Epidemiology and ethnic distribution of multidrug-resistant tuberculosis in southern Israel, 1992–1997: the impact of immigration. Chest 2000; 117: 738–43.

82. Talbot EA, Moore M, McCray E, Binkin NJ. Tuberculosis among foreign-born persons in the United States. J Am Med Assoc 2000; 284: 2894–900.

83. Centers for Disease Control and Prevention. Trends in tuberculosis – United States, 2005. MMWR Morb Mortal Wkly Rep 2006; 55: 305–308.

84. Raviglione MC, Gupta R, Dye CM, Espinal MA. The burden of drug-resistant tuberculosis and mechanisms for its control. Ann N Y Acad Sci 2001; 953: 88–97.

85. Nitta AT, Knowles LS, Kim J et al. Limited transmission of multidrug-resistant tuberculosis despite a high proportion of infectious cases in Los Angeles County, California. Am J Respir Crit Care Med 2002; 165: 812–17.

86. Davies PDO, Grange JM. Factors affecting susceptibility and resistance to tuberculosis. Thorax 2001; 56 (Suppl. II): II23–9.

87. Caminero JA, Pena MJ, Campos-Herrero MI et al. Epidemiological evidence of the spread of a Mycobacterium tuberculosis strain of the Beijing genotype on Gran Canaria Island. Am J Respir Crit Care Med 2001; 164: 1165–70.

88. Pfyffer GE, Straessle A, van Gorkum T et al. Multidrug-resistant tuberculosis in prison inmates, Azerbaijan. Emerg Inf Dis 2001; 7: 855–61.

89. Dye C, Williams BG, Espinal MA, Raviglione MC. Erasing the world's slow stain: strategies to beat multidrug-resistant tuberculosis. Science 2002; 295: 2042–6.

90. Roche PW, Antic R, Bastian I et al. Tuberculosis notifications in Australia, 2004. Commun Dis Intell 2006; 30: 93–101.

91. Heath TC, Roberts C, Winks M, Capon AG. The epidemiology of tuberculosis in New South Wales 1975–1995. Int J Tuberc Lung Dis 1998; 2: 647–54.

92. Das D, Baker M, Venugopal K, McAllister S. Why the tuberculosis incidence rate is not falling in New Zealand. N Z Med J 2006; 119: U2248.

93. Das D, Baker M, Calder L. Tuberculosis epidemiology in New Zealand: 1995–2004. N Z Med J 2006; 119: U2249.

94. Geng E, Kreiswirth B, Driver C et al. Changes in the transmission of tuberculosis in New York City from 1990 to 1999. N Engl J Med 2002; 346: 1453–8.

95. Weis SE, Slocum PC, Blais FX et al. The effect of directly observed therapy on the rates of drug resistance and relapse in tuberculosis. N Engl J Med 1994; 330: 1179–84.

96. STOP TB Partnership, World Health Organization. Global plan to stop TB 2006–2015. Geneva: World Health Organization, WHO/HTM/STB/2006.35, 2006.

97. World Health Organization. The stop TB strategy. Geneva: World Health Organization, WHO/HTM/STB/2006.37, 2006.

98. Zignol M, Wright A, Jaramillo E et al. Patients with previously treated tuberculosis no longer neglected. Clin Infect Dis 2007; 44: 61–4.

99. Schwoebel V, Lambregts-van Weezenbeek CS, Moro ML et al. Standardization of antituberculosis drug resistance surveillance in Europe. Recommendations of a WHO and IUATLD Working Group. Eur Respir J 2000; 16: 364–71.

100. Loddenkemper R. The need for antituberculosis drug resistance surveillance in Europe. Eur Respir J 2000; 16: 195–6 (editorial).

101. Helbling P, Altpeter E, Raeber PA et al. Surveillance of antituberculosis drug resistance in Switzerland 1995–1997: the central link. Eur Respir J 2000; 16: 200–202.

102. Styblo K, Bumgarner J. Tuberculosis can be controlled with existing technologies: evidence. Tuberc Surveill Res Unit Prog Rep 1991; 2: 60–72.

103. Borgdorff MW, Veen J, Kalisvaart NA et al. Defaulting from tuberculosis treatment in the Netherlands: rates, risk factors and trend in the period 1993–1997. Eur Respir J 2000; 16: 209–13.

104. Pai M, Menzies D. Interferon-γ release assays: What is their role in the diagnosis of active tuberculosis? Clin Infect Dis 2007; 44: 74–7.

105. Dewan P, Grinsdale J, Kawamura M. Low sensitivity of a whole-blood interferon-γ release assay for detection of active tuberculosis. Clin Infect Dis 2007; 44: 69–73.

106. Enarson DA, Fanning EA, Allen EA. Case finding in the elimination phase of tuberculosis: high risk groups in epidemiology and clinical practice. Bull Int Union Tuberc Lung Dis 1990; 65: 73–4.

107. Hardie RM, Watson JM. Screening migrants at risk of tuberculosis. Br Med J 1993; 307: 1539–40.

108. Hopewell P, Pai M. Tuberculosis, vulnerability and access to quality care. J Am Med Assoc 2005; 293: 2790–3.

109. Hawker JI, Bakhshi SS, Ali S, Farrington CP. Ecological analysis of ethnic differences in relation between tuberculosis and poverty. Br Med J 1999; 319: 1031–4.

110. Haddad M, Wilson T, Ijaz K et al. Tuberculosis and homelessness in the United States, 1994–2003. J Am Med Assoc 2005; 293: 2762–6.

111. Rieder HL, Cauthen GM, Comstock GW, Snider DE. Epidemiology of tuberculosis in the United States. Epidemiol Rev 1989; 11: 79–98.

112. Reyes H, Coninx R. Pitfalls of tuberculosis programmes in prisons. Br Med J 1997; 315: 1447–50.

113. Chaves F, Dronda F, Cave MD et al. A longitudinal study of transmission of tuberculosis in a large prison population. Am J Resp Crit Care Med 1997; 155: 719–25.

114. Aerts A, Hauer B, Wanlin M, Veen J. Tuberculosis and tuberculosis control in European prisons. Int J Tuberc Lung Dis 2006; 10: 1215–23.

115. Drobniewski F, Balabanova Y, Nikolayevsky V et al. Drug-resistant tuberculosis, clinical virulence, and the dominance of the Beijing strain family in Russia. J Am Med Assoc 2005; 293: 2726–31.

116. Tala E, Kochi A. Elimination of tuberculosis from Europe and the world. Eur Respir J 1991; 4: 1159–60 (editorial).

117. Nisar M, Williams CSD, Ashby D, Davies PDO. Tuberculin testing in residential homes for the elderly. Thorax 1993; 48: 1257–60.

118. Stead WW, Lofgren JP, Warren E, Thomas C. Tuberculosis as an endemic and nosocomial infection among the elderly in nursing homes. N Engl J Med 1985; 312: 1483–7.

119. Zevallos M, Justman J. Tuberculosis in the elderly. Clin Geriatr Med 2003; 19: 121–38.

120. Styblo K. The impact of HIV infection on the global epidemiology of tuberculosis. Bull Int Union Tuberc Lung Dis 1991; 66: 27–32.

121. World Health Organization. Strategic framework to decrease the burden of TB/HIV. Geneva: World Health Organization, WHO/CDS/TB/2002.296, 2002.

122. Menzies D. Tuberculosis crosses borders. *Int J Tuberc Lung Dis* 2000; 4: S153–9.

123. Valway SE, Greifinger RB, Papania M *et al.* Multi-drug resistant tuberculosis in the New York state prison system, 1990–91. *J Infect Dis* 1994; 170: 151–6.

124. Centers for Disease Control and Prevention. Prevention and control of tuberculosis in correctional and detention facilities: recommendations from CDC. *MMWR Morb Mortal Wkly Rep* 2006; 55: 1–44.

125. IUATLD/WHO. Control of tuberculosis in healthcare settings. Joint statement by the IUATLD and the WHO. *Tuberc Lung Dis* 1994; 75: 94–5.

126. Riley RL, Mills CC, Nyko W *et al.* Aerial dissemination of pulmonary tuberculosis. A two year study of contagion in a tuberculosis ward. *Am J Hyg* 1959; 70: 185–96.

127. Malasky C, Jordan T, Potulski F, Reichman LB. Occupational tuberculous infections among pulmonary physicians in training. *Am Rev Respir Dis* 1990; 142: 505–507.

128. Condos R, Schluger N, Lacouture R, Rom W. Tuberculosis infections among house staff at Bellevue Hospital in an epidemic period. *Am Rev Respir Dis* 1993; 147 (Suppl. A) 124.

129. Redwood E, Anderson V, Felton CP *et al.* Tuberculin conversion in hospital employees in a high tuberculosis prevalence area. *Am Rev Respir Dis* 1993; 147 (Suppl. A): 119.

130. Menzies D, Fanning A, Yuan L, Fitzgerald M. Tuberculosis among healthcare workers. *N Engl J Med* 1995; 332: 92–8.

131. Jensen P, Lambert A, Iademarco M, Ridzon R. CDC guidelines for preventing the transmission of *Mycobacterium tuberculosis* in health-care settings, 2005. *MMWR Morb Mortal Wkly Rep* 2005; 54: 1–141.

132. Schwartzman K, Loo V, Pasztor J, Menzies D. Tuberculosis infection among healthcare workers in Montreal. *Am J Respir Crit Care Med* 1996; 154: 1006–12.

133. Meredith S, Watson JM, Citron KM *et al.* Are healthcare workers in England and Wales at increased risk of tuberculosis? *Br Med J* 1996; 313: 522–5.

134. Diel R, Seidler A, Nienhaus A *et al.* Occupational risk of tuberculosis transmission in a low incidence area. *Respir Res* 2005; 6: 35.

135. Franchi A, Richeldi L, Parrinello G, Franco G. Room size is the major determinant for tuberculin conversion in health care workers exposed to a multidrug-resistant patient. *Int Arch Occup Environ Health* 2007; 80: 533–8.

136. Raitio M, Tala E. Tuberculosis among healthcare workers during three recent decades. *Eur Respir J* 2000; 15: 304–307.

137. Blumberg H, Leonard M, Jasmer R. Update on the treatment of tuberculosis and latent tuberculosis infection. *J Am Med Assoc* 2005; 293: 2776–84.

138. Iseman MD. Treatment of multidrug-resistant tuberculosis. *N Engl J Med* 1993; 329: 784–91.

139. Deutsches Zentralkomitee zur Bekämpfung der Tuberkulose. Richtlinien zur medikamentösen Behandlung der Tuberkulose im Erwachsenen- und Kindesalter. *Pneumologie* 2001; 55: 494–511.

140. Moro ML, Errante I, Infuso A *et al.* Effectiveness of infection control measures in controlling a nosocomial outbreak of multidrug-resistant tuberculosis among HIV patients in Italy. *Int J Tuberc Lung Dis* 2000; 4: 61–8.

141. Tuberculosis Coalition for Technical Assistance. *International standards for tuberculosis care (ISTC).* The Hague: Tuberculosis Coalition for Technical Assistance, 2006: 1–57.

142. Centers for Disease Control and Prevention. Update: Guidelines for the investigation of contacts of persons with infectious tuberculosis. *MMWR Morb Mortal Wkly Rep* 2005; 54: 1–37.

143. Shaw JB, Wynn-Williams N. Infectivity of pulmonary tuberculosis in relation to sputum status. *Am Rev Tuberc* 1954; 69: 724–32.

144. Deutsches Zentralkomitee zur Bekämpfung der Tuberkulose. Richtlinien für die Umgebungsuntersuchung bei Tuberkulose. *Gesundheitswesen* 1996; 58: 657–65.

145. Diel R, Forßbohm M, Loytved G *et al.* Empfehlungen für die Umgebungsuntersuchungen bei Tuberkulose. *Pneumologie* 2007; 61: 440–55.

146. Deutsches Zentralkomitee zur Bekämpfung der Tuberkulose. Empfehlungen zur Infektionsverhütung bei Tuberkulose. Frankfurt/Main: pmi Verlagsgruppe, 1996: 1–24.

147. Schaberg T, Hauer B, Haas W *et al.* Latent tuberculosis infection: recommendations for preventive therapy in adults in Germany. *Pneumologie* 2004; 58: 255–70.

148. Mazurek G, Jereb J, LoBue P *et al.* Centers for Disease Control and Prevention. Guidelines for using the QuantiFERON®-TB Gold Test for detecting *Mycobacterium tuberculosis* infection, United States. *MMWR Morb Mortal Wkly Rep* 2005; 54: 49–55.

149. Sagebiel D, Hauer B, Haas W *et al.* Future supply of tuberculin in Germany. *Bundesgesundheitsblatt Gesundheitsforschung Gesundheitsschutz* 2005; 48: 477–82.

150. Rieder HL. Theoretische und praktische Überlegungen bei Anwendung des Tuberkulintests. *Pneumologie* 1997; 51: 1025–32.

151. Schluger N. Challenges of treating latent tuberculosis infection. *Chest* 2002; 121: 1733–5.

152. Lalvani A, Pathan AA, Durkan H *et al.* Enhanced contact-tracing and spatial tracking of *Mycobacterium tuberculosis* infection by enumeration of antigen-specific T cells. *Lancet* 2001; 23: 2017–21.

153. Mazurek GH, LoBlue PA, Daley CL *et al.* Comparison of a whole-blood interferon gamma assay with tuberculin skin testing for detecting latent *Mycobacterium tuberculosis* infection. *J Am Med Assoc* 2001; 286: 1740–7.

154. Mori T, Sakatani M, Yamagishi F *et al.* Specific detection of tuberculosis infection. An interferon-γ-based assay using new antigens. *Am J Respir Crit Care Med* 2004; 170: 59–64.

155. Pai M, Riley L, Colford J. Interferon-γ assays in the immunodiagnosis of tuberculosis: a systematic review. *Lancet Infect Dis* 2004; 4: 761–76.

156. Lee J, Choi H, Park I *et al.* Comparison of two commercial Interferon-gamma assays for diagnosing *Mycobacterium tuberculosis* infection. *Eur Respir J* 2006; 28: 24–30.

157. Kunst H. Diagnosis of latent tuberculosis infection: The potential role of new technologies. *Respir Med* 2006; 100: 2098–106.

158. Ferrara G, Losi M, Meacci M *et al.* Routine hospital use of a new commercial whole blood interferon-γ assay for the diagnosis of tuberculosis infection. *Am J Crit Care Med* 2005; 172: 631–5.

159. Richeldi L. An update on the diagnosis of tuberculosis infection. *Am J Crit Care Med* 2006; 174: 736–42.

160. Ewer K, Deeks J, Alvarez L *et al.* Comparison of T-cell-based assay with tuberculin skin test for diagnosis of *Mycobacterium tuberculosis* infection in a school tuberculosis outbreak. *Lancet* 2003; 361: 1168–73.

161. Arend S, van Meijgaarden K, de Boer K *et al.* Tuberculin skin testing and *in vitro* T cell responses to ESAT-6 and culture filtrate protein 10 after infection with *Mycobacterium marinum* or *M. kansasii. J Infect Dis* 2002; 186: 1807.

162. Kobashi Y, Obase Y, Fukuda M *et al.* Clinical reevaluation of the QuantiFERON TB-2G test as a diagnostic method for differentiating active tuberculosis from nontuberculosis mycobacteriosis. *Clin Infect Dis* 2006; 43: 1540–6.

163. Rangaka M, Wilkinson K, Seldon R *et al.* The effect of HIV-1 infection on T cell based and skin test detection of tuberculosis infection. *Am J Respir Crit Care Med* 2007; 175: 514–20.

164. Hauer B, Loddenkemper R, Detjen A *et al.* Interferon-γ assays – description and assessment of a new tool in the diagnosis of tuberculosis. *Pneumologie* 2006; 60: 29–44.

165. Crawford J. Genotyping in contact investigations: a CDC perspective. *Int J Tuberc Lung Dis* 2003; 12: S453–7.

166. Small PM, McClenny NB, Singh SP *et al.* Molecular strain typing of *Mycobacterium tuberculosis* to confirm cross-contamination in the mycobacteriology laboratory and modification of procedures

to minimize occurrence of false-positive cultures. *J Clin Microbiol* 1993; **31**: 1677–82.

167. Driscoll JR, Lee PA, Jovell RJ *et al.* How and why we fingerprint tuberculosis. *RT, J Resp Care Pract* 2001; 2/3.

168. van Soolingen D, Borgdorff MW, De Haas PE *et al.* Molecular epidemiology of tuberculosis in the Netherlands: a nationwide study from 1993 through 1997. *J Infect Dis* 1999; **180**: 726–36.

169. Moro ML, Gori A, Errante I *et al.* An outbreak of multidrug-resistant tuberculosis involving HIV-infected patients of two hospitals in Milan, Italy. *AIDS* 1998; **12**: 1095–102.

170. Verver S, Warren R, Beyers N *et al.* Rate of reinfection tuberculosis after successful treatment is higher than rate of new tuberculosis. *Am J Respir Crit Care Med* 2005; **171**: 1430–35.

171. Alland D, Kalkut GE, Moss AR *et al.* Transmission of tuberculosis in New York City: an analysis by DNA fingerprinting and conventional epidemiologic methods. *N Engl J Med* 1994; **330**: 1710–16.

172. Small PM, Hopewell PC, Singh SP *et al.* The epidemiology of tuberculosis in San Francisco: a population-based study using conventional and molecular methods. *N Engl J Med* 1994; **330**: 1703–709.

173. Diel R, Ruesch-Gerdes S, Niemann S. Molecular epidemiology of tuberculosis among immigrants in Hamburg, Germany. *J Clin Microbiol* 2004; **42**: 2952–60.

174. Diel R, Meywald-Walter K, Gottschalk R *et al.* Ongoing outbreak of tuberculosis in a low-incidence community: a molecular-epidemiological evaluation. *Int J Tuberc Lung Dis* 2004; **8**: 855–61.

175. Maguire H, Dale J, McHugh T *et al.* Molecular epidemiology of tuberculosis in London 1995-7 showing low rate of active transmission. *Thorax* 2002; **57**: 617–22.

176. van Rie A, Warren R, Richardson M *et al.* Exogenous reinfection as a cause of recurrent tuberculosis after curative treatment. *N Engl J Med* 1999; **341**: 1174–9.

177. Veen J. Microepidemics of tuberculosis: the stone-in-the-pond principle. *Tuberc Lung Dis* 1992; **73**: 73–6.

178. Styblo K, Meijer J, Sutherland I. The transmission of tubercle bacilli – its trend in a human population. Tuberculosis Surveillance Research Unit Report No. 1. *Bull Int Union Tuberc* 1969; **42**: 1–104.

179. Cain K, Haley C, Armstrong L *et al.* Tuberculosis among foreign-born persons in the United States: achieving tuberculosis elimination. *Am J Respir Crit Care Med* 2007; **175**: 75–9.

180. Ormerod P, Skinner C, Moore-Gillon J *et al.* Control and prevention of tuberculosis in the United Kingdom: Code of practice 2000. Joint Tuberculosis Committee of the British Thoracic Society. *Thorax* 2000; **55**: 887–901.

181. Rieder HL. Interventions for tuberculosis control and elimination. Paris: IUATLD, 2002: 1–251.

182. American Thoracic Society, Centers for Disease Control, American Academy of Pediatrics. Treatment of tuberculosis and tuberculosis infection in adults and children. *Am J Respir Crit Care Med* 1994; **149**: 1359–74.

183. Enarson DA, Rieder HL, Arnadottir T, Trébucq A. *Management of tuberculosis. A guide for low income countries*, 5th edn. Paris: IUATLD, 2000: 1–89.

184. Bourdin Trunz B, Fine P, Dye C. Effect of BCG vaccination on childhood tuberculous meningitis and miliary tuberculosis worldwide: a metaanalysis and assessment of cost-effectiveness. *Lancet* 2006; **367**: 1173–80.

185. de Roux A, Rieder H, Sagebiel D, Uphoff H. Vaccinations in pneumology: Pneumococci, influenza, and BCG. *Pneumologie* 2007; **4**: 47–62.

186. Tala-Heikkilä M, Tuominen JE, Tala EO. Bacillus Calmette–Guérin revaccination questionable with low tuberculosis incidence. *Am J Respir Crit Care Med* 1998; **157**: 1324–7.

187. Fine PE. Variation in protection by BCG: Implications of and for heterologous immunity. *Lancet* 1995; **436**: 1339–45.

188. Infuso A, Falzon D. European survey of BCG vaccination policies and surveillance in children, 2005. *Eurosurveillance* 2006; **11**: 6–11.

189. Ormerod P, Campbell I, Novelli V *et al.* Chemotherapy and management of tuberculosis in the United Kingdom: recommendations 1998. Joint Tuberculosis Committee of the British Thoracic Society. *Thorax* 1998; **53**: 536–48.

190. Adal KA, Anglim AM, Palumbo CL *et al.* The use of high-efficiency particulate air-filter respirators to protect hospital workers from tuberculosis. *N Engl J Med* 1994; **331**: 169–73.

191. Miller SL, Macher JM. Evaluation of a methodology for quantifying the effect of room air ultraviolet germicidal irradiation on airborne bacteria. *Aerosol Sci Technol* 2000; **33**: 274–95.

192. Ko G, First MW, Burge HA. The characterization of upper-room ultraviolet germicidal irradiation in inactivating airborne microorganisms. *Environ Health Perspect* 2002; **110**: 95–101.

193. Wells W. *Airborne contagion and air hygiene.* Cambridge, MA: Harvard University Press, 1955.

194. Riley R, Knight M, Middlebrook G. Ultraviolet susceptibility of BCG and virulent tubercle bacilli. *Am Rev Respir Dis* 1976; **113**: 413–18.

195. Nardell DA. Use and misuse of germicidal UV air disinfection for TB in high-prevalence settings. *Int J Tuberc Lung Dis* 2002; **6**: 647–8.

196. Talbot EA, Jensen P, Moffat HJ, Wells CD. Occupational risk from ultraviolet germicidal irradiation (UVGI) lamps. *Int J Tuberc Lung Dis* 2002; **6**: 738–41.

197. Espinal MA, Laserson K, Camacho M *et al.* Determinants of drug-resistant tuberculosis: analysis of 11 countries. *Int J Tuberc Lung Dis* 2001; **5**: 887–93.

198. Porco T, Lewis B, Marseille E *et al.* Cost-effectiveness of tuberculosis evaluation and treatment of newly-arrived immigrants. *BMC Public Health* 2006; **6**: 157.

199. Klewer J, Seelbach H, Kugler J. What do medical students know about the epidemiology of tetanus and tuberculosis in Germany? A comparison of epidemiologic knowledge regarding a rare and a prevalent infectious disease. *Gesundheitswesen* 2000; **62**: 30–33.

200. World Health Organization. *Tuberculosis: a manual for medical students.* Geneva: World Health Organization, WHO/CDS/TB/96.272, 2003.

201. Holland SM. Cytokine therapy of mycobacterial infections. *Adv Intern Med* 2001; **45**: 431–52.

202. Small PM, Perkins MD. More rigour needed in trials of new diagnostic agents for tuberculosis. *Lancet* 2000; **356**: 1048–9.

203. Sharma M, Al-Azem A, Wolfe J *et al.* Identification of a predominant isolate of *Mycobacterium tuberculosis* using molecular and clinical epidemiology tools and *in vitro* cytokine responses. *BMC Infect Dis* 2003; **3**: 3.

204. Johnson J, Ssekasanvu E, Okwera A *et al.* Randomised trial of adjunctive interleukin-2 in adults with pulmonary tuberculosis. *Am J Respir Crit Care Med* 2003; **168**: 185–91.

205. Wallis R, Song H, Whalen C, Okwera A. TB Chemotherapy: Antagonism between immunity and sterilization. *Am J Respir Crit Care Med* 2004; **19**: 771–2.

206. Wallis R, Vinhas S, Johnson J *et al.* Whole blood bactericidal activity during treatment of pulmonary tuberculosis. *J Infect Dis* 2003; **187**: 270–8.

207. Greinert U, Ernst M, Schlaak M, Entzian P. Interleukin-12 as successful adjuvant in tuberculosis treatment. *Eur Respir J* 2001; **17**: 1049–51.

208. O'Brian R, Spiegelman M. New drugs for tuberculosis. *Clin Chest Med* 2005; **26**: 327–40.

209. Andries K, Verhasselt P, Guillemont J *et al.* A diarylquinolone drug active on the ATP synthase of *Mycobacterium tuberculosis*. *Science* 2005; **307**: 223–7.

210. TB Alliance. Global alliance for TB drug development. www.tballiance.org. Last accessed 27 December 2006.

211. van Embden JD, Cave MD, Crawford JT *et al.* Strain identification of *Mycobacterium tuberculosis* by DNA fingerprinting: recommendations for a standardized methodology. *J Clin Microbiol* 1993; **31**: 406–409.

212. Moore D, Evans C, Gilman R *et al.* Microscopic observation drug-susceptibility assay for the diagnosis of TB. *N Engl J Med* 2006; **355**: 1539–50.

213. Riska PF, Jacobs WR, Alland D. Molecular determinants of drug resistance in tuberculosis. *Int J Tuberc Lung Dis* 2000; **4**: S4–S10.

26

Control of tuberculosis in high-prevalence countries

JAYANT N BANAVALIKER

If the number of victims which a disease claims is the measure of its significance, then all diseases, particularly the most dreaded infectious diseases, such as bubonic plague, Asiatic cholera, etc., must rank far behind tuberculosis.

Robert Koch, 24 March 1882

GLOBAL EPIDEMIOLOGY AND HIGH-PREVALENCE COUNTRIES

Tuberculosis (TB) has affected mankind for nearly 5000 years. In 1892, Robert Koch discovered the causative organism of tuberculosis – *Mycobacterium tuberculosis*. In the 1920s, Calmette and Guérin introduced the bacille Calmette–Guérin (BCG) vaccine and in the 1940s, Waksman found the miracle drug – streptomycin. In spite of all this, the formidable foe is still going strong.

In March 1993, the problem of TB being insurmountable, the World Health Organization (WHO) declared TB a global emergency.[1]

In 2005, an estimated 8.8 million new cases of TB were detected, 7.4 million were in Asia and sub-Saharan Africa. TB is still a major cause of death worldwide, a total of 1.6 million people died of TB, including some 195 000 of them who were infected with HIV.[2] The global prevalence of TB is estimated to be 14.6 million.[3]

According to WHO, TB prevalence and death rates have been falling globally. In 2005 in the six WHO regions (African region, America, Eastern Mediterranean region, European region, South East Asia region and Western Pacific region), the incidence of TB was stable or on the decline and had reached a peak worldwide.

Between 1980 and 2005, 90 million TB patients have been reported to the WHO-assisted programme world-wide. In 199 countries, 5 million cases of TB (new and relapsed) were reported in 2005. Under the DOTS programme, implemented in 187 countries throughout the world in 2005, 2.3 million new smear-positive pulmonary cases were reported and 2.1 million patients were registered for treatment in 2004.

An estimated US$10 billion is spent annually on global TB control and of this US$3 billion is spent by developing countries on TB control in their own countries.

Though the rate at which people developed TB in 2005 was static or even declined slightly compared to 2004, the actual number of TB cases continued to rise slowly. This can be attributed to the expanding world population. The rate at which new cases of TB developed in 2005 was slightly lower than the growth in the global population, but the actual number of cases in 2005 was 8 787 000 as compared to 8 718 000 in 2004.

Asia has the highest burden of TB in the world. India, China and Indonesia account for nearly half the global TB burden (Figure 26.1). The WHO South East Asia region (SEARO), covering 11 countries with a total population of 1.6 billion, has one-third of all TB cases in the world. In 2005, of the estimated 5 million prevalent cases of TB in this region, nearly 3 million were new cases with an incidence rate of 182 per 100 000 population. More than half a million people continue to die of TB annually in this region, i.e. one person every minute.[4]

The economic impact of TB in high-burden countries is considerable (Table 26.1). The morbidity and mortality (75 per cent of TB deaths) occur in the age range of 15–54 years, which is the group that is the most economically productive. TB results in an estimated 4–7 per cent of gross domestic product (GDP) loss and depletes the economies of the poor developing countries by a total of US$12 billion per year.[5]

Table 26.1 Estimated tuberculosis burden 2005 in high-prevalence countries.

Countries	Population in 1000s	Incidence				Prevalence		Mortality		High prevalence in incident TB cases (%)
		All forms		Smear positive		All forms		All forms		
		No. 1000s	Per 10⁵ population per year	No. 1000s	Per 10⁵ population per year	No. 1000s	Per 10⁵ population per year	No. 1000s	Per 10⁵ population per year	
India	1 103 371	1852	168	827	75	3299	299	322	29	5.2
China	1 315 844	1319	100	593	45	2737	208	205	16	0.5
Indonesia	222 781	533	239	240	108	584	262	92	41	0.8
Nigeria	131 530	372	283	162	123	704	536	100	76	19
Bangladesh	141 822	322	227	145	102	575	406	66	47	0.1
Pakistan	157 935	286	181	129	82	468	297	59	37	0.6
South Africa	47 432	285	600	116	245	242	511	34	71	58
Ethiopia	77 431	266	344	118	152	423	546	56	73	11
Philippines	83 054	242	291	109	131	374	450	39	47	0.1
Kenya	34 256	220	641	94	276	321	936	48	140	28
DR Congo	57 549	205	356	90	156	311	541	42	73	17
Russian Federation	143 202	170	119	76	53	214	150	28	20	6.2
Viet Nam	84 238	148	175	66	79	198	235	19	23	3.0
UR Tanzania	38 329	131	342	56	147	190	496	29	75	29
Brazil	186 405	111	60	49	26	142	76	15	7.5	14
Uganda	28 816	106	369	46	158	161	559	26	91	30
Thailand	64 233	91	142	41	63	131	204	12	19	7.6
Mozambique	19 792	89	447	37	185	118	597	24	124	50
Myanmar	50 519	86	171	38	76	86	170	8	15	7.1
Zimbabwe	13010	78	601	32	245	82	631	17	130	60
Cambodia	14 071	71	506	32	226	99	703	12	87	6.0
Afghanistan	29 863	50	168	23	76	86	288	10	35	0.0

Source: WHO Report 2007; Global tuberculosis control, surveillance, planning, financing; Geneva: World Health Organization 2007.

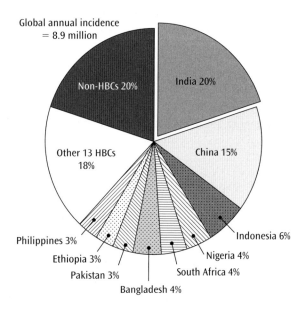

Figure 26.1 Data demonstrating that India has the highest tuberculosis burden globally, accounting for one-fifth of the global incidence. From Ref. 2. HBC, high-burden country.

A total of 22 countries account for almost 80 per cent of the global TB burden and are commonly known as high-burden countries (HBCs). They are Afghanistan, Bangladesh, Brazil, Cambodia, China, Democratic Republic of Congo, Ethiopia, India, Indonesia, Kenya, Myanmar, Nigeria, Pakistan, Peru, the Philippines, the Russian Federation, South Africa, Thailand, Tanzania, Uganda, Vietnam and Zimbabwe.

In the various WHO regions, the African region (23 per cent), the South East Asia region (35 per cent) and the Western Pacific region (25 per cent) accounted for the 83 per cent of all new and relapse cases in 2005.

The 22 high-prevalence countries (HPCs) or high-burden countries have shown improvement in their parameters of TB control. The African continent has 12 HBCs, which is largely due to high-prevalence of HIV in these countries.

DOTS coverage has been steadily increasing since 1995. All the 22 HBCs have adopted the DOTS programme. In India, the country with highest number of TB cases, the DOTS programme known as the Revised National TB Control Programme (RNTCP), covered the entire country by March 2006. Similarly, in 18 countries of the total 22 HBCs, 90 per cent of the population follows the DOTS programme. The coverage of DOTS was less extensive in the Russian Federation (83 per cent), Afghanistan (81 per cent), Brazil (68 per cent) and Nigeria (65 per cent).

The three WHO regions with the highest rate of case detection was South East Asia, the Americas and the Western Pacific. The increase in cases detected between 2004 and 2005 was less than in the preceding year.

The DOTS programme detected an estimated 53 per cent of all new cases and 60 per cent of new smear-positive cases in 2005. The point estimate of 60 per cent detection rate of smear-positive cases under the DOTS programme in 2005 is 10 per cent below the target of 70 per cent case detection.

A total of 67 countries met the 70 per cent target of case detection by the end of 2005. Of the additional new smear-positive cases reported compared to those in 2004, 39 per cent were in China and 17 per cent in India under the DOTS programme in 2005. Sadly, in 2005, China and India still accounted for an estimated 27 per cent of all undetected new smear-positive cases. In fact, Nigeria accounted for 59 per cent of all cases not detected by the DOTS programme in 2005.

Amongst the innumerable diseases which ravage developing countries, TB ranks number one. Africa, Asia and the 'poorer' Western countries have a high-prevalence of TB which paradoxically can be cured with the most effective available antituberculosis chemotherapy. Yet it still remains the disease which ends a large number of lives, economically depletes the family of its meagre resources and drives them more and more down the poverty line.

SOCIAL AND ECONOMIC FACTORS FOMENTING TB IN HIGH-PREVALENCE COUNTRIES

The high burden of TB in many developing countries makes TB control a priority.

There are several factors which have made TB a problem in HPCs. TB has a severe impact on socioeconomic development and is exacerbated by poor hygiene, criminal behaviour and drug addiction, which are rampant in slums and poor housing conditions. Overcrowded rooms increase the chance of transmission of disease, while poor nutrition reduces body resistance to ward off the disease.

Population

In any country, a large population, coupled with economic deprivation, is an additional factor for poverty and TB. A large population leads to higher financial needs, worse living conditions, less living space and overcrowding, which leads to easy transmission of contagious communicable diseases like TB.

India, Indonesia and Bangladesh are three countries that contribute the major share of TB cases in the world.[6]

A study at the Tuberculosis Research Centre, Chennai, India, indicated that TB may cause 300 000 children to become orphans and 100 000 Indian women to be rejected by their families each year.[7]

India, with its vast population and diversity, has been long regarded as one of the greatest challenges for TB control.[8]

Poverty

The relationship between TB and poverty is intricate and complex. It impoverishes people suffering from it and the cycle continues to increase the number of those who are poor. TB perpetuates and exacerbates poverty. It affects families economically and undermines development. The burden of suffering and economic loss caused by TB in the developing world is enormous. The direct and indirect economic costs of the TB epidemic costs India at least US$3 billion each year. It includes the loss of 100 million work days and more than US$100 million is incurred by the patients directly.[9]

Researchers at the Tuberculosis Research Centre in Chennai found that an average patient suffering from TB incurs a total expenditure of US$99 (£48) on diagnosis and treatment. This is a prohibitive amount for a daily wage labourer who might hope to earn the equivalent of US$200–400 (£97–195) per year. In another study in Andhra Pradesh, India, Ramana et al.[10] found that on an average, rural TB patients spent US$30 (£14) per month on TB diagnosis and treatment, while urban patients spent US$15 (£7) per month.

The relationship between TB and poverty is complex and the situation is worsened by socioeconomic decline. Collapse of health and social support in Russia after 1990 led to a rapid rise in TB, with rates increasing by 7 per cent per year in the Russian Federation, Ukraine and other countries of the former Soviet Union.[11]

The other problem leading to poverty is indebtness. An Indian study showed that more than two-thirds of households went into debt to cover the cost of treatment of TB. The average family debt incurred by patients because of TB amounted to US$120 million.

Poverty continues to be the key underlying factor for spread of TB. Due to poverty, patients are less well educated, live in appalling, unhealthy environments, are malnourished and are unaware of problems relating to health and disease. In fact, poverty and TB is a vicious cycle.

In the 22 HBCs or HPCs, 80 per cent of the population have a per capita income of less than US$760 (£370). It is estimated that over 50 per cent of new TB patients are living on less than US$2 (£0.98) per day. Affluent countries too have economically weaker areas. The incidence of TB in Afro-Americans and non-whites in San Francisco is comparable with Botswana, which is a HBC. A report by the World Bank[12] revealed a link between poverty, food, income and access to health-care facilities in 60 000 poor people from 60 countries. Within countries, e.g. in Chiapas, a Mexican state with a high poverty level, the incidence of TB is twice as high as the national average. Poverty even affects the health-seeking behaviour of the patient. They do not attend the centres due to the cost of transportation involved, resulting in cessation of treatment and subsequent worsening of disease. In a Chinese study, financial constraints were identified as contributing to 45 per cent of the cause of treatment delays. Similarly, in countries such as India where women are not the bread-winners of the family, they report late for diagnosis as compared to men. The associated stigma with TB can cause lowering of social position and power. Studies from Vietnam reveal isolation and/or rejection of women affected with TB.[13]

Due to concern about the effect of poverty on TB, the WHO's World TB Day theme in 2002 was 'Stop TB Fight Poverty'.

A major contributing factor is the global indifference to TB, which is predominantly a disease of the poor and destitute. In 1908, Leonard Williams, critical of the attitude of fellow medical practitioners toward TB commented, 'The crusade against consumption may be said to have degenerated into a pious opinion that the [tuberculosis] bacillus resembles the socialist in being a very wicked and obtrusive person whose existence it is well that people of refinement should forget'. The words sound prophetic even after 100 years.[14]

Education

Education forms an integral part of the overall development of personality. It imparts an ability to think, to decide and reform. Illiteracy breeds ignorance, inferiority and stunts the development of personality. Stigma relating to TB has it genesis in ignorance and illiteracy. Though the fact that TB is curable is well known, in those countries where the literacy rate is low, control of TB is difficult due to the stigma that TB is incurable and is a hereditary disease. In India and other countries where TB is stigmatized, young girls do not come to centres for treatment as it might jeopardize their prospects of getting married. Such tradition is more prevalent in rural India where the literacy rate is extremely low.

Poor awareness and knowledge about the disease due to lack of basic education plays another important role, which leads to improper diagnosis and delay in treatment. A study from India has shown that 8 per cent of rural and 13 per cent of urban children were taken out of school when either of the parents developed TB.[7]

Public health services

The complexity of the subject of the health of those who constitute the motor which turns the wheel of economy

and prosperity is well known. Governments aim to keep their people healthy and for this an efficient health service is the main requisite. The cost of the health service should be relatively less important consideration, as long as the economy can tolerate the burden. In the developed and affluent countries of the world, there are extremely good public health services, which is one of the reasons that there is effective control of TB, for example in Norway and Denmark. However, where the public health services are poor as in African and Asian countries, diseases like TB are difficult to control, due to the perennial short supply of financial as well as material resources both at central and state level.

Inadequate funding, shortage of essential drugs and lack of equipment are some of the factors leading to the failure of the well-planned National TB Control Programme of India, which was started in 1962.

Another dilemma for public health-oriented health services is to choose between integrated (horizontal) and specialized (vertical) strategies. Vertical programmes are more efficient because it is easier to supervise and improve them. However, they are extremely expensive, have less coverage of the population and are sometimes not in accord with the perceived needs of the people. The National TB Programme of India is a good example of this difficult choice, especially when cost is crucial in limiting the ravages of the diseases which the programme aims to bring under control. However, as Karl Styblo has pointed out, 'In many developing countries tuberculosis has been so "perfectly" integrated into the general health service that nobody cares about it'.[15] This should be a word of caution for all health planners and programmers.

In HBCs such as India, the TB control programme has been running vertically. They have specifically designated staff with allotted work relating to TB only and there are separate TB control programme officers at state and central governmental level.

However, in some countries, the TB services run within general health facilities and the staff are well trained in the tenets of TB control. Thus, there is hardly any difference between separate TB control units at one end and the TB programme integrated into the general health system at the other. Strengthening the health system is one of the important components of the Stop TB Strategy 2006. There is, therefore, a growing need for the TB programme in the HBCs to strengthen the various aspects of health management, human resources, financial management, logistics delivery and information systems.

The general health system, the National TB Programme and proper links with the private sector could in future enhance the effectiveness of TB control.

At present, strengthening of the public heath system is the priority for all the countries with a high-prevalence of TB. The diagnosis and treatment of TB should be fully integrated into the public health system of most countries. Usually, antituberculosis drug management is integrated into the general drug management system, while the function of the

National TB Programme is quality control of sputum smear microscopy, monitoring and evaluation of the programme.

There is a need for collaboration with the various agencies involved in general health-care planning and coordination amongst the various health development frameworks at central, state and district level. Examples of this include a poverty reduction strategy paper (PRSP), sectorwise approach programme (SWAP) and medium-term expenditure frameworks (MTEFs). TB control now covers other aspects such as a practical approach to lung health (PAL); public–public and public–private mix (PPM) approach, an international standard for TB care,[16] the Patient Charter for Tuberculosis Care and Community TB Care. All of the HPCs have some form of PPM activity in progress.

On the other hand there is a danger that the tendency towards public health sector reform may lead to exclusively peripheral responsibility and patients having to pay for the treatment. As stated by Sir John Crofton, the USA, the richest country in the world, has demonstrated in New York the sort of disaster that can occur when a previously successful service is subsequently neglected.[8]

Priority for TB

TB has ravaged mankind for thousands of years. Hence it has become a part of life and therefore the importance accorded to other diseases, such as cardiac diseases, has not been given to TB. The other factor is that it is a 'poor man's disease'. There are a few advocates for TB sufferers as there is no powerful lobby for better TB care. TB still carries a significant stigma that makes it more invisible as a health problem.[17]

However, TB is no longer a separate area of work but integrated into the strategic objective on HIV/TB and malaria control. The Global Fund for AIDS, TB and Malaria is an example of the priority for AIDS and malaria as well.

Political commitment

The funds allocated for TB over the years in most developing countries has been meagre. One of the reasons is lack of strong political commitment in not only developing countries but also in developed countries, leading to neglect of the disease and a sharp rise in the number of cases. In 1990, the Commission on Health Research for Development stated that, 'The magnitude of the tuberculosis problem is matched only by its relative neglect by the international community'.[18]

Private practitioners

Private practitioners of health belonging to any system, allopathic or otherwise, have close contact with the patients.

Private practitioners form a major proportion of medical services. Most poor countries have large and expanding private medical sectors. Private medical sectors extend from corporate hospitals at one end, to the small nursing home and clinics run by renowned or smaller private practitioners at the other. In developing countries like India, traditional private practitioners or 'quacks' practicising traditional and alternative medicine run successful practices as they are cheap, available in any rural or urban area and are often extremely popular. In India, 80 per cent of households use the private sector for treatment of minor illnesses and 75 per cent of households prefer to visit private sectors for major illness.[19]

For management of TB, the first point of contact in most poor countries is the private practitioner; for example, in India 50 per cent of TB patients are managed by the private sector.[20]

A WHO survey in Mexico revealed that one-third of patients who died of TB were treated by private practitioners.[21]

The management of TB by private practitioners is based on chest x-ray. Sputum for smear microscopy or culture examination is taken less, hence many people in the private sector are not treated according to scientific norms. This is more likely in rural and semi-urban areas where the patients tend to be illiterate, superstitious and amenable to all types of treatment.

It cannot be denied that the private sector is a force to be reckoned with in TB control. Due to their presence in all areas, the private practitioner is valuable to TB control, as he/she is residing in the community. Accessibility and acceptability is therefore easier. They can play a pivotal role in the early detection of a case, ensuring efficient case-holding, minimal default, better compliance due to faith in the private practitioner and better treatment outcome.

The WHO made a global assessment of the participation of private practitioners in the TB programme in 23 countries of the six WHO regions. The role of private practitioners in countries with low, medium and high-prevalence of TB was reviewed. The report highlighted the perception of collaboration of the government at one end and the private practitioners at the other. A comparison was made of the productive involvement of the private sector in TB activities resulting in better TB control. For example, the New York City Tuberculosis Bureau was compared to largely unorganized, less regulated activity in poor countries.[22]

In economically deprived nations, private practitioners can play a meaningful role by being given greater autonomy in the operation of the DOTS programme.

In Ahmedabad and Jamnagar, in the state of Gujarat, India, private practitioners were independently running the DOTS centre in their clinics, while in another city, Delhi, the private practitioners prominently displayed boards stating their association with the Government in free treatment of TB under DOTS.[23]

In India, the Indian Medical Association (IMA) has formed a national cell for the RNTCP and identified coordinators at national and state level. The IMA is a strong medical body in India basically formed of private practitioners, and holds regular meetings and an annual conference. Other organizations, such as the National College of Chest Physicians of India, are formed by specialists in the field of TB and pulmonary medicine. Currently over 14 500 private practitioners are involved in RNTCP.[24]

TB, being a chronic disease, becomes a target for exploitation in various developing countries. Often, the patient spends a great deal of money to receive treatment. Uplekar and Rangan[25] have reported a study of 102 private practitioners in Mumbai. These doctors used 10 different antituberculosis drug combinations in 80 different regimens of varying duration. This not only complicated the regimens of treating simple cases of pulmonary TB, but sharply increases the cost of the medicines to the patients who were often poor. Often, due to the high cost of the antituberculosis drugs, the patients abandon the treatment half way through the course and this leads to drug resistance.

Under the public private mix, the number of private practitioners is critical. Private practitioners belonging to the various systems have been trained and indicated as the 'DOTS provider' in the area. In HBCs such as India, traditional private practitioners are more popular within rural, semi-urban communities. Thus, the success of the DOTs programme is enhanced by these doctors being part of the programme.

Pandemic of HIV/AIDS

Human immunodeficiency virus/acquired immunodeficiency syndrome (HIV/AIDS) is the modern world's principal pandemic. The HIV-propelled emergence of drug-resistant TB is now a cause for serious concern in several countries.[26] Though the association of TB and HIV has long been known, implementation of joint activities were started only in the past 5 years. Initially, in the implementation of the DOTS programme, it was felt that the component of HIV/AIDs might deter the prospective TB patient from approaching TB centres as HIV/AIDS was more stigmatized than TB. However, with the induction of efficient antiretroviral drugs for HIV, the support of various agencies, international donors and the stigma of TB gradually waning, the concept of management of TB and HIV together is gaining importance, especially in the African region.

The WHO policy on collaboration with TB/HIV activities is as follows:[2]

1 The organizational structure should be such that TB/HIV management is part of it.
2 All patients with HIV should be tested for TB. If they test positive, then immediate treatment under DOTS should be instituted and if latent TB is detected than isoniazid prevention therapy (IPT) should be started.

3 All patients suffering from TB should undergo HIV counselling and voluntary testing. If tested positive for HIV then cotrimaxazole preventive therapy (CPT) is given and if the factors point to a serious form of HIV then antiretroviral therapy (ART) may be given.

'We cannot win the battle against AIDS if we do not also fight TB. TB is too often a death sentence for people with AIDS', commented Nelson Mandela at the 2004 XV International AIDS Conference, in Bangkok. TB is often the first disease that an HIV-infected person contracts. An HIV-positive person is six times (50–60 per cent lifetime risk) more likely to develop TB disease once infected as compared to 10 per cent lifetime risk in an HIV-negative person.

The worst affected areas for TB and HIV are Eastern and Southern Africa, South East Asia and the Russian Federation.

Where the HIV infection rate is high, so is TB.

In 2005, South Africa with 0.7 per cent of the world's population had 19 per cent of co-infection, while 10 per cent of co-infected cases were in India. In Africa, the situation is worsening. The African region accounted for 61 per cent of TB and HIV co-infection in 2005. At the same time, in Swaziland, 75 per cent of TB patients were HIV-positive. In 2005, the South East Asia region with a population of approximately 6.26 million had an estimated 2.6 million infected with HIV. Approximately two-thirds of these cases were in India.

The trend of HIV and TB is changing in HPCs (Figure 26.2), such as Thailand, and in four southern states in

TB incidence per 1 00 000

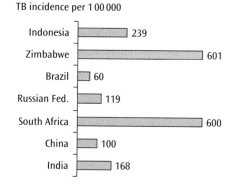

HIV prevalence in TB

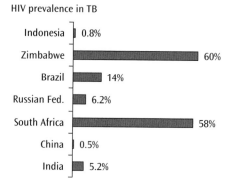

Figure 26.2   Deadly duo (incidence of tuberculosis and HIV in high prevalence countries).

India, the HIV prevalence appears to be decreasing gradually. However, in countries such as Bangladesh and Indonesia, the incidence of HIV is rising amongst high-risk groups, also increasing the incidence of TB.[4]

In the subregion of Africa with high HIV prevalence, TB and HIV prevalence which started to rise in 1990 had started to fall in 2005. Even the peaks in the incidence of the two diseases may show a lag phase. For example, Zimbabwe had the maximum estimated HIV prevalence in 1997, while the highest TB case notification was reported in 2002.

The burden of HIV infection in India is estimated to be 5.22 million (about 0.9 per cent of the adult population), making it the country with the highest number of TB cases in the world. This, in turn, fuels the increase in TB cases. There is, therefore, a need to scale up the TB-HIV collaborative activities.

While TB is curable HIV/AIDS is not, and the treatment time for TB is limited while for people with HIV/AIDS it is life long. Drugs for the treatment of TB are at present affordable, while those for HIV/AIDS are expensive and beyond the reach of many millions of poor. When patients with HIV infection are managed in the same facility as those with TB, it is essential to have effective infection control measures as there is high risk of nosocomial transmission of TB.[27]

In some African counties, for example Kenya, Malawi and Rwanda, HIV testing in TB patients has increased. CPT is being provided to 80 per cent of HIV-positive cases and ART has been instituted in 30 per cent of TB-HIV cases. In fact, the number of patients on ART in the African region increased 40-fold between 2003 and 2005. CPT is also provided at the periphery of health services, while ART, which is expensive, is available in hospital and only a few areas have it.[2]

The progress of screening HIV cases for TB has been slow, but in countries like Botswana, it is being carried out effectively and IPT is provided on a large scale. Death in TB-HIV co-infection is common and it has been observed that in Africa the death rate in smear-positive cases was higher in 2004 than in other WHO regions, probably due to high HIV prevalence.

In India, coordination activities in states with a high-prevalence of HIV (Andhra Pradesh, Karnataka, Maharashtra, Manipur, Nagaland and Tamil Nadu) were scaled up. From January to December 2006, the number of patients referred from ICTC to RNTCP increased by 114 per cent compared to 2005. Provision of ART to HIV-positive TB patients is provided in 85 centres in India.[24]

MULTIDRUG-RESISTANT TUBERCULOSIS

Multidrug-resistant TB (MDR-TB) is defined as resistance to isoniazid and rifampicin, with or without resistance to other antituberculosis drugs. The emergence of a strain of *M. tuberculosis* resistant to antimicrobial agents is a world-wide issue. Development of drug resistance is largely a reflection of poor management of TB cases and poses a threat to TB control in HPCs.

The phenomenon of a drug-resistant strain of TB currently accounts for 10 per cent of all new TB infections. The management of MDR-TB is very expensive for resource-poor countries. The causes of drug resistance are due to lapses on the part of the patient, the health system or the drug itself. The available data show 1–3 per cent MDR-TB amongst new cases and 13–17 per cent amongst the treated cases in India.[24]

Under the Stop TB Strategy and Global Plan, control of MDR-TB would include drug-resistant surveys and treatment of MDR-TB as a standard component of all TB control programmes.

The Green Light Committee (GLC) constituted by the WHO approves the management of MDR-TB under the DOTS-Plus strategy.[28] In 2006, the GLC approved 53 projects for more than 25 000 MDR-TB patients in 42 countries, which include most of the countries with a high-prevalence of TB.[2] In 2007, under the global plan, it is estimated that 20 000 in 2006 and 36 000 MDR-TB cases will be treated according to the international standard. The number of reported MDR-TB cases continues to grow due to better diagnostic methods. The proportion of treated cases under the GLC is expected to rise from 35 per cent in 2006 to 47 per cent in 2007.

In the HBCs, the number of GLC-approved, DOTS-Plus programmes are rapidly increasing largely due to funding from the Global Fund for AIDS, Tuberculosis and Malaria (GFATM) and following the guidelines of the Stop TB Strategy, these DOTS-Plus programmes are being integrated into the National TB Control activities.

In GLC-approved projects, the treatment success rate for MDR-TB patients is 57 per cent. A few have reported higher treatment success rates averaging 70 per cent (77 per cent amongst new cases and 69 per cent in previously treated cases).[29]

The global incidence of MDR-TB cases has been estimated at over 400 000, of which many are inadequately treated, undiagnosed and not treated at all. The first priority in any country remains prevention of acquired drug resistance through effective implementation of DOTS.

With the challenge of a growing pool of patients with MDR-TB, high-burden countries require better national laboratories with efficient quality control to diagnose patients with MDR-TB. In this regard, the RNTCP in India aims to establish a network of accredited quality-assured intermediate reference laboratories (IRLs). It is planned to have at least one accredited IRL in each of the large states by 2009–10 and 24 state IRLs will be established in India by the end of RNTCP phase II (2010–11). The laboratory will be under the National Reference Laboratories (NRLs). At present there are three NRLs in Chennai, New Delhi and Bangalore.[24]

The continuous supply of reserve-line TB drugs has to be ensured for proper management of MDR-TB. By the end of 2006, UNITAID will increase by three countries the areas to receive second-line antituberculosis drugs. UNI-TAID offers long-term support through sustainable and predictable funding and facilitates access to high-quality antituberculosis drugs and diagnostics for HIV and TB.[2]

Economic constraints, manpower shortages, unimaginative implementation of DOTS, inefficient TB infection control measures even in health-care settings, and inadequate TB drug resistance surveillance are leading to further problems of extreme drug-resistant TB (XDR-TB), largely in countries with a high-prevalence of TB.

XDR-TB is defined as TB that is resistant to rifampicin and isoniazid, as well as two other drugs (a member of the fluroquinolone class and at least one of the three amino-glycosides (capreomycin, kanamycin and amikacin)).

The outbreak of XDR-TB in Tugela Ferry, a rural town in Kwazulu Natal province of South Africa occurred in 2005. A total of 53 of the 1539 patients surveyed were extensively drug resistant (XDR). Of these 53, 52 patients died; all of them tested HIV positive. There was a median survival of 16 days from the time of diagnosis.[30]

The emerging threat of XDR-TB is not limited to South Africa but as reported by Dr Paul Nunn, one or more cases have been found in at least 28 countries. Two-thirds of these cases are from China, India and Russia. Globally about 6 per cent of resistant TB cases are resistant to some second-line drugs – 15 per cent in the former Soviet Union.[31]

The new strain (XDR-TB) is virtually untreatable and the spread of this form of TB poses a serious threat to the control programmes of TB and could even reverse recent gains in the field. The expense of controlling such a public health problem is immense.[32]

ADVENT OF DOTS

The Director General of the WHO declared on 24 March 1997 that 'the DOTS strategy represents the most important public health breakthrough of the decade, in terms of lives which will be saved'.[33] DOTS is the most effective strategy available for controlling the TB epidemic today. Even though DOTS is an important breakthrough, the principles of DOTS are not new. It is a product of India's long and distinguished tradition of TB research. Many principles of the DOTS strategy which are now in operation were first documented in India, but sadly it is a classic example of research material not being applied where it is most needed.

The Tuberculosis Research Centre, Chennai, India, had established the necessity and feasibility of treatment supervision in the community and the efficiency of directly observed intermittent treatment. Simultaneously the National Tuberculosis Institute, Bangalore, documented the efficacy and feasibility of case detection by sputum microscopy in the 1960s. It showed that technicians in the periphery can perform sputum microscopy if they are given minimal training and regular supervision. The scheme recommended the use of sputum microscopy as the primary tool for diagnosis of TB. Furthermore, it demonstrated that even with limited facilities most TB patients make use of the care at health facilities, indicating that active case finding is not necessary.[34]

All these aspects formed the essential principles underlying the DOTS strategy, which were later developed and propagated by Dr Karl Styblo, Scientific Director of the International Union against TB and Lung diseases. He combined these components into a powerful treatment system, affordable for developing countries and which ensured monitoring, supervision and accountability for every patient. Styblo found 'that a well-organized outpatient chemotherapy scheme, especially if provided free of charge, will attract symptomatic patients from far and wide'.[35] He showed that this system could provide effective TB treatment and would be affordable for developing countries.[11] In Tanzania, where Styblo first tested his system, cure rates increased from 30–40 per cent to 80 per cent. Even more impressive was the fact that these results were achieved for a very small additional cost. In addition, DOTS has been shown to be highly cost-effective.

The DOTS or the Revised National TB Control Programme in India is the second largest such programme in the world. To date, the programme has trained over half a million staff within the health system, evaluated more than 24 million people with suspected TB, examined more than 100 million sputum slides, treated more than 6.7 million patients and prevented almost 1.2 million TB deaths.[24]

The components of DOTS

The various components of DOTS are given in Table 26.2. The DOTS strategy takes sound technology – the successful components of TB control – and packages it with good management practices for widespread use through the existing primary health-care network.

It has proved to be a successful, innovative approach to TB control in countries such as China, Bangladesh, Vietnam, Peru and countries of West Africa.

The technical, logistical, operational and political aspects of DOTS work together to ensure its success and applicability in a wide variety of contexts. Case detection and diagnosis is through the sputum microscopy of the acid-fast bacilli (AFB). Sputum smear microscopy is the most cost-effective, reliable, rapid method of screening suspected cases of pulmonary TB, especially in developing countries which have a high burden of TB cases. Out of all TB cases, 50–60 per cent are sputum smear-positive pulmonary, 35–40 per cent are sputum smear-negative pulmonary cases and 10–15 per cent extrapulmonary cases.[36]

The goal of the programme is that all suspects having respiratory symptoms should have three sputum smears examined by microscopy and all patients diagnosed with TB be registered and treated.

Table 26.2 Technical, logistical, operational and political aspects of DOTS.

Technical	Case detection and diagnosis
	Standardized short-course treatment
	Direct observation of Treatment
	Recording and reporting of progress and cure
Logistical	Regular and effective drug supply to the patient
	Backup of Laboratories for microscopy work
	Supervision and training of health care workers
Operational	Flexibility in implementation of technical aspect

Short-course chemotherapy (SCC) is the treatment regimen using a combination of effective antituberculosis drugs for a duration of 6–8 months. The treatment can be given on a daily regimen or intermittently (three times weekly) as in China and India.

There are several barriers to the implementation of the DOTS programme and their potential solutions for health-care workers and the community are outlined in Table 26.3.[37]

The recording and reporting system is elaborate and time-consuming, but a small amount of paperwork ensures accountability to the health service. The sample forms and formats of the tuberculosis laboratory registers, patient treatment cards, quarterly reports on new cases and relapses of TB and quarterly reports on results of treatment of pulmonary TB patients registered 12–15 months earlier which are used in India are shown in Figures 26.3–26.9 (pp. 466–475).

DISTRICT TB REGISTERS

The register is used to monitor progress and treatment outcome of all patients in the district. In India, one health worker and a laboratory technician are responsible for one centre per 100 000 population and five such centres constitute one TB unit. Each district TB centre covers between 500 000 and 1 million people. Supervision is one of the most critical elements of DOTS. Each unit is supervised by a supervisory TB worker and a supervisory laboratory worker.

THE LABORATORY REGISTERS

The laboratory registers are maintained in each centre by the laboratory technician and the operation of the laboratory is monitored by supervisory staff. All the TB suspects submit two spot samples and one overnight sample of sputum at the centre and, depending on the result, the treatment is instituted. At the end of the intensive phase (2 months), nearly 85–90 per cent of all new smear-positive cases normally become sputum smear-negative. Conversion of smear positivity to smear negativity after the initial 2 months is the most effective way of assessing if the patient has regularly taken the treatment or requires more drugs.

THE PATIENT TREATMENT CARDS

The patient cards are provided in each centre. The card records basic epidemiological, clinical information and drugs administered. Each person diagnosed to be suffering from TB along with his/her sputum status (smear-positive or smear-negative), pulmonary or extrapulmonary disease is recorded on the patient treatment card. This card provides information

Table 26.3 Barriers to effective tuberculosis control programme and possible solutions.

	Tuberculosis control programme	Health-care workers	Patient and community
Sociocultural barriers	Qualitative studies Health education and information	Training on communication with patients	Studies on perception and attitude to care Involvement of support Identification of special groups (migrants, displaced individuals, refugees, etc.) and assessment of needs
Economic barriers	Integration of tuberculosis control into public health-care services		Free diagnostic and care services
Geographical and environmental barriers	Decentralization of diagnostic and treatment services		Diagnostic and treatment services accessible to remote areas Community-based care
Health system barriers	Ensure health-care delivery at district level Ensure adequate supervision	Capacity strengthening	Choice of treatment (DOTS) supporter

REVISED NATIONAL TUBERCULOSIS CONTROL PROGRAMME

Tuberculosis Register

Quarter : _____ Year : _____

TB. No.	Date of regis- tration	Name (In full)	Sex M / F	Age	Complete address	Name of Treatment Centre	Date of starting treatment	Regimen/ Category	Disease class Pulm./ xpulm. (P/EP)	Type of Patient						
										New case (N)	Relapse (R)	Trans- fer (T)	Failure (F)	Treat- ment after default (D)	Other (O)	

SUMMARY								
New smear-positive		Relapse		Smear-negative		Extra-pulmonary		
M	F	M	F	M	F	M	F	

Figure 26.3 Tuberculosis register.

on regularity of the patient in coming to the centre, taking the DOT, any treatment interruption and the measures taken to ensure adherence to the treatment. Finally, the card records the outcome at the end of continuation phase: cured (if the sputum smear is negative) or completed (if no sputum sample is available at the end of 6 or 8 months). The patient identity card, given to the patient, acts as a reminder to the patient about visits to the centre and all relevant information regarding the centre and sputum status.

QUARTERLY REPORTING

Quarterly reporting provides simple but revealing information pertaining to various indicators of treatment progress and treatment success.

Finally, cohort analysis is undertaken to evaluate the effectiveness of the TB control activity in the district, city, state or country. Cohort analysis is a key management tool referring to the systematic follow up of the patient and his outcome.

Stop TB strategy

In 2006, the Stop TB strategy was introduced.[38] The strategy is an extension of the original DOTS strategy (Table 26.4). The strategy addresses several issues connected with TB which were not clearly outlined when DOTS was ini-

Table 26.4 Components of the Stop TB strategy.

1. Pursuing high-quality DOTS expansion and enhancement
2. Adressing TB/HIV, MDR-TB and other challenges
3. Contributing to health system strengthening
4. Engaging all care providers
5. Empowering people with tuberculosis within communities
6. Enabling and promoting research

tially introduced. Thus an extension of DOTS, the Stop TB strategy has incorporated issues of TB/HIV, MDR-TB, issues relating to prisons and other high-risk groups, strengthening the health system through innovative measures to yield more coverage and provide quality TB care. The Stop TB strategy envisages more active community participation and community ownership of the programme. Finally, the strategy hopes to encourage operational research and future resources aimed at newer diagnosic techniques and more research into new drugs for the treatment and prevention of TB.

CHALLENGES IN THE DOTS PROGRAMME

Treatment observation

Treatment observation is not simply the supervision of patients taking antituberculosis drugs. The treatment

REVISED NATIONAL TUBERCULOSIS CONTROL PROGRAMME   II

Tuberculosis Register

Sputum examination								Date when treatment was stopped						Remarks
Pretreatment		End of I.P.*		2 months in C.P.**		End of treatment		Cured	Treatment completed	Died	Failiure	Defaulted	Transferred out	
0 months		2 or 3 months		4 or 5 or 6 months		6 or 7 or 8 or 9 months								
Smear	Lab No.	Smear	Lab No.	Smear	Lab No.	Smear	Lab No.							

* I. P. Intensive Phase

** C.P. Continuation Phase

Type of patient	Cured	Treatment completed	Died	Failure	Defaulted	Transferred
New smear-positive						
New smear-negative						
New extra-pulmonary						
Relapse (smear-positive)						
Failure (smear-positive)						
Treatment After Default (smear-positive)						
Others treated with CAT II						

Figure 26.3   Continued

observation succeeds by building a human bond between the patient and the treatment organizer as the patient is constantly in touch with him/her for the total duration of his/her treatment period. The treatment observation should be taken as a service to the patient and if there is a good link between the two will ensure a high cure rate, thereby protecting the family of the patients and the community at large and ensuring success of the programme.

Supervision and monitoring

The key to success of the programme lies in effective supervision at all levels. Monitoring and supervision is a process of detecting any problem in the implementation of the programme, introducing remedial methods and helping the staff to improve their performance. There are various key areas where supervision can be a matter of routine, and is both effective and vital. These areas include laboratory work, direct observation, patient categorization, drug storage, record keeping and reporting. Supervision in the RNTCP in India is carried out at every level – supervisory staff includes the senior TB supervisor and senior TB laboratory supervisor responsible for an area with a population of 500 000, who in turn are supervised by the medical officers of the units. Thus, from the subunit to district, state and national level an efficient system exists whereby monitoring and supervision is effectively performed.

Default (treatment interruption)

One of the major impediments in the control of TB worldwide is default (treatment interruption). It has been repeatedly proven that at least one-third of patients do not take the full course of medicines, even if the medicines are available without cost, treatment is convenient and adequate health education is given.[39,40] Various attempts have been made to assess the extent of the problem of treatment interruption by patients and to determine the reasons for this. These include low literacy rate, low monthly income, large family size, loss of wages, inconvenient clinic timings, long waiting hours and non-availability of medicines. Other reasons cited include impolite behaviour of staff,[41] social belief, social stigma,[42] poor knowledge about disease amongst patients and inadequate understanding of the treatment regimes.[43]

Discontinuation of treatment for TB may be due to disappearance of symptoms, such as pyrexia and loss of appetite, and the return of a sense of general well-being. These factors occurring after 6–8 weeks of effective antituberculous treatment cause the patient to leave the medication half way through treatment. 'It is only natural to enjoy the recovery and stop taking medication'.[44]

A recent report stated that the default rate amongst those treated by the DOTS strategy programme was less than one-quarter compared to those treated in a non-DOTS, unsupervised programme (11 and 58 per cent,

REVISED NATIONAL TUBERCULOSIS CONTROL PROGRAMME

Laboratory Register

Year _____

Lab Serial No.	Date	Name (in full)	Sex M / F	Age	Complete address (for new patients)	Name of Referring Health Centre	Reason for Examination*		Results			Signature	Remarks
							Diagnosis	Follow-up	1	2	3		

* If sputum is for diagnosis, put a tick (✓) mark in the space under 'Diagnosis'.
If sputum is for follow-up of patients on treatment, write the patient's TB no. in the space under 'Follow-up'.

Figure 26.4   Laboratory register.

respectively). The default rate of patients in short-course therapy with directly observed strategy was 10 per cent compared with 39 per cent for patients not on directly observed treatment.[45]

Adherence/compliance

Compliance to treatment is the key word in the management and outcome of TB. Other terms, such as 'adherence'[46] and 'concordance'[47] have been introduced to signify that the action on the part of the patient to take treatment and continue it until the end of the course depends on multiple factors. Smith[48] has propounded the 'hold chain' model (Figure 26.10, page 476)). The hold chain model for adherence is a summation of directly observed therapy, effective therapy education, quality service, training and supervision, and logistics. This intricate link is delicate and any break in the link would result in loss of treatment concordance. Thus, the term 'hold' refers to 'not to holding the patient on treatment, but to holding the health service together'.

In a study in Kathmandu, Nepal,[49] regarding factors affecting patient adherence to DOTS, availability of daily health education and knowledge about TB treatment was an important factor in compliance. The reasons for non-adherence were due to not being told to take treatment regularly (35.6 per cent) and the patient thinking they were cured prematurely (25.4 per cent). Other factors of non-adherence were long distance, resulting in increased travel cost (6.8 per cent), non-friendly TB staff (3.4 per cent), inconvenient opening of DOTS (15.2 per cent) and side effects of TB drugs (13.6 per cent).

Similar opinion is expressed in other studies in Malaysia,[50] Ethopia,[51] Tanzania,[52] Gambia[53] and India.[54] A study in South Africa[55] has reported regular interaction by voluntary work and TB staff improved compliance to DOTS treatment. In the USA,[56] detention for non-adherence by patients has also been used as a deterrent for the patient to prevent treatment interruption.

Alcoholics, drug addicts, the destitute and the homeless are more prone to abandon treatment before completion. Patients who fall into these groups are difficult to tackle, hence 'soft' and 'hard' tactics are used for maintenance of regular treatment.

Motivation of patients by those who have already completed treatment, reminder cards and regular, frequent and intensive supervision by health workers may contribute to lowering treatment interruption and increase the patient adherence to treatment.[57]

There is no single factor or strategy to improve the treatment adherence, but there is no doubt that treating the patient as a VIP (a user friendly approach) would go a long way in curing the patient.

It has been observed that achieving treatment adherence is not an easy task, both for the patient and the provider, but the dreadful outcome of worsening disease, continued infectiousness and multidrug resistance can result from non-adherence to treatment.

ISSUE IN CONTROL OF TB IN HIGH-PREVALENCE COUNTRIES

Advocacy, communication and social mobilization

The sustainability of any programme lies with acceptance by the community. The community must own the programme for a better, more efficient outcome. The community and health workers must work in close cooperation for improved, productive interaction. Advocacy, communication and social mobilization involves a large area which interconnects the entire TB control network with the aim of improving the TB control strategy. These links include the health provider, community volunteer, mass media, non-governmental organizations and such related sectors as education, communication economics, professional societies, political authorities (national, state, local) and TB patients' associations.

Involvement and training of medical professionals and bodies and creating partnership with various medical and other bodies to build influence, monitor health policies and increase the sustainability of the social mobilization activity is important. Any activities carried out should be assessed for their impact on the community.[58]

Food supplement

Food support is implemented in various countries as an incentive for the patient to attend the TB centres. The World Food Programme (WFP) has been providing food to all TB cases in Cambodia since 1998. Food is also provided to TB patients in hospital.

In Malawi, Zambia and Uganda, food is provided to TB patients during their visit to TB centres and their weight is monitored for the effect of food on their general health.

Food assistance is provided by WFP as a regular food ration to TB patients in hospital in Chechnya and Burkina Faso. In Lesotho, Sudan and Tajikistan, only those patients who are considered food insecure usually benefit from food assistance.

In India, Rama Krishna Mission, a non-governmental organization provides food to all patients attending their TB centres in a slum area of New Delhi. The measure has increased compliance to treatment (unpublished data).

The WFP is a UNAIDS lead agency in nutrition and dietary support for people living with HIV in food-insecure situations. The WFP has HIV programmes in 53 countries and supports TB programmes in 20 countries. The first objective of the WFP, food assistance in the Stop TB strategy, is to help patients in food-insecure households to meet their nutritional needs during the period of treatment. The choice of the beneficiaries depend on an assessment of the local food security situation, objective of the food support, socioeconomic characteristics of potential beneficiaries, the logistics

REVISED NATIONAL TUBERCULOSIS CONTROL PROGRAMME

Treatment Card

TB01

State : _____ City/District : _____

Name : _____ Sex :M ☐ F ☐ Age : _____

Complete Address : _____

Code district/subdistrict _____

Patient TB No./year : _____

Health Unit : _____

Name of DOT provider : _____

Name and Address of Contact Person : _____

Disease Classification

☐ Pulmonary

☐ Extra-pulmonary

Site : _____

Type of Patient

☐ New ☐ Relapse

☐ Transfer in ☐ Failure

☐ Treatment after default ☐ Other (Specify) _____

Month	Date	Lab. No.	Smear result	Weight
0				
2/3				
4/5/6				
6/7/8/9				

1. INITIAL INTENSIVE PHASE—Prescribed regimen and dosages:

Tick (✓) the appropriate Category below :

Category I ☐

New Case

(pulmonary smear-positive, seriously ill smear-negative, or seriously ill extra-pulmonary)

Category II ☐

Retreatment

(relapse, failure, treatment after default)

Category III ☐

New case

(pulmonary smear-negative, not seriously ill, or extra-pulmonary, not seriously ill))

Write number of tablets or dose of streptomycin in the boxes below :

3 times / week | 3 times / week | 3 times / week

H R Z E | H R Z E S | H R Z

H: Isoniazid   R:Rifampicin   Z:Pyrazinamide   E:Ethambutol   S:Streptomycin

Tick (✓) appropriate date when the drugs have been swallowed under direct observation. :

Month Day	1	2	3	4	5	6	7	8	9	10	11	12	13	14	15	16	17	18	19	20	21	22	23	24	25	26	27	28	29	30	31

(a)

Figure 26.5 Treatment card. (a) Initial intensive phase; (b) continuation phase.

II. CONTINUATION PHASE
(See Guidelines)

II

Prescribed regimen and dosages

Category I ☐

New Case

(pulmonary smear-positive, seriously ill smear-negative, or seriously ill extra-pulmonary)

Write number of tablets per dose in the boxes below :

3 times / week

H	R

Category II ☐

Retreatment

(relapse, failure, treatment after default)

3 times / week

H	R	E

Category III ☐

New case

(pulmonary smear-negative, not seriously ill, or extra-pulmonary, not seriously ill)

3 times / week

H	R

Enter 'X' on date when the first dose of drugs has been swallowed under direct observation and draw a horizontal line (X ———) to indicate the period during which medicine will be self-administered.

Month / Day	1	2	3	4	5	6	7	8	9	10	11	12	13	14	15	16	17	18	19	20	21	22	23	24	25	26	27	28	29	30	31

Remarks :

(b)

Figure 26.5   Continued

Treatment Outcome					
Cured	Tr Completed	Died	Failure	Deflt.	Trans. Out

REVISED NATIONAL TUBERCULOSIS CONTROL PROGRAMME
TUBERCULOSIS IDENTITY CARD

District T. B. No.

Regd. No. _____ Date _____

Name _____

Complete Address _____

_____

Sex : M _____ F _____ Age _____ Wt. _____ Kg.

Health Centre _____

_____

REMEMBER

1. Take care of your card.
2. Bring the card on every visit.
3. Pegular intake of all medicines as per doctor's advice for 6-8 months ensure full cure.
4. Premature stoppage of medicine or irregular treatment may lead to recurrence and treatment failure.
5. Untreated you may infect many others.

Disease Classification
Pulmonary _____
Extrapulmonary _____
(Site) _____
Sputum _____

Date Treatment Started :

Date	Month	Year

Type of Patient
New _____ Relapse _____
Transfer in _____ Other _____
Treatment _____ (Specify) _____
After Default _____ Failure _____

Type of Treatment

Cat-I	Cat-II	Cat-III

Drugs Patient is Receiving :
Initial Intensive Phase

_____

_____

_____

Continuation Phase

_____

_____

Appointment Dates

Figure 26.6 Tuberculosis identity card.

capacity needed for food delivery and available resources.

Funds

The total cost of TB control in the 22 countries with a high-prevalence of TB was US$644 million in 2002 and the projected budget for 2007 is US$1.7 billion. The Russian Federation and South Africa has the highest share (US$ 829 million). China, India, Brazil and Indonesia are the other four countries with the maximum budget for TB control. These six countries account for 78 per cent of the total cost of TB control amongst 22 HBCs. The budget per patient, which includes the cost of the antituberculosis drug and all line items, is variable. In India, Pakistan and Ethiopia, the budget per patient is less than US$100, while in the Russian Federation it is US$1000 per patient.

The budget for the National Tuberculosis Programme (NTP) increased sharply from 2002 to 2007. In 2007, the total budget estimated for the HBCs is US$1.25 billion as compared to US$509 million budgeted in 2002. Funding for the NTP budget for 2007 is US$1 billion which had increased by US$592 million since 2002. Among all 22 HBCs, Kenya and Vietnam have projected their budget for 2007 and it is less than that in 2002.

The GFATM has funds allocated to all HBCs and this amounts to US$168 million. Thus, the total fund in 2007 is US$758 million (61 per cent) provided by the national government and US$241 million (19 per cent) funding provided by donors – resulting in a funding gap of 20 per cent (US$ 251 million). The funding deficit is in Afghanistan, Cambodia, Democratic Republic of Congo, Kenya, Mozambique, Myanmar and Pakistan.[2]

REVISED NATIONAL TUBERCULOSIS CONTROL PROGRAMME

Quarterly Report on Programme Management and Logistics
District Level

Name of the District:_____   Quarter:_____

Number of Tuberculosis Units planned in the District: _____   Year:_____

Number of Tuberculosis Units operational in the District: _____

Total population of the District: _____

Population of the District covered by the RNTCP: _____

The following reports are enclosed (Tick [✓] to indicate that report is enclosed)

☐ Quarterly Report on Case-Finding (number of TB Units reporting*: _____)

☐ Quarterly Report on Sputum Conversion (number of TB Units reporting*: _____)

☐ Quarterly Report on Treatment Outcomes (number of TB Units reporting*: _____)

* If any TB Unit did not report, list name(s) and report(s): _____

Supervisory Activities by the Staff of the DTC

Type of Unit	Number in the District	Number participating in the RNTCP	Number of these visited during quarter
TB Unit			
Government Hospital			
Sanitorium/TB Hospital			
PHC			
CHC			
BPHC			
Microscopy Centre			
Treatment Centre			
Patient's Home			
Other:_____			

Microscopy Activities (all Tuberculosis Units Including the DTC)

(a)	Number of new adult outpatient visits in health facilities	
(b)	Out of (a), number of chest symptomatic **patients** whose sputum was examined for diagnosis	
(c)	Out of (b), number of smear-positive **patients** diagnosed	

Treatment Initiation (all Tuberculosis Units Including the DTC)

(d)	Of the number of smear-positive patients diagnosed (c), the number who reside within the district	
(e)	Of the smear-positive patients diagnosed who reside within the district (d), number put on DOTS	
(f)	Of the number of smear-positive patients diagnosed who reside within the district (d), number put on treatment other than DOTS	
(g)	Initial defaulters among smear-positive patients diagnosed and residing within the district (g = d − e − f)	

Activities of Community Volunteers

Number of Community Volunteers engaged during quarter: _____

Number of Community Volunteers paid during quarter: _____

Total amount paid to Community Volunteers during quarter: Rs _____

Figure 26.7 Quarterly report on programme management and logistics: district level.

REVISED NATIONAL TUBERCULOSIS CONTROL PROGRAMME

Quarterly Report on New and Retreatment Cases of Tuberculosis

Patients registered during _____ quarter* of 19_____

Name of Reporter:_____

Name of area _____ No.#_____

Signature:_____

Date of completion of this form

				1	9	
d	d	m	m			

Block 1: All patients registered in the quarter

Pulmonary tuberculosis						Extra-pulmonary tuberculosis (4)		Total (5)		
Smear-positive				Smear-negative (3)						
New cases (1)			Relapses (2)							
M	F	Total	M	F	M	F	M	F	M	F	Total

Block 2: Smear-positive New cases only: from Column (1) above

Age-group (years)															Total		
0–14		15–24		25–34		35–44		45–54		55–64		65 and above					
M	F	M	F	M	F	M	F	M	F	M	F	M	F	M	F	Total

Block 3: All patients started on treatment

Type of patient	Category I		Category II		Category III		Total
	smear-positive	smear-negative extra-pulmonary	smear-positive	smear-negative	smear-negative	extra-pulmonary	
New							
Relapses							
Failures							
Treatment After Default							
Others							
Total							

Notes: *Quarters: 1st quarter   January, February, March
2nd quarter   April, May, June
3rd quarter   July, August, September
4th quarter   October, November, December

#Number   Identification number of the area

12/97

How to fill in the form

Block 1: New cases and relapses of tuberculosis registered during_____ quarter of (year)_____ (*Fill in the quarter and the year.*)

Column (1):   Smear-positive new cases   Patients with sputum smear-positive pulmonary tuberculosis who have never recieved anti-tuberculosis treatment or have recieved treatment for less than 4 weeks.

Column (2):   Smear-positive relapses   Patients with sputum smear-positive pulmonary tuberculosis who were declared cured by a Medical Officer but have now got the disease.

Column (3):   Smear-negative cases   Patients with pulmonary tuberculosis with 3 sputum samples negative for AFB, in whom the diagnosis of tuberculosis was made by means other than sputum microscopy.

Column (4):   Extra-pulmonary tuberculosis   Patients with tuberculosis of organs other than the lungs.

Column (5):   Total   Males   Add all male patients in columns 1+2+3+4
Females   Add all female patients in columns 1+2+3+4
Total   Add all patients (males+females) in columns 1+2+3+4

Block 2: Smear-positive new cases: from Column (1) above.

In this block enter the patients already recorded in Block 1, Column (1) according to their sex and age group. If the exact age of the patient is not known at the time of his/her registration it should be estimated to the nearest 5 years (e.g. 15, 20, 25, etc.).

Block 3: This gives category-wise break up of treatment regimens for new patients (both smear-positive and smear-negative), relapses, failures, return to treatment after default (TAD), and patients who are classified as Others.

Figure 26.8   Quarterly report on new and retreatment cases of tuberculosis.

Paediatric tuberculosis

Children constitute a major proportion of the population, especially in South East Asian countries. TB is prevalent in children, though it is generally less infectious than in adults. Yet it is a primary cause of morbidity and mortality. Serious forms of TB, such as tubercular meningitis, are still prevalent in poor countries and causes death or serious disability. It is estimated that in India 6–8 per cent of all new TB cases occur in the paediatric age group; mainly in the 1- to 4-year age group.[24]

The source of infection to children is sputum smear-positive adults who disseminate the disease to their children. The diagnosis of TB is difficult as children swallow the sputum and so the bacterial yield is low. Because

REVISED NATIONAL TUBERCULOSIS CONTROL PROGRAMME

Quarterly Report of Sputum Conversion of
New Cases, Relapses and Failures

Patients registered during

_____ quarter of 19_____

Name of area: _____

No._____

Name of Reporter: _____   Signature: _____

Date of completion of this form: | | | | | 1 | 9 | | |

d   d   m   m

Complete this proforma for sputum smear-positive patients. The total number should be the same as in the Quarterly Report on New and Retreatment Cases of Tuberculosis.

Total number of new sputum-positive patients	Sputum at 2 months			Sputum at 3 months		
	Negative	Positive	N.A.	Negative	Positive	N.A.

Total number of smear-positive relapse patients	Sputum at 3 months		
	Negative	Positive	N.A.

Total number of smear-positive failure patients	Sputum at 3 months		
	Negative	Positive	N.A.

N.A. – Not available; sputum examination was not done.

12/97

Figure 26.9   Quarterly report of sputum conversion of new cases, relapses and failures.

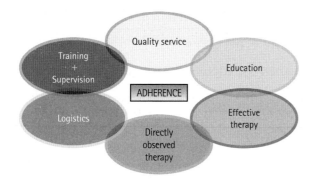

Figure 26.10 The hold chain. (1) Quality service: appropriate, accessible, acceptable, equitable, efficient and effective service; (2) Training and supervision: to ensure that all health workers develop and maintain the skills needed to manage patients with tuberculosis; (3) Logistics: The system that ensures a continuous and uninterrupted supply of medicine to all treatment centres; (4) Directly observed therapy: a means of ensuring a continuous supply of treatment is made available to the patient together with the encouragement and information to assist him/her take that treatment until cured; (5) Effective therapy: drugs that rapidly render the patient non-infectious and cure them, without producing significant adverse effects. (6) Education: empowering patients, their relatives, and their communities with understanding about their disease, its cure and its prevention.

children are less infectious than adults, the management of TB is accorded low priority in the 22 HBCs.

The Mantoux test, or tuberculin skin test, still remains a major tool in the diagnosis of paediatric tuberculosis.

Public–private partnership

The PPM has been accepted by the HBCs as a link between TB control and the general health system. Eleven HBCs (Bangladesh, China, Democratic Republic of Congo, India, Indonesia, Kenya, Mozambique, Myanmar, Philippines, Tanzania and Vietnam) have implemented the programme. Only the Russian Federation is yet to involve the private sector. These activities yield excellent results, as they are not only improving access to care for the poor but also reducing total costs to the patient.[59]

Future of TB control programme in high-prevalence countries

Three important issues will dominate the future of TB in HBCs.

1   Newer diagnostic techniques: a sputum smear-positive case of TB infects 10–15 people every year. Late diagnosis of the disease not only increases the morbidity of the case, but also increases the dissemination of the disease;

hence, the need for early diagnosis. A rider to the problem is the sputum smear-negative patient. The diagnosis of such a person and to provide early treatment to stop the disease from advancing further. A rapid and accurate diagnostic tool for TB could save up to 625 000 lives each year.[60] An accurate and authentic (highly specific and sensitive) method is needed, which is convenient to use (even by an untrained health worker) and inexpensive, so that it can be widely used in endemic countries. The present diagnostic criteria have certain limitations. The sputum microscopy for AFB can only demonstrate the bacilli in 50 per cent of cases. The conventional culture method uses Lowenstein– Jensen media and shows positivity on culture after 6 weeks. Radiometric diagnostic methods are expensive and not readily affordable for the poor patient.

The tuberculin skin test cannot differentiate between infection and disease and in countries with a high-prevalence of TB, the value of the tuberculin skin test is diminished as the infection rate in these countries is high. x-Rays as a diagnostic tool are non-specific and subjective. Radiographically, TB can mimic any lung disease. The need for better and newer diagnostic techniques grows as the problem of HIV rises. Sputum for AFB in the HIV-infected patient is usually negative and the tuberculin skin test gives a low positive rate due to the patient's depressed immune state. Compounding this is the problem of MDR-TB and XDR-TB in HIV patients. The rising problem of drug resistance can be limited by early diagnosis, early treatment and cure. The Foundation for Innovative New Diagnostics (FIND) created by the Bill and Melinda Gates Foundation is working on the evaluation and demonstration of new molecular techniques and demonstration projects for the liquid culture mycobacterium growth indicator tube (MGIT) system. In addition, rapid antigen detection is based on identification of lipoarabinomannan (LAM) in urine and trials are going on in Tanzania. Evaluation of interferon-γ release assays is another area of investigation. Fluorescence microscopes are being developed to improve the smear test to make them more sensitive. These sensitive, low-cost, user-friendly fluorescent microscopes will not be available until 2009. In Bangladesh, Peru and Tanzania, feasibility studies with loop-mediated isothermal amplification (LAMP) techniques are being tested on a pilot basis. Sadly, the funds available for a new test in 2005 was a meagre US$16.5 million.[61]

2   Newer antituberculosis drugs: if the problem of compliance, drug default, long duration of treatment, issue of drug side effects, compatibility with HIV drugs and fear of drug resistance is to be avoided, then it is imperative to have newer antituberculosis drugs. If the present duration of antituberculosis drugs (first-line DOTS) taken for 6 months is reduced to a period of weeks to 3–4 months, then it will go a long way towards increasing compliance and adherence to the treatment.

Further, certain drugs, such as rifampicin, interact with antiretroviral drugs (nevirapine) which are commonly used in economically poor countries. Such a combination may promote resistance or if doses are not adjusted may lead to toxicity. In such situations, newer antituberculosis drugs which do not interact with any antiretrovirals could be used in Africa and South East Asian nations, where HIV and TB is rampant. Finally, it should be borne in mind that the standard four-drug regimen has a cure rate of 95 per cent. Hence, any new drug discovered should have high efficacy and be extremely safe for use anywhere.

3 Vaccines: the only vaccine to prevent TB was developed 86 years back by Albert Calmette and Camilla Guérin. This vaccine is a live attenuated form of *Mycobacterium bovis*. The vaccines have been extensively use worldwide and 100 million doses are given to children each year. It has reduced mortality by about 90 per cent in vaccinated children.[62] BCG vaccine protects children from severe forms of TB – haematogenous, miliary or disseminated TB. In 2002 alone, BCG prevented an estimated 30 000 cases of meningeal TB during infancy.[63,64] However, the protective effect of the vaccine diminishes within 10–15 years and a booster dose does not confer any additional benefit.[65] In 2006, the WHO Global Advisory Committee on Vaccine Safety reviewed evidence from South Africa and Argentina and reported that in infants infected with HIV, the risk of BCG vaccination outweighs the benefits.[66] Better understanding of host immunity to TB, the development of modified ways to stimulate immune response through the use of adjuvant therapies, the identification of TB genes, as well as antigens and better ways of exposing the antigen to the immune system through vectors have led to new strategies to develop a more efficient vaccine for TB. All

Table 26.5 Goals, targets and indicators for TB contol.

Millennium development goal 6

Combat HIV/AIDS, malaria and other diseases

Target 8	Have halted by 2015 and begin to reverse the incidence of malaria and other major diseases
Indicator 23	Prevalence and death rates associated with tuberculosis
Indicator 24	Proportion of tuberculosis cases detected and cured under DOTS

the vaccines being investigated are designed to keep the infection latent. New approaches would prevent the bacteria from gaining a foothold in the lungs at all.

FINAL WORD

The WHO has expanded the framework to provide targets for all United Nation's Millennium Development Goals (MDGs) (Table 26.5).[67]

The targets are based on the assumption that achieving 70 per cent case detection and 85 per cent cure rate will reduce the prevalence of infectious smear-positive cases of TB, thereby reducing further cases and mortality. In 1991, it was believed that when the targets have been achieved, a decline in annual TB incidence rate of 5–10 per cent per year would result in the absence of HIV.

In 2005, 22 countries achieved the target, including China, the Philippines and Vietnam (Figure 26.11). If the global TB incidence rate is falling then the MDG 6 (target 8) has been achieved, 10 years before the 2015 deadline.[2]

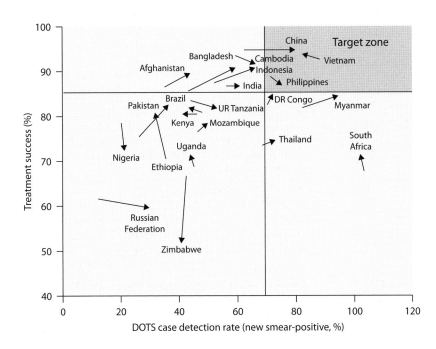

Figure 26.11 DOTS progress in high-burden countries, 2004–2005. Treatment success refers to cohorts of patients registered in 2003 and 2004 and evaluated by the end of 2004 and 2005, respectively.

Table 26.6 Stop TB Partnership targets.

By 2005	At least 70% of people with sputum smear-positive tuberculosis will be diagnosed (i.e. under the DOTs strategy) and at least 85% cure. These are targets set by the World Health Assembly of the WHO.
By 2015	The global burden of tuberculosis (per capita prevalence and death rates) will be reduced by 50% relative to 1990 levels.
By 2050	The global incidence of tuberculosis disease will be less than one case per million population per year.

The Stop TB partnership has set targets (Table 26.6) with the aim of reducing by 50 per cent the TB prevalence and death rate by 2015, in comparison to the rate estimated for 1990 (the baseline for all MDGs).[68]

The Global Plan to Stop TB includes cases with and without HIV. In 2015, the target prevalence and death rate are estimated to be approximately 150 and 15 per 100 000 population, respectively, and stated that the mortality from TB would be less than 1 million. The ultimate goal by 2050 is the elimination of TB as a public health problem.[69] This can be achieved by reducing the incidence of all forms of TB to one case per million population or less by 2050.[70]

Finally, the second Global Plan to Stop TB (2006–15)[71] envisages the utilization of all health systems in an attempt to achieve the targets laid down, with the hope of reflecting the sentiments expressed by Robert Koch in his 1882 lecture at the University of Berlin:

I have no business to live this life if I can not eradicate this horrible scourge from mankind.

LEARNING POINTS

- In 1993, WHO declared TB to be a global emergency. Twenty two HBCs have been highlighted; they have 80 per cent of the world burden of TB.
- The association between TB and poverty is strong but complex. In high-income countries, the average estimated incidence of TB is 10 per 100 000; in low-income countries it is 20 times higher.
- India is implementing the largest TB control programme in the World. A total of 110 000 patients are put on DOTS every month.
- DOTS comprises government commitment to sustained TB control strategies, case detection by sputum smear microscopy among symptomatic patients self-presenting to health services, directly observed therapy with short-course regimens, a regular uninterrupted supply of drugs and a standardized recording and reporting system.

- Treatment observation is not just supervised swallowing. It succeeds by building a bond between the patient and the observer.
- The key to success is effective supervision at all levels.
- There is a need for extension and strengthening of the DOTS programmes globally.
- TB-HIV combination is one of the most challenging aspects of TB treatment.
- MDR-TB and XDR-TB pose a major public health hazard in the developing world. The WHO has introduced the DOTS-Plus programme for the treatment of MDR-TB.
- Funds must be made available from affluent countries to help poorer nations.
- TB cannot be eradicated by one country alone. It is a world problem and therefore can only be solved by a world programme.

REFERENCES

1. World Health Organization. *Report on TB epidemic. TB is a global emergency.* Geneva: World Health Organization, WHO/TB/94.177, 1994.
2. World Health Organization. *Report 2007, Global tuberculosis control surveillence, planning, financing.* Geneva: World Health Organization, WHO/HTM/TB/2007.376, 2007.
3. World Health Organization. Fact sheet No. 104. Geneva: World Health Organization, 2006.
4. World Health Organization. *Tuberculosis control in the South East Asia region.* The regional report. WHO project No. ICP TUB 001. New Delhi: World Health Organization Regional Office for South East Asia, 2006.
5. World Health Organization. *Tuberculosis disease report: The global fund to fight AIDS, TB and malaria.* Geneva: World Health Organization, 2006.
6. World Health Organization. Tuberculosis in South East Asia – 50 years Commemorative Series. Geneva: World Health Organization, 1998.
7. Rajeshwari R, Balasubramanium R, Muniyandi M *et al.* Socio-economic impact of tuberculosis on patient and family in India. *Int J Tuberc Lung Dis* 1999; **3**: 869–77.
8. Crofton J. Good news from India. *Int J Tuberc Lung Dis* 2000; **4**: 189–96 (editorial).
9. World Health Organization. *Research for action. Understanding and controlling tuberculosis in India.* New Delhi: World Health Organization Regional Office for South-East Asia, 2000.
10. Ramana GNY, Naidu BMCS, Murthy KJR. Mapping of TB treatment provided at selected sites in Andhra Pradesh State, India. Geneva: World Health Organization, WHO/TB/97.233, 1997.
11. World Health Organization. *Global tuberculosis control. WHO Report 2000.* Geneva: World Health Organization, WHO/CDS/TB/2000.275, 2000.
12. World Bank. *Voices of the poor: Can anyone hear us?* New York: World Bank, 2000.
13. Hanson C. Tuberculosis, poverty and inequity: a review of the literature and other issues. Geneva: Stop TB Partnership, World Health Organization, 2002.
14. Zumla A, Grange JM. Doing something about tuberculosis. *Br Med J* 1999; **318**: 956 (editorial).
15. Styblo K. Tuberculosis in developing countries. *Ethiop Med J* 1983; **21**: 101–22.

16. Hopewell PC, Pai M, Maher D, Uplekar M, Raviglione MC. International standards for tuberculosis care. *Lancet Infect Dis* 2006; **6**: 710–25.

17. Frieden TR. Can tuberculosis be controlled? *Ind J Tuberc* 1998; **45**: 65–72.

18. Commission on Health Research for Development. *Health research: essential link to equity in development*. New York: Oxford University Press, 1990.

19. National Council of Applied Economic Research. *Household survey of health care institution and expenditures*. New Delhi: NCAER, Working paper no. 53. 1995.

20. Pathania V, Almedida J, Kochi A. *TB patient and project health care provider in India*. Geneva: World Health Organization, WHO/TB/97-233.1997, 1997

21. World Health Organization. *Tuberculosis control in Mexico, joint programme review*. Geneva: World Health Organization, WHO/TB/96.202, 1995.

22. World Health Organization. *Involving private provider and communicable diseases control; issues, interventions and emerging policy framework for tuberculosis*. Geneva: World Health Organization, WHO/CDS/TB/2006, 2006.

23. Uplekar M, Pathania V, Raviglione M. Private practitioners and public health; weak links in tuberculosis control. *Lancet* 2001; **358**: 912–16.

24. TB India 2007. *RNTCP status report*. New Delhi: Central TB Division, Directorate General of Health Services, Ministry of Health and Family Welfare, 2007.

25. Uplekar MW, Rangan S. Private doctor and tuberculosis control in India. *Tuber Lung Dis* 1993; **74**: 332–7.

26. Narain JP, Pontali E, Tripathi S. Symposium on HIV and TB. Epidemiology and control strategies. *Ind J Tuberc* 2002; **49**: 3–9.

27. Steinbrook R. Tuberculosis and HIV in India. *New Engl J Med* 2007; **356**: 1198–9.

28. World Health Organization. *Guidelines for the programmatic drug resistance tuberculosis*. Geneva: World Health Organization, WHO/HTM/TB/2006.361, 2006.

29. Nathanson E, Lambregts-van Weezenbeek C, Rich ML *et al.* Multidrug resistant tuberculosis management in resource limited setting. *Emerg Infect Dis* 2006; **12**: 1389–97.

30. Gandhi NR, Moll A, Sturm AW *et al.* Extensively drug resistant tuberculosis as a cause of death in patients co infected with tuberculosis and HIV in rural area of South Africa. *Lancet* 2006; **368**: 1575–80.

31. Editorial. Extreme tuberculosis. *New York Times* 14 September 2006.

32. World Health Organization. Report of the meeting of the WHO global task force on XDR TB. Geneva: World Health Organization, WHO/HTM/TB/2006.XXX, 2006.

33. World Health Organization. WHO calls for immediate use of new tuberculosis breakthrough (press release). Geneva: World Health Organization, WHO/24:1997:1-2, 1997.

34. Banerji D, Anderson S. A sociological study of awareness of symptoms amongst persons with pulmonary tuberculosis. *Bull World Health Organ* 1963; **29**: 665–83.

35. Styblo K. *Epidemiology of tuberculosis*. Jena: VEB Gustav Fisher Verlag, 1984.

36. Fox, W. Self-administration of medicaments. A review of published work and a study of the problems. *Bull Int Union Tuberc* 1961; **31**: 307–31.

37. Lienhardt C, Rustomjee R. Improving tuberculosis control; an interdisciplinary approach. *Lancet* 2006; **369**: 949–50

38. Raviglione MC, Uplekar MW. WHO's new Stop TB strategy. *Lancet* 2006; **367**: 952–5.

39. Grzybowski S. Drugs are not enough: failure of short course chemotherapy in a district of India. *Tuber Lung Dis* 1993; **74**: 145–6.

40. Rouillon A. Problem raised by the organization of an efficient ambulatory treatment for tuberculosis patient. *Bull Int Union Tuberc* 1972; **47**: 68–93.

41. Liefooghe R. Perceptions and social consequences of tuberculosis; a focus group study of tuberculosis patients in Sialkot, Pakistan. *Soc Sci Med* 1995; **41**: 1685–92.

42. Barnhoorn F, Adriaanse H. In search of factors responsible for non compliance amongst tuberculosis patients in Wardha District, India. *Soc Sci Med* 1992; **34**: 291–306.

43. Frieden T (ed.). *Toman's tuberculosis: Case detection, treatment and Monitoring – questions and answers*, 2nd edn. Geneva: World Health Organization, 2002.

44. Frieden TR. Directly observed treatment short course (DOTS). The strategy that ensures cure of tuberculosis patients. In: Sharma SK, Mohan A (eds). *Tuberculosis*. New Delhi: JP Brothers, 2001: 536–46.

45. Iseman MD, Cohn DL, Sharbaro JA. Directly observed treatment of tuberculosis. We can't afford not to try it. *N Engl J Med* 1993; **328**: 576–8.

46. Sumartojo E. When tuberculosis treatment fails: a social behavioural account of patient adherence. *Am Rev Respir Dis* 1993; **147**: 1311–20.

47. Milburn HJ, Cochrane GM. Treating the patient as decision maker is not always appropriate. *Br Med J* 1997; **314**: 1906.

48. Smith I. Directly observed therapy. In: Sharma SK, Mohan A (eds). *Tuberculosis*. New Delhi: JP Brothers, 2001: 547–57.

49. Bam TS, Gunneberg C, Chamroonsawasdi K *et al.* Factors affecting patient adherence to DOTS in urban Kathmandu, Nepal. *Int J Tuberc Lung Dis* 2006; **10**: 270–6.

50. O'Boyle SJ, Power JJ, Ibrahim MY, Watson JP. Factors affecting patient compliance with antituberculosis chemotherapy using directly observed treatment shortcourse strategy (DOTS). *Int J Tuberc Lung Dis* 2002; **6**: 307–12.

51. Tekle B. Defaulting from DOTS and its determinants in three districts of Aris Zone in Ethiopia. *Int J Tuberc Lung Dis* 2002; **6**: 573–9.

52. Wandwalo ER, Morkve O. Knowledge of disease and treatment among tuberculosis patient in Mwanza, Tanzania. *Int J Tuberc Lung Dis* 2000; **4**: 1041–6.

53. Harper M, Ahmadu FA, Ogden JA *et al.* Identifying the determinant of tuberculosis control in resource poor countries: insight from a qualitative study in the Gambia. *Trans R Soc Trop Med Hyg* 2003; **97**: 506–10.

54. Barnhoorn F, Driaanse H. In search of factors responsible for noncompliance among tuberculosis patient in Wardha district, India. *Soc Sci Med* 1992; **34**: 291–306.

55. Peltzer K, Onya H, Seoka P *et al.* Factors at first diagnosis of tuberculosis associated with compliance with the directly observed therapy (DOTS) in the Limpopo province, South Africa. *Curationis* 2002; **25**: 55–67.

56. Burman WJ, Cohn DL, Rietmeijer CA *et al.* Short term incarceration for the management of noncompliance with tuberculosis. *Chest* 1997; **112**: 57–62.

57. Volmink J, Garner P. Systematic review of randomized control trials of strategies to promote adherence to tuberculosis treatment. *Br Med J* 1997; **315**: 1403–406.

58. International Union against Tuberculosis and Lung Diseases. *Social mobilisation of nongovernmental organisations in TB control*. New Delhi: The Union, 2005.

59. Floyd K, Arora VK, Murthy KJ *et al.* Cost and cost effectiveness of PPM-DOTS for tuberculosis control: evidence from India. Bull World Health Organ 2006; **84**: 437–85.

60. Keeler E, Perkins MD, Small P *et al.* Reducing the global burden of tuberculosis: the contribution of improved diagnostics. *Nature* 2006; **S1**: 49–57.

61. Camp R, Jefferys R, Swan T, Syed J. *What's in the pipeline: New HIV drugs, vaccines, microbicides, HCV and TB therapies in clinical trials*. New York: Treatment Action Group (TAG), 2006.

62. Anderson P, Doherty TM. The success and failure of BCG: Implications for a novel tuberculosis vaccine. *Nat Rev Microbiol* 2005; **3**: 656–62.

63. Girard MP, Fruth U, Kieny MP. A review of vaccine research and development tuberculosis. *Vaccine* 2005; 30: 5725–31.

64. Trunz BB, Fine P, Dye C. Effect of BCG vaccination on childhood tuberculous meningitis and miliary tuberculosis worldwide; a meta-analysis and assessment of cost effectiveness. *Lancet* 2006; **367**: 1173–80.

65. Young D, Dye C. The development and impact of tuberculosis vaccines. *Cell* 2006; **124**: 683–7.

66. Hesseling AC, Marais BJ, Gie RP *et al.* The risk of disseminated bacille Calmette-Guérin (BCG) disease in HIV-infected children. *Vaccine* 2006; **25**: 14–18.

67. Dye C, Maher D, Weil D *et al.* Targets for global tuberculosis control. *Int J Tuberc Lung Dis* 2006; **10**: 460–62.

68. Dye C, Watt CJ, Bleed DM *et al.* Evolution of tuberculosis control and prospects of reducing tuberculosis incidence, prevalence and death globally. *J Am Med Assoc* 2005; **293**: 2767–75.

69. Stop TB Partnership. *Washington commitment to Stop TB.* First Stop TB Partners Forum, 22–23 October 2001. Geneva: World Health Organization, 2001.

70. Institute of Medicine. *Ending neglect the elimination of tuberculosis in the United States.* Washington DC: Institute of Medicine, 2000.

71. Stop TB Partnership and World Health Organization. *Global plan to Stop TB 2006–2015.* Geneva: World Health Organization, WHO/HTM/STB/2006.35, 2006.

27

The role of the specialist TB nurse

SUSAN JAMIESON

INTRODUCTION

It is said that 'there is nothing new under the sun' (*Ecclesiastes* 1:9) and so it would seem when considering the role of the community tuberculosis (TB) nurse. The names may change, as different health authorities and NHS trusts reorganize their practice, indeed many are themselves undergoing dramatic changes, but whatever title is used, a good TB nurse will have organizational skills, interpersonal skills and an ability to deliver excellent patient-centred care based on national guidance. TB is no respecter of persons, although poverty continues to be a factor,[1] but patients come from every walk of life and culture, and the service should be adaptable enough to give whatever level of support is needed in order to achieve the gold standard of TB prevention and control. Given finance and political will, eradication of this age-old disease is not impossible. A TB service may be delivered differently depending upon geography, culture, economics, politics and local rate of infection, but throughout the world the basic principles remain the same.

This chapter will discuss the central role of the TB nurse in each of these areas, which may translate to worldwide contexts in its aspirations, but is written from the perspective of a nurse working in a small team in a UK city with a TB infection rate of 16/100 000.

EASY ACCESS TO THE TUBERCULOSIS SERVICE

It is important that all those to whom a suspected TB case presents are aware of the pathway to TB screening in their area. A referral to a general chest clinic may well be delayed by a backlog of work by medical secretaries, appointments departments, full or cancelled clinics, etc. A central TB unit or clinic staffed by a designated TB team can take referrals from all sources, both medical and non-medical, and effectively triage referrals. The nurse may have knowledge of, or investigate the contact with, a TB case and ensure that screening is necessary for the type/site of disease and that the timing is appropriate. The worried-well can be reassured and for those who need urgent screening, this may be initiated without delay. This may involve arranging sputum collection or tuberculin skin testing (Mantoux) before their appointment with a physician with TB expertise. For those who are symptomatic, fast-tracking to a clinic or admission to hospital for investigations will be necessary.

Figures 27.1 and 27.2 show a referral form and a protocol giving details of the criteria for referral. The signs, symptoms and risk indications of TB are clearly set out as an aide-mémoire for those who use this method of referral, which is designed for use in a primary care setting and by other agencies whose knowledge may be less but who have contact with those who do not regularly access primary care, such as workers with the homeless.

Referral forms are useful but they are simply a tool. We cannot afford to miss early diagnosis of a possible TB case because a form is not completed. We need to be alert to early warnings from our colleagues in radiology and laboratory services, in other clinics, in primary care, nursing and residential homes, in hostels for the homeless or refugees, even in the casual remark of existing patients or a member of the public.

Preliminary screening or bacille Calmette–Guérin (BCG) catch-up sessions can be arranged in the local community which yield a higher take up rate (see An effective screening programme for higher-risk groups).

REFERRAL to LIVERPOOL PCT COMMUNITY TB SERVICE

ABERCROMBY HEALTH CENTRE, GROVE ST, LIVERPOOL L7 7HG
Tel 0151 709 1840   Fax 0151 709 6725   E-Mail sue.jamieson@liverpoolpct.nhs.uk

| Name

DOB

NHS Number	Address & Telephone	GP Details

Referred by..Designation..Date..................

REASON FOR REFERRAL		FOR TB SERVICE USE
Symptomatic

Cough lasting 4 weeks or more
Haemoptysis
Weight Loss
Night Sweats
Abnormal Chest X-Ray
Other | details | Date received |
| Positive Skin Test | result in mm

? Previous BCG | |
| Contact of Pulmonary TB | Details if poss | |
| New Entrant to UK
from? | date of arrival | |
| BCG Request
Baby from higher risk group
Under 16 from higher risk group | details | |

Figure 27.1   Form to be completed for patients referring to the TB service.

RAPID DIAGNOSIS AND COMMENCEMENT OF TREATMENT

Having accessed the service, those who are found to have TB should be commenced on treatment as soon as possible. For those with smear-positive disease, every day delayed might mean transmission to others. Where further investigations are required before the start of treatment, for example to obtain material that may be stained and cultured, the nurse will need to be available to reassure the anxious patient and their contacts and give advice on their level of infectiousness or lack thereof. TB still holds fear and stigma for many people and the nurse's input in these early stages is vital. The most important element in helping a patient to complete treatment is the relationship built between patient and their nurse. This is recognized in the latest UK guidelines.[2]

The on-going responsibility may be delegated in some cases, but the first encounter will be vital and provide a point of reference for the patient.

In the first weeks of treatment, a patient has to come to terms with having a disease which they or others fear, a treatment regime which they may find difficult stretching out for months ahead, an interference with the way they practise contraception[3] or conduct their social activities,[4] and minor or serious reactions to the drugs. In addition to all this, the realization that others will be inconvenienced by screening at the least or that infection may have passed to their friends and families, is a major source of concern. A further cause of concern may be the request for them to

Protocol For Referral to the Liverpool Tuberculosis (TB) Service

The purpose of this protocol is to aid in the swift detection and treatment of Tuberculosis and to provide easy access to The Liverpool TB Service.

The following Groups may be referred directly to the TB Service:

➢ Those exhibiting signs and symptoms of TB.
➢ Those found to have a positive Mantoux test.
➢ Those at a higher risk of TB who require screening.
  ○ Contacts of TB.
  ○ New Arrivals to the city from countries having a high incidence of TB.
➢ Children and young people for whom BCG is recommended.

HOME VISITS

❖ For urgent cases the TB Specialist Nurse will visit at home within a few days and if necessary arrange a clinic appointment the following week.
❖ Home/hostel visits can be arranged for screening of urgent cases who would find attending clinic difficult, although they may be required to attend clinic for a chest x-ray later.
❖ The TB Specialist Nurse routinely visits patients with Tuberculosis who are on treatment.
❖ The TB Specialist Nurse will visit patients on preventative Tuberculosis treatment if required.

• Please send referral forms by fax, post or e-mail.
• Referral forms can be photocopied or obtained by post or e-mail.
• Information/rationale of this protocol is available from the TB Service.
• The TB Service can be contacted by health professionals or the public for advice.

Figure 27.2   Protocol for referral to the TB service.

undergo HIV testing as the co-morbidity is explained; so it becomes apparent that the nurse's friendliness, knowledge and skills will be tested to the full. The nurse has to be able to relate to people of all social classes, all ages, all levels of understanding with whatever challenges they are facing. An early rapport needs to be established between nurse and patient as co-workers who are journeying together to eventual cure. To this end, a virtual contract is made with the level of care required assessed according to risk of defaulting affected by lifestyle, previous TB history or history of non-concordance for other conditions.

A LEVEL OF CARE THAT SUPPORTS THE PATIENT TO COMPLETION OF TREATMENT

Patient contact at diagnosis and commencement of treatment is essential for all cases and well worth whatever time is necessary to ensure the patient fully understands the treatment, possible adverse effects, expected course of the disease and implications for his/her contacts. Follow-up visits will need to be tailored to the patient and range from the occasional encouraging phone call to daily visits. The former group will typically be in regular employment, attend clinic appointments and phone his/her key worker if there is a problem. Those needing intensive support in

---

Box 27.1: Directly observed treatment (DOT)

Supervised treatment should be considered when there is
• a previous history of TB;
• previous treatment failure;
• drug resistance, especially multidrug-resistant (MDR)-TB;
• homelessness;
• alcohol or substance abuse;
• a need for support due to age and comprehension;
• a cultural or other resistance to taking regular medication.

---

the community will be receiving directly observed treatment (DOT) (Box 27.1), which may include an injectible drug as part of the regime. Where possible, an intermittent (three times weekly) regimen is usually the best way forward. This not only frees up nurse time, but is less restrictive for the patient who may want to lie in or go out for the day. Even 3 days a week is a big commitment for many and care should be taken to arrange a time for DOT that is least disruptive and most likely to have a successful outcome. The constraints of clinics, staff and location will need to be addressed, but patients can quickly appreciate the nurse's efforts to accommodate their needs and compromises are possible. In this way, nurse and patient build up a partnership which is more likely to effect good concordance than a demand to be in a certain place at a certain time. As treatment progresses and the medication is reduced in the continuation phase, a gradual withdrawal with transfer of responsibility from nurse to patient is often possible. Drugs supplied in blister packs or put out weekly into a dosette box are useful measures in this period which is usually well into the continuation phase of treatment.

> The approach to TB treatment should be to 'step down' with proven good adherence, rather than to 'step up' when problems develop.[5]

As the nurse gets to know the patient and visits their home, other health, social and housing issues may emerge or be shared. The nurse becomes a trusted friend and advocate and can play an important part in signposting another service, organizing a joint visit with social services or supporting a request for improved housing. The building up of relationships, though immeasurable, plays an important part in keeping the patient on track, with the patient far less likely to simply stop treatment or miss clinic appointments.

Time and interest invested in the patient (or simply the shock of contracting TB) sometimes produces a change in lifestyle and reduction of, or even abstention from, alcohol, cigarettes or illegal substances. When this happens, it is enormously rewarding, but when, as is more usually the case, no such change occurs, the nurse must continue to maintain a non-judgemental approach. The risks associated with TB medication and alcohol or drug abuse should be explained and the patient should be seen regularly to monitor liver function should signs and symptoms occur.

With the increase in the number of patients needing DOT, the TB nurse will need to be creative in enlisting help. Most community pharmacies are equipped with a private area/cubicle where patients can take their medicine discretely. For those already receiving methadone under supervision, TB treatment can also be monitored if the pharmacist is willing to take on this additional responsibility. Where the patient is in supported living, a support worker may be willing to help or, if the patient is receiving daily visits by another health professional, an agreement to supervise TB treatment may be possible. However, in making these arrangements, the nurse must first discuss with the patient, what would be best for them; they may not wish to disclose their condition to a third party. The TB nurse has the responsibility for supervision of medication and must ensure that those undertaking this task on her behalf understand the possible side effects; they should be able to contact the nurse in case of default or suspected adverse reactions. The nurse must also continue to maintain contact with the patient.

AN EFFECTIVE SCREENING PROGRAMME FOR HIGHER-RISK GROUPS

TB contacts

Contact tracing yields 1 per cent of active disease[6] and up to 10 per cent latent TB infection (LTBI). These figures are much higher when immunocompromised contacts are exposed.[7] Those found to have a recently acquired infection, but not disease, are recommended to have preventative treatment, thus reducing the pool of LTBI and therefore the number of future cases, making this active case-finding worthwhile. Young people who have been screened and are free of infection are given BCG vaccination. The TB nurse will discuss contact screening with a newly diagnosed case as soon as possible, explaining the possibility of transmission from them and if possible find the source of transmission to them. Although a source is infrequently found, this sends out a clear message that there is no blame attached to them as the index case. Only close contacts of cases of smear-negative pulmonary TB and extrapulmonary TB need to be included whilst close and casual contacts of smear-positive pulmonary and upper respiratory tract TB should be screened. Close contacts would be defined as those living in the same house or spending considerable time with the index case, such as a partner or colleague working in close proximity.[8] Attention is paid to any vulnerable contacts such as young children and immunosuppressed individuals, who should be screened along with any symptomatic contacts within 1 week. It is important that contacts have access to information regarding their particular circumstance by being given assurance that they may call the TB nurse for advice. The TB nurse's role in deciding the who, when and how of contact screening is very important in ensuring that the appropriate contacts attend for screening and the worried well are reassured that they do not need screening immediately or at all.

The UK guidelines[8] show the recommended action for contact screening (Figure 27.3). Although the use of interferon-γ testing is included, it has not become a routine investigation in many contact clinics although it may be

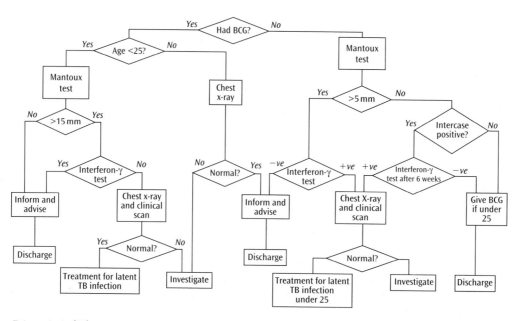

Figure 27.3 Tuberculosis (TB) contact tracing algorithm.

specially requested if indicated; infection with HIV may be one such indication.

It is advised[9] that before large contact screening exercise is undertaken such as in a school, the TB diagnosis should be confirmed by rapid laboratory diagnostics.

When dealing with such episodes it is advisable to distribute information and arrange an open meeting or an advice line to assure possible contacts that their risk is being assessed and they will be offered screening if necessary.

It may be practical to arrange on-site screening such as an interview or questionnaire and a Mantoux test. Those showing symptoms, tuberculin positivity or having increased risk factors to TB can be seen at the clinic. Having had contact with the nurse, those advised to have further investigations are unlikely to default, whilst those not needing a clinic appointment do not feel they have been neglected.

Children of smear-positive TB cases should be given a Mantoux test at the earliest opportunity. If negative, this should be repeated in 6 weeks and BCG given if appropriate.

Some contacts may have been infected, as suggested by positive Mantoux or interferon-γ testing, but have a normal chest x-ray (CXR). These individuals, if under the age of 35 years, may be offered preventative treatment. For children and young adults, this is strongly recommended. Although serious adverse effects are very rare in this group, the TB nurse should ensure that they fully understand the diagnosis of a LTBI, their treatment and possible adverse effects. They should be given written information[8] and a contact telephone number to call should they have any concerns. Treating LTBI plays an important role in TB control and those receiving treatment are supported by the TB nurse, although this element is not usually factored into the level of specialist nurses recommended.

New entrants

New entrants may be long-stay visitors, overseas students, work permit holders, or family members/dependants of any of these groups. They may also be individuals or families who have planned their immigration and often have an address where they know they will live. Others may be refugees or asylum seekers who will need an increased level of support. UK guidelines advocate screening those people who have entered the UK from an area of high TB incidence (40/100 000). This is approached in various ways by different TB services and according to the circumstances of the new entrant. It is usually more convenient for students and health-care workers to be screened by occupational health services who will refer strong tuberculin reactors and any exhibiting signs and symptoms of TB to the chest clinic. Asylum seekers may be living in a hostel or induction centre where partial screening to check history of contact, signs and symptoms and a skin test is a useful way to identify those who may need further investigation. This system addresses the difficulty that many new entrants face

if simply called up for a clinic appointment. Is the appointment in a language that is understood? Can the individual negotiate or afford public transport in a strange country? Has he/she been moved to a different address by the time the referral is received and processed? Whilst this preliminary screening is more productive in screening new entrants and enabling BCG vaccination to be given if appropriate, it does not strictly adhere to the latest National Institute for Health and Clinical Excellence (NICE) guidelines in that all new entrants should have a CXR or have had a recent CXR (Figure 27.4).[8]

Homeless

This group has also been shown to be at a higher risk of developing TB[10] by reason of failure or delay in accessing health services, lowered immunity associated with poor nutrition, alcohol or drug abuse and contact in homes or hostels in which there may be overcrowding. The TB nurse works with those giving support to this group, to raise awareness of signs and symptoms, accept referrals, provide opportunities for screening at a time and place that is easy and accessible and if necessary arrange further investigations and/or hospital admission. There is an excellent information leaflet from the Health Protection Agency[11] giving advice and indicating the referral pathway.

Many areas have nurses and/or health units working with the homeless, new entrants, HIV-positive individuals, students and health-care workers. It is prudent to work with colleagues who may be better placed to identify possible TB symptoms opportunistically and to carry out preliminary screening. A good working relationship will encourage colleagues to phone for advice or make a referral (Figure 27.1).

EDUCATION

Colleagues who carry out such preliminary screening will need to understand the basic principles of TB and be competent to perform Mantoux testing. The rewards of having nurses who are able and willing to take on this additional activity is well worth the time and energy invested in their training. Other colleagues will see far fewer potential cases, but if they are aware of the signs and symptoms and means of getting further advice, they will play an important part in preventing TB transmission by swift action. So the TB nurse will give talks and presentations to nurses, GPs, staff from residential and nursing care homes and any other interested party. Most TB services will be aware of cases that should have been picked up sooner by GPs, Accident and Emergency Departments, clinics, etc., where delay has meant progression of the disease and transmission to more contacts.[12]

Education for the public is most important. A new patient will want to know as much as possible about their condition and their cure will be effected by treatment concordance. This in turn is more likely to succeed when the

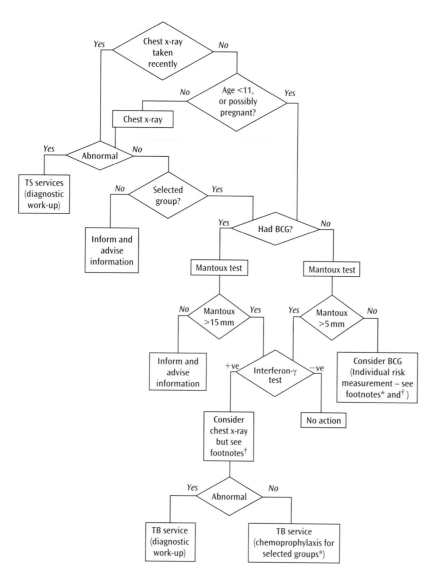

Figure 27.4   New entrant screening algorithm.

*Select new entrants for further screening if they are any of the following:
 • age <16;
 • age 16–65 from sub-Saharan Africa or a country with incidence greater than 500 per 100 000.
†Timing of chest x-ray and/or BCG may be dependent on pregnancy status. Interpret existing chest x-ray if one
  has been taken recently.

patient understands the importance of uninterrupted chemotherapy. The NICE guidelines[13] recognize the TB nurse's role in education thus: 'This key worker should facilitate education and involvement of the person with TB in achieving adherence'.

Contacts who do not understand TB may be unwilling to come for screening, may become over-anxious or may shun the index case. The 'advise and inform' following screening is essential and verbal information with accompanying leaflet serves to reassure the contact for the present and warn them for the future. The importance of this final step in screening has increased in importance since a series of follow-up appointments for contacts is no longer recommended.

Education for those in higher-risk groups is vital. New entrants from countries with a high TB incidence[14] who are screened and found clear may have a false sense of security and fail to seek help if TB symptoms occur in the future. Surveillance figures show that 75 per cent of TB cases are found in individuals who are non-UK born.[15] Information must be given verbally and in writing, if possible in the patient's first language.

A GOOD RECORD-KEEPING/SURVEILLANCE SYSTEM

The TB nurse is in the best position for ensuring that full and accurate records are kept and relevant information passed to the Health Protection Agency. From this information, national data are produced which is important to the epidemiology of TB locally, nationally and internationally. Systems in place can be audited and practice enhanced according to outcome. An example of this would be that mentioned earlier where it was found that non-attendance at clinics by new entrants was costly and time-consuming and a higher level of screening would be achieved if it were taken to the clients.

London, which bears the highest burden of TB in the UK, operates a TB register which is proving highly effective. The register allows TB treatment centres to share patient information, thus improving and coordinating the care of TB patients across London. The London Health Committee recommends that this system should be developed into a National TB Database[16] and this would certainly enhance the systems currently in operation on a local level and dispense with need for paper surveillance forms.

For the nurse's current case load, accurate records must be kept to monitor treatment and starting date, laboratory reports, visits, problems and action taken. A weekly multi-disciplinary team meeting is an excellent way to ensure an exchange of information between nurse, chest physician, microbiologist and the infectious diseases team thus providing a joined-up TB service and an opportunity to learn from each other.

CONCLUSIONS

Over the last 30 years a variety of patient groups have been seen to benefit from specialist nurses who have experience and expertise in their particular condition. In the case of TB, a disease as old as the hills, nurses have long specialized in the care of its victims and its prevention and control. They have recognized the need to address social and economic problems, issues of stigma, isolation and education. They have embraced the advances of vaccination and chemotherapy, and they have responded to evolving needs of co-infection, drug resistance and non-concordance. The public health dimension has meant that nurses have been innovative in case-seeking and passionate in seeing a patient through from notification to cure. The TB nurse works contextually, his/her aims being little different to his/her peers worldwide which is apposite. We are on a world mission to stop TB and we each do what we can in our own place. Thankfully the UK NICE guidelines recognize that we must have global involvement; it is to be hoped that local, national or world politics do not thwart our best efforts.

> ### LEARNING POINTS
>
> - A TB service must be easily accessible to referrers and referees. The TB nurse can effectively triage referrals to ensure swift action for those who may have the disease.
> - Nurse involvement from diagnosis is important in building a relationship which will have a positive effect in the patient's journey.

> - An appropriate level of support including DOT increases completion rates.
> - The TB nurse organizes screening clinics for recent TB contacts, new entrants and those found by other agencies or health professionals to be symptomatic or having a positive Mantoux test/suspicious CXR. Flexibility in initial TB screening will lessen the number of those who do not attend.
> - Preventative treatment for LTBI is important in reducing future cases. Although adverse drug effects are less common in this group, the TB nurse will offer support and advice.
> - In a low-prevalence country, both public and health professionals need to be reminded to think TB.
> - The TB nurse is ideally placed to contribute to statistical data for local, national and international epidemiology.

REFERENCES

1. Nhelma B. Achieving global targets: the need for a pro-poor approach to TB control. The EQUI-TB Knowledge Programme, 2003.
2. NICE. Clinical diagnosis and management of tuberculosis, and measures for its prevention and control. London: National Institute for Health and Clinical Excellence: March 2006. www.hpa.org.uk/tbknowledge/resources/PDFs/NICE/CG033quickrefguide
3. British National Formulary. 7.3.1 Interaction of rifampicin with hormonal contraception. www.bnf.org.
4. Stockley IH (ed.). Stockley's drug interactions. London: Pharmaceutical Press.
5. Health Protection Agency. Outbreak of isoniazid-resistant MTB in North London 1999–2004. Executive summary report, key points and recommendations. www.hpa.org.uk/london.
6. Nice Clinical Guidance. CG33 Tuberculosis. London: Royal College of Physicians, 2006.
7. www.who.int/mediacentre/factsheets/fs104/en.
8. NICE. Clinical diagnosis and management of tuberculosis, and measures for its prevention and control. London: National Institute for Health and Clinical Excellence, 2006.
9. Joint Tuberculosis Committee of the British Thoracic Society. Control and prevention of tuberculosis in the United Kingdom: code of practice 2000. Thorax 2000;55(11):887–901.
10. Story A, Gorton S, Glyn-Jones J, Hayward A. TB & Housing. Meeting the needs of homeless & 'hard to reach' TB patients in London, London: London Regional Public Health Group and Strategic Health Authority, 2004.
11. TB & Homelessness Guidance for homeless service managers www.hpa.org.uk/tbknowledge/resources
12. www.brit-thoracic.org.uk/article27
13. Tuberculosis: Quick Reference Guide. Clinical diagnosis and management of tuberculosis, and measures for its prevention and control. London: National Institute for Health and Clinical Excellence, March 2006 http://www.hpa.org.uk/tbknowledge/resources/PDFs/NICE/CG033quickrefguide.pdf
14. www.hpa.org.uk/infections/topics_az/tb/epidemiology/who_table1.htm
15. www.hpa.org.uk/infections/topics_az/tb/data
16. www.london.gov.uk/assembly/reports/health/tb.rtf

28

Global Plan to Stop TB, 2006–2015

SARAH ENGLAND, MARCOS ESPINAL AND MARIO RAVIGLIONE

INTRODUCTION

The Global Plan to Stop TB, 2006–2015 is a pathway towards the United Nations Millennium Development Goals and the Stop TB Partnership's targets for 2015. It sets the course towards eliminating tuberculosis (TB) by 2050. It comprises three main components: general strategic direction, regional scenarios and more specific strategic plans in eight areas of work. Its credibility is built on the success of the first Global Plan to Stop TB 2001–2005, and it is based on epidemiological and financial models. In 2015, we should be able to look back on the global plan and say 'that's what really helped us to move forward … it was a catalyst for action, an accelerator of change'.

This chapter sets out the context of the plan within a global partnership, the main elements of the plan, challenges to implementation, and next steps. It is not a summary of the content of the plan, but rather aims to provide the reader with a sense of the main objectives and strategic

---

Box 28.1: The medical professional within the Stop TB Partnership

Medical professionals fit into the Stop TB Partnership in several ways. A number of professional organizations are Stop TB partners as are organizations representing medical and nursing students. There are many academic institution partners which include medical professionals involved in research. Some private sector corporations are partners which employ medical professionals involved in workplace TB programmes. Medical professionals, working for non-governmental organizations, may be partners through their organizations. In addition, medical professionals may be Stop TB partners through a national Stop TB partnership, a regional Stop TB organization, or as individuals through the Stop TB list at global level.

There are three main ways in which independent medical professionals and those in the corporate sector are explicitly addressed in the work of the Partnership. One is through the subgroup of the DOTS Expansion Working Group that is concerned with public–private mix DOTS (PPM DOTS). The other is through the workplace TB initiatives of the private sector constituency of the Partnership. This group has developed workplace TB control guidelines together with the World Health Organization and the International Labour Organization. Third, individuals may be members of national Stop TB partnerships or other similar organizations at national or subnational levels, or they may join the global Partnership as individuals and be included on its list. More broadly speaking, any medical professional who is following the ISTC can be counted as a contributor to the goals and targets of the Partnership. The purpose of the ISTC is to describe a widely accepted level of care that all practitioners, public and private, should seek to achieve in managing patients who have, or are suspected of having, TB.[1]

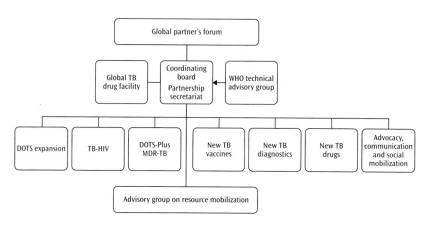

Figure 28.1   Structure of the Global Stop TB Partnership.

focus of the partnership over the period 2006–15, as detailed in the plan. The Learning Points at the end of this chapter highlight the ways medical professionals fit into the Stop TB Partnership and how they can contribute to the implementation and financing of the Second Global Plan to Stop TB.

BACKGROUND

A global consensus on strategy and implementation planning

The Global Plan represents a consensus among thousands of stakeholders in the global TB community. This consensus, together with the backing of the World Health Organization (WHO), is the source of its power and legitimacy. The consensus concerns the core strategy – the Stop TB Strategy – underpinning the plan, the targets it is designed to achieve, and the means of reaching those targets. Such a consensus, extending across more than 500 organizations, has important implications for TB control. First, it means that countries shouldering heavy burdens of TB disease have a clear framework which they can use to structure their national plans, with the confidence of knowing that this framework is robust and fully defensible. Second, it means that TB stakeholders can present a united front in advocating support for the plan and its financing; and third, the unity of the partners on issues of strategy and planning means that time and resources can be devoted to implementation rather than on further debate.

The Partnership: structure and function

The Global Stop TB Partnership is the forum through which the Global Plan's structure and content were determined and by which consensus on the strategy and plan were reached. Its principal function is coordination of all stakeholders in the global movement to eliminate TB as a public health problem. Partnership policy on non-technical issues is determined by its Coordinating Board, which comprises representatives of the main constituencies of the

Partnership (e.g. governments, non-governmental organizations, multilaterals, affected communities, etc.). Technical policy is determined by the WHO with the advice of its TB Strategic and Technical Advisory Group (STAG), an assembly of internationally recognized TB experts convened by the Stop TB Department of the WHO. Both the WHO and the STAG hold seats on the Coordinating Board.

The Coordinating Board has the main function of coordination and consensus building. The secretariat is responsible for ensuring that the decisions of the Coordinating Board are implemented. The secretariat is housed and administered by the WHO at its Geneva headquarters. It is headed by an executive secretary who is appointed by the WHO in close consultation with the Coordinating Board.

The strategic plans of the component parts of the Global Stop TB Partnership, the secretariat and the seven working groups (DOTS Expansion, Working Group on DOTS-Plus for multidrug-resistant TB (MDR-TB), TB/HIV Advocacy, Communication and Social Mobilization, and the three working groups focused on the development and implementation of new TB drugs, TB diagnostics and TB vaccines) are the central elements of the Global Plan (Figure 28.1). DOTS is the first component of the WHO Stop TB Strategy. It is the internationally recognized strategy for delivering the basics of TB case-finding and treatment. It comprises five elements: political commitment, case detection through quality assured bacteriology, short-course chemotherapy ensuring patient adherence to treatment, adequate drug supply, and sound reporting and recording systems.

The first Global Plan to Stop TB, 2001–2005

The early 1990s witnessed increasing concern over TB as a global public health issue. Nearly forgotten for two decades in the developed world after the advent of effective chemotherapy in the late 1940s, TB was resurging on the wave of the HIV epidemic. TB control targets were set by the World Health Assembly (WHA) in 1991 and TB was declared a global emergency in 1993.[2] These targets were to 'attain a global target of cure of 85 per cent sputum-positive patients under treatment and detection of 70 per cent of cases by the year 2000'.[3] At the WHA 2000, this target date was extended to 2005 and the Stop TB Partnership was founded in 2000 as a tool of the international community in accelerating its efforts to reach the targets.

In that year and in early 2001, several planning initiatives were under way, including the Global DOTS Expansion Plan. It became evident that these efforts would have maximum impact on the governments of countries shouldering high burdens of TB, as well as on donors if they were consolidated into one overarching and coherent plan with fully costed components. While recognizing and acknowledging that the DOTS package was essential, it was also becoming clear that more than DOTS expansion was required to Stop TB in the new century. Research for the development of new tools and adaptation of DOTS to the challenges of HIV-TB and MDR-TB were recognized as critical to achieving the WHA targets. These four areas formed the core of the first Global Plan.[4]

Therefore, the Partnership initiated work on a document that would build on the DOTS Expansion Plan and other planning elements. It aimed to attract, mobilize and unite partners to take action against TB, provide a framework to push forward work in TB control, care and research, focus efforts on the areas of highest priority, gain visibility for the TB issue, and mobilize resources. The first Global Plan to Stop TB was launched at the first Stop TB Partners' Forum hosted by the World Bank in Washington DC in 2001.

Progress on the first global plan

Within 3 years of the launch of the first Global Plan to Stop TB, the Partnership grew rapidly to 280 organizations. By this time, national TB control strategies were in place for all of the 22 high-burden countries, the Global Drug Facility – an initiative governed and housed by the Stop TB Partnership Secretariat to increase access to high-quality TB drugs for DOTS implementation – was well established and had served over 1.9 million people in 49 countries with first-line TB treatment at significantly lowered drug costs.[5] Guidelines for collaborative TB/HIV projects were published. Through the Green Light Committee, more people had access to life-saving second-line drugs to treat people suffering from MDR-TB and drug costs were reduced by as much as 90 per cent.[6] A pipeline of TB drug candidates was identified, a structure to spur the development of new diagnostics was established, and two vaccine candidates entered phase I clinical trials.[7]

By 2006, the end of the first Global Plan period, there were more than 500 partners in the Global Stop TB Partnership.[8] There was a functional Stop TB Partnership in the Western Pacific region, a newly launched Stop TB Partnership in the European region, and efforts to establish regional partnerships in the Eastern Mediterranean and African regions. National partnerships were active in Brazil, Canada, Ghana, Indonesia, Iran Italy, Mexico, Pakistan, Sudan and Uganda.

In terms of the WHA targets, data from 2005[9] indicate that globally a 60 per cent case detection and 84 per cent cure rate were achieved, representing – especially for the cure rate – a near miss. The detection target was reached in 57 countries and the cure rate target was reached in 60 countries. Over 26 million patients were treated through the DOTS strategy in 11 years.

By 2006, we also began to see the impact of the Global Fund to Fight AIDS, TB and Malaria (GFATM). The contribution of the Fund to TB is substantial, with a high rate of success for TB proposals. In the GFATM proposal round 6, the Technical Review Panel (TRP) reviewed 55 TB components. Sixty-two per cent of TB proposals that were reviewed by the TRP were recommended for funding (34/55) – the highest ever success rate. The Stop TB Partnership technical assistance coalition (TBTEAM), coordinated by the WHO, supported 48 countries in the proposed development process in this round. Of those supported by these TB experts, 71 per cent were successful (34/48). Approved TB proposals constitute 40 per cent of the number of all HIV, TB and malaria proposals approved in round 6 (34/85).[10]

In part, this success rate is due to the work of the technical agencies within the Partnership together with the National TB Programmes in endemic countries.

To date, the work on TB-HIV has for the most part comprised the development by the TB-HIV working group of a policy framework to support countries in putting collaborative TB/HIV activities into action and monitoring them.[11] As of 2006, 21 countries reported having developed a joint TB-HIV plan.[12]

As of October 2006, 40 projects involving close to 23 000 patients were approved for treatment with second-line drugs against MDR-TB.[13] This is in contrast to the period before the first Global Plan in which fewer than five pilot projects for second-line drug deployment were approved through the Green Light Committee (GLC) mechanism in its first year of functioning. These projects are in countries of which many are now receiving support for their MDR operations through the GFATM. Of the 22 countries with the highest burdens of TB, 11 had carried out nationwide TB drug resistance surveys by 2006.[13] The growth in approvals of GLC-sponsored programmes of MDR-TB management in the period from 2000 to 2006[13] is illustrated in Figure 28.2. This growth represents the growing recognition that second-line treatment can be taken on responsibly in resource-poor settings without undue risk of losing the efficacy of these second-line drugs, provided the TB programmes are performing well.

By the end of the first Global Plan period, the New Diagnostics Working Group had carried out a number of activities encompassing technology screening, market research, development support, product development, evaluation and demonstration studies, impact modelling and reviews of regulatory issues.[14] The New Drugs Working Group has put together a coordinated portfolio

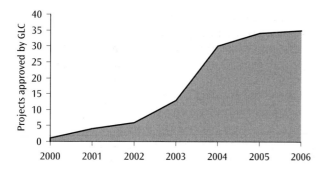

Figure 28.2   Scaling up of programmatic multidrug-resistant tuberculosis (MDR-TB) treatment through the Green Light Committee (GLC).

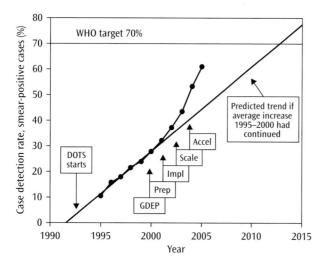

Figure 28.3   Trend of tuberculosis case detection rate.

of candidate compounds, the so-called 'pipeline'. This pipeline included 16 classes of compound in the discovery phase, the earliest phase of drug development, five compounds in preclinical trials, and six compounds in clinical testing.[15] The Vaccines Working Group had largely achieved its goal to have five vaccine candidates in phase I trials as four candidates were in phase I in 2005 and four others followed in 2006.[16]

The results of the advances in TB control, care, political commitment and financing since the first global plan was launched in 2001 are demonstrated in the graph of TB case detection (Figure 28.3).[17] This graph indicates a marked change in the trajectory of the rate of change of TB case detection rate from approximately 2001.

The launch of the second global plan in 2006 was a much needed boost to the global movement to stop TB. The strong results of the implementation of the first Global Plan inspired high-level support of the second plan at its launch by policy-makers, current and former heads of state, senior public servants, heads of agencies and heads of private foundations.

However, 2006 was not a year to rest on laurels. A cluster of cases of extensively drug-resistant TB (XDR-TB) was

identified in South Africa, leading to heightened concern regarding continued underinvestment in TB control and care, and the associated health systems requirements.[18]

THE SECOND GLOBAL PLAN

Why a 10-year plan?

First and foremost, the 10-year time-frame was chosen to coincide with that of the United Nations Millennium Development Goals. Millennium Development goal 6 is to combat HIV/AIDS, malaria and other diseases. Target 8 under goal 6 is to have halted and begun to reverse the incidence of these diseases. Under goal 6, indicator 23 is prevalence and deaths associated with TB and indicator 24 is the proportion of TB cases detected and cured under DOTS.[19]

Following the declaration of the Millennium Development Goals, the Stop TB Partnership identified two targets with the same 10-year horizon:

- to reduce TB prevalence by 50 per cent compared to the 1990 estimated baseline of approximately 300/100 000 and
- to reduce deaths due to TB by 50 per cent compared to the 1990 estimated baseline of approximately 30/100 000, both by 2015.

These are ambitious targets, not least because the HIV/AIDS epidemic peaked after 1990 and the MDR-TB problem worsened in this period, driving the TB epidemic along with them. These targets reflect a halving of rates which were already considerably lower than those in 2006. The Second Global Plan to Stop TB is therefore intended to be the road map by which the Partnership navigates towards these targets over a 10-year period.

Approach to planning and process

The development of the Second Global Plan to Stop TB was a consensus-based highly consultative process with the direct involvement of hundreds of public health specialists through presentations at key TB meetings, through the Stop TB Coordinating Board, through STAG and through the Partnership's working groups and secretariat. Thousands of people were consulted on the draft outline through the Partnership of listserv and the web site. The outline itself was devised following a survey of the impact of the first Global Plan and a needs assessment which sought to determine the uses to which partners wished to put the second Global Plan. Once feedback on a draft outline was incorporated, it was presented together with a proposed development process to the Stop TB Coordinating Board for endorsement. A steering committee and writing committee were established and these worked to guide the process and to put the pieces together, respectively. The process was coordinated by the Stop TB Partnership secretariat.

The basic approach was to work backwards from a scenario in which the 2015 targets were met in order to determine what disease control targets would have had to be achieved from 2006 onwards in seven of eight epidemiological regions. These targets were later adjusted for realism, with the result that the plan does not actually take us to the 2015 targets in all epidemiological regions. The regional scenarios and the general strategic approaches outlined in the first part of the plan were the basis of strategic plans from each of the seven working groups and the Partnership secretariat. Summaries of these strategic plans appear in the third part of the Global Plan. The elements of the Plan have been meticulously costed. Current and expected flows of funds have been calculated and the remaining resource gap quantified.

STRATEGIC DIRECTIONS

The Stop TB Strategy

The first Global Plan was centred on DOTS and its adaptation to TB-HIV and MDR-TB, with additional attention paid to research and development. The second Global Plan is underpinned by a more comprehensive strategy that embraces DOTS, but moves beyond a purely public health viewpoint to include health system strengthening in general and a human rights approach that provide for universal access, private sector and community involvement, and other innovations, while mainstreaming responses to new threats, full partner engagement, service innovations and

research. This is a significant paradigm shift for a community that has historically been predominantly concerned with the public health implications of smear-positive (contagious) TB, rather than with the rights of all individuals affected by the disease. The Stop TB Strategy developed by the WHO is depicted in Figure 28.4.

The Global Plan takes into account the impact of cross-cutting issues including health systems, poverty, children and gender. The Plan includes considerations of how health systems barriers and poverty contribute to the TB epidemic. It also seeks to determine and define the responsibilities of the TB community in addressing these constraints. It recognizes the special needs of the poor, children and those who may be marginalized or subject to reduced health services access for other reasons, such as gender inequities.

A few examples of the results that can be expected following full funding and implementation of the global plan are as follows:[20]

- an additional 14 million lives saved as compared to the no-DOTS expansion scenario and 50 million people treated under the Stop TB Strategy;
- second-line drug treatment for 800 000 people with MDR-TB;
- antiretroviral therapy for 3 million people co-infected with HIV and TB;
- improved quality of care through the Stop TB Strategy;
- meaningful involvement of patients and communities in TB care and control;
- rapid sensitive diagnostic tests for use at the point of care and a predictive test to identify people who are at highest risk of progressing from latent to active TB infection;

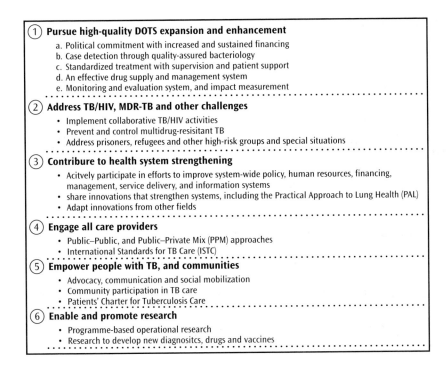

Figure 28.4   The Stop TB Strategy.

(1) **Pursue high-quality DOTS expansion and enhancement**
   a. Political commitment with increased and sustained financing
   b. Case detection through quality-assured bacteriology
   c. Standardized treatment with supervision and patient support
   d. An effective drug supply and management system
   e. Monitoring and evaluation system, and impact measurement

(2) **Address TB/HIV, MDR-TB and other challenges**
   • Implement collaborative TB/HIV activities
   • Prevent and control multidrug-resisitant TB
   • Address prisoners, refugees and other high-risk groups and special situations

(3) **Contribute to health system strengthening**
   • Acitvely participate in efforts to improve system-wide policy, human resources, financing, management, service delivery, and information systems
   • share innovations that strengthen systems, including the Practical Approach to Lung Health (PAL)
   • Adapt innovations from other fields

(4) **Engage all care providers**
   • Public–Public, and Public–Private Mix (PPM) approaches
   • International Standards for TB Care (ISTC)

(5) **Empower people with TB, and communities**
   • Advocacy, communication and social mobilization
   • Community participation in TB care
   • Patients' Charter for Tuberculosis Care

(6) **Enable and promote research**
   • Programme-based operational research
   • Research to develop new diagnositcs, drugs and vaccines

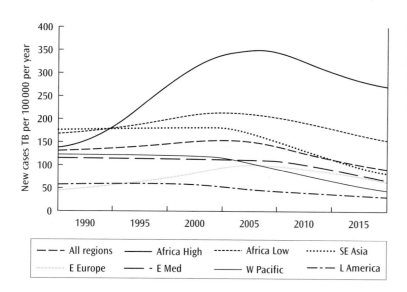

Figure 28.5 The predicted trajectory of tuberculosis incidence rates by region assuming full implementation of the Global Plan. A significant decrease in incidence is expected worldwide from approximately 2005. This will result in the prevention of 30 million cases of tuberculosis.[20]

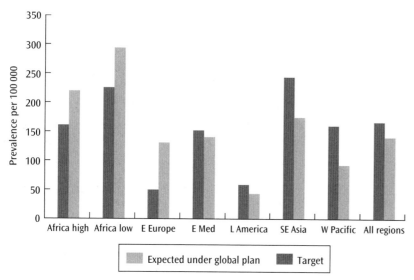

Figure 28.6 The expected impact of the Plan on death rates by region.[20]

- a new TB drug by 2010 and a new 1- to 2-month regimen effective against MDR-TB and compatible with antiretroviral therapy in approximately 10 years;
- a new safe and effective and affordable TB vaccine;
- a higher profile for TB on development agendas.

A full summary table of expected results is available in the Global Plan document.[20] More precise epidemiological outcomes are described under Global and regional scenarios.

GLOBAL AND REGIONAL SCENARIOS

The Global Plan to Stop TB 2006–2015 was conceived to serve as a road map towards the Millennium Development Goals and Partnership targets for 2015. Therefore, an attempt was made to construct realistic scenarios in which the targets were reached globally and in each of eight epidemiological regions. The scenarios are built on optimistic but realistic assumptions on the rate of scale-up of TB interventions and on their impact on the epidemic. The

scenarios include estimates of the costs of these interventions and the associated technical support. The steps in generating the scenarios were as follows:

- defining and costing intervention packages;
- estimating the magnitude and pace of scaling up of activities;
- estimating TB control outcomes and impact; and
- estimating the cost of DOTS expansion, DOTS-Plus and TB/HIV.

The scenarios do not take into account the possibility of socioeconomic change or innovations in TB tools, but health system constraints have been considered in making the assumptions.

The methodology used in developing the scenarios is described elsewhere.[21] For the purpose of this exercise, eight epidemiological regions were created which were: (1) Africa, high HIV prevalence; (2) Africa, low HIV prevalence; (3) American region including Latin American countries, but not established market economies; (4)

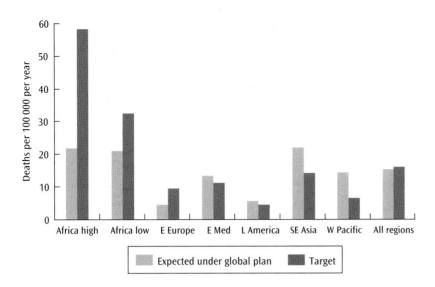

Figure 28.7 The expected impact of the Plan on prevalence by region.[20]

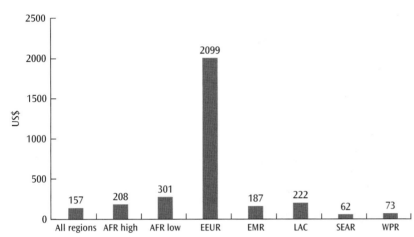

Figure 28.8 The cost per disability-adjusted life year (DALY) saved in the different regions based on the projected costs and impacts. The high cost per DALY in the Eastern European region is due to higher rates of hospitalization and the expenses associated with the treatment of multidrug-resistant tuberculosis.

Eastern Mediterranean region (including North Africa); (5) Eastern European region including Central Asia, but not including established market economies; (6) South East Asian region; (7) Western Pacific region, excluding established market economies; and (8) established market economies and central Europe. Of these regions, all except the established market economies (which have very low TB prevalence rates) were used as the basis of the scenarios.

The key outputs of the modelling exercise were the predictions of impact on TB prevalence, TB incidence, death rates due to TB, and cost-effectiveness of the planned interventions in terms of cost per DALY (disability-adjusted life year – a measure of the amount of human suffering averted by the intervention or set of actions) saved. Total costs of the interventions have also been estimated.

The modelling results indicated that global targets would be met, but that on a regional basis it would not be feasible to halve prevalence or the death rate due to TB in the region of Africa that suffers from high HIV prevalence, nor in the Eastern European epidemiological region that includes Central Asia. Additional measures that might be attempted in these regions in order to reach the targets are unlikely to be feasible (Figures 28.5–28.8).

Note that the targets are not expected to be met in a realistic scenario by 2015 in either of Africa or Eastern Europe (including Central Asia).

The Global Plan provides a summing up of the regional scenario results:[20]

Plans for implementation of TB control during the period are ambitious, realistic and shaped to individual country needs. In those countries – in Asia, Latin America and parts of the Eastern Mediterranean – where success is already being built, the need is to consolidate that success, sustain progress and lay the foundation for eventual elimination of TB. Long-term investment and commitment are essential.

In Africa and Eastern Europe, where success remains elusive because of HIV or multidrug-resistant TB and wider societal and health system issues, emergency action is critical. As in other regions, the constraints cannot be overcome by the Stop TB Partnership alone, however effective. Collaboration with the HIV programmes is essential. More generally, to reach the targets and bridge the unacceptable gaps between regions, the Stop TB Partnership will engage with other partners in the African and Eastern European regions and with the international financial institutions to seek increased political commitment and to address health system, infrastructure and economic barriers to the full-scale implementation of core strategies to address TB, TB/HIV and multidrug-resistant TB.

PARTNERSHIP ACTION TO ACHIEVE THE GOALS

Partnership action to achieve the Millennium Development Goals and the Stop TB Partnership's own targets is described in the Global Plan in the form of summaries of the strategic plans of the seven working groups and of the Stop TB Partnership secretariat. These working groups are DOTS Expansion, DOTS-Plus for MDR-TB, HIV/TB, New TB Diagnostics, New TB Drugs, New TB Vaccines and Advocacy Communication and Social Mobilization. Of these, the DOTS Expansion Working Group Strategic Plan is the cornerstone, laying out the foundation for TB control and care and forming the foundation of work by the DOTS-Plus for MDR-TB, HIV/TB and Advocacy Communication and Social Mobilization working groups. Deployment of new tools such as diag-

nostics, drugs and vaccines, as they become available will rely on the interplay of the implementation-oriented groups with those who have developed the technologies.

DOTS Expansion Working Group Strategic Plan

The DOTS Expansion Working Group Strategic Plan[17] has been developed to address the following key challenges as stated in the plan document:

- The rapid scale up of DOTS coverage has put high demand on programme management, supervision and quality control.
- TB diagnosis and treatment still relies on relatively old and imperfect technologies.
- True access to quality services is still poor in many settings.
- There is still limited awareness of TB in communities worldwide.
- Large parts of the health systems in most countries are still not supporting DOTS implementation.
- There are limited resources for external technical assistance to countries, now benefiting from large sums from new financial mechanisms.

The Plan itself uses the Stop TB Strategy elements as its cornerstone and sets global targets for a number of key

Table 28.1 DOTS expansion implementation status at 2005, 2010 and 2015 and milestones.[22]

	2005	2010	2015
DOTS coverage	All HBCs covered, except Brazil and Russia	Full DOTS coverage	→
DOTS quality improvement	Considerable investments and achievements, especially in SEAR and WPR	Completed in all priority countries in Africa, AMR, AMR and EUR	Completed in all countries
PPM DOTS	Piloted in most HBCs and limited scale up in a few HBCs and other countries	Scale up completed in key countries and started in most HBCs and other priority countries	Scale up completed. 3.8 billion people covered
Community DOTS	Widely used in a number of countries mainly in AFR, SEAR and WPR	Full scale up completed to cover whole population in Africa and most other HBCs/priority countries	Scale up completed in all relevant areas, covering 1.9 billion population
PAL	A few countries have pilot projects	Scale up started in selected countries, predominantly in EMR, EUR and AMR	Scale up completed in all relevant areas, covering 2 billion population
Culture and DST	Widely used in EUR but need quality improvement. Very limited in other regions	At least 50% of the population in all regions live in areas with cultures and DST services	Scale up completed covering more than 5 billion population

AMR, WHO region of the Americas; DST, drug sensitivity testing; EMR, WHO Eastern Mediterranean region; EUR, WHO European region (includes Central Asia); HBC, high-burden country; PAL, practical approach to lung health; PPM, public–private mix; SEAR, WHO South East Asian region; WPR, WHO Western Pacific region.

indicators capturing the main elements of the strategy. These targets are to be met through the implementation of approaches, such as traditional DOTS expansion, DOTS quality improvement, public–private mix DOTS (PPM DOTS), community care and engagement, practical approach to lung health (PAL), and improved capacity for culture and drugs sensitivity testing (DST). Milestones for the implementation of these approaches are shown in Table 28.1.

The Plan uses models to estimate the level of effort required to implement these approaches at a sufficiently high scale in order to reach the impact level demanded by the Millennium Development Goals and Partnership targets. The cost of this level of scale up of activities has been calculated using the results of this modelling exercise. The Plan further outlines the monitoring plan, lists priorities for action and sets out the terms of reference, structure and function of the working group itself.

DOTS-Plus for the MDR-TB working group strategic plan

The strategic plan of DOTS-Plus for the MDR-TB working group lays out its vision, objectives, targets and milestones, expected impact and estimated costs. Its vision is

to integrate drug resistance surveillance (DRS) and the management of MDR-TB as routine components of TB control providing access to diagnosis and treatment for all TB patients and by all health care providers. This is in line with the new comprehensive approach to global TB control. As a result, all MDR-TB management measures will be implemented in collaboration with DOTS expansion and strengthening activities and also in line with the activities of the other Stop TB working groups.[22]

Although the work does not start from zero, it is a fact that very few people with MDR-TB, about 2 per cent, are treated according to WHO guidelines.

In order to achieve its vision, the working group has identified the following objectives:[22]

1 By 2015, representative data on the global magnitude of MDR-TB, reliable trends from high MDR-TB prevalence countries and data on the relationship between MDR-TB and HIV/AIDS should be available.
2 By 2015, all regions should provide DST for all previously treated TB patients. In the Eastern European region, DST will also be provided for all new cases and in the Latin American, South East Asia and Western Pacific regions, DST should be provided for 20 per cent of new TB patients, targeting those people at increased risk of having MDR-TB.
3 By 2015, all detected MDR-TB patients should be treated with quality-assured second-line drugs in line

with WHO guidelines (17 per cent of the estimated culture-positive MDR-TB cases in 2010 and 56 per cent in 2015).
4 By 2015, further reductions in the price of second-line drugs should be achieved, as well as additional production of quality-assured second-line drugs by manufacturers based in high MDR-TB burden countries.
5 Technical direction and strategic planning for the management and coordination of global MDR-TB surveillance and control through the Stop TB working group on DOTS-Plus for MDR-TB should be provided, in close collaboration with the other Stop TB working groups, including those on new drugs and diagnostics.

The plan identifies key risk factors that may challenge the achievement of these objectives and a model has been used to estimate the level of effort required for scaling up work in this area, the expected impact and costing.

TB/HIV working group strategic plan

As stated in the TB/HIV working group strategic plan, the document 'lays out the activities that need to be undertaken by the WG and its partners over the next 10 years to achieve the 2015 targets under the following four objectives:

1 scale up and expand collaborative TB/HIV activities;
2 develop and coordinate implementation of research to improve the prevention, early diagnosis and rapid treatment of TB in people living with HIV and incorporate results into global policy;
3 increase political and resource commitment to collaborative TB/HIV activities;
4 contribute to strengthening health systems to deliver collaborative TB/HIV activities.'[11]

Again, the plan elaborates on objectives and activities and plans for scaling up efforts in order to reach the Partnership's targets and the millennium development goals. Impact and costs are modelled and risks are described.

Advocacy, communication and social mobilization

The Working Group on Advocacy, Communication and Social Mobilization (ACSM) has two subgroups, one focused on global action and the other on country level action. The objectives of the group as described in the plan are as follows:[20]

1 help to mobilize the financial resources required to fully fund the global plan;
2 encourage a higher profile of TB on policy agendas;
3 increase political and social support for TB control policies recommended by WHO;

4 engage policy-makers and others to secure greater political support for TB control;

5 build the capacity of national TB programmes and partnerships, and other key actors to develop and implement ACSM plans;

6 build the capacity of civil society and affected communities in donor and endemic countries to advocate for the fight against TB;

7 promote exchange of information between the working groups and the sharing of ACSM-related lessons and experiences;

8 build ACSM indicators and monitoring and evaluation mechanisms into institutional monitoring and evaluation systems.

The Global Plan targets and milestones for ACSM are:

• by 2010, civil society TB advocacy organizations or coalitions will be functioning in 20 donor countries and 40 endemic countries;

• by 2015, the ACSM working group will have helped to mobilize US$56 billion;

• by 2015, multisectoral, participatory ACSM methodology will be a fully developed component of the WHO Stop TB Strategy;

• by 2015, all priority countries will be implementing effective and participatory ACSM initiatives;

• by 2008, at least 10 endemic countries will have developed and will be implementing multisectoral, participatory ACSM initiatives and generating qualitative and quantitative data on the contribution of ACSM to TB control;

• by 2010, at least 20 priority countries will be implementing multisectoral, participatory ACSM initiatives, and monitoring and evaluating their outcomes.

New tools working groups

The new tools working groups are New TB Diagnostics, New TB Drugs and New TB Vaccines. There is a section of the Global Plan dedicated specifically to the strategic plans of these three groups. The preamble summarizes the place of new tools in achieving the mission of the Partnership:[20]

The Plan has a two-track approach to Stop TB: maximizing the benefit of applying the existing tools for TB control, while at the same time developing the new tools (diagnostics, drugs and vaccines) that are so urgently needed. Innovation is key to both these approaches. The Plan encompasses innovative methods of expanding access to quality TB care. The Plan also encompasses the innovation of research and development in making available the new, improved tools to Stop TB.

Until recently, TB as a global health issue suffered from a lack of investment in the development of innovative tools to stop TB. Full funding of the Plan will transform this situation, as new diagnostics, drugs and vaccines become increasingly available. The dramatic breakthrough to eliminate TB by 2050 depends on these innovative tools.

Innovation is the key to progress, through maximizing the benefit from existing tools and promoting the development of new tools to stop TB.

The New Diagnostics Working Group objectives as reported in the plan are:

1 address existing gaps in knowledge that are obstructing development of new diagnostic tools;

2 development and evaluation of a portfolio of new diagnostic tools and demonstration of impact;

3 implementation of new diagnostic tools and ensuring access.

Expected results of the new tools working groups are shown in Table 28.2 below. For each of these objectives, a set of targets and indicators have been developed by the Working Group as well as a timetable for introduction of new diagnostic tests.

Table 28.2 Expected results of the new tools working groups.[20]

	By 2006	By 2010	By 2015
Vaccines	Five candidates in phase I trials	Nine candidates in phase II trials; at least two vaccines in phase IIb or 'proof of concept' trials by 2008; beginning of phase III trials	Four phase III efficacy trials carried out. One safe, effective, licensed vaccine available by 2015
Drugs	27 new compounds in the TB pipeline	One or two drugs registered for TB indication; treatment shortened to 3–4 months	Seven new drugs registered for TB indication; regimen revolutionized; clinical testing of drugs that can shorten treatment to 1–2 months
Diagnostics	Rapid culture for case detection and DST in demonstration phase	Point of care, rapid culture, improved microscopy. Phage detection (+DST) and simplified NAAT introduced	Predictive test for LTBI in demonstration phase

DST, drug sensitivity; LTBI, latent tuberculosis infection; NAAT, nucleic acid amplification test.

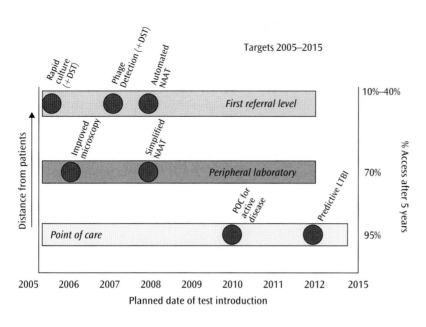

Figure 28.9 Targets for introduction of tests, leading to sustainable adoption, 2006–15.[20] LTBI, latent tuberculosis infection; POC, point of care.

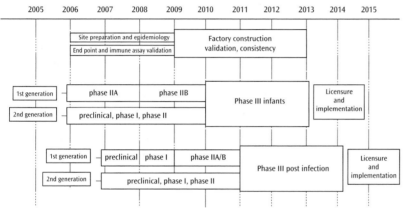

Figure 28.10 Timelines for tuberculosis vaccine development 2006–15.[20]

The ultimate aim is a diagnostic test available at the point of care which can identify people with latent TB infection who are at greatest risk of developing active TB (Figure 28.9).

The objectives of the Working Group for New TB Drug Development are:[20]

1 identify and validate drug targets for persistent and latent disease;
2 ascertain mechanisms of action of drugs in the global portfolio to generate complementary or even synergistic combinations effective against TB;
3 develop a sustainable portfolio of new drug candidates that meet the drug profile criteria;
4 develop animal models that can be used to predict the activity and side effects of compounds, and validated surrogate markers that are broadly adopted by TB drug developers;
5 build clinical trial sites and initiate and conduct clinical trials that meet regulatory requirements and the highest ethical standards. Develop biomarkers, surrogate endpoints and testing programmes to speed future clinical development programmes;

6 establish harmonized regulatory guidelines, including fast-track approval for TB drug developers.

The working group aims to introduce a new TB drug in 2010. By 2015, a new TB treatment regimen should be within reach, offering the promise of a cure within 1–2 months of the start of treatment, effective against MDR-TB and compatible with antiretroviral treatment.[20]

The Working Group on New TB Vaccines aims to have 'a safe, effective, licensed vaccine available at reasonable cost by 2015' (Figure 28.10).[20] It aims to achieve this goal through the following objectives:[20]

1 maintain and improve BCG vaccination programmes;
2 discovery and translation research ('keeping the pipeline filled');
3 facilitate preclinical development;
4 build capacity at vaccine trial sites;
5 ensure availability of vaccine production capacity/scale up;
6 perform clinical trials;
7 provide an enabling infrastructure.

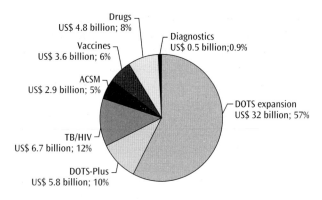

Figure 28.11 Total Global Plan costs by working group area of responsibility. ACSM, advocacy, communication and social mobilization.

The Stop TB Partnership Secretariat

The main areas of work of the Partnership secretariat are managing the partnership in response to the coordinating board, resource mobilization, advocacy and TB drug supply. Its objectives over the period of the Global Plan are as follows:[20]

1 promote accountability, flexibility and coordination in the management of partnership resources;

2 stimulate the mobilization of sufficient resources to enable the implementation of the Global Plan to Stop TB (2006–2015);

3 ensure the effective functioning, growth, dynamism and catalyzing effect of the global TB drug facility in global TB control;

4 facilitate relationships between and with existing partners and strengthen our coalition by reaching out to new or potential partners;

5 build skills, resources and capacity at regional and national level to enable successful partnerships to be developed;

6 place TB on the global development agenda, while at the same time mainstreaming pro-poor approaches into TB control;

7 take TB beyond the existing reach and scope of traditional disease control programmes by catalyzing new opportunities and promoting the aims and objectives of the Global Plan to Stop TB (2006–2015);

8 monitor and evaluate the impact of the secretariat and Partnership in delivery of the Global Plan to Stop TB (2006–2015).

FINANCING THE PLAN

Financial modelling has identified the total cost for full implementation of the Global Plan as US$56.1 billion over the 10-year period (Figure 28.11). From this analysis it is apparent that the greatest share of cost is for DOTS expansion in countries heavily affected by TB. Specifically, financing for countries' national TB programmes and associated efforts is estimated at US$44.3 billion.

Of the total projected cost of Global Plan implementation, approximately 45 per cent is expected through current and pledged funding flows, largely the domestic budgets of affected countries (Figure 28.12). The overall financial gap is US$31 billion.

CHALLENGES IN IMPLEMENTATION

Finances aside, the main constraints to full implementation of the Global Plan to Stop TB will be familiar to anyone working in public health. These are a lack of political commitment to honour commitments. There is a lack of 'boots on the ground' to put plans into action in affected countries, partly due to a lack of engagement by partners, but also due to the health workforce crisis, i.e. the qualitative and quantitative deficiencies related to human resources capable of implementing control efforts in non-

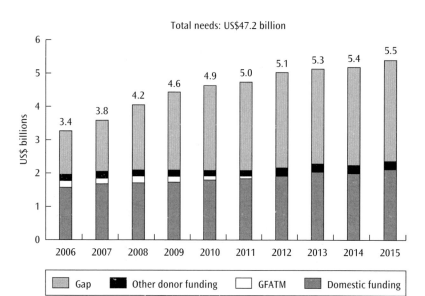

Figure 28.12 The breakdown of the projected costs for programme implementation in affected countries, illustrating the proportion of the total cost that is expected to be borne by the countries themselves, the proportion that is expected from the Global Fund to Fight AIDS, TB and Malaria (GFATM) and other donors, and the remaining gap.

endemic countries. Constraints associated with the health systems infrastructure, as well as basic infrastructure outside the health sector need to be addressed concurrent with plan implementation if access to quality TB care is to be made universal. Finally, there is increasing competition for resources among public health initiatives, among development initiatives and among humanitarian causes. We will need to think creatively and fully engage all Stop TB Partners to meet these challenges.

DOES THE PLAN GO FAR ENOUGH?

The Global Plan to Stop TB, 2006–2015 is meant to be optimistic but achievable. In the interests of realism, it may fall short on ambition. It may be criticized for not going far enough in its demands on the international community. For example, it does not call for universal access to drug sensitivity testing in order to detect drug-resistant TB before a patient endures treatment failure and may infect others. As a result, only a total of 800 000 MDR-TB patients may be treated according to international standards in the decade, while yearly about 400 000 new MDR-

TB cases are estimated to arise. In fact, the working group on MDR-TB has agreed to revise its strategic plan to call for universal access. The international community may decide that the Global Plan does not go far enough, does not ask enough and leaves too many patients underserved. However, the targets and goals set in the Global Plan are not meant to be limits to endeavour, but rather goal posts along the way to the ultimate goal of a world free of TB. Therefore, it is up to countries with high burdens of TB disease to tailor their national plans to the specific needs of their populations, using the Global Plan as a framework to inspire, motivate and guide, rather than to limit.

NEXT STEPS: COUNTRY-LED ACTION

Besides the continued functioning of the working groups and the implementation of their strategic plans, the success of the Global Plan rests on action in affected countries.

Tables 28.3 and 28.4[23] illustrate the state of country-led action regarding the six elements of the Stop TB Strategy in the 22 countries which together shoulder 80 per cent of the world's TB disease burden. The data were compiled

Table 28.3 Countries with a plan in line with the second Global Plan (GP2).

Country	DOTS		TB/HIV, MDR-TB				HSS		
	Plan in line with GP2	No. culture facilities	% TB patients HIV tested	% HIV⁺ TB patients on ARV	DRS complete	GLC project	HRD TB plan linked to HRH plans	Integrated staff at facility level	PAL activities
Afghanistan	Yes	0	HIV		No	No	Yes	No	Planned
Bangladesh	Yes	2			No	Approved	No	No	No
Brazil	Yes	137			Yes	No	Yes	Yes	Planned
Cambodia	Yes	3			Yes	Approved	No	Yes	Planned
China	Yes	317	47	85	Yes	Review	Yes	Yes	No
Congo	Yes	1	3		Yes	Approved	Yes	Yes	No
Ethiopia	No	1			Yes	No	No	No	No
India	Yes	5	2	1	Yes	Review	Yes	Yes	No
Indonesia	Yes	41	3	29	Yes	No	Yes	Yes	Planned
Kenya	Yes	1	3		Yes	Approved	No	Yes	Planned
Mozambique	Yes	1			No	No	Yes	Yes	No
Myanmar	Yes	2	15	20	Yes	Preparation	Yes	Yes	Planned
Nigeria	Yes	3			No	No	No	No	No
Pakistan	Yes	3	2	31	No	No	Yes	Yes	Planned
Philippines	Yes	3	11		Yes	On-going	No	No	No
Russia	Yes	159			Yes	On-going	Yes	No	No
South Africa	Yes	16	22	33	Yes	No			Yes
Thailand	Yes	80			Yes	No	No	Yes	Planned
Uganda	Yes	2	8		No	No		Yes	Yes
Tanzania	No	3	4	28	Yes	No		Yes	Planned
Vietnam	Yes	30			Yes	Preparation	Yes	Yes	Yes
Zimbabwe	No	1			No	No	Yes	Yes	No

ARV, antiretrovirals; DRS, drug resistance surveillance; GLC, Green Light Committee; HRD, human resource development; MDR-TB, multidrug-resistant tuberculosis; PAL, practical approaches to lung health.

Table 28.4   Country status in terms of scaling up the PPM approach to engaging private medical practitioners in the national TB programme, familiarity with ISTC, familiarity with the patients' charter and the degree to which there is community involvement in TB control and care.

Country	Engage all care providers		Empower people with TB and communities		Operational research
	PPM scale up	Familiar with ISTC	Familiar with patients' charter	Country with community involvement (%)	Examples
Afghanistan	No	No	No	7	TB/HIV prevalence survey
Bangladesh	Yes	No	Yes	50	Health-seeking behaviour in Dhaka
Brazil	No	No	Yes	40	Evaluation of information system
Cambodia	No	Yes	Yes	70	HIV seroprevalence survey, KAP
China	Yes	Yes	No	0	Diagnosis and treatment of smear-negative patients
Congo	Yes	No	No	0	TB/HIV prevalence
Ethiopia	No	Yes	Yes	30	Isoniazid preventive therapy
India	Yes	Yes	Yes		PPM cost evaluation
Indonesia	Yes	Yes	Yes	10	TB/HIV seroprevalence survey, DRS
Kenya	Yes	No	Yes	25	Diagnosis (future)
Mozambique	Yes	Yes	Yes	5	DRS, prevalence survey (future)
Myanmar	Yes	Yes	No	20	Effectiveness of FDCs
Nigeria	No	Yes	Yes	25	Smear-negative diagnosis (future)
Pakistan	No	Yes	No	30	Treatment adherence and default tracing
Philippines	Yes	Yes	Yes	25	Public–public DOTS effectiveness
Russia	No	Yes	No	0	Drug resistance
South Africa	No				
Thailand	No	Yes	No	5	M&E in select provinces
Uganda	No	Yes	No	100	Diagnosis of smear-negative patients
Tanzania	No	Yes	Yes	5	Tuberculin survey
Vietnam	Yes	Yes	No	80	Service quality at commune level
Zimbabwe	No	No	Yes	25	DRS

DRS, drug resistance surveillance; ISTC, International Standards for TB Care; PPM, public–private mix; TB, tuberculosis.

from a 2006 WHO questionnaire distributed to the countries and may not always reflect reality, but it is probably the best approximation available today of the situation in these countries.

The data indicate that 15 of the 22 countries with the highest TB disease burdens on the planet do not have a national TB plan in line with the Global Plan to Stop TB, 2006–2015, in all the areas of DOTS, TB-HIV, MDR-TB and health systems strengthening. Completion of this planning process through country-led processes with more fully-engaged partners is therefore an urgent priority. This must be paired with high level advocacy both in endemic countries and globally in order to generate the political commitment and resources that are needed to implement global, regional and national plans. Implementing plans means scaling up quickly, while assuring quality, learning from new experiences and maintaining accountability and transparency.

Table 28.3 indicates whether the countries have a plan in line with the second Global Plan (GP2), the number of culture facilities for drug sensitivity testing, the percentage of TB patients who are offered HIV testing, the percentage of HIV-positive TB patients on antiretroviral therapy, whether the country has completed a TB drug resistance

survey (DRS), whether there is a Green Light Committee (GLC) project in the country for the provision of second-line drugs to treat MDR-TB, whether there is a plan for TB human resource development (HRD) linked to human resources for health plans, whether there are TB-specific staff at the health facility level or whether TB services are integrated with other aspects of the health system at that level, and whether there are PAL activities in the country.

Table 28.4 indicates the status of the country in terms of scaling up the public–private mix approach to engaging private medical practitioners in the national TB programme (PPM), familiarity with the International Standards for TB Care (ISTC), familiarity with the patients' charter and the degree to which there is community involvement in TB control and care.

NEXT STEPS: MONITORING GLOBAL PLAN IMPLEMENTATION

Progress in implementation of the Stop TB Strategy at country level is monitoring to a large extent by the WHO and reported in its annual Global TB Report.[24] At its eleventh

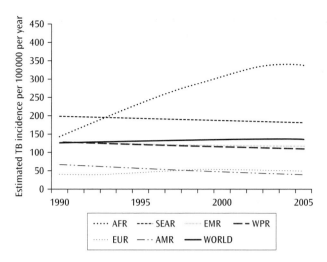

Figure 28.13 A possible slowing of the incidence rate in Africa and Asia and hence globally.[25] AFR, Africa; AMR, Americas; EMR, Eastern Mediterranean Region; EUR, Europe, SEAR, South East Asia.

meeting in Jakarta, Indonesia in November 2006, the Stop TB coordinating board agreed in principle to a process for monitoring Global Plan implementation by the working groups at global level. This will most likely take the form of informal reporting to the coordinating board twice a year at its meetings, in addition to more formal reporting against an agreed template based on the indicators and milestones of the working groups' strategic plans.

MEETING THE MILLENNIUM DEVELOPMENT GOAL TARGET FOR TB

Given the results of country-level epidemiological monitoring, reaching the millennium development goal target for TB seems feasible. In part, TB incidence may be slowing as a possible result of the passing of the peak of the HIV epidemic in Africa (Figure 28.13).

However, turning the TB epidemic around will require full financing and implementation of the Global Plan, including its use as a framework for robust, funded, country-owned plans to implement the Stop TB Strategy.[9] Health system constraints must be addressed including the need for sound monitoring and evaluation in the context of good programme management. Ultimately, a world free of TB can only come into being if we continue to innovate. We will need to develop new and better tools to fight the disease such as diagnostics, drugs and vaccines, and new approaches to TB control and care.

CONCLUSIONS

The Global Plan to Stop TB makes clear that progress towards the elimination of TB relies on both investments to maximize the impact of currently available tools for TB control, and the rapid development and application of new tools such as drugs, diagnostics and vaccines. These investments must be joined with study of the socioeconomic determinants that cause TB to be prevalent in a society. Better understanding of these contributors to disease will be essential to accelerating the elimination of TB.

LEARNING POINTS

What can medical professionals do to implement the Global Plan to Stop TB?

The Global Plan can be used as a framework within which regional, national, organizational, community and individual efforts can be situated. As a medical professional, you may already be a member of the partnership through your professional organization, or you may choose to join a national partnership as an individual. There are a number of things you as a medical professional can do to help reach the 2015 targets:

- Make a commitment to implement the Stop TB Strategy and the International Standards for TB Care.
- Post the TB patient's charter in your clinic or hospital.
- Join the Stop TB Partnership at national, regional and/or global level.
- Read the Global Plan to Stop TB, the regional plan and the national plan to Stop TB and find your role.
- Set targets for your organization's role in stopping TB in the context of a national plan to stop TB or promote the development of a national plan if none exists.
- Help ensure access to quality treatment by taking action and by supporting advocacy efforts.
- Organize a local stakeholders meeting to work out what your community can do to implement the plan.
- Help mobilize the resources to fully fund the plan: US$56 billion over the 10 years will result in 50 million TB patients treated and 14 million additional lives saved, as well as new diagnostics, drugs and vaccines, resulting in better TB control, healthier communities and less poverty.
- Help ensure that quality TB care reaches all TB patients.
- Participate in or promote research to develop new improved tools and approaches to combat TB.
- Use the Global Plan as a tool to persuade all stakeholders to fulfil their commitment to stop TB, perhaps through a national partnership or by forming a national partnership where there is none.
- Take part in or initiate advocacy campaigns such as the Call to Stop TB, shown in the annex to this chapter.
- Send a donation to the Stop TB Trust Fund or one of the Stop TB Partner organizations.
- Find more information on the Stop TB website: www.stoptb.org.

ANNEX

THE CALL
TO STOP TB

Figure 28.14 The Call to Stop TB. Reproduced with permission from the Stop TB Partnership.

"WE CALL ON WORLD LEADERS, GOVERNMENTS, ORGANIZATIONS, CIVIL SOCIETY, CORPORATIONS AND INDIVIDUALS TO ENDORSE, FULLY FUND AND IMPLEMENT THE GLOBAL PLAN TO STOP TB 2006–2015"

BECAUSE EACH YEAR NEARLY 2 MILLION PEOPLE DIE AND 9 MILLION PEOPLE BECOME SICK WITH TB AND BECAUSE TB INFECTS ONE-THIRD OF THE WORLD'S POPULATION.

BECAUSE TB IS A GLOBAL PANDEMIC AND AN EMERGENCY IN AFRICA AND THE EUROPEAN REGION.

BECAUSE TB IS THE BIGGEST KILLER OF PEOPLE WITH HIV/AIDS AND MULTI-DRUG RESISTANT FORMS OF TB ARE A THREAT AROUND THE GLOBE.

BECAUSE TB IS CURABLE.

BECAUSE THE STOP TB STRATEGY IS GETTING RESULTS.

BECAUSE 14 MILLION MORE LIVES CAN BE SAVED OVER THE NEXT 10 YEARS.

BECAUSE TREATING AND CURING PEOPLE WITH TUBERCULOSIS PREVENTS THE SPREAD OF THE DISEASE, REDUCES POVERTY, STRENGTHENS HEALTH SYSTEMS, ENGAGES ALL CARE PROVIDERS AND EMPOWERS THOSE AFFECTED.

BECAUSE NEW VACCINES, DRUGS AND DIAGNOSTICS TO STOP TB ARE URGENTLY NEEDED.

BECAUSE ACCESS TO TB TREATMENT IS A HUMAN RIGHT.

BECAUSE TB CAN BE ELIMINATED BY 2050 IF WE TAKE ACTION NOW.

FOR THESE 10 REASONS, WE COMMIT OURSELVES, THROUGH OUR ACTION, TO A WORLD FREE OF TB.

ACKNOWLEDGEMENTS

Thanks to Richard Maggi for his help in preparing the manuscript.

REFERENCES

1. Tuberculosis Coalition for Technical Assistance. *International standards for tuberculosis care (ISTC)*. The Hague: Tuberculosis Coalition for Technical Assistance, 2006.
2. World Health Organization. WHO declares tuberculosis is a global emergency. Press release, 1993.
3. World Health Assembly. *Resolutions and decisions. Resolution WHA 44.8*. Geneva: World Health Organization, WHA44/1991/REC/1, 1991.
4. World Health Organization. *The Global Plan to Stop TB 2000–2005*. Geneva: World Health Organization, WHO/CDS/STB/2001.16, 2001 (www.stoptb.org/globalplan).
5. Kumaresan J, Smith I, Arnold V, Evans P. The global TB drug facility: innovative global procurement. *Int J Tuberc Lung Dis* 2004; **8**: 130–38.
6. Gupta R, Kim JY, Espinal M *et al.* Responding to market failures in tuberculosis control. *Science* 2001; **10**: 1049–51.
7. World Health Organization. Progress report on the global plan to stop tuberculosis. Geneva: World Health Organization, WHO/HTM/STB/2004.29, 2004 (www.stoptb.org/globalplan)
8. Stop TB Partners Directory. www.stoptb.org/partners.
9. Dye C. Did we reach the 2005 targets, will we reach the MDGs? DOTS Expansion Meeting, Paris, 30 October 2006 (www.stoptb.org/wg/dots_expansion/meetings).

10. Stop TB Partnership 11th Coordinating Board Meeting. Summary sheet agenda item 2.06-13.0 Global fund progress and challenges, 30 November 2006, Jakarta, Indonesia.

11. Stop TB HIV/TB Working Group. Strategic plan 2006–2015, 22 pp. (www.stoptb.org/globalplan/docs_splans).

12. Reid A, Scano F, Getahun H et al. Towards universal access to HIV prevention, treatment, care, and support: the role of tuberculosis/HIV collaboration. Lancet Infect Dis 2006; 6: 483–95.

13. Tupasi T. Progress in implementing the Stop TB Strategy and the Global Plan to Stop TB. DOTS Expansion Meeting, Paris, 30 October 2006 (www.stoptb.org/wg/dots_expansion/meetings).

14. Stop TB New Diagnostics Working Group. Strategic plan 2006–2015, 17 pp. (www.stoptb.org/globalplan/docs_splans).

15. Stop TB Partnership Working Group on New TB Drugs. Strategic plan 2006–2015, 18 pp. (www.stoptb.org/globalplan/docs_splans).

16. Stop TB Partnership Working Group on New TB Vaccines. Strategic plan 2006–2015, 7 pp. (www.stoptb.org/globalplan/docs_splans).

17. DOTS Expansion Working Group. Strategic plan 2006–2015. Geneva: World Health Organization, WHO/HTM/TB/2006.370, 2006 (www.stoptb.org/globalplan/docs_splans).

18. CDC. Worldwide emergence of Mycobacterium tuberculosis with extensive resistance to second-line drugs. MMWR Morb Mortal Rep Wkly 2006; 55: TK–TK.

19. United Nations General Assembly Resolution A/RES/55/2, 18 September 2000. Agenda item 60 (b). United Nations Millennium Declaration.

20. The Global Plan to Stop TB 2006–2015. Actions for life towards a world free of tuberculosis. Geneva: World Health Organization, WHO/HTM/STB/2006.35, 2006 (www.stoptb.org/globalplan).

21. The Global Plan to Stop TB 2006–2015. Methods used to estimate costs, funding and funding gaps. Geneva: World Health Organization, WHO/HTM/STB/2006.38, 2006 (www.stoptb.org/globalplan/docs_main).

22. Stop TB Working Group on DOTS-Plus for MDR-TB. Strategic plan 2006–2015. (www.stoptb.org/globalplan/docs_splans).

23. Raviglione M. Moving ahead with the Stop TB Strategy, where are we today? DOTS Expansion Meeting, Paris, 30 October 2006 (www.stoptb.org/wg/dots_expansion/meetings).

24. World Health Organization. Global tuberculosis control report. Geneva: World Health Organization, WHO/HTM/TB/2006.362, 2006 (www.who.int/tb/publications/global_report/2006).

25. Raviglione M. Progress in meeting 2005 targets and challenges to meet 2015 goals. DOTS Expansion Meeting, Vancouver, Canada, 22 February 2007.

PART **8**

RELATED ASPECTS

29

Environmental mycobacteria

JOHN BANKS AND IAN A CAMPBELL

INTRODUCTION

In addition to *Mycobacterium tuberculosis* and *Mycobacterium bovis*, other species of mycobacteria may cause human disease. Variously referred to as mycobacteria other than tuberculosis (MOTT), opportunist, non-tuberculous, atypical, anonymous and environmental mycobacteria, these organisms are ubiquitous in nature and have been isolated from sources including soil, dust, water and milk, as well as a variety of animals and birds.[1–4] In humans, they are usually low-grade pathogens. The significance of an isolate can therefore be doubtful and it is necessary to establish criteria which determine significance and the need for treatment. The type of specimen from which the organism is isolated, the number of isolates, the degree of growth and the identity of the organism are important considerations. The clinical presentation and predisposing factors in the patient are also helpful in determining significance. Disease usually occurs in patients with pre-existing lung disease or states of immunodeficiency, but is found less in patients with no obvious predisposing condition. Genetic factors may play a part.[5,6] For *Mycobacterium kansasii*, there is an association with occupational dust exposure.[7,8] Infection is most probably acquired from the environment, although the source and portal of entry may differ between individuals. If it occurs at all, cross-infection is extremely rare (an example was presumed to have occurred when a father and son in the same household both had *M. kansasii* infection).[9] Notification of cases is not therefore necessary.

Over 80 species of environmental mycobacteria have been identified.[10] Those that are potentially pathogenic are shown in Table 29.1. Clinicians should be aware of non-

Table 29.1 Major environmental mycobacteria that may cause human disease.

Species	Major sites of infection
M. avium[a]	Pulmonary
M. intracellulare[a]	Pulmonary/lymph gland
M. scrofulaceum[a]	Pulmonary
M. kansasii	Pulmonary
M. xenopi	Pulmonary
M. malmoense	Pulmonary
M. fortuitum	Soft tissues/surgical wounds
M. chelonei	Soft tissues/surgical wounds
M. ulcerans	Skin
M. marinum	Soft tissues/surgical wounds

[a]*M. avium*, *M. intracellulare* and *M. scrofulaceum* are also referred to as MAIS.

pathogenic species that are occasionally isolated from the sputum and other clinical specimens, but are rarely of clinical significance. These include *Mycobacterium gordonae*, *Mycobacterium gastri*, *Mycobacterium terra*, *Mycobacterium triviale*, *Mycobacterium non-chronogenicum* and *Mycobacterium flavescens*.[11–15]

M. kansasii is the most common species encountered in Western Europe, Texas and the upper central states of North America[12,15] and the *M. avium intracellulare* complex (MAC), known also as *M. avium intracellulare scrofulaceum* (MAIS), predominates in south-eastern USA, Western Australia and Japan, where the prevalence of pulmonary infection caused by MAC is approximately 10 per cent of that resulting from *M. tuberculosis*.[15,16] Geographical patterns of disease also appear within the

UK. Before the AIDS epidemic, *M. kansasii* was the most common species encountered in Britain, but infection in London and south-east England was predominantly caused by *M. xenopi*.[17] Of 533 clinically confirmed new cases of environmental mycobacterial infections recorded by the Regional Mycobacterium Laboratory in the south-east of England (Dulwich), 37 per cent were due to *M. xenopi*, 28 per cent to *M. kansasii*, 20 per cent to MAC and 8 per cent to *M. fortuitum* or *M. chelonei*.[18] In Scotland, *M. malmoense* predominates. For a time the problem of disseminated infection caused by MAC in patients infected with HIV altered these patterns of disease, but with the advent of highly active antiretroviral therapy (HAART) the picture is reverting.

Diagnosis depends on identification of the infecting mycobacteria using standard culture medium, as well as special methods, e.g. temperature range, oxygen preference, sensitivity pattern, pigment production, ability to hydrolyse Tween 80,[19] gas–liquid and thin-layer chromatography,[20] DNA probes (MAC, *M. kansasii* and *M. gordonae*)[21] and polymerase chain reaction (PCR) with reverse hybridization (*M. kansasii*, *M. malmoense*, *M. xenopi*, *M. chelonae*, *M. fortuitum*, *M. avium* and *M. intracellulare*).[22] Combining these molecular methods with the use of automated liquid culture techniques (BACTEC or MB/BacT) can speed up diagnosis by as much as 2 weeks. Differential skin testing is not reliable for diagnosis because of the non-specificity of mycobacterial antigens, which results in cross-reactivity between different mycobacterial species. Hypersensitivity to purified protein derivative (PPD) from MAC, for example, can arise as a result of infection with a wide range of mycobacterial species and does not specifically indicate MAC infection.[23] Similarly, skin testing using multiple types of PPD does not discriminate between infection caused by *M. tuberculosis* and *M. kansasii*[24] and is no substitute for the isolation and identification of the infecting mycobacteria.

Many sites of infection have been reported, including soft tissue, bone, joint and genitourinary tract, but pulmonary disease, lymphadenitis and disseminated infection are the most common and most important clinical problems.

PULMONARY DISEASE

The species that most often cause disease in the lungs are *M. kansasii*, MAC, *M. malmoense* and *M. xenopi*, with prevalence varying geographically and in relation to the prevalence of HIV. Patients may present with an acute or subacute illness that is clinically and radiologically identical to that caused by infection with *M. tuberculosis*. Symptoms, which may develop over several weeks, include cough, sputum, night sweats, haemoptysis, breathlessness, malaise and loss of weight. Occasionally, disease is discovered in an asymptomatic patient. The infiltrate and cavities seen on the chest x-ray are indistinguishable from those

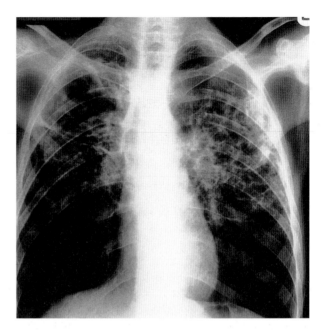

Figure 29.1 Chest x-ray showing extensive pulmonary disease caused by *M. xenopi* in an elderly man.

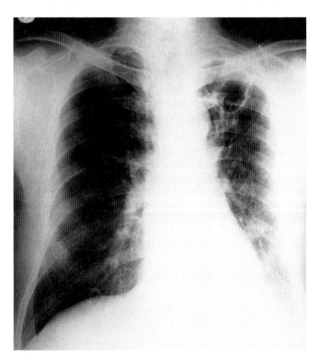

Figure 29.2 Chest x-ray showing a single cavity in the left apex in a 60-year-old man. *M. malmoense* was isolated from the sputum on repeated occasions.

caused by *M. tuberculosis* and between the various environmental species (Figures 29.1 and 29.2), cavitation occurring in 60–90 per cent of patients with these infections.[25–31] Pleural effusion, hilar and/or mediastinal lymphadenopathy are rare. Although infection may occur in previously healthy individuals, most patients have coexisting lung disease, commonly chronic bronchitis and emphysema, bronchiectasis or pneumoconiosis and are middle-aged to elderly men.[27,29–31] Not surprisingly, many patients are thought to have tuberculosis (TB) when acid-fast bacilli are seen on sputum smear and the correct diagnosis is confirmed only some weeks later on the results of culture. Pulmonary disease is eventually diagnosed when positive cultures are obtained from specimens of sputum obtained more than 7 days apart in a patient whose chest x-ray suggests mycobacterial infection and who may or may not have symptoms of pulmonary infection.

Although diagnosis is usually straightforward in patients who present with an acute pattern of disease, it may be more difficult when infection pursues a more chronic, insidious course developing over a period of months or even years. In these patients, weight loss and cachexia, which often accompany respiratory symptoms, may be attributed to coexistent pulmonary disease and not to mycobacterial infection. The chest x-ray can be difficult to interpret, often showing chronic, apparently indolent abnormalities which may also be attributed to other causes, e.g. post-tuberculous fibrosis. Mycobacteria isolated from the sputum of such patients may be thought to represent colonization of previously damaged lung rather than signifying active infection.

Disease is likely if multiple colonies of the same strain of mycobacteria are repeatedly isolated in the absence of other pathogens from symptomatic patients whose chest x-rays show abnormalities consistent with mycobacterial disease.[32,33] A single isolate from sputum that cannot be repeated is unlikely to be of any significance. Two positive cultures of M. kansasii[34] or M. malmoense[35] obtained on separate occasions usually signify genuine disease, but some authors suggest that three or four isolates of M. xenopi or MAC should be obtained in order to establish a diagnosis.[36,37] Colonization should not be lightly dismissed since transformation to invasive disease may occur unpredictably, sometimes following years of apparent quiescence.[38] Patients with MAC in their sputum do not always develop progressive disease, but can do so with a fatal outcome,[39] whilst disease caused by M. kansasii has progressed insidiously in some patients over several years in the absence of new symptoms at the time of diagnosis.[40] If doubt exists about the significance of repeated isolates, it is probably wise to treat the patient with antimycobacterial drugs.

SUPERFICIAL LYMPH NODE DISEASE

This occurs predominantly in the cervical lymph nodes of children, more often between the ages of 1 and 5 years. Often a single node is involved and may be 'hot' or 'cold'. When more than one node is involved, these tend to be unilateral rather than bilateral. There is little systemic upset, the affected glands are usually painless and non-tender,[41,42] and there is rarely any accompanying constitu-

tional illness. The chest x-ray is usually clear. These infections are caused primarily by MAC or M. malmoense. A diagnosis is made by resection of the involved glands, with specimens sent for culture for mycobacteria. Histological appearances are indistinguishable from those caused by M. tuberculosis. Treatment is by total excision of the affected node(s). Antimycobacterial chemotherapy is not indicated,[33,41–43] unless disease recurs when chemotherapy for 18 months to 2 years with rifampicin and ethambutol (possibly supplemented by isoniazid or clarithromycin) should be considered after further excision. Aspiration of the node, or incision and drainage, should be avoided because such procedures may leave a discharging sinus which can persist for many years, and sometimes even lead to ugly scarring.

DISEASE AT OTHER EXTRAPULMONARY SITES

Infection with M. fortuitum or M. chelonei usually occurs as a skin or soft-tissue infection following penetrating trauma or surgery, giving rise to recurrent abscess and fistula formation. Sternotomy wounds have become a particularly common site of infection.[44–47] Inoculation of the skin by M. marinum may occur following abrasions acquired in contaminated swimming pools or aquaria.[48] The initial lesion, which is often papular but which may later form a superficial ulcer, is known as the 'swimming pool' or 'fish tank' granuloma. The skin may also be infected by M. ulcerans, giving rise to chronic, indolent, necrotic ulcers known as 'Buruli ulcers', most commonly seen in central Africa.[49] Bone, joint and genitourinary tract infections have been reported, but these are rare.

Wound infections with M. fortuitum or M. chelonei should be treated by surgical debridement combined with ciprofloxacin and an aminoglycoside or imipenem.[33,44–47] Clarithromycin may have a place in combination therapy for these infections.[50] Skin lesions caused by M. marinum often heal spontaneously, although successful treatment has been reported using cotrimoxazole[51] or tetracycline.[52] Wide surgical excision with skin grafting is the treatment of choice for skin infection by M. ulcerans.[53]

There is no evidence from clinical trials to indicate how long chemotherapy should be continued for these infections. A minimum of 6 months seems sensible, but it may be necessary to prolong treatment for up to 2 years if the response to initial treatment is suboptimal.[33]

TREATMENT OF PULMONARY DISEASE

There is no general agreement about the treatment of pulmonary disease caused by environmental mycobacteria and many different approaches to treatment have been advocated. This lack of consensus reflects the paucity of large clinical trials assessing treatment and subsequent reliance upon results from small, non-comparable, retrospective or prospective series. Recommendations about treatment have been hampered by inappropriate comparisons with the treatment of TB. For example, the use of chemotherapy for the treatment of *M. kansasii* infection was originally questioned because patients remained sputum culture positive and showed persistent cavities on the chest x-rays after a few months of treatment with isoniazid, paraminosalicylic acid (PAS) and streptomycin.[54–57] Because this compared unfavourably with the prompt bacteriological and radiological response seen in patients with TB given the same treatment, drug therapy was discouraged in favour of surgical treatment.[58] The apparent failure of chemotherapy was attributed to drug resistance. Subsequent reports, however, showed that despite poor *in vitro* drug susceptibility successful treatment was possible in 85 per cent of patients when the duration of chemotherapy was prolonged beyond that normally considered adequate for TB.[59–61] Poor *in vitro* drug susceptibility to conventional antimycobacterial drugs did not predict treatment failure, but indicated a need to prolong treatment for 18–24 months. Clearly, criteria of *in vitro* drug susceptibility that govern the treatment of infection caused by *M. tuberculosis* do not usually apply to disease caused by other mycobacterial species. Confirmation of this has come from the recent prospective study conducted by the British Thoracic Society (BTS).[29–31,62]

M. kansasii

Important drugs in the regimen are rifampicin and ethambutol.[63] In a recent large prospective study of 9 months' therapy, treatment failed in only one of 173 patients. The patient who failed to respond admitted to poor compliance with treatment. Of 154 patients entering the post-chemotherapy follow-up period, 15 (9.7 per cent) developed positive cultures in the 51 months after the end of chemotherapy. Relapse in eight of these was influenced by factors such as lack of compliance with treatment, malnourishment, corticosteroid therapy, severe bronchiectasis and the development of carcinoma. In a further three patients, positive cultures were accompanied by fresh changes on the chest x-ray on the side other than that originally involved, or in a lobe different from the lobe originally involved. Relapse rate was not influenced by age, sex, coexisting disease, extent of original pulmonary involvement, cavitation or whether isoniazid had been part of the initial regimen and all 15 patients responded to further chemotherapy with rifampicin and ethambutol.[27] Another prospective study of 40 patients has been reported, using a regimen of ethambutol, rifampicin and isoniazid for 12 months. In the follow-up period, which varied between 3 and 5 years, a relapse rate of 2.5 per cent was noted.[64] A retrospective study of 471 patients in Czechoslovakia treated for 9–12 months with various antimycobacterial regimens reported an 8 per cent relapse rate in a period of follow up

ranging from 1 to 7 years.[65] Although the mortality from other causes in patients who develop *M. kansasii* pulmonary infection is high (10–25 per cent) less than 1 per cent die because of the *M. kansasii* pulmonary infection.[27,63–65]

Current knowledge would suggest that treatment with ethambutol and rifampicin for 9 months would be sufficient for most patients, but for those with overtly compromised immune defences therapy should probably be continued for 15–24 months or until the sputum has been negative on culture for 12 months. If patients fail to respond to ethambutol and rifampicin then the addition of prothionamide or streptomycin should be considered. The role of clarithromycin, if any, remains to be assessed by prospective, comparative (preferably randomized) clinical trials. Non-compliant patients should be followed up indefinitely and relapses retreated with 15–24 months of ethambutol and rifampicin.[33]

MAC (MAIS)

The outcome of treatment for MAC infection is less predictable than that for *M. kansasii*. Poor *in vitro* susceptibility to conventional antimycobacterial drugs tested singly and failure of chemotherapy in some patients has led to recommendations for surgical treatment whenever possible.[66] Good results following surgical treatment for pulmonary MAC have been reported, with conversion to sputum culture negative occurring post-operatively in 93–100 per cent of those patients and relapses occurring in only 5 per cent during prolonged follow up.[66,67] Results in other series have been less impressive, with 33 per cent of patients ultimately relapsing post-operatively.[68] Surgery may not be feasible in most patients with coexistent lung conditions or those with extensive lung involvement secondary to mycobacterial infection. Medical treatment is the only therapeutic option for most patients.

As with earlier reports describing chemotherapy in patients with *M. kansasii* infection, chemotherapy for MAC infection may have failed in many cases because treatment was not continued for long enough. In more recent series, successful results were achieved in 60–94 per cent of patients given combinations of rifampicin, ethambutol, isoniazid and streptomycin for at least 18 months.[39,69] *In vitro* drug susceptibility did not predict the eventual clinical response, but did correlate in some studies with the time taken to convert sputum culture to negative.[70,71] Both the initial response to treatment and relapse following cessation of chemotherapy may be influenced by the severity of the coexisting pulmonary disease. Ninety-four per cent of patients in one study who were not breathless at the start of treatment responded to rifampicin, isoniazid and ethambutol given for 18 months and only 6 per cent relapsed during follow up.[69] In another study, 91 per cent of patients with moderately advanced cavitating disease responded to treatment with three or more standard antimycobacterial drugs, compared with only 64 per cent of those with advanced disease given the same treatment.[72] Although treatment with five or six drugs has been recommended,[73-75] there have been no comparative studies to show that such multiple regimens are more effective than those comprising fewer drugs, whilst second- or third-line drugs, or regimens with four or more drugs, are associated with toxicity and non-compliance.[39]

In the first BTS prospective trial, rifampicin combined with ethambutol or alternatively rifampicin, ethambutol and isoniazid were given for 2 years. Patients were followed for 3 years after the end of chemotherapy by which time 36 per cent of the 75 had died, only three deaths being primarily attributable to MAC disease. Respiratory failure, ischaemic heart disease, pneumonia and lung cancer accounted for the majority of deaths. Of the 28 per cent who either had positive cultures at the end of treatment or had relapsed post-chemotherapy, fewer had received triple therapy but more of the deaths occurred in that treatment group. Age, male sex, involvement of more than one lung zone and low initial body weight were independent predictors of death. In all, a third of patients either failed treatment, relapsed or died because of the MAC disease. Twenty-three (31 per cent) were known to be alive and cured at the end of 5 years. Drug toxicity was minimal.[29,62] These results were comparable with the best reported to date, but better regimens are clearly needed.

A more recent BTS trial assessed the places of clarithromycin, ciprofloxacin and immunotherapy with *M. vaccae* in 170 patients.[76] Immunotherapy did not improve the outcomes at 5 years of 2 years' triple therapy with rifampicin, ethambutol and either clarithromycin or ciprofloxacin (REClari versus RECipro). All-cause mortality was higher with REClari (48 per cent) than with RECipro (30 per cent), but there was no difference between the two regimens in the numbers of deaths attributed to MAC disease (2 versus 3 per cent). Overall, 19 per cent either failed treatment, relapsed or died because of MAC disease, with no statistically significant difference between the regimens. Nor was there any difference in the numbers who completed treatment as allocated and were known to be alive and cured at 5 years (24 versus 23 per cent). These outcomes were much the same as found in the previous BTS trial, except for drug toxicity which was twice as common with these regimens compared with the regimens used in the earlier trial.[29,62,76]

The experience of the last 25 years indicates that first-line treatment should be with rifampicin and ethambutol for 2 years. In those who fail to respond or who relapse, one or more of isoniazid, ciprofloxacin, clarithromycin or streptomycin can be added and continued until the sputum culture has been negative for at least 12 months. In some patients, chemotherapy does not cure the disease but is sufficient to keep it in check and in these circumstances can be continued indefinitely. Resection of the affected lobe should be considered in those who fail to respond to chemotherapy and where surgery is thought to be technically feasible.[33]

M. xenopi

Patients treated with combinations of rifampicin, ethambutol and isoniazid usually show clinical improvement and convert to sputum culture negative while receiving treatment, despite the organism's poor *in vitro* sensitivity to these agents tested singly.[77,78] Unfortunately, relapse may occur in up to 25 per cent of patients following cessation of treatment. Other patients can develop progressive disease while receiving treatment with drugs such as ethionamide and cycloserine, even though these agents appeared highly effective when tested singly *in vitro*.[77,79] Drug toxicity and poor compliance with treatment were thought to have contributed to poor outcome in some patients. Surgical treatment has been effective in controlling the disease in small numbers of patients, but has been associated with a high rate of post-operative complications and may not be feasible because of coexisting pulmonary conditions. In the BTS's earlier prospective trial of 2 years of rifampicin and ethambutol or 2 years of rifampicin, ethambutol and isoniazid, 12 per cent were still culture positive at the end of treatment or relapsed after completing treatment. Only seven (17 per cent) of the 42 patients were known to be cured and 26 per cent known to be alive at 5 years. The death rate of 69 per cent was very high, but only 7 per cent died primarily from the *M. xenopi* disease. Lung cancer, pneumonia, respiratory failure not attributable to *M. xenopi*, ischaemic heart disease and stroke were the major causes of mortality.[31,62] In the more recent BTS trial of REClari versus RECipro for 2 years, with or without initial immunotherapy with *M. vaccae*, the overall death rate (38 per cent) was lower and only one of the 34 patients in the trial died because of their mycobacterial disease.[76] Overall, mortality was higher with RECipro than REClari. Five patients (15 per cent) failed to convert to culture negative or relapsed, much the same as the figure in the earlier study. Twelve (34 per cent) were alive and cured at 5 years, six REClari and six RECipro. Again, there was little, if any, difference in outcome when compared with the previous BTS trial,[31,62] other than more frequent drug toxicity in the recent study. Immunotherapy conveyed no advantages in outcome.[76] In the two retrospective studies, the death rates were 30–40 per cent, but patients were followed up for variable periods, usually shorter than 5 years.[77,79] More attention to improving nutrition and to prevention and treatment of co-morbid conditions, and early referral of suitable patients for surgery should have some effect on mortality, but better regimens are urgently needed. In the meantime, 2 years of rifampicin and ethambutol remains the recommended regimen,[33] with the option of adding clarithromycin, isoniazid or ciprofloxacin in those patients whose response is unsatisfactory.

M. malmoense

Until 2001, few reports had described the response to treatment.[35,80] Rifampicin, ethambutol and isoniazid taken for 18–24 months were effective in the patients in one series, although the rate of relapse could not be determined because follow up was relatively short.[80] Including ethambutol in the regimen appears to be important as its withdrawal has been followed by clinical deterioration in some patients. As was the case with MAC, the use of second- or third-line drugs, or regimens containing four or five drugs, was associated with poor tolerance and poor results of treatment.[35] In the first BTS trial, 10 per cent of 106 patients remained positive on culture at the end of treatment or relapsed after treatment for 2 years with either rifampicin and ethambutol or rifampicin, ethambutol and isoniazid.[30,62] Sixty-three (59 per cent) were known to be alive at 5 years of whom 44 (42 per cent of the original 106 entries) were cured. Only four of the 36 deaths were attributable primarily to the *M. malmoense*. The pattern of diseases causing the other deaths was much like that seen with MAC and *M. xenopi*.[29,31] In the two retrospective studies, the overall death rates were much as found in the first BTS study.[35,80] In all, 14 per cent of the patients had a poor outcome of their mycobacterial disease (failure of treatment, relapse or death because of *M. malmoense*). Involvement of more than one zone of the lung and resistance to ethambutol were independent predictors of death, whilst increase in weight during the second year of chemotherapy predicted survival.[30] The second BTS trial examined the roles of clarithromycin, ciprofloxacin and immunotherapy with *M. vaccae* as adjuncts to rifampicin and ethambutol.[76] As with MAC, immunotherapy did not improve on the effects of the two triple-therapy regimens, REClari and RECipro. Poor outcome at 5 years (death due to *M. malmoense*, failure of treatment and relapse) was noted in 7 per cent overall, with no difference between the two regimens. More REClari patients completed treatment as allocated and were known to be alive and cured (38 per cent) than did those on RECipro (20 per cent). All-cause mortality was higher with RECipro (56 per cent) than with REClari (42 per cent). Unwanted effects were encountered with much the same frequency (20 per cent) with either regimen, a frequency twice that seen with RE and REH in the first BTS trial, but other outcome measures were much the same.[30,62,76] Thus, the current BTS recommendation of rifampicin and ethambutol for 2 years as first choice for the treatment of *M. malmoense* pulmonary disease still stands,[33] with the option of adding isoniazid and/or clarithromycin if the response is not satisfactory.

M. chelonei and *M. fortuitum*

These infections are infrequent in the UK. Reports on efficacy of treatment are anecdotal: successful treatment with ciprofloxacin or ofloxacin has been reported.[81,82] Because single-agent treatment may permit the emergence of quinolone-resistant strains, Wallace *et al.*[83] suggest that treatment should include a second drug, such as amikacin, imipenem, doxycycline, clarithromycin or a sulphonamide,

which have also occasionally been reported as effective for these conditions. Rifampicin, ethambutol and clarithromycin should form the basis of the regimen, perhaps with the addition of a quinolone.[33] Duration of therapy for these organisms, as well as for the other rarer environmental mycobacterial pulmonary infections, should not be less than 24 months. Surgery, if technically feasible, may be an option.

EFFECT OF THE AIDS EPIDEMIC

In HIV-positive patients, infection with environmental mycobacteria is not usually limited to the lungs but is frequently bacteraemic. Patients usually have pronounced immunodeficiency and complain more of general malaise, fever, sweating, weight loss and diarrhoea than of pulmonary symptoms. Skin lesions, lymphadenopathy and hepatosplenomegaly are the most common findings. The chest x-ray is usually abnormal and may show mediastinal lymphadenopathy, pulmonary nodules or patchy alveolar infiltrates, cavitation being uncommon.[84] Diagnosis is usually made from blood or stool cultures or on histology of biopsies of lymph nodes, liver, skin or bone marrow.[84–87]

In this population, MAC occurs more commonly than the other species:[88] after diagnosis of AIDS, disseminated MAC was found in 14 per cent at 1 year, 25 per cent at 2 years and 36 per cent at 3 years.[89] Prior to the use of HAART, response to chemotherapy was usually transient and prognosis dismal.[87,90] Restoring immunocompetence with that regimen has resulted in a decline in the incidence of MAC disease and an increase in survival during and after treatment with antimycobacterial therapy. On starting HAART, patients may develop malaise, fever, new or enlarging lymph nodes and worsening of skin lesions – the immune reconstitution inflammatory syndrome (IRIS).[91]

Various combinations of antimycobacterial drugs have been tried in patients with AIDS and environmental mycobacterial infection, but poor design and/or small sizes of the published studies limit the deductions that can be made from the results.[91] If a decision is taken to treat the mycobacterium, then ethambutol and a rifamycin should be used. If the organism is *M. kansasii*, prothionamide should be added and chemotherapy continued until the patient has been culture negative for at least 12 months. For MAC, *M. malmoense* or *M. xenopi*, lifelong ethambutol and a rifamycin should be given, plus one or more of clarithromycin, ciprofloxacin, streptomycin or, for MAC, isoniazid.[33] Rifabutin, which interacts with clarithromycin to cause uveitis and will also reduce serum fluconazole levels, has not been convincingly shown to be more effective than the cheaper rifampicin, although it is easier to use with viral protease inhibitors.[91] Properly controlled, prospective, well-designed clinical trials are much needed in this population of patients.

Prophylactic chemotherapy with rifabutin has been shown to reduce the frequency of disseminated MAC infection in patients with AIDS and CD4 counts

<200 mm³, but did not significantly prolong survival.[92] Another study has suggested that cotrimoxazole may have a useful prophylactic effect.[93] Azithromycin and the combination of azithromycin and rifabutin were better than rifabutin alone in preventing MAC infection, although survival was not affected. Unfortunately, this study did not include a placebo arm.[94] In a placebo-controlled, prospective study, clarithromycin (500 mg orally, twice daily) was superior to placebo in preventing MAC infection (6 versus 16 per cent) and in prolonging survival (68 versus 59 per cent), but resistance to clarithromycin developed in over 50 per cent.[95] It remains to be seen whether such resistance can be avoided by using clarithromycin in combination with other antimycobacterial drugs. Monotherapy with rifamycins in prophylaxis for these infections should be avoided because of the possibility of an adverse effect on drug resistance in *M. tuberculosis*, which is a common pathogen in the AIDS population.[33]

IN VITRO DRUG SENSITIVITY TESTS FOR ENVIRONMENTAL MYCOBACTERIA

In contrast to infection caused by *M. tuberculosis*, drug resistance defined by standard laboratory tests does not correlate with the clinical response to treatment in patients with infection caused by environmental mycobacteria.[29–31,35,39,62,77,78,80] There are several possible explanations for this discrepancy. *In vitro*, the minimum inhibitory concentrations (MICs) that predict the clinical response to treatment are known for *M. tuberculosis*, but not for other mycobacterial species. It has become customary to classify environmental mycobacteria as being drug resistant if their MICs exceed those that have been established for drug-sensitive strains of *M. tuberculosis*.[96] This assumes that all mycobacteria species have the same critical MICs as *M. tuberculosis*, which is unlikely, considering that the basic mechanisms of drug resistance differ between species. Isoniazid resistance for *M. tuberculosis* usually occurs by a single mutational step and is dependent on the loss of catalase peroxidase activity,[97–99] yet MAC shows natural resistance to isoniazid despite possessing catalase peroxidase activity.[74] It is inappropriate, therefore, to use MICs established for *M. tuberculosis* as yardsticks to define drug resistance for MAC. Environmental mycobacteria are undoubtedly less sensitive than strains of *M. tuberculosis* to conventional antimycobacterial drugs *in vitro*, but this may simply indicate the need to prolong treatment in order to achieve a successful therapeutic result.

Drug resistance cannot be defined simply by relating *in vitro* MICs to serum drug concentrations because serum levels do not always reflect drug concentrations achieved within tissues or macrophages. For example, concentrations of ethambutol in normal and caseous lung tissue are 3–10 times higher than plasma levels.[100] Even higher concentrations are achieved within alveolar macrophages,[101,102] yet concentrations required to kill phagocytosed bacilli are lower than bactericidal concentrations required in culture medium.[103] Intracellular levels of rifampicin, clarithromycin and ciprofloxacin are also several times higher than their respective serum levels.[104] These high intracellular concentrations, coupled with the enhanced bactericidal action of the drugs within macrophages, may account for the effect of some drugs in treatment despite their poor action in culture medium.

Synergy may account for the effectiveness of some drugs in treatment. Drug combinations *in vitro* have been shown to be more effective than single agents against *M. kansasii*, MAC, *M. xenopi* and *M. malmoense*.[105–112] The particular efficacy of rifampicin and ethambutol can be explained on theoretical grounds: rifampicin acts against mycobacteria by inhibiting bacterial DNA-dependent RNA polymerase, thereby blocking transcription.[113,114] Rifampicin-resistant strains of *M. tuberculosis* have a resistant polymerase.[115] In contrast, rifampicin resistance with environmental mycobacteria results from a failure of the drug to penetrate the bacterial cell wall.[116] The RNA polymerase of rifampicin-resistant strains belonging to MAC is in fact highly sensitive to rifampicin, but is protected by the cell wall permeability barrier. Ethambutol, even in low concentrations, induces morphological changes in the bacterial cell wall *in vitro*,[117] probably by interfering with mycolic acid and phospholipid synthesis.[117,118] This action on the cell wall might facilitate access of rifampicin into the cell, thus exposing its rifampicin-sensitive polymerase. A similar mechanism operating *in vivo* would explain the effectiveness of these two drugs in treatment.

SUMMARY

The treatment of infection caused by environmental bacteria, in particular MAC, *M. xenopi* and *M. malmoense*, remains a clinical challenge. Physicians are often left confused about which treatment to use in the face of seemingly conflicting recommendations in the literature.[33,76,91,119] These issues can be resolved only by conducting large, prospective studies assessing and comparing different approaches to treatment.

LEARNING POINTS

- Nomenclature still contested:
  - mycobacteria other than tuberculosis (MOTT);
  - non-tuberculous mycobacteria;
  - environmental mycobacteria;
  - opportunist mycobacteria;
  - atypical mycobacteria;
  - anonymous mycobacteria.
- Infection is from the environment, not from another human source.

- Environmental mycobacteria are an increasingly common cause of disease caused by acid fast bacteria in older patients in the UK.
- Symptoms tend to be more chronic and insidious than those from *M. tuberculosis*, but these diseases cannot be separated on the basis of symptomatology and radiographic findings alone: they are distinguishable from TB only by culture.
- Pulmonary diseases due to environmental mycobacteria usually occur in older patients with chronic lung disease such as previous *M. tuberculosis*, chronic bronchitis and emphysema and bronchiectasis.
- *In vitro* sensitivity testing is a poor guide to *in vivo* effect of drug therapy.
- First-line treatment for pulmonary disease should be rifampicin and ethambutol. If necessary, isoniazid (MAC and *M. malmoense*), clarithromycin (*M. malmoense* and *M. xenopi*) and ciprofloxacin can be added or substituted.
- Soft-tissue infections are best managed with surgery, as are superficial lymph node infections in children.
- MAC infection is associated with HIV infection.

ACKNOWLEDGEMENTS

The authors thank Elizabeth Lyons for typing the manuscript.

REFERENCES

1. Chapman JS. The ecology of the atypical mycobacteria. *Arch Environ Health* 1971;**22**: 41–6.
2. Chapman JS, Bernard JS, Speight M. Isolation of bacteria from raw milk. *Am Rev Respir Dis* 1965; **91**: 351–5.
3. Marks J, Jenkins PA. The opportunist mycobacteria – 20 year retrospect. *Postgrad Med J* 1971; **47**: 705–9.
4. McSwiggan DA, Collins CH. The isolation of *M. kansasii* and *M. xenopi* from water systems. *Tubercle* 1974; **55**: 291–7.
5. Levin M, Newport MJ, D'Souza S *et al.* Familial disseminated atypical mycobacterial infection in childhood: a human mycobacterial susceptibility gene? *Lancet* 1995; **345**: 79–83.
6. Gelder CM, Hart KW, Williams OM *et al.* Vitamin D receptor gene polymorphisms and susceptibility to *M. malmoense* pulmonary disease. *Infect Dis* 2000; **181**: 2099–102
7. British Thoracic and Tuberculosis Association. Opportunist mycobacterial pulmonary infection and occupational dust exposure: an investigation in England and Wales. *Tubercle* 1975; **56**: 295–310.
8. Marks J. Occupation and *M. kansasii* infection in Cardiff residents. *Tubercle* 1975; **56**: 311–3.
9. Penny ME, Cole RB, Gray J. Two cases of *Mycobacterium kansasii* infection occurring in the same household. *Tubercle* 1982; **63**: 129–30.
10. Tortoli E. Impact of genotypic studies on mycobacterial taxonomy: the new mycobacteria of the 1990s. *Clin Microbiol Rev* 2003; **16**: 319–54.
11. Runyon EH. Ten mycobacterial pathogens. *Tubercle* 1974; **55**: 235–401.
12. Jenkins PA. Non-tuberculous mycobacterial disease. *Eur J Respir Dis* 1981; **62**: 69.
13. Clague H, Hopkins CA, Roberts C, Jenkins PA. Pulmonary infection with *Mycobacterium gordonae* in the presence of bronchial carcinoma. *Tubercle* 1975; **66**: 61–6.
14. Tsukamura M, Kita N, Otsuka W, Schimoide H. A study of the taxonomy of the mycobacterium non-chromogenicum complex and report of six cases of lung infection due to mycobacterium non-chromogenicum. *Microbiol Immunol* 1983; **27**: 219–36.
15. Selkon JB. Atypical mycobacteria: a review. *Tubercle* 1969; **50** (Suppl.): 70–8.
16. Edwards FGB. Disease caused by 'atypical' (opportunist) mycobacteria: a whole population review. *Tubercle* 1970; **51**: 285–95.
17. Marks J, Schwabacher H. Infection due to *M. xenopi. Br Med J* 1965; **1**: 32–3.
18. Grange JM, Yates MD. Infections caused by opportunist mycobacteria: a review. *J R Soc Med* 1986; **79**: 226–9.
19. Marks J. Classification of mycobacteria in relation to clinical significance. *Tubercle* 1972; **53**: 259–64.
20. Parez JJ, Faville-Dufaux M, Dossogne JL, de Hoffman E, Pouthier F. A faster identification of mycobacteria using gas–liquid and thin layer chromatography. *Eur J Clin Microbiol Infect Dis* 1994; **13**: 717–25.
21. Reisner BS, Gatson AM, Woods GL. Use of Gen-Probe Accuprobes to identify *Mycobacterium avium complex, Mycobacterium tuberculosis complex, Mycobacterium kansasii,* and *Mycobacterium gordonae* directly from Bactec TB broth cultures. *J Clin Microbiol* 1994; **32**: 2995–8.
22. Padilla E, Gonzalez V, Manterola JM *et al.* Comparative evaluation of the new version of the INNO-LiPA Mycobacteria and GenoType Mycobacterium assays for identification of Mycobacterium species from MB/BacT liquid cultures artificially inoculated with Mycobacterial strains. *J Clin Microbiol* 2004; **42**: 3083–88.
23. Wijsmuller G, Erikson P. The reaction to PPD-Battey. A new look. *Am Rev Respir Dis* 1974; **109**: 29–40.
24. Hyde Cl. Skin testing with multiple PPD antigens in the differential diagnosis of mycobacterial disease. *Chest* 1974; **66**: 108–109.
25. Christensen EE, Dietz GW, Ahn CH *et al.* Initial roentgenographic manifestations of pulmonary *Mycobacterium tuberculosis, M. kansasii,* and *M. intracellularis. Chest* 1981; **80**: 132–6.
26. Evans AJ, Crisp AJ, Colville A, Evans SA, Johnston IDA. Pulmonary infections caused by *Mycobacterium malmoense* and *Mycobacterium tuberculosis*: comparison of radiographic features. *AJR* 1993; **161**: 733–7.
27. Research Committee, British Thoracic Society. *Mycobacterium kansasii* pulmonary infection: a prospective study of the results of nine months of treatment with rifampicin and ethambutol. *Thorax* 1994; **49**: 442–5.
28. Evans AJ, Crisp AJ, Hubbard RB *et al.* Pulmonary *Mycobacterium kansasii* infection: comparison of radiological appearances with pulmonary tuberculosis. *Thorax* 1996; **51**: 1243–7.
29. The Research Committee of the British Thoracic Society. Pulmonary disease caused by *Mycobacterium avium-intracellulare* in HIV-negative patients: five year follow-up of patients receiving standardized treatment. *Int. J Tuberc Lung Dis* 2002; **6**: 628–34.
30. The Research Committee of the British Thoracic Society. Pulmonary disease caused by *Mycobacterium malmoense* in HIV-negative patients: five year follow-up of patients receiving standardized treatment. *Eur Respir J* 2003; **21**: 478–82.
31. The Research Committee of the British Thoracic Society. Pulmonary disease caused by *Myocbacterium xenopi* in HIV-negative patients five year follow-up of patients receiving standardized treatment. *Respir Med* 2003; **97**: 439–44.

32. Diagnostic standards and classification of tuberculosis and other mycobacterial diseases. *Am Rev Respir Dis* 1981; **123**: 343–58.

33. Subcommittee of the Joint Tuberculosis Committee of the British Thoracic Society. Management of opportunist mycobacterial infections: Joint Tuberculosis Committee guidelines 1999. *Thorax* 2000; **55**: 210–18.

34. Harris GD, Johanson WG Jr, Nicholson DP. Response to chemotherapy of pulmonary infection due to *Mycobacterium kansasii*. *Am Rev Respir Dis* 1975; **112**: 31–6.

35. Banks J, Jenkins PA, Smith AP. Pulmonary infection with *Mycobacterium malmoense* – a review of treatment and response. *Tubercle* 1985; **66**: 197–203.

36. Ahn CH, Nash DR, Hurst GA. Ventilatory defects in atypical mycobacteriosis, a comparison study with tuberculosis. *Am Rev Respir Dis* 1976; **113**: 273–9.

37. Yamamoto M, Ogura Y, Sudo K, Hibino S. Diagnostic criteria for disease caused by 'atypical' mycobacteria. *Am Rev Respir Dis* 1967; **96**: 773–8.

38. Banks J. Treatment of pulmonary disease caused by non-tuberculous mycobacteria. MD thesis, University of Manchester, 1988.

39. Hunter AM, Campbell IA, Jenkins PA, Smith AP. Treatment of pulmonary infection caused by mycobacteria of the *Mycobacterium avium-intracellulare* complex. *Thorax* 1981; **36**: 326–9.

40. Francis PB, Jay SJ, Johanson WG Jr. The course of untreated *Mycobacterium kansasii* disease. *Am Rev Respir Dis* 1975; **111**: 477–87.

41. Prissick FH, Masson AM. Cervical lymphadenitis in children caused by chromogenic mycobacteria. *Can Med Assoc J* 1956; **75**: 798–83.

42. MacKellar A. Diagnosis and management of atypical mycobacterial lymphadenitis in children. *J Paediatr Surg* 1976; **11**: 85–9.

43. White MP, Bangash H, Goel KM, Jenkins PM. Non-tuberculous mycobacterial lymphadenitis. *Arch Dis Child* 1986; **61**: 368–71.

44. Wallace RJ, Musser JM, Howell SI *et al.* Diversity and sources of rapidly growing mycobacteria associated with infections following cardiac surgery. *J Infect Dis* 1989; **159**: 708–16.

45. Hanson P, Thomas J, Collins J. *Mycobacterium chelonae* and abscess formation in soft tissues. *Tubercle* 1987; **68**: 297–9.

46. Wallace RJ Jr, Swenson JM, Silcox VA *et al.* Spectrum of disease due to rapidly growing mycobacteria. *Rev Infect Dis* 1983; **5**: 657–79.

47. Rappaport W, Dunington G, Norton I *et al.* The surgical management of atypical mycobacterial soft tissue infections. *Surgery* 1990; **108**: 36–9.

48. Greenberg AE, Kupka E. Swimming pool injuries, mycobacteria, and tuberculosis-like disease. *Publ Health Rep* 1957; **72**: 902.

49. Meyers WM, Shelly WM, Connor DH, Meyers EK. Human *Mycobacterium ulcerans* infections developing at sites of traumatised skin. *J Trop Med Hyg* 1974; **23**: 91.

50. Wallace RJ Jr, Tanner D, Grennin PJ, Brown PA. Clinical trials of clarithromycin for cutaneous (disseminated) infection due to *Mycobacterium chelonei*. *Ann Intern Med* 1993; **119**: 482–6.

51. Black MM, Eykyn SJ. The successful treatment of tropical fish tank granuloma (*Mycobacterium marinum*) with co-trimoxazole. *Br J Dermatol* 1977; **97**: 689–92.

52. Izumi AK, Hanke CW, Higaki M. *Mycobacterium marinum* infections treated with tetracycline. *Arch Dermatol* 1977; **113**: 1067–8.

53. Glynn PJ. The use of surgery and local temperature elevation in *Mycobacterium ulcerans* infection. *Aust N Z J Surg* 1972; **41**: 312–17.

54. Lester W Jr, Botkin J, Colton R. An analysis of 49 cases of pulmonary disease caused by photochromogenic mycobacteria. Transactions of the 17th Conference on Chemotherapy and Tuberculosis, VA Armed Forces, Cleveland, Ohio, 1958: 289–97.

55. Jenkins DE, Bahar D, Chofnos I *et al.* The clinical problem of infection with atypical acid fast bacilli. *Trans Am Climat Assoc* 1959; **71**: 21–33.

56. Christianson LC, Dewlett HJ. Pulmonary disease in adults associated with unclassified mycobacteria. *Am J Med* 1960; **29**: 980–91.

57. Phillips S, Larkin JC Jr. Atypical pulmonary tuberculosis caused by unclassified mycobacteria. *Ann Intern Med* 1964; **60**: 401–8.

58. Corpe RF, Runyon EH, Lester W. Status of disease due to unclassified mycobacteria. A statement of the Subcommittee on Unclassified Mycobacteria of the Committee on Therapy. *Am Rev Respir Dis* 1963; **87**: 459–61.

59. Pfuetze KH, Bo LV, Reimann AF *et al.* Photochromogenic mycobacterial pulmonary disease. *Am Rev Respir Dis* 1965; **92**: 470–5.

60. Pfuetze KM, Nuchprayoon CV, Berg JS, Pamintuan R. Present status of open negative cavities due to photochromogenic mycobacteria among co-operative patients. *Am Rev Respir Dis* 1966; **94**: 467.

61. Lester W. Unclassified mycobacterial disease. *Am Rev Med* 1966; **17**: 351–60.

62. Research Committee of the British Thoracic Society. First randomized trial of treatments for pulmonary disease caused by *M. avium-intracellulare, M. malmoense* and *M. xenopi* in HIV-negative patients: rifampicin, ethambutol and isoniazid versus rifampicin and ethambutol. *Thorax* 2001; **56**: 167–72.

63. Banks J, Hunter AM, Campbell IA, Smith AP. Pulmonary infection with *Mycobacterium kansasii* in Wales, 1970–9: review of treatment and response. Thorax 1983; **38**: 271–4.

64. Ahn CH, Lowell JR, Ahn SS *et al.* Short course chemotherapy for pulmonary disease caused by *Mycobacterium kansasii*. *Am Rev Respir Dis* 1983; **128**: 1048–50.

65. Kaustovi J, Chmelik M, Ettlova D *et al.* Disease due to *Mycobacterium kansasii* in the Czech Republic: 1984–89, *Tuberc Lung Dis* 1995; **76**: 205–209.

66. Corpe RF. Surgical management of pulmonary disease due to *Mycobacterium avium intracellulare*. *Rev Infect Dis* 1981; **3**: 1064–7.

67. Moran JF, Alexander LG, Staub EW *et al.* Long-term results of pulmonary resection for atypical mycobacterial disease and thoracic surgery. *Am Thorac Surg* 1983; **35**: 597–604.

68. Rosenzweig DY. Pulmonary mycobacterial infections due to *Mycobacterium intracellulare* and *avium* complex. *Chest* 1979; **75**: 115–19.

69. Engbaek EC, Vergmann B, Bentzon MW. A prospective study of lung disease caused by *Mycobacterium avium/Mycobacterium intracellulare*. *Eur J Respir Dis* 1984; **65**: 411–18.

70. Etzkorn ET, Aldarondo S, McAllister CK *et al.* Medical therapy of *Mycobacterium avium intracellulare* pulmonary disease. *Am Rev Respir Dis* 1986; **134**: 442–5.

71. Horsburgh CR Jr, Mason UG III, Heifets LB *et al.* Response to therapy of pulmonary *Mycobacterium avium intracellulare* infection correlates with results of *in vitro* susceptibility testing. *Am Rev Respir Dis* 1987; **135**: 418–21.

72. Tsujumura N, Ichiyama S, Takuaya M. Superiority of enviomycin or streptomycin over ethambutol in initial treatment of lung disease caused by *Mycobacterium avium* complex. *Chest* 1989; **95**: 1056–8.

73. Yaeger H Jr, Raleigh JW. Pulmonary disease due to *Mycobacterium intracellulare*. *Am Rev Respir Dis* 1973; **108**: 547–52.

74. Lester TW. Drug resistant and atypical mycobacterial disease. Bacteriology and treatment. *Arch Intern Med* 1979; **139**: 1399–401.

75. Lester W, Moulding T, Fraser RI *et al.* Quintuple drug regimens in the treatment of Battey-type infections. Transactions of the 20th Pulmonary Disease Research Conference, VA Armed Forces, Cleveland, Ohio 1969: 83.

76. Research Committee of the British Thoracic Society. Clarithromycin vs ciprofloxacin as adjuncts to rifampicin and

ethambutol in the treatment of opportunist mycobacterial pulmonary disease and an assessment of the value of immunotherapy with *M. vaccae*. *Thorax* (in press).

77. Banks J, Hunter AM, Campbell IA *et al*. Pulmonary infection with *Mycobacterium xenopi*: review of treatment and response. *Thorax* 1984; **39**: 376–82.

78. Smith MJ, Citron KM. Clinical review of pulmonary disease caused by *Mycobacterium xenopi*. *Thorax* 1983; **38**: 373–7.

79. Contreras MA, Cheung OT, Sanders DE *et al*. Pulmonary infection with non-tuberculous mycobacteria. *Am Rev Respir Dis* 1988; **137**: 149–52.

80. France AJ, McLeod DT, Calder MA, Seaton A. *Mycobacterium malmoense* infections in Scotland: an increasing problem. *Thorax* 1987; **42**: 593–5.

81. Burns DN, Rohatgi PK, Rosenthal R *et al*. Disseminated *Mycobacterium fortuitum* successfully treated with combination therapy including ciprofloxacin. *Am Rev Respir Dis* 1990; **142**: 468–70.

82. Yew WW, Kwan SYL, Wong PC, Lee J. Ofloxacin and imipenen in the treatment of *Mycobacterium fortuitum* and *Mycobacterium chelonae* infections. *Tubercle* 1990; **71**: 131–3.

83. Wallace RJ Jr, Bedsole G, Sumpter G *et al*. Activities of ciprofloxacin and ofloxacin against rapidly growing mycobacteria with demonstration of acquired resistance following single drug therapy. *Antimicrob Agents Chemother* 1990; **34**: 65–70.

84. Horsburgh CR Jr, Mason UG, Farhi DC, Iseman MD. Disseminated infection with *Mycobacterium avium intracellulare*. A report of 13 cases and a review of the literature. *Medicine* 1985; **64**: 36–48.

85. Wall B, Edwards FF, Kiehn TE *et al*. Continuous high grade *Mycobacterium avium intracellulare* bacteraemia in patients with the acquired immuno-deficiency syndrome. *Am J Med* 1985; **78**: 35–40.

86. Marinelli DL, Albelda SM, Williams DM *et al*. Non-tuberculous mycobacterial infection in AIDS: clinical, pathologic and radiographic features. *Radiology* 1986; **160**: 77–82.

87. Hawkins CC, Gold JWM, Whimbey E *et al*. *Mycobacterium avium* complex infections in patients with acquired immunodeficiency syndrome. *Ann Intern Med* 1986; **105**: 184–8.

88. Centres for Disease Control, US Dept Health and Human Services. Diagnosis and management of mycobacterial infection and disease in persons with human immunodeficiency virus infection. *Ann Intern Med* 1987; **106**: 254–6.

89. Flegg PJ, Laing RVS, Lee C *et al*. Disseminated disease due to *Mycobacterium avium* complex in AIDS. *Q J Med* 1995; **88**: 617–26.

90. Horsburgh CR Jr, Havlik JA, Ellis GA *et al*. Survival of patients with acquired immunodeficiency syndrome and disseminated *Mycobacterium avium* complex infection with and without anti-mycobacterial chemotherapy. *Am Rev Respir Dis* 1991; **144**: 557–9.

91. Pozniak AL, Miller R, Lipman M *et al*. British HIV Association treatment guidelines for TB/HIV infection, February 2005 (www.bhiva.org).

92. Nightingale SD, Cameron DW, Gordin FM *et al*. Two controlled trials of rifabutin prophylaxis against *Mycobacterium avium* complex infection in AIDS. *N Engl J Med* 1993; **329**: 828–33.

93. Fraser I, MacIntosh I, Wilkins EG. Prophylactive effect of co-trimoxazole for mycobacterium avium complex infection: a previously unreported benefit. *Clin Infect Dis* 1994; **19**: 211 (letter).

94. Havlir DV, Dube MP, Sattler FR *et al*. Prophylaxis against disseminated *Mycobacterium avium* complex with weekly azithromycin, daily rifabutin or both. *N Engl J Med* 1996; **335**: 392–8.

95. Pierce M, Crampton S, Henry D *et al*. A randomised trial of clarithromycin as prophylaxis against disseminated *Mycobacterium avium* complex infection inpatients with advanced acquired immunodeficiency syndrome. *N Engl J Med* 1996; **335**: 384–91.

96. Marks J. A system for the examination of tubercle bacilli and other mycobacteria. *Tubercle* 1976; **57**: 207–25.

97. Middlebrook G. Isoniazid resistance and catalase activity of tubercle bacilli. *Am Rev Tuberc* 1954; **69**: 471–2.

98. Dunbar FP, McAllister E, Jeffries MB. Catalase and peroxidase activation of isoniazid susceptible and resistant strains of mycobacteria and tuberculosis. *Am Rev Tuberc* 1959; **79**: 669–71.

99. Youatt J. A review of the action of isoniazid. *Am Rev Respir Dis* 1969; **99**: 729–49.

100. Djurovic B, DeCroix G, Daumet P. L'ethambutol chez l'homme. Etude comparative des taux seriques erythrocytaires et pulmonaries. *Nouv Presse Med* 1973; **2**: 815–16.

101. Johnson JD, Hand WL, Frances JB *et al*. Antibiotic uptake by alveolar macrophages. *J Lab Clin Med* 1980; **95**: 429–39.

102. Liss RH. Anti-mycobacterial activity of ethambutol in human pulmonary mononuclear phagocytes. *Prax Clin Pneumol* 1983; **37**: 485–6.

103. Crolle HA, Svarvaro JA, Judson FN, May MH. The effect of ethambutol on tubercle bacilli within cultured human macrophages. *Am Rev Respir Dis* 1985; **132**: 742–5.

104. Ellner JJ, Goldberger MJ, Parenti DM. *Mycobacteria avium* infection and AIDS: a therapeutic dilemma in rapid evolution. *J Infect Dis* 1991; **163**: 1326–35.

105. Tsang AY, Bentz RR, Schork MA, Sodeman TM. Combined vs single drug studies of susceptibilities of *Mycobacterium kansasii* to isoniazid, streptomycin and ethambutol. *Am J Clin Pathol* 1978; **138**: 816–20.

106. Zimmer BL, DeYoung DR, Roberts GD. *In vitro* synergistic activity of ethambutol, isoniazid, kanamycin, rifampicin and streptomycin against *Mycobacterium avium intracellulare* complex. *Antimicrob Agents Chemother* 1982; **22**: 148–50.

107. Nash DR, Steingrube BA. Selecting drug combinations for the treatment of drug resistant mycobacterial diseases. *J Clin Pharmacol* 1982; **22**: 297–300.

108. Heifets LB. Synergistic effect of rifampicin, streptomycin, ethionamide and ethambutol on *Mycobacterium intracellulare*. *Am Rev Respir Dis* 1982; **125**: 43–8.

109. Kuze F. Experimental chemotherapy in chronic *Mycobacterium avium intracellulare* infection in mice. *Am Rev Respir Dis* 1984; **129**: 453–9.

110. Banks J, Jenkins PA. Combined versus single antituberculous drugs on the *in vitro* sensitivity patterns of non-tuberculous mycobacteria. *Thorax* 1987; **42**: 838–42.

111. Hoffner SE, Svenson SV, Kallenius G. Synergistic effects of antimycobacterial drug combinations on *Mycobacterium avium* complex determined radiometrically in liquid medium. *Eur J Clin Microbiol* 1987; **6**: 530–5.

112. Hoffner SE, Hjelm U, Kallenius G. Susceptibility of *Mycobacterium malmoense* to antibacterial drugs and drug combinations. *Antimicrob Agents Chemother* 1993; **37**: 1285–88.

113. Sippal A, Hartmann G. Mode of action of rifampicins on the RNA polymerase reaction. *Biochem Biophys Acta* 1968; **157**: 218–9.

114. Wehrli W, Knusel R, Schmid K, Staehelin M. Interaction of rifampicin with bacterial RNA polymerase. *Proc Natl Acad Sci USA* 1968; **61**: 667–73.

115. Tsukamura M. The pattern of resistance development to rifampicin in *Mycobacterium tuberculosis*. *Tubercle* 1972; **53**: 111–17.

116. Hui J, Gordon N, Kajioka R. Permeability barrier to rifampicin in mycobacteria. *Antimicrob Agents Chemother* 1977; **11**: 773–9.

117. Kilburn JO, Greenberg J. Effect of ethambutol on the viable cell count in *Mycobacterium smegmatis*. *Antimicrob Agents Chemother* 1977; **11**: 534–40.

118. Takayama K, Armstrong EL, Kunugi KA, Kilburn KO. Inhibition by ethambutol of mycolic acid transfer into the cell wall of *Mycobacterium smegmatis*. *Antimicrob Agents Chemother* 1979; **16**: 240–2.

119. Griffith DE, Aksamit T, Brown-Elliot BA *et al*. An official ATS/IDSA statement: diagnosis, treatment and prevention of non-tuberculous mycobacterial diseases. *Am J Respir Crit Care Med* 2007; **175**: 367–416.

30

Animal tuberculosis

DIRK U PFEIFFER

INTRODUCTION

Apart from humans, infection with bacterial organisms belonging to the *Mycobacterium tuberculosis* complex (MTB) can potentially affect a wide spectrum of mammalian species. Nowadays, their public health relevance is typically attributed to infection with *M. tuberculosis*, to the extent that many diagnostic laboratories will not differentiate it from the other members of the complex: *Mycobacterium africanum*, *Mycobacterium bovis* or *Mycobacterium microti*. Amongst the latter, *M. bovis* is the most important in animal species, whereas *M. tuberculosis* is almost insignificant. Tuberculosis (TB) caused by *M. bovis* used to be a more important human health hazard, particularly during the nineteenth century. However, the introduction of pasteurization of milk together with fairly effective disease control in cattle has reduced the incidence of human infection with *M. bovis* in the developed countries to a negligible level. Disease control in cattle has not been effective where a significant wildlife reservoir is present, but even in these countries the public health infection risk is considered to be extremely low. Many countries around the world justify their continuing effort towards control and eradication of animal TB not just by the zoonotic potential, but also by the threat of restrictions on the international trade of livestock and their products, resulting from a country having endemic animal TB infection.

Apart from *M. tuberculosis* and *M. bovis*, *Mycobacterium avium* is worth noting as an important cause of TB in animals.[1] This ubiquitous opportunistic pathogen can affect a wide range of species. It is most common in birds, but generally considered to be less common in livestock species. It has special significance because the main diagnostic tool for detection of cattle infected with *M. bovis*, the tuberculin test, cross-reacts to infection with *M. avium*.[2]

HISTORY

Animal TB was first recognized in cattle. The first confirmed description of *M. bovis* infection in cattle is based on a report by Columella in the year 40 AD. In seventeenth and eighteenth century Germany 'Perlsucht' (a term referring to the grape-like lesions) was considered a symptom of syphilis ('the French disease'), which resulted in strict procedures for the disposal of the affected animals. When this misconception was corrected, the control measures were removed. It was considered possible to eat meat from tuberculous animals and there were then no obstacles in the way of the spread of the disease. It was not until Robert Koch identified *M. bovis* that the relationship between 'Perlsucht' and lung TB in cattle was established.[3]

As a result of Robert Koch's insistence that *M. bovis* would not be pathogenic in man, it took a number of years before it was generally accepted that it can cause all of the forms of TB which *M. tuberculosis* is able to produce.[4] Another misconception resulting from Koch's statements was that *M. bovis* could only be transmitted to humans via the alimentary route.[5] Only when detailed examinations revealed that between 0.5 and 8.5 per cent of human cases of pulmonary TB in Great Britain were due to *M. bovis* was this hypothesis disproved.[6]

Based on the tuberculin skin test, the first disease control programme which was successfully implemented was Bang's eradication scheme in Denmark in 1892. At that time, such a programme based on tuberculin testing of every animal had not been considered economically feasible in Germany. In 1912, Robert von Ostertag's eradication scheme, which relied on the detection of animals with open lesions, was introduced in Germany on a voluntary basis.[7] The scheme was discontinued in 1939, because it was found that reactor rates were higher in herds which took part in the programme. The USA started with an eradication programme in 1916 and the UK in 1934.[8] In 1952, a compulsory TB control scheme was introduced in West Germany which was based on identification of infected cattle using the tuberculin test. The number of TB-free herds increased from 9.9 per cent in 1952 to 99.7 per cent in 1961. By 1975, such good progress had been made in Germany that it was possible to reduce cattle herd testing to once every 3 years. Since then, the number of infected herds has steadily decreased, but the number of reactors within infected herds has increased.[3] In many industrialized countries, similar programmes were conducted at the same time. However, while it was often possible to reduce reactor rates to low levels, in a number of countries it was not possible to completely eradicate the disease. Factors responsible included the imperfect specificity of the tuberculin test, the reintroduction of disease into TB-free herds through animal trade or wildlife reservoirs of infection, but also transmission from *M. bovis*-infected humans.[9]

AETIOLOGY

Mycobacteria can be grouped according to clinical importance into strict pathogens which include the MTB complex, opportunistic pathogens including *M. avium* and various rare pathogens. Traditionally, mycobacteria have been differentiated using phenotypic characteristics, but these have now been complemented by genotypic methods.[1] The latter include polymerase chain reaction restriction fragment length polymorphism (PCR-RFLP) methods and desoxyribonucleic acid sequencing. This has led, for example, to differentiation of *M. avium* and *M. avium* spp. *paratuberculosis* from *M. intracellulare* which used to be grouped together as *M. avium-intracellulare* complex.

It used to be thought that after the domestication of cattle, a mutation occurred in the bovine bacillus to create the human type.[10] However, the recent finding that the genome sequence of *M. bovis* is shorter than *M. tuberculosis* suggests that it is more likely that *M. bovis* had evolved from an ancestor of *M. tuberculosis*, possibly *M. canettii*.[11,12]

PATHOGENESIS

Most mammalian species are susceptible to infection with mycobacteria and specifically *M. bovis*.[13] Schließer[3] combined his own data comparing the susceptibility to infection of different livestock and laboratory animal species

Table 30.1 Susceptibility of various animal species to selected mycobacterial species.

Species	M. bovis	M. tuberculosis	M. avium
Man	+	+	0
Rhesus monkey	++	++	+/–
Chimpanzee	++	++	0
Cattle	+	0	+/–*
Sheep	+	0	+/–*
Goat	+	0	+/–*
Pig	+	+	+/–
Horse	+/–	0	+/–
Dog	+/–	+/–	0
Cat	+	+/–	+/–
Guinea pig	++	++	+/–*
Rabbit	++	0	+
Mouse	+/–	+/–	+/–
Rat	0	0	0
Birds	0	0	++

0, not susceptible; +/–, poorly susceptible; +/–*, local reaction; +, susceptible; ++, highly susceptible.
From Ref. 3.

with information originally presented by Rich[14] (see Table 30.1). These results were based on experimental work with the organisms, but they cannot alone explain the differences in the infection prevalence found in these species. In this context, it is important to recognize that being susceptible to infection does not necessarily mean that an animal becomes clinically diseased and/or is capable of transmitting infection.

The host response to infection with MTB organisms varies considerably between infected species,[13] but also depends on variation in immune responses between individuals of the same species. It may express itself as a generalized spread of infection including visible pathological change, as localized macroscopic or microscopic pathology or not show any macroscopic change and remain confined to lymphoid tissue. The development of macroscopic tuberculous lesions requires that the infectious organisms can proliferate in the host tissue, and that they induce a host-specific immune response resulting in the classic granuloma. The different stages of the pathogenesis of animal TB have been defined as follows, based on a schema originally developed for human TB.[15] First, the primary complex develops at the infection site during the early stages of the infection period. It is considered to occur in most species, but may not be detected when disease has developed to the next stage. A strong host response may be capable of stopping the disease process and lead to encapsulation and calcification of the primary complex. This is often observed with intestinal *M. avium* infections in the intestinal lymph nodes in pigs. In cattle, during the early infection period *M. bovis* may lead to generalization described as miliary TB. The early infection period is followed by the post-primary period focusing on specific organ systems. This phase occurs only in cattle, rarely in goats and pigs. It is characterized by lesions in defined organ systems such as lung or udder, and eventually leads to 'open' TB. Recovery of the animal during this phase is unlikely. The final phase is the generalization period, which mainly occurs in cattle, and rarely in small ruminants. It results from a breakdown in the host's immune response. Haematogenous spread is common during this phase, eventually leading to fever, loss of body condition and apathy and finally to the death of the animal.[3] A comprehensive comparison of *M. bovis* pathogenesis between different animal species is provided in Lepper and Corner[13] as well as Thoen and Barletta.[12]

EPIDEMIOLOGY

M. bovis

The occurrence of *M. bovis* in a biological system is influenced by a multitude of factors, including, for example, livestock management practices and the density of particular host species. Focusing on the species, it is important to distinguish between host species that are capable of maintaining infection within their population, i.e. maintenance (or reservoir) hosts, and those which can become infected but are not very effective at transmitting it between themselves, i.e. spillover hosts.[16] Disease management methods are used to change a maintenance into a spillover host. This has been successfully achieved with cattle in many countries around the world, as a result of disease control campaigns. Continuing infection presence in such cases typically results from the presence of another maintenance host, such as infected wildlife species (see Figure 30.1). It therefore has to be emphasized that an understanding of the linkages and interfaces which allow effective transmission between the different host species is important when designing effective control programmes.

The transmission dynamics of *M. bovis* infection in humans have changed considerably from prehistoric times to the present, mainly as a result of civilization. The importance of aerogenous as well as alimentary transmission from cattle to humans is now being emphasized. Milk represents an ideal medium for alimentary transmission, as a result of its high fat content which increases absorption into the lymph system. In the absence of pasteurization, bacteria contained in milk products can remain infectious for extended periods of time. This can be up to 100 days in butter and 322 days in certain types of cheese.[3] As long as consumption of raw milk from infected cattle was common, particularly in children, infection and progressive disease caused by *M. bovis* was therefore more likely to occur in children than in adults. Depending on the stage of pathogenesis, meat from tuberculous animals may constitute a significant risk of infection if available for consumption. *M. bovis* has even been isolated from minced meat.[3]

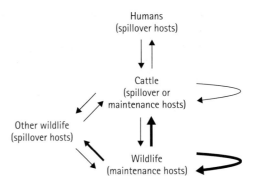

Figure 30.1 Systems diagram representing the *Mycobacterium bovis* infection flows between different host species in a biological system (thickness of arrows reflects relative magnitude of infection risk).

The risk of aerogenous infection has long been underestimated, but it may well be higher in a shed with tuberculous cattle due to the potentially high levels of dust and other aerosol particles than in a hospital with TB cases.[17] Infection by direct contact would be a risk factor for certain occupations such as farmers, abattoir workers and veterinarians. Transmission between humans and from humans to cattle is possible but relatively uncommon.[5]

As species identification in many countries, particularly in the developing world, is not carried out routinely, it is difficult to estimate the present contribution of *M. bovis* to total TB morbidity and mortality in humans.[8] Table 30.2 shows official reporting statistics for Europe. It indicates that about 0.5 per cent of reported TB cases are associated with *M. bovis* infection, but it can reach as much as 5 per cent as in the case of Cyprus. The source of these infections is often difficult to determine. As an example, based on epidemiological analysis of 50 human cases of *M. bovis* infection identified in the UK between 1997 and 2000, Gibson *et al.*[18] report that 59 per cent of 22 cases had some contact with farmed livestock. However, the source of infection was not determined in the vast majority of these cases. The same paper mentions a single case of occurrence of transmission of *M. bovis* between humans on a farm. The information about *M. bovis* occurrence in developing countries is scarce, but probably accounts for less than 10 per cent of all human TB cases.[19,20] The occurrence of AIDS and TB in humans has been termed 'the cursed duet'.[21] Both diseases can interact, for example AIDS patients latently infected with *M. bovis* develop clinical TB, or the other way around.

Intensification of livestock husbandry during the last 100 years resulted in increased herd sizes, higher stocking densities and greater numbers of cattle movements which facilitated transmission and spread of infectious diseases. As early as 1868, Villemin[22] had observed higher prevalence of TB in housed cattle compared with those kept continuously on pasture. In intensive production systems, bovine TB is more common in dairy cattle than in beef cattle as a result of increased opportunities for contact. It

Table 30.2 Human tuberculosis cases in Europe in 2004 by *M. tuberculosis* complex species.

Geographic area/ country	M. tuberculosis		M. bovis		M. africanum		Unknown/not done		Total
	No.	(%)	No.	(%)	No.	(%)	No.	(%)	
EU and West									
Austria	165	(28.2)	4	(0.7)	0	(0.0)	417	(71.2)	586
Belgium	945	(99.7)	3	(0.3)	0	(0.0)	0	(0.0)	948
Cyprus	17	(89.5)	1	(5.0)	0	(0.0)	1	(5.3)	19
Czech Republic	644	(96.7)	2	(0.3)	0	(0.0)	20	(3.0)	666
Denmark	289	(99.3)	2	(0.7)	0	(0.0)	0	(0.0)	291
Estonia	187	(41.4)	0	(0.0)	0	(0.0)	265	(58.6)	452
Finland	285	(99.3)	0	(0.0)	0	(0.0)	2	(0.7)	287
Germany	3411	(78.6)	54	(1.2)	13	(0.3)	860	(19.8)	4338
Hungary	114	(100.0)	0	(0.0)	0	(0.0)	0	(0.0)	114
Ireland	185	(88.5)	4	(1.9)	0	(0.0)	20	(9.6)	209
Italy	1289	(66.0)	6	(0.3)	11	(0.6)	648	(33.2)	1954
Latvia	1156	(100.0)	0	(0.0)	0	(0.0)	0	(0.0)	1156
Lithuania	1592	(100.0)	0	(0.0)	0	(0.0)	0	(0.0)	1592
Luxembourg	31	(100.0)	0	(0.0)	0	(0.0)	0	(0.0)	31
Malta	8	(100.0)	0	(0.0)	0	(0.0)	0	(0.0)	8
Netherlands	724	(95.4)	13	(1.7)	8	(1.1)	14	(1.8)	759
Portugal	13	(0.6)	1	(0.0)	0	(0.0)	2078	(99.3)	2092
Slovakia	347	(97.2)	0	(0.0)	0	(0.0)	10	(2.8)	357
Slovenia	231	(100.0)	0	(0.0)	0	(0.0)	0	(0.0)	231
Sweden	365	(98.6)	4	(1.1)	1	(0.3)	0	(0.0)	370
Subtotal EU	12 898	(74.3)	94	(0.5)	33	(0.2)	4335	(25.0)	17 360
Andorra	6	(100.0)	0	(0.0)	0	(0.0)	0	(0.0)	6
Iceland	8	(100.0)	0	(0.0)	0	(0.0)	0	(0.0)	8
Norway	246	(100.0)	0	(0.0)	0	(0.0)	0	(0.0)	246
Switzerland	422	(88.3)	5	(1.0)	7	(1.5)	44	(9.2)	478
Total EU and West	13 580	(75.0)	99	(0.5)	40	(0.2)	4379	(24.2)	18 098
Centre									
Albania	201	(100.0)	0	(0.0)	0	(0.0)	0	(0.0)	201
Bosnia and Herzegovina	1123	(99.8)	0	(0.0)	0	(0.0)	2	(0.2)	1125
Romania	13 324	(100.0)	0	(0.0)	0	(0.0)	0	(0.0)	13 324

Source: EuroTB 2006; note that data were not available for all EU countries.

may also be the result of the different age structures, given that prevalence increases with age and dairy cattle are usually kept longer than beef cattle.[3] In extensive cattle production systems around the world, TB is usually less prevalent. However, in some situations (Africa, Australia), high incidences have been reported in range cattle. This may be related to aggregation of animals around watering points.[2]

Studies in Northern Ireland suggested that within- and between-herd transmission through aerosolized secretions may be of continued importance in the epidemiology of bovine TB. It was found that in cattle infected with *M. bovis*, lung lesions and nasal excretion occurred frequently and could be diagnosed from 2 months after the last negative tuberculin test.[23,24] Analysis of cattle herd TB breakdown data from Great Britain shows that TB is rarely transmitted to neighbouring herds. It was suggested that the presence of non-reacting excreting cattle was more

likely to affect within-herd transmission and that the introduction of infection through purchases of tuberculous cattle is an important risk factor.[25]

Other domestic species affected significantly by *M. bovis* infection are farmed deer. In 1978, TB infection was reported from farmed red deer in New Zealand.[26] With intensification of deer farming, it became the most important bacterial disease in farmed deer in New Zealand.[27,28] It has been suggested that deer kept under farm conditions may be more susceptible to *M. bovis* infection than cattle. Depending on a range of behavioural and environmental factors, extensive lesions can develop rapidly which in turn result in increased probability of spread within a herd.[29] Recognizing the threat of TB to the deer farming industry, New Zealand, Denmark and Great Britain have all embarked on TB control or eradication programmes. They are mainly based on tuberculin skin testing and subsequent slaughter of reactor animals. Owing to the presence of endemic infection in wildlife in New Zealand and in the UK the eradication of TB in farmed deer may be difficult to achieve.[29] Tuberculous captive deer have been implicated in New Zealand as a source of infection for possums which are an important wildlife reservoir for bovine TB.[30]

Prevalence of TB infection in small ruminants is believed to be linked to the disease frequency in other hosts such as cattle. In industrialized countries, detection of tuberculous lesions in small ruminants is less common when disease levels within the cattle population decreases. In extensive animal husbandry systems, transmission probabilities are low, resulting in low overall prevalence.[3] In some instances, prevalence levels of up to 10 per cent have been observed in sheep flocks in New Zealand.[31,32] It has been postulated that sheep TB is less common than cattle TB in countries with wildlife reservoirs of infection, because sheep behaviour is such that there is less opportunity for contact with an infection source.[33] Similarly, goat flocks can become infected, largely as a result of exposure to a maintenance host.[34]

Disease levels in domestic pigs also usually reflect the incidence in local cattle populations. In 1921, 12 per cent of pigs slaughtered under federal inspection in the USA were found to have tuberculous lesions.[35] In the midwest of the USA, it was possible to trace 96 per cent of swine carcass condemnations for TB to feeding of unsterilized skim milk or other dairy products or to keeping them together with cattle. Prevalence in pigs is thought to increase with age. The principal route of infection in the pig is the digestive tract, by consumption of milk or milk products, kitchen and abattoir scraps, and excreta from tuberculous cattle.[36] Transmission between pigs is considered epidemiologically insignificant, as lesions usually remain localized and pigs are slaughtered at an early age. High disease levels in cattle can result in prevalence of up to 20 per cent in local pig populations.[2]

Occasional incidents have been reported where dogs or cats became infected with M. bovis. As scavenging animals, they can be exposed to infection particularly from consumption of carcasses from diseased animals. In one study, tuberculous lesions were found in four of nine dogs and 24 of 52 cats on farms with M. bovis infection in the USA.[37] In New Zealand, between 1974 and 1992 a total of 73 domestic cats were found to be infected with M. bovis by the national Animal Health Laboratory, but only two isolates were found in dogs. It is unlikely that domestic dogs and cats represent an epidemiologically significant factor in the dynamics of TB infection.[38,39]

TB has been known as a serious clinical disease in wild mammals in captivity for more than a century.[40] It is widely distributed in captive wild mammal populations in the USA, where outbreaks caused by infection with M. bovis have been reported mainly from zoos, game parks and primate colonies.[41] In European countries, sporadic incidents of bovine TB in wild mammals were mainly reported before eradication of cattle TB was achieved.[3]

Evidence from various countries in the world shows that significant levels of TB infection can be found in wild or feral species such as buffalo, goats, pigs, deer, badgers and brush-tailed possums under specific epidemiological circumstances.[27] The risk which these reservoirs of infection constitute for domestic animals and man is difficult to estimate. Biet et al.[42] produced a summary table of the epidemiological characteristics of M. bovis infection in various wild animal species.

Although various wild and feral species can become infected with M. bovis, the most important wild animal reservoir hosts so far discovered are the European badger (Meles meles), the Australian brush-tailed possum (Trichosurus vulpecula Kerr) and various species of deer.[27]

Badgers are an important reservoir of reinfection for cattle in the UK and Ireland.[43,44] The disease is considered to be endemic in badger populations in some areas of both countries.[44] Most badgers get infected via the respiratory route. Infected animals can survive for extended periods of time.[45,46] It is thought that transmission to cattle occurs via contamination of pasture and contact with moribund badgers.[47] The justification and effectiveness of control methods for the disease in badgers are contentious, particularly the use of badger population reduction.[48,49]

In New Zealand, Australian brush-tailed possums, which were introduced to the country in the nineteenth century, are a major reservoir species for M. bovis infection, but not in their native Australia. In the presence of this source of infection, eradication of bovine TB from the cattle population is unlikely to succeed. Traditional methods of disease control such as test-and-slaughter of cattle and culling of possums have not proved adequate to achieve effective control of TB in either the cattle or the possums. Possum TB occurs in spatial clusters of prevalence between 5 and 30 per cent.[50] Tuberculous lesions occur primarily in lungs, as well as in axillary and inguinal lymph centres.[51] The respiratory route is considered to be a major transmission path between possums.[52]

Bovine TB used to be endemic in feral water buffalo populations of the Australian Northern Territory.[53] A prevalence of 0.02 was found in 11 322 buffalo examined during routine post-mortem examination at two abattoirs during 1979.[53] The large proportion of cases with sole or predominant involvement of the thoracic organs suggests that as in cattle the respiratory route is the most important transmission path in feral buffalo.[54]

In 1963, TB was reported from wild African buffalo in Ruwenzori National Park, Uganda[55] at 10 per cent prevalence amongst 52 buffaloes from a random sample and 38 per cent of 64 animals which were selected based on being in poor condition. M. bovis was identified in 12 of 14 cases. Most cases appeared to be infected by respiratory transmission and no lesions were seen which could be ascribed to alimentary infection. The close herding habits of wild buffaloes and their propensity for wallowing in tight groups in small mud holes facilitate droplet transmission.[56] African buffalo are maintenance hosts of M. bovis in

Kruger National Park with up to 90 per cent infection prevalence in some herds, and more than 50 per cent of herds infected. Lions and other carnivores are also affected, but are considered to be spillover hosts.[57]

Tuberculous lesions have been found at prevalence levels of up to 50 per cent in wild bison populations in Canada.[58,59] The lesion distribution suggested that infection occurs primarily via the respiratory route.

Infection with *M. bovis* has been reported from a number of free-ranging deer species.[27,29] In Michigan, infection in wild white-tailed deer populations occurring at a state-wide prevalence of less than 1 per cent is the primary reason preventing eradication of infection in cattle.[60] Transmission of infection is thought to be the result of congregation of animals at winter feeding places.

Wild pigs have been found to be infected with *M. bovis* at significant levels in a number of countries. Infection prevalence between 19 and 54 per cent has been reported from Australia's Northern Territory and New Zealand.[61,62] This relatively high prevalence may have been the result of pigs living in close association with swamp buffalo as the maintenance host. At the end of each dry season, hundreds of old buffalo die, thereby providing food and a potential source of infection with *M. bovis* given the high incidence of TB in wild buffalo in the Northern Territory. Wild pigs are likely to be spillover hosts for *M. bovis* and not a significant source of infection for cattle.[61]

Woodford[56] found that bovine TB infection was endemic in the warthog population of Ruwenzori National Park, Uganda. He concluded that the disease must have been introduced with domestic cattle.

Feral goats were found with TB prevalence levels of up to 31 per cent within individual groups in areas with endemic TB in New Zealand.[63] The epidemiological significance of bovine TB in feral goats is generally considered to be minimal. In most cases, it is related to the presence of a reservoir of infection in another species, such as the Australian brush-tailed possum in New Zealand.

Infection in wild carnivorous species has to be expected in areas where TB is endemic in important infection reservoir species, such as for example brush-tailed possums in New Zealand or African buffalo in South Africa. High infection prevalence levels have been reported from some lion populations in South Africa's national parks. Wild ferret populations have been found with 18 per cent prevalence in some locations of New Zealand compared with less than 2 per cent in feral cats and wild stoats.[64] Hedgehogs have also been found with tuberculous lung lesions from *M. bovis* infection.[65] In most of these situations, the scavenging/predator species is most likely to be a spillover host.[66]

Mycobacteria other than *M. bovis*

M. avium occurs in pigs and birds mainly as a result of environmental exposure.[67] Cats and dogs are rarely found to be infected with *M. avium*.[68] They can also become infected with *M. tuberculosis*, typically as a result of exposure to infected humans.[38] It has also been suggested that *M. tuberculosis* infection might be an emerging disease in free-ranging wild animals.[69] These authors described outbreaks amongst mongooses in Botswana and suricates in South Africa. Non-human primates and elephants in captive populations can become reservoirs of *M. tuberculosis* infection.[70]

DIAGNOSIS

For a long time, the most commonly used diagnostic methods for TB have been the tuberculin skin test, gross and histologic examination, as well as bacteriological culture. All are used as standard tools in cattle TB control programmes around the world. A presumptive diagnosis of *M. bovis* in cattle is typically based on the result of the tuberculin skin test, clinical history, clinical or gross necropsy findings. Diagnoses are confirmed by histopathological results, histochemical or immunohistochemical staining, or by *in situ* hybridization with *M. bovis*-specific probes.[71]

The tuberculin delayed-type hypersensitivity skin test reaction depends on the cell-mediated immune response of the host which in turn is influenced by the stage of pathogenesis. Purified protein derivative is used as the antigen in this test, and it is derived from *M. bovis* or *M. avium* culture. In cattle, it can be applied in the caudal fold, as a single or as a comparative intradermal cervical test. The tests are read 72 hours after intradermal injection through measurement of skin thickness.[72] de la Rua-Domenech *et al.*[73] reviewed different studies for the single and comparative tuberculin tests, and they report sensitivities and specificities as ranging between 50–100 per cent and 75–100 per cent, respectively.[74,75] Despite its variable performance characteristics, it has been a cornerstone of many successful disease control campaigns. This is largely due to the fact that its comparatively poor sensitivity can be overcome by interpreting the test at the herd level. That means that as long as there are multiple infected animals within the herd, the test should detect at least one of them in a whole herd test. Research is under way to identify peptide cocktails which have higher sensitivity than current tuberculin tests, and are not compromised by bacillus Calmette–Guérin (BCG) vaccination.[76]

In vitro diagnostic methods used to be based on only gross and histological examination or bacteriological culture, but a number of molecular methods techniques have been developed over the last 10 years. Routine abattoir gross lesion inspection focuses on the detection of granulomatous lesions in lymph nodes, particularly those associated with the respiratory tract. It is acknowledged that this method may fail to detect up to half of the animals with lesions.[77] Histological examination is based either on fluorescence microscopy or Ziehl–Neelsen staining. Relative to bacteriological culture, its sensitivity is reported to vary between 22 and 78 per cent, and specificity around 99 per cent.[78] These methods are still used as the main diagnostic tools for confirmatory TB diagnosis in cattle in many countries, particularly in the developing world. Bacteriological culture is still the definitive diagnosis, and its sensitivity has been described to be as good as animal inoculation. It is particularly important for species differentiation. It has the disadvantage that it takes up to 8 weeks, for example, for *M. bovis* to grow in culture. Immunodiagnostic assays have been developed as faster alternatives to culture, but also to remove the need for an examination after 72 hours as is necessary with the tuberculin test. Amongst these, antibody-based diagnostic methods have generally not provided satisfactory sensitivity and specificity.[75,79] The exception is an ELISA test developed for deer in New Zealand that is reported to reach sensitivity of up to 85 and 95 per cent when used in combination with lymphocyte transformation and tuberculin skin tests, respectively.[80] The first cell-mediated immunity-based diagnostic methods measured T-cell reactivity as lymphocyte transformation tests, but they had the disadvantage that they were too complex, costly and slow to be able to replace tuberculin testing.[81] It is now accepted that enzyme immunoassays based on detection of the cytokine interferon-γ can perform as well as the tuberculin skin test, although their specificity can be inferior.[73–75,81,82]

Molecular diagnostic methods are used particularly as investigative epidemiological tools. The whole genomic technique restriction-endonuclease analysis has been applied in an assessment of the likelihood of transmission between wildlife, domestic and human *M. bovis* TB in New Zealand.[83,85] However, this technique is considered too complex and requires subjective interpretation. Since then, a wide range of partial genomic techniques methods have been developed, of which IS*6110*-RFLP and spoligotyping have been amongst the most commonly used techniques.[86] These techniques are being used increasingly to assist in epidemiological investigations.[87,88]

TREATMENT

Similar to the situation in humans, mycobacteria are difficult to treat. They are facultative intracellular parasites and can survive within host macrophages for long periods of time.[89] Combinations of isoniazid with rifampicin or streptomycin have been used successfully as long-term treatments of TB cases in monkey colonies.[90,91] However, the high risk of infection for humans and other animals during therapy of animals infected with *M. bovis* combined with the risk of the development of resistant strains has led to treatment being discouraged for animal species.[3] Countries which aim to eradicate *M. bovis* will not allow treatment of livestock species.[2]

CONTROL METHODS

Specific disease control programmes have been developed for *M. bovis* and they are based on test-and-slaughter of domestic cattle and farmed deer populations. Animals reacting to the tuberculin test are typically culled and movement of animals for reasons other than slaughter would not be allowed until the herd has been tested negative.[71] In addition, abattoir surveillance based on postmortem inspection of carcasses is used, but its sensitivity has been reported to be less than 50 per cent.[77] This type of disease control programme works very effectively, as long as no wildlife reservoir species is present, such as badgers in the UK and Ireland, possums in New Zealand and white-tailed deer in Michigan. In the case of badgers and possums, disease occurrence in cattle could only be decreased by reducing the population density of the wildlife reservoir host species.[66,92] In the national parks of South Africa, a capture test-and-slaughter policy is currently used to control infection in buffalo populations. Selective depopulation is not considered appropriate, since there are indications that other species, such as greater kudu, may also act as maintenance host in these ecosystems.[93] Since population reduction as a control method has become less acceptable to society, alternative control tools are currently being developed. These include vaccination of the wildlife reservoir species and possibly cattle.[94] The existing BCG vaccine has shown potential when evaluated in cattle and possums as part of experiments and field studies.[95–97] If used in cattle, it will cause positive reactions to the tuberculin skin test which cannot be differentiated from natural infection. For this reason, its use is not being considered in most countries of the world, but it may be of use in developing countries to limit the spread of infection.[94] Recent years have seen advances that may lead to the development of vaccines against *M. bovis* infection for cattle which will be sufficiently effective and not interfere with diagnostic testing.[98]

CONCLUSION

Despite several decades of control efforts, animal TB caused by *M. bovis* is of continued importance, mainly as a result of the presence of wildlife reservoir species in some countries. Better diagnostic methods are being developed to replace the tuberculin skin test. However, eradication will only ever be achieved if vaccines become available that can be used with domestic and in particular wildlife populations. It has also become clear that effective disease control requires a satisfactory understanding of the epidemiology of animal TB in an ecosystem, including identification of maintenance and spillover hosts, and the quantitative importance of different transmission mechanisms within and between species.

LEARNING POINTS

- *M. bovis* is the most important organism of the *M. tuberculosis* complex infecting animals, whereas *M. tuberculosis* is almost insignificant.

- *M. bovis* is no longer a health hazard in humans where milk pasteurization is carried out.
- TB in cattle was first described in the first century.
- Cattle eradication schemes, for the elimination of TB began in the USA in 1916, the UK in 1934 and in West Germany in 1952.
- In contrast to previously held theories that *M. tuberculosis* developed from *M. bovis*, gene sequencing suggests that because the *M. bovis* genome is shorter, it is more likely that this evolved from *M. tuberculosis*.
- The highest incidence of *M. bovis* in Europe is in the Republic of Ireland (4.2 per cent). The reason for this is not clear.
- TB in small ruminants is believed to be linked to disease in cattle.
- Household pets may become infected with *M. bovis*, but this is unlikely to be epidemilogically significant.
- Badgers are the most important species for the reinfection of cattle in the UK and Ireland. In New Zealand, Australian brush-tailed possums perform a similar role.
- A presumptive diagnosis of TB in animals is based on a positive skin test. It is confirmed by histopathology.
- Countries which aim to eliminate animal infection by *M. bovis* will not allow treatment of animals.
- Control is based on a test-and-slaughter policy.

REFERENCES

1. Rastogi N, Legrand E, Sola C. The mycobacteria: an introduction to nomenclature and pathogenesis. *Rev Sci Tech* 2001; **20**: 21–54.
2. Radostits OM, Gay CC, Blood DC, Hinchcliff KW. *Veterinary medicine – A textbook of the diseases of cattle, sheep, pigs, goats and horses*, 9th edn. London: WB Saunders, 2000.
3. Schließer T. Mycobacterium. In: Blobel H, Schließer T, eds. *Handbuch der bakteriellen Infektionen bei Tieren*. Stuttgart: Gustav Fischer Verlag, 1985: 155–280.
4. Collins CH, Grange JM. A review: The bovine tubercle bacillus. *J Appl Bacteriol* 1983; **55**: 13–29.
5. Grange JM, Collins CH. Bovine tubercle bacilli and disease in animals and man. *Epidemiol Infect* 1987; **92**: 221–34.
6. Griffith AS. Bovine tuberculosis in man. *Tubercle* 1937; **22**: 33–9.
7. von Ostertag R. Die Bekämpfung der Tuberkulose des Rindes. Berlin: Schoetz, 1913.
8. Pritchard DG. A century of bovine tuberculosis 1888–1988: Conquest and controversy. *J Comp Pathol* 1988; **99**: 357–99.
9. Schliesser Th. Zur Geschichte und Entwicklung der Rindertuberkulose-Bekaempfung. *Zbl Bakt Hyg, I Abt Orig A* 1982; **251**: 326–40.
10. Stead WW, Eisenach KD, Cave MD *et al.* When did *Mycobacterium tuberculosis* infection first occur in the new world ? *Am J Respir Crit Care Med* 1995; **151**: 1267–8.
11. Brosch R, Gordon SV, Marmiesse M *et al.* A new evolutionary scenario for the *Mycobacterium tuberculosis* complex. *Proc Natl Acad Sci U S A* 2002; **99**: 3684–9.
12. Thoen CO, Barletta RG. Pathogenesis of *Mycobacterium bovis*. In: Thoen CO, Steele JH, Gilsdorf MJ (eds). *Mycobacterium bovis infection in animals and humans*, 2nd edn. Ames, IA: Blackwell, 2006: 49–53.
13. Lepper AWD, Corner LA. Naturally occurring mycobacterioses of animals. In: Ratledge C, Stanford J (eds). *Immunological and environmental aspects*. London: Academic Press, 1983: 417–521.
14. Rich AR. *The pathogenesis of tuberculosis*, 2nd edn. Springfield, IL: Charles C Thomas, 1951.
15. Nieberle K. *Tuberkulose und Fleischhygiene*. Jena: Gustav Fischer Verlag, 1938.
16. Morris RS, Pfeiffer DU, Jackson R. The epidemiology of *Mycobacterium bovis* infections. *Vet Microbiol* 1994; **40**: 153–77.
17. Jensen KA. Bovine tuberculosis in man and cattle. *Advances in the control of zoonoses*. WHO/FAO Seminar on Zoonoses, Vienna, November 1952. Geneva: World Health Organization, 1953: 11.
18. Gibson AL, Hewinson G, Goodchild T *et al.* Molecular epidemiology of disease due to *Mycobacterium bovis* in humans in the United Kingdom. *J Clin Microbiol* 2004; **42**: 431–4.
19. Cosivi O, Grange JM, Daborn CJ *et al.* Zoonotic tuberculosis due to *Mycobacterium bovis* in developing countries. *Emerg Infect Dis* 1998; **4**: 59–70.
20. Zinsstag J, Kazwala RR, Cadmus I, Ayanwale L. *Mycobacterium bovis* in Africa. In: Thoen CO, Steele JH, Gilsdorf MJ (eds). *Mycobacterium bovis infection in animals and humans*, 2nd edn. Ames, IA: Blackwell, 2006: 199–210.
21. Chretien J. Tuberculosis and HIV. The cursed duet. *Bull Int Union Tuberc Lung Dis* 1990; **65**: 25–8.
22. Francis J. *Tuberculosis in animals and man*. London: Cassell, 1958.
23. McIlroy SG, Neill SD, McCracken RM. Pulmonary lesions and *Mycobacterium bovis* excretion from respiratory tract of tuberculin reacting cattle. *Vet Rec* 1986; **118**: 718–21.
24. Neill SD, O'Brien JJ, McCracken RM. *Mycobacterium bovis* in the anterior respiratory tracts in the heads of tuberculin-reacting cattle. *Vet Rec* 1988; **122**: 184–6.
25. Dunnet GM, Jones DM, McInerney JP. *Badgers and bovine tuberculosis – Review of policy*. London: Her Majesty's Stationery Office, 1986.
26. Beatson NS. Tuberculosis in Red Deer in New Zealand. Biology of deer production. *R Soc N Z Bull* 1985; **22**: 147–50.
27. De Lisle GW, Mackintosh CG, Bengis RG. *Mycobacterium bovis* in free-living and captive wildlife, including farmed deer. *Rev Sci Tech* 2001; **20**: 86–111.
28. Griffin JFT, Mackintosh CG. Tuberculosis in deer: Perceptions, problems and progress. *Vet J* 2000; **160**: 202–19.
29. Clifton-Hadley RS, Wilesmith JW. Tuberculosis in deer: a review. *Vet Rec* 1991; **129**: 5–12.
30. Livingstone PG. Cattle TB – an update on the situation in New Zealand. *Surveillance* 1988; **15**: 3–7.
31. Davidson RM, Alley MR, Beatson NS. Tuberculosis in a flock of sheep. *Vet Rec* 1981; **29**: 1–2.
32. Cordes DO, Bullians JA, Lake DE, Carter ME. Observations on tuberculosis caused by *Mycobacterium bovis* in sheep. *N Z Vet J* 1981; **29**: 60–2.
33. Allen GM. Tuberculosis in sheep – a rare disease. *Surveillance* 1988; **15**: 8–9.
34. Edington J. Tuberculosis in a South Canterbury goat flock. *Surveillance* 1989; **16**: 22–3.
35. Myers JA, Steele JH. *Bovine tuberculosis – Control in man and animals*. St Louis, MI: Warren H Green, 1969.
36. Acha PN, Szyfres B. *Zoonoses and communicable diseases common to man and animals*, 2nd edn. Washington, DC: Pan American Health Organization, 1989.
37. Snider WR, Cohen D, Reif JS *et al.* Tuberculosis in canine and feline populations – Study of high risk populations in Pennsylvania, 1966–1968. *Am Rev Respir Dis* 1971; **104**: 866–76.
38. Snider WR. Tuberculosis in canine and feline populations – Review of the literature. *Am Rev Respir Dis* 1971; **104**: 877–87.

39. De Lisle GW, Collins DM, Loveday AS et al. A report of tuberculosis in cats in New Zealand, and the examination of strains of Mycobacterium bovis by DNA restriction endonuclease analysis. N Z Vet J 1990; 38: 10–13.

40. Thoen CO, Karlson AG, Himes EM. Mycobacterial infections in animals. Rev Infect Dis 1981; 3: 960–72.

41. Stetter MD, Mikota SK, Gutter AF et al. Epizootic of Mycobacterium bovis in a zoologic park. J Am Vet Med Assoc 1995; 207: 1618–21.

42. Biet F, Boschiroli ML, Thorel MF, Guilloteau LA. Zoonotic aspects of Mycobacterium bovis and Mycobacterium avium-intracellulare complex (MAC). Vet Res 2005; 36: 411–36.

43. Wilesmith JW. Epidemiological features of bovine tuberculosis in cattle herds in Great Britain. J Hyg 1983; 90: 159–76.

44. Krebs JR, Independent Scientific Review Group. Bovine tuberculosis in cattle and badgers. London: MAFF, 1997.

45. Clifton-Hadley RS, Wilesmith JW, Stuart FA. Mycobacterium bovis in the European badger (Meles meles): Epidemiological findings in tuberculous badgers from a naturally infected population. Epidemiol Infect 1993; 111: 9–19.

46. Wilkinson D, Smith GC, Delahay RJ et al. The effects of bovine tuberculosis (Mycobacterium bovis) on mortality in a badger (Meles meles) population in England. J Zool 2000; 250: 389–95.

47. Benham PFJ, Broom DM. Interactions between cattle and badgers at pasture with reference to bovine tuberculosis transmission. Br Vet J 1989; 145: 226–41.

48. Griffin JM, Williams DH, Kelly GE et al. The impact of badger removal on the control of tuberculosis in cattle herds in Ireland. Prev Vet Med 2005; 67: 237–66.

49. Woodroffe R, Donnelly CA, Jenkins HE et al. Culling and cattle controls influence tuberculosis risk for badgers. Proc Natl Acad Sci U S A 2006; 103: 14713–7.

50. Pfeiffer DU, Hickling GJ, Morris RS et al. The epidemiology of Mycobacterium bovis infection in brushtail possums (Trichosurus vulpecula Kerr) in the Hauhungaroa Ranges, New Zealand. N Z Vet J 1995; 43: 272–80.

51. Jackson R, Cooke MM, Coleman JD, Morris RS. Naturally occurring tuberculosis caused by Mycobacterium bovis in brushtail possums (Trichosurus vulpecula): I Pathogenesis. N Z Vet J 1995; 43: 306–14.

52. Jackson R, Cooke MM, Coleman JD et al. Naturally occurring tuberculosis caused by Mycobacterium bovis in brushtail possums (Trichosurus vulpecula): III. Routes of Infection and excretion. N Z Vet J 1995; 43: 322–7.

53. Hein WR, Tomasovic AA. An abattoir survey of tuberculosis in feral buffalo. Aust Vet J 1981; 57: 543–7.

54. McCool CJ, Newton-Tabrett DA. The route of infection in tuberculosis in feral buffalo. Aust Vet J 1979; 55: 401–2.

55. Woodford MH. Tuberculosis in wildlife in the Ruwenzori National Park, Uganda (Part I). Trop Anim Health Prod 1982; 14: 81–8.

56. Woodford MH. Tuberculosis in wildlife in the Ruwenzori National Park, Uganda (Part II). Trop Anim Health Prod 1982; 14: 155–60.

57. Hilsberg S, van Hoven W. Tuberculosis in wild animals in Africa: a review with special reference to the Kruger National Park. Infect Dis Rev 1999; 1: 248–52.

58. Choquette LPE, Gallivan JF, Byrne JL, Pilipavicius J. Tuberculosis and some other pathological conditions in bison at Wood Buffalo and Elk Island National Parks in the fall and winter 1959–60. Can Vet J 1961; 2: 168–74.

59. Tessaro SV, Forbes LB, Turcotte C. A survey of brucellosis and tuberculosis in bison in and around Wood Buffalo National Park, Canada. Can Vet J 1990; 31: 174–80.

60. O'Brien DJ, Schmitt SM, Fierke JS et al. Epidemiology of Mycobacterium bovis in free-ranging white-tailed deer, Michigan, USA, 1995-2000. Prev Vet Med 2002; 54: 47–63.

61. Corner LA, Barrett RH, Lepper AWD et al. A survey of mycobacteriosis of feral pigs in the Northern Territory. Aust Vet J 1981; 57: 537–42.

62. Wakelin CA, Churchman OT. Prevalence of bovine tuberculosis in feral pigs in Central Otago. Surveillance 1991; 18: 19–20.

63. Sanson RL. Tuberculosis in goats. Surveillance 1988; 15: 7–8.

64. Ragg JR, Moller H, Waldrup KA. The prevalence of bovine tuberculosis (Mycobacterium bovis) infections in feral populations of cats ((Felis catis), ferrets (Mustela furo) and stoats (Mustela erminea) in Otago and Southland. N Z Vet J 1995; 43: 333–7.

65. Lugton IW, Johnstone AC, Morris RS. Mycobacterium bovis infection in New Zealand hedgehogs (Erinaceus europaeus). N Z Vet J 1995; 43: 342–5.

66. De Lisle GW, Bengis RG, Schmitt SM, O'Brien DJ. Tuberculosis in free-ranging wildlife: detection, diagnosis and management. Rev Sci Tech 2002; 21: 317–34.

67. Thorel MF, Huchzermeyer HF, Michel AL. Mycobacterium avium and Mycobacterium intracellulare infection in mammals. Rev Sci Tech 2001; 20: 204–18.

68. De Lisle GW. Mycobacterial infections in cats and dogs. Surveillance 1993; 20: 24–6.

69. Alexander KA, Pleydell E, Williams MC et al. Mycobacterium tuberculosis: an emerging disease of free-ranging wildlife. Emerg Infect Dis 2002; 8: 598–601.

70. Montali RJ, Mikota SK, Cheng LI. Mycobacterium tuberculosis in zoo and wildlife species. Rev Sci Tech 2001; 20: 291–303.

71. Cousins DV. Mycobacterium bovis infection and control in domestic livestock. Rev Sci Tech 2001; 20: 71–85.

72. Francis J, Choi CL, Frost AJ. The diagnosis of tuberculosis in cattle with special reference to bovine PPD tuberculin. Aust Vet J 1973; 49: 246–51.

73. de la Rua-Domenech R, Goodchild AT, Vordermeier HM et al. Ante mortem diagnosis of tuberculosis in cattle: A review of the tuberculin tests, gamma-interferon assay and other ancillary diagnostic techniques. Res Vet Sci 2006; 81: 190–210.

74. Monaghan ML, Doherty ML, Collins JD et al. The tuberculin test. Vet Microbiol 1994; 40: 111–24.

75. Adams LG. In vivo and in vitro diagnosis of Mycobacterium bovis infection. Rev Sci Tech 2001; 20: 304–24.

76. Cockle PJ, Gordon SV, Hewinson RG, Vordermeier HA. Field evaluation of a novel differential diagnostic reagent for detection of Mycobacterium bovis in cattle. Clin Vaccine Immunol 2006; 13: 1119–24.

77. Corner LA, Melville L, McCubbin K et al. Efficiency of inspection procedures for the detection of tuberculous lesions in cattle. Aust Vet J 1990; 67: 389–92.

78. Petersen KF, Urbanczik R. Mikroskopische und kulturelle Methoden für die Laboratoriumsdiagnose der Tuberkulose. Kurzer historischer Überblick. Zbl Bakt Hyg , I Abt Orig A 1982; 251: 308–25.

79. Amadori M, Tameni S, Scaccaglia P et al. Antibody tests for identification of Mycobacterium bovis-infected bovine herds. J Clin Microbiol 1998; 36: 566–8.

80. Griffin JFT, Cross JP, Chinn DN et al. Diagnosis of tuberculosis due to Mycobacterium bovis in New Zealand red deer (Cervus elaphus): Using a composite blood-test and antibody-assays. N Z Vet J 1994; 42: 173–9.

81. Wood PR, Rothel JS. In vitro immunodiagnostic assays for bovine tuberculosis. Vet Microbiol 1994; 40: 125–35.

82. Wood PR, Corner LA, Rothel JS et al. A field evaluation of serological and cellular diagnostic tests for bovine tuberculosis. Vet Microbiol 1992; 31: 71–9.

83. Collins DM, Lisle de GW. DNA restriction endonuclease analysis of Mycobacterium bovis and other members of the tuberculosis complex. J Clin Microbiol 1985; 21: 562–4.

84. Collins DM, Lisle de GW. DNA restriction endonuclease analysis of Mycobacterium bovis and other members of the tuberculosis complex. J Clin Microbiol 1985; 21: 562–4.

85. Baker MG, Lopez LD, Cannon MC et al. Continuing Mycobacterium bovis transmission from animals to humans in New Zealand. Epidemiol Infect 2006; 134: 1068–73.

86. Durr PA, Hewinson RG, Clifton-Hadley RS. Molecular epidemiology of bovine tuberculosis – I. *Mycobacterium bovis* genotyping. *Rev Sci Tech* 2000; **19**: 675–88.

87. Gopal R, Goodchild A, Hewinson G et al. Introduction of bovine tuberculosis to north-east England by bought-in cattle. *Vet Rec* 2006; **159**: 265–71.

88. Costello E, Flynn O, Quigley F et al. Genotyping of *Mycobacterium bovis* isolates from badgers in four areas of the Republic of Ireland by restriction fragment length polymorphism analysis. *Vet Rec* 2006; **159**: 619–23.

89. Barrow WW. Treatment of mycobacterial infections. *Rev Sci Tech* 2001; **20**: 55–70.

90. Ward GS, Elwell MR, Tingpalapong M, Pomsdhit J. Use of streptomycin and isoniazid during a tuberculosis epizootic in a rhesus and cynomolgus breeding colony. *Lab Anim Sci* 1985; **35**: 395–9.

91. Wolf RH, Gibson SV, Watson EA, Baskin GB. Multidrug chemotherapy of tuberculosis in rhesus monkeys. *Lab Anim Sci* 1988; **38**: 25–33.

92. Morris RS, Pfeiffer DU. Directions and issues in bovine tuberculosis epidemiology and control in New Zealand. *N Z Vet J* 1995; **43**: 256–65.

93. de Lisle GW, Bengis RG, Schmitt SM, O'Brien DJ. Tuberculosis in free-ranging wildlife: detection, diagnosis and management. *Rev Sci Tech* 2002; **21**: 317–34.

94. Skinner MA, Wedlock DN, Buddle BM. Vaccination of animals against Mycobacterium bovis. *Rev Sci Tech* 2001; **20**: 112–32.

95. Aldwell FE, Pfeffer A, De Lisle GW et al. Effectiveness of BCG vaccination in protecting possums against bovine tuberculosis. *Res Vet Sci* 1995; **58**: 90–95.

96. Buddle BM, Keen D, Thomson A et al. Protection of cattle from bovine tuberculosis by vaccination with BCG by the respiratory or subcutaneous route, but not by vaccination with killed *Mycobacterium vaccae*. *Res Vet Sci* 1995; **59**: 10–16.

97. Corner LAL, Norton S, Buddle BM, Morris RS. The efficacy of bacille Calmette–Guérin vaccine in wild brushtail possums (*Trichosurus vulpecula*). *Res Vet Sci* 2002; **73**: 145–52.

98. Vordermeier M, Hewinson RG. Development of cattle TB vaccines in the UK. *Vet Immunol Immunopathol* 2006; **112**: 38–48.

PART 9

CONCLUSIONS

31

Conclusions

PETER DO DAVIES, PETER F BARNES AND STEPHEN GORDON

INTRODUCTION

In the Conclusions of the third edition, we said:

Since the publication of the second edition of *Clinical Tuberculosis* in 1998, there have been substantial developments in the fight against tuberculosis. Thanks to the Global Drugs Fund (GDF) provided by WHO the cost of drugs to the poorest users can be zero. The argument that treatment for tuberculosis is not affordable no longer holds.[1] Governments and Non-Governmental Organizations (NGOs) with a potentially large patient base can apply for free drugs to WHO through the web. By competitive purchasing, the cost of a curative course of antituberculosis chemotherapy is no more than $20.

Substantial amounts of funding have now materialized through the Global Alliance for TB Drug Development. But what has been given still represents only a fraction of what is required to develop new drugs and vaccines. Pharmaceutical companies are moving, if somewhat slowly into new TB drug research, but the incentives will have to be humanitarian rather than profit based.

The problem is that nothing much has changed in the 5 years since we wrote those words. Still the global fund is not receiving sufficient resources, even to reduce the increase in new cases of tuberculosis (TB). The total amount of funding made available would not be enough to fund the development of a single drug under normal pharmaceutical development let alone new vaccines and diagnostics.

EPIDEMIOLOGY

Figures for 2005 from the World Health Organization (WHO) suggest that TB case rates may have peaked across the globe, but due to the increase in the population total cases are still rising.

Current approximate figures are that 8–9 million new cases of TB occur each year and about 1.9 million deaths. This makes TB the second biggest cause of death from infection after HIV/AIDS. Eighty per cent of cases occur in the 22 high-burden countries with India providing about a quarter of all cases (Figures 31.1 and 31.2).

Although TB was increasing across the globe, between 2000 and 2005 the increase was estimated to be as little as 1.7 per cent a year. The most rapid increase was seen in areas affected by HIV, particularly sub-Saharan Africa and increasingly South and South East Asia. The second most rapid increase was seen in countries of the former Soviet Union, where economic collapse has resulted in social conditions favouring the spread of TB, particularly within the prison system. Judging from trends in case notifications and from mathematical modelling, the global TB epidemic is on the threshold of decline. The incidence rate per capita was growing during the 1990s, but had stabilized or begun to fall by 2005. However, because the populations of the countries heavily affected by TB are still growing, the total number of new TB cases arising each year was also still slowly increasing in 2005.

In some middle- and high-income countries, such as the UK, there has been an increase due to migration from high-prevalence areas. This increase was 10.8 per cent between 2004 and 2005, the sharpest increase since the war

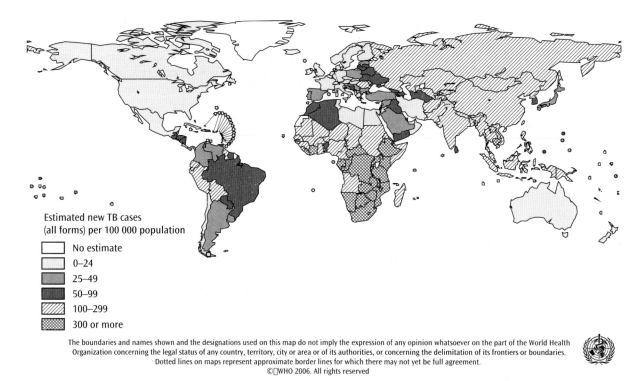

The boundaries and names shown and the designations used on this map do not imply the expression of any opinion whatsoever on the part of the World Health Organization concerning the legal status of any country, territory, city or area or of its authorities, or concerning the delimitation of its frontiers or boundaries. Dotted lines on maps represent approximate border lines for which there may not yet be full agreement.
©WHO 2006. All rights reserved

Figure 31.1 Estimated rates of tuberculosis (TB) across the world by country.

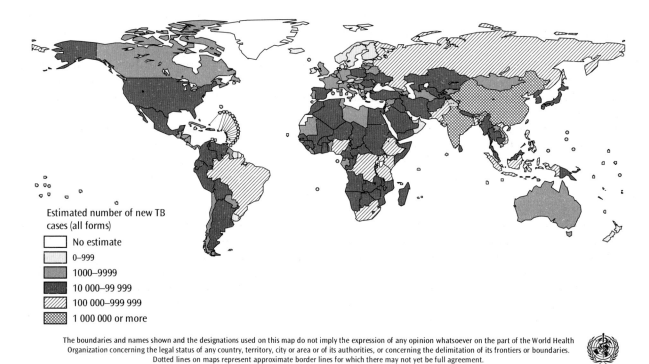

The boundaries and names shown and the designations used on this map do not imply the expression of any opinion whatsoever on the part of the World Health Organization concerning the legal status of any country, territory, city or area or of its authorities, or concerning the delimitation of its frontiers or boundaries. Dotted lines on maps represent approximate border lines for which there may not yet be full agreement.
© WHO 2006. All rights reserved

Figure 31.2 Estimated number of cases of tuberculosis (TB) by country.

years. In others countries, such as Hong Kong, an increasingly elderly population developing reactivated disease from remote infection probably plays a part.

Although DOTS has played the most important role in bringing TB under control where it has been properly applied, it is not sufficient to eliminate TB on its own. This is especially true in areas of high HIV prevalence. Additional means such as active case finding and preventive therapy will be needed to eliminate TB.

Mycobacterium tuberculosis is a relatively inefficient organism at causing disease in infected individuals. Only about 1 in 10 of those infected go on to develop disease. This pathogen/host factor may be exploitable in the development of preventive therapy or vaccination. With one-third of the world's population infected, the opportunity for disease control in this area could be massive if it could be afforded.

The causes for the decline in cases in Europe from the middle of the nineteenth century for a hundred years until specific chemotherapy became available are disputed. Improved living conditions probably played a major part and it may be that until mass poverty is alleviated TB will remain a problem in large areas of the world and therefore a continuing problem for all medical services to a greater or lesser degree.

MICROBIOLOGY AND DIAGNOSIS

TB is a disease caused by a member of the *M. tuberculosis* complex and the diagnosis can only be confirmed by isolating the bacterium from the patient. Where resources are sufficient, methods of speeding up identification of mycobacteria and sensitivity testing have improved remarkably, principally due to molecular based methods. Liquid media using such methods as BACTEC has decreased culture times from 4–6 weeks to 2–3 weeks. Nucleic acid amplification methods can reduce this to just a few days. Nucleic acid amplification tests are most effectively used in patients with positive sputum acid-fast smears and in those with negative smears in whom the clinical suspicion of TB is moderate or high. Because isolated rifampicin resistance remains uncommon, rifampicin resistance is generally a good indicator of multidrug-resistant TB. Several molecular techniques permit identification of mutations in the *rpoB* gene that confer rifampicin resistance, allowing detection of multidrug-resistant organisms in sputum samples in as little as 48 hours. In well-resourced countries, this enables rapid institution of appropriate treatment and infection control measures. The development of MODS (microscopic observation for drug sensitivity) offers a reasonably inexpensive technique for identifying growth and sensitivity of the organism quickly at a price which looks affordable to poorly resourced settings.

The tuberculin skin test (TST) is the primary means used to detect latent tuberculosis infection in richer countries. However, the skin test suffers from many logistical disadvantages and is relatively non-specific, with false-positive reactions resulting from bacillus Calmette–Guérin (BCG) vaccination and exposure to environmental mycobacteria. New blood tests to detect *M. tuberculosis* infection are based on production of interferon-gamma by effector memory T cells that recognize *M. tuberculosis*-specific antigens that are absent from BCG and most environmental mycobacteria. Of the two available interferon-gamma release assays (IGRAs), the QuantiFERON-TB Gold test is simpler to perform, but the T-SPOT.TB test may be more sensitive in immunosuppressed people. IGRAs are more objective and specific than the TST, and

they perform as well as or better than the TST in people with recent TB infection, children and immunocompromised patients. The major factors preventing their widespread adoption is physician lack of familiarity with the tests, combined with the higher cost of materials used for performing IGRAs. However, compared to the TST, the blood test reduces the personnel costs associated with interpretation of a skin test, and the cost of evaluating and treating false-positive TST results.

GENOTYPING

One of the most important tools for TB control which has emerged from the molecular revolution is the development of genotyping to distinguish different *M. tuberculosis* strains. This allows us to trace strains as they cause community outbreaks and as they spread globally, increasing our understanding of the natural history of the disease. Genotyping, combined with detailed epidemiologic investigations, has demonstrated that recent infection contributes substantially to TB morbidity in industrialized nations. The transmission dynamics of TB have been found to vary in different cities, and many different locations, such as homeless shelters, bars and jails. These can serve as major foci of TB transmission. Furthermore, transmission outside the home and through casual contact have been found to be more important than was previously believed. Second episodes of TB are now known to be due to exogenous reinfection rather than reactivation in a substantial proportion of patients in locations where the disease is common.

Genotyping studies have suggested that contact investigations should focus more heavily on locations frequented by TB patients and on casual contacts in addition to the standard emphasis on household and other close contacts. Population-based genotyping can evaluate the efficacy of TB control programmes, as the incidence of recent infection should decline with effective control measures. With the advent of rapid genotyping methods that can be performed on clinical samples, a TB outbreak can be identified during its evolution rather than retrospectively, facilitating institution of appropriate preventive measures. Unfortunately, because of lack of funding and logistical issues, genotyping has not been incorporated into most TB control programmes.

IMMUNOPATHOGENESIS

Infection with *M. tuberculosis* can lead to latent tuberculosis infection (LTBI), primary tuberculosis or reactivation tuberculosis many years after infection. The course of infection depends on interactions between the host innate and adaptive immune response and *M. tuberculosis*. Innate immunity is mediated by macrophages, dendritic cells, natural killer cells and epithelial cells. Recent studies have shown that classic findings linking vitamin D to antituberculosis immunity may be mediated by the antimycobacterial effects of vitamin D, which induces macrophages to produce the antimicrobial peptide cathelicidin, which in turn kills intracellular *M. tuberculosis*. Adaptive immunity is mediated by T_H1 T cells, which produce interferon-γ. The most critical T_H1 cells are CD4$^+$ cells that produce interferon-γ to activate macrophages. CD8$^+$ T cells also contribute to adaptive immunity, primarily by lysing infected cells. T_H2 cells that produce interleukin (IL)-4 can interfere with immunity to TB. These cells are induced by chronic parasitic infections, which may favour progression of TB infection to disease. Regulatory T cells (Tregs) are a recently discovered subpopulation of T cells that dampen immune responses and prevent excessive tissue damage from overexuberant inflammatory responses. In autoimmune and infectious diseases, Tregs can suppress immunity through production of IL-10 and transforming growth factor-β, and through cell-to-cell contact. The role of Tregs in the immune response to TB is currently unclear. Excessive Treg activity may result in immunosuppression and reactivation of TB. Alternatively, Tregs may be beneficial by limiting tissue damage during active TB.

Immune responses in TB are compartmentalized to sites of disease, such as the lungs and the pleural space. Local immunity is characterized by enhanced *M. tuberculosis* antigen-specific T_H1 responses, while systemic T_H1 responses are suppressed. The characteristic tissue response to TB involves formation of granulomas, which are composed primarily of macrophages and T cells. Tumor necrosis factor (TNF)-α is important in granuloma formation and immune defenses against TB and the use of TNF-α inhibitors to treat autoimmune diseases markedly increases the risk of reactivation of TB.

The clinical manifestations of TB are influenced by the immunologic status of the host. People with intact immunity are more likely to develop marked inflammatory reactions that result in extensive pulmonary infiltrate and cavitary disease. In contrast, immunosuppressed individuals, such as those with HIV infection, are more likely to have limited interstitial infiltrates, mediastinal adenopathy and extrapulmonary disease, particularly lymph node and miliary TB.

The members of the *M. tuberculosis* complex differ from each other by the presence or absence of genomic segments called regions of difference (RD). All strains of *M. tuberculosis* have a gene segment called RD1, which is also present in *M. bovis*, but absent from BCG. RD1 is believed to encode important virulence genes, including the early secreted antigenic target, 6 kDa, a secreted protein which lyses infected cells and results in spread of infection from cell to cell. This protein is also an important target of the immune response and the IGRAs discussed above to detect TB infection are based in part on the T-cell response to this protein.

M. tuberculosis has evolved to avoid human antimycobacterial defenses and to survive in a harsh intracellular environment. Sequencing the *M. tuberculosis* genome revealed that an unusually large number of genes encode enzymes that are involved in lipid metabolism, most of which control synthesis of the complex lipid-rich cell wall that provides a first line of defence against the environment. Macrophages engulf mycobacteria in phagosomes that eventually fuse with lysosomes, resulting in a bactericidal acidic environment. However, mycobacterial lipids arrest phagosome maturation and prevent fusion with lysosomes. Mycobacterial proteins also inhibit the capacity of macrophages to present antigens to T cells, limiting their ability to respond to mycobacterial infection. There has been increasing appreciation that *M. tuberculosis* strains differ in their virulence and induction of host immunity. Some strains divide more rapidly than others in human macrophages, and some strains elicit production of lower concentrations of IL-12 and TNF-α by macrophages, resulting in less effective immune responses.

CLINICAL DISEASE

Increasing globalization has brought some advantages in terms of unifying case definitions of TB. However, there is still a divide between those who are able to carry out culture for *M. tuberculosis* and those who cannot, i.e. the vast majority. For the former, a proven case of TB is one from whom *M. tuberculosis* has been isolated. The latter group depend on sputum smear result and response to treatment for case definition. Even in developed countries, an appreciable proportion of cases are not proven, especially of non-respiratory cases.

With the decline in case numbers, in some developed countries there is a tendency to overlook the diagnosis of TB. In 2001, the UK suffered an unprecedented number of outbreaks of TB as a result.[2] The diagnosis of a potentially infectious case of TB is easy, provided it is considered. Sputum smear positivity to the appropriate stain, Zhiel–Neelsen or phenol auramine, is all that is required. The diagnosis in children, who because of the nature of primary disease less frequently produce bacteria-laden sputum remains problematic. Newer techniques of diagnosing infection, such as IGRAs, may help in the future, but only for better resourced settings.

There is a rise of non-respiratory presentations of TB across the world. In poorer nations, this is principally because HIV, by reducing immunocompetence, allows dissemination of *M. tuberculosis* throughout the body. In the developed world, it is increasing as a higher proportion of cases arise in ethnic minority groups. The reason for higher non-respiratory rates in these groups is not usually HIV related, but may be caused by some factor related to immigration, such as acquired vitamin D deficiency.

As well as causing an increase in cases and especially non-respiratory cases, HIV makes the diagnosis of respiratory disease more difficult. This is because by destroying immunity to *M. tuberculosis* in the human host, HIV removes the delayed type hypersensitivity (DTH) effect, which is principally responsible for creating cavitation with resultant very high bacterial loads. The HIV-positive respiratory patient is therefore less likely to be smear positive than the HIV-negative patient. In the resource-poor setting where HIV prevalence is high, diagnosis of these patients is therefore made difficult.

As cases increase worldwide, clinicians must be made aware that no one is absolutely immune from TB and the diagnosis should always be considered.

TREATMENT

Little has changed in the field of treatment even over the last two decades. The 'best buy' still remains isoniazid, rifampicin, pyrazinamide and ethambutol for 2 months or until sensitivity results are available, whichever is the longer. Then isoniazid and rifampicin should be given together for a further 4 months. Where culture and sensitivity testing is not carried out, the sputum smear must be repeated at 2 months and if still positive the four-drug regimen should be continued for a further month.

If possible, combination therapy should be given provided the drugs have proven bioavailability.

Category II or retreatment cases must be given streptomycin as a fifth drug in the intensive phase of treatment. These should be continued for 2 months or 3 if the sputum remains positive and then reduced to isoniazid, rifampicin and ethambutol for the 6-month continuation phase. Recently, US guidelines for treatment of patients with cavitatory disease who remain culture-positive after 2 months have been modified to extend the duration of the continuation phase from 4 months to 7 months.

There is some dispute as to whether these regimens, designed for pulmonary disease, can be applied to extrapulmonary disease. Where controlled trials exist for disease at these sites; spinal, lymph gland, pericardial and genitourinary (GU) disease, 6 months of treatment has been shown to be sufficient. For tuberculous meningitis, there is also some evidence that 6 months is sufficient, but most doctors treating this form of disease would prefer to treat for a full 12 months.

The new challenge in terms of treatment for TB is that outlined by Farmer in Chapter 18, DOTS and DOTS-Plus. There is a danger that using only four and then five drugs in the treatment of TB in developing countries can amplify drug resistance. There has, therefore, been a call to provide the more expensive second-line drugs in these settings, so that patients can receive appropriate therapy for drug-resistant disease.

NEW DRUG DEVELOPMENT

For the first time in 40 years, several new drugs with promising attributes have entered the clinical development pipeline for the treatment of TB. At present, these are the fluoroquinoloes (moxifloxacin and gatifloxacin), but newer drugs such as diarylquinolones are also approaching the time for clinical studies. With good fortune, one or more of these agents will fulfil or exceed its potential demonstrated in animal models and provide a new cornerstone for the treatment of TB. Additional candidates are percolating up through discovery and preclinical development programmes. Despite the apparent robustness of this portfolio, many challenges must be overcome before any of these new drugs contributes meaningfully to the control of TB. Beyond bringing a new drug to market, defining the most appropriate use of new agents and assuring the availability and reliability of the best new regimens in the areas that need them most, will require an unprecedented level of cooperation between drug sponsors, those who conduct clinical trials, funding agencies and national treatment programmes.

DOTS AND THE CONTROL OF TB IN DEVELOPING COUNTRIES

It must always be emphasized that DOTS consists of five elements: government commitment and funding, good drug supply, good record keeping, good microscopy and directly observed therapy. Sometimes it is only the last, which is emphasized.

Though DOTS has received its share of criticism, there can be no doubt that in developing countries it remains the only realistic method of ensuring cure. In developed countries where completion rates fall below 85 per cent, it should be applied.

No special medical qualifications are required to carry out DOTS, but a firm commitment and understanding of the reasons are necessary (Figure 31.3).

DRUG RESISTANCE AND DOTS-PLUS

Farmer makes a compelling case for DOTS being a cause of amplifying drug resistance, which is already present. In other words, where there is resistance to one or two drugs the standard DOTS regimen when given to a patient, may increase resistance so that the organism becomes resistant to four or even five drugs. In this situation, it has previously been felt that the cost of second-line drugs is too great and the patient with MDR-TB in resource-poor settings is in effect abandoned, so that cheaper first-line drugs can be afforded for patients with fully susceptible disease.

Farmer argues that the cost of not treating the MDR cases initially will increase the costs of treatment in the long run as untreated MDR-TB cases spread their infection and disease to others. Intense political pressure has reduced the cost of many second-line drugs enormously, so that this is no longer the major barrier to second-line treatment. The problem is in developing the necessary clinical expertise and infrastructure to manage such patients. The DOTS-Plus model, which Farmer has

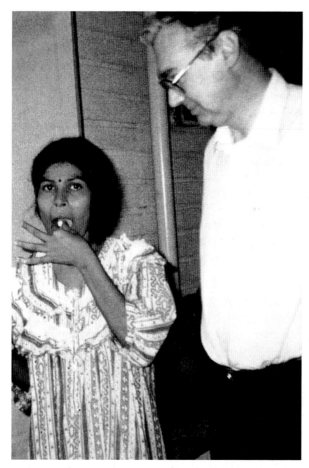

Figure 31.3 The editor as a DOTS worker, Mumbai, February 1998.

developed in Peru, is a good example of how the management of MDR-TB in the resource-poor setting can be achieved.

Drug resistance and MDR-TB is created by medical mismanagement. Thanks to increased awareness and improvement in expertise and in techniques to identify drug resistance, the rapid increase in MDR disease, which was expected in many developed countries just a few years ago, does not seem to have materialized. It is certainly an enormous problem in parts of the former Soviet Union, particularly the prison service. It is probably an increasing problem in the Indian subcontinent, but data here are scarce. Only persistent vigilance will keep it that way.

THE CONTROL OF TB IN WELL-RESOURCED NATIONS

The increase in TB in many developed countries has often caught provision of staff, particularly specialist nurses and clerical support, understrength. Sometimes governments have been slow to provide resources for adequate control measures to be brought into place. The USA during the

1970s and 1980s showed how the destruction of the TB control infrastructure turned a problem into a crisis.

The increase in cases is often confined to specific areas where immigrants tend to live. Specific targeting of these areas must therefore be a priority.

Some centres have good success rates with self-administered treatment. Treatment should only be undertaken if full social and medical support can be given to the patient. Though directly observed therapy should be considered for all patients, if cure/completion exceeds 85 per cent the system of patient supervision is working whatever the method used. The overwhelming majority of patients can be treated at home. Inpatient treatment may sometimes be required to ensure compliance. If facilities are made sufficiently 'patient friendly', the need for compulsory detention is almost always avoidable.

Monitoring of drug resistance so that specific measures can be taken to counter any increase is vital. Drug-resistant TB should be treated at specialist centres, which have access to negative pressure rooms. Monitoring of outcomes should be standard practice.

The screening of high-risk groups particularly new immigrants needs to be monitored for cost-effectiveness. Most individuals coming from overseas do not arrive with active disease, but may develop disease soon after arrival. Local health professionals therefore need to be made aware of the risk.

Methods of DNA fingerprinting are useful in tracing outbreak pathways and can be vital in analysing nosocomial (hospital-acquired) infection so that improved infection control methods can be implemented.

Lack of experience in diagnosing and managing TB has led to a number of outbreaks in some developed countries. It is important that sufficient training in TB is provided both at undergraduate and graduate level for medical and allied health professionals.

TB AND HIV/AIDS

HIV is now the most important cause of the increase in TB worldwide and is a contributory factor to the increase in a number of industrialized countries.

The presence of HIV substantially alters the epidemiology and clinical presentation of TB. The risk of infection leading to disease is increased by about 100-fold. Repeated infections causing second or subsequent episodes of disease are common.

The characteristic patterns of disease particularly radiographically are altered as HIV destroys both the cell-mediated immune protection and the delayed-type hypersensitivity in the host (Chapter 18, DOTS and DOTS-Plus). Extrapulmonary presentations are more common than pulmonary. HIV will probably become increasingly important in presentations of TB all over the world. The clinician diagnosing and treating TB must remain well informed and on guard.

The treatment of HIV/AIDS with highly active anti-retroviral therapy (HAART) is now routine in developed countries. This has reduced mortality and morbidity by up to 90 per cent. The debate is whether treatment could and should be afforded for patients in developing countries. One thing is certain: if mechanisms are not in place to treat TB (a 6-month regimen), they will not be in place to treat HIV/AIDS, which may require a lifetime of therapy.

The drug–drug interactions caused by the co-treatment of TB and HIV is a potential minefield. Details are set out in Chapter 12 (Clinical pharmacology), but the best advice must be to treat one infection at a time if possible. The standard four-drug regimen of isoniazid, rifampicin, pyrazinamide and ethambutol which provides the quickest cure for TB should be used.

Paradoxical reactions (apparent worsening) may occur as HAART is given to TB patients on treatment, due to reconstitution of the immune process: the immune reconstitution inflammatory syndrome (IRIS).

PREVENTION

It is in the field of prevention that the widest areas of disagreement occur. At one extreme is the USA, which shuns BCG but uses preventive therapy very aggressively. On the other are most developing countries, which can only afford BCG and struggle even to treat and cure infectious cases.

Bacillus Calmette–Guérin

A very clear defence of BCG is given by Rieder (Chapter 24, BCG vaccination). Most studies show a benefit when given to children as early as possible in life especially against disseminated or meningeal disease. BCG should therefore continue to be given to infants in high-prevalence countries. In countries with a low incidence, the benefits are less clear and the possible complication of interpreting the tuberculin skin test is often cited as a reason for not giving BCG.

Yet even in low-prevalence countries there are some groups, which are of high risk, such as children born to immigrants from high-prevalence countries who would clearly benefit from neonatal BCG.

Since the last edition was published some notable changes have occurred in the UK. The very useful multi-pronged Heaf test has had to be discontinued as the manufacturers have withdrawn it. Second, on 6 July 2005 it was announced that routine BCG given to 13-year-olds would be stopped. It must have seemed odd to the general public that the vaccine against TB was being stopped just when TB was increasing across the land. What was more difficult to explain was that BCG given to the 13-year British age group was protecting the population with the lowest and still declining incidence of TB, rendering the programme completely cost-ineffective.

It is probably of benefit to continue to vaccinate high-risk groups. The decision to discontinue vaccination must be made country by country and will probably be influenced by political, as much as scientific, considerations.

New antituberculosis vaccines

The explosion of knowledge of the human immune response to *M. tuberculosis* has led to the development of several antituberculosis vaccine candidates. The most promising ones are genetically modified strains of *M. bovis* BCG or vaccinia virus that produce immunogenic mycobacterial proteins, or subunit vaccines composed of immunogenic proteins. These vaccines are being tested in human phase I and phase II trials.

Preventive treatment

Preventive therapy, either of young children at risk from infection, or others who have been infected to prevent the development of disease, latent tuberculosis infection (LTBI), is increasingly being practised in countries where it can be afforded. As Zellweger points out (Chapter 22, Preventive therapy), national programmes lacking the resources to provide short-course chemotherapy for cases should not consider a general LTBI treatment programme.

With approximately one-third of the world's population infected with the tubercle bacillus, the potential for continued disease and transmission is enormous.

This is particularly true in the presence of HIV, which increases the risk of infection proceeding to disease by about 100-fold. Amongst HIV-positive individuals, isoniazid LTBI treatment significantly reduced the incidence of HIV disease, AIDS and death in tuberculin test-positive participants.

There is some disagreement among developed countries as to which drugs to use. Isoniazid alone for at least 6 months has been the best researched by clinical trials. However, compliance is a problem and it seems counterproductive to treat LTBI for the same time as active disease. A placebo-controlled study of daily LTBI therapy among silicotic patients in Hong Kong suggested that rifampicin alone for 3 months was of comparable efficacy to 3 months of rifampicin plus isoniazid and isoniazid alone for 6 months. The 3-month isoniazid/rifampicin combination is the regimen preferred in the UK. We personally feel a sense of unease in giving rifampicin alone as treatment in any situation. It is much too precious a drug to be given 'unprotected', that is without a combination with another drug, such as isoniazid.

Because of theoretical considerations of the sterilizing effect of rifampicin and pyrazinamide and the efficacy of this combination in the mouse model, the USA has recently adopted its use. However, there has been an unexpectedly high morbidity. For this reason it will not be possible to use this combination as widely as had been hoped.

The lack of an age cut-off in the American guidelines may be a factor in the high morbidity. In the UK, guidelines do not recommend giving preventive therapy to those older than 35 years.

Whether this is appropriate or not is open to debate. One fact which is not in dispute is that over the last decade the USA has been considerably more successful in bringing down its TB rates than virtually any other country. This may be an effect of the number of immigrants entering a country and the relative rates in their countries of origin. Yet even among the white indigenous population of the USA rates have declined from 8/100 000 in 1991and are now less than 2 compared with comparative figures of a decline from 5.5 to 4 in the UK.[3]

The best regimen for the prevention of MDR LTBI is still open to debate until clinical trial results are available. In the absence of any experimental data, the combination of pyrazinamide plus ciprofloxacin was favoured by a group of experts.

Recent information demonstrating enhanced sterilizing activity against *M. tuberculosis* from newer fluoroquinolones, such as moxifloxacin, suggests that monotherapy with such an agent might provide for highly effective and well-tolerated treatment of latent MDR LTBI.

THE FUTURE

Were it not for HIV infection we would probably have the means to control and virtually eliminate TB within three or four generations. Through DOTS, it has been shown possible to bring rates rapidly down by achieving 75 per cent detection and 85 per cent cure. Even the relatively inefficient 6-month treatment regimen can achieve cure. Dye has shown that MDR-TB does not appear to be the overwhelming threat once feared and once proper control is established in hot-spot areas, such as Russia, even current drugs can achieve cure and elimination.

The development of the Global Fund against HIV, Tuberculosis and Malaria shows that at least we have made a start as a global community. Though insufficient funds are currently forthcoming, with increasing public awareness there must be optimism that resource targets will be met.

However, the overwhelming problem, quite literally, is HIV infection. Many African health structures and economies are already devastated by the HIV TB pandemic. The increasing threat as HIV crosses Asia and Eastern Europe is posing monumental problems in health care, particularly TB control. These changes in TB epidemiology make the development of new drugs and vaccines imperative. We are told that there may be a new drug within 10 years. No date has been guessed at for a new vaccine, but it will surely take even longer. In the meantime, we shall just have to manage with what we have. We can certainly improve the efficiency with which we use what means we have at our disposal. If HAART becomes available to even the poorest, the prospects for control would be improved but the responsibility of the medical services to see that we do not lose precious drugs by creating drug resistance will be considerably increased.

Even if there are no new drugs or vaccines for TB on the horizon, there are continuing advances in diagnostics. Recent studies show that IGRAs to detect T cell-specific responses to *M. tuberculosis* antigens provide a more accurate test for infection than the tuberculin skin test. This represents a significant improvement on a test, which has just celebrated its 110th birthday, while incidentally providing a silver lining to the cloud of England's biggest point outbreak of TB.[4]

REFERENCES

1. www.stoptb.org/GDF.
2. Watson JM, Moss F. TB in Leicester: out of control, or just one of those things? *Br Med J* 2001; **322**: 1133–4.
3. www.cdc.gov/nchstp/tb/faqs/qa.
4. Ewer K, Deeks J, Alvarez L *et al.* Comparison of T-cell-based assay with tuberculin skin test for a diagnosis of *Mycobacterium tuberculosis* infection in a school tuberculosis outbreak. *Lancet* 2003; **361**: 1168–73.

Subject Index